Fourth Edition

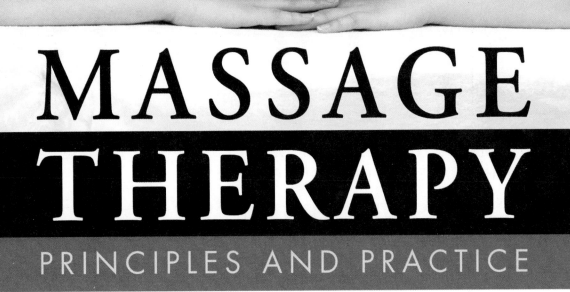

MASSAGE
THERAPY

PRINCIPLES AND PRACTICE

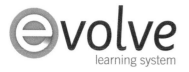

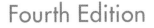

Fourth Edition

MASSAGE THERAPY

PRINCIPLES AND PRACTICE

SUSAN G. SALVO, BEd, LMT, NTS, CI, NCTMB
Co-Director and Instructor
Louisiana Institute of Massage Therapy
Lake Charles, Louisiana

ELSEVIER
SAUNDERS

3251 Riverport Lane
St. Louis, Missouri 63043

Vice President and Publishing Director: Linda Duncan
Executive Editor: Kellie White
Senior Developmental Editor: Jennifer Watrous
Editorial Assistant: Emily Thomson
Publishing Services Manager: Julie Eddy
Senior Project Manager: Andrea Campbell
Design Direction: Kim Denando

Printed in Canada

Last digit is the print number: 9 8 7 6 5 4 3 2 1

This book is dedicated to

Chris and Suzanne Salvo

During the creation of any book, the author receives support, in one way or another, from various family members. Some proofread, some babysit, while others bring you coffee or rub your tired neck and shoulders as a loving gesture. Some contributions are so monumental that they change the face, appearance, and appeal of the book.

Two such family members, Chris and Suzanne Salvo, have been this book's photographers extraordinaire. Their beautiful images have been a major selling point for the past decade—combining stunning graphics with brilliant instruction. The photographic images in the second, third, and now fourth edition bring the content to life and support the student's learning process. It has been such a wonderful experience to work with such dedicated people. The fact that Chris is my brother and Suzanne is my sister-in-law is a bonus.

Chris and Suzanne, thanks for everything!

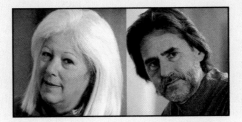

And you who want to see more of their work, check out
http://salvophoto.com/

CONTRIBUTORS

LAURA ALLEN, BA, LMBT, NCTMB
Approved Provider of Continuing Education under
the NCBTMB
Rutherfordton, North Carolina
Biographical Sketch

SANDRA K. ANDERSON, BA, LMT, NCTMB
Co-Owner, Tucson Touch Therapies
Tucson, Arizona
Test Your Knowledge, Glossary

CELIA BUCCI, MA, LMT
Chicago, IL
Biographical Sketches, Case Studies

JUDITH DELANY, LMT
Director and Certified NMT Instructor
NMT Center
St. Petersburg, Florida
Clinical Massage

MEGAN LAVERY, LMT, BS
Faculty and Board of Directors, Zero Balancing Health
Association
Faculty, Natural Health Institute of Bowling Green
Bowling Green, Kentucky
Therapeutic Relationships

RITA S. LEBLEU, LMT, MA
Rhetorical and Interpersonal Communication
DeQuincy, Louisiana
Biographical Sketches

**SANDY GROVER MASON, BA, LMBT 4403, CMT,
AMTA, NCTMB**
Clinical Education Coordinator and Instructor, Therapeutic
Massage
Forsyth Technical Community College
Owner, Body Therapeutic
Winston-Salem, North Carolina
Appendix: SOAP Notes

MONICA J. RENO, LMT
Continuing Education Provider
Touch Education, LLC
Lady Lake, Florida
Clinical Massage

HAYLEY A. SALVO
Bachelors in Journalism, Magna Cum Laude
The English Centre
Málaga, Spain
Biographical Sketches

JOELLEN M. SEFTON, PhD, ATC, CMT
Director, Warrior Research Center/Warrior Athletic
Training Program Director
Neuromechanics Research Laboratory, Department of
Kinesiology
Auburn University
Auburn, Alabama
Research Literacy, Effects of Massage Therapy

RALPH R. STEPHENS, BSEd, LMT, NCTMB
Owner, Ralph Stephens Seminars, LLC
Cedar Rapids, Iowa
Seated Massage

H. MICHEAL TARVER, PhD
Dean, College of Arts and Humanities
Professor of History, Arkansas Tech University
Russellville, Arkansas
History of Massage

KENNETH G. ZYSK, PhD, DPhil
Associate Professor
Institute for Cross-Cultural and Regional Studies
Department of Asian Studies
University of Copenhagen
Copenhagen, Denmark
Energy-Based Bodywork Therapy: Shiatsu and Ayurveda

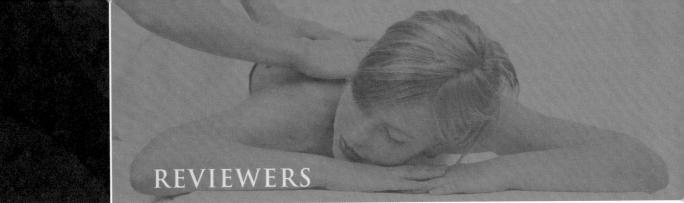

REVIEWERS

LAURA ALLEN, BA, LMBT, NCTMB
Approved Provider of Continuing Education under the
NCBTMB
Rutherfordton, North Carolina
*Self-Care; Body Mechanics, Client Positioning, and
Draping; Massage Techniques, Joint Mobilizations,
and Stretches*

ROBIN B. ANDERSON, LMT, NCTBM, CPT-ACE
Outpatient Rehabilitation Department
Franklin Square Hospital
Baltimore, Maryland

ROBYN ANTHONY, LMT
Orlando, Florida
*Foot Reflexology, Seated Massage, Introduction to
the Human Body*

SANDRA K. ANDERSON, BA, LMT, NCTMB
Co-Owner, Tucson Touch Therapies
Tucson, Arizona

KATHLEEN S. BECKER, RN BSN, MeD, MSN
Professor of Nursing
St. Louis Community College at Forest Park
St. Louis, Missouri
Special Populations and Pregnancy, Integumentary System

PATRICIA BERAK, NCTMB, CHt, BHSA, MBA
Program Director of Massage Therapy and BHSA
Baker College of Clinton Township
Clinton Township, Michigan

ROBERT D. BERNAUER, Jr., MD
McNeese State University
Lake Charles, Louisiana
*Introduction to the Human Body, Kinesiology, Nervous
System, Endocrine System, Reproductive System,
Digestive System*

DONALD A. BISSON, RRPr
Ontario College of Reflexology
New Liskeard, Ontario, Canada
Foot Reflexology

WILHELMINA M. BLANK, MEd, NCTMB
Founder, Director
Pennsylvania Myotherapy Institute
Abbottstown, Pennsylvania

MICHAEL A. BREAUX, LMT
Co-Owner, Louisiana Institute of Massage Therapy
Past Chairman, Louisiana State Board of Massage Therapy
Lake Charles, Louisiana
Therapeutic Relationships

DANA BREEN, LMT
Stillpoint Massage Therapy
Chicago, Illinois
Research Literacy

CELIA BUCCI, MA, LMT
Chicago, IL
Tools of the Trade

BELINDA BURNSIDE, MOST, BAppSc
Royal Melbourne Institute of Technology
Melbourne, Australia
Former Instructor of Physiology
Sky Hill Institute
Petaluma, California

JILL BURYNSKI, LMBT, NCTMB
Instructor, Director of Continuing Education
North Carolina School of Advanced Bodywork
Owner & Lead Instructor
Living Sabai Continuing Education
Asheville, North Carolina

**TERRY MAHAN BUTTARO, PhD, APN-BC,
GNP-BC, FAANP**
Assistant Clinical Professor
Simmons College
Boston, Massachusetts
Treatment Planning

SUSIE BYRD, MTI
Director and Massage Therapy Instructor
Neuromuscular Therapist
The Edge School of Massage Therapy
Fayetteville, Arkansas
Therapeutic Relationships

JUDI CALVERT
CEO, Hands-On Trade Association
Massage Historian
Spokane, Washington
History of Massage

MICHELLE CARBONNEAU, BA, LMT,
    Certified Yoga Instructor
Director of Education
Massage and Anatomy Instructor
Hawaii Healing Arts College
Honolulu, Hawaii
Tools of the Trade; Hydrotherapy and Spa

MARCELA M. COLLINS, MS, LMT, NCBTMB
Tennessee Massage Licensure Board Member
Balance Sanctuary-Holistic Health & Wellness
Clarksville, Tennessee

DENISE CUGINI, BBA, LMT
Beacon Wellness Arts Center
Petaluma, California
Therapeutic Relationships

JUDITH DELANY, LMT
Director and Certified NMT Instructor
NMT Center
St. Petersburg, Florida

GAUTAM J. DESAI, DO, FACOFP, CPI
Board Certified, Family Medicine
Medical Acupuncture
Associate Professor, Department of Family Medicine
Kansas City University of Medicine and Biosciences
    College of Osteopathic Medicine
Kansas City, Missouri
Digestive System, Urinary System

SATTARIA S. DILKS, DNP, APRN
Psychiatric Nurse Practitioner
Associate Professor, McNeese State University
Lake Charles, Louisiana
Therapeutic Relationships

ADAM FIORE
Academic Advisor, NHC Institute
Montreal, Québec

SANDY FRITZ, MS, NCTMB
Founder, Owner, Director, and Head Instructor
Health Enrichment Center School of Therapeutic
    Massage and Bodywork
Lapeer, Michigan
Clinical Massage

RICHARD W. GOGGINS, MS, CPE, LMP
Director of Ergonomics Services
Save Your Hands! Injury Prevention and Ergonomics
    Solutions for Manual Therapists
Coconut Creek, Florida
*Self-Care; Body Mechanics, Client Positioning,
    and Draping*

RICHARD M. GOLD, LAc, PhD
President and Senior Instructor
International Professional School of Bodywork
San Diego, California
Energy-Based Bodywork Therapy

JULIE A. GOODWIN, BA, LMT
Instructor, Cortiva Institute-Tucson and Arizona School of
    Acupuncture and Oriental Medicine
Tucson, Arizona
*Therapeutic Relationships; Effects of Massage Therapy;
    Massage Techniques, Joint Mobilizations, and
    Stretches; Special Populations and Pregnancy; Clinical
    Massage; Introduction to the Human Body*

KIMBERLY E. GORAL, MS, LMT
Boston, Massachusetts

LAURIANN GREENE, CEAS
President/Consultant
Save Your Hands! Injury Prevention and Ergonomics
    Solutions for Manual Therapists
Coconut Creek, Florida
*Self-Care; Body Mechanics, Client Positioning,
    and Draping*

MIRRA GREENWAY, BS, LMT, NCTMB
Founder/Executive Director, MTIM/Massage Therapy
    Institute of Missouri; The Greenways Wellness
    Services; GreenMassage Organization
Secretary, AMTA-MO Chapter
Columbia, Missouri
*Tools of the Trade; Massage Techniques, Joint
    Mobilizations, and Stretches; Treatment Planning*

JEANNE deMONTAGNAC-HALL, BS, LMT, MT
Owner and Instructor
VITAL TOUCH® Massage Therapy
West Chester, Ohio

LAURA STJERN HANSEN BA/S LMP. LAMP
Owner, New Horizon School of Massage
Richland Washington
Respiratory System

ROBERT HARRIS, HND, RMT, CLT-LANA
Director and Senior Instructor, Dr. Vodder School—
    International
Victoria, British Columbia, Canada
Lymphatic System and Immunity

MEGHAN HART, LMT, BCST
Instructor, University of Spa & Massage Therapy
Springfield, Illinois
Nervous System

PATRICIA M. HOLLAND, MC, LMT
Instructor and Dean of Students, Cortiva Institute—Tucson
Owner and Practitioner, Mindful Touch Therapeutic
    Massage
Tucson, Arizona
Therapeutic Relationships; Seated Massage

GLENN M. HYMEL, EdD, LMT
Professor of Psychological Sciences & Former Chair
Department of Psychological Sciences, Loyola University
New Orleans, Louisiana
Research Literacy

RHONDA LEJEUNE JOHNSON, RN, MSN, EdD
Assistant Professor of Nursing, College of Nursing
McNeese State University
Lake Charles, Louisiana
Endocrine System, Reproductive System

MELINDA ANN KEELING, LMT
Lead Instructor for the Massage Therapy Program,
    Pima Medical Institute
Mesa, Arizona
*Self-Care; Massage Techniques, Joint Mobilizations,
    and Stretches*

LESLIE KORN, PhD, MPH, LMHC, RPP, NCB
Director, Center for Traditional Medicine
Olympia, Washington
Energy-Based Bodywork Therapy

KATHY LEE, LMT, BS Business Administration
Director of Career Services, Cortiva Institute
Tucson, Arizona
Business, Marketing, Accounting, and Finance

TERRI L. LEVIEN, PharmD
Clinical Associate Professor, College of Pharmacy
Washington State University Spokane
Spokane, Washington

ALEXEI LEVINE, MPT, PT, LMT
Director, The Massage School
Easthampton, Massachusetts
Body Mechanics, Client Positioning, and Draping

NIKI LIN, BS, CPT, LMT
Owner, RPM Pilates and Massage
Orlando, Florida
*Foot Reflexology, Seated Massage, Introduction to
    the Human Body*

DAVID MARQUART, BA, CMT
Corporate Director for Massage Therapy Programs
Education Department
Centura College
Virginia Beach, Virginia

MICHAEL MATTHEWS, LMT
Instructor/Massage Therapy Program Director
Tennessee Technology Center Division
Chattanooga State Community College
Chattanooga, Tennessee

ANNIE MORIEN, PhD, PA-C, LMT
Florida School of Massage
Gainesville, Florida
Integumentary System

CHRISTOPHER A. MOYER, PhD
Assistant Professor of Psychology, University of
    Wisconsin-Stout
Menomonie, Wisconsin
Research Literacy

ERIC A. MUNN, BS, CMT
Director, Department of Massage Therapy
Fortis Institute
Wayne, New Jersey

JOSEPH E. MUSCOLINO, DC
Instructor, Purchase College, State University of
    New York
Purchase, New York
Owner, The Art and Science of Kinesiology
Stamford, Connecticut
Muscular System, Skeletal System

PATRICIA C. NUOVO, BA, Naturopath, LMT, CFP
Regent and Instructor, Sky Hill Institute of Wholistic
    Healing Arts
Petaluma, California

JENNIFER OPFER, BS, LMT, NCBTMB, MBLEX
Medical Instructor, Pittsburgh Technical Institute
Oakdale, Pennsylvania

ANGELA K. PALMIER, LMT, NCTMB
Resource ETC LLC
Smithton, Illinois
Research Literacy

GRANT PARKER, BSc, Dip Ed, RMT, DC
Qualicum Beach, British Columbia, Canada
Muscular System, Skelatal System, Kinesiology

MONICA F. PHILLIPS, MA, LMBT, ATRC
Director/Instructor, Gaston College
New Hope Therapeutic Massage
Gastonia, North Carolina

KEVIN PIERCE, LMT, MBA
National Director, Massage Therapy Programs
Anthem Education Group
Orlando, Florida
Cardiovascular System; Lymphatic System

SHARON PUSZKO, LMT, PhD
Owner/Director/Educator of Daybreak Geriatric
    Massage Institute
Daybreak Geriatric Massage Institute
Continuing Education Provider
Offices, Indiana, Florida, and California
*Special Populations and Pregnancy; Integumentary
    System; Urinary System*

JOHN C. QUINDRY, PhD, FACSM
Director, Cardioprotection Laboratory
Department of Kinesiology, Auburn University
Auburn, Alabama
Research Literacy, Effects of Massage Therapy

MONICA J. RENO, LMT
Continuing Education Provider
Touch Education, LLC
Lady Lake, Florida
*Clinical Massage; Effects of Massage Therapy; Body
    Mechanics, Client Positioning, and Draping;
    Treatment Planning; Business, Marketing, Accounting,
    and Finance; Appendix*

JEFF RIACH
CEO, Oakworks, Inc.
New Freedom, Pennsylvania
Tools of the Trade

LAURA C. RICHARDSON, MEd
Instructor, Gentle Healing School of Massage
Cranbury, New Jersey

NANCY C. ROBBINS, MSN, CFNP, CDE
Family Nurse Practitioner
Sentara Family Medicine—First Colonial
Virginia Beach, Virginia
Infection Control and Emergency Preparedness

ELAN SCHACTER, LMT, RMT
Charlotte, North Carolina
Hydrotherapy and Spa

MICHAEL J. SHEA, PhD
Shea Educational Group, Inc.
Juno Beach, Florida
Therapeutic Relationships

ELAINE STILLERMAN, LMT
MotherMassage
Brooklyn, New York
Special Populations and Pregnancy

**VICTORIA JORDAN STONE, Certified Massage
    Therapist, BA, MA, MFA, Registered Yoga Instructor**
Academic Coordinator, Blue Ridge School of Massage
    & Yoga
Blacksburg, Virginia

SHAWNA STRICKLAND, PhD, RRT-NPS, AE-C
Director, Respiratory Therapy Program
University of Missouri
Columbia, Missouri
Respiratory System

DONALD R. THIGPEN, DC, BS, CMT
Certified Instructor of Human Anatomy, Physiology,
    and Pathology
Certified Spinal Decompression Practitioner
Chiropractic Physician
Center for Chiropractic and Rehabilitation, LLC
Texas Chiropractic College
Louisiana Institute of Massage Therapy
McNeese State University
Lake Charles, Louisiana
Clinical Massage

KATHLEEN VINTALORO, NCTMB
Primary Instructor, Warren County Community College
Washington, New Jersey

JANET K. VIZARD, MA, LMT, NCTMB
Lead Faculty, Therapeutic Massage Program
Pima Community College
Tucson, Arizona
Massage Techniques, Joint Mobilizations, and Stretches

DENNIS M. WALKER, MD
Practitioner, Orthopaedic Specialists
Lake Charles, Louisiana
Clinical Massage

CHARLES B. WOODARD, MD, FACC, FAHA
Lake Charles Memorial Hospital
Lake Charles, Louisiana
Cardiovascular System

FOREWORD

Massage therapy is becoming a mature health care field. This maturity is evident in the publication of the *Massage Therapy Body of Knowledge* in May 2010. That document details the confluence of massage therapy as an art form and massage therapy as a science. This is demonstrated by new science revealing that human nervous systems and vascular systems are built for empathy, compassion, and altruistic love. The art and science of touching someone with such empathy and compassion is what is most necessary in today's massage therapy education. This textbook by Susan Salvo addresses these profound changes in the massage therapy profession and places it at a level with other major disciplines in both the biomedical and alternative health care communities. This book fully integrates the Massage Therapy Body of Knowledge into a coherent narrative for the beginning student and others in the field. It takes the reader step by step through the vital knowledge, skills, and abilities necessary to practice successfully in the 21st century. By using this book, massage therapy schools will be able to fully prepare their students for a successful career in massage therapy.

This comprehensive textbook, *Massage Therapy: Principles and Practice*, reaches every level of massage therapy. It is an essential starting text for the new practitioner and fully informs experienced practitioners of the very latest developments in the field. Susan has identified key topics in all areas of massage therapy necessary for upgrading as well as updating the field in light of the current science and understanding, especially the musculoskeletal system and the therapeutic relationship. This is nothing short of a monumental effort.

My own experience as a licensed massage therapist began in a federally funded massage school in Miami, Florida, in 1975. I was placed in a European style spa for wealthy South American clients as my first job. I worked in a tiny windowless room and was called a "masseur." Gradually over several decades I became a massage therapist through continuing education and the evolution of the field. With the efficacy of the massage therapy profession now supported by significant findings in the research, the entire massage therapy community can be considered as having achieved parity with all other major health care professions. This textbook is the portal to this important paradigm shift in massage therapy.

The value of loving therapeutic touch has been more than demonstrated in the past decade, starting with the fact that infants spend up to 60% of their time being held by caregivers. Infants can detect whether that caregiver is holding and contacting them with loving kindness. This capacity can be impaired and create lifelong issues for many people, even with the well-trained touch from the loving intention of a massage therapist. Skills imparted in this book will help the nervous systems and bodies of such clients to rehabilitate, and others with symptoms affecting their musculoskeletal system to stabilize. The dilemma of the contemporary client is having a body under constant stress and being unable to manage or integrate the type of trauma occurring regularly at every level of our society.

It is no wonder that the massage therapy profession has grown so large and so strong in the past several decades. It is through this army of massage therapists in the United States that the opportunity to heal the body is greatly enhanced and is a cause for me to be very optimistic about the future of our society. Susan Salvo is also an optimist and has a grasp of what the human body needs and she provides precise instructions on how to do so for massage therapists. She is a leader in the field and her book represents a turning point for massage therapists in the direction of integrating loving kindness and science into a single discipline.

MICHAEL J. SHEA, PhD
Shea Educational Group, Inc.
Juno Beach, Florida

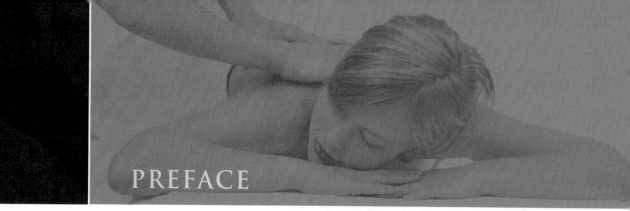

Massage works miracles. There's the miracle "cure" of reducing pain in a runner's hip just before an event. There's the wonder of de-stressing the harried mother of twins with a scrub, a soak, and a massage. There's the look of peace as the businessman's brow unfurrows during a session of Asian bodywork. One of my favorite miracles is what massage does to attitude. A first-time client may come in the door with a combination of excitement and apprehension, wearing that "Oooh, I've never done this before" look. But after the massage, he is smiling and saying, "Why did I wait so long to try this?" Sometimes the miracle comes from the emotional release of a client who just needs to talk or cry.

As therapists, we not only facilitate these miracles, we too are changed by them. Most major religions contain stories of miracles. Many of the miracle stories are based on doctrines of love for our fellow man. Touch is often used as part of the process. This is true for Judeo-Christian teaching, Buddhism, Islamic belief, Native American lore, and even the old pagan mythologies.

Regardless of our personal ideologies, beliefs, and differences, we can all participate in miracles through the use of touch. The one common belief is that touch is a powerful and transformational experience. And so we go out into the world much like the monks, missionaries, and prophets. We are disciples of touch, working miracles and changing the world one person at a time.

This textbook and other professional projects I've been involved in are my contributions to the profession I love.

Each edition combines:

- Tried and true techniques
- Current research studies
- The latest educational technologies
- The best art and photography available
- Tips for learning complex concepts
- A common-sense approach

By taking each chapter to the classroom for test runs, we have expanded, deleted, and revised until the finished product is one that is friendly to the eye, meets the needs of students and instructors, and produces massage therapists for the clients of tomorrow.

As always, I have requested the assistance of expert contributors and feedback from a team of reviewers to help achieve these goals. It's a tradition I'd like to continue and expand with the use of the Internet and social networking. I'd love to hear YOUR feedback and suggestions.

Who Will Benefit From This Book?

Students will benefit from the user-friendly nature of this book. This text is based on the fusion of massage and anatomic science, focusing on their commonalities. The stunning photography and detailed illustrations provide both instruction and inspiration to the learner, and the format of the book is readable and engaging.

Instructors will appreciate the straightforward writing style and visually appealing presentation. The book content, combined with your unique teaching style, will help your students master the foundational knowledge, skills, and abilities for their career in massage therapy. I have infused cutting-edge, practical information and my professional insight into this broad, in-depth, and engaging resource, giving you and your students everything you need during school.

Established massage therapists can use the text as a method of updating their knowledge, studying for advanced certificate exams, and as a resource, desk reference, and teaching tool for clients.

Organization

This textbook is divided into two units.

In **Unit One**, we explore the history of massage, including current events. These are exciting times. The massage timeline includes formation of the FSMTB, MTF, MTBOK, and the upcoming advanced certification by NCBTMB. Then we look at therapeutic relationships before heading into equipment, body mechanics, and massage techniques. Infection control and treatment planning are discussed as well as modalities of hydrotherapy, foot reflexology, clinical massage, seated massage, and Eastern approaches. We finish the unit with a hefty dose of business material.

Topics of anatomy and physiology are featured in **Unit Two**. All body systems are discussed with significant coverage given to kinesiology, which includes bones, muscles, and their movements.

Distinctive Features of This Book

Interweaving massage with the anatomical sciences—The anatomy and physiology chapters explore each body system, explaining the structure and function of the key components in relevant terminology. Woven into the anatomy chapters are their associated pathologies along with precautions, contraindications, and massage adaptations. The anatomy and physiology chapters are written from a massage therapist's point of view. This book incorporates a general knowledge of anatomic science while focusing on aspects that are most important to the massage therapist.

Emphasis on research—Research supports the efficacy of massage therapy. Each anatomy chapter features a "Spotlight on Research." These boxes include summaries of recent relevant research studies of massage therapy that are supported with evidence-based practices. This edition also features a chapter on research literacy and effects of massage and hot and cold applications that are supported by research.

SPOTLIGHT ON RESEARCH

Research suggests that massage therapy may:

- Increase serotonin and dopamine, important chemicals relating to depression, pain, fatigue, and other conditions
- Decrease motor neuron pool excitability
- Improve sleep
- Decrease stress, depression, and anxiety
- Activate parasympathetic response and increase relaxation
- Enhance brain wave activity
- Improve cognitive and memory functioning
- Reduce spasticity, increase muscle flexibility and motor function
- Improve social interaction in persons with cerebral palsy
- Improve functional abilities, range of motion, and muscle strength in persons with spinal cord injury
- Reduce pain and increase nerve conduction velocity in persons with carpal tunnel syndrome
- Decrease fidgeting and improve mood in persons with attention deficit–hyperactivity disorder
- Reduce touch aversion and other stereotypic behaviors in persons with autism
- Reduce agitation, resisting, and other stereotypic behaviors in persons with dementia and Alzheimer disease
- Improve daily functioning and improve sleep in persons with Parkinson disease
- Decrease anxiety and depression and improve self-esteem and body image in persons with multiple sclerosis

Biographies—We have included biographies and candid interviews with the most respected authorities and pioneers of massage therapy and bodywork. New biographies focus on individuals who may not be well known on a national level, but are out in communities touching the lives of others through massage. Be sure and peruse the biography index in the back of this book for a complete list of bios.

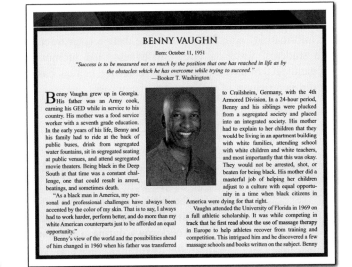

BENNY VAUGHN

Born: October 11, 1951

"Success is to be measured not so much by the position that one has reached in life as by the obstacles which he has overcome while trying to succeed."
—Booker T. Washington

Benny Vaughn grew up in Georgia. His father was an Army cook, earning his GED while in service to his country. His mother was a food service worker with a seventh grade education. In the early years of his life, Benny and his family had to ride at the back of public buses, drink from segregated water fountains, sit in segregated seating at public venues, and attend segregated movie theaters. Being black in the Deep South at that time was a constant challenge, one that could result in arrest, beatings, and sometimes death.

"As a black man in America, my personal and professional challenges have always been accented by the color of my skin. That is to say, I always had to work harder, perform better, and do more than my white American counterparts just to be afforded an equal opportunity."

Benny's view of the world and the possibilities ahead of him changed in 1960 when his father was transferred to Crailsheim, Germany, with the 4th Armored Division. In a 24-hour period, Benny and his siblings were plucked from a segregated society and placed into an integrated society. His mother had to explain to her children that they would be living in an apartment building with white families, attending school with white children and white teachers, and most importantly that this was okay. They would not be arrested, shot, or beaten for being black. His mother did a masterful job of helping her children adjust to a culture with equal opportunity in a time when black citizens in America were dying for that right.

Vaughn attended the University of Florida in 1969 on a full athletic scholarship. It was while competing in track that he first read about the use of massage therapy in Europe to help athletes recover from training and competition. This intrigued him and he discovered a few massage schools and books written on the subject. Benny

Self-assessment questions—We want you to pass your tests. Giving you anatomy information and teaching you massage techniques is not enough if you cannot pass licensing exams. We have included self-assessment questions at the end of each chapter to assist the student in self-evaluation, as well as studying for and taking tests. Yes, there is a skill involved and if you know and understand that skill, your test-taking ability will improve. We call it becoming "test-wise." Hence, you can use this book as a study guide to prepare for and successfully pass state and/or national examinations.

MATCHING I

Place the letter of the answer next to the term or phrase that best describes it.

A.	2000	E.	Health	I.	Nutrient
B.	3500	F.	Intellectual	J.	Strenuous
C.	Calorie	G.	Macronutrients	K.	Stress
D.	Exercise	H.	Micronutrients	L.	Wellness

_____ 1. The physical activity classification Bonnie Prudden places the massage therapy profession in

_____ 2. Condition of physical, mental, emotional, and social well being and the absence of disease

_____ 3. Amount of calories the United States Food and Drug Administration (FDA) says most adults require to accomplish their daily activities

_____ 4. The category of nutrients that includes vitamins, minerals, and water; also called the *no-calorie group*

_____ 5. An expression of health in which an individual is aware of, chooses, and practices healthy choices, creating a more successful and balanced life

_____ 6. Unit of energy-producing potential received from the food that is eaten

_____ 7. University of Nebraska's wellness model includes emotional, environmental, occupational, physical, social, spiritual and this other dimension

_____ 8. Substance that provides nourishment and affects metabolic processes such as cell growth and repair

_____ 9. The key to a healthier life, according to the American College of Sports Medicine and the American Heart Association

_____ 10. The body's response to any demand placed on it, whether it is emotional, mental, physical, or chemical

_____ 11. Amount of calories in one pound

_____ 12. This category of nutrients includes proteins, carbohydrates, and fats; also called the *calorie group*

Case Studies—Every chapter includes a case study—a vignette of a person involved in a situation related to massage therapy. Each case study presents the student with several questions to ponder. Most often, there is more than one dilemma so the situation must be thought about from several different angles. Each possible solution has consequences. Often the best solution is the one with the fewest negative consequences. The therapist will be faced with many decisions in the course of a day. Case studies are valuable sources of information, stimulating dialogue between instructors and students, fostering open-mindedness, and promoting humanity. All of the case studies presented are factual, based on the experiences of real massage therapists.

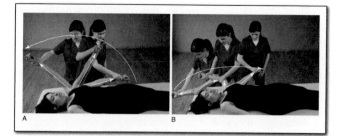

CASE STUDY

Up in Smoke

Susan was the mother of four children and the wife of a loving husband. For their fifteenth wedding anniversary, Susan's husband bought her a massage with her therapist, Delilah. He had been laid off work recently and saved up to give this anniversary gift to his wife. She had been stressed because of a recent diagnosis of a chronic illness. He would stay home with the children while she relaxed.

Susan was diagnosed with chronic obstructive pulmonary disease, specifically, chronic bronchitis. She had smoked for 20 years and it had taken its toll on her lungs. Susan's doctor instructed her to avoid cigarette smoke. She was currently on a drug regimen to quit smoking and it was successful.

When Susan arrived for her appointment, she was ready for tranquil moments. The receptionist greeted her and asked her to have a seat and that Delilah would be with her shortly.

When Delilah called Susan to the massage room, she was anticipating the smell of clean linens, soothing music, and an inviting atmosphere. To her surprise, there was an overwhelming stench of cigarette smoke in the room and on Delilah's clothes. Delilah greeted her with a welcoming smile and asked Susan about her health since her last visit. Susan informed her of the recent diagnosis. She told Delilah about the avoidance of cigarette smoke. Delilah, who was a cigarette smoker, thought nothing of this as she did not smoke in the building.

Critical thinking questions—Each chapter also features critical thinking questions. These questions will require you to actively and skillfully conceptualize, analyze, synthesize, evaluate, and apply information. Responses are generated from reasoning, reflection, experience, or discussion.

CRITICAL THINKING

What is meant by the proverb, "Physician, heal thyself," and how can massage therapists apply this principle to their practice?

Chat Room—This feature is a place where I share additional information, expound on important concepts, offer suggestions and recommendations, present historical facts, and suggest tips for remembering test material.

CHAT ROOM

Providing a safe service also means that our work environment is barrier-free and accessible to all, including persons with disabilities. Therapists should also have a plan outlining what to do in an emergency. This includes a fire evacuation plan, and a designated safe area in which to retreat during events such as tornados or earthquakes.

New figures—This edition features more than 675 high-quality photographs and illustrations to help clarify difficult concepts in vibrant detail. Most of the new images are from my brother, photographer Chris Salvo, and his lovely partner and wife, Suzanne Salvo. Many of the new figures are innovative "motion" photographs that demonstrate technique sequence in greater clarity than traditional images.

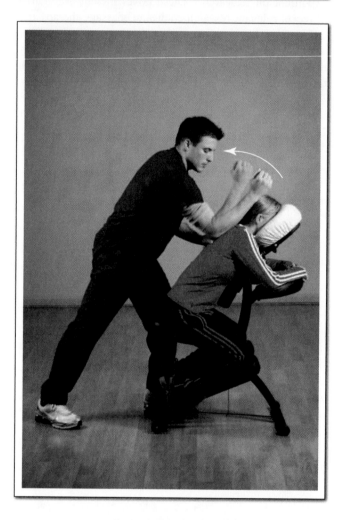

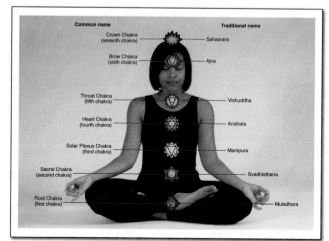

Inspirational quotes—Besides providing intellectual stimulation, one of our goals is to have the book inspire students cognitively, emotionally, and spiritually. This is accomplished through the use of insightful and thought-provoking quotations throughout the book.

> *"Too often we underestimate the power of a touch, a smile, a kind word, a listening ear, an honest compliment, or the smallest act of caring, all of which have the potential to turn a life around...."*
> —Leo Buscaglia

Pathologic conditions—We've include more than 200 different pathologies grouped according to their body system and affected structure. For ease of use, we've also reduced the specifics of each pathology by making the discussions of massage precautions and suggestions more succinct. For greater in-depth instruction, we recommend our companion textbook, *Mosby's Pathology for Massage Therapists* by Susan Salvo.

---

massaged, even though both groups of babies had the same number of feedings and averaged the same intake per feeding. The massaged babies were also more active and alert and left the hospital six days earlier than non-massaged babies. The massaged babies were also more socially active and more responsive, and had better coordination and motor skills, compared with the nonmassaged babies.

In 1992 Dr. Field formally established the Touch Research Institute (TRI) at the University of Miami School of Medicine through a start-up grant from Johnson & Johnson. The TRI is devoted solely to the study of touch and its application in both science and medicine. Research efforts continue today. The TRI has researched the effects of massage therapy in all stages of life, from newborns to senior citizens. In these studies, the TRI has shown that touch therapy has many positive effects on health and well-being.

> *"Writing a novel is like driving a car at night.*
> *You can see only as far as your headlights,*
> *but you can make the whole trip that way."*
> —E. L. Doctorow

DERMATOLOGIC PATHOLOGIES

Bacterial Skin Infections

Acne. Acne is an inflammatory bacterial infection of hair follicles and their associated sebaceous glands. It is marked by the presence of pimples with localized redness. Acne laden skin often appears greasy. Scars may develop if the condition becomes chronic.

Massage over the infected area is contraindicated.

Impetigo. Impetigo is a bacterial infection that occurs mainly around the mouth, nose, and hands (Figure 22-10). The infection is highly contagious and is easily spread by direct contact or by handling contaminated objects such as eating utensils, toothbrushes, towels, and bed (or massage) linens.

Massage is postponed until the affected area has completely healed as impetigo is highly contagious.

Folliculitis. Folliculitis is an infection that occurs when bacteria (usually staphylococci) enter hair follicles damaged by friction, such as from shaving or clothing. It can occur anywhere in hair-bearing skin, but is seen mainly in the groin, axillae, or the bearded areas of males. It often resembles acne.

Local massage is contraindicated because massage will further irritate follicles, which would increase inflammation.

Boils. Boils, or furuncles, are infected skin glands or hair follicles. Pain increases as the boil enlarges (which can be as large as a golf ball). Eventually, the abscess bursts. Once drainage occurs, the boil heals. This sequence of events takes about 2 weeks.

Local massage is contraindicated because massage will make the inflammation worse and may spread the infection.

Fungal Skin Infections

Ringworm. Ringworm is a fungal infection of the skin. This condition usually affects nonhairy parts of the face, trunk, and limbs (Figure 22-11). Ringworm is characterized by red, raised, round or oval scaling areas, creating a ringed appearance.

Since ringworm is contagious, massage is contraindicated until lesions have completely disappeared.

Athlete's Foot. Athlete's foot is a fungal infection of the foot. It is characterized by skin discoloration with a ridge of red tissue. The skin may flake, crack, and bleed, or ooze clear fluid. The infected foot often appears dry and has an unpleasant or musty odor.

Massage over the infected area is contraindicated. Although athlete's foot is not easily spread by contact with infected linens, treat massage linens as contaminated.

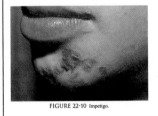

FIGURE 22-10 Impetigo.

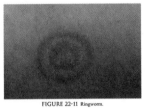

FIGURE 22-11 Ringworm.

Additional Learning Aids

It's All Greek to Me—These tables help you decipher the language of anatomy, physiology, and pathology. Medical and scientific terms all have the same origins. If you know that *cyto* is Greek for *cell*, it is easier to learn terms such as cytoplasm or osteocyte.

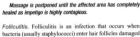

IT'S ALL GREEK TO ME	
arachnoid	*Gr.* spider; shaped
autonomic	*Gr.* self; law
axon	*Gr.* axis
baroreceptor	*Gr.* weight; *L.* to receive
Broca area	Broca, French surgeon (1824-1880)
cauda equina	*L.* tail-like; horse
cerebellum	*L.* little brain
cerebrum	*L.* brain
chemoreceptor	*Gr.* chemical; *L.* to receive
cochlea	*L.* snail shell
conduction	*L.* to lead together
corpus callosum	*L.* body; hard or callused
cortex	*L.* bark or rind
cyton	*Gr.* cell
dendrites	*Gr.* treelike
diencephalon	*Gr.* two or second; brain
dura mater	*L.* hard or tough; mother
encephalic	*Gr.* brain
filum terminale	*L.* threadlike; at the end
ganglion	*Gr.* knot
gyri	*Gr.* circle
incus	*L.* anvil
internuncial	*L.* between; together, amid; messenger
intrafusal	*L.* within; spindle
macula	*L.* spot
mechanoreceptor	*Gr.* machine; *L.* to receive
medulla oblongata	*L.* marrow or middle; long
meninges	*Gr.* membrane
myelin	*Gr.* marrow
neurilemma	*Gr.* sinew; husk
neuro	*Gr.* sinew
neuroglia	*Gr.* sinew; glue
neurotransmitter	*Gr.* sinew; *L.* a sending across
nociceptor	*L.* hurt; to receive
node of Ranvier	Ranvier, French pathologist (1835-1922)
oligodendrocyte	*Gr.* little; tree; cell
parasympathetic	*Gr.* by the side of, sympathetic
photoreceptor	*Gr.* light; *L.* to receive
pia mater	*L.* tender, soft; mother
plexus	*L.* braid
presbyopia	*Gr.* old man; eye
proprioceptor	*L.* one's own; a receiver

Charts and tables—This feature summarizes important information such as nutrition for fast, easy reference at a glance.

BOX 22-1

Abnormal Moles

Abnormal moles should be avoided in massage and then reported to the client. Encourage your client to have abnormal moles medically evaluated as they may be malignant melanomas, a deadly skin cancer. **ABCDE** is a method of mole assessment to determine abnormal moles, which stands for:

Asymmetry. Asymmetry means that if a line were drawn down the middle, there would be not be two equal halves. Common moles are symmetrical and round. Malignant moles are asymmetrical.

Border. The edges or borders of early melanomas are uneven, often containing scalloped or notched edges.

Color. Different shades of brown or black are often the first sign of a problem. Common moles are evenly shaded brown.

Diameter. Common moles are usually less than one-quarter inch in diameter (6 mm), the size of a pencil eraser. Early melanomas tend to be larger.

Evolving. Common moles do not change much, if at all. Malignant moles evolve or change over a period of time, and may rapidly increase in size, indicating metastasis.

In addition, any lesion that does not heal properly may indicate malignancy.

TABLE 23-1 Examples of Neurotransmitters

NEUROTRANSMITTER	LOCATION	FUNCTION
Acetylcholine (ACh)	Found in neuromuscular junctions and in many parts of the brain	Can be excitatory or inhibitory; vital for stimulating muscle contraction; also involved with memory
Epinephrine	Found in several areas of the CNS and in the sympathetic division of the ANS	Can be excitatory or inhibitory; mediates the "fight or flight" response; hormonelike action when secreted by the adrenal medulla
Norepinephrine	Found in several areas of the CNS and in the sympathetic division on the ANS	Similar to epinephrine, can be excitatory or inhibitory; also a hormone secreted by the adrenal medulla. This hormone mediates several physiologic and metabolic responses related to sympathetic arousal (fight or flight); also involved in dreaming, mood regulation, and emotional responses
Dopamine	Found in the brain and ANS	Mostly inhibitory and involved in emotions, moods, and motor control regulation; also implicated in attention and learning
Serotonin	Found in several regions of the CNS	Mostly excitatory and important for sensory perception, mood regulation, and normal sleep
Histamine	Found in the brain	Mostly excitatory and involved in, body temperature regulation, and water balance; histamine stimulates inflammatory responses when not acting as a neurotransmitter
Enkephalins	Found in several regions of the CNS, the retina, and the intestinal tract	Mostly inhibitory and action is similar to that of opiates as a pain-reducing agent
Endorphins	Found in several regions of the CNS, the retina, and the intestinal tract	Mostly inhibitory and action is similar to that of opiates as a pain-reducing agent
Gamma-aminobutyric acid (GABA)	Found in the brain	Mostly inhibitory
Substance P	Found in the brain, spinal cord, pain pathways, and the intestinal tract	Mostly excitatory and transmits pain information

Key terms and glossary—Key terms are bolded throughout the textbook. They can also be located in the glossary for easy access to definitions.

Mini-Labs—These short lab sessions within chapters are skill-building activities designed so that left-brained and right-brained techniques reinforce each other. Direct student participation enhances the learning process by stimulating creativity and imagination.

MINI-LAB

Touching With Intent

1. Work with a partner.
2. Assign one person to be the giver and one person to be the receiver. Sit facing each other.
3. The receiver extends his or her hands, palms up. The giver places his or her hands on the receiver's hands, palm down. Both the giver and the receiver close their eyes.
4. The giver becomes unfocused, disinterested, and mentally distracted as the receiver stays relaxed for 2 minutes.
5. After that time, the giver becomes very aware, interested, and concerned about the receiver. This attitude is maintained for 2 minutes.
6. Reverse roles and repeat.
7. Reflect on your experience and share it with your partner. Did you notice any differences when the attitudes changed? Does intent alter how touch is received? How can you use this information during a massage therapy session?

DVD—The bound-in DVD guides you through 2 hours of specific massage techniques, routines, procedures, and client interactions. These videos can also be viewed on the Evolve website. A play-button icon will appear in the text whenever a pertinent video clip is available, to help you save time and study more efficiently.

Be sure to avoid enlarged lymph nodes. However, if you possess advanced certification in manual lymphatic drainage or lymphatic massage, your education has made you familiar with workable and non-workable conditions. Superficial lymph nodes are located in the groin (inguinal nodes), in the armpits (axillary nodes), and in the neck (cervical nodes). When palpated, enlarged lymph nodes feel hard, similar to a tablet or capsule under the skin.

Absolute Contraindication

Absolute contraindications occur when receiving massage might put you or your client at serious health risk or the client's condition could be made worse with massage. Examples are a:

- Reported disease that is highly contagious
- Client who has widespread infection or inflammation
- Client who has fever
- Chronic disease that is in exacerbation
- Client who is in a state of medical emergency

When a client presents with an absolute contraindication, massage is not advised. When the client's disease resolves, is in a state of remission, or is cleared by the physician who managed the medical emergency, the client can then receive massage.

Treatment Modifications

In many cases, all that is needed are a few adaptive measures or treatment modifications. The type and extent of disease, as well as the client's health status, determine modifications to treatment. More on treatment planning and medication use (e.g., pain killers, hypoglycemics) can be found in Chapter 10. Chapter 11 is devoted to treatment modification for special populations (e.g., elderly or pregnant client).

Most treatment modifications are either positional or procedural. Examples of *positional modifications* are (1) use of a seated or semireclining position, (2) avoidance of the prone position, and (3) placement of a supportive cushion under the right pelvis and trunk to tilt the lower body to the left in cases of advanced pregnancy.

Examples of *procedural* or *modifications of technique* are (1) use of lighter-than-normal pressure, (2) avoiding percussion or joint mobilizations, and (3) assisting the client off the massage table. The last modification may be needed if your client is taking blood pressure medication, is pregnant, or is elderly and frail.

CHAT ROOM

Chronic diseases often have stages of remission and exacerbation. During *remission*, signs and symptoms subside or disappear. Also called flare-ups or relapses, *exacerbation* ushers in an increase in sign and symptom severity. Example of diseases with remission and exacerbation are multiple sclerosis and rheumatoid arthritis. Be sure to postpone massage in cases of disease exacerbation.

" A musician must make music, an artist must paint, a poet must write, if he is to be ultimately at peace with himself."
—Abraham Maslow

INFECTION CONTROL FOR MASSAGE THERAPISTS

As a massage therapist, you are at a slightly higher risk for contracting infection by direct contact or inhalation of infected respiratory droplets. Massage therapists who are hospital-based or who work with individuals who are sick or injured are at increased risk for contracting and spreading disease. Infection control decreases the risk of disease transmission in all settings.

So what are some ways infection can spread? You may unknowingly massage over an infectious rash in a treatment room with low lighting and spread the infection from one part of the client's body to another. Fluid from a boil may seep and enter broken skin. A client with a cold sore may touch the lip; then, after massaging your client's now infected hand, you may touch your own face. Additionally, infection can be spread through contact with contaminated linens, massage tools, and open containers of massage lubricant.

In December 1991, the Occupational Safety and Health Administration (OSHA) supported and helped pass federal legislation that requires all health care providers to adhere to a plan that helps prevent transmission of pathogens, namely human immunodeficiency virus (HIV), hepatitis B virus (HBV), and other blood-borne pathogens.

From this legislation, the Centers for Disease Control and Prevention (CDC) established *universal precautions*. Under universal precautions, blood and certain body fluids of all patients are considered potentially infectious.

In 1996, CDC published new guidelines for health care providers called *standard precautions*. These new guidelines expounded on original universal precautions, which dealt mainly with blood-borne pathogens. Standard precautions represent a wider range of infection control measures such as glove use when touching mucous membranes and guidelines for hand sanitation. Standard precautions for massage therapists include:

- Hand hygiene
- Using disposable gloves
- Laundering contaminated linens appropriately
- Disinfecting contaminated massage equipment and tools
- Dispensing uncontaminated massage lubricant
- Personal hygiene
- Maintaining a clean and sanitary office and treatment environment

In some circumstances, state law or employers require massage therapists to be immunized against diseases such as rubella, rubeola, diphtheria, tuberculosis, and hepatitis B. Some employers of massage therapists, such as

Internet support—Sprinkled throughout the text, you will find Evolve boxes indicating that additional material is available online. The Evolve website for this text has been radically expanded to include activities, flash cards, drag-and-drop exercises, video clips, student tips, a collection of additional graphic images, weblinks to other resources and, because you requested it, a mock national certification exam. These enhanced online resources make chapter review and exam preparation easy and engaging. A list of all resources is included at the end of each chapter. Log in to your student account on the Evolve website and view animations of the cardiac cycle, arterial and venous blood flow, blood pressure, and more.

E-RESOURCES

ⓔvolve

http://evolve.elsevier.com/Salvo/MassageTherapy

- Chapter challenge
- Flash cards
- Photo gallery
- Technique videos
- Additional information
- Downloadable forms
- Weblinks

New and Expanded

Kinesiology chapter—This all-new chapter thoroughly covers the topics of bones, bony markings, and muscles—their origins, insertions, actions, and innervations. It includes more than 170 images of individual muscles and vibrant 3-D illustrations of muscle groups to help you accurately identify, locate, and palpate muscles.

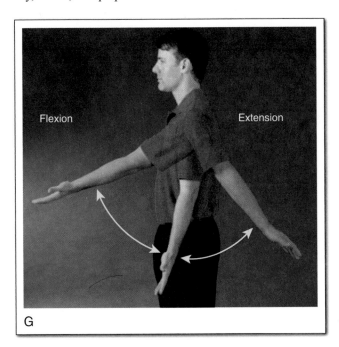

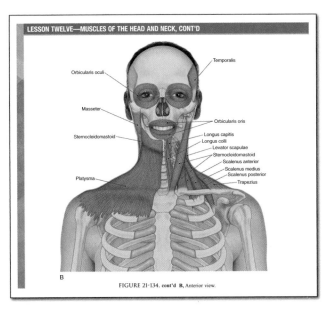

FIGURE 21-134. cont'd **B**, Anterior view.

Clinical massage chapter—This chapter broadens your career potential with detailed information on trigger points, posture, gait, and rehabilitation for working in physician-referred practices, multidisciplinary clinics, and sports injury environments.

Special populations chapter—Completely revised and expanded, this chapter focuses on pregnancy massage, infant massage, and working with children and adolescents, the elderly, and hospice patients. Clients with disabilities and impairment are discussed, including clients who are wheelchair-bound. This chapter also features suggestions when working with clients who are struggling with addiction.

Research literacy chapter—This chapter demonstrates the importance of research-based massage practice and guides you through the process of acquiring, reading, interpreting, and applying the latest scientific information. This and other content areas reflect the most essential massage therapy topics as identified by the Massage Therapy Body of Knowledge (MTBOK). In recent years, research and evidence-based practice is a central focus of professional organizations, which have also strongly encouraged their members to carry out investigations to provide evidence supporting or rejecting the use of specific modalities.

Research-based massage effects chapter—This new chapter discusses the effects of massage by body system. The experiments used to support these massage effects are annotated (157 to be exact), allowing students to locate and read the published studies themselves. The pain cycle and gate control theory are also featured, as well as indications for specific conditions and populations.

Hydrotherapy and spa chapter—Because one third of therapists are now employed in spas, this chapter has been updated and reorganized to include heat and cold applications, bath and shower techniques, types of exfoliations and body wraps, and specialized methods such as hot stone massage, shirodhara, and watsu. As a bonus, we have expanded the section on aromatherapy.

Business chapter—This chapter has been expanded to better prepare you for today's job market and appeal to potential employers and clients using digital media and social networking tools.

Self-help chapter—This new chapter discusses health and wellness models and includes suggestions for physical activity, basic nutrition principles, nutrients such as vitamins and minerals, and stress reduction techniques. This information can be used for client education or as a guide for the therapist as he or she pursues a healthy lifestyle.

Infection control and medical emergency preparedness—This revised and expanded chapter now includes the most current information on standard precautions, local and absolute contraindications, and hand hygiene. First aid measures and safe procedures to follow in cases of medical emergencies are also included such as choking, hypoglycemia, insulin shock, stroke, heart attack, and seizures.

Therapeutic relationships—This expanded chapter includes emphasis on interpersonal skills and guidance in ethical decision making. This chapter takes the topic of boundaries to a whole new level.

Treatment planing chapter—The scope of practice discussion has been moved to this chapter to help therapists better understand their professional boundaries while devising treatment plans. This chapter also addresses concepts of health literacy. As you may know, I'm a big supporter of treatment planning and advocate the use of assessment domain as a way of gathering pertinent client information. The PPALM system is featured in this chapter. This chapter also features a table of frequently used medications, their side effects, and massage considerations. Because much of our population have medical conditions managed by medications, understanding their effects has become increasingly important.

SOAP note appendix—Also included in this edition is additional information on SOAP documentation.

For Instructors

TEACH—TEACH resources will continue to support the instructor's needs. The **TEACH Instructor Resource** is designed to help instructors prepare for classes and will reduce lesson plan preparation time, give new and creative ideas to promote student learning, and help make full use of a rich array of resources.

Evolve—Instructors will also find the following on the Evolve website:

- Test bank in ExamView format with 1200 questions
- Answer keys to self-test questions in the book
- Downloadable forms such as PPALM, intake, and student surveys
- Image collection in JPG and PowerPoint, containing all images from the book
- Supplemental collection of images not found in the book
- Teaching tips for each chapter
- Testing and grading information
- Crossword puzzles for handouts
- Much more!

For Students

Evolve—Students will find the following on the Evolve website:

- Client consultation and technique video clips
- Audio glossary
- Image collection (same as instructor site)
- Downloadable forms
- Activities including drag-and-drop exercises, muscle drawing activities, and games
- Mock National Certification Exam
- Weblinks

SUSAN G. SALVO
www.facebook.com/susansalvo
www.LaMassageSchool.com

ACKNOWLEDGMENTS

I would like to acknowledge the following individuals and companies who assisted me in writing and developing this edition:

Rebecca Savich at ABC Table Works
Laura Allen
Sandra Kauffman Anderson
Jeanine Utzman Babineaux
David Ballard
William Barry
Jennifer Behn
Chelsea Breaux
Jennifer Breaux
Jessica Breaux
Michael Breaux
Celia Bucci
Lisa Bunch
Elaine Calenda
Andrea Campbell
Danielle R. Caraway (aromatherapy)
Dave Carlson, Artist
Karyn Chabot
Teena Cole
Barb Cousins
Susie Ogg Cormier
Bill Curet
Judith DeLany
Tari Dilks
Mary Donker
Catherine Dupuis
Tish Ecker
Cindy Ellender
Facebook.com—Friends and Colleagues
Alice Funk
Julie Goodwin
Tricia Grafelman
Christy Granger
Lauriann Greene
Robert Harris
Chip Hines (MTBOK)
Mike Hinkle
James Hollingshed
Francis Johnson
Karen Kinslow
Colleen Kruse (MRF)
Karen Kubek (AMTA)
David Lauterstein
Kathie Lea
Rita LeBleu
Whitney Lowe
Megan Lavery
Sandy Grover Mason
Massage Professionals.com—Friends and Colleagues
Maria and Wayne Mathias
Joey Erwin Mazzera
Cherie Monlezun
Eric Munn
Joseph Muscolino
Nicole Owen (Biotone)
Grant Parker
Debra Persinger (Federation)
Monica Reno
Jeffrey Riach (Oakworks)
Hayley Salvo
Suzanne and Chris Salvo
Diego Sanchez
Jennifer Schaaf
JoEllen Sefton
Lisa Severn (Oakworks)
Randall Short
Ralph Stephens
Elaine Stillerman
H. Micheal Tarver
Georgia Tetlow
Donald Thigpen
Annie LaCroix Tiedeman
Emily Thomson
Michelle Vahlkamp (AMTA)
Jennifer Wagley (NCBTMB)
Dennis Walker
Tracy Walton
Jennifer Watrous
Ruth Werner
Freda Whalen Plues
Kellie White
Anne Williams (ABMP)
Maggie Woosley
Michelle Zenz (AMTA)
Kenneth Zysk

A final word of appreciation: Over the years this book has evolved and gained popularity basically because of "the look" created by the teamwork of the editorial staff and contributors. For this fourth edition, that look is attributed to the photography and illustrations. This is a combination of the photography talents of Chris and Suzanne Salvo with the illustrations from Joe Muscolino's book *The Muscular System Manual*. I highly recommend that it be included in the library of every serious massage therapist. Thank you, Dr. Muscolino, and thanks again to Chris and Suzanne.

SUSAN G. SALVO

CONTENTS

UNIT ONE

FOUNDATIONS FOR PRACTICE, BASIC AND COMPLEMENTARY METHODS, AND BUSINESS PRACTICES

UNIT TWO
ANATOMY AND PHYSIOLOGY

FOUNDATIONS FOR PRACTICE, BASIC AND COMPLEMENTARY METHODS, AND BUSINESS PRACTICES

CHAPTER 1

History of Massage

H. Micheal Tarver, PhD, and Susan G. Salvo, BEd, LMT, NTS, CI, NCTMB

"Travel is fatal to prejudice, bigotry, and narrow-mindedness."
—Mark Twain

LEARNING OBJECTIVES

After completing this chapter, the student should be able to:

- Define the term *massage*.
- Name major figures in the development of medicine and specifically in massage therapy.
- Discuss ancient views and uses of massage, incorporating both Eastern and Western cultures.
- Explain the role of the European Renaissance and Enlightenment on the massage therapy profession.
- Distinguish the contributions of Pehr Henrik Ling from those of later physicians and therapists.
- Reconstruct the development of massage.
- Discuss the current events of the massage therapy profession.

http://evolve.elsevier.com/Salvo/MassageTherapy

INTRODUCTION

The history of massage and healing touch is long and multifaceted, with currently more than 80 different methods of massage and *bodywork*; the latter is a generic term used to describe any therapeutic or personal self-development practice that may include massage, healing touch, movement, or energetic work. However, the terms *massage* and *bodywork* are frequently used interchangeably. Archaeological and historical evidence indicates that massage and bodywork have been practiced for thousands of years in all regions of the globe.

Massage is instinctive and intuitive. It is a natural response to rub our aches and pains, whether or not we are familiar with the "whys" behind these actions.

Massage, or **massage therapy,** is the manual and scientific manipulation of the soft tissues of the body for the purpose of establishing and maintaining health and promoting wellness. The therapist uses a wide variety of techniques to assist a client in fulfillment of his or her therapeutic goals. Examples of client goals are relaxation, injury rehabilitation, management of symptoms during a long-term illness, and enhancing personal growth.

Client therapeutic goals are established thorough treatment planning, which incudes an intake process.

In modern health care, massage has taken on an important role. It has been shown to be beneficial in reducing stress, enhancing blood flow, decreasing pain, promoting sleep, reducing swelling, enhancing relaxation, and increasing the oxygen capacity of the blood (see Chapter 6). Massage has also been recognized for alleviating certain cancer treatment side effects and postoperative pain.

In this chapter, we will briefly examine the history of massage from its earliest records to the present (Figure 1-1). This historical perspective will take us down the path that leads us to where we are as a profession currently and will instill a sense of connection with those who preceded us. Some names will be familiar, and others will be quite foreign. You need not memorize every name mentioned in the following pages, although some are important enough that you should know them (ask your instructor). What the names, with their different nations of origin, tell us is that the development of massage was a global endeavor; people from around the world contributed to the knowledge base that transformed massage from folk remedy to medical treatment.

It should be noted that from the beginning of this chapter, the word *massage* is used to refer to soft tissue manipulation, even though the term did not come into use until the middle of the nineteenth century. The origin of the word massage is unclear, but it can be traced to numerous sources: the Hebrew word *mashesh,* the Greek roots *masso* and *massin,* the Latin root *massa,* the Arabic root *mass'h,* the Sanskrit word *makeh,* and the French word *masser.*

THE PREHISTORIC WORLD

In prehistoric times (i.e., before written records), evidence supports the position that several groups around the world practiced massage. Archaeologists have found artifacts that depict the use of massage in many world cultures. Although no direct prehistoric evidence verifies the use of massage for medical reasons, the indirect evidence clearly implies that it was used in this manner. For example, European cave paintings (c. 15,000 BC) depict what appears to be the use of massage. In this period, extensive pictorial records show the use of massage.

> *"Time is a great teacher, but unfortunately it kills all its pupils."*
> —Hector Berlioz

---

evolve *Log on to the Evolve website for Massage Therapy: Principles & Practice, ed. 4, at* http://evolve.elsevier.com/ Salvo/MassageTherapy *and register for student resources that accompany this text. Select a password to use each time you log on. Once the registration process is complete, peruse all the Evolve assets at your disposal.* ∎

THE ANCIENT WORLD

In the ancient East, a concern with illness has been documented in China for several millennia, and records have revealed that the practice of massage goes back as early as 3000 BC. However, in the period between the second century BC (200 to 101 BC) and the first century AD (AD 1 to 100), Chinese medicine began to take on its basic shape. Manuscripts found in China dating from the second century BC discuss massage as one of the treatments for illnesses. However, acupuncture was not mentioned in Chinese medical writings until 90 BC.

Using their knowledge of massage and later acupuncture, the Chinese developed a style of massage that they termed *amma, amna,* or *anmo.* **Amma** is regarded as the original massage technique and the precursor to all other therapies, manual and energetic. The Chinese had developed the art of massage so well that they were the first to train and employ massage therapists who were blind.

As early as the first century AD, various schools of medical thought had been founded and had already begun to produce diverging ideas. These various ideas and beliefs were compiled under the name of the mythical Yellow Emperor and became the classic scripture of traditional Chinese medicine, the *Huang-ti nei-ching.* Although the exact date of the original writing of the work is unknown, it was already in its present form by approximately the first century BC. The work, commonly known as *Nei Ching,* contained descriptions of healing touch procedures, herbal

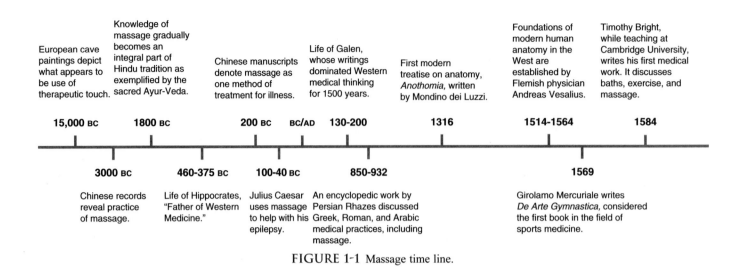

European cave paintings depict what appears to be use of therapeutic touch.

Knowledge of massage gradually becomes an integral part of Hindu tradition as exemplified by the sacred Ayur-Veda.

Chinese manuscripts denote massage as one method of treatment for illness.

Life of Galen, whose writings dominated Western medical thinking for 1500 years.

First modern treatise on anatomy, *Anothomia*, written by Mondino dei Luzzi.

Foundations of modern human anatomy in the West are established by Flemish physician Andreas Vesalius.

Timothy Bright, while teaching at Cambridge University, writes his first medical work. It discusses baths, exercise, and massage.

15,000 BC   1800 BC   200 BC   BC/AD   130-200   1316   1514-1564   1584

3000 BC   460-375 BC   100-40 BC   850-932   1569

Chinese records reveal practice of massage.

Life of Hippocrates, "Father of Western Medicine."

Julius Caesar uses massage to help with his epilepsy.

An encyclopedic work by Persian Rhazes discussed Greek, Roman, and Arabic medical practices, including massage.

Girolamo Mercuriale writes *De Arte Gymnastica,* considered the first book in the field of sports medicine.

FIGURE 1-1 Massage time line.

medicines, acupuncture, and their uses. Some debate is ongoing over the actual date of this work, with some historians arguing that it was written around 2760 BC. By AD 700, a Chinese ministry of health and a public health system were established.

By the sixth century AD, the use of massage was well established in China and had found their way into Japan. In general, the Japanese methods of massage were basically the same as those of the Chinese. In Japan, amma was practiced for many centuries. Eventually it evolved into shiatsu, literally meaning finger pressure, a term first coined in the early 1900s.

Shiatsu is a Japanese method based on the same traditional Chinese medicine concepts as acupuncture, namely that energy flows in the body in streams called channels or meridians. When these channels become blocked or depleted, pain and discomfort result. Acupuncturists use needles at specific points to balance the flow of energy; shiatsu therapists use their fingers, thumbs, forearms, elbows, and even their knees and feet to balance the client's energy. Shiatsu can be performed generally on each channel, or at specific points called *tsubo*. Tsubos are openings into the channels. As with the Chinese, the medieval Japanese employed blind massage therapists.

In addition to Chinese and Japanese, other Asian cultures practiced massage. On the Indian subcontinent, the practice of massage has also existed for more than 3000 years. Knowledge of massage had probably been brought to India from China, and it gradually became an integral part of Hindu tradition, as exemplified by the inclusion of massage in the sacred practice of Ayurveda (c. 1800 BC). The Ayurveda, literally meaning *code of life,* deals with rebirth, renunciation, salvation, the soul, the purpose of life, the maintenance of mental health, and the prevention and treatment of diseases.

As for medicine, the most important Ayurvedic texts are the *Samhitas.* A later work, the *Manav Dharma Shastra* (c. 300 BC), also mentions massage. In addition to the previously mentioned Eastern cultures, the Polynesians have also been documented as practicing massage.

The concept of health and medicine in the West began to take shape during the seventh and sixth centuries BC. During that time, the legendary Greek physician Æsculapius (Asclepius) evolved into a god who was responsible for the emerging medical profession. His holy snake and staff still remain the symbol of the medical profession. In Greece, around 500 BC, various ideas of healing and treatments were merged into a *techne iatriche,* or healing science. During this process, two individuals, Iccus and Herodicus, concerned themselves with exercise and the use of gymnastics.

Among the followers of this new science was Hippocrates of Cos (460 to 375 BC) (Figure 1-2). With his emphasis on the individual patient and his belief that the healer should take care to avoid causing any additional harm to the patient, Hippocrates is generally recognized as the father of modern Western medicine. Although we know little about him,

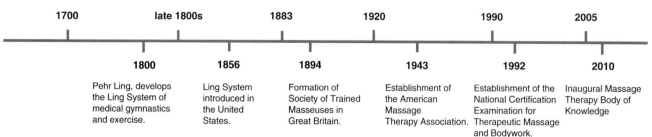

In Italy, Giovanni Borelli has analyzed the phenomenon of muscular contraction. In England, William Harvey demonstrates that blood circulation is impelled by the beat of the heart. These discoveries enhance the acceptance of massage as therapeutic.

Dr. Douglas Graham publishes several books on the history of massage.

Hartvig Nissen opens the Swedish Health Institute.

Chartered Society of Massage and Medical Gymnastics is founded.

Establishment of the Massage Therapy Foundation.

Formation of the Federation of the State Massage Therapy Boards.

1700   late 1800s   1883   1920   1990   2005

1800   1856   1894   1943   1992   2010

Pehr Ling, develops the Ling System of medical gymnastics and exercise.

Ling System introduced in the United States.

Formation of Society of Trained Masseuses in Great Britain.

Establishment of the American Massage Therapy Association.

Establishment of the National Certification Examination for Therapeutic Massage and Bodywork.

Inaugural Massage Therapy Body of Knowledge

FIGURE 1-1, cont'd

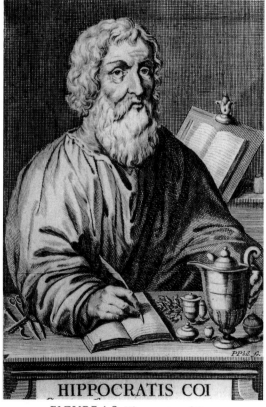

FIGURE 1-2 Hippocrates of Cos.

Hippocrates is reputed to have been a fine clinician, a founder of a medical school, and the author of numerous books, although most of the works attributed to him were written by other members of the Hippocratic school. These works are collectively known as the *Corpus Hippocraticum,*

which summarized much of what was known about disease and medicine in the ancient world. During the four centuries after the development of the *techne iatriche,* several debates occurred within the healing profession, one of which placed great stock in the value of massage.

In his essay *On Joints,* Hippocrates wrote, "μολλ^ων ^εν π^ειρον σ^ει τον ιητρον, αταρ ση και ανατριψιοζ"

("The physician must be skilled in many things and particularly friction," section IX, lines 25-26).

Hippocrates also noted that after reduction of a dislocated shoulder, friction should be done with soft, gentle hands (section IX, lines 31-33). Obviously, Hippocrates was a proponent of massage.

During the transitional period between Greek and Roman dominance in the ancient world, a few individuals helped pass on the medical knowledge of the Greeks and incorporated it into Roman medicine. One such individual was Aulus Celsus, who is regarded by many researchers to be the first important medical historian. His *De Medicina* is an outstanding account of Roman medicine, and it bridges the gap between his times and those of Hippocrates. During this period, massage had gained such acceptance that Julius Caesar (c. 100 to 44 BC) used it to help his epilepsy.

A group of Greek physicians residing in Rome, known as the Methodists, supported a simplistic view of healing and restricted their treatments to bathing, diet, massage, and a few drugs. The founder of this school of thought was Asclepiades. Among his many contributions to Roman medicine was a treatise on friction (massage) and exercise. Although the work is no longer in existence, Aulus Aurelius Cornelius Celsus (c. 25 BC to AD 50) cited it in his writings on friction.

"There are no rules here. We're trying to accomplish something."
—Thomas Edison

A later follower of Hippocratic medicine was Galen of Pergamon (c. AD 130 to 200). Galen was a Roman physician who studied medicine in Alexandria (Egypt) and became the personal physician to the Roman emperor Marcus Aurelius. In at least 100 treatises, Galen combined and unified Greek knowledge of anatomy and medicine; his system continued to dominate medicine throughout the Middle Ages and until relatively recent times. Among his many works, Galen's *De Sanitate Tuenda* considers exercise, the use of baths, and massage. After the Roman Empire divided into eastern and western halves, the decline in learning was much more rapid and severe in the Roman West than in the Greek East (Byzantium).

Farther east of the Romans, the ancient Slavs reportedly used massage. In the Americas, the Mayas and Inca have been documented as practicing joint manipulation and massage. The Inca also used the application of heat in their treatments of joint disorders through the use of the leaves of the chilca bush. They had a higher success rate for *trepanation,* a surgical procedure involving the removal of a segment of the skull, in 2000 BC than the Europeans did in AD 1800. In addition, records indicate that the Cherokees and Navajos used massage in their treatments of colic and to ease labor pains.

"Do not go where the path may lead, go instead where there is no path and leave a trail."
—Ralph Waldo Emerson

THE MIDDLE AGES

After collapse of the Roman Empire (AD 476), Western medicine experienced a period of decline. In reality, it was only because of the writing efforts of a few Western physicians (e.g., Oribasius, Alexander of Tralles) that ancient medical knowledge of the Greeks and Romans was preserved. After decline of the Roman Empire, the Hippocratic-Galenic tradition survived in the Greek-speaking East. Then after the fall of Alexandria (AD 642), knowledge of Greek medicine spread throughout the Arabic world.

After expansion of the Islamic world in the seventh and eighth centuries, a comprehensive body of Greco-Roman medical doctrine was adopted, together with extensive Persian and Hindu medical knowledge. One such example of this synthesis of knowledge was an encyclopedic work *(Kitabu'l Hawi Fi't-Tibb)* by the Persian physician Rhazes (Abu Bakr Muhammad ibn Zakariya al-Razi) (c. AD 850 to 932), which discussed Greek, Roman, and Arabic medical practices, including massage. Another important work was by the Persian physician Abu-Ali al-Husayn ibn-Sina (AD 980 to 1037), generally known as Avicenna. He authored numerous medical books that remained the standard until the seventeenth century.

Avicenna's *Canon of Medicine* was an especially famous medical text, one that compiled the theoretical and practical medical knowledge of the time. The work illustrates tremendous influence of Galen on the medical knowledge of this era; the text makes numerous references to the use of massage. In fact, by the end of the ninth century, almost all of Galen's lengthy medical texts had been translated into Arabic. In fact, if it wasn't for these Middle Eastern translations, much of the ancient Greek and Roman information would have been lost. The Muslims simply incorporated Greco-Roman medical knowledge into the Islamic framework. Through Latin translations of these Arabic authors, most of the knowledge of Greek medicine was revived in the Christian West (i.e., Europe).

⊖volve *As you know, the Odyssey tells the story of Odysseus' return from the Trojan War. Log on to Evolve to view a Bas-Relief depicting Odysseus receiving massage.* ■

For the most part, Western medical practitioners of the Middle Ages abandoned massage in favor of other treatments. Massage did, however, remain an important procedure for folk healers and midwives, and massage was passed on as a healing art form. Subsequently, no early compilation of these techniques and procedures was undertaken.

During the course of the later Middle Ages, the collection, preservation, and transmission of classical medical knowledge occurred. After the twelfth century, medieval medical knowledge in the West expanded, thanks in part to the existing works by the Muslims, who had earlier translated Greek and Latin medical texts into Arabic.

By the thirteenth century, medical knowledge had advanced to the point that three major European centers (Montpelier and Paris, France, and Bologna, Italy) were offering degrees in medicine. In 1316, Mondino dei Luzzi wrote *Anothomia,* the first modern treatise on anatomy.

"Books are the DNA of civilization."
—Anonymous

THE EUROPEAN RENAISSANCE AND ENLIGHTENMENT

The Renaissance (c. 1250-1550) was an exciting period in the history of medicine and medical treatments. The word *renaissance* means rebirth. With the revival of classical Greek learning during the Renaissance, Western medicine was revitalized by new translations of old Greek and Latin texts. Among the newly revived texts was Aulus Celsus's *De Medicina,* which came into circulation again, thanks to the newly invented printing press (thank your Johannes Gütenberg [c. 1450]). The Flemish physician, Andreas Vesalius (1514-1564) established the foundations of modern human anatomy (in the West) during this time. His *De Humani Corporis Fabrica* (1543) is considered one of the most important studies in the history of medicine. In addition, the Swiss physician Philippus von Hohenheim (1493-1541), better known as Paracelsus, laid the foundations of chemical pharmacology, as opposed to herbal remedies.

New surgical procedures were also established, particularly those by the French military surgeon Ambroise Paré (c. 1510-1590). In addition to inventing several surgical instruments, Paré was among the earliest modern physicians to discuss the therapeutic effects of massage, especially in orthopedic surgery cases. Paré even went so far as to classify various types of massage movements.

---

evolve Log on to the Evolve website to see illustrations of Galen of Pergamon and Ambroise Paré. ■

Two other notable Renaissance physicians were Girolamo Mercuriale (1530-1606) and Timothy Bright (c. 1551-1615). Mercuriale spent several years in Rome examining manuscripts of ancient writers. His extensive knowledge of the attitudes of the Greeks and Romans toward diet, exercise, and their effects on health and disease is evident in *De Arte Gymnastica* (1569), considered to be the first book in the field of sports medicine.

This book compiled history of gymnastics up to that time, synthesizing all that had been written on the use of exercise (for both the purpose of health and the treatment of disease). Bright's first work (c. 1584) was divided into two parts, *Hygienina on Restoring Health* and *Therapeutica on Restoring Health*. In these works, Bright discussed baths, exercise, and massage, and he began teaching his ideas to students at Cambridge University in Cambridge, England.

About the sixteenth century we see two important East Asian works that dealt with massage. The Chinese published *Chen-chiu ta-ch'eng*, which contained a chapter on pediatric massage, and the Japanese published *San-tsai-tou-hoei*, which mentioned both passive and active massage procedures.

By the end of the seventeenth century, Western medicine had experienced a revolution in both ideas and knowledge. In Italy, Giovanni Alfonso Borelli (1608-1679) carried out extensive anatomical dissections and had analyzed the phenomenon of muscular contraction.

In England, William Harvey (1578-1657) had demonstrated that blood circulation in animals is impelled by the beat of the heart through arteries and veins. This discovery enhanced the acceptance of massage as a therapeutic measure.

Another crucial development during the seventeenth century was the realization of the necessity to compile complete clinical descriptions of disease, generally at bedsides, and to develop specific remedies for each specific disease. In this area, the English physician Thomas Sydenham (1624-1689) was most prominent. At the same time these scientific advances were being made, massage was reemerging as a therapy that was acceptable to the medical profession and as a therapeutic practice for health and disease.

The European Renaissance and Enlightenment era also had an impact on Western medicine. What emerged was an optimistic outlook concerning the role and benefits of the field of medicine. The widely held belief asserted that health was a natural state to be attained and preserved.

Within this new philosophy, massage came to be viewed as a popular treatment in Europe. Simon André Tissot (1728-1797) published several works on gymnastic exercises that recommended massage for various diseases and gave indications for its use. The eighteenth century also saw the creation of new medical systems that incorporated the anatomical, physiological, and chemical discoveries of the previous 200 years. Some people believed that the gathering and dispensing of this new knowledge would add prestige to the medical profession and help weed out the quacks.

"Oftentimes, when people think about history, they think of it as something that's passed. However, the only really important history is the history that's still alive, that's affecting us today."
—David Lauterstein

THE MODERN ERA

The era of modern massage began in the early nineteenth century when a wide variety of authors were advocating massage and developing their own systems.

The most important of these writers was Pehr Henrik Ling (1776-1839), a Swedish physiologist and gymnastics instructor (see Ling biography in this chapter). Through his experiences at the University of Lund and the Swedish Royal Central Institute of Gymnastics, Ling developed his own system of medical (or Swedish) gymnastics and exercise, known as the *Ling System, Swedish Movements,* or *Swedish Movement Cure.* The primary focus of Ling's work was on gymnastics or movements applied to the treatment of disease and injury. According to Ling, his Swedish gymnastics was a therapeutic system by which we—by means of influencing movement—overcome discomfort that has arisen through abnormal conditions.

Ling's system consists of three primary movements: active, passive, and duplicated. *Active movements* were those performed by the patient (e.g., exercise). *Passive movements* were movements of the patient performed by the therapist (e.g., stretching, joint mobilizations). *Duplicated movements* were those performed by the patient with the cooperation of the therapist (e.g., active assistive movements). As part of duplicated movements, the therapist may oppose (restrain) the patient's movements (active resistive movements). Other terms used to describe Swedish gymnastics are remedial gymnastics, table stretches, and range-of-motion exercises.

Massage was viewed as a component of Ling's overall system. He blended massage with physiology, which was just emerging as a science. Shortly thereafter, the term Swedish massage was used to describe the massage component of Ling's system. Rightly so, Ling is regarded as the father of Swedish massage. While he did not invent massage, he can be credited with helping develop it into a formal treatment modality. His followers used massage strokes in tandem with the movements described previously. Swedish massage and Swedish gymnastics were noted to improve circulation, relieve muscle tension, improve range of motion, and promote general relaxation. This system eventually led to the development of physical therapy as a profession. In the early years, massage was a major component of physical therapy. In later years, physical therapy and massage therapy diverged into two separate professions.

From 1813 to 1839, Ling taught these techniques at the Royal Central Institute of Gymnastics in Stockholm, Sweden, which he founded with government support. His students were responsible for spreading his ideas throughout the world. Among the more important cities with established schools that were teaching Ling's methods were St. Petersburg, London, Berlin, Dresden, Leipzig, Vienna and Paris. Within 12 years of his death (1839), 38 institutions in Europe were teaching the Swedish movements system. Among these students were numerous medical physicians who became convinced of the usefulness of massage and therapeutic exercise in the practice of medicine. Medical physicians could complete Ling's Swedish gymnastics program in 1 year, as compared with 2 to 3 years for non-physicians. As more physicians were trained, massage became more and more acceptable as a traditional medical procedure and practice.

"A story should have a beginning, a middle, and an end... but not necessarily in that order."
—Jean-Luc Godard

Another key individual in the history of massage was the Dutch physician Johann Mezger (1838-1909). Mezger is responsible for making massage a fundamental component of physical rehabilitation. He has also been credited with the introduction of the still-used French terminology to the massage profession (e.g., effleurage, pétrissage, tapotement). The French translated several of the Chinese books on massage, and this effort probably explains why French terminology to describe massage techniques has become so common in massage texts such as this one. Also, French was considered the international language in the nineteenth century.

Mezger, being a physician, was much more able than Ling to promote massage using a medical and scientific basis. In this regard, Mezger was quite successful in getting

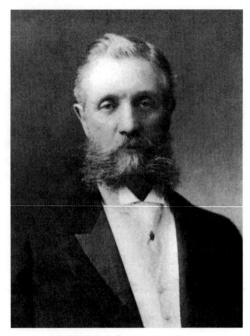

FIGURE 1-3 Hartvig Nissen.

the medical profession to accept massage as a bona fide medical treatment for disease and illness. A significant number of European physicians began to use massage therapy and to publish scientifically its positive effects. What occurred was the inclusion of the art of massage in the science of medicine.

Two brothers, Drs. George Henry Taylor and Charles Fayette Taylor, introduced the Swedish movement system into the United States in 1856. The Taylors had studied the techniques in Europe and returned to the United States, where they opened an orthopedic practice with a specialization in the Swedish Movements. The two physicians published many important works on Ling's system. George Taylor wrote the first American textbook on the subject in 1860 entitled *An Exposition of the Swedish Movement Cure.*

A third prominent American follower of the Swedish movement system was Douglas O. Graham. Not only was Dr. Graham a practitioner of the system, but from 1874 to 1925, he also authored several works on the history of massage.

Another prominent figure in the United States was Hartvig Nissen (Figure 1-3), who in 1883 opened the Swedish Health Institute for the Treatment of Chronic Diseases by Swedish Movements and Massage (Washington, D.C.). In 1888 Nissen presented the paper *Swedish Movement and Massage,* which was subsequently published in several medical journals. The result of publication was numerous letters from physicians who wanted to know more about Ling's system, and this inquiry led him to publish *Swedish Movement and Massage Treatment* in that same year. Taken together, Nissen's book and Graham's *A Treatise on Massage, Its History, Mode of Application and Effects* (1902) are generally credited with arousing interest in the U.S. medical profession in the benefits of massage.

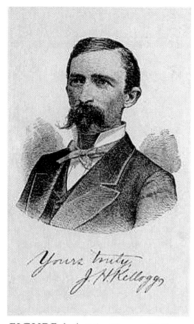

FIGURE 1-4 John Harvey Kellogg.

While the Taylor brothers, Graham, and Nissen were convincing the medical community of the benefits of massage and gymnastics, several other individuals were busy convincing the general public. Among the most famous of these individuals was John Harvey Kellogg (1852-1943) of Battle Creek, Michigan. He wrote numerous articles and books on massage and published *Good Health,* a magazine that targeted the general public (Figure 1-4). Some books Kellogg wrote, such as the *Art of Massage: A Practical Manual for the Nurse, the Student and the Practitioner*, were not published until after he died in 1943. Efforts by men such as Kellogg helped popularize massage in the United States.

The end of the nineteenth and beginning of the twentieth centuries witnessed important changes in the use of massage, the most important of which was the development of the field of physical therapy. Physical therapy, which developed from physical education, was responsible for training of women to work in hospitals, where they used massage and therapeutic exercise to help patients recover.

World War I provided countless opportunities for the use of massage therapy, exercise, and other physiotherapeutic methods (electrotherapy and hydrotherapy) in efforts to rehabilitate injured soldiers. During the course of treating war casualties, the earlier ideas of Just Lucas-Championniere (1843-1913) were important. Dr. Lucas-Championniere advocated the use of massage and passive-motion exercises after injuries, especially fractures.

By the beginning of the twentieth century, massage had begun to be used throughout the West. Once the procedures of massage were accepted, what developed was the profession of massage. In Great Britain, several women who realized the need for the standardization and professionalization of their trade formed *The Society of Trained Masseuses* (1894). The organization was successful in several key areas: establishing a massage curriculum; accrediting massage schools, which had to undergo regular inspections; requiring qualified instructors for the massage classes; and establishing a board certification program. By the end of World War I (1918), the Society had nearly 5000 members.

In 1920 the Society merged with the Institute of Massage and Remedial Exercise, and the new group became known as the *Chartered Society of Massage and Medical Gymnastics.* This new group also took some important steps at professionalism. Among the new membership requirements were physician referrals and the issuance of certificates of competence to persons who passed the required tests. By 1939 the membership in the organization numbered approximately 12,000.

After World War I, medical organizations such as the American Society of Physical Therapy Physicians also formed. In the 1920s and 1930s, programs for physical therapists were becoming standardized, while at the same time physicians were being trained in the field. In 1926 John S. Coulter became the first full-time academic physician in physical medicine at the Northwestern University Medical School in Evanston, Ill. By 1947 the field of physical therapy and rehabilitation was established as a separate medical specialty.

Although many masseurs and masseuses frowned on the encroachment of the medical profession on their art form, the events just described can be viewed with excitement. By the early part of the twentieth century, the Western medical profession had begun to realize what the Chinese and masseurs and masseuses had long preached: Massage had an important place in the treatment of illnesses and diseases. The professionalism of medical gymnastics (now called *physical therapy*) simply meant that, in addition to learning the art of massage, the therapist needs also to acquire the scientific background necessary to understand human anatomy, physiology, and pathology. As this textbook illustrates, the authors and contributors also believe in a well-educated, well-trained massage therapist.

As the health care system in the United States became influenced by biomedicine and technology in the early 1900s, physicians began assigning massage duties to nurses because massage therapy is labor intensive and time-consuming. In the 1930s and 1940s, nurses lost interest in massage and abandoned the art.

As technology and medical advances caught up with the profession, a simple massage became decreasingly crucial on its own; it became one procedure in the arsenal of rehabilitation. As a consequence, the British Chartered Society of Massage and Medical Gymnastics changed its name to the Chartered Society of Physiotherapy.

In 1943, postgraduates from the College of Swedish Massage in Chicago created the American Association of Masseurs and Masseuses (AAMM). The AAMM changed its name to the American Massage and Therapy Association

PEHR HENRIK LING

Born: 1776; died: 1839. Father of Swedish massage.

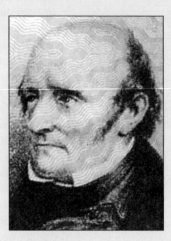

Born in Smaaland, one of the southern provinces of Sweden, Pehr Henrik Ling led an interesting life. After being expelled from school for disciplinary problems, Ling traveled through Europe and eventually returned to Sweden, where he learned fencing (the art of using a sword). In 1804 he accepted a post at the University of Lund, where he taught fencing and gymnastics. At the same time, he studied anatomy and physiology. In his teaching of fencing techniques, he noted that the movements he often wanted his pupils to make were hindered by motions that the student had learned from habit. Ling therefore resolved to teach the movements of the body in a systematic manner. For Ling, this training was important for military concerns, and he viewed fencing as an important part of gymnastics. What he meant was that soldiers could be taught to use weapons and move muscles in ways that were new to them.

At the same time, Ling also developed what is referred to as *Swedish gymnastics,* through which we—by means of influencing movements—overcome discomfort that has arisen through abnormal conditions. These gymnastics were composed of only a few stretching movements done by the student alone (active movements), performed by another pupil while the student relaxed (passive movements), or performed by the student with the cooperation of the pupil (duplicated movements such as active assistive and active resistive). In Ling's system, very little, if any, mechanical apparatus was involved.

In 1813 Ling opened the Swedish Royal Central Institute of Gymnastics, where he further developed his own system of medical gymnastics and exercise, known as the *Ling System, Swedish Movements,* or the *Swedish Movement Cure.* The primary focus of Ling's work was on gymnastics applied to the treatment of disease and injury. Massage (later known as Swedish massage) was viewed as a component of Ling's overall system.

Ling was not a physician, and his system of Swedish gymnastics was bitterly opposed by many people within the medical profession during much of his lifetime. However, many of his students were physicians, and these individuals spread his teachings and began to publish success stories of his techniques in respectable medical journals. Ling's influence was so great that, by 1851, 38 schools located throughout Europe were teaching his system of gymnastics and massage.

After years of failing health, Pehr Henrik Ling died in 1839. His legacy is seen today throughout the health professions, especially in the teachings of massage therapy, physical therapy, kinesiology, and gymnastics.

in 1958 and then again changed its name to the American Massage Therapy Association (AMTA) in 1983.

Over time, the AMTA evolved to represent the professional masseurs and masseuses, preferably called *massage therapists.* It is the second largest massage therapist organization, with 58,000 members in 51 chapters (all 50 states and Washington, D.C.), as well as members in 18 countries.

⊘volve *Log on to the Evolve website and access the additional resources for Chapter 1. View the membership pin of the American Association of Masseurs and Masseuses from the 1960s, the current logo of the American Massage Therapy Association, and the current logo of the American Bodywork and Massage Professionals.* ■

NEW METHODS

The Associated Bodywork and Massage Professionals (ABMP) was founded in 1987 as an organization that would include not only massage therapists but also all current and emerging bodywork styles. As of 2010, it has grown to more than 70,000 members and is currently the largest organization that serves massage therapists. The most significant difference between the two organizations is that AMTA's board is elected and ABMP's board is appointed.

> *"When you steal from one author, it's plagiarism; if you steal from many, it's research."*
> —Wilson Mizner

CURRENT EVENTS

In the last 25 years, massage has risen in popularity in the United States. Especially important in this rise are the individuals looking for alternative and complementary therapies (e.g., nutrition, physical activities, herbal remedies, acupuncture, acupressure, massage) to supplement their medical treatments and create a positive impact on their health. Massage has been shown to be beneficial for many people and has become a respected and much-used allied health care profession.

As a consequence of this increase in massage popularity, the profession has also grown. In 1988 the AMTA pushed for the development of national certification, which came in 1992 with the independent National Certification Board of Therapeutic Massage and Bodywork (NCBTMB) and the development of a national certification examination.

NCBTMBs examination was originally a single examination, encompassing both Eastern and Western principles. In 2005, a second examination was offered, one that focused solely on Western principles.

In 2010, NCBTMB launched advanced certification for the massage and bodywork professions. This offered the therapist a way to achieve credentialing far above minimum requirements. Currently, requirements to sit for this examination is that the applicant possesses a current license or certificate to practice to massage therapy or bodywork and he or she document at least 2000 hours in the field. These hours can come from a number of sources such as in a school setting, continuing education, client sessions, teaching and publication, work with related boards, committees, or even educational administration.

In 1990, the AMTA established the American Massage Therapy Association Foundation to further advance massage by supporting scientific research. In 2004, the foundation shortened its name to the Massage Therapy Foundation and became an independent organization, no longer under the AMTA. Along with massage research, the foundation includes services such as education and community outreach.

Another important event in massage history is the establishment of the Touch Research Institute in 1992 by Dr. Tiffany Field at the University of Miami School of Medicine. The Institute's team of researchers is the first in the world to study solely the effects of touch therapy and its application in science and medicine and the treatment of disease. Much of their research has shown that touch therapy has numerous beneficial effects on health and well-being.

The Federation of State Massage Therapy Boards was formed in 2005 to address the need for a valid and reliable licensing examination and the desire to bring commonality in licensing requirements to assist with reciprocity and professional mobility. To this end, the Federation developed the Massage & Bodywork Licensing Examination (MBLEx), which was released in 2008.

In 2008, organizations tied to the massage therapy profession came together to discuss the development and adoption of a single body of knowledge. A profession's body of knowledge is generally described as a compendium of what an individual must know and/or be able to do to successfully accomplish work in a specific field. This document would serve the profession as a living resource of competencies, standards, and values that would inform and guide domains of practice, licensure, certification, education, accreditation, and research.

Most bodies of knowledge are produced by the professional association for that field. Since massage therapy does not have a single professional association, a stewardship group was formed from five of the major organizations in the field: American Massage Therapy Association (AMTA), Associated Bodywork & Massage Professionals (ABMP), Federation of State Massage Therapy Boards (FSMTB), Massage Therapy Foundation (MTF), and National Certification Board for Therapeutic Massage & Bodywork (NCBTMB).

In 2009, this Stewardship group appointed an independent task force to create the inaugural Massage Therapy Body of Knowledge (MTBOK), which was released in 2010.

To date, approximately 80 massage methods have been classified. Although space limitations prohibit detailed discussions of these procedures, a listing of several styles has been compiled on the *Evolve* website. These styles have been categorized according to their primary approach on the human body, mind, and spirit. Most of these styles were developed in the United States since 1960.

By no means is this study of massage history complete and exhaustive. A detailed history of massage would take volumes and entail years of research. However, this chapter should have provided a thorough sense of how the profession developed and in what direction it appears to be headed.

E-RESOURCES

ⓔvolve

http://evolve.elsevier.com/Salvo/MassageTherapy
- Chapter challenge
- Flash cards
- Photo gallery
- Additional information
- Weblinks

BIBLIOGRAPHY

American Massage Therapy Association: *A short history: the American Massage Therapy Association* (website): http://www.amtamassage.org/about/history.htm. Accessed March 3, 2010.

American Massage Therapy Association: *Advancing the massage therapy profession for 60 years* (website): http://www.amtamassage.org/about/history.html. Accessed March 3, 2010.

Basham AL: The practice of medicine in ancient and medieval India. In Leslie C, editor: *Asian medical systems*, Berkeley, Calif, 1976, University of California Press.

Buikstra JE: Diseases of the pre-Columbian Americas. In Kiple KF et al, editors: *The Cambridge world history of human disease*, New York, 1993, Cambridge University Press.

Calvert RN: *The history of massage: an illustrated survey from around the world*, Rochester, Vt, 2002, Healing Arts Press.

Castiglioni A: *A history of medicine*, New York, 1947, Alfred A Knopf. (Translated by EB Krumbhaar.)

Coulter J: *Physical therapy*, New York, 1932, Paul B Hoeber.

Eisenberg D et al: Trends in alternative medicine use in the United States, 1990-1997: results of a follow-up national survey, *JAMA* 280(18):1569-1575, 1998.

Federation of State Massage Therapy Boards: FSMTB history (website): http://www.fsmtb.org/html/about/history.html. Accessed October 19, 2009.

Fryback P, Reinert B: Alternative therapies and control for health in cancer and AIDS, *Clin Nurse Spec* 11(2):64-69, 1997.

Goldberg J et al: The effect of therapeutic massage on H-reflex amplitude in persons with a spinal cord injury, *Phys Ther* 74(8):728-737, 1994.

Hernandez J: *A history of massage therapy*, California Hematology Oncology Medical Group (website): http://www.chomg.com/history_of_massage_therapy.html. Accessed March 3, 2010.

Hippocrates: *Hippocrates, vol iii, on wounds in the head, in the surgery, on fractures, on joints, mochlicon*, Cambridge, Mass, 1928, Harvard University Press. (Translated by ET Withington.)

Liddel L: *The book of massage: the complete step-by-step guide to Eastern and Western techniques*, New York, 1984, Simon & Schuster.

Massage Therapy Body of Knowledge: Version 1 (website): http//www.mtbok.org/. Accessed September 30, 2010.

Massage Therapy Body of Knowledge: Resources (website): http://www.mtbok.org/resources.html. Accessed October 19, 2009.

Massage Therapy Foundation: About the foundation (website): http://www.massagetherapyfoundation.org/about.html# Accessed October 7, 2007.

McMillan M: *Massage and therapeutic exercise*, Philadelphia, 1921, WB Saunders.

Means PA: *Ancient civilizations of the Andes*, New York, 1931, C Scribner and Sons.

Meintz SL: Alternatives and complementary therapies: whatever became of the back rub? *RN* 58(4):49-501, 1995.

Mulliner MR: *Mechano-therapy: a textbook for students*, Philadelphia, 1929, Lea & Febiger.

Nissen H: *Practical massage in twenty lessons*, Philadelphia, 1905, FA Davis.

Rahman F: *Health and medicine in the Islamic tradition: change and identity*, New York, 1987, Crossroad Press.

Rops MS: *Identifying and using a Field's body of knowledge*, Washington, DC, 2002, ASAE Foundation.

Salmon JW, editor: *Alternative medicine: popular and policy perspectives*, New York, 1984, Tavistock.

Solomon W: What is happening to massage? *Arch Phys Med* 31:521-523, 1950.

Unschuld PU: History of Chinese medicine. In Kiple KF et al, editors: *Cambridge world history of human disease*, New York, 1993, Cambridge University Press.

U.S. Department of Health and Human Services: *Acute pain management in adults: operative procedures-quick reference guide for clinicians*, Rockville, Md, 1992, The Department.

U.S. Department of Health and Human Services: *Management of cancer pain: adults-quick reference guide for clinicians*, Rockville, Md, 1994, The Department.

Veith I, Huang T: *Nei ching su wen*, Baltimore, 1949, Williams & Wilkins.

Wanning T: Healing and the mind/body arts: massage, acupuncture, yoga, tai chi, and Feldenkrais, *AAOHN J* 41(7):349-351, 1993.

White J: Touching with intent: therapeutic massage, *Holist Nurs Pract* 2(3):63-67, 1988.

Wide AG: *Handbook of medical and orthopedic gymnastics*, New York, 1905, Funk and Wagnall.

Zyzk KG: *Religious healing in the Veda, with translations and annotations of medical hymns in the Rgveda and the Atharvaveda and renderings from the corresponding ritual texts*, Philadelphia, 1985, American Philosophical Society.

MATCHING

Place the letter of the answer next to the term or phrase that best describes it.

A. 3000 BC
B. Amma
C. Arte Gymnastica
D. Ayurveda

E. China
F. Hippocrates of Cos
G. Pehr Henrik Ling
H. Massage

I. Johann Mezger
J. Middle 1900s
K. Nei-ching
L. Swedish gymnastics

_____ 1. What is the manual and scientific manipulation of the soft tissues of the body?

_____ 2. Records have revealed that the practice of massage goes back as early as _____.

_____ 3. What is the original massage technique?

_____ 4. In what country did the first written accounts of therapeutic rubbing (massage) originate?

_____ 5. Who is the father of modern Western medicine?

_____ 6. What is the classic scripture of traditional Chinese medicine?

_____ 7. Who is regarded as the father of Swedish massage?

_____ 8. When did the term *massage* first come into use?

_____ 9. What is the sacred practice of the Hindu tradition; means *code of life*?

_____ 10. The individual whose efforts led to the use of French terminology to describe massage techniques.

_____ 11. The work generally credited as being the first book in the field of sports medicine.

_____ 12. According to Ling, a therapeutic system by which we, by means of influencing movement, overcome discomfort that has arisen through abnormal conditions.

CASE STUDY

Professionalism

While not exactly a case study, this activity will help to familiarize yourself with the organizations that inform and serve our profession.

Use the Internet to look up the following organizations.

- American Massage Therapy Association [http://www.amtamassage.org/]
- Associated Bodywork and Massage Professionals [http://www.abmp.com/home/]
- Federation of State Massage Therapy Boards [http://www.fsmtb.org/]
- National Certification Board for Therapeutic Massage and Bodywork [http://www.ncbtmb.org/]
- Massage Therapy Foundation [http://www.massagetherapyfoundation.org/]
- Massage Therapy Body of Knowledge [http://www.mtbok.org/]

Locate information regarding their history and current events. Write a brief paragraph about each organization and share it with your class.

Instructors, feel free to create an online discussion and ask students to post their findings.

CRITICAL THINKING

Why might it be important for a massage therapist to understand the history of the profession?

CHAPTER 2

Therapeutic Relationships

Megan E. Lavery, LMT, BS, and Susan G. Salvo, BEd, LMT, NTS, CI, NCTMB

"Good fences make good neighbors."
—Robert Frost

LEARNING OBJECTIVES

After completing this chapter, the student should be able to:

- Define the therapeutic relationship.
- State interpersonal skills of the therapeutic relationship.
- Contrast and compare legal and ethical issues.
- Contrast and compare disclosure with confidentiality.
- Define boundaries and state their importance in the therapeutic relationship.
- Identify characteristics of healthy boundaries.
- List and describe types of boundaries.
- Discuss boundary management.
- Point out common mistakes that may lead to crossing boundaries.
- Compare and contrast client neglect and client abuse.
- Discuss reasons and ways to avoid conflicts of interest.
- Compare and contrast transference and countertransference.
- Define dual relationship, identifying reasons they exist, and reasons why they are problematic.
- Define and give examples of sexual misconduct.
- Discuss sexual risk management and steps to take when a session is terminated.
- Outline possible consequences of sexual misconduct by the therapist.
- Discuss steps taken when allegations of sexual misconduct by a fellow therapist emerge.

http://evolve.elsevier.com/Salvo/MassageTherapy

INTRODUCTION

Many massage students and therapists know that interpersonal skills help form an important relationship between them and their clients. This relationship, or therapeutic relationship, is the basis of all treatment approaches regardless of their specific aim. During a client's initial contact with us, he or she needs to feel that we are reliable, trustworthy, consistent, and will respect confidentiality. The client needs to also feel that the relationship will be conducted within appropriate and clear boundaries. As the Robert Frost quotation reminds us, fences, a type of physical boundary, can enhance our relationships with others. Boundaries in all relationships impart a sense of self, establish personal space, and a sense of protection.

The therapeutic relationship is a creative process and distinct to each therapist. While this relationship serves the best interest of the client, each person brings his or her own uniqueness to the relationship. Each person brings his or her own uniqueness to the therapist-client relationship. Historically, this process was referred to as the *therapeutic use of self*. The efficacy of the therapeutic relationship can be substantiated scientifically. Research has found repeatedly that development of a positive alliance (i.e., therapeutic relationship) is one of the best predictors of positive outcomes in therapy.

THE THERAPEUTIC RELATIONSHIP

For massage therapy to be effective and beneficial, a therapeutic relationship needs to form between the massage therapist and the client. This relationship can span anywhere from a single session to throughout the client's lifetime.

The **therapeutic relationship** is the relationship between therapist and client that seeks to support his or her therapeutic goals. Regardless of its length, the therapeutic relationship serves the needs and best interests of the client. It is also dependent on our ability to gather client information, correlate it with our knowledge of health and illness, and then apply it within a client-centered session.

This chapter offers guidance in navigating the therapeutic relationship, which involves recognizing what does and does not belong in this experience. More specifically, this chapter focuses on the interpersonal skills aspect of the therapeutic relationship. These interpersonal skills involve ethical behavior, professional boundaries, confidentiality, and conflict resolution. But first, we explore the framework of interpersonal skills, which includes our capacity for empathy, acceptance, safety, trust, respect, and acknowledgment of a power differential (Figure 2-1).

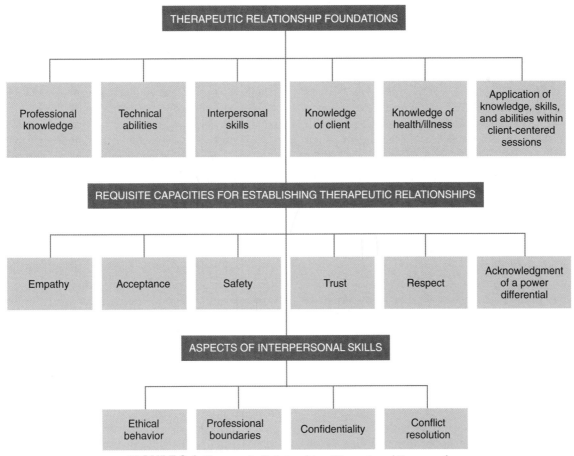

FIGURE 2-1 Therapeutic Relationships: Elements and Framework.

Empathy

Empathy is the ability to understand the unique world of another. Empathetic listening involves trying to understand the other person, not just knowing many facts about that person. With empathy, the therapist can experience the client's world as if it were their own, without mistaking it for their own. The client may perceive our empathy both verbally and nonverbally such as during quiet moments of back massage.

When obtaining health or medical information, a client may disclose facts more fully if the therapist has empathy. And because we have a better understanding of the client, we can formulate more appropriate and realistic treatment plans.

In some cases, this process may also reveal client needs and treatment goals that are not within our scope of practice, generating a referral to better serve the client. Even in instances when we cannot directly help a client with his or her therapeutic goals, empathy demonstrates a deeper level of understanding and acceptance, which helps a client feel less alone and more cared for.

Acceptance

The therapist accepts the client for who he or she is, including physical, mental, spiritual, and emotional aspects. Acceptance includes valuing, highly regarding, or esteeming clients for who they are. *Unconditional positive regard*, a term coined by American psychologist Carl Rogers (1961), describes acceptance for the client that does not depend on the client's behavior. It is valuing clients because their humanity warrants your care.

Acceptance also has implications in regards to treatment progress. While we have established therapeutic goals, fulfillment of those goals is dependent on factors out of our control. So when we truly accept a client, we also accept their progress or lack of progress. For example, while reassessing a client's range of motion after treatment, avoid thoughts or statements such as "I wish he would stretch more," or "she would hold less stress in her body if she would meditate." Accept them fully for who they are right now and let go of thoughts that reduce your acceptance of them.

Acceptance is also demonstrated legally as we gain consent for therapy, stating that we cannot discriminate, specifically in regards to race, nationality, gender, religion, or sexual preference. Acceptance and nondiscrimination help promote an emotionally safe environment for the client.

Safety

Safety, which is freedom from danger, has several implications in the therapeutic relationship. First, working within our scope of practice is a safety measure as this represents an understanding and respect for the legal parameters of our professional activities. To practice safely, we must understand concepts of anatomy and physiology, pathology, and when and how to adapt or postpone treatment with regard to various life stages, conditions, and injuries.

Client safety also involves the establishment and maintenance of professional boundaries. Through boundaries and a relationship that is predictable, we create a sense of safety and security for the client.

Safety has its roots in communication. Time is spent communicating with clients about treatment planning. Time is also spent discussing boundary related issues such as dual relationships, which are avoided to ensure the sanctity of the therapeutic relationship. This reinforces to the client that we will protect and safeguard the therapeutic relationship. A feeling of safety may also lead to clearer communication and better identification of client goals.

CHAT ROOM

Providing a safe service also means that our work environment is barrier-free and accessible to all, including persons with disabilities. Therapists should also have a plan outlining what to do in an emergency. This includes a fire evacuation plan, and a designated safe area in which to retreat during events such as tornados or earthquakes.

Trust

Trust is a willingness to be vulnerable to the actions of another. Trust is earned by the responsible acts of both parties and trust grows when risk taking is met with responsible behavior.

Clients may feel vulnerable; they often come to us in pain or under considerable stress. Lying on our table or sitting in our chair is an act of trust. If the client's expectation is fulfilled, he or she is likely to put their trust in you again. A history of trust often results in better therapeutic outcomes for the client.

If the therapist's demeanor, dress, or speech is inconsistent with the professionalism that the client expects, then the client can become alarmed and mistrustful of the competence of care (see Appearance section) (Figure 2-2). Trust can be easily upset not only by important issues but also by seemingly insignificant things. For example, it is best not to tell a client that he or she can contact you anytime. Although you may be sincere in wanting to help the client, you may not be comfortable receiving a phone call or text message at 3:00 AM. A careless statement may mislead the client, weaken trust, and possibly damage the therapeutic relationship.

To be perceived as a trustworthy and dependable professional, you must be willing to behave consistently in a professional manner.

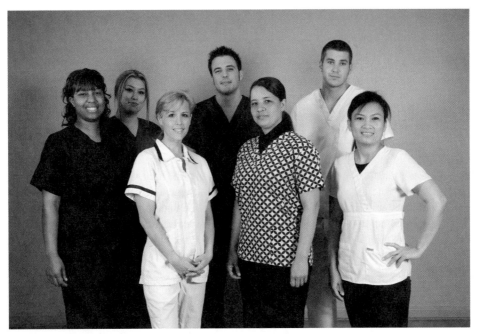

FIGURE 2-2 The massage therapist is a professional in demeanor, dress, and speech.

Respect

Respect refers to a consideration or thoughtfulness exhibited by words and actions. A therapist must respect the inherent worth of both the client and the therapeutic relationship.

Respect is demonstrated during the informed consent process as we explain the *who, how, why,* and *when* of treatment, and is reinforced when we respond to questions the client has. Respect is demonstrated as we protect client information. Finally, respect is demonstrated as we modify massage in response to pressure being requested by the client.

Professional boundaries also demonstrate respect to our clients, to our profession, and to ourselves. We are also respectful of client boundaries, valuing their personal space, their privacy, their time, and any financial restrictions they may have. Draping the client can be viewed as an act of respect.

We also demonstrate respect for the client and for the relationship when we acknowledge and do not abuse the power differential that is intrinsic to this relationship (discussed next).

Lastly, we show respect to other professionals, both fellow therapists and other health care providers, by not denigrating other therapists or methods. And we show respect to other professions by not performing services for which we are not licensed (such as joint manipulations, prescriptive exercise, or counseling, all of which are under the practice of chiropractic, physical or occupational therapy, and psychotherapy, respectively.) We can show respect to clients, the therapeutic relationship, and to other professionals when we refer clients to the appropriate health care provider.

We also show respect for the diversity of different cultures found throughout the globe. What may be commonplace to us may be highly inappropriate to others. If you are unsure about particular cultural norms, such as woman receiving massage from a specific gender, find out through reliable sources before your client arrives, when possible.

Power Differential

All therapeutic relationships come with an inherent power differential. One person, the *client,* has a particular need and comes for help to another person, the *therapist,* who has knowledge, skills, and abilities in that specific area. Clients usually lie down undressed and the therapist is positioned above them, creating an impression of authority. Even though treatment planning is a co-creative process, we have knowledge and skills clients need, which puts them in a position of vulnerability. This vulnerability puts us in a position of power.

This imbalance of power is a natural occurrence and, in and of itself, is not a problem. Problems may arise when this power is misused to serve our interests rather than those of the client. Any time a power differential exists in a relationship and the person who wields the greater power does not recognize or respect the boundaries of the other, client abuse and client neglect can occur. The law holds the professional to a higher standard of behavior because of this power differential. The power differential does not empower the client to say *no* easily to the therapist.

Another aspect of the power differential is that the therapist needs to be comfortable in the position of power. If the therapist has self-esteem issues, or does not acknowledge the power inherent in their role, then he or she may not be able to maintain professional boundaries (Box 2-1).

BOX 2-1

In the Service of Life

In recent years the question *how can I help?* has become meaningful to many people. But perhaps there is a deeper question we might consider. Perhaps the real question is not how can I help, but *how can I serve?*

Serving is different from helping. Helping is based on inequality; it is not a relationship between equals. When you help you use your own strength to help those of lesser strength. If I am attentive to what is going on inside of me when I am helping, I find that I am always helping someone who is not as strong as I am, who is needier than I am. People feel this inequality. When we help we may inadvertently take away from people more than we could ever give them; we may diminish their self-esteem, their sense of worth, integrity, and wholeness. When I help I am very aware of my own strength. But we do not serve with our strength, we serve with ourselves. We draw from all of our experiences. Our limitations serve, our wounds serve, even our darkness can serve. The wholeness in us serves the wholeness in others and the wholeness in life. The wholeness in you is the same as the wholeness in me. Service is a relationship between equals.

Helping incurs debt. When you help someone they owe you one. But serving, like healing, is mutual. There is no debt. I am as served as the person I am serving. When I help I have a feeling of satisfaction. When I serve I have a feeling of gratitude. These are very different things.

Serving is also different from fixing. When I fix a person I perceive them as broken, and their brokenness requires me to act. When I fix I do not see the wholeness in the other person or trust the integrity of the life in them. When I serve, I see and trust that wholeness. It is what I am responding to and collaborating with.

There is distance between ourselves and whatever or whomever we are fixing. Fixing is a form of judgment. All judgment creates distance, a disconnection, an experience of difference. In fixing there is an inequality of expertise that can easily become a moral distance. We cannot serve at a distance. We can only serve that to which we are profoundly connected, that which we are willing to touch. This is mother Teresa's basic message. We serve life not because it is broken but because it is holy.

If helping is an experience of strength, fixing is an experience of mastery and expertise. Service, on the other hand, is an experience of mystery, surrender, and awe. A fixer has the illusion of being causal. A server knows that he or she is being used and has a willingness to be used in the service of something greater, something essentially unknown. Fixing and helping are very personal; they are very particular, concrete, and specific. We fix and help many different things in our lifetimes. but when we serve we are always serving the same thing. Everyone who has ever served through the history of time serves the same thing. We are servers of the wholeness and mystery in life.

The bottom line, of course, is that we can fix without serving. And we can help without serving. And we can serve without fixing or helping. I think I would go so far as to say that fixing and helping may often be the work of the ego, and service the work of the soul. They may look similar if you are watching from the outside, but the inner experience is different. The outcome is often different, too.

Our service serves us as well as others. That which uses us strengthens us. Over time, fixing and helping are draining and depleting. Over time we burn out. Service is renewing. When we serve, our work itself will sustain us.

Service rests on the basic premise that the nature of life is sacred, that life is a holy mystery which has an unknown purpose. When we serve, we know that we belong to life and to that purpose.

Fundamentally, helping, fixing, and service are ways of seeing life. When you help, you see life as weak. When you fix, you see life as broken. When you serve, you see life as whole. From the perspective of service, we are all connected: All suffering is like my suffering and all joy is like my joy. The impulse to serve emerges naturally and inevitably from this way of seeing.

Lastly, fixing and helping are the basis of curing, but not of healing. In 40 years of chronic illness I have been helped by many and fixed by a great many others who did not recognize my wholeness. All that fixing and helping left me wounded in some important and fundamental ways. Only service heals.

by Rachel Naomi Remen, MD

"In the Service of Life," adapted from a talk given by Rachel Naomi Remen at IONS fourth annual conference, first appeared in the *Noetic Sciences Review*, (Spring 1996, issue number 37), published by the Institute of Noetic Sciences (IONS), and is reprinted with permission of IONS (www.noetic.org), all rights reserved. Copyright 1996.

> *"The quality of the therapeutic relationship has consistently been shown to be more important than the therapist's clinical outlook."*
> —Kalman Glantz and John Pearce

LEGAL VERSUS ETHICAL ISSUES

Legal issues are associated with laws, rules, and regulations. The primary purpose of massage therapy laws is to protect the public from injury. This is done by providing rules for obtaining and maintaining licensure. Ideally, laws promote smooth functioning of a society. If laws are broken, then civil or criminal liabilities may occur. Upon conviction, the therapist may be fined, imprisoned, have his or her license revoked, or suffer other penalties as determined by the courts.

Ethical issues are associated with human duty, appropriate right conduct, and responsibility. Professional ethics are the values and ideals that a particular profession creates for itself, setting the standards of conduct for its members. If these principles and standards are not followed, the professional is in violation and may be suspended or evicted from the professional society of which he or she is a member, as decided by peers.

Thus not renewing a state license and continuing to practice massage is illegal. Offering stone massage after only watching a video is unethical, but not illegal.

Can an issue be both illegal and unethical? Yes. An example of this is a breach of confidentiality (discussed next). And in some states any issue that is unethical is also considered illegal. For example, your state licensing law may include a provision that all licensed massage therapists adhere to the state massage board's code of ethics. Therefore, any action that is listed in the code of ethics as unethical (such as dating a client, or providing services without adequate training) would also be illegal and could result in a fine or suspension of license.

DISCLOSURE AND CONFIDENTIALITY

From the initial contact and throughout the therapeutic relationship, clients will reveal not only their past and current medical information and treatment goals, they will also share with us their thoughts and feelings. Honest and open sharing of personal knowledge, as well as ideas and insights, is known as **disclosure**. Over time, your client will reveal more about him or herself if emotional safety is perceived.

Personal information shared by the client is closely guarded by the therapist. Nondisclosure of privileged information is called **confidentiality**. A breach of confidentiality is both illegal and unethical. Self-disclosure of information by the client and confidentiality of this information are important aspects of the therapeutic relationship.

Every client has the right to and guarantee of privacy within the therapeutic relationship. This means that your client's name and any information shared by the client as well as details of his or her treatments are not to be divulged to a third party. And while you cannot disclose aspects of treatment or the therapeutic relationship, your client can certainly tell family and friends details of the session and his or her perception of the quality of care received.

Even in social situations, protect your client's confidentiality. Name-dropping is rarely impressive and only reveals us as therapists who do not protect a client's privacy. Telling a third party that someone is your client is never a good idea; doing so risks offending the client, breaks trust, and is illegal.

In situations when the therapist receives a referral from a client, avoid sharing information regarding the common acquaintance with either client. This means not telling either client when the other was last in for an appointment, even if you are asked directly. Let's take this concept one step further; if you are treating a married couple separately,

refrain from answering questions about the other. Avoid answering even caring questions such as "Was my wife's neck range of motion better when you saw her yesterday?" Your reply might be "Due to confidentiality I can't share information about a client with anyone other than that client. I hope you understand" or "I can't answer that, but I'm sure your wife can."

In social settings that include both you and your client, avoid initiating a conversation with him or her. Perhaps make eye contact, smile, and give a nod of politeness. If the client initiates a conversation, do not to reveal information if other people are nearby. Because many social settings exist in which both you and your client may be present, you may wish to discuss how these situations will be handled beforehand, perhaps as part of your initial visit during discussions of informed consent (see Chapter 10). Take time to explain your policy regarding privacy and confidentiality.

Respecting confidentiality also means that treatment rooms are in a private setting and should be soundproof so that people standing or passing the room cannot hear conversations in the treatment room. Client intake and interviews are conducted in private, never in public areas.

Many clients want to have some sense of who we are as people. They are disclosing their personal history, as well as letting us massage them. They may feel more comfortable knowing something about the person with whom they are in a relationship. This may lead to personal questions about you.

Some experts in the field of psychotherapy, ethics, and massage recommend that we disclose very little about our personal selves, letting us be a blank slate so the relationship is entirely about the client. There is also concern that too much personal information can lead to transference (discussed later in the chapter).

However, others argue that giving clients some personal information can help them relax and feel comfortable, knowing we are human. Appropriate information might include how long we have lived in the area and why we moved here. Clients will often want to know if the therapist has a family, for no reason other than to know something about you as a person.

Especially important is not disclosing your personal experience related to a similar problem. This may lead to your client's minimizing his or her own experience as yours may be perceived as more significant. For example, if your client is grieving after the death of a parent, and you share your own experience of a parent that died the previous year, the client may feel overly concerned about your feelings, and discontinue talking about their own grief. This may prevent your client from having their needs met because they are concerned with taking care of you.

Exceptions to the Rule

Professional confidentiality is limited by two factors: (1) the therapist's obligation to the law and (2) the therapist's obligation to others.

Regarding the therapist's *obligation to the law,* client records can be subpoenaed by court order.

Regarding the therapist's *obligation to others,* releasing his or her records to other health care providers (e.g., physicians, physical or occupational therapists, chiropractors) may be in the client's best interest when working as part of the client's health care team. Our professional experience and opinion may be needed to develop an overall treatment plan for the mutual client. Be sure to obtain the client's written consent before releasing the record (see Chapter 10). Other third-party involvement can include a translator for someone with a language barrier, a relative who has power of attorney for a disabled client, or an insurance company that requests client information so reimbursement can be made.

Other examples where therapists can legally breach confidentiality include when there is a threat to self or others, when there are suspicions of child or elder abuse or neglect, or when a medical emergency exists. In some states massage therapists are mandatory reporters when there is suspected child or elder abuse or neglect. In these cases, failure to report child or elder abuse or neglect may result in criminal or civil liability.

BOUNDARIES

Boundaries are parameters indicating a border or limit. A **boundary,** with regard to relationships, delineates differences between clients and therapists. Boundaries define our personal and professional space, our emotional separateness, our sense of autonomy, how we conduct our business affairs, and how we establish and maintain different kinds of relationships. Hence, boundaries in personal relationships are different than those in therapeutic relationships.

Boundaries help to clarify each person's role in the therapeutic relationship such as individual responsibilities, expectations, and limitations. Boundaries are established and maintained through communication. Communicating with clients about boundaries is vital, given that all interactions occur at boundaries—yours and theirs—where you, the *therapist*, end and where your *client*, begins. Boundaries are part of all healthy relationships, they create a sense of predictability. In therapeutic relationships, this predictability helps promote feelings of safety and trust.

When we identify types of boundaries (i.e., physical, intellectual, emotional), they are more easily maintained. And the more awareness and respect we have for our own boundaries, the more we can respect the boundaries of others. By doing so, we instill a sense of dignity and respect to our clients, to our profession, and to ourselves.

Unintentional or intentional neglect or abuse is more likely in relationships without clear boundaries.

The irony is that good boundaries cannot be experienced from a book. We all have past experiences of boundaries, beginning in early childhood, and these were role modeled to us by family and friends. Hopefully, these were examples of good boundaries and healthy relationships. If so, we know

firsthand how it feels to be with someone who is clear and careful with boundaries. If not, the process of establishing and maintaining healthy boundaries may be challenging. In these cases, consider approaching individuals who you feel have healthy boundaries and ask them to be role models and mentors. Additionally, a mental health counselor may also be helpful in exploring boundaries.

The analogy of a cell might be helpful when visualizing boundaries. Imagine that you are surrounded by a semipermeable membrane. This membrane lets nutrients in and keeps toxic materials out. This membrane also defines the cell's existence by separating it from other cells. Healthy cells also have an innate intelligence; it knows it is a brain cell and that brain cells and liver cells are different types.

Another analogy of healthy boundaries is an intact immune system, which helps to maintain the boundary of the body's unique individuality, distinguishing what is me and removing what is *not* me.

Characteristics of Healthy Boundaries

Healthy boundaries possess certain characteristics including:

Awareness. You have to be aware of a boundary to define and maintain it. To keep this awareness, you must be able to think clearly at all times. This means avoiding mood-altering substances such as recreational drugs or alcohol before and during professional practice.

Congruency. Boundaries must be congruent and compatible with your core values. If there is a conflict between the two, boundaries will be difficult, if not impossible, to maintain.

Mutuality. Being in a therapeutic relationship and having healthy boundaries is only part of the picture. You must respect mutually the boundaries of another in and outside your professional life.

Protection. Boundaries also provide protection, safeguarding the individual's sense of self-worth and uniqueness. Conversely, healthy boundaries also enhance and protect the self-worth and uniqueness of others.

Flexibility and Adaptability. Boundaries are inherently flexible and adaptive to different people and different situations. The boundaries you have with friends and family are different than those you have with clients. Evaluate your own boundaries periodically and be willing to create more rigid or flexible boundaries as needed.

TYPES OF BOUNDARIES

There are many types of boundaries. Next, we will examine the major types of boundaries within therapeutic relationships, which include physical, intellectual, and emotional boundaries. Then we will look at boundaries related to time, location, appearance, and finances. These boundaries are also important aspects of a professional practice as they demonstrate our commitment to integrity.

Physical Boundaries

Physical boundaries create a safe space around us. They help define the who, when, where, how and under what circumstances we feel safe with touch. Each person has a slightly different amount of personal space surrounding their body that feels safe to them. In American culture, the distance is approximately 3 feet. If we stand closer than the person's "comfort zone" it may feel invasive to them. Conversely, if we stand further away, it may feel like we are being distant. Touching without the person's consent is a violation of the physical boundary. Even with consent, touching that does not feel good is also a boundary violation.

Boundaries are flexible; they can adapt to different situations. While most Americans like to have 3 feet around them, they allow people closer in certain situations. Have you ever noticed that when a line starts, say at a movie theater, people tend to line themselves up a normal personal distance of a few feet apart? And as the line grows longer, the distance between people gets smaller. Over time, we might find we are standing within inches of the person in front of us, and it does not bother us. This is an example of boundaries being flexible.

In massage relationships, physical boundaries change quickly. When we greet our clients in the waiting room, we stand a normal distance from them, shaking hands. Once we have started the intake process we may sit closer (Figure 2-3). When they are on the massage table, we stand within inches of them, and are touching them. At this point the physical boundary is literally skin to skin. But, once the massage is complete, it is important to return to a more normal distance. Just because the client has allowed physical boundaries to shrink to allow touching during the massage

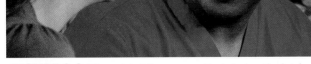

FIGURE 2-3 Therapist sitting near a client during the intake.

does not mean that it would be appropriate to continue touching them when he or she is not on the massage table.

During treatment planning, therapeutic goals are established. Based on this information, you will disclose areas that merit focused attention and any areas that will be avoided (i.e., local contraindications). We are essentially setting boundaries of the session. Others aspects of the session that need clear boundaries are:
- How deep an area is worked
- How long an area is worked
- Consent for working in sensitive areas such as the abdomen, buttocks, female pectoral areas
- What part of your body touches the client
- Not touching the client inadvertently with your clothing or body parts not engaged with the massage (be careful how you lean against the table)
- Use of scents or aromas
- How your client is draped
- How the draped is moved
- Refraining from working under a drape
- Making sure your client knows that he or she can keep on any clothes they wish
- Making sure your client knows he or she is empowered to speak up if they feel uncomfortable with anything during the session.

Hugging. Some massage therapists like to hug clients on their arrival or departure. But hugging also represents a physical boundary. Some questions that need consideration are:
- How do you know you have the client's permission to give them a hug? Was it spoken or unspoken?
- Does the client initiate the hug?
- How long does the hug last?
- What is the norm for your geographic area?
- What type of work setting are you in?
- Do you hug only opposite gender (or same gender) clients?
- Do you hug only attractive clients?
- Do you hug only young clients?
- Do you hug only clients who you find unintimidating?
- If you hug some clients and not others, what determines who you hug?

Answers to these questions will help you formulate your own hugging policy. Some massage therapists go by a general rule of thumb of hugging only clients who request one. Other therapists avoid hugging any clients, feeling that other health care providers do not hug their clients. Whatever your choice, hugs should respect the client's physical boundary and not be forced upon them.

Intellectual Boundaries

Intellectual boundaries encompass our beliefs, thoughts, and ideas. When others agree with us, we tend to feel safe, to feel validated, and to feel close to the person we see like-minded. Conversely, when we find our beliefs, thoughts, and ideas challenged or rejected, we may feel vulnerable. When the person challenging us is an authority figure, we may feel especially vulnerable, perhaps reverting to how we felt when a grade school teacher scorned us when we did not produce the "right" answer.

Do you show respect for your client's intellectual boundaries? Do items in your office challenge a client's beliefs? Posters, calendars, or art prints that espouse your philosophy, may be challenging or even offensive to a client with different beliefs. This is especially true with regards to political, religious, or spiritual beliefs. Even our choice of art could be offensive if they depict nudity or sensuality.

Additionally, think about how you offer information to clients. Do you disregard their personal beliefs or ideas? Or do you offer information in a way that is tailored to each client, which takes into consideration their ideas and builds on them? Do you ask the client if they are interested in, or want, the information before it is presented?

If we impose our political, religious, or spiritual beliefs on our clients who do not share them, we are violating their intellectual boundary.

Emotional Boundaries

Boundaries that revolve around our feelings must also be considered while in therapeutic relationships. As stated previously, a characteristic of healthy boundaries is a sense of protection; they help client's feel safe. While clients, after feeling safe, share their feelings with you, they may also feel vulnerable and exposed. Recall a time you have cried unexpectedly in front of someone. How did you feel? Were you concerned that the person would judge you, or think less of you?

When clients share their feelings with us, they are showing their trust in the therapeutic relationship. To earn trust, we safeguard client information, including their feelings and expressions of those feelings. For example, if a client shares their emotions with us in one session, refrain from bringing it up in subsequent sessions. This demonstrates respect for a client's emotions. We will not mention the event unless they bring it up or unless it directly impacts the session. For example, if your client had an emotional release while your were massaging his or her feet, it would be appropriate to gain consent before working on that area again (Box 2-2).

The same is true for clients who make a physical connection with their emotions. An example of a client making these connections are statement such as "I almost ran out of my office today," followed by "I had suppressed the urge to run and still feel tension in my legs." Ask the client if the area mentioned should be addressed or avoided during the session. This puts the focus back on the client's body while acknowledging and respecting their emotional boundary.

BOX 2-2

Scope of Practice: Massage Therapy, Psychotherapy, and Emotional Release

Clients will share their thoughts and feelings with us. Clients may have emotions surface unexpectedly during a session (see Chapter 11). The surfacing of emotions may lead to their expression. The most common form of expression is crying.

If your client begins to cry during a session, approach the situation with acceptance. If the client seems uncomfortable crying in front of you, is it within our scope of practice to reassure the client with statements such as "Crying is normal," "You are in a safe place," "I am comfortable with your tears." Come up with a phrase that works for you and your client in this situation. When the client has finished crying, helping him or her feel more grounded with statements such as "Take a few deep breaths," and "Feel the massage table beneath you," are also within our scope. Again, find phrasing that works for you and your client.

Not within the scope of practice are:
- Encouraging clients to share emotional content
- Processing the emotions
- Delving for deeper held emotions
- Offering unsolicited "insights" or advice
- Intentionally evoking emotional responses in the client

Anytime the focus of the massage session becomes more about the client's emotions than about the body, this boundary has been crossed. A good guideline when it comes to the client's emotions is *seek not, forbid not.*

Another reason we do not cross the emotional boundary with clients is that massage therapists are not trained to differentiate between emotional experiences that are helpful to the client and those that are harmful. There is mounting evidence that release-based cathartic therapies may feel good in the moment but have no lasting benefits for the health and well-being of the client. More than no benefits, these cathartic releases are often harmful to the healing process, even frequently retraumatizing to the client. Even if a massage therapist is cross trained in a recognized form of body psychotherapy, such work requires a different license to practice in which massage therapy would not be employed. This will be discussed in the Dual Licensure and Dual Roles section.

Time Boundaries

Unlike personal relationships in which time is usually flexible, we have a contract with the client for our time. The client has essentially rented our time for the length of the session. It is our job to focus fully on them during this time. Ways to show respect for the client and for time boundaries include:

— Being ready when the client arrives with music playing (if appropriate) and clean linens on the massage table
— Beginning and ending the session on time

— Focusing on the client during the session and avoiding distracting activities such as talking or texting on your phone or conversing with other clients in the waiting room

Different therapists have different views about when to start the clock for the client's session. For some therapists, the clock starts ticking when the massage begins, after the client intake and interview. Other therapists start the clock when they begin the client intake and interview. Which ever you chose, be sure to communicate your policy/procedure regarding treatment time to your client so he or she may plan accordingly. It would be confusing to the client, and shows lack of respect for time boundaries, when a 1-hour massage lasts 60 minutes during one session, 75 minutes the next, and 55 minutes during another session. Other time issues to consider are:

- What if your client is running late?
- What if you are running late?
- Would you allow sessions to run over time? Under what circumstances? Would you ask the client if it is OK?
- What if your client arrives early? What if you are ready to begin? What if you are not ready to begin?

Other aspects of time boundaries include how we handle cancellations and no-shows. These are violations of the time boundary and possibly impact financial boundaries. Consider:

- Do you have a policy for cancellations?
- How far ahead do you expect clients to cancel?
- Do you charge the full amount or a partial amount for cancellations?
- Do you charge for no-shows?
- Do you have any policy or leniency for emergencies?
- What happens if you miss an appointment?

And a final aspect of time boundaries is during what hours you schedule appointments.

- Do you have set office hours?
- Do you ever bend this rule?
- Under what circumstances?
- Do you charge extra for after-hours or off-day appointments?

CHAT ROOM

Legal statutes do a good job of outlining our scope of practice. However, situations can arise in everyday practice that creates confusion and "muddying the waters" of scope of practice. Massage therapists need to have solid and impeccable boundaries regarding the type of service they offer a client. Although the mind, body, and spirit cannot be separated in their physiologic functioning, massage therapists must be absolutely sure that their treatments, advice, and focus remain on the soft tissue of the body. We can recognize the imprint that the emotions make on the fascial structures of the body, but we should not intentionally use techniques that evoke an emotional response in the client, nor engage in exercises whose primary purpose is to address the human psyche directly.

Location Boundaries

Provide professional services in an appropriate setting. Social settings are not regarded as appropriate places to perform professional activities. This is not only true for practicing therapists but for students as well. If someone asks you to rub his or her sore neck, and you are not in your office, then you might say, "Right now, I'm not working, and I can do a better job at my office. Why don't we schedule an appointment for you?" This sets clear boundaries about both your location and your time (in this case your time off).

Avoid giving your professional opinion or advice during social events. You can be held accountable for professional advice given in social settings. You may not have all information when this advice is given, and it may be contraindicated in that particular person's case. Instead, offer a business card and request that he or she call you during business hours.

Your office space should be clean, professional, and barrier-free (see Chat Room on p. 16 regarding other important safety considerations). Many massage therapists work out of their homes. In these cases it is even more important that the location project professionalism. Ideally your client entrance and work area is not part of your home's living space. If this is not possible, be sure these areas are clutter-free, with little or no personal items. Also if you work out of your home, you need to be aware of boundaries that govern zoning and city, county or state regulations (discussed in Chapter 17).

If you do out-calls, ask about space designated for the massage in advance. Ask about where you are to park (you don't want to have to carry your table three blocks). It is best for the safety of the therapist to have a policy regarding out-calls for clients whom you do not know. This might include calling a third party to inform them when you arrive at the out-call location and that you will call as you are leaving. Be sure that the third party knows where you are and has the name and phone number of the new client. As this is a violation of the normal client confidentially, it is important to inform the client when booking the session that this is your policy and get the client's consent to share their name and phone number for this purpose only. Ideally the third party would be another professional that you work with. If you work alone, it could be a supervisor, or another massage therapist. Try to avoid having the third party be a friend or family member, as that will create a dual relationship (dual relationships are discussed later in this chapter).

Appearance

Professional appearance is another important aspect of the therapeutic relationship because it helps to instill a sense of trust. Dress and grooming should be consistent with other professionals in your locality, and for the type of setting in which you work (Figure 2-4). What is appropriate for working in a day spa in Boston may be very different than what is appropriate when working a triathlon in Hawaii.

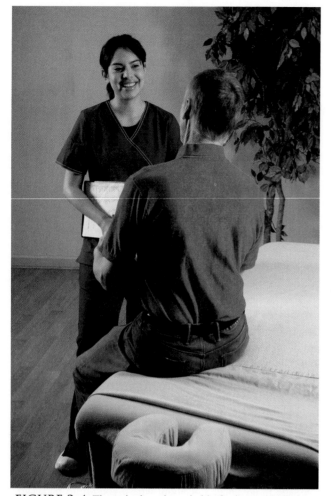

FIGURE 2-4 Therapist in attire suitable for her work setting.

In any setting your appearance should be clean and neat, no scents or odors, nails trimmed and hair held back from the face. Your clothing should be such that it will not drape or hang on the client during the session yet it should not be so tight fitting as to be revealing, or so low cut as to show cleavage on women.

Tattoos, body art, and body piercing are becoming more common. While this represents personal choice, therapists who have visible body art might consider how clients might view them. A 20-year-old client from Los Angeles might view body art differently than a 60-year-old client from Tulsa. Body art could have a negative impact on a job interview or during the initial contact with a new client; your professionalism might be called into question. Because of this, weigh all pros and cons when considering alterations in your appearance.

Financial Boundaries

Money is an important part of our practice. We are professionals whose expertise is of value to our clients. We offer our time, focused attention, and expertise in exchange for money. If you are uncomfortable with money or have money issues, it may affect how you establish and enforce financial boundaries.

The therapeutic relationship is also a business relationship in which we have boundaries regarding fee schedules and payment procedures. Be sure to inform new clients of your fees, when payment is due, what forms of payment are accepted, and any other polices such as how situations of insufficient funds will be handled. Even if this information is imparted when the initial appointment is made, be sure to mention it again when obtaining consent for treatment (informed consent is discussed in Chapter 10). As fees and payment polices change, inform existing clients well in advance and perhaps post a notification in your office.

Some therapists have sliding fee scales, allowing clients to pay different amounts depending upon the client's ability. This can become a boundary issue when money gets in the way of the therapist being fully present in the therapeutic role. Imagine how it would feel if a client who was getting a discount came in one week all excited about their upcoming Caribbean vacation or their new expensive car. What if the therapist herself had not had a vacation for a few years for financial reasons?

Also think about how you will handle payment arrangements when receiving massage from fellow therapists. Will you offer and/or expect a professional discount? Will you trade for services? What if you charge more for an hour than does your fellow therapist? How will you address the difference in fees for the same time spent, if at all? If you are trading services, when will trades be scheduled? What will happen if the therapist you are trading with has just scheduled the third session with you and you have only received one session from her? Will you stop trading until the session number is equal or will you expect payment for the third session? Ideally, these types of situations should be discussed before they occur, mutually agreeing on how they will be handled.

BOUNDARY MANAGEMENT

After boundaries are established, they need to be managed throughout the course of the therapeutic relationship. Clear communication about boundaries during the initial session and consequences for crossing them will reduce or eliminate misunderstandings. When boundaries are unclear or when we continually bend or disregard boundaries, we may be viewed as unprofessional, which can harm or even destroy the relationship.

It is helpful to remember that our role as a massage therapist never goes away. We are massage therapists in the office. We are still massage therapists when we are grocery shopping or at the movie theater. When our clients see us in these settings, we must still exhibit professionalism.

Boundary violations vary widely and range from mild inconsiderateness to the more serious sexual misconduct. Boundary management extends from our clients to other massage therapists and health care providers and may include responsible acts of confronting a fellow therapist when we hear rumors of unethical or illegal conduct. Steps to take when we hear of misconduct by a fellow therapist are discussed later.

Learning to Say "No"

Maintaining healthy boundaries means learning how to say no. If you have clearly stated your professional boundaries, kindly but firmly restate them when clients request that you bend the rules on their behalf. And if you find yourself bending your own policies, ask yourself why. Are you trying to save your client? Do you want to be considered a nice person? Do you feel uncomfortable disappointing others? Answers to these questions will help you with self-evaluation.

In fact, periodic self-evaluation is an important part of boundary management. As stated previously, congruency is a characteristic of healthy boundaries. How you feel about yourself must be congruent, or match, your boundaries. If there is conflict, boundaries will be difficult, if not impossible, to maintain. As you inventory your own personal needs, ask yourself if they are met in appropriate ways; make any needed changes. We need to be clear about our intentions, focusing on the client and putting his or her therapeutic goals before our own needs. The therapeutic relationship is not a place to have personal needs met because doing so opens the door for dual relationships and countertransference. And you, the professional, are held accountable for any negative consequences resulting from lack of boundary management.

Professional Distance

Professional boundaries create a healthy, professional distance between the client and the therapist. In fact, the distance helps make the therapeutic relationship a safe place for the client's experience. Let us consider Chapter 11 of the *Tao Te Ching*:

> *Thirty spokes share the wheel's hub;*
> *It is the center hole that makes it useful.*
> *Shape clay into a vessel;*
> *It is the space within that makes it useful.*
> *Cut doors and windows for a room;*
> *It is the holes which make it useful.*
> *Therefore profit comes from what is there;*
> *Usefulness from what is not there.*
> —Lao Tsu

When space, or distance, is provided for clients to relax and be themselves, healing is more likely to occur. If we fill up the space with too much conversation, with our own agendas, or with our own concerns, then the client does not have the opportunity to come out from behind his or her wall (a wall of muscular tension).

Professional distance also displays another characteristic of healthy boundaries, protection. The distance we maintain demonstrates that we value and will protect the therapeutic relationship by not entering into dual relationships with our clients (see Dual Relationships section). Professional distance, similar to the pauses in a symphony, is often where peace, sanctity, and oneness are experienced. This is one of the gifts of the therapeutic relationship; a gift that is not often acknowledged.

"When we work from a place of compassion, it is a place of non-judgment, non-comparison, without the need to understand. With compassion we are not entrained in the drama of the client's story, we are just with them. This is love, which resides in the heart."
—Fritz Frederick Smith

Crossing Boundaries: Common Mistakes

Following is a list of common mistakes therapists make when professional boundaries are crossed. Being forewarned is being forearmed; therefore by examining these pitfalls, you may prevent them.

Lack of Proper Training and Experience. Avoid the *weekend workshop warrior syndrome*, which is representing yourself as qualified in a specific technique or method without proper training and experience. The syndrome involves taking a workshop and then promoting yourself as skilled in your new specialty without proper certification. Doing so may result in injury to the client. While practice is necessary to hone a new skill, caution is required in the time interim between training and certification. When practicing a new technique, gain client consent, stating both its benefits and potential risks. Also state how use of the new technique may help the client achieve his or therapeutic goals.

Intentionally Evoking an Emotional Release. Playing psychotherapist by using techniques that are designed to intentionally evoke an emotional release is another common mistake. We endanger our clients both mentally and emotionally not only when we provoke emotions, but also when we attempt to verbally process emotional material that naturally surfaces during a session. An academic degree and separate license are needed to practice individual counseling or psychotherapy. Additionally, acting the role of psychotherapist shows disrespect not only for the client, but for all mental health professions as well. Be sure to have contact information of several counselors and/or psychotherapists when referral is appropriate. For more information, see Box 2-2.

Asking a Client to be Your Friend. This issue is common enough to deserve a lengthy discussion under the Dual Relationships section. By refraining from moving the therapeutic relationship into a friendship, we avoid the dangers of client abuse, client neglect, dual relationships, transference, and countertransference (see appropriate sections later in the chapter).

Making Comments About a Client's Appearance. Comments about a client's appearance may seem harmless at first. But if your client has been traumatized by physical, emotional, or sexual abuse, he or she may misread the comment or gesture as abusive and perhaps seductive. Comments of this nature may interfere with a client's progress. Clients who have or are recovering from eating disorders may also be hurt by comments about their appearance. For example, after hearing a compliment about their shoes, clients with low self-esteem may feel as if nothing else about them was worth complimenting. Comments about a client's appearance are best avoided.

Ignoring Contraindications. Avoid working on clients who have contraindications to massage (see Chapter 9). This may be difficult if you work in a setting in which refusing to work on a client is discouraged (i.e., salon or day spa). Perhaps you have an overwhelming urge to help the client and believe the benefits outweigh the harm massage may cause. However, contraindications for massage do exist. In most cases, massage can be modified by client positioning, avoidance of select techniques, or an area of the client's body. In some cases, massage is best postponed. Be sure to discuss your reasons for massage modifications or postponement with your client during treatment planning (see Chapter 10). When a client needs service or evaluation outside of our scope of practice, be sure to refer him or her to the appropriate provider.

Client Neglect and Abuse

When any professional, whether a physician, attorney, minister, or massage therapist, does not recognize or respect the rights and boundaries of the client, the result may be client abuse or client neglect. As mentioned previously, all therapeutic relationships include a power imbalance, with the professional having more power than the client.

Client neglect is defined as *unintentional* physical or emotional harm resulting from therapist's insensitivity or lack of knowledge. An example of client neglect is a therapist who mistakes a cyst for a trigger point, causing cyst rupture through direct prolonged pressure. Another example is a therapist who, rather than providing emotional support for the client who is crying, oversteps his or her training and slips into a counselor role. In both examples, the therapist did not intend to harm the client, yet it happened.

Negligent treatment is often spawned by ignorance or lack of forethought. Ways to avoid client negligence are (1) stay within your scope of practice, (2) have strong professional boundaries (3), continue your own education, and (4) develop a cautious and professional attitude.

Client abuse is defined as physical or emotional harm sustained from *deliberate* acts of the therapist. An abusive therapist is one who consciously takes advantage of a client emotionally, physically, mentally, sexually, or financially. Let's explore these more closely.

Emotional Abuse. The potential for emotional abuse exists in all relationships in which there is an imbalance of power. Abuse happens when the person who wields the greater power does not recognize or respect the boundaries of the other. In therapeutic relationships, the therapist has the more powerful or authoritative position. The client enters into the relationship because the therapist has particular knowledge, skills, and abilities. The client may feel vulnerable both physically and emotionally because he or she is usually lying down and draped, whereas the therapist is standing and clothed. In many instances, when someone removes his or her clothing, he or she may feel emotionally naked and vulnerable. Because of this vulnerability, careless statements have the potential to impact the client deeply, as well as show lack of respect for the client's emotional boundary. For example, telling your client that he or she is the "tightest person I have ever worked on" may seem harmless, but the client may take it that a person of authority has declared that something is wrong with them.

Physical Abuse. Although rare, physical abuse may include disregarding the client's request for lighter pressure because you believe that *more pressure is better*. If a client becomes bruised or injured as a result of deep or prolonged massage, you may be liable, and the client may file battery charges. If you discover that your client bruises easily (e.g., taking platelet inhibitors, is elderly, or inactive), discuss the potential for bruising and obtain written consent before proceeding with a deeper, more vigorous massage.

Sexual Abuse. Sexual abuse may be physical, verbal, or nonverbal. Examples of sexual abuse range from verbal advances to leaning your body against your client during the massage. For more discussion, see the section on dating clients (under Dual Relationships) and the section on sexual misconduct.

Financial Abuse. Financial client abuse is taking advantage of a client's resources. It may be charging more than the standard rate simply because the therapist knows the client is in a high-income bracket. Accepting expensive gifts or access to a client's living quarters for a weekend is financially abusive. For more discussion on client tips and gifts, see Chapter 17.

Make a list of five or more situations to create fire drills. These situations can be repeats of past unpleasant experiences or situations that constitute the most uncomfortable scenarios between a client and therapist you can imagine. For example, it might be that a client has a seizure on the table, you accidentally undrape a client, or someone makes a pass at you.

Act out each situation with a classmate in front of the class. Once the situation is complete, ask the class and/or instructor for other options. Revise the fire drill strategies if necessary. This activity will help you become more prepared to handle difficult situations.

CONFLICT AND CONFLICT RESOLUTION

When boundaries become vague or nonexistent, conflicts can arise. Conflicts can also result when client expectations are not met; you do not start a massage on time, you do not adequately address an area the client says is problematic, or you cancel a client's appointment for the third time this month.

The key to reducing conflict is to have boundaries communicated clearly and to role model healthy boundaries. But in all relationships, conflicts will occur naturally and can provide opportunities for exploration and perhaps a deeper understanding of why boundaries and communication are important aspects of professional practice.

A brief look at healthy and unhealthy strategies is located in Table 2-1. Creativity is also needed in conflict resolution, but guidelines are important as they provide a frame of reference.

- Communicate clearly.
- Identify and accept the problem.
- Communicate with *I* messages instead of *you* messages; *you* messages can be perceived as blaming the other party.
- Have healthy boundaries, which are essential to conflict resolution.
- Look for solutions that are in the best interest of the client and the relationship.
- Be open to a variety of solutions.
- Do not take problems and differences personally.
- Let each party keep his or her respect and dignity.
- Take full responsibility for your own behavior.
- Separate issues from people.
- Avoid power plays.
- Pick your battles carefully, asking yourself if this issue will matter in 5 or 10 years.
- Save ultimatums for absolute nonnegotiables or late-stage negotiations.
- Do not waste time negotiating nonnegotiables.
- Take time out when angry emotions are running high; step back and look at the problem before reacting.
- Look for the gift or the lesson after the conflict is resolved.

How Disgruntled Clients Are Handled

It is important to take action immediately when a client is unhappy with the service being provided. Be willing to listen carefully and sincerely to the complaint without interjecting opinions or becoming defensive. Once the client has completely stated his or her position, ask, "What would you like for me to do?" Comply within reason. Sometimes, the best course of action is to offer a dissatisfied client a refund or gift certificate for a future session, even if no negligence exists on the part of the therapist. Giving an immediate refund to a client without question may save a therapist a mountain of aggravation later.

TABLE 2-1 Healthy and Unhealthy Conflict Resolution Strategies

STRATEGY	ACTION	BY
Fight	Trying to impose one's preferred solution on the other party	Insisting, blaming, criticizing, accusing, shouting
Submit	Lower aspirations and settle for less than one would have liked	Giving in or giving up Agreeing to simply end the conflict Surrendering to what the other wants
Flee	Choose to leave the scene of the conflict	Ceasing to talk Leaving physically, cognitively, and/or emotionally Changing the topic
Freeze	Choose to wait for the other's next move	Waiting Doing nothing
Problem solve	Pursue alternatives that satisfy both sides; develop a win-win strategy	Talking, listening, gathering information, thinking, generating options, resolving

---

INCIDENT REPORT FORM

Date:_____ Client's name_____

Time:_____ Therapist's name:_____

Place:_____

Therapist's perceptions of incident:

Individual's involved in the incident:

Actions taken:

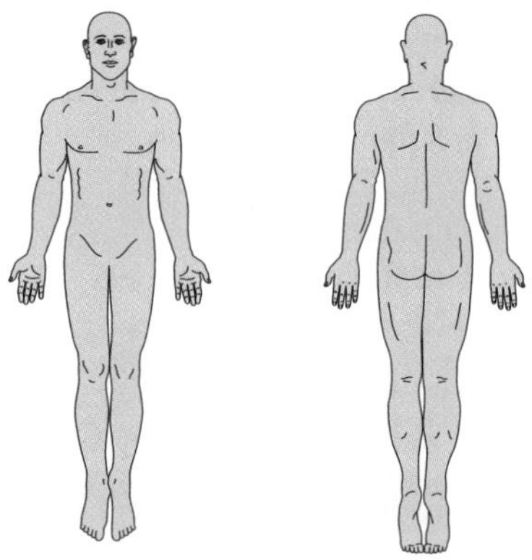

_____   _____
Signature of Massage Therapist   Date

Reviewed and resolved:

Date:_____ Time: _____

Place:_____

FIGURE 2-5 A sample incident report form.

Incident Reports

Any incident that involves a client and unusual activity should be documented. Regardless of how small or unusual the incident, a report should be completed and retained to document these occurrences (Figure 2-5). Incident reports may involve a client who slips and falls, a client who misplaces belongings, or a client that has made sexual advances. The incident report should include the date, time, and exact location of the occurrence; who was present; and what steps were taken to alleviate the problem. If physical injury was involved, the report should include the condition of the client when he or she departed from your establishment. The report should state facts, not feelings. Statements should be obtained from anyone present during the incident.

> evolve *Log on to the Evolve website and access Chapter 2 on your student account to print out an incident report form for use as mentioned above.* ■

Conflicts of Interest: Therapists as Salespersons

One of the characteristics of therapeutic relationships is a power differential, with the professional or authoritative person in the more powerful position. As stated earlier, this imbalance of power is a natural occurrence and, in and of itself, is not a problem. Conflicts may arise, however, when this power is misused and seeks to serve the interests of the therapist rather than the client. If conflicts of interests arise, ask yourself and answer honestly the question, "Whose interest am I really serving?"

A common scenario is when the therapist is selling products. In this situation, the therapist may be faced with choosing between what is in the best interest of his or her finances and what is in the best interest of the client. Therein lies a possible conflict; can we be objective when we are making a profit on the sale? Even without direct monetary gain, the therapist responsible for the sale may receive points leading to fulfillment of established work goals such as increased commission or promotion.

Selling anything to clients other than professional services for which we have contracted creates a dual relationship; you are *therapist* and *salesperson*. And dual relationships are often problematic. A power differential exists and we have some degree of influence in the relationship. Is the client really free to refuse the offer? Might the client make the purchase to please the therapist? Perhaps the sales pitch simply feels funny to the client. This awkwardness may lead the client to schedule his or her next massage appointment with a therapist who does not sell products.

Suppose a client has an allergic reaction to the supplement or herbal cream that you sold. What would happen if your client believed he or she did not gain the benefits you said to expect? How would these and similar issues be handled? Be sure to consider these and other possibilities before selling products to your massage clients. As you can see, selling products may damage the therapeutic relationship.

In some work settings, you may be expected to sell products. There are varying opinions in the profession as to how to handle sales in these situations. In some settings, the product is visible and you do not mention it unless asked. In other settings, you may be expected to approach the client about purchasing products. Be sure to discuss product sales with your employer and understand his or her expectation before accepting a position. If possible have another employee, such as the receptionist, handle the actual sale. Be aware that any situation that involves selling of retail items may put stress on the therapeutic relationship.

TRANSFERENCE AND COUNTERTRANSFERENCE

Transference and countertransference exhibit themselves in all relationships: therapeutic, personal, and professional. Psychotherapists have long been taught about these frequent experiences of personalization that takes place between counselors and their clients. Sigmund Freud was the first to describe it. Even though massage therapists are not counselors, we may encounter transference and countertransference and therefore should be able to recognize and manage them.

As you explore these concepts, remember that transference and countertransference influence relationships in ways that, under certain conditions, may be helpful to everyone concerned. Transference and countertransference are, by their nature, both complex and interrelated. They can also be quite normal. Therapists will remind clients of other people in their lives, past and present. Clients will remind therapists of people in their own lives. Power differentials, a component of therapeutic relationships, play a role in amplifying transference.

When a client feels unconsciously or consciously that the therapist is someone other than a health care provider, the result is transference. Conversely, the therapist may experience countertransference if he or she feels that the client is more than just a client. Transference can sometimes produce a powerful love (positive transference) or destructive hatred (negative transference), both of which are based on misperceptions.

This information presented next will give you a deeper understanding about transference and countertransference and reiterates that clear boundaries, a key component of therapeutic relationships, can minimize their negative affects. It can be helpful to receive supervision when these types of issues arise in your practice.

Transference

Transference occurs when the client *transfers* feelings, thoughts, and behaviors related to a significant person in his or her early life (e.g., parents) onto the therapist. During transference, the therapist now assumes a more significant role in the client's subconscious mind. Transference may occur when needs not being met in the client's personal relationships are now being met by you and the therapeutic relationship. These may be touch needs, the need for attention, listening, validation, and the feelings of nurturing that massage can bring. Vulnerability felt by the client may bring on feelings of transference. Transference may also be about past unresolved feelings and patterns of behavior.

During transference, the client begins to personalize the therapeutic relationship. Instead of seeing the therapist as a professional providing a service, the client's sees and relates to the therapist as if he or she were a significant person from their past. For example, if you begin to remind the client of her father, the client's perception of you may change, leading to a change in behavior. In this situation, client behavior will depend on the paternal relationship she had. Did your client have a loving, nurturing relationship with her father or was it filled with violence or abandonment? During positive transference, your client may bring you raisin cookies that her father liked, do things her father expected, and want to be treated as the special daughter "client," such as spending extra time on her or scheduling appointments outside your normal office hours. The client experiencing positive transference is not likely to question your actions (even ones that deserve questioning) and may invite you to lunch or ask personal questions to encourage a more personal relationship.

But when you do not reciprocate by treating this client special, she may feel hurt or even angry. And if you happen to make the client feel special by preferential treatment, transference may continue and even intensify. After all, who wouldn't be willing to bend the rules for a client who brings us gifts and does us favors, right? But this may lead to further client distortions and confusion of the true nature of the therapeutic relationship.

A client, particularly a needy client, may develop a romantic infatuation on the therapist. Clients bring a variety of feelings, including pain, both physical and emotional, to the massage table. A therapist who represents unrealistically the epitome of kindness, sensitivity, and warmth may inadvertently fill the client's unmet emotional needs. It is not hard to fathom a needy client wanting to be friends with his or her therapist. The therapist is, in most cases, kind, thoughtful and willing confidant; this type of person is perhaps missing in the client's life.

Keep in mind that you cannot control how your clients think. When you recognize transference, reduce its impact on the relationship by developing awareness and understanding of how it can affect the therapeutic relationship. Then avoid behaviors that encourage or intensify transference, and have good boundaries. Successful navigation of these waters requires maturity, integrity, and ethical professionalism. Once again, seek supervision when needed.

Countertransference

Countertransference occurs when the therapist brings unresolved emotional issues or personal needs into the therapeutic relationship; it runs *counter*, or in the opposite direction of, transference, from the therapist to the client. But similar to transference, countertransference can stem from unresolved feelings, thoughts, and perceptions about someone from the therapist's past, but not always. And as with transference, countertransference is unconscious. The therapist is not aware, at first, that they are transferring thoughts and feelings onto the client.

Countertransference can occur when you have trouble maintaining professional distance and detachment from a client. Detachment is not thinking less of a client but rather thinking of a client less. These feelings may be caused by the attention from a client's transference. You may find yourself taking a personal interest in the client or it can occur when you play along with and acting on a client's romantic infatuation. Countertransference can also occur when the client reminds you of someone significant from your past and you start treating the client differently, perhaps less professionally.

Countertransference can also occur when you see many aspects of yourself in your client. For example, your client may be of the same age, recently divorced, or have children with ages similar to your children. Because of these similarities, you may believe your the client will be best served by the same type of work or solutions that helped you. Remember, both transference and countertransference involve seeing a person as someone else; not who they truly are. Countertransference may prevent you from ascertaining your client's unique history and therapeutic goals, then acting in his or her best interest.

So how do you know countertransference is occurring? Signs are:

- Having intense feelings, positive or negative, toward a client
- Becoming angry or depressed when a client cancels an appointment
- Becoming impatient, angry, or depressed when a client is not progressing with treatment
- Being argumentative with a client
- Seeking to or becoming involved in a client's personal life
- Thinking excessively about the client between appointments
- Making excuses for a client's inappropriate behavior
- Giving a particular client additional time during each appointment
- In extreme cases, romantic and sexual fantasizing
- Ignoring or relaxing professional boundaries

So what can you do if you find yourself suddenly in countertransference? Begin by taking a closer look at what might be causing it. Are your getting your needs met? If not, how can you begin doing so outside the therapeutic relationship? Does your client remind you of someone significant in your life? As stated previously, awareness is vital to healthy boundaries, and self-awareness is key to averting countertransference. If you fail to identify reasons behind countertransference, this pattern may continue or repeat itself with other clients. Consider seeking the guidance from a colleague or mental health counselor. This will help you identify areas of unmet needs and develop appropriate ways of getting them met.

If it is too difficult to reverse countertransference, the best course of action may be to terminate the therapeutic relationship and refer the client to another therapist. Caution is advised during termination of the relationship because the client may feel it as rejection. Again, seek guidance from a trusted source before talking with the client if you are unsure how to proceed.

Finally, professional distance may reduce or eliminate countertransference and is an important part of boundary management. Be sure to leave personal needs and emotional burdens outside the treatment room to serve the highest good of the client.

> *"Attachment is the great fabricator of illusions; reality can be attained only by someone who is detached."*
> —Simone Weil

Seductive Client

Some clients are highly manipulative and experts at making the therapist feel special or creating situations in which the therapist feels compelled to get involved. These seductive clients seem to know how to throw us off balance and create an illusion that a special relationship with them is not inappropriate or unethical. These clients seem to know the right buttons to push. And they are indifferent to the emotional damage they cause.

Patterns of behavior exhibited by seductive clients usually come from wounds inflicted in early childhood. He or she learns that the best way to get needs met is by manipulating others seductively, which boosts their self-esteem. These patterns of behavior are not about sexual seduction, it is more about receiving positive affirmation of their self-worth when they seduce someone into a relationship with them. The more forbidden the relationship, the more they win. These signs are indeed red flags of a strong transference. This kind of transference is highly volatile, it can change quickly from attraction and delight to disappointment and rage. Seductiveness is not about affection, love, or sex; it is about dominance, control, selfishness, and aggression.

The best way to deal with seductive clients is to have strict boundaries and to address quickly any boundary violations as they occur. Some therapists find it difficult to maintain healthy boundaries with a seductive client. If you have a hard time saying "No" to people because of being afraid to hurt other's feelings, or do not have clear boundaries, managing boundaries with a seductive client may be challenging. You may find yourself in countertransference and spend significant time thinking and obsessing about the client's seductive acts. However, the smallest blunder or *slip of the hand* can turn the therapeutic relationship into a

nightmare. Countertransference with a seductive client needs to be discussed with a professional counselor or trusted, mature, unbiased colleague who will give you a good dose of reality.

DUAL RELATIONSHIPS

Ideally, massage therapists work with an attitude of professionalism, objectivity, and nonjudgment. They keep their focus on clients and client goals. Our professionalism and ability to focus on our clients may be thwarted when we enter into dual relationships with them. Dual relationships occur when we have more than one type of relationship with a client; more than just a therapeutic relationship.

When we have more than one type of relationship with a client, a complex interweaving of roles occurs and maintaining professional boundaries can be challenging. Treating all clients the same is difficult if some are friends and others are not. Conflicts may arise unintentionally, boundaries become blurred, and the potential for client abuse and neglect is heightened. You cannot promise that entering into a dual relationship with your client will not affect the therapeutic relationship; no one can make that kind of promise.

In therapeutic relationships, each person has realistic expectations of the other. Our clients expect us to perform our professional duties and responsibilities. We expect our clients to keep their appointments and to comply with our office polices regarding payment and behavior. But when we have additional roles with each other, such as a client who is also our real estate agent, it changes our roles and brings in a new set of expectations.

When professional boundaries blur, trouble is often around the corner. Remember, the therapeutic relationship is not equal. A power differential exists, similar to a parent-child or teacher-student relationship. The client looks to the therapist to help achieve therapeutic goals, whether it is stress relief, pain relief, or just a little TLC.

Given the complexity of dual relationships, how can they be managed ethically? NCBTMB's standards of practice remind us to avoid relationships that can impair professional judgment (http://www.ncbtmb.org/about_standards_of_practice.php). Good boundaries will help us manage these relationships and help us be clear about which role we are in. We want to avoid wearing more than one hat at a time (see next section). When our role is that of therapist, be a therapist. When our role is that of friend, be a friend. When our role is that of family member, be a family member.

Strangely, one of the reasons therapists initiate dual relationships is that they are convenient. A potential friend is right in front of you. Or in the case of a friend, a potential client is right in front of you.

Maintaining boundaries and ethics is not the client's responsibility. The power differential makes it nearly impossible for a client's behavior to be unethical. A professional license denotes professional responsibility, accountability, and adherence to a code of ethics. The person in the professional role is held responsible for any negative consequences of dual relationships.

Most Common Dual Relationship: Friendship

In addition to our roles as therapists, what other interpersonal roles are possible? Can a therapist become friends with a client? What about a client who becomes a business partner? What if a therapist becomes romantically or sexually involved with the client? Should a therapist rent property or borrow money from a client? Imagining how a romantic, sexual, or business relationship might evolve from the therapeutic relationship is not difficult. Let us explore the most common dual relationship: *friendship*.

If a client becomes our friend, we now assume two roles in the client's life. Being exclusively in one single role when more than one exists is difficult; for example, being solely in the role of therapist when your client is also a friend. Imagine how hard it would be *not* to chat with a friend during a massage. Self-disclosure to a client (now friend) will create a different atmosphere during the sessions. You and your client-friend may treat scheduled appointments as opportunities to develop further your friendship. Massage sessions may become social affairs rather than professional events. You may become careless, not keeping the focus on the client. Whose interest is being served now?

So how do therapeutic relationships differ from friendships? In a friendship, the relationship is ideally 50/50; a certain amount of give and take exists between parties. In a friendship, your friend knows as much about you as you know about your friend. This type of familiarity is not the case in therapeutic relationships; it is not an equal partnership. A power differential exists. In therapeutic relationships, you know much more about your clients than they know about you.

Besides, can we really call what develops between a client and a therapist a friendship? Nina McIntosh examines this question in her book, *Educated Heart*. Do we go to our client's offices, remove our clothing, lie on their desks, get a massage, and pay for their time? This scenario occurs rarely if at all. McIntosh also states that we typically do not show our clients what she calls our *lower selves*, the part of us reserved for only those closest to us. Negative aspects of our lower selves include our pettiness, neediness, jealousies, idiosyncrasies, and quirks. Ideally, we project our *higher selves* in professional settings. Positive aspects of our higher selves include empathy, compassion, and altruistic loving kindness. Because of this projection, clients often see only our higher selves.

Turning clients into friends may also interfere with our relationships with other clients. How would you feel if your therapist Michael was friends with his client Mary and not with you? If not hurt, you may question his professional boundaries.

Social networking sites such as Facebook and MySpace have brought the complexities of dual relationships to a new level. Now, it is easy for clients to know more about you including your likes, dislikes, relationship status, and sometimes your personal schedule. Participation in this social environment can make boundary management with our clients trickier. The Internet can be a tremendous boon for marketing and networking, as long as we are cautious about what we post. It is best to regard social networking sites as an open public folder in which its contents can be read by everyone.

Maintaining professional boundaries is difficult with someone with whom we have a close relationship. Despite this fact, friendships with clients routinely develop. However, as we examine dual relationships in the context of intimacy, we can further differentiate between friendships and professional relationships.

Intimacy. So what is an intimate relationship? How does an intimate relationship differ from a therapeutic relationship? *Intimacy* is close personal association in which the following elements exist: choice, mutuality, reciprocity, trust, and delight.

Choice. We choose to be in the relationship; it cannot be forced.

Mutuality. Both parties agree mutually to enter into and maintain the relationship.

Reciprocity. Over time, I will receive as much from the relationship as I give to it.

Trust. Both parties have confidence in and reliance on each other's role in the relationship.

Delight. The relationship brings joy to both parties.

The feelings and experiences of intimacy are generally reserved for those whom we are closest, usually family and friends.

Therapeutic relationships are similar to intimate relationships. Choice and mutuality exist, or the relationship would not exist. Trust is necessary to initiate the relationship and is maintained as each party keeps their promises. Both parties may experience delight because the therapeutic relationship should be a pleasant experience. Because of these similarities, some clients may confuse an intimate relationship with a therapeutic relationship.

A key element missing in therapeutic relationships is *reciprocity*. Recall that the roles of client and therapist are not equal, we do not ask our clients to attend to our emotional and physical needs. In intimate relationships, boundaries are relaxed and become permeable; the lives of both parties are revealed. In a therapeutic relationship, you do not disclose openly personal information, nor share personal history (Figure 2-6).

Some therapeutic relationships feel close, but we have seen that they are not the same as intimate relationships. Each party is receiving something of worth from the relationship, but it is not equal or reciprocal. This is as it should be, and helps keep the safety of the therapeutic relationship intact.

NINA McINTOSH

Born: May 27, 1943, died: July 18, 2010

"Being professional is just an educated way of being kind."

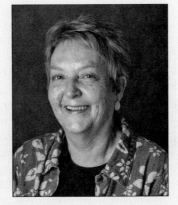

Nina McIntosh was the author of *The Educated Heart,* the first book about ethics and boundaries written specifically for massage therapists. McIntosh self-published the first edition of *The Educated Heart* in 1999, and it was quickly adopted by massage therapy schools across the country and in Canada. In 2005, after the book had been through numerous reprints, it was bought by Lippincott Williams & Wilkins, and the second edition was published.

Nina McIntosh was born in Memphis, Tenn., where she lived until she moved to New Orleans to attend the Newcomb College of Tulane University. She graduated 1965 with a BA in Psychology. After being employed as a social worker in New Orleans for 3 years, she continued her education at the graduate school at Tulane School of Social Work and earned an MSW degree.

Her professional career began in earnest in 1970 when she moved to Denver and worked as a psychiatric social worker. Nina recalls those years as the time she first encountered—and began her lifelong fascination with—professional boundaries. While working in a psychiatric hospital, she found it distressing that the staff was discouraged from touching the patients, and she felt strongly that the "body" part of the body/mind was being neglected, much to the patient's detriment.

McIntosh became curious about alternative methods of health care, and went to what is now the Boulder College of Massage Therapy in 1978. A few years later, she became a Certified Rolfer at Rolf Institute in Boulder. During her years as a Rolfer, she traveled extensively and settled for a while in the San Francisco Bay area. In 1998, McIntosh came full circle when she moved home to Memphis to care for her aging parents while maintaining a part-time Rolfing practice. After her parents' death in 1995, McIntosh found the time and the inspiration to write *The Educated Heart*. In 2004, she relocated to Asheville, N.C. After she retired from Rolfing, McIntosh continued to remain active in the bodywork community and she wrote about professional ethics. In the past few years, her interest in the psychological component of therapeutic bodywork has led her to study at Rosen Method Center Southwest in Santa Fe, N.M.

Her column on ethical boundaries, "The Heart of Bodywork," appeared in *Massage & Bodywork* magazine for most of a decade. For more than 15 years, she continued to teach workshops on ethics around the country, do private consulting for massage schools and practitioners, and market her popular home study course.

The third edition of McIntosh's *The Educated Heart* was released in March 2010. It continues to be a best-seller and one of the most popular books about professional ethics. It provides the framework for establishing and maintaining the integrity of the therapeutic relationship through the careful observance and nurturing of the boundaries of both client and therapist. The book is an easy read and engaging to reader's with its conversational style, McIntosh's dry wit, and plenty of real-life examples of the boundary dilemmas that all bodyworkers are likely to encounter at some point—along with her seasoned advice for handling those situations we all wish we didn't have to find ourselves in. It is an invaluable resource for anyone who practices in the somatic field.

McIntosh was diagnosed with Amyotropic Lateral Sclerosis (Lou Gehrig Disease) in 2009, and despite of her illness, still had the desire to care for others. She was active in her church and served on the handicap accessibility committee there, persuading them to put in an elevator so those in wheelchairs could go anywhere within the building. She struck up a friendship with a man who had been unjustly incarcerated on death row for more than 15 years, and who was released after DNA evidence cleared him. She was his supporter and advocate. She maintained her sense of humor even after she was no longer able to speak. She bore her physical challenges with dignity and strength.

In June of 2010, she was honored with the Aunty Margaret Humanitarian Award at the World Massage Festival in Berea, Kentucky. She was unable to travel; Laura Allen accepted the award on her behalf. She modestly said, "I don't think I'm much of a humanitarian." She definitely was. Nina McIntosh died on July 18, 2010. She will live on for years to come through *The Educated Heart*.

Intimate Relationships

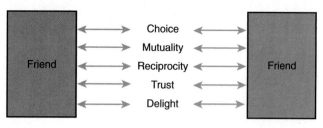

Therapeutic Relationships

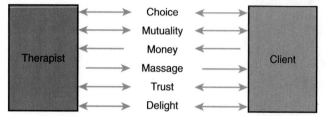

FIGURE 2-6 Intimate versus therapeutic relationships.

What About Friends Who Become Clients?

What about friends who become clients? Is this arrangement okay? What are possible concerns?

For a therapeutic relationship to occur from a friendship, professional boundaries must be established, just as with all clients. Both parties need to understand their individual positions and responsibilities. You, the therapist, will provide a service for which your friend, the client, will pay a fee. During the session, keep the conversation and focus on the client.

In some cases, it is better if your friend goes to a massage therapist with whom there is no previous relationship. Remember that the therapeutic relationship is designed to serve the client. A friend may not be willing or able to give you the authority you deserve, receive full benefit from the session, or take your work seriously as he or she would with another therapist who is not also a friend.

While in school, students often massage their friends for practice. Consider letting your friends know that, after licensure, a fee will be attached. If you know what the fee will be, let them know early on so they will be prepared to pay the requested fee. This time is also a great opportunity for you to practice being in the role of the therapist with professional boundaries intact, to treat practice sessions as you would in professional settings.

What About Working With Family Members?

What about family members who become clients? Is this arrangement okay? What are possible concerns?

Working with spouses, children, or other family members can be even more complicated than working with friends. Even though they are family members, a therapeutic

relationship must exist while performing professional services. Just like in all other therapeutic relationships, both parties need to understand their individual roles and responsibilities. Keeping clear boundaries is more challenging with family, yet vitally important. That said, it can be a source of great joy to work with family members, particularly when they are in pain or need our services. However, if the relationship is a strained one, that will further complicate the therapeutic relationship. There is a tendency to carry over any family dynamic into the therapeutic relationship. For example, if you have always wanted your sister's approval, you may use the massage as a way to gain it. This places a strain and unrealistic expectations on the therapeutic relationship, removing the focus from the sister client, to your needs.

Other considerations, for both family members and friends, may include:

- Do you charge your family members? If so, is your fee schedule different?
- Do you expect family members to scheduled appointments? Will you handle missed appointments differently than you do clients who are not family members?
- Are you willing to work on family members outside normal office hours?
- If you work with one family member and not another, will this negatively impact family dynamics? If so, how?

Dating Clients

Another complicated situation is moving the therapeutic relationship into a romantic or sexual one. Some *Code of Ethics,* such as the NCBTMB's, recommend discontinuing the client-therapist relationship for a minimum of 6 months before the new relationship begins (http://www.ncbtmb.org/about_code_of_ethics.php). It needs to be stressed that this time period should be considered a minimum. In many cases, 6 months is not enough. In fact, there will be cases where no amount of time is adequate.

Issues that need consideration include: the length of time both parties were in the therapeutic relationship; the level of client disclosure while in the relationship; and whether transference occurred and if the client still sees the therapist in a power or authoritative role, which is usually unconscious. When the latter occurs, it may be difficult for the client to feel equal in a new relationship with the therapist.

Compare the level of disclosure with a client who you have been seeing for 2 weeks for a hamstring strain and a client you have been seeing weekly for 3 years, during which time he went through a divorce and lost a parent. It is easy to imagine that the second client may lean on you more for emotional support. In fact, you may have become a major part of his support network. In this case, no amount of time will put the two of you on equal footing because of the deep bond your client experienced. The client may always see you as his savior, even as you establish a new relationship.

The decision to date an ex-client should be considered carefully. Such situations can easily damage the therapist's relationship with other clients, damage reputations, and raise a red flag of its own within the therapist's profession. The best and safest decision is most often to not go out with ex-clients.

Dual Licensure and Dual Roles

In some cases, a licensed massage therapist also holds another license to practice in a different profession. When this occurs, the person with dual licenses refrains from wearing *two hats* simultaneously. For example, if acting in the capacity of mental health counselor, provide only those services within that particular scope of practice. When the massage therapist who is also a licensed counselor gives a massage, provide only the services within that particular scope of practice.

Keep in mind that all professions have their independent codes of ethics. The code of ethics for a licensed mental health counselor for example will be different from the code of ethics for a massage therapist. In cases of an individual's possessing more than one professional license, the profession with the strictest code of ethics prevails and becomes the standard of conduct for the individual in *every* therapeutic relationship.

If you possess a dual license, consider informing both licensing boards and ask them to contact you if they have any questions or concerns.

SEXUAL MISCONDUCT

Sexual misconduct involves any sexual contact between a therapist and client as well as any sexualizing of the therapeutic relationship. It can range from innocent comments made about your client's body to sexual harassment to offering clients sexual services. The sensual pleasure inherent in massage is one of its greatest assets, but it is also one of its most obvious liabilities and can lead to situations of abuse, romantic seduction, and exploitation. Given that our profession uses touch as its primary therapeutic tool, therapists need to be prepared for the possibility of their touch being misinterpreted. And while the intention behind touch is professional and therapeutic, the client may experience an emotional or sexual response.

Since therapists may have to deal with these issues, talking about them early is best, such as while you are in school. If we ignore sexual issues, they will not disappear. Through talking about these issues, we obtain the *know-how* to make sound judgments and good decisions. Class discussion is important in that students learn not only from the instructors experience but from classmates as well. William Greenberg, the former grievance chairman for the American Massage Therapy Association, states that complaints filed

against therapists for sexual misconduct have decreased recently. Greenberg attributes this reduction to the fact that schools are giving more instruction on boundaries in general and sexual boundaries in particular.

Feelings are just feelings. They are impermanent. Sometimes clients are sexually attracted to their therapists; sometimes therapists are sexually attracted to their clients. This does not mean that these feeling must be acted on. Infatuations typically have a short lifespan of hours or days. Some of us are uncomfortable dealing with issues of sexuality, and therefore supervision can be helpful when they arise in the therapeutic relationship. The potential for sexual misconduct is in every profession, not just in massage.

Negative Perception of Massage

Some people still believe that massage is a euphemism for prostitution. Much of this illusion is perpetuated by movies, television shows, magazines, newspapers, telephone books, and prostitutes who use the term *massage parlor* to describe their place of business. While it is changing, it is still true that in some parts of country *massage* and *massage therapist* are presented side by side in lists of services, the former often are used to describe unlicensed individuals who offer adult entertainment. Some print media do not separate the two entities; for example, an ad featuring Tootsie's tantric or erotic massage next to a legitimate ad for massage therapy.

To further perpetuate the myth, society sexualizes touch. In fact, sometimes the only way some people are touched is when engaging in sex. Massage is used and often taught as a kind of foreplay in courses intended for couples.

As massage therapy becomes mainstream and available everywhere from the airport to hospitals, the negative perceptions will fade out. However, it is important to address the subject, empowering students to skillfully and respectfully respond to negative perceptions about massage, whether from potential clients or the public at large.

Examples of Sexual Misconduct

Examples of sexual misconduct that may lead to client abuse are:

- Engaging in verbal or physical flirtatious behavior, including comments made about a client's body or clothing
- Gestures or expressions that are seductive in nature or sexually demeaning
- Looking at a client seductively
- Telling sexual jokes
- Failure to ensure privacy through proper draping
- Entering the room before the client is completely draped or dressed
- Conversations about sexual problems, sexual performance, preferences, or fantasies initiated or involving either the therapist or client

- Unnecessary examination or treatments near female breasts or the pelvic area
- Filming the client without his or her permission
- Asking a client for a date
- Masturbation by therapist or client
- Intercourse
- Rape

Sexual Risk Management

Because massage had a negative connotation and our society often sexualizes touch, it is important that we are proactive; an ounce of prevention is worth a pound of cure. There are many things we can do to minimize or alleviate misunderstandings in regards to our touch being misinterpreted. And even with preventative measures, closeness felt by a client may lead to misunderstandings and false accusations. We are touching people, sometimes with the gentleness and attentiveness that might be commonly shared with a lover.

You may have clients who are survivors of sexual abuse. These individuals are often hypersensitive to seduction and are more likely than others to misinterpret the therapist's intent. Conversely, some people with abuse in their past dissociate (a kind of numbing both mentally and physically) and are unable to detect or stop the therapist's inappropriate behavior because they feel they were unable to stop it from happening before. Therapists who are survivors themselves may not realize that they are being sexually inappropriate with a client.

As with other professions, most complaints are made by female clients against male therapists. With this fact in mind, men are more at risk than women for being unjustly accused of sexual misconduct. Although every therapist should be watchful and alert with regard to sexual boundaries, male therapists need to take extra precautions. Precautions for both male and female are:

- Avoid terms of endearment (e.g., honey, dear sweetie) because they may be misread by the client
- When advertising, avoid words such as *release, available anytime, open 24 hours, my place or yours, total relaxation, complete relaxation, full service, full body massage,* and *happy endings.*
- When booking an appointment for a new client, ascertain his or her treatment goals. Note the prospective client's demeanor, tone of voice, and language he or she uses when making the initial appointment and note if you are uncomfortable.
- Do not work in a secluded office with clients whom you do not know.
- Do not schedule new clients late in the day or while no one will be in the office.
- Realize problems associated with a home office. Leading a client through your home to the bedroom area (now a treatment room) can make a client feel uneasy and may give mixed messages.

- Out-calls deserve special consideration. Screen clients carefully. Perhaps accept out-call requests with people who have been referred by someone you know and trust.
- Avoid sexual signals that you may be inadvertently sending, such as wearing tight or revealing clothing to work or for one particular client. When you start dressing for work as though you are going on a date, you are asking for trouble.
- When work on or near the female breast is clinically indicated, obtain separate written consent. Work should be conducted in this area over the sheet. It is strongly recommended that only female therapists work on a female client's breast. If a male therapist is massaging near a female client's breast, ask another female to be present in the room as a safeguard. Know and adhere to your state's laws regarding massage on female breasts.
- Be aware of body contact during the massage. Pay attention to the way you lean into your client's body. Be conscious of what part of your body touches the client during strokes, joint manipulations, and stretches.

Erections. There are several ways to manage situations that involve erections. You can simply ignore the erection because it may be a reflex response. Or you can ask questions that serve to distract the client from thoughts or feelings leading up to the erection. For example, "Tell me about your mother?" or "What type of work did your father do when you were a child?" Even if you do not know his parents, you can ask. Referencing parents often stops any erections stimulated by reflex response.

Or you can ask him to roll over and then continue the massage. Be sure to avoid any areas that might restimulate this response, such as the lower abdomen, inner thighs, and lumbosacral region.

If your client has an erection followed by inappropriate behavior, he is sexualizing the massage. Examples of inappropriate behavior may be subtle or overt and include noises such as moaning; repetitive rhythmic movements that often involve his pelvis, touching his pelvic area, or removing some or all of the drape. Other examples are sexually suggestive jokes, comments, or questions while he has the erection; touching you; or propositioning you for sex.

If you have discussed how these situations will be addressed when gaining consent for therapy (see Chapter 10; Right of Refusal), then proceed with those actions, such as terminating the session (see Terminating a Session section). If measures taken in these situations were not discussed previously, consider removing your hands from the client, stepping back and toward the door, and saying something like "I do not like the way in which you are behaving (talking). If you do not stop immediately, I will end this session." If he agrees to stop, you may continue with the massage if you feel comfortable. However, if you feel uncomfortable or if he makes excuses about his behavior or tries to minimize your reaction to his behavior, it is best to terminate the session. You have the right to refuse massage to a client who makes you feel uncomfortable, unsafe, or who continues to sexualize the massage once warned.

Terminating a Session

Rarely does a massage therapist have to terminate a session because of some inappropriate statement or action by the client. The decision should not be taken lightly, but once the decision has been made, it needs to be carried out. Here are some guidelines when terminating a massage while in session.

- Remove your hands from the client; step back and toward the door.
- Tell the client that the massage is over.
- Inform the client that you will wait outside while he or she gets dressed.
- Avoid answering questions until the client is dressed and out of the massage room.
- If the circumstances leading to the session are extreme, or if the therapist works alone and becomes frightened, either:
  - Call 911 and stay on the telephone until the client leaves, or
  - Lock yourself in a room as a safety measure until the client has left.

Document events leading to the session termination and what actions were taken (see Figure 2-5). This information can be used as a reference should the situation become libelous. If the situation involved sexual improprieties, then document statements verbatim or describe actions that gave that impression. If you feel fear as a result of the session termination, some form of intervention should be taken such as filing a police report. Filing a report is also appropriate if you feel sexually harassed or stalked by the client.

Consequences of Behavior

Every massage therapist must contemplate possible consequences of his or her own inappropriate behavior, particularly sexual misconduct. If a therapist intentionally or unintentionally violates a client sexually, the client's realization of what occurred rarely happens during the session. Most often, only after the massage does the client reflect on events and the therapist's inappropriateness. One can see how most acts of sexual misconduct by a therapist go unaddressed. The violated client may be silent regarding the event or blames him or herself for what happened.

Inappropriate behavior and sexual misconduct are forms of client abuse. One of the themes of this chapter has been how the therapist may take advantage of the more powerful positions in the therapeutic relationship to meet their own needs.

When a therapist violates the boundaries, consequences associated with the violation are often of corresponding severity. Possible consequences include:

- Loss of income
- Loss of reputation
- Loss of marriage
- Loss of friendships
- Loss of relationship with peers and colleagues
- Loss of license
- Loss of membership in professional organizations
- Loss of insurance coverage
- Lawsuits for damages
- Criminal charges
- Fines
- Attorney's fees
- Court costs
- Time in jail

Behind any sexual misconduct lies a blatant disregard of ethics, morals, and disregard for the entire profession of massage therapy. There is no excuse for sexual misconduct. Remember that the therapist is *always* responsible and liable for his or her actions, even if the client initiates the situation. The client cannot be consenting because the therapist has the power in the relationship.

Do not depend on professional liability insurance to cover any damages; most policies do not cover damages resulting from sexual misconduct.

> *"Our deeds determine us, as much as we determine our deeds."*
> —George Eliot

Sexual Misconduct of a Colleague

If we hear of a fellow therapist who has engaged in sexual misconduct, we have a professional responsibility to take action. The first step is to contact the therapist and let him or her know what is being said. Also offer observations made by you related to the alleged misconduct. Listen objectively to how the therapist responds.

If the therapist confirms the allegation and wishes to change the inappropriate behavior, suggest that he or she refer the client to another therapist.

If the therapist confirms the allegation and does not wish to discontinue the inappropriate behavior and act in the best interest of the client, then the next step is to file a complaint with the proper authorities. This is often the state board that regulates licensure and professional affiliations of which the therapist is a member.

In many states, there is "duty to report" misconduct by other therapists. This means if we have first hand knowledge (i.e., witnessed it ourselves, or told by the offending therapist) of misconduct, then we are required to file a complaint with the state licensing board. If we fail to do so, we are in violation of the law. If the allegations are second-hand (i.e., told by a client or fellow therapist) our role is to encourage the victim to file a complaint. Licensing boards and professional organizations are most able to act when they have a complaint filed by the victim. Some boards and organizations do allow anonymous complaints, but these are not as strong as ones filed by victims, and are harder to take action on.

Remember that sexual misconduct by a therapist shows disrespect for her professional role. Such a therapist is not concerned about boundaries, is indifferent to the emotional damage caused, and shows a lack of concern for the client's well-being. This behavior must be stopped.

E-RESOURCES

Ⓔvolve

http://evolve.elsevier.com/Salvo/MassageTherapy

- Chapter challenge
- Flash cards
- Photo gallery
- Additional information
- Downloadable forms
- Weblinks

BIBLIOGRAPHY

American Massage Therapy Association: *Code of ethics*, (website): http://www.amtamassage.org/About-AMTACore-Documents/Code-of-Ethics.html. Accessed August 28, 2010.

American Massage Therapy Association: *Standards of practice*, (website): http://www.amtamassage.org/About-AMTA/standards.html. Accessed August 29, 2010.

Baron RA: *Psychology*, ed 2, Boston, 1992, Allyn and Bacon.

Baur S: *The intimate hour*, New York, 1997, Houghton Mifflin.

Benjamin B, Sohnon-Moe C: *The ethics of touch*, Tucson, 2005. SMA.

Benjamin P: *Professional foundations for massage therapists*, Upper Saddle River, NJ, 2009, Pearson Prentice Hall.

Carnes P: *Out of the shadows: understanding sexual addiction*, ed 3, Minneapolis, 2001, Hazelden Publishing & Educational Services.

Dimond B: *The legal aspects of complementary therapy practice: a guide for health care professionals*, New York, 1998, Churchill Livingstone.

Fritz S, Grosenbach MJ, Paholsky K: Ethics and professionalism, *Massage Mag* Jan/Feb 46, 1997.

Fritz S: *Mosby's fundamentals of therapeutic massage*, ed 4, St Louis, 2009, Mosby.

Gill S: Safety for the massage professional: How to avoid those ticking time bombs (website): http://www.massagetherapy.com/articles/index.php/article_id/524/Safety-for-the-Massage-Professional%3A-How-To-Avoid-Those-Ticking-Time-Bombs. Accessed October 21, 2010.

Greene E, Boodrich-Dunn B: *The psychology of the body*, Philadelphia, 2004, Lippincott Williams & Wilkins.

Hamric AB, Spross JA, Hanson CM: *Advanced practice nursing: an integrative approach*, ed 3, Philadelphia, 2004, Saunders.

Hedricks G: *A year of living consciously: 365 daily inspirations for creating a life of passion and purpose*, New York, 2000, HarperCollins.

Ignatavicius DD: *Medical-surgical nursing: critical thinking for collaborative care*, ed 5, St Louis, 2005, Mosby.

Johanson G, Kurtz R: *Grace unfolding, psychotherapy in the spirit of the Tao-te Ching*, New York, 1994, Crown Publishing Group.

Kasl CD: *Women, sex and addiction: a search for love and power*, New York, 1989, Ticknor and Fields.

Kellogg T: *Sex and sexuality: a workshop*, Dallas, 1998, self-published.

Kurtz R: *Body-centered psychotherapy: the Hakomi method*, Mendocino, Calif, 1990, LifeRhythm Books.

LaRowe K: *The therapeutic relationship*, Compassion Fatigue (website): http://compassion-fatigue.com/Index.asp?PG=89. Accessed August 30, 2010.

MTBOK: *Massage therapy body of knowledge*, (website): www.mtbok.org. Accessed August 12, 2010.

McIntosh N: *The educated heart: professional guidelines for massage therapists, bodyworkers, and movement therapists*, ed 3, Baltimore, Lippincott Williams & Wilkins (in press).

Mehrabian A: *Silent messages: implicit communication of emotions and attitudes*, ed 2, Belmont, Calif, 1980, Wadsworth.

Miller-Keane, O'Toole MT: *Miller-Keane encyclopedia and dictionary of medicine, nursing, and allied health*, ed 7, St Louis, 2005, Mosby.

National Certification Board for Therapeutic Massage and Bodywork: *Code of ethics*, (website): http://www.ncbtmb.org/about_code_of_ethics.php. Accessed August 29, 2010.

National Certification Board for Therapeutic Massage and Bodywork: Standards of practices, (website): http://www.ncbtmb.org/about_standards_of_practice.php. Accessed September 2, 2010.

Natural Wellness: *Ethics: therapeutic relationships*, Montgomery, NY, 2004, self-published.

Ogden P: *Boundaries II or somatic psychology*, Boulder, Colo, 1995, Hakomi Integrative Somatics.

Odgen P: *Trauma and the body: a sensorimotor approach to psychotherapy*, New York, 2006, WW Norton & Co.

Roberts B: *Boundaries and the massage therapist: a workshop*, Lake Charles, La, 1999, self-published.

Rogers C: *On becoming a person*, New York, 1961, Houghton Mifflin.

Shea M: *Biodynamic craniosacral therapy*, vol 2, Berkley, Calif, 2008, North Atlantic Press.

Shea M: Personal conversations and personal writings 2009-2010.

Siegal D: *The developing mind: how relationships and the brain interact to shape who we are*, New York, 1999, Guilford Press.

Singer R Jr: *The therapeutic relationship is the most important ingredient in successful therapy*, SelfGrowth (website): www.selfgrowth.com. Accessed August 1, 2010.

Sohnen-Moe C: *The ethics of touch: the hands-on practitioner's guide to creating a professional, safe, and enduring practice*, Philadelphia, 2004, Lippincott Williams & Wilkins.

Torres LS: *Basic medical techniques and patient care for radiologic technologists*, ed 4, Philadelphia, 1993, JB Lippincott.

Tsu L: *Tao Te Ching*, New York, 1972, Vintage Books (Translated by G Feng and J English).

Varcarolis EM, Halter MJ: *Essentials of psychiatric mental health nursing: a communication approach to evidence-based care*, St. Louis, 2008, Saunders.

Webster's new world college dictionary, Springfield, Mass, 1995, G and C Merriam.

Whitfield CL: *Boundaries and relationships: knowing, protecting and enjoying the self,* Deerfield, Fla, 1993, Health Communications.

Wold GH: *Basic geriatric nursing*, ed 4, St Louis, 2008, Mosby.

Yardley-Nohr T: *Ethics for massage therapists*, Philadelphia, 2007, Lippincott Williams & Wilkins.

MATCHING I

Place the letter of the answer next to the term or phrase that best describes it.

A. Boundaries
B. Client abuse
C. Client neglect
D. Confidentiality

E. Countertransference
F. Disclosure
G. Dual relationships
H. Empathy

I. Intimacy
J. Power differential
K. Sexual misconduct
L. Transference

_____ 1. Personal needs, or unresolved feelings, thoughts and perceptions a therapist has about someone else which become assigned to the client

_____ 2. Aspect of the therapeutic relationship in which the therapist has a position of authority and the client is the more vulnerable position

_____ 3. Any sexual contact between a therapist and a client as well as any sexualizing of the therapeutic relationship.

_____ 4. Limits we establish between ourselves and others with regard to various aspects of our lives

_____ 5. The subconscious tendency of the client to assign feelings, thoughts and behaviors related to a significant person in his or her early life to the therapist

_____ 6. Nondisclosure of privileged information

_____ 7. Relationships that exist between the therapist and a client in addition to the therapeutic relationship

_____ 8. Close personal association involving choice, mutuality, reciprocity, trust, and delight

_____ 9. Physical or emotional harm sustained from deliberate acts of the therapist

_____ 10. Honest and open sharing of personal knowledge as well as ideas and insights

_____ 11. Ability to understand the unique world of another

_____ 12. Unintentional physical or emotional harm resulting from therapist's insensitivity or lack of knowledge

MATCHING II

Place the letter of the answer next to the term or phrase that best describes it.

A. Conflict
B. Emotional boundaries
C. Ethical issues
D. Incident report
E. Intellectual boundaries

F. Legal issues
G. Physical boundaries
H. Respect
I. Seductiveness
J. Trust

K. Unconditional positive regard
L. Weekend workshop warrior syndrome

_____ 1. Willingness to be vulnerable to the actions of another

_____ 2. Boundaries that encompass a person's beliefs, thoughts and ideas

_____ 3. Boundaries that encompass a person's feelings

_____ 4. Boundaries that help create a safe space around a person; help define the who, when, where, how and under what circumstances the person feels safe with touch

_____ 5. Behavior used by one person that seems designed to make another person feel special but in reality is meant to manipulate and control the other person

_____ 6. Struggle that can result when boundaries are vague or nonexistent or client expectations are not met

_____ 7. Respect for the client that does not depend on the client's behavior; valuing clients because their humanity warrants the therapist's care

_____ 8. Report that documents any unusual activity involving a client

_____ 9. Syndrome involving a therapist representing himself or herself as qualified in a specific technique or method without having the proper training and experience

_____ 10. Situations associated with human duty, appropriate right conduct, and responsibility

_____ 11. Situations involving laws, rules and regulations

_____ 12. Consideration or thoughtfulness exhibited by words and actions

CASE STUDY

Client Gifts

Chastity, a massage therapist, had a marriage that was coming to an end. She worked in a contract labor setting for another massage therapist, Jill. To minimize expenses, Chastity was looking for a cheaper apartment. Chastity had had a difficult time with the separation, and the stress was evident to many of her clients. One client, Bill, had questioned her until she had finally divulged her dilemma. That night, Bill talked the problem over with his wife, Marjorie, and then offered to let Chastity stay at their camp on the river, rent free, until she got back on her feet financially. Chastity was so excited to finally get a break. When Jill came in to close the books for the day, Chastity was bubbling over and proceeded to tell her boss about her new living arrangements. Jill was quiet for a moment and then said, "Chastity, we need to talk."

Jill's view was that accepting free rent from a client, especially one of the opposite gender, was an unethical decision. "What will you do if he just shows up and lets himself in unexpectedly?" Jill asked. "What if he asks for legitimate favors? Aren't you going to feel somewhat indebted?"

Jill tried to get Chastity to understand her point of view, but Chastity just became sullen and eventually hostile. "I thought you'd be happy for me," cried Chastity, barely able to hold back the tears.

Despite the fact that Chastity had been a loyal and productive employee for several years, Jill told her that she had to make a choice-find another living arrangement or find a new job.

If you were Chastity, how would you analyze the situation ethically? How would you approach Jill for further dialogue on the subject? What would your decision be in regard to the situation?

If you were Jill, what would you do to put yourself in Chastity's place?

What, if any, compromise would you be willing to make?

If Chastity chooses to stay, what kind of dialogue might prevent further similar occurrences?

If Chastity chooses to leave, what kind of references would you give to a prospective employer?

CRITICAL THINKING

How does an ethical code differ from a set of standards for practice?

Tools of the Trade

LEARNING OBJECTIVES

After completing this chapter, the student should be able to:

- Discuss reasons to obtain a massage table from a reputable manufacturer.
- Identify and discuss massage table features.
- Apply fabric care to the massage tabletop and table accessories and identify conditions or substances that damage fabric.
- Identify ways to disinfect table and accessory vinyl.
- Discuss table accessories, such as face rests and bolsters, used during massage.
- Discuss choices of massage linens and how to disinfect them when needed.
- State how to choose a massage lubricant and dispense it to prevent cross-contamination.
- Discuss massage lubricant storage and shelf life.
- Create a list of supplies needed for practice as well as furnishings for the massage room.
- Understand the importance of the massage environment while stating several essential elements.
- Identify guidelines to provide a safe and barrier-free facility.

INTRODUCTION

Your career as a massage therapist depends not only on your education, knowledge, and skills, but also on your ability to use wisely the tools of the trade. As with any other skilled artisan, you will use tools of your trade during the massage session. Your tools include your massage table (or massage chair), related accessories, linens, lubricants, and even the environment where the massage takes place.

In this chapter, we will open up your toolbox and examine each instrument. Practical suggestions are included to assist you in making decisions when choosing equipment and accessories or when designing a room. We will also discuss proper maintenance of these items and such as fabric care. Lastly, we will look at safety considerations for your massage equipment and your massage room.

But first, let us examine massage tables.

MASSAGE TABLES

A massage table is the most important item you will purchase (it is second only to your massage education in importance). Think of it as an investment that will last you most of your career. If fact, a good massage table will outlast the life of your automobile, so choose wisely. You and your table will be together a long time.

The most popular massage tables are portable tables and account for 95% of all sales by table manufacturers, with prices ranging from $200 to $600. Portable massage tables are hinged in the middle to be folded in half and carried from one location to another (Figure 3-1), resembling an over-sized suitcase.

The primary advantage of these tables is their portability—they are easily transported for off-site visits or set up and taken down if you have multiple office locations.

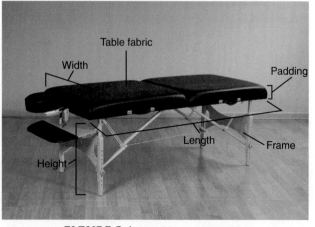

FIGURE 3-1 Portable massage table.

SELECTING A TABLE MANUFACTURER

You must feel totally confident in your equipment. It will most likely be a major expenditure, especially when purchased with accessories. Make every effort to obtain professional-grade equipment for the comfort, safety, and security for both you and your clients.

Purchasing a table package from a reputable, well-established company is important for several reasons. First, these companies tend to provide great customer service. Next, most established table manufacturers offer a trial period and, if you are not satisfied, will refund your money once the table is returned. Third, these massage product companies offer the best warranties, usually 5 years and up. Last, if the table must be sold as used, their products will be easier to sell, will hold their value, and will bring a better price.

One more thing to mention; massage table packages purchased by department stores or membership shopping clubs may seem like a deal at the time, but if your face rest or table leg breaks, it is unlikely you will be able to purchase a single accessory or replacement part from the retailer or from the manufacturer. When dealing with reputable massage table manufacturers, you can purchase replacement parts or accessories that fit your table (or chair) at any time.

Find out where the tables offered by the table manufacturer are made. Products made in the United States most often have better construction and overall quality than those in other countries where manufacturing standards are not as stringent.

CHAT ROOM

It may be interesting to note that, in the massage table industry, there is no standard for determining weight ratings for portable tables. When consumers (in this case, massage therapists) are looking for a strong and safe massage table, they must rely on the weight ratings provided by individual manufacturers. The more reputable the manufacturer is, the more you can trust their weight ratings. As with most things in life, you get what you pay for.

Over 2000 years ago, the Romans had a saying that still rings true today "Caveat emptor": "Let the buyer beware."

CHAT ROOM

When your table arrives, see if the table information is located underneath. If not, your table will come with a packing slip listing the table model, dimensions, color, and manufacturer's address and telephone number. Make a copy of the packing slip and attach it to the bottom of your table with a sheet of adhesive laminate. This information is needed when ordering additional equipment or supplies such as table pads or linens.

MASSAGE TABLE FEATURES

Most massage table manufacturers offer several choices such as width, height, length, framing, padding, and fabric. One guiding principle is that the massage table should suit your body, and the accessories should accommodate the multitude of clients' bodies you will encounter. For example, tall clients might need an 8-inch bolster. Let us examine table features.

Width

Most massage tables sold are between 28 and 33 inches wide. In most cases, portable table width depends on the height of the therapist transporting the table. Short therapists might consider a narrow table because it is easier to lift and carry when folded. Tall therapists do fine with a wide table.

Unfortunately, wide tables may make reaching across the table and applying pressure difficult for the therapist because of the loss of leverage. Conversely, narrow tables often make large-framed clients feel uneasy when lying supine (face up) because their arms tend to hang off the sides. Additionally, when performing a side-lying massage on a pregnant client, a wider table is preferred.

CHAT ROOM

My table is a 33 inches wide with a super deluxe table pad (4 inch). Wider tables more easily accommodate clients with special needs (try doing a side lying massage on a pregnant woman in her eighth month on a 28-inch table). Also, as I age, I find myself using the extra width to "perch" myself on the table while I massage. The super-soft padding is preferred by the majority of clients and provides comfortable prone, or face down, positioning in cases of breast tenderness (a frequent female client complaint). A soft table pad also allows me to easily work beneath the client (I slip my hand between the client's back and the tabletop). This technique is best utilized while I sit on a stool (my favorite accessory).

Height

The height range is usually between 22 and 34 inches. Adjustment is achieved, usually in 1-inch increments, by lengthening or shortening the four table legs. Aluminum table legs are made of nested tubes and adjustments can be made quickly by pushing in a spring-loaded button and adjusting the leg length. Wooden table legs are made in two sections held together by a tongue and groove system and one or two bolts. Height adjustments to wooden tables require unscrewing the knob(s), repositioning the table leg, and rescrewing the knob(s) to lock the leg in place.

Length

Most massage tables are either 72 or 73 inches long. Because most therapists use face rests and bolsters, a 6-foot-or-taller client will have ample room because a face rest adds 10 to 12 inches to table length, and a 6- or 8-inch-high bolster will shorten the client's leg length when placed under the knees or ankles.

Frames

Table frames, as well as its understructure, provide table support. These are typically made of wood, aluminum, or a combination of the two materials. Portable tables that are predominately wood tend to be a little heavier when carried than metal frames.

More petite therapists might purchase aluminum-frame tables because they are easier to transport. Aluminum tables also have the advantage of quicker leg adjustments as mentioned previously. Although some therapists rarely change table height, clients' girth varies enough to make leg adjustability a consideration. This circumstance is especially true when working on the fourth, fifth, or sixth client of the day, when energy conservation and proper body mechanics (or lack thereof) become a major concern.

Padding

If you ask clients what they remember most about being on your massage table, they will often mention table padding. It should be very comfortable, adapting to and supporting your client's body. When selecting table padding, consider its density, loft, and durability. Let us examine these areas.

Density. Most foam pads are divided into three grades of density: light, medium, and high. High-density generally has better *memory*, or ability of the foam to return to its original height after being disturbed by pressure. Most high-quality tables use medium- to high-density foam as they are more durable and last longer.

Loft. Foam thickness, or loft, typically ranges from 1.5 (firm) to 4 inches (ultra plush). Therapists who use deep-pressure techniques often like firmer padding as the client will not sink into the table pad as pressure is being applied. In this instance, a firmer padding prevents loss of therapist's energy when downward pressure is applied. Thick padding is best for client comfort and for therapists who apply techniques under the client's body.

Durability. In general, table pads on high-quality tables will 10 years or more. Foam padding has a cellular structure that breaks down over time. However, some of the newer foams, such as AeroCel and UltraCell, are highly resilient and maintain their loftiness for the entire life of your table. Also,

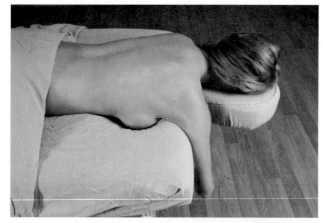

FIGURE 3-2 Table pad for breast comfort.

switch the end you use for the client's head on a regular basis to help extend the life of your table pad. An easy way to do this is to switch the end you use for the face rest, or rotate the table 180° monthly.

Some tables also have a recess for breast comfort (Figure 3-2). These special table pads may or may not have a method of changing the depth of the recess.

Table Fabric

Table fabric is the skin or covering of your table and accessories. Lower-quality tables are covered with vinyl and higher quality tables are covered with polyurethane fabrics (which do not contain polyvinyl chlorides [PVCs]). Both fabrics are long lasting and easy to clean. But like skin, these fabrics can be injured. For example, it can be punctured by keys, hairpins, jewelry, and pet (cat) claws.

Vinyl and polyurethane fabrics are smooth and linens may slip on their slick surfaces. This can be remedied by placing a fitted table pad, a fitted sheet, or a flat sheet (with corners tied in knots) on the table before dressing the table with massage linens.

▌MINI-LAB

If you are fortunate enough to have table models from different companies displayed at your school, try these tests before you finalize your purchase.

1. *One-knee test.* While kneeling down on the table, place your weight on one knee. If you feel the bottom, your client might too.
2. *The bounce.* Sit upright on the table and gently bounce up and down. Notice if and how much the table flexes as you land. Your table should offer slight resistance as you bounce.
3. *Table rock.* As you sit on one end of the table, grasp the side of the table and rock it back and forth to check for lateral stability. If the table wobbles, it lacks integrity (or knobs need to be tightened). Also, listen for noises; the table should be quiet.
4. *Ready, set, go!* Fold the massage table, and close it securely. Holding it by the handles, lift the table and take about 10 steps. Unfold the table and set it up on its four legs, noticing the ease or difficulties you encounter.

TABLE FABRIC

Your table fabric is like the skin on your body. It looks great in the beginning and will show signs of age over time. There are a few things you can do to make it look better longer. Also important is how to disinfect your table fabric when it comes into direct contact with infectious agents.

Keep It Covered

Keeping your table covered at all times is the best way to ensure your fabric will last. When your table is unfolded and set up, use a mattress cover or a single fitted or tied flat sheet over it. While in transit, be sure to keep it in a carry case. Keeping table fabric unblemished without a carry case is nearly impossible when moved about—from the massage room to the car, to the client's home or office, back to the car, back to the massage room, and so on. Additionally, keep a stowed table enclosed in its carry case.

Keep It Cool

Table fabrics are similar to fine wine; they do not like wide temperature ranges. Extreme hot or cold (above 95°F or below 32°F) will damage your table and accessory fabric. Examples of damage are brittleness, cracking, and stretch marks. Do not stow your table in your car, near heaters, or in direct sunlight.

If your table has been exposed to extreme temperatures, allow it to return to room temperature before use. Weight placed on hot or cold table fabric may cause permanent damage.

Cleaning Table and Accessory Fabric

Most cleansers and detergents are too strong and when used full strength rather than diluted, will damage your table and accessory fabric. Recommended products include a 4:1 diluted solution of green Windex, 409, Fantastik, or any nonabrasive, nonalcohol-based cleanser. Some therapists use vinegar as a natural cleanser. Citrus oil–based cleaners should be avoided because they will degrade most polyurethane fabrics.

Chlorine bleach is often used when disinfecting, but avoid these agents for general cleaning such as when removing oil smudges and fingerprints from fabrics.

Disinfecting Table and Accessory Fabric

Disinfection is needed when your table or accessory fabric comes into contact with unidentifiable substances or body fluids. To disinfect, wipe the surface with a 1:10 diluted solution of household bleach. Be sure to wear disposable gloves. Disinfect only when needed because overuse of these substances can erode fabrics' protective topcoat, which is designed to keep it soft, supple, and resilient.

Suggestions for cleaning and disinfecting should be regarded as general guidelines. Contact the company that manufacturers your table and ask for their approved product list.

"One day, someone showed me a glass of water that was half full. And he said, 'Is it half full or half empty?' So I drank the water. No more problem."
—Alejandro Jodorowsky

TABLE ACCESSORIES

Accessories add comfort to your clients and help to protect and transport your table. Examples of accessories are face rest, arm self, and bolsters. Included in this section are stools, carry cases, table carts.

Face Rest

A face rest, or face cradle, allows clients to keep their heads and necks relatively straight while lying prone (face down). See Figure 3-3, *B* for position of a face rest while a client is

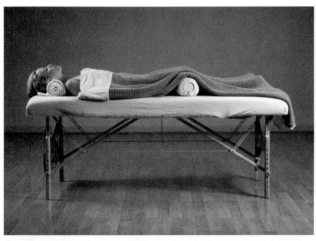

A

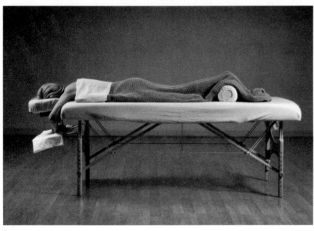

B

FIGURE 3-3 Bolsters placed in the supine **(A)** and prone **(B)** positions. Note the use of a face rest and arm shelf in (B).

prone. A face rest consists of two parts: a crescent-shaped cushion and a frame. The cushion is generally attached to the frame by loop-and-pile fasteners, which enable the cushion to be widened or narrowed (accommodating a range of facial structures) or even removed.

Facial comfort of your clients is important while they are prone. Face rest cushions can be filled with foam padding or even contain water balls. If possible, lay on a few types to test for comfort before you make your final selection.

The frame is attached to the table through support rods that insert into grommets at either one end or both ends of the table. Occasionally, switch the face rest from one end of the table to the other to reduce uneven wear on the table pad.

The face rest, which is usually the same fabric as the table, adds approximately 10 to 12 inches to the table's length when inserted into the table.

Standard face rests allow the head and neck to be in one position—parallel to the tabletop. Adjustable frames allow the neck to be flexed for client comfort and easy access of the posterior head and neck for the therapist. Adjustable frames can be folded down when not in use.

Some adjustable face rests frames can be locked into a U shape, allowing clients to lie prone on the floor with comfortable breathing space. This may be needed when performing massage in a regular chair or on the floor.

CHAT ROOM

Your preference of face rest frame may be the determining factor in your decision on which table to purchase. Face rest frames are *not* universal, and will fit only tables made by the same company. If you are unhappy with your face rest, you will likely be unhappy with your entire table.

While we are on the subject … about once a week, remove the cushion from your face rest frame, reshape it with a few firm squeezes and place it back on the frame. Over time and usage, the cushion will migrate laterally and needs periodic reshaping.

Arm Shelf

The arm shelf, providing a place for arms to rest while a client is in the prone position, is a small platform suspended below the face rest. See Figure 3-3, *B* for arm shelf position while the client is prone. Arm shelves that attach to the table frame are more stable than those suspended from the face rest by fabric straps. However, because the former is attached to the table frame, these arm shelves are usable at only one end of the table.

It should be noted that your arm shelf and perhaps your face rest may break if your client pushes down on them with his or her hands while lifting up and turning over. The prevent this mishap, instruct your clients to scoot down on the table first before instructing them to turn over.

Bolsters and Cushions

Bolsters and cushions enhance client comfort and relaxation by providing support for the neck, knees, and ankles (Figure 3-3). A bolster placed behind the knees while supine often reduces lower back strain by decreasing a lordotic curve. Bolsters placed in front of the ankles while your client is prone helps to relieve hip, knee, and foot strain. These cushions come in a variety of sizes and shapes—tubular, square, rectangular, wedged, and wavy—and can be made of foam or stuffed with feathers or grains such as buckwheat or flaxseed.

Be sure to use a protective drape over the bolster and launder the drape after each use.

Some therapists slide the bolster under the bottom sheet instead of using a separate protective drape. This process is more difficult if the bottom sheet is fitted rather than flat.

A soft, tubular pillow or rolled up towel is used behind the neck while your client is supine (see Figure 3-3, *A*). Neck muscles and joints will relax more easily if they can rest against a cushion.

The most popular knee and ankle bolster height is 6 inches, but 3 and 8 inch heights are also available. Flat-bottomed bolsters stay in place better than full round bolsters.

In addition to the aforementioned bolsters, keep four to six standard-size bed pillows and pillowcases on hand for client support while in a side-lying position.

Many table manufacturers offer advanced positioning systems for side lying and prone positioning. These often provide increased client comfort and stability and better ergonomics (or comfort and safety) for the therapist.

Stool

My favorite table accessory, a stool, allows you to sit comfortably when performing head, neck, hand, foot massage (Figure 3-4), or even back and shoulder massage while your client is supine. Ideally, your stool will have a height adjustment feature, ranging from hydraulics to manual rotation.

A stool is a multitask item; you can use it as an arm shelf for your clients (be sure to cover the stool with a drape) or as a storage table on wheels (put your massage lubricant on the seat and push it with your foot where you need the stool to go).

Some therapists use a large inflatable physioball as a stool. Saddle stools are also available, which may help you to sit in a more ergonomically correct position.

Carrying Case

A carrying case protects table fabric from damage while being transported; it also has padded handles and straps, making the table easier to lift and carry. Most cases have several deep zippered pockets for storing items.

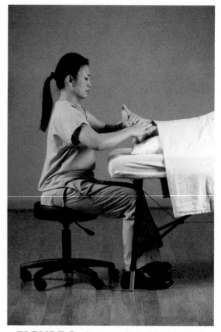

FIGURE 3-4 Therapist using a stool.

Table Carts

If you move your table often, a cart can save your back and shoulders from aches and injury and help conserve your energy. Carts allow your table to be easily rolled instead of lifted and carried. Be sure that your table can be lifted with the cart attached as steps are typically encountered while transporting your table.

Most carts can be attached to a folded table by an adjustable quick-clip strap. Once the cart is attached, the table can be easily pushed or pulled.

---

evolve *Log on to the Evolve website and, after accessing your student account, view additional images of equipment used by therapists in Chapter 3 Additional Resources.* ∎

▌MINI-LAB

Obtain a 3-inch bolster, a 6-inch bolster, and an 8-inch bolster. Lie in the supine position and place the 3-inch bolster behind your knees for 1 minute. Next, place the 6-inch bolster behind your knees for 1 minute. Then, place the 8-inch bolster behind your knees for 1 minute. On a sheet of paper, note the differences you feel in your back, hips, knees, ankles, and feet. Repeat the procedure, but this time lie in the prone position and place the bolsters under your ankles for 1 minute. Again, noting the differences in specific body joints, jot down your findings on a sheet of paper. This exercise will help you understand why bolsters are used in massage practice.

MASSAGE LINENS

Sheets

Massage linens include a top and bottom sheet for the table, bolster covers, face rest covers, and pillowcases (any cloth that touches your client). Popular fabrics are flannel, cotton, cotton blends, and percale. Many therapists purchase twin sheet sets, which include fitted and flat sheets and a standard pillowcase (the pillow case can serve as a cover for your bolster or the face rest). Some therapists prefer the use of two twin flat sheets because these offer greater versatility for draping and bolstering. A flat sheet as the table drape can be pulled up over the client for quick warming or for secure draping in side-lying positions. Also, bolsters can be easily inserted and removed beneath a flat sheet when used as the table drape.

White, off-white, or soft pastels sheet colors wash and wear better than darker sheet colors; the latter shows stains more easily.

Be cognizant of the weight and thickness of the sheets. Many less expensive fabrics such as cotton-polyester blends are thin and transparent (which means you can see through them). And less expensive fabrics typically do not hold up well with repeated washings.

Towels

Some therapists use bath-size towels or bath sheets to drape their clients. They are thicker and heavier than sheets and provide easy access to the abdomen on women when a towel is used over the breasts. Other reasons therapists use towels are easy maneuverability over sheets.

Blankets and Table Warmers

As the body relaxes, blood pressure lowers, circulation returns to the core, and basal body temperature decreases. Because of this, clients may become chilled. A chilled client will not relax easily.

Blankets and table warmers help ensure that your client will stay warm while he or she relaxes. Table warmers are placed on the table beneath all other coverings. Turn the table warmer on before your client arrives, starting at a low setting. After a few minutes, inquire about client comfort and make setting adjustments as needed.

You can also use a woven cotton or woolen blanket for added warmth. Like the table warmer, use a blanket at the start of the session, before the client relaxes and becomes chilled (See Figure 3-3, *A*). Along with warmth, the weight of the blanket adds comfort and a sense of security for the client. Because of this, heavier fabrics are preferred over lightweight fleece. Be sure your blankets are machine washable.

The blanket does not replace the top drape. Instead, place the blanket *over* the top drape. Be sure to fold the client drape over the blanket edge that is near the client's face.

MASSAGE LINEN CARE

All linens used during the massage must be laundered after use. Replace linens whenever they become stained, odorous, or threadbare. Remember that even clean linens that are stained or smell rancid appear unclean to clients.

If Linens Become Contaminated

Linens that have come into contact with a contaminant must be disinfected. Examples of how this occurs include a client sneezing onto your face rest, a scab from a fresh wound rubs across the sheet and leaks blood, or if a nursing mother leaks breast milk.

If your massage linens become contaminated, follow these steps.

1. Wash and dry your hands.
2. Remove linens with gloved hands.
3. Wash linens in hot water; use laundry detergent and ¼ cup of household bleach. Dry linens using hot air.
4. After donning a new pair of disposable gloves, clean the table and accessory fabric with soap and water, and then disinfect it with a 1:10 solution of household bleach and paper towels.
5. Discard the gloves and paper towels.
6. Finally, rewash and dry your hands.

TYPES OF LUBRICANTS

Types of lubricant are creams, butters, oils, gels, and lotions (Figure 3-5). Some massage methods use powders such as cornstarch. Additionally, liniments may be used to enhance the therapeutic effect of massage.

The primary purpose of a massage lubricant is to reduce friction between your hands (forearms and elbows) and the client's skin.

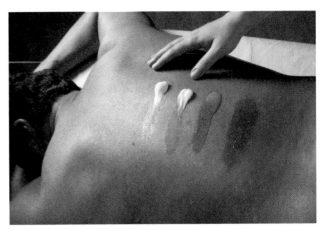

FIGURE 3-5 Lubricant choices. From left to right: butter, cream, gel, and oil.

This section will discuss types of lubricants, pros and cons of each choice, safe dispensing and other application considerations, and its storage for best shelf life.

Cream

Massage cream is currently the best-selling massage lubricant and has been so since the early 1990s. Creams are moisturizing and hydrating, and are more emollient than other lubricants. Because of this, creams have a staying power almost equal to that of massage oils and gels.

Because creams are thick, they are less likely to spill out of their container (think about the mess when you drop a container of oil). Cream is also less likely to stain your (and your client's) clothing and massage linens.

Butter

Butters, which are made from fruit, nuts, or seeds, are thicker than creams. Like creams, butters are hydrating and moisturizing and have an excellent rapport with the skin.

The three most common butters are cocoa, jojoba, and Shea. *Cocoa butter*, also known as theobroma oil, is obtained from cacao seed and is commonly found in stick form. African *Shea butter* is extracted from the tree's fruit (called nuts). *Jojoba* is a liquid wax and is taken from the desert shrub's seeds; it is chemically similar to the skin's oil (called sebum). Butters take a little time to get used to; body temperature will cause them to melt, so use sparingly.

Oil and Gel

Oils and gels are excellent value. Because of their superior quality, nut and seed oils are preferred. Because clients may have allergies to nuts and seeds, you should have a hypoallergenic alternative. Sesame, grape, and hemp seed oils are well tolerated.

Additives such as vitamin E are often used. Vitamin E, an antioxidant, also acts as a preservative, which is important because of oil's quick rancidity.

Gels have a relatively longer shelf life and do not contain alcohol or mineral oil, so they are excellent for sensitive skin types. But avoid using oils and gels on clients who have oily skin.

One drawback of oil or gel is the accidental (and inevitable) spill that spells disaster on walls or flooring.

Clothing does not fare well after an oil encounter. If you use oil or gel, suggest that your client bring a change of old clothes to wear after the session.

Some massage oil manufacturers sell a product to be added to the wash to help remove the appearance and smell of oil from linens. These products have mixed reviews (some therapists say they work and others say they do not work).

Some therapists mix their oil or gel with lotion in a 50/50 solution.

Lotion

Lotions do not have the staying power of oils, gels, or creams and are quickly absorbed in the skin.

Most companies formulate lotions to be used in two different settings: rehabilitation and spa.

Therapists who specialize in rehabilitative methods and treat specific injuries and conditions prefer a *deep-tissue lotion* because it offers the least amount of glide and the most control. Lotions are tackier than other lubricants because they absorb quickly. This quality creates a slight drag on the skin.

Hydrating lotions are preferred by therapists who work in spa settings and are used as the final or finishing treatment in a three-step spa procedure (i.e., exfoliation, mineralization, and hydration).

Powder

Powder or cornstarch is used when doing lymphatic massage and massage during a pregnant woman's labor. It affords limited friction reduction but does not leave a greasy residue. Powdered lubricants do not work well on areas with a lot of body hair.

Be careful when applying powder because particles can enter nasal passages and cause the client or therapist to sneeze or cough.

Liniment

Not really a lubricant, liniments are used as analgesics (agents that reduce pain) and to create the sensation of heat (and sometimes cold). All liniments are *rubefacient*, which means they redden the skin because the ingredients cause irritation. As reddening occurs, the skin's vessels dilate and claim to increase local blood supply.

Avoid using liniments on a client's hands and feet, near mucous membranes, or before heat or cold applications.

CHOOSING A LUBRICANT

Several factors must be considered when choosing a lubricant. These include its ingredients, possible skin reactions, its effect on your massage linens, and its cost.

Ingredients

Ingredients such as cold-pressed vegetable, nut, and seed oils and plant essences are good for the skin, whereas ingredients such as mineral oil and isopropyl alcohol can clog pores and deplete skin nutrients.

There has been a growing concern about the use of parabens in massage products. These products are widely used, but may mimic the hormone estrogen, which is known to play a role in the development of breast cancers. In response to the growing concern, most massage product manufacturers are removing them from their product lines.

Stearyl and cetyl alcohols are also found in many massage products. These products are used as emulsifiers and stiffening agent and although do not nourish the skin, are found safe. Also, keep in mind that whichever product you choose, your hands and thus your skin will be in continual contact with it and your lubricant should be as high a quality as you can afford.

Skin Reaction

Your client may have a negative skin reaction to the lubricant. This is more common in fair-complexioned individuals.

During the initial massage consultation, inquire about allergies to nuts or other products that are ingredients in massage lubricants. Keep a copy of all ingredient lists on hand, and allow the client to read the ingredient list for prior approval.

Because lubricant sensitivity cannot always be predetermined, keep a hypoallergenic lubricant handy to use when the need arises.

CHAT ROOM

If a product is hypoallergenic, it underwent lengthy testing and the majority of the subjects in the study were unaffected. It does not mean that the product will not cause allergic reactions; it's just less likely than with nonhypoallergenic products. Many massage lubricants contain nut oils, such as peanut and almond. Avoid these products if your client is allergic to these or any other ingredient in the product. A common-sense measure is to ask your client to review a list of lubricant ingredients before applying it to the skin. Because lubricant sensitivity cannot always be predetermined, keep a hypoallergenic lubricant on hand to use when the need arises.

Scented lubricants increase the likelihood of allergic reactions.

Scented Versus Unscented

Massage lubricants are available as scented or unscented. Unscented lubricants can be scented with the addition of essential oils (discussed in Chapter 12). Custom scents can be created by combining more than one essential oil.

Before using a scented lubricant, place a small amount on the back of your client's hand and allow him or her to smell it. Once approved, proceed with the massage.

If not approved, select another scent or suggest unscented.

CHAT ROOM

I use scented massage creams. I have a spring/summer scent (lavender and tangerine) and an autumn/winter scent (lavender and sandalwood). But I always keep an unscented, hypoallergenic cream on hand, just in case.

Linen Reaction

Lubricants with high oil content are more likely to stain linens. These linens also emit an unpleasant, rancid odor over time. Be sure to replace oil-stained or rancid-smelling linens with new ones.

Cost

Cost will depend on your preference and your pocketbook. Quality costs. If you subscribe to a business philosophy of *only the best for your clients,* then you are likely to invest in a more expensive lubricant. Typically, the most expensive lubricants are butters and creams—with oils and gels the least expensive. However, therapists who use oils and gels tend to replace their linens more frequently.

DISPENSING LUBRICANT

Dispensing massage lubricant from an open container contaminates the lubricant if the same container is used for multiple clients. To prevent cross-contamination, use either a single-use container or a pump/flip-top dispenser. Refillable tubes that must be squeezed to dispense the product may also be used.

The dispenser can be placed on the massage table between the client's knees for easy access and to prevent it from being accidentally knocked off the table during massage.

Lubricant containers become contaminated with each use and must be washed between clients.

Holsters that suspend dispensers from straps are available; they allow dispensers to be worn round the therapist's waist or hips. Keep in mind that these too become contaminated with each use and must be washed between clients.

How Much Lubricant

When applying lubricant on the client's skin, place the proper amount in your hands, warming it by rubbing the fingers and palms together. Avoid applying lubricant directly on the client's skin. Apply lubricant only on the area you will be massaging, never on adjacent areas.

If too much lubricant is accidentally used, wipe off the excess.

The amount of lubricant you use will depend on:

Emolliency. The more emollient the lubricant is, the less lubricant and reapplications are needed. Creams, butters, oils, and gels are more emollient than lotions.

Skin Dryness. Dry skin requires more lubricant and reapplication than nondry skin.

Body Hair. Areas with a plethora of body hair require more lubricant and reapplication than skin without hair. Additionally, when working in hairy areas of the body, use linear rather than circular movements because they are less likely to mat and tangle hair.

Intention. In relaxation and wellness massage, the therapist primarily uses gliding strokes, and a reasonable amount of lubricant is needed. Specific massage, such as that used in sports and rehabilitation, requires the therapist to grasp and manipulate superficial layers of skin and fascia. Only a small amount of lubricant is needed and thinner, more tacky lubricants are preferred.

In general, excessive amounts of lubricant will reduce tissue manipulation, and inadequate amounts increase friction and will pull and irritate the skin. Experience will teach you how much to use in which circumstance. Less is better; adding more lubricant is easier than removing it.

Lubricant Storage and Shelf Life

Once purchased, store all massage lubricants (with the exception of powder) in a cool, dark location out of direct sunlight. In these conditions, lubricants can last up to 18 months.

The product's shelf life can be extended up to an additional year with refrigeration or freezing; allow them to return to room temperature before use.

SUPPLIES

Supplies are items such as paper towels and drinking cups that are bought and used often. They are needed to provide the massage and assist with a clean, sanitary, and comfortable massage environment. Some massage supplies are used for the massage itself; others are convenient personal care items such as hair spray, contact lens solution, and cotton balls.

Use the checklist provided on the *Evolve* website when shopping for supplies. Blank lines have been added to the checklist for additional items you wish to include in your massage office. Bottled water may be supplied either for personal use or for client use.

©volve *Log on to the Evolve website and access your student account. Print out the Massage Supply Checklist under Chapter 3 Additional Resources and use it when stocking your massage room with supplies.* ■

"It isn't what you know when you start, but what you learn when you get out there."
—Carol Kresge

FURNISHINGS

The furnishings for the massage room require brief mention. These items help create the proper atmosphere where the massage takes place. These items include a mirror, clock, wastebasket, supply cabinet, chair, a place for your client's clothes and personal items, and wall decor. Window treatments, light sources, and floor and wall treatment also deserve discussion. The massage room is an important element of the massage experience. It says a little about you and a little about how you feel about your work.

Mirror

A mirror is essential for massage rooms. Clients use mirrors to groom themselves after a massage. Therapists use full-length mirrors to aid in posture assessment. Mirrors also reflect light or room objects and can be used to make a space appear larger.

Clocks

Wall or desk clocks help to keep you on a schedule, and they help regulate timed treatments such as ice packs or body masques. The clock should be quiet and visible to you rather than your client, for whom it may be a distraction.

Wastebasket

A wastebasket is needed in the massage room for used paper towels, facial tissue, gloves, and other disposable items. Most state laws require the wastebasket to close with a lid. Lidded wastebaskets with foot pedals are preferred to those with lids that need to be lifted by hand for sanitation reasons.

Supply Cabinet

A supply cabinet is needed to stow massage linens, supplies, and lubricant. Hinged doors are preferred to open shelving if items need to be out of sight. Cabinets or closets fitted with louvered doors allow stowed items access to open air and allow music from hidden speakers to move through slats. Be sure that shelf tops are covered with an easy-to-clean material such as laminate (e.g., Formica).

Chairs

A chair provides a place for the client to sit while removing and putting on trousers, stockings, shoes, and socks. Depending on available space and personal taste, choose a simple straight-back chair, a plush and oversized chair, a chaise lounge, or ottoman. If you have a rolling stool for your own use, be sure to point out the chair for client use to avoid liability issues.

Place for Personal Items

Clients will need a place to put their personal items, such as removed garments, eyeglasses, jewelry, and cell phones. A place can be provided for these items such as wall hooks, a coat tree, a freestanding locker, or a valet.

If your client leaves the area where their personal items are stowed, be sure they are secured with only the client having access to the key. Or provide a small dish or basket for smaller items such as keys, pocket change, wallet, eyeglasses, wristwatches, and jewelry. In this way, clients can easily take their personal property with them if they move from one location to another.

MASSAGE ROOM ENVIRONMENT

Before you design and furnish your massage room, think about the image you want to project. Who you are and how you perceive your work will play a role in how your massage room looks and feels. If sports and rehabilitative massage is your forte, your room may look clinical, filled with anatomical charts, medical reference books, and white massage linens. It may also contain a single free-standing locker for clients' garments. A sports massage therapist is more likely to own a portable massage table to be used when his or her services are needed at sports events.

A massage therapist who focuses on relaxation and wellness may have a softer warmer environment. There may be soft, indirect lighting. The walls may be painted in earth colors and soothing music playing. A hint of lavender might be detected in the air.

The atmosphere of your massage room sets the tone for your client's experience. Ideally, you want a space that is quiet, private, serene, and easy to heat or cool. The room should be free of pet dander, as well as tobacco and cleaning solution odors. Supplies such as bolsters, blankets, lubricants, and pillows should be within your reach during the session but not where they can create an obstacle for the client. Convenient access to a toilet is desirable.

Remind your clients to turn off their cell phones (unless the client insists). Be sure to turn off your own cell phone. If there are other therapists in adjacent rooms, ask them to do the same to provide a relaxing environment for everyone.

A dinner party metaphor is often used to explain the importance of atmosphere. When planning, preparing, and serving a meal for a special guest, adjustments are made to make the dining experience extraordinary. The table is set using clean, attractive linens. The host pulls out the fine china and crystal and polishes the silverware. A special flower arrangement is placed in the room. Soft music plays in the background, and the lights are dimmed. Give clients the same care and consideration by treating them as honored guests.

The importance of ambiance cannot be overstated. The Chinese symbol for space is the Japanese symbol for gates. Open the gates to relaxation and healing by creating a space where these can occur. The atmosphere should begin when the client drives up to the office and should be maintained all the way to the massage room. Atmospheric considerations include lighting, music, temperature, and room color. Examples are listed here to stimulate your imagination and to help with goal setting.

CHAT ROOM

When receiving massage from other therapists, be aware of *everything*. This includes the therapist's appearance, his or her punctuality, the office ambience, the massage table, the room layout—not just the massage itself. So many things play a part in the massage experience.

Light

Lighting serves several purposes and requires differing amounts. First, enough lighting must be provided so clients can fill out paperwork, remove garments, safely maneuver around the room, get on and off the massage table, dress, and exit the office. Adequate lighting is needed for you to assess the skin's condition before and during the massage, but subdued lighting is needed during the massage to assist in client relaxation.

Natural light, or sunlight, is often the best light source. Room light from a window is easily adjusted. Window glass can also be tinted.

During overcast days or after dusk, indirect lighting can be used. Indirect indicates that the light source is obscured from view by shades or baffles. This effect can be achieved with floor or table lamps, recessed ceiling lights in the room's corners, or a string of lights placed strategically in the room. To illuminate a dark area, use a nightlight behind a large object such as an oversized vase.

Many therapists enjoy candlelight in their massage rooms. Although candles are unbeatable for creating a relaxing ambiance, they are also a fire hazard. Regardless of how careful you are, candle wax spills, and soot deposits occur on shelves and walls. Most insurance available to massage therapists does not cover the use of fire for candles, incense, or ear candling. Be sure to check your specific terms of coverage. If you like candle light, consider flameless candles.

Music

Music hath charms to soothe a savage breast (William Congreve, c. 1697), and although clients are not savages, they do respond to music. Music is art for the ears. Music for massage helps clients relax (if the music is soft and slow), and will help you maintain a soothing rhythm when applying massage movements.

STEVEN HALPERN, PhD

Born: April 18, 1947

"Composing music to support relaxation and healing during massage is different than composing music merely for entertainment."

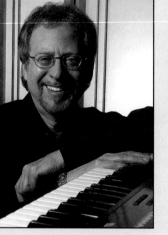

As the true pioneer in the field of relaxation music, Steven Halpern is far from being simply a gifted musician. His eternal thirst for knowledge has benefited the field of massage therapy, and any therapist who has used any of his music can attest to this undeniable fact. His extensive research has taken music to a scientific level and beyond.

After an early career in jazz/rock and old school R&B, Halpern began composing a new kind of soothing, relaxing music. His Inner Peace series of recordings create sacred space by invoking an aura of timelessness and peace. His music evokes the innate 'relaxation response.' It's based on the rhythm of a deep breath, and supports greater rapport between client and therapist.

During college in the late 1960s, Halpern's curiosity about music led to his revolutionary research on the effects of certain rhythms on the human body. At the time, it was practically a virgin field. Few schools would allow such research, but fortunately Halpern was introduced to the University of California at Sonoma, where he had access to biofeedback equipment and conducted investigations on the effects of music using subtle rhythms, gentle tones, and nontraditional harmonics. The result has been the hallmark of his approach to composition. "One of the most fundamental responses of the human organism is that it is easily rhythm entrained to an external rhythmic stimulus," he says. "In other words, if there is a steady beat, your heart and pulse will naturally synchronize to that rhythm." As he says, "Trying to relax to music with a fast beat is like drinking three cups of coffee and trying to relax. The 'audio caffeine' makes it virtually impossible."

This theory instantly made Halpern's music popular with massage therapists and clients. After hearing this new type of music, people actually hired him to play live as they were receiving massages. Many massage professionals claimed that as a result of listening to his music, clients were actually relaxing before a hand was even placed on them. Thus therapists received much less resistance from clients, which, in turn, resulted in making therapists' work much easier.

Although music is important, Halpern reminds us not to forget about other forms of sound. Having a great deal of control over his or her environment, a therapist needs to be aware of the noises that are often taken for granted. Halpern says that he is amazed at how many therapists have a loud ticking clock or a noisy air conditioner. These factors should be addressed before music can even be considered. Many of us have conditioned ourselves to block out certain sounds. Halpern states, "Mother Nature gave us eyelids. She didn't give us earlids or body-lids." Whether we are consciously aware of it, a person's entire body is picking up and responding to all sounds.

Halpern notes that "listening to truly relaxing music can help choreograph a state of flow in which the massage therapist naturally tunes into the strokes that are most appropriate for that client. As both individuals resonate and entrain to the music, healing energy flows more freely, because that is the state I am in when I am recording. New research is confirming this fact; in the meanwhile, to receive the benefits, all you have to do is play the music during your session."

Halpern encourages massage professionals to add the healing power of music to their healing bodywork. His most popular recordings for massage are "Chakra Suite," "Ocean Suite," "Relaxation Suite," "Paradigm Shift," and "Music for Sound Healing."

Keep an assortment of music selections on hand. Some therapists allow clients to bring their own music selections to the session. Although music, as with room décor, is a matter of taste, most therapists prefer a slow, even melody. Most classical selections are not appropriate because of the ebb and flow of crescendos and decrescendos.

Be cautious of New Age music because many selections contain jumpy melodies. Some music stores include a music category called *minimalism,* which is suitable for massage. Nature sounds such as waves breaking on the shore, whale songs, and thunderstorms, combined with orchestral music, are good choices (as long as no surprising screeches or cackling birds are heard). However, trickling water sounds may stimulate the urge to void in some clients. Also, be sure and listen to the entire music selection before you play it during massage to ensure there are no surprises.

Wall Decor

Wall decor serves several purposes in a massage practice. They provide ambiance, educational reference, or instill a sense of professionalism.

When choosing wall decor for ambiance, consider color and content. Warm or soft colors such as peach and beige are calming and tranquil. Bright, intense colors such as red and yellow are stimulating. Nature scenes such as waterfalls, ocean waves, and open meadows provide a relaxing environment. Visual art is music for your eyes. Keep it simple; if it is too busy, it may distract from the massage experience. Make a brief statement, not an exclamation.

Anatomical and trigger point charts or meridian charts are often used as wall decor. These provide quick reference for locating relevant structures such as muscles, trigger points, and acupoints. Charts are also used for educating clients about anatomy, trigger points, and areas of referred pain. Charts also create a more clinical atmosphere. Many anatomical chart companies offer desktop flip charts that can be stored on a bookshelf and referred to as needed.

Framed diplomas, certificates, and awards portray professional accomplishment and success, instilling a sense of confidence in clients by demonstrating not only achievement, but your commitment to your profession. When applicable, include photos of yourself receiving awards or giving lectures.

Window Treatments

Window treatments include blinds, shades, and draperies and are available in a wide variety of styles and colors. Fabric-covered blinds are more attractive than the vinyl and aluminum versions, but they are more expensive. Window coverings serve many important functions such as for decoration, sound and light reduction, and for visual privacy. Drapes made from heavy fabrics will absorb sound better than blinds or sheers.

Window treatments can either block or filter light. I prefer light blocking material and use lamp light when more light is needed such as when performing a client intake or when the client is getting on or off the table.

Flooring

A nonslip surface such as carpet is the best choice for flooring in a massage room. As an insulator, carpet provides warmth and sound absorption. Carpeted floors create a measure of client safety; oily feet create a liability risk on smooth flooring. If the massage room happens to have smooth flooring, carpet or a carpet remnant can then be cut to fit the room. A throw rug creates a tripping or slipping hazard. Wiping lubricant off client's feet at the end of the session reduces stains on carpet and decreases the slip effect on the client's feet.

CHAT ROOM

Along with heavy draperies and carpet flooring, I have also used insulation to soundproof interior walls. My husband has also replaced all hollow-core doors with solid-core doors to help keep noise from seeping in while I am giving a massage.

"Where the spirit does not work with the hand, there is no art."
—Leonardo da Vinci

Temperature

A comfortable temperature for a massage room is approximately 72° to 75°F. A lot depends on your clients. For example, women who are pregnant or who are perimenopausal prefer a room temperature that is cooler.

If your room is too cool, your client may find it difficult to relax. This is because, as the massage progresses, your client's pulse rate, respiration rate, and blood pressure decrease as blood returns to the body's core. When this occurs, basal body temperature drops, and your client may then become chilled.

As a proactive measure, use a blanket or electric heating pad to keep your clients comfortably warm. See the prior section on blankets for more information.

However, you may be warm because you are expending energy. To keep cool, wear cotton clothing because these fabrics breathe (allow air to move through it). Additionally, a small oscillating fan placed on the floor and directed at your feet is helpful.

Color

Colors can be divided into two categories: warm and cool.

Warm colors, which include reds, browns, yellows, and oranges are cozy, but can be overly stimulating if a bright shade is used.

Cool colors, such as blues, violets, and greens, are soothing but can make a room feel too cool, depending of the shade of the color. Hence, a brown can be dark and dreary or light and airy. White is the absence of color, and black is the combination of all colors.

Ⓔvolve *After logging on to your Evolve student account, download and print out the massage room layouts for a massage practice located in Chapter 3 Additional Resources. Using a new sheet of drawing paper, design your ideal massage room.* ∎

MINI-LAB

Choose an annual date (such as New Year's Day or the anniversary of your massage school graduation) and reevaluate your massage room. This means not only looking for things that need to be repaired or replaced, but also things that need tweaking. For example, get a massage in your own massage room. While lying on your table, notice what you see, hear, and smell. Make changes if needed. Be sure to "accentuate the positive and minimize the negative."

SAFETY GUIDELINES

This chapter would not be complete without a discussion on safety considerations of your massage equipment and facility. The following is a list of suggestions for providing a treatment facility that is safe and accessible for all clients.

- Comply with all state and municipal building fire and safety codes.
- Establish and maintain current liability insurance coverage. The original or copy of this policy must be kept on the premises at all times and made available for inspection.
- Maintain an operative fire extinguisher and heat or smoke detectors on the premises. Fire extinguishers must be located at eye level, near an exit route, and in clear view (ratings specified by the city ordinance).
- Have a fire escape route posted in the office and clearly mark all building exits.
- Provide safe and unobstructed human passage in the public areas. Safe passage includes level flooring. Omit area rugs because they can be a slipping or tripping hazard.
- Choose only nonslip flooring.
- Bathrooms should be accessible to individuals with disabilities and should include a wheelchair-height lavatory with lever-style faucets. Grab bars should be located near the toilet for transferring to and from the toilet seat.

- Use lever-style door handles.
- Have a designated handicapped-accessible parking space. Slopes, not steps, are needed between the parking space and the building. The space should be marked with the international symbol for accessibility. Exterior ramps should be designed so that they drain well and do not hold water.
- Public telephones should have an adjustable volume control.
- The street address should be outside the building in clear view, which will make locating your business easier for emergency assistance (see Chapter 9).
- Maintain all equipment used to perform massage services in safe condition, which includes checking and tightening your massage table hinges, knobs, and locks before each business day.

E-RESOURCES

Ⓔvolve
http://evolve.elsevier.com/Salvo/MassageTherapy
- Chapter challenge
- Flash cards
- Photo gallery
- Downloadable forms
- Weblinks

BIBLIOGRAPHY

Beck MF: *Theory and practice of therapeutic massage*, ed 4, Albany, NY, 2005, Thomson Delmar Learning.

Foster MA: *Somatic patterning: how to improve posture and movement and ease pain*, Longmont, Colo, 2004, Educational Movement Systems Press.

Fritz S: *Mosby's fundamentals of therapeutic massage*, ed 4, St Louis, 2009, Mosby.

Fritz S: *Mosby's essential sciences for therapeutic massage*, ed 3, St Louis, 2009, Mosby.

Greene L: *Prevention tips*, Save Your Hands (website): http://www.saveyourhands.com. Accessed May 10, 2010.

Greene L: *Save your hands! The complete guide to injury prevention and ergonomics for manual therapists*, ed 2, Coconut Creek, Fla, 2008, Gilded Age Press.

Hollingshed J: Research and development manager, 2005, Oakworks, Inc.

Owen N: 2010, Biotone Professional Products.

Prudden B: *Pain erasure*, New York, 1980, M Evans.

Riach J: Chief Executive Officer, 2010, Oakworks, Inc.

Salvo SG: *Massage online for Mosby's pathology for massage therapists*, ed 2, St Louis, 2010, Mosby.

Schaff J: Massage Market Director, 2005, Oakworks, Inc.

Severn L: Account Executives, 2010, Oakworks, Inc.

Stillerman E: *Prenatal massage: a textbook of pregnancy, labor, and postpartum bodywork*, St Louis, 2008, Mosby.

MATCHING I

Place the letter of the answer next to the term or phrase that best describes it.

A. 18 months
B. 10 years
C. Cross-contamination
D. Crème
E. Household bleach
F. Hypoallergenic
G. Isopropyl alcohol
H. Jojoba
I. Foam memory
J. Mineral oil
K. Reduce friction
L. Vitamin E

_____ 1. Used in a 1 : 10 diluted solution to disinfect table or accessory fabric if it becomes contaminated

_____ 2. Lubricant that is a liquid wax

_____ 3. Lubricant or lubricant ingredient avoided because it is carcinogenic

_____ 4. The length of time massage lotions and creams can last if they are stored in a cool, dark place out of direct sunlight

_____ 5. The primary purpose of using massage lubricant

_____ 6. A type of product that is less likely to cause allergic reactions

_____ 7. What can happen if dispensing lubricant from an open container is then used for multiple clients

_____ 8. Ability of the massage table foam pad to return to its original height after being disturbed by pressure

_____ 9. Used in 1 : 7 diluted solution to disinfect table or accessory fabric if it becomes contaminated

_____ 10. Length of time table pads on high quality tables last

_____ 11. Added to massage oils as a preservative

_____ 12. The best-selling massage lubricant since the early 1990s.

MATCHING II

Place the letter of the answer next to the term or phrase that best describes it.

A. Behind the knees
B. Charts
C. Cool colors
D. Face rest
E. Loft
F. Non-slip surface
G. Polyurethane fabrics
H. Sheets, flat or fitted
I. Under the ankles
J. Vinyl fabrics
K. Warm colors
L. Window treatments

_____ 1. The most commonly used drape over the table top

_____ 2. Serve as decoration, sound and light reduction, and for visual privacy

_____ 3. Where to place a bolster while the client is supine to reduce lower back strain

_____ 4. What the flooring should be in a massage room

_____ 5. Cozy, but can be overly stimulating if a bright shade of these colors are used

_____ 6. Soothing but can make a room feel too cool, depending on the shade of colors

_____ 7. Often used as table fabric for lower quality tables

_____ 8. Allows clients to keep their heads and necks relatively straight while lying prone on a massage table

_____ 9. Where to place a bolster while the client is prone to help relieve hip, knee and foot strain

_____ 10. Used for quick reference for locating relevant body structures and for educating clients about anatomy, trigger points and areas of referred pain

_____ 11. Often used as a table fabric for higher quality tables

_____ 12. A term used to describe thickness of foam used as padding on massage tables

CASE STUDY

Lost Possessions

Tiffany owns and operates a massage therapy business, Southern Comfort, in her hometown. She has two associate therapists, Juanita and Suzanne, who work with her. One of the salon's most frequent clients, Rebecca, the wife of the town's mayor, scheduled a massage with Juanita at 10 AM. Rebecca was feeling happy, sad, and tired. For the last few months, she had been planning her only daughter's wedding. The wedding was this past weekend, and Rebecca was ready to unwind.

That afternoon, Rebecca telephoned to report that she left her wedding ring in the massage room. She described the ring to Tiffany as a very expensive platinum and diamond solitaire that was given to her by her husband on their 10-year wedding anniversary. After a brief conversation, a highly emotional Rebecca claimed that she does not remember putting it on her finger after the massage.

Tiffany searched the massage room and was unable to locate the ring. Rebecca came by and searched the massage room as well. She even emptied her purse onto the massage table; both Rebecca and Tiffany looked for the ring. Tiffany looked at the appointment book and noticed that both therapists used the massage room after Rebecca's massage. Tiffany told Rebecca that she would ask both Suzanne and Juanita if a ring was found in the massage room and that she would call Rebecca if it were found.

If you were Tiffany, how would you approach Suzanne and Juanita about the missing ring?

If Rebecca sounded accusatory, how should Tiffany deal with the situation professionally?

If you were Rebecca, how would you react to Tiffany's current plan of action?

CRITICAL THINKING

Why is the atmosphere of the massage studio so important to an effective practice? Are a massage therapist's skill and appearance enough?

CHAPTER 4

Self-Care: Health, Wellness, Nutrition, and Stress Reduction

"You cannot give what you do not have."
—Milton Trager

LEARNING OBJECTIVES

After completing this chapter, the student should be able to:

- State reasons why health and wellness are important elements when practicing massage therapy as a career.
- Contrast and compare the seven elements of wellness.
- List the current recommendations of physical activity (time allotment and frequency) and what types of activities your physical fitness program might include.
- Perform basic strengthening and stretching activities designed to help prepare the hands, arms, and shoulders of massage therapists.
- Define nutrition, diet, and essential nutrients.
- Contrast and compare macronutrients with micronutrients and list examples of each.
- Understand the importance of dietary fiber and list several sources.
- Design a personalized weekly dietary plan based on principles of proper nutrition.
- Discuss the importance of stress reduction for both yourself and your clients.
- List at least three stress reducing activities.

http://evolve.elsevier.com/Salvo/MassageTherapy

INTRODUCTION

The opening quote says it all. Because you cannot give what you do not have, a massage therapist should take good care of him or herself. This chapter discusses the multifaceted topic of self-care and includes proper nutrition, regular physical activity, and stress reduction. The concept of self-care is expanded to include a wellness model featuring emotional, intellectual, and spiritual realms. If you have an implemented successful program of health-promoting activities, great; let this chapter serve to affirm what you are already doing.

But for those of us who need a little guidance, let this chapter be the beginning of a life-long commitment to yourself, to your career, and to your community.

A prudent therapist subscribes to habits that promote health and wellness. These habits help to obtain and maintain stamina needed to perform multiple massages during the course of your workday. These habits also demonstrate your commitment to your profession and clientele by making the statement that he or she cares about one's own personal health.

As massage therapists, our bodies are considered the primary tool of our profession. Caring for our bodies is a form of insurance; practicing self-care is essential for your career longevity. As you will see in the next section, massage is a strenuous occupation. On Bonnie Prudden's occupational scale, it is on par with a professional athlete and dancer; two occupations that demand attention to health and wellness. Education is the first step and there are a multitude of resources available. Remember, you cannot give what you do not have. Managing your health is the best gift you can give yourself and your clients.

Many therapists work well into their fifth, sixth, or even their seventh decade of life. While the natural aging process will affect us, we can choose to age gracefully by remaining physically active, using stress management techniques, eating properly, and incorporating other principles of health and wellness into our lives.

MASSAGE CAN BE STRENUOUS

When you give a massage, you are expending energy—and lots of it. During class trades, students who are massaging often comment on how warm the room feels while their classmates on the table are chilly. During student clinics, if you are not in shape, you may feel like you have worked out in the gym. Massage is physically demanding on you, the therapist.

Bonnie Prudden, in her book, *Pain Erasure: The Bonnie Prudden Way* (1980), classifies occupations into five categories based on the degree of physical activity involved to perform required tasks. These categories are (1) *sitting,* (2) *standing,* (3) *walking,* (4) *active,* and (5) *strenuous* occupations (Box 4-1). Prudden lists massage therapist in the strenuous category because of the expenditure of physical energy

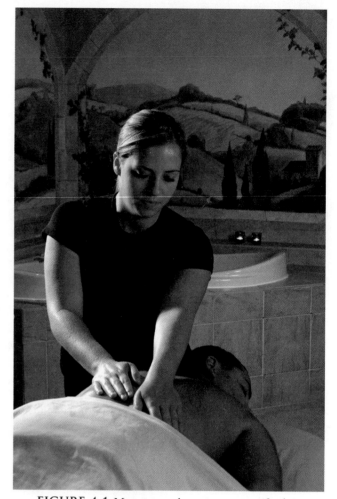

FIGURE 4-1 Massage can be a strenuous profession.

and the use of torque (twisting and turning motions that occur in the torso). She also states that strenuous occupations often result in back pain. Because of the physical nature of our work, prescribing to a plan of health and wellness can prepare and maintain your body and mind for your work (Figure 4-1).

The information in Box 4-1 can also be used when determining areas in your client's body prone to stress and strain. For example, if your client is an accountant (a sitting occupation), he or she will most likely have trigger points in the upper and lower back. Knowing your client's occupation will help you focus on actual or potential problem areas.

HEALTH AND WELLNESS

Health is a condition of physical, mental, emotional, and social well-being and the absence of disease. René Dubos, often quoted in nursing education, says, "The states of health or disease are the expressions of the success or failure experienced by the organism in its efforts to respond adaptively to environmental challenges." In other words, health is often

BOX 4-1

Occupations and Related Pain Hazards*

SITTING	STANDING	WALKING	ACTIVE	STRENUOUS
Accountant	Bank teller	Detective	Carpenter	Athlete
Administrator	Barber and beautician	Flight attendant	Carpet layer	Construction worker
Anesthetist	Bartender	Librarian	Electrician	Dancer
Architect	Butcher	Nurse	Farmer	Diver
Artist	Cafeteria server	Orderly	Fireman	Heavy equipment operator
Author	Clerk	Postal carrier	Forester	Linesman
Bookkeeper	Cook	Real estate agent	Maintenance person	Longshoreman
Bus, truck, and cab driver; chauffeur	Dental hygienist	Restaurant wait staff	Mason	Martial arts instructor
Computer programmer	Dentist	Security guard	Mechanic	Massage therapist
Crane operator	Electrologist		Painter	Miner
Dispatcher	File clerk		Photographer	Steel worker
Draftsman	Machinist		Plumber	
Editor	Physician		Police officer	
Educator	Sales clerk		Sailor	
Engineer	Surgeon		Ski instructor	
Executive	Teacher		Soldier	
Jeweler	Veterinarian		Sports coach	
Lawyer				
Pilot				
Psychiatrist				
Secretary				
Student				

Sitting

Sitting occupations often put trigger points in the chest, shoulders, and upper and lower back. Because the body is constantly bent, the groin may be involved. If excessive weight impairs circulation, then the legs and buttocks, which are constantly compressed against chairs, become involved.

Standing

Occupations requiring long hours of standing in one place contribute to the risk of low back pain. The upper back is also in danger, as are the arms, shoulders, and neck. Swelling may also occur in the feet and ankles.

Walking

Occupations requiring ordinary walking are not at risk. However, when the walking includes carrying (postal carrier or restaurant wait staff), the back is in danger.

Active

Active occupations all entail danger. For example, carpenters damage their elbows and experience tennis elbow, the plumber working with pipe threaders and large wrenches puts trigger points in the chest muscles, the mason strains the back, and the ski instructor damages the legs and lower back.

Strenuous

Strenuous occupations often result in back pain, and the injuries often involve torque, such as the ladder that gets away, the barrel that rolls the wrong way, or anything that pulls the torso with a twisting motion.

*Occupations classified by kind or degree of physical activity required.
Modified from Prudden B: *Pain erasure: the Bonnie Prudden way,* Lanham, MD, 1980, M. Evans & CO.–The Rowman & Littlefield Publishing Group.

a reflection of how well our bodies adapt to our environment. Good health helps our bodies adapt to change.

When attending massage school, your instructor will address the physical, mental, and emotional demands inherent in any service or health care profession. During student clinics, massage students are expected to use what they have learned in school as well as their critical thinking skills to address client goals and make safe practice decisions. However, student clients also give massage students the experience of the physical demands of working on several clients within a day. It can feel as if students are training for an athletic event.

Prepare for your career by making health a priority. A healthy body will give you the energy you need for your clients and will decrease the likelihood of injury because it is easier to maintain good body mechanics when core muscles are toned and strong. Being a health care provider can be mentally and emotionally draining. Plan for this consequence with stress reducing activities geared toward pleasure and fun.

Wellness is a more expansive concept of health and includes important dimensions that infuse our lives such as environmental and spiritual health. **Wellness** is an expression of health in which an individual is aware of, chooses, and practices healthy choices, creating a more successful and balanced life. It is important to take responsibility for your own health and wellness.

It is important for you to enjoy yourself while striving for wellness; the choices you make will reflect your own uniqueness. For example, you might benefit psychologically more from a brisk walk in the park alone (or with your dog) than an hour in the gym surrounded by people. Your wellness program should fit your personality.

"You can't turn back the clock, but you can wind it up again."
—Bonnie Prudden

Wellness Model

The University of Nebraska developed a seven-element wellness model that includes emotional, environmental, intellectual, occupational, physical, social, and spiritual dimensions. Let us examine briefly these elements. Figure 4-2 is based on that model.

Emotional. Involved with the awareness of and acceptance for our feelings and emotions and the feeling and emotions of others. Be sure to honor your emotions by expressing them appropriately. Perhaps keep a journal, talk with a

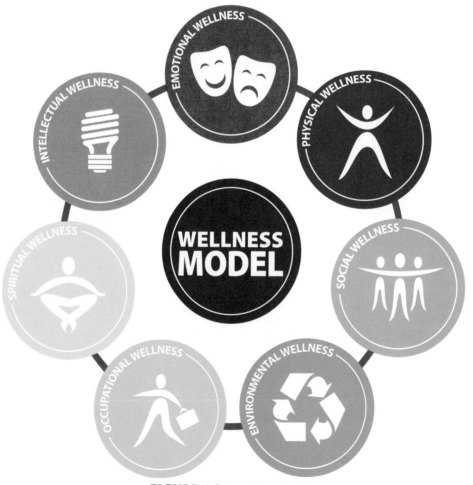

FIGURE 4-2 A wellness model.

counselor, or join a peer support group. Emotional health also encompasses relationships.

Environmental. Recognizing our interdependence with the environment and with nature. This includes activities such as recycling and conservation as well as spending time in state and national parks.

Intellectual. Embracing new ideas and developing ourselves through reading, surfing the Internet, attending lectures, traveling and learning about new places, and keeping current with information on healthy living. Go to art galleries, museums, worship services, and concerts. Read a book, write poetry, or see a foreign film. Talk about religion and politics with someone who has differing philosophies.

Occupational. Choosing a satisfying career and/or contributing to society through volunteer efforts. As massage therapist, this may also mean receiving regular massage sessions.

Social. Participating in social arena by establishing and maintaining personal friendships and getting involved in community events, such as celebrations and festivals. Laugh. Surround yourself with positive, happy people. Go to a comedy club. Tell stories with old friends. Watch a Monty Python or a Marx Brothers movie.

Spiritual. Experiencing a connection with a higher power and contemplative acts, such as meditation and prayer. This also encompasses pondering the meaning and purpose of human existence with or without religious affiliation.

Physical. Establishing and maintaining health through proper nutrition, regular physical activity, adequate sleep, and avoidance of harmful habits. Examples include limiting your intake of salt, sugar, caffeine, and alcohol and avoid all forms of tobacco use. Physical health also involves personal hygiene, and regular medical and dental examinations.

PHYSICAL WELLNESS

Therapists need physical strength, stamina, and endurance to perform the number of massages he or she is comfortable doing in a single day, and to be able to withstand the rigors of whatever amount of time the massage is. Then, therapists need enough energy for themselves, their family, and friends. This is best achieved through healthy habits that include physical activity, nutrition, and stress reduction. Let us look more closely at these elements.

Physical Activity

According to the American College of Sports Medicine and the American Heart Association, physical activity, or exercise, is called the *key to a healthier life*. Their current recommendations are *30 to 60 minutes of moderate physical*

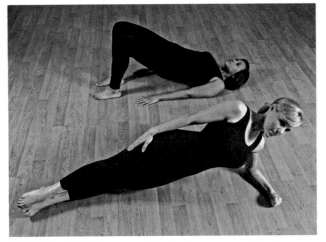

FIGURE 4-3 Women participating in core strengthening exercises.

activity daily. Examples of moderate physical activity are walking, biking, swimming, and gardening.

A physical fitness program often includes (1) cardio or endurance training, (2) stretching and balance poses, (3) core strengthening exercises (Figure 4-3), and (4) strength training.

Regular physical activity is important at any age. But as we age, it becomes even more important. Being physically active will reduce the risk of falls, a common cause of disability among seniors.

It is highly recommended that you consult your physician or other qualified health care provider before beginning any exercise program. He or she can determine what type of activity, the frequency, and intensity that is appropriate for you as some programs need to be catered to health issues.

Some benefits of regular physical activity include:

- Improves self-esteem and mood
- Weight management
- Increases bone density
- Manages blood pressure
- Boosts high-density lipoproteins (HDLs or good cholesterol)
- Increases energy
- Improves sleep
- Lowers your risk of heart disease, diabetes, gallstones, and some cancers
- Improves sex life

MINI-LAB

Evaluate your own personal fitness plan. See if any changes are in order. If you do not currently subscribe to a plan, design one for yourself and take appropriate steps to put it in action.

"The greatest discovery of my generation is that a human being can alter his life by altering his attitudes."
—William James

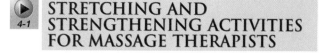

STRETCHING AND STRENGTHENING ACTIVITIES FOR MASSAGE THERAPISTS

The following exercises are designed to help you prepare your hands, arms, and shoulders for the physical exertion involved in massage therapy. Add additional movements as you see fit. Remember to breathe as you move.

Warm-up

Rub your palms and fingers together to generate friction and warmth; then rub vigorously the backs of your hands and arms. Shake your hands and fingers at the wrists, and then drop your hands to your sides and roll your shoulders forward for 10 repetitions (Figure 4-4, *A*). Reverse the

direction, and rotate your shoulders backward. This warm-up is effective for preparing the hands right before a massage or before other hand-developing exercises.

Finger Stretch

Touch your finger and thumb pads together as you keep your wrists apart. Next, spread your fingers apart. Press and release pressure while maintaining contact (Figure 4-4, *B*). Repeat the press-and-release sequence 20 times.

Hand Swishing

Press your palms and fingers together at chest level with fingertips pointing up to your chin. Rotate your elbows until fingers are pointing downward toward the toes and then

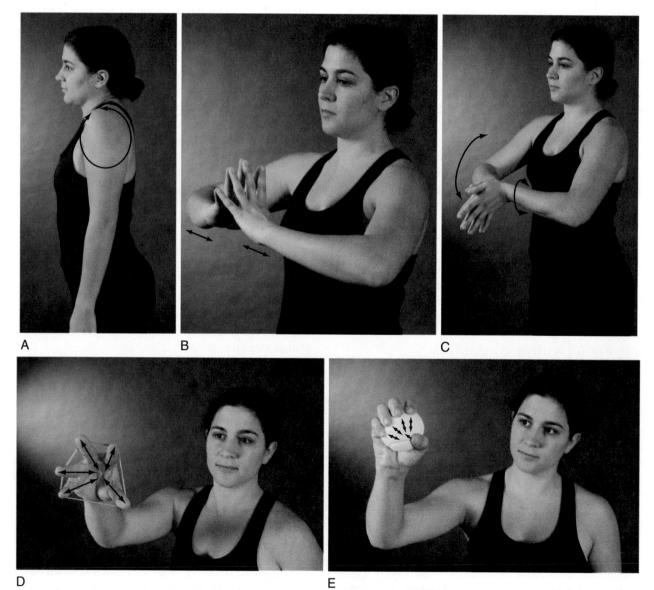

FIGURE 4-4 A, Therapist rolling shoulders. **B,** Finger stretch. **C,** Hand swishing. **D,** Rubber band stretch. **E,** Ball squeeze.

reverse back to the starting position. This motion should be playful, quick, and vigorous (Figure 4-4, *C*). NOTE: Shoulders remain fixed during the movement.

Wrist Circles

Begin with your arms at your sides. Flex your elbows 90 degrees, lifting your hands in front of you to chest level. With your fingers relaxed and extended, circle wrists in one direction for 10 revolutions, and then reverse the direction for 10 revolutions. Repeat wrist circles in both directions, but this time, close your hands into a fist. Perform 10 revolutions in both directions.

Rubber Band Stretch

Place a thick rubber band around the outside of the fingers at the level of the nail. Stretch the rubber band as you move the fingers apart (Figure 4-4, *D*). Repeat 10 times. Switch hands and repeat. If you find this exercise too much of a strain, use a thinner rubber band.

Ball Squeeze

Place a tennis ball or racquetball in the palm of your hand, and wrap your fingers around it. Squeeze the ball firmly for 5 seconds (Figure 4-4, *E*). Repeat 10 times. Switch hands and repeat.

Reach and Pull

Start with your open palms at your sides. Pull your hands up to chest, height, closing the palms into fists. Without stopping, continue the upward thrust of your hands over your head, extending your fingers out and inhaling simultaneously. Reverse the direction, bringing your arms back down. Close your hands as you pass your chest, and reopen them as they reach your sides, exhaling forcefully. Keep your pace slow and your movements graceful. Repeat the sequence 5 times, but stop immediately if you become lightheaded.

⊖volve *Log on to your student account and retrieve images related to this section in Chapter 4 on Preparing for the Massage. Create two other activities and share them with your classmates.* ∎

NUTRITION

Proper nutrition is vital to good health. By definition, **nutrition** is the way our bodies take in and use, or assimilate, food. Nutrients obtained from proper nutrition give us energy, help with the growth and repair body tissues, and regulate body functions. *Diet,* in contrast, is the food (and

drink) consumed to supply the processes of nutrition. Diet directly affects a body's nutrition, which has an impact on overall health. An individual's nutritional needs vary throughout life. Factors such as age, gender, activity levels, and disease are important considerations when calculating proper diet. Determining what and how much to eat is the first step in proper nutrition.

A **nutrient** is a substance that provides nourishment and affects metabolic processes such as cell growth and repair. The body produces some nutrients such as cholesterol in adequate amounts, making dietary supplements unnecessary.

Some nutrients, called *essential nutrients*, are produced by the body in insufficient amounts or not produced at all. Essential nutrients must be obtained by foods we eat (or by supplementation). Examples of essential nutrients are carbohydrates, proteins, fats, minerals, and vitamins.

Essential nutrients can be divided into two groups; macronutrients (required in large amounts) and micronutrients (required in small amounts).

Macronutrients are nutrients that provide us with energy through calories. Because of this, macronutrients are often referred to as the "calorie group." Examples of macronutrients are proteins, carbohydrates, and fats.

Micronutrients are needed throughout life but in small quantities for good health. Vitamins and minerals fall into this category. Because micronutrients lack caloric value, they are referred to as the "no-calorie group." Despite the low levels required for health, micronutrient deficiencies affect approximately one in three people. Some texts list water as a nutrient.

Protein

Proteins are composed of chains of amino acids. Amino acids are also called the building blocks of proteins. The body uses about 24 amino acids; 8 are essential (i.e., must be supplied by diet). These are the main building blocks of the body. Proteins assist in the body's growth and energy needs. They also help build and repair tissues and blood as well as help form antibodies to fight infection.

Good sources of proteins are both animal and plant sources such as meat, fish, poultry, eggs, milk, cheese, beans, peas, and nuts.

Two types of proteins are complete and incomplete. *Complete proteins* contain all eight essential amino acids and are found in animal sources. Plant proteins are often deficient in one or more amino acids; however, combining multiple plant proteins can provide all of the essential amino acids. Beans and grains together can make a complete protein.

Carbohydrates

Carbohydrates are also known as saccharides or sugars. The hierarchy from simple to complex is monosaccharides, disaccharides, and polysaccharides. *Monosaccharides,* or simple sugars, are glucose (blood sugar), fructose (fruit sugar), and galactose (milk sugar). *Disaccharides*, the union of two monosaccharides and include sucrose (table sugar), lactose (milk sugar), and maltose (malt sugar). *Polysaccharides*, or trisaccharides (carbohydrates containing three or more simple sugar molecules), include dextrins, glycogen (stored glucose), cellulose, and gums.

Carbohydrates are the most common source of energy for the body. They help generate adenosine triphosphate (ATP), provide dietary fiber, and satisfy hunger.

Most sources are plant-based such as breads, cereals, potatoes, corn, beans, peas, fresh fruits, sugar, syrup, and honey.

Fats

Fats are a subgroup of lipids called triglycerides. Fats can be unsaturated or saturated. The distinction is simple; at room temperature *unsaturated fats* are liquid, whereas *saturated fats* are solid.

Fats are also an energy source (carbohydrates are the preferred source), but fats act more as an energy reserve and are stored for later use. Fats also protect and insulate the body.

Good sources of fats are animal and plant sources, such as nuts, seeds, oils, butter, cream, fatty meats, avocados, and other fatty foods.

Vitamins

Vitamins are essential for metabolic reactions in the body. They are either soluble by water or fat. *Water-soluble vitamins* are absorbed easily and excreted within hours. Examples of water-soluble vitamins are the B vitamins and vitamin C.

Fat-soluble vitamins are absorbed slowly and often reside in the liver and fat cells. Examples of fat-soluble vitamins are A, D, E, and K.

See Table 4-1 for an overview of vitamins including its function, sources, and recommended daily intake.

Minerals

Minerals are chemical elements found in nature and divided into two categories: macro (bulk) minerals such as calcium and micro (trace) minerals such as iron.

Minerals are vital in regulating many body functions. They act as coenzymes (iron can transport oxygen), support organs (potassium supports kidney function), build bone (calcium), and aid healthy growth and development (zinc). Minerals often work with vitamins to perform bodily functions. Good sources can be found in both plant and animal products, such as vegetables, meats, dairy, and soy.

See Table 4-2 for a list of a few mineral examples. Included are its atomic letters as designated by the periodic table.

Water

Water, the most important nutrient, regulates body temperature and transports all the other nutrients. The body is roughly 70% water (this statistic varies according to the source). Water intake must balance water lost through urination, sweating, and respiration. If water loss exceeds water intake by as little as 5%, the body becomes dehydrated. If water loss exceed water intake by 10%, many bodily functions fail to proceed at their normal rates. Although a rare occurrence, a 20% loss of water is often fatal and may be seen with severe burns and untreated severe vomiting or diarrhea.

Although all water comes essentially from the same source, the important factor is purity. The Environmental Protection Agency (EPA) governs tap water standards. The Food and Drug Administration (FDA) sets the standards for bottled water based on the EPA's recommendations. Tap water quality will vary by location but must adhere to the EPA's standards. Every region of the United States produces annual reports on tap water quality, available online. Bottled waters offer a consistent product and are often chosen for taste reasons.

The standard calculation for daily water intake is half ounce per pound of body weight (e.g., 128 lb = 64 oz [gallon] of water per day). Soda, coffee, sports drinks, and tea do not count toward this total. Bottled water has become the fastest growing beverage market. There are many brands now in five categories: artesian (water from well tapping), mineral (water with natural minerals), purified (water produced by distillation or other suitable processes), sparkling (water with higher CO_2 levels), and spring (water from an underground source that naturally flows to the surface).

▌MINI-LAB

Write down everything you put into your mouth for 24 hours. Your list should include its calories, macronutrients, and micronutrients. Using the *MyPyramid Plan* link at *www.mypyramid.gov*, find out what the recommended daily allowance is for you. Then compare your list with the recommendations and see how you fare. Make adjustments where needed.

Dietary Fiber

Dietary fiber, or roughage, is found in the walls of plant cells. Fiber is essential to human health, even though enzymes in the digestive tract cannot break it down.

There are two types of fiber: soluble and insoluble. *Soluble fiber* mixes with water to form a gel that slows digestion in the stomach and intestine, resulting in a lower absorption rate of starches and sugars and reduces cholesterol levels. Good sources of soluble fiber include dried beans and peas, oats, barley, and fruits.

Insoluble fiber acts as a laxative and gives stool its bulk, helping it move quickly through the digestive tract. Good

TABLE 4-1 Vitamins

VITAMINS	FUNCTIONS	SOURCES	RDV*
Vitamin A (retinol)	Acts as an antioxidant, supports immune system function, promotes healthy eyes, helps maintain skin smoothness and clarity, and helps control bone growth.	Liver, spinach, sweet potatoes, pumpkin, collard greens, and milk.	900 µg/700 µg
Vitamin B complex	Once considered a single vitamin, there are now more than 20 types of B vitamin. The B complex refers to eight B vitamins: B_1, B_2, B_3, B_5, B_6, B_7, B_9, and B_{12}.		
B_1 (thiamine)	Promotes proper heart function and helps convert carbohydrates and fat into energy.	Pork, whole grains, spinach, wheat germ, and fortified cereals.	1.2 mg/1.1 mg
B_2 (riboflavin)	Promotes red blood cell formation and helps prevent cataracts.	Asparagus, organ meats, milk, yogurt, almonds, soybeans, and fortified cereals.	1.3 mg/1.1 mg
B_3 (niacin)	Promotes adrenal gland production, assisting in expelling toxins, and helps maintain muscle tone.	Beets, chicken, turkey, veal, salmon, tuna, sunflower seeds, and peanuts.	16 mg/14 mg
B_5 (pantothenic acid)	Promotes red blood cell production, aids in the breakdown of fats and carbohydrates for energy, and helps maintain a healthy digestive tract.	Brewer's yeast, corn, tomatoes, egg yolks, beef, duck, sweet potatoes, whole grains, and lobster.	5 mg/5 mg
B_6 (pyridoxine)	Promotes healthy nerve and brain function, aids in the production of DNA and RNA, and helps the proper absorption of vitamin B_{12}.	Brown rice, whole grain flour, bran, shrimp, lentils, fish, and nuts.	1.3 mg/1.3 mg
B_7 (biotin, vitamin H)	Aids in the metabolism of carbohydrates, fats, and amino acids.	Brewer's yeast, organ meats, nut butters, soybeans, legumes, and cooked eggs (raw egg white can interfere with biotin absorption).	30 µg/30 µg
B_9 (folic acid)	Aids in the production of DNA and RNA, and is crucial for proper brain development and function.	Spinach, whole grains, orange juice, wheat germ, asparagus, salmon, avocado, root vegetables (carrots, potatoes), and milk.	400 µg/400 µg (600 µg during pregnancy)
B_{12} (cobalamin)	Promotes proper iron function, and regulates red blood cell formation.	Fish, dairy, organ meats (liver, kidney) eggs, beef, and pork.	2.4 µg/2.4 µg
Vitamin C (ascorbic acid)	Acts as an antioxidant, helps the body resist infection, promotes adrenal gland function, aids in collagen production, and can reduce high blood pressure and cholesterol.	Citrus fruits (oranges, limes), strawberries, broccoli, and sweet red peppers.	90 mg/75 mg
Vitamin D (cholecalciferol)	Promotes bone development, helps absorb and metabolize calcium, and aids the immune system.	Fortified milk, fish liver oils, and sun exposure (sunlight helps skin to synthesize vitamin D).	5 µg/5 µg
Vitamin E (tocopherol)	Powerful antioxidant, repairs tissue, reduces blood pressure, promotes sperm development, helps prevent cataracts, and increases maternal circulation during pregnancy.	Almonds, peanuts, sunflower seeds, spinach, avocado, oils (wheat germ, safflower), and carrot juice.	15 mg/15 mg
Vitamin K	Aids in blood clotting and maintains bone health. Bacteria found in the intestines produce this vitamin.	Beef liver, green tea, spinach, dark green lettuce, asparagus, broccoli, and kale.	120 µg/90 µg

*RDV, Recommend daily values and includes both adult male and female values (e.g., 10 mg/6 mg).
µg, microgram; mg, milligram.

sources of insoluble fiber include fruits, vegetables, and whole grains.

Determining Dietary Needs

Food nutrients within packaged foods are listed on nutrition labels. Understanding how to read and use the information is vital for planning proper food intake. In this section, we will discuss how to read nutrition labels and what to look for when planning a limited calorie diet.

A *calorie* is a unit of energy-producing potential you receive from the food you eat. In the United States, a calorie is equal to the heat energy needed to raise the temperature of 1 kg of water by 1° C. It is also referred to as a kilocalorie (kcal). Macronutrients each have set caloric values: fat has 9 kcal, and protein and carbohydrates both have 4 kcal. As stated earlier, micronutrients such as vitamins and water do not have any caloric value.

The General Guide to Calories, developed by the FDA, determines an individual's daily caloric needs to be 2000 kcal. This number is the basis for percentages found on nutrition labels. This means on average an adult requires 2000 calories to provide the energy needed to accomplish their daily activities.

TABLE 4-2 Minerals

MINERALS	FUNCTIONS	SOURCES	RDV*
Calcium (Ca)	Supports the development and maintenance of strong bones and teeth, and promotes heart, nerve, and muscle function. To properly function, calcium requires other nutrients, such as vitamin D.	Cheese, ice cream, yogurt, broccoli, almonds, Swiss chard, and milk.	1000 mg/1000 mg
Potassium (K)	Essential for proper kidney function and supports normal heart function and aids digestive function.	Unprocessed foods, including meat, fish, vegetables (especially potatoes), fruit (especially avocados, bananas, and orange juice), dairy, and whole grains.	2000 mg/2000 mg
Iron (Fe)	Attaches to the hemoglobin in red blood cells, thereby delivering oxygen to the tissues.	Liver, lean red meat, fish, poultry, oysters, whole grains, dried beans, legumes, fortified breads and cereals.	18 mg/18 mg (27 mg during pregnancy)
Zinc (Zn)	Acts as an antioxidant promotes proper immune system function, and helps regulate appetite, taste, and smell. It is essential for normal growth and development and supports most aspects of reproduction.	Oysters, red meats, poultry, cheese, shellfish, legumes, whole grains, and mushrooms.	11 mg/8 mg

*RDV, Recommend daily values and includes both adult male and female values (e.g., 10 mg/6 mg).
mg, milligram.

Many factors will determine a specific individual's daily caloric needs: age, gender, weight, height, lifestyle, and exercise. Calculators are available online to determine your caloric needs (*http://nutritiondata.com/calories-burned.html* and *http://health.discovery.com/tools/calculators/basal/basal.html*). Bear in mind that these calculations are based on the average healthy adult. They do not take into consideration special needs or medical conditions and diseases.

Maintaining Weight and Weight Loss

Once your caloric needs are established, your current weight can be maintained with a diet based on that number. By reading nutrition labels and paying close attention to serving size, you can plan a healthy diet without gaining weight.

To lose weight, one needs simply to consume less than his or her base caloric need. One pound is equal to 3500 calories, so to lose one pound per week, a person can cut back 500 calories per day.

Although we live in a society overwhelmed with fad diets, "miracle" pills, and radical surgeries, weight loss comes down to a simple math equation: expend more energy than you take in. This can be accomplished by taking in fewer calories (dieting) or expending more energy (physical activity), or a combination of both. Simply put: eat less and move more. This is true for the average healthy adult.

Nutrition Labels

It is important to remember that when limiting your caloric intake, the body must still obtain the proper amount of nutrients. Although supplements are available, balancing your diet with foods rich in vitamins and minerals is recommended. Consult the nutrition label to ensure you are selecting the best food for your needs; items are often not as healthy as one might think.

Let us look a how to read a nutrition label (Figure 4-5). Our example is one of peanut butter (one of my favorites). The first thing on the label is serving size. Portion control is vital. Most canned foods contain at least two servings, but are often eaten by one person.

Calories are listed next. Peanut butter is considered a moderate calorie. The general rule: 40 kcal is low, 100 kcal is moderate, and 400 kcal is high.

Macronutrients are the next section. One serving of peanut butter, only 2 tablespoons, would count for a quarter of your daily fat allowance. To balance this, your next meal may need to include leaner options.

Micronutrients come next on the label. This food choice contains vitamin E, vitamin B (riboflavin and niacin), and iron.

The bottom portion is a standard footnote that must be on all labels. It simply serves as a reference.

> *"When health is absent…*
> *Wisdom cannot reveal itself*
> *Art cannot become manifest*
> *Strength cannot be exerted*
> *Wealth is useless and*
> *Reason is powerless…"*
> —Heraphiles, 300 BC

Food Pyramid

Another useful tool in diet planning is the Food Pyramid. It was developed by the U.S. Department of Agriculture (USDA) in 1992 to illustrate five major food groups and identify the number of servings from each group that are

Nutrition Facts

Serving Size 2 Tbsp (31g)
Servings Per About 16

Amount Per Serving

Calories 190   Calories from Fat 130

	% Daily Value*
Total Fat 17g	25%
Saturated Fat 3g	16%
Trans Fat 0g	
Cholesterol 0mg	0%
Sodium 70mg	3%
Total Carbohydrate 31g	2%
Dietary Fiber 2g	9%
Sugars 3g	
Protein 8g	
Vitamin E	15%
Riboflavin	2%
Niacin	20%
Iron	4%

* Percent Daily Values are based on a 2,000 calorie diet. Your Daily Values may be higher or lower depending on your calorie needs.

		Calories:	2,000	2,500
Total Fat	Less than		65g	80g
Sat Fat	Less than		20g	25g
Cholesterol	Less than		300mg	300mg
Sodium	Less than		2,400mg	2,400mg
Total Carbohydrate			300g	375g
Dietary Fiber			25g	30g

FIGURE 4-5 Nutrition label for peanut butter.

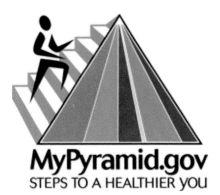

Grains – Make half your grains whole
Vegetables – Vary your veggies
Fruits – Focus on fruits
Oils – Know your fats
Milk – Get your calcium-rich foods
Meats & Beans – Go lean on protein

FIGURE 4-6 Food pyramid.

needed daily to provide a healthy, well-balanced diet. In 2005 the USDA unveiled MyPyramid, the pyramid's new look (Figure 4-6). It was redesigned to include an emphasis on physical activity and a new customizable edge, offering 12 different versions.

The five major groups have remained consistent, but serving suggestions are more tailored for each of the 12 versions. The look now includes color coding for each group and a slogan. The bottom width of the colored bands denotes the comparative amount required daily. The figure climbing the steps represents the importance of daily physical activity. Visit www.MyPyramid.gov for more resources, including videos and games.

Special Considerations: Vegetarianism

Vegetarian diets can meet all the nutritional recommendations by consuming a variety of foods to meet their daily caloric needs. Vegetarianism can be a very healthy choice;

grains, vegetables, and fruits tend to represent the majority of food consumed, which is exactly what MyPyramid suggests. A vegetarian diet usually results in higher than average amounts of most nutrients with a few exceptions. Meat can be a primary source of protein, iron, calcium, zinc, and vitamin B_{12}, so vegetarians may need to focus on these nutrients. All of these can be obtained through adherence to a vegetarian diet, mostly through beans, nuts, vegetables, and fortified foods.

The food industry has never been more accommodating to the vegetarian diet. For nearly every meat and dairy product, there is a soy or vegetable equivalent. Technology has advanced so that many vegetarian products look and even taste like their counterpart. Most restaurants have vegetarian options, or can make the necessary modifications to provide one. Asian and Indian restaurants especially tend to offer such options.

Special Considerations: Pregnancy and Breast-feeding

Studies have shown that diet can weigh considerably in the outcome of a pregnancy. The standard MyPyramid recommendations are a good foundation for healthy diet planning through pregnancy, allowing consideration for the changing caloric needs of the mother. Consulting a physician is vital for any pregnant woman concerning the proper dietary plan.

While macronutrient needs may generally remain consistent, nearly all micronutrients will require a higher recommended daily value (RDV) than the standard. It is often hard to achieve this nutrition through diet alone. Iron and folic acid intake are especially important; the increase of both is considerable (RDVs for pregnancy are 27 mg of iron, as compared with the standard 18 mg and 600 µg of folic acid as compared with the standard 400 µg). Prenatal vitamins are routinely recommended to supply the additional needs of pregnancy and nursing.

CHAT ROOM

Physical activity and proper nutrition are vital to overall health, and as massage therapists, it is our duty to recognize that relationship. We are health care providers, and as such our clients will often seek our advice on health topics. While we must be careful not to out-step the boundaries of our practice (and nutritional counseling is outside of a massage therapist's scope of practice), any suggestions made must be with an understanding of nutrition and its role in bodily health.

"Keep working on yourself, because the more you invest in yourself, the more you invest in your ability to serve others."
—Barry Green

STRESS REDUCTION

Most of us are on the go 24/7 and live stress-filled lives. This lifestyle takes its toll on our health. Heart rate, blood pressure, immune response, breathing, digestion, and muscle tension are all affected. Chronic stress produces a sustained increase in stress hormones that trigger inflammation throughout the body. Reducing stress is an important part of an overall health program.

Stress is the response of the body to any demand placed on it. It can be emotional, mental, physical, or chemical, all of which require a response from the body. Some stress is healthy and desired. For example, if you need to study for an examination (mental stress), you make time to study (healthy response to stress). Stress is also an essential part of sports training. For example, if you plan to run a marathon (physical stress), you make time to prepare for the event (healthy response to stress).

Your body can adapt to some stress, especially when coupled with a healthy response. But when stress is repeated, prolonged, or coming from numerous sources, your body may be unable to adapt and may respond by breaking down and not working properly.

According to the *Journal of the American Medical Association,* most stress diseases are related to psychological stress. What is psychological stress? Good question. *Psychological stress* occurs when an individual perceives that the demands of life exceed his or her capacity. So much of psychological stress revolves around our perceptions. In other words, stress can be symbolic rather than an actual threat.

The Chinese word symbol for stress combines symbols for danger and peril (Figure 4-7). Stress can be the impetus and motivation to use stress reduction techniques to create a more balanced life and to learn more about ourselves.

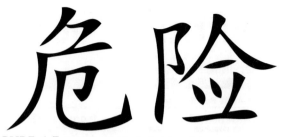

FIGURE 4-7 Chinese symbols that translate as danger or peril. Stress is dangerous for our health.

Breathe

Deep breathing is an effective relaxation tool. Within your nervous system, there are two branches with specialized functions. These branches innervate the visceral organs. One branch is more stimulatory and generates a fight or flight alarm reaction (sympathetic); the other is inhibitory and brings the body back to homeostasis or normal functioning (parasympathetic). Sympathetic arousal is also called the *stress response*; parasympathetic arousal is also called *rest and digest*. Chapter 23 features a more complete discussion.

You can stimulate either reaction through breathing. So you can control, to a certain degree, your reaction to stress. Breathing that induces relaxation is slow and deep and involves your abdomen.

Try this: expand your abdomen as you breathe in through your nose, hold a few seconds, and then release the breath out through your mouth. Pause a few seconds before the next inhalation. Repeat as desired.

Also, watch and imitate how babies and cats breathe. Their bellies expand as they inhale. This may feel awkward at first, but can be very relaxing once you become accustomed to it.

So when you feel anxious and your heart is racing and you feel like your head is going to explode, stop and take several deep abdominal breaths and say hello to the relaxation response.

Activities such as tai chi, yoga, and meditation are excellent for reducing stress by quieting the mind and promoting full deep breathing.

Laughter is a wonderful stress management tool. It promotes deep breathing, reduces muscular tension, and stimulates the production of endorphins, the body's natural pain killers.

Filing Dots

This activity combines deep breathing with a visual trigger.

First, identify items at locations you see everyday that may cause stress. Examples of items are the speedometer or rear view mirror of your car, your checkbook or debit/credit card, your cell phone or wrist watch, refrigerator (if you tend to eat when stressed), or even the front door to your home or office. If you cannot identity specific stressors, choose locations that you notice six or more times per day.

Next, place a red filing dot on each of the locations. Colorful stickers or stars can be used rather than filing dots.

When you see one of your stickers, pause and take three deep breaths. It will take about 30 seconds; just enough time to activate your relaxation response.

We cannot always change the stress-producing events around us, but we can change how we respond to them.

After about 2 weeks, reevaluate your sticker locations. If you do not notice them at least six times per day, move some around.

After doing this technique for a month, you should notice a significant drop in your stress level.

CHAT ROOM

These stress-reducing techniques are also great to teach your clients.

Journaling

Journaling, or writing, has the potential to change the way you perceive stressors. It brings clarity to thoughts and feelings. Journaling mirrors inner processes and assists you in looking at and evaluating decisions you make throughout the day. If you are pleased with the outcomes, then repeat the decisions. If you are not pleased, then make appropriate modifications.

Instead of a paper journal, create a blog (read only by yourself). Use it to express yourself. Write yourself letters about the things you want to do or places you want to see.

Journaling, whether it is on paper or on the screen, will help you diffuse a stressful day.

Affirmations

Oftentimes, stress occurs because of the attitudes we have about ourselves and our lives. Attitudes come from our beliefs; most beliefs are unconscious. As fate would have it, most beliefs are acquired during childhood. You grow up in a certain environment where you acquire a certain set of beliefs; these beliefs reflect your attitudes.

Beliefs help us make sense of the world and they are also there for our protection. Some beliefs are inherited from our parents. This occurs more readily when parents express their ideas as absolutes rather than opinions. Repetition aggravates this affect.

Some of our beliefs and attitudes are not in our service. They may be causing some of the stress in our lives. Those are the ones we might want to change. So how do you change your attitude? One way is with positive affirmations.

An affirmation is a positive statement. Writing, saying, or even thinking about affirmations is a way to reduce stress and to bring positive change into your life.

When you select your affirmation(s), write it down on several pieces of paper. Then put it on places you see often (like the filing dots activity mentioned previous). When you see the statement, say it aloud with passion. You may repeat it several times. Passion and repetition are what helps keep your statement real. Use positive affirmations to reduce the stress in your life.

Examples of positive affirmations are:
- Peace and prosperity are mine.
- I am a successful massage therapist.
- I am safe and secure; I am confident; I feel wonderful.
- I will be more patient and loving to my family today.

And, of course, there is the serenity prayer. The short version is:

> *God, grant me*
> *the serenity to accept the things I cannot change,*
> *the courage to change the things I can,*
> *and the wisdom to know the difference.*
> —Rev. Reinhold Niebuhr

Prioritize

Stress can also occur when you lose sight of things that are important to you. You fill your day with activities that are meaningless and have little time for things you value.

One way to reduce stress is to prioritize. On a sheet of paper, write down the five most important things in your life. When anyone (or anything) requests two of your biggest commodities, which are often your time and your money, see if it is in line with your priorities. If it is not, then it is time to say "no thanks." Because the *"things that matter most should never be at the mercy of the things that matter least,"* Goethe said.

Review the list annually, such as on New Years Day or perhaps on your birthday. Your priorities will change over time. For example, health may not be on a priority list when an individual is in the second decade of life, but may be high on the list when in the fifth or later decade of life.

Enjoy Yourself

Another reason people experience excess stress in their lives is that they stop doing things they enjoy. Tom Hanks, playing Forrest Gump in the movie with the same name, says, *"You know, some times you do something for no reason at all."* Yet the mere thought of doing something without a reason makes many of us feel uneasy.

Self-indulgence and pampering oneself are nurturing, frivolous, and directionless activities we do for ourselves because we enjoy them. Often, these activities are tarnished with guilt because they are without purpose. We exercise and eat right because it is good for us. Pleasurable activities just plain feel good and are more akin to play.

On a piece of paper, write down 10 things you enjoy doing. Be sure to leave a little space between each item.

MARY ANN FOSTER

Born: November 13, 1956

"Be the change you want to see in the world."
–Mahatma Ghandi

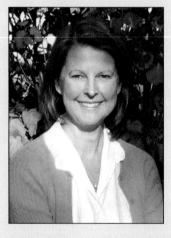

Movement patterns have fascinated Mary Ann Foster since she was a child. She realized that if she could imitate someone's gait and posture just right, she might better understand how they feel and how they view the world, giving her insight into what it would be like to be that person. One of eight children, Foster's mother made general massage a part of daily life. The integration of movement patterning and bodywork has been the foundation of her study and practice since 1981.

A resident of northeast Ohio, Foster was profoundly affected by the 1970 shootings at Kent State University, when the Ohio Army National Guard opened fire on students protesting the U.S. invasion of Cambodia and the Vietnam war. She enrolled at Kent State in 1976 where, in addition to studying education and dance, Foster took lessons through The Center for Peaceful Change, a program in peace and conflict resolution developed to memorialize the massacre. It was here that Foster got her first taste of humanistic psychology, alternative healing, and movement analysis.

She left Kent State University in 1979 to devote herself to the study of dance and movement. During this time, Foster suffered debilitating muscle spasms resulting from several childhood injuries, car accidents, and working her body too hard for too long. It was through her long healing process that her study of Laban movement analysis and Bartenieff movement fundamentals were particularly inspiring. She began to more specifically focus on the benefits of incorporating hands-on therapy with movement patterns to improve efficiency and core support.

It was also during this period that Foster decided to study massage therapy. She graduated from the Seattle Massage School and the Boulder School of Massage Therapy, and went on to study Rolfing® movement integration, craniosacral therapy, Hakomi bodywork, and Body-Mind Centering®. Foster also studied somatic psychology and earned a bachelor's degree in Healing Arts from Naropa University.

Foster's passion, as she describes it "…boils down to a fascination with the architectural design of the human body and its incredible repertoire of movement patterns." This passion and years of research resulted in her 2004 publication *Somatic Patterning: How to Improve Posture and Movement and Ease Pain*. Somatic patterning is a multidimensional approach that integrates somatics, patterning, and kinesiology into body mechanics and bodywork, providing a holistic model for structural therapy that gives organization and direction to each massage stroke. Somatic patterning embraces the idea that the human body has a perfect design that, when experienced by the practitioner or the client, moves the individual toward greater harmony and balance in the body and mind. "As a result of somatic patterning, I feel great in my own body and mind, physically, emotionally, and mentally. I feel far better now than I felt when I was in my twenties."

Foster authored sections on classroom management, teaching anatomy and physiology, and teaching body mechanics for the text *Teaching Massage*. She has been the co-author of "Talk about Touch," a recurring column in *Massage and Bodywork* magazine, since 2008. Her current objective is to bring structural integration and developmental movement principles into massage therapy as an organizing principle. "I expected the holistic paradigm of structural integration would have long ago been integrated into basic massage skills. Movement studies, whether basic kinesiology, sports, dance, or yoga, begin to fill this gap, although making the translation to table work is still missing. I wrote *Somatic Patterning* to figure out the basic precepts of the somatic therapies. Now I'm working on translation the somatic patterning precepts into the language of kinesiology."

Next, cut the paper into strips until you have 10 strips; each strip contains something you enjoy doing. Fold the strips in half and then in half once more. Place the folded strips in a Ziploc bag (or other container).

When you are feeling stressed out, reach inside your bag and pull out a strip. After reading, do the thing you enjoy.

Here are a few self-indulgent confessions:

- Lynda (mother and housewife)—stealing time to read a noneducational, sometimes trashy, purely fictional novel.
- Tina (consultant)—eating outdoors.
- Jackie (executive officer)—a facial and a massage.
- Susan (massage therapist and mother)—comfortable lounge wear.
- Lloyd (social worker)—going to the movies and watch two or three feature films, back-to-back, while eating more than his share of chocolate-covered raisins.
- Betty Joe (grandmother)—finger painting.

If someone asked you what you enjoy doing, what would you tell them?

CHAT ROOM

One reviewer for this edition stated that, after reading this section, she closed her eyes and began thinking about things she enjoyed. She felt relaxed almost immediately.

MINI-LAB

After looking over all the suggestions for stress reducing activities, select ones you particularly like and make them part of your overall health plan.

E-RESOURCES

Evolve

http://evolve.elsevier.com/Salvo/MassageTherapy

- Chapter challenge
- Flash cards
- Photo gallery
- Stress-busting tips for massage students
- Additional information
- Educational animation
- Weblinks

▶ **DVD**

- 4-1: Preparing for the massage

BIBLIOGRAPHY

ACSM: Physical activity guidelines (website): http://www.acsm.org/AM/Template.cfm?Section=Home_Page&TEMPLATE=CM/HTMLDisplay.cfm&CONTENTID=7764. Accessed May 9, 2010.

Applegate EJ: *The anatomy and physiology learning system*, ed 3, Philadelphia, 2006, Saunders.

Cohen S, Janicki-Deverts D, Miller GE: Psychological stress and disease, *JAMA* 298:1685-1687, 2007.

CNPP: *2005 food pyramid guideline* (website): http://www.mypyramid.gov/. Accessed October 13, 2009.

Damjanov I: *Pathophysiology for the health-related professions*, ed 3, Philadelphia, 2006, Saunders.

EMS Press: http://www.emspress.com/html/introductions.html. Accessed December 17, 2009.

Environmental Protection Agency: *Drinking water and health* (website): http://www.epa.gov/safewater/faq/pdfs/fs_healthseries_bottlewater.pdf. Accessed October 13, 2009.

Frazier MS, Drzymkowski JW: *Essentials of human diseases and conditions*, ed 3, Philadelphia, 2004, Saunders.

Gallaher D: Present knowledge in nutrition, University of Maryland Medical Center (website): http://www.umm.edu/altmed/ConsSupplements/Fibercs.html. Accessed October 13, 2009.

Gould BE: *Pathophysiology for the health professions*, ed 3, Philadelphia, 2006, Saunders.

Greene L: *Save your hands! the complete guide to injury prevention and ergonomics for manual therapists,* ed 2, Coconut Creek, Fla, 2008, Gilded Age Press.

Jacob S, Francone C: *Elements of anatomy and physiology*, Philadelphia, 1989, WB Saunders.

Larson E, Mayur T, Laughon BA: Influence of two hand washing frequencies on reduction in colonizing flora with three products used by health care personnel, *Am J Infect Control* 23:17, 1989.

Louisiana State Department of Social Services: *Uniform federal accessibility standards accessibility checklist*, Baton Rouge, La, 1995, United States Architectural and Transportation Barriers Compliance Board.

Mardis A: A look at the diet of pregnant women, USDA (website): http://www.cnpp.usda.gov/Publications/NutritionInsights/Insight17.pdf. Accessed October 13, 2009.

Mayo Clinic: Exercise: seven benefits of regular physical activity (website): http://www.mayoclinic.com/health/exercise/HQ01676. Accessed October 15, 2009.

Pliszka M: The truth about antibacterial soaps, *Twins* Mag Jan/Feb: 38-39, 2006.

Prudden B: *Pain erasure*, New York, 1980, M Evans.

Salvo SG: *Mosby's pathology for massage therapists*, ed 2, St Louis, 2009, Mosby.

Simon H: Vitamins: highlights, University of Maryland Medical Center (website): http://www.umm.edu/patiented/articles/vitamins_carotenoids_phytochemicals_000039.htm. Accessed October 13, 2009.

Somatic Patterning: http://www.somatic-patterning.com/html/author.html. Accessed December 17, 2009.

Thibodeau G, Patton K: *Anatomy and physiology*, ed 6, St Louis, 2006, Mosby.

Thibodeau G, Patton K: *Structure and function of the body*, ed 12, St Louis, 2004, Mosby.

Torres LS: *Basic medical techniques and patient care for radiologic technologies*, Philadelphia, 1993, JB Lippincott.

Tortora GJ: *Introduction to the human body: the essentials of anatomy and physiology*, ed 5, Hoboken, NJ, 2000, John Wiley & Sons.

USDA: Dietary guidelines for Americans 2005 (website): http://www.health.gov/dietaryguidelines/dga2005/document/pdf/DGA2005.pdf. Accessed October 14, 2009.

USFDA: How to understand and use nutritional facts labels (website): http://www.cfsan.fda.gov/~dms/foodlab.html. Accessed October 15, 2009.

MATCHING I

Place the letter of the answer next to the term or phrase that best describes it.

A. 2000
B. 3500
C. Calorie
D. Exercise

E. Health
F. Intellectual
G. Macronutrients
H. Micronutrients

I. Nutrient
J. Strenuous
K. Stress
L. Wellness

_____ 1. The physical activity classification Bonnie Prudden places the massage therapy profession in

_____ 2. Condition of physical, mental, emotional, and social well being and the absence of disease

_____ 3. Amount of calories the United States Food and Drug Administration (FDA) says most adults require to accomplish their daily activities

_____ 4. The category of nutrients that includes vitamins, minerals, and water; also called the *no-calorie group*

_____ 5. An expression of health in which an individual is aware of, chooses, and practices healthy choices, creating a more successful and balanced life

_____ 6. Unit of energy-producing potential received from the food that is eaten

_____ 7. University of Nebraska's wellness model includes emotional, environmental, occupational, physical, social, spiritual and this other dimension

_____ 8. Substance that provides nourishment and affects metabolic processes such as cell growth and repair

_____ 9. The key to a healthier life, according to the American College of Sports Medicine and the American Heart Association

_____ 10. The body's response to any demand placed on it, whether it be emotional, mental, physical, or chemical

_____ 11. Amount of calories in one pound

_____ 12. This category of nutrients includes proteins, carbohydrates, and fats; also called the *calorie group*

MATCHING II

Place the letter of the answer next to the term or phrase that best describes it.

A. Carbohydrates
B. Diet
C. Essential
D. Fats

E. Fat-soluble vitamins
F. Food Pyramid
G. Incomplete
H. Insoluble fiber

I. Protein
J. Soluble fiber
K. Water-soluble vitamins
L. Water

_____ 1. A, D, E, and K are examples of this vitamin group

_____ 2. Substance that slows digestion in the stomach and intestine, resulting in a lowered absorption rate of starches and sugars and reduced cholesterol levels

_____ 3. Good sources of this macronutrient include meat, fish, poultry, eggs, milk, cheese, beans, peas, and nuts

_____ 4. The most important nutrient; regulates body temperature and transports all the other nutrients

_____ 5. Not only a type of energy source, but acts more as an energy reserve and are stored for later use

_____ 6. Term used to describe a type of nutrients that must be obtained by food or by supplementation because the body either does not produce them in sufficient amounts or does not produce them at all

_____ 7. Acts as a laxative and gives stool its bulk, helping to move it more quickly through the digestive tract

_____ 8. B and C are examples of this vitamin group

_____ 9. The body's most common energy source

_____ 10. Food and drink consumed to supply the processes of nutrition

_____ 11. Illustrates five major food groups and identifies the number of servings from each

group that are needed daily to provide a healthy, well-balanced diet

_____ 12. Term used to describe proteins that do not contain all eight essential amino acids

CASE STUDY

More than Just an Accident

Margaret was a recent graduate from the Gulf Coast School of Massage. She acquired her state license and began her practice at a well-established chiropractic clinic. Margaret massaged the physicians' patients before their spinal adjustments. The patients loved the massage, and the physicians loved that the patients reported improving more quickly with the addition of the massage before the spinal adjustments.

Mark was Margaret's next client. It was Mark's first massage at the clinic. He was a car sales associate uptown and was recently involved in a minor car accident. Mark's chiropractor gave clearance for him to begin receiving massages. Because Margaret was asked to address his back, neck, and shoulders only, Mark left on his trousers.

When Margaret reentered the massage room, Mark was lying prone with the sheet draped across his back and legs. Margaret lowered the sheet and observed a large portion of his back covered with red circles. The edges of the circles were slightly elevated, and she noticed a slight odor to his skin.

Should Margaret continue with the massage?

Should Margaret ask the client or his physician about the circles?

When should she make the inquiry?

Should she consult the physician before, after, or during the massage?

CRITICAL THINKING

What is meant by the proverb, "Physician, heal thyself," and how can massage therapists apply this principle to their practice?

CHAPTER 5

Research Literacy

JoEllen M. Sefton, PhD, ATC, CMT

LEARNING OBJECTIVES

After completing this chapter, the student should be able to:

- Define research.
- Discuss types of research.
- Explain the scientific method.
- Identify parts of a scientific article.
- Explain why research is important to the massage profession.
- Demonstrate research literacy skills.
- Discuss ways research is funded and the importance of professional involvement.

"There are a number of very important irreversibles to be discovered in our universe. One of them is that every time you make an experiment you learn more; quite literally, you can not learn less."
—Buckminster Fuller

http://evolve.elsevier.com/Salvo/MassageTherapy

INTRODUCTION

Sarah, a new client, comes to you to reduce her lower back pain. You develop a treatment plan and after just one session, she is feeling some relief. After three sessions, she is pain free. During the third session, after telling you how much better she feels, she looks up and asks "How exactly does massage work?" What do you tell her?

Clients seek out massage therapy for many reasons such as relaxation and stress reduction,[1,2] after injury or surgery, to decrease the discomfort of cancer treatments,[3,4] to combat depression and anxiety,[5-7] to deal with past physical and emotional trauma,[8] and to gain body awareness.[8,9] While massage therapy has been used for thousands of years,[10] we have only recently begun to understand HOW it works. We know that massage assists with depression and anxiety,[5,11,12] improves joint range of motion,[7,13] and improves infant birth weight[14,15] but *how*? If we do not know how these effects are produced, how can we be certain we are using the best methods and techniques to achieve optimal results for our clients? How can we ask insurance companies or clients to pay, or physicians to prescribe a therapy when we cannot explain exactly how the treatment works?

Research is the answer. The word *research* may strike fear into the hearts of massage therapists, but do not be afraid … research is simply a way to find the answers to these questions. Researchers are a curious group of people who like to solve puzzles and answer perplexing questions. The research methods that we are going to learn about in this chapter help to ensure that the answers we get are accurate. The scientific method can be intimidating, but it is important for the therapist to understand the general research process as it applies to their work.

This chapter will discuss how researchers go about finding answers to important questions. It will give you a better understanding of research, help you locate research articles, and understand parts of a research paper. When we are done, you will be able to better answer your clients' questions. And you may decide to discover some of the answers yourself.

WHAT IS RESEARCH?

Research is a way to solve a puzzle using prescribed methods, with the goal of discovering new facts or revising current theories. How do we find these new facts and how do we ensure the answers we find are correct? Researchers/scientists follow a process called the *scientific method*. The scientific method is a group of techniques used to investigate questions and develop new knowledge through the gathering of evidence (i.e., observable, measurable, or empirical), experimentation, and testing theories or hypothesis. Based on the rules of science, the scientific method helps to develop studies or investigations that reveal new information and relationships between cause and effect. How these studies are developed and performed is very important to ensuring

that the results are correct. Let us look at an actual example that happened to some graduate students at a university several years ago where failure to adhere to scientific method resulted in a slippery research dilemma.

Two biology graduate students developed a study to look at how exercise influenced leg muscles in frogs. After each day's exercise (called a *treatment* in research lingo), they chose a frog to test (a *subject/participant*) from the group of frogs. Each frog was tested once, and then removed from the group of frogs in the study (the *sample population*).

The study was almost done when a fellow researcher came to watch the process. He asked an important question—how do you choose which frog to test? The students were just grabbing the first frog that they could catch. The researcher then asked "so, you are catching the slow, lazy frogs first. The stronger frogs that jump more and are harder to catch will remain until the end of your study; won't that affect your results?" This simple experimental design flaw meant that their information, or *data,* was biased and could not be used because the slow lazy frogs were tested first and the stronger active frogs remained until the end of the study. Because the study was testing muscle strength and activity, the data was flawed.

If the graduate students had randomly chosen a frog by numbering the frogs, putting the numbers on slips of paper in a bowl, choosing a number, and then catching the selected frog, their data would have been fine and they could have finished their study confident that their facts, or *results*, would be true and accurate. By careful experimental design following the scientific method, researchers attempt to ensure that their study provides the correct solutions to the puzzle.

TYPES OF RESEARCH

There are many different types of research and they can be group into several categories. Two general categories are (1) basic research and (2) clinical or applied research. Each type is important when answering some of the questions about how massage works. Other important types include case studies, case reports, survey research, epidemiological research, and many others.

Basic Research

Basic research seeks to find fundamental information at the molecular, cellular, or tissue level and is typically conducted in a laboratory. For example, if you tell your client, Sarah, that massage therapy is thought to work through changing how brain neurotransmitters are released, research providing this type of information would be considered basic research. Knowledge gained from basic research can be used to develop applied research questions, optimize protocols, or develop translational research programs. It may first appear that basic research has no direct application to a massage treatment; however, we just need to look deeper into the process. For example, if a researcher learns that pressure on a collagen strand changes the molecular composition, that may provide a direct link to how massage reduces scar tissue (*mechanism of action*).

Clinical or Applied Research

Clinical or applied research uses investigations, or *research studies*, to examine questions on a functional level. Most research investigations into massage therapy fall into this category. For example, if you tell your client, Sarah, that massage therapy is thought to work through increasing blood flow to muscles,[16,17] this knowledge could come from an applied research study.

Research studies investigate specific measurements (called *outcome or **dependent variables***) such as heart rate or blood flow after a massage treatment. ***Independent variables*** in a study are things that the researcher controls or manipulates; such as the time measurements are taken (e.g., pretest and posttest measurements), or the treatment group (i.e., massage group versus the control group).

The experimental design helps to ensure the resulting data tell the correct story. Part of a good research design includes a control group that is not treated or receives a pretend treatment (called a *sham treatment*) or an alternative therapy (i.e., heat or cold) that is being compared with the treatment of interest (i.e., massage therapy). This enables the researcher to conclude that any significant results are a result of the massage treatment, and not simply from being a part of a study. There are many factors that may influence the outcome variables. For example, the simple act of testing blood pressure may cause blood pressure to increase. The relaxation felt from lying on a massage table may reduce stress levels and change outcome variables. All these factors must be taken into account when researchers attempt to understand how massage therapy works. A control group shows the researcher how the study itself might influence the study measures being assessed.

Another important effect is the *placebo effect*. If a participant believes a treatment or a drug will be beneficial, that belief can produce changes in the outcome measures. It is thought that the placebo effect accounts for at least 15% of all changes in experimental measures in drug studies. As massage therapists we understand the importance of the mind/body connection and how this can be involved in healing. In research, we need to take this into account when designing studies and understanding the results.

Most social, psychological, and educational research comes under applied research. As such, investigators attempt to understand why people do what they do, and discover what factors (called *variables*) might affect their actions. For example, we may want to find out (*research question*) why more women seek out massage therapy treatment; what determines if a new client will continue therapy; or how treatment price influences clientele.

Another problem, especially with clinical research, is that there are often influencing factors we cannot control called *extraneous variables and confounding variables*. This is especially true when doing research in complementary and alternative medicine (CAM). For example, you are conducting a 6-week research study to assess the effects of a 20-minute massage treatment for neck pain. All of your participants have had a history of muscular neck pain lasting at least 4 weeks. What if one of your participants slept in position that aggravated the pain, another was going through a particularly stressful time at work that aggravated her pain, and a third person decided to take long hot baths at night and was feeling better? All of these things could affect your results. These are examples of confounding variables that may influence your data. During the design of the study, we try to anticipate and account for confounding variables through the use of good research design and control groups. Larger groups help to balance out the effects resulting from these uncontrollable influences. Because of this, large numbers of participants are often needed and much time is spent asking questions about their health and outside activities before and during the study (called *participant inclusion/ exclusion criteria*). In the case of the example given above, the neck pain caused by a poor night of sleep would violate the study inclusion criteria. That subject would either be eliminated from study consideration or would be tested at a later date.

Additional Types of Research

There are many other ways to group research and many other types of investigations. One common category is *analytical research*, which includes in-depth investigations into complex issues and mechanisms. This would include historical research, philosophical research, and research reviews and synthesis (summaries of research that has already been completed). Another category is *descriptive research,* which typically includes survey and interview studies (In Sarah's case, research showing clients experiencing a decrease in lower back pain after massage would be a survey study). Case studies and reports, job analysis, observational and developmental studies, correlational studies (looking at relationships between variables such as massage and heart rate) and epidemiologic research (projects such as large studies assessing population trends in health and wellness), all look to answer a different research question. Each type of research study is important in providing information about our profession and improving our knowledge base. What is important is to choose the correct type of research study to answer the research question.

> *"Research is what I'm doing when I don't know what I'm doing."*
> —Wernher von Bruan

THE SCIENTIFIC METHOD

Scientific method defines the protocols used to create new knowledge, gathering information through observation and data collection, and testing a *research hypothesis* (Figure 5-1). The scientific method consists of a series of steps used to determine the *research question*, our theory about what will happen (the *hypothesis*), and the steps taken to test the hypothesis (called the *experimental design*). This becomes a circular process. We:

- Read the literature and develop a question
- Develop a theory as to what the answer might be
- Develop a way to test this theory and a hypothesis
- Test this in a study
- Analyze the results and determine whether our theory was correct
- Adjust our theory (if we were wrong) or develop a new question (if we are right) and
- Start over with another question

As we saw with the frog study, a simple flaw in the experimental design can ruin a study and render the conclusions worthless. In this example the problem was discovered early. What if these results were published and the flaw was never discovered? What if the results of a study indicate that we should change the way we do a treatment, but there was a flaw in how the data was obtained, a flaw in the use of the scientific method? This can and does happen, every research study has limitations. A good study will list these limitations near the end of the article. However, studies are published with serious flaws. This is one reason it is important to learn to read the literature with a critical eye, and to understand the research process. Becoming an informed massage therapy research consumer will enable you to determine which studies have serious limitations, and which ones provide new knowledge that you should incorporate into your practice.

CHAT ROOM

We have seen what a flawed study looks like (the frog study), how about an example of a great study? Researchers looked at the effects of touch and massage therapy in brain development in one of the few basic research studies conducted in this area. This study used both an animal model and preterm infants to examine changes in brain development and activity at both the cellular and organ level (basic research). This study found improved brain development in infants and identified a mechanism responsible for this change. Published in a premiere neurological scientist-reviewed journal (see later discussion), studies such as this go a long way toward increasing the body of knowledge for massage therapy.[18] See the abstract of this article in Box 5-1 to learn more about this study.

Over centuries of conducting studies and through much trial and error, scientists have identified some basic rules for the research process—developing the scientific method as we know it today. We will go into more detail about this process throughout this chapter, but essentially the process of the scientific method is:

1. Combine your observations, experience, and knowledge with that of other researchers (through a literature search) to develop a foundation of knowledge;
2. Use this knowledge to form a testable research question;
3. Based on your study rationale, develop a prediction as to the results; and
4. Test your theory in a well designed study.

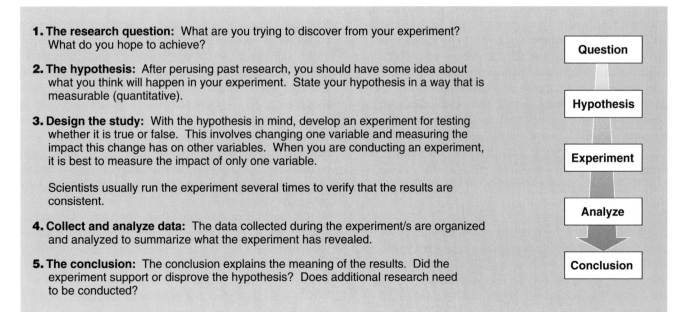

1. **The research question:** What are you trying to discover from your experiment? What do you hope to achieve?

2. **The hypothesis:** After perusing past research, you should have some idea about what you think will happen in your experiment. State your hypothesis in a way that is measurable (quantitative).

3. **Design the study:** With the hypothesis in mind, develop an experiment for testing whether it is true or false. This involves changing one variable and measuring the impact this change has on other variables. When you are conducting an experiment, it is best to measure the impact of only one variable.

Scientists usually run the experiment several times to verify that the results are consistent.

4. **Collect and analyze data:** The data collected during the experiment/s are organized and analyzed to summarize what the experiment has revealed.

5. **The conclusion:** The conclusion explains the meaning of the results. Did the experiment support or disprove the hypothesis? Does additional research need to be conducted?

Question

Hypothesis

Experiment

Analyze

Conclusion

FIGURE 5-1 The scientific method.

How can we ensure that the results of a study can be trusted? We look at specific aspects of the data and how they were collected. A measure that is *reliable* indicates that we would achieve the same results if we performed the study again. *Accuracy* indicates how close our result is to the actual value of what we are measuring. For example, our thermometer is inaccurate if it measures a temperature of 93° F today, and the actual temperature is 95.7° F. You can see how the accuracy of our equipment would be important to obtain correct results. Finally, we need to know if our measures are *valid*. There are many types of research validity, but we need to know if we are measuring what we think we are measuring. For example, if we give an examination to our foreign language massage students is it measuring their anatomy knowledge, or their ability to read and process English? Is the examination a valid measure of their knowledge of the human body? Any problem with reliability, accuracy, or validity means we may not be able to trust the result of a study.

The Research Question

Developing a good research question is an important, yet difficult, part of the scientific process. To begin, ask yourself, what exactly do you want to know? A well-designed research question can make or break the study. A simple question such as *how does massage affect blood flow* is really not as simple as it appears, there are many factors involved in blood flow. Do you want to know how massage affects arterial blood flow, venous blood flow, or peripheral blood flow? Do you care about blood flow to the skin or to the muscles? Do you want to look at a specific massage technique such as effleurage, or do you want to look at a 20-minute clinical session? How will you measure blood flow?

All of these things need to be determined as you write your research question. While this can be the most challenging part of the process, it can also be the most fun. It is like developing the plot (research question) to the mystery novel; you then have to write the story (experimental design) that helps you discover that the butler did it (results).

A great research question is specific and succinct: How does a 20-minute clinical massage of the neck and shoulders change peripheral blood flow in the trapezius muscle in healthy adults? Now *this* is a well-defined question we can answer. Now we can proceed to developing our hypothesis.

The Hypothesis

The hypothesis (*pl.* hypotheses) is the expected result of your study based on your background research and knowledge. A hypothesis must be testable. It is important to research the literature (via peer reviewed journals) to understand what has been done in the past. Previous work is important to help us determine what we think will happen as a result of the study. Each time we do research we add to this knowledge base. Think of what we have learned in the past 20 years about massage. What will we know in 20 more years? Thoroughly understanding the previous research is vital to creating a proper study design.

Additionally, we do not want to test a lot of different measures (*variables*) for no real scientific reason in an effort to find *something* that looks important (a *statistically significant outcome*). This approach is not considered good science, and often leads to incorrect conclusions.

Good science is said to be "hypothesis driven" in that there is a scientific rationale for undertaking the investigation and an expected outcome is postulated. Finally, it is very important to understand that a study never *proves* a hypothesis; it can only support or reject the hypothesis.

Designing the Study

Once we have determined a research question, reviewed the relevant literature, and developed a hypothesis, it is time to carefully develop a research study to test the hypothesis and answer the research question. This process requires knowledge of statistics, research methods, and experimental design procedures; as well as knowledge in your specific area of investigation (e.g., massage therapy and the physiology of blood flow).

It can be difficult to find all of this expertise in one individual, thus research is often conducted by research teams. This approach allows each individual to focus in their area of expertise, as well as taking advantage of different points of view that typically combine to make a stronger research project.

It is important to remember, however, that a research project does not have to be complex to provide important data. Some of the most elegant and important studies were simple ones. Important knowledge is also gained through survey studies, case studies, and case reports. So do not read this section and think that you can never get involved in research. All massage therapists can contribute to improving our knowledge base.

An important part of developing a research study is doing preliminary work to test your procedures, techniques, and equipment. This simple step can prevent fatal flaws in design and save time and money. Equipment used in the study must be tested to ensure that it is valid and reliable. If a researcher develops a new piece of equipment or a new procedure, the validity and reliability of these must be assessed in a separate study. In this case, if the testing equipment results cannot be reproduced, then your study results are meaningless.

It is also important to carefully define terms. *Operational definitions* state exactly how a variable is measured, manipulated, or defined. For example: what does "massage therapy" mean in our study? We must define the term so that anyone reading published findings of the study understands exactly how it was performed and be able to repeat the study if desired. This is especially true for those terms associated with measurements or expressing ideas in psychological or social research. For example, what does it mean that a client *prefers* a specific treatment? If you were studying client preferences about massage, you would have to define "prefers" (called a *conceptual definition*) so those who read your research results would understand precisely what you mean. If we were measuring postural balance after a massage therapy treatment we would have to define how balance was measured; was your participant standing on one or two legs and what type of measurement did we used to determine balance?

There are many different experimental designs; one is the *clinical trial*, which is a controlled look at the safety and effectiveness of a treatment using human subjects. Clinical trials come after preliminary studies have assessed basic information about a procedure, drug, or device. There are many different types of clinical trials: observational, intervention, screening, treatment, diagnostic, and other types. The type most frequently discussed is the *randomized, controlled trial*. This provides such a high level of evidence that any treatment effect found during the trial has a high probability of real.

A precise series of steps called *methods* (or *protocols* or *procedures*) is developed before testing (*data collection*). These methods must be followed uniformly for each participant and anyone helping with the study (the *investigators*) must adhere to this protocol. The methods are written step-by-step like a recipe so another investigator could follow it and produce comparable results.

Some massage protocols are developed to test the real world application of massage. This can mean simply specifying that 10 minutes of massage will be completed on the neck and shoulders. Another may look at one specific technique, such as the effect of compression on blood flow. The specific methods used will be detailed in the final experimental write up submitted for publication at the study conclusion.

Before data are collected on human subjects, we must have our methods reviewed by the institution where we work (called the *Institutional Review Board*) to ensure that our participants will be treated safely and ethically. The IRB approves the study and monitors the process for any incidents that occur that might affect the well-being of the participants.

Collecting the Data

Data are collected while the experiment is being conducted. This may involve gathering numerical data or by recording field notes or actual transcripts from participants. During data collection, it is important that all investigators know, understand, and follow the research protocols outlined in the methods exactly, without deviation. In this way, the data will be an accurate representation of the effect of the independent variables on the study measures.

Analyzing the Data

After all of the data are collected, the investigators analyze it and discover the results of their work. The data are usually

---

CHAT ROOM

The Review Committee and Informed Consent

Any study involving human or animal participants must have a committee that approves, monitors, and reviews the scientific, ethical, and regulatory aspects of the research process. These committees have various names such as an Institutional Review Board (IRB), an Ethical Review Board, or an Independent Ethics Committee.

Human subject research is not only limited to studies where a researcher draws blood or conducts a massage on a participant. If a researcher conducts a survey, interacts with a person, receives identifiable information (e.g., medical records), conducts a survey over the Internet, or if the study includes any private information, a person would normally expect not to be public (hidden video), IRB approval must be obtained.

Members of an IRB committee are designated by federal regulations, including such criteria as (1) having a five-member minimum, (2) possessing members who are familiar with any vulnerable populations studied (prisoners, pregnant women, minors, etc.) so that their rights may be adequately protected, (3) including both men and women who are not from the same profession (e.g., all physicians), and (4) at least one scientist, one nonscientist, and one member not affiliated with the sponsoring organization (this person is often a member of the clergy).

Informed consent must be obtained from all participants. Informed consent indicates that the person agrees to participate in a research study and is thoroughly informed on what will be involved. This includes the potential risks and benefits, what they will have to do during the study, what will be done with their personal information, and that they can stop the study at any time. Informed consent is also discussed in Chapter 10.

---

entered into a computer database and the researchers must determine what it means (i.e., which relationships are significant and which are not).

There are many ways to do this. Looking at the data in different ways will tell the researchers different things. A specialist in analysis, or a *statistician*, may be brought in to perform this part of the study. A good statistician will understand the research question and develop an analysis process specifically designed to answer the research question. The statistician will also help the researchers understand or *interpret* the results and develop graphs and charts that help to explain the outcomes.

Data analysis will determine whether the original hypothesis was supported (called a statistically significant finding) or rejected (results were not statistically significant). Statistically significant simply means that it is unlikely that any differences found after treatment were the result of chance. It does not mean that the treatment was proven effective.

Another factor to consider is whether the change found after the treatment is *clinically significant*. A change resulting from a massage treatment could be found to be statistically significant, but the question the massage therapist should ask is does the treatment produce a clinical effect for my client. If the treatment increased range of motion at the shoulder by one degree it could be statistically significant. However, will a one-degree increase in shoulder flexion affect your client's life? If not, the study would be clinically insignificant.

It is also important to understand that a rejected hypothesis is not a failed study. Often researchers learn as much from insignificant results as they do from those that are statistically significant. For example, if a study shows no effect of massage on weight loss this would not be a "failed study;" this would provide important information for therapists to provide to their clients.

Study results, significant or not, are important to publish. They can save other researchers time and money and generally help us to improve our overall knowledge base.

The Conclusion

The research team then develops a conclusion based on the results or *findings*. It is important to understand that this conclusion is limited to specifically what was tested. For example, if a study found that massage therapy increased range of motion in the neck of healthy adults, it could not be concluded that massage therapy also would increase range of motion in the back, or produce changes in children. The conclusion must be carefully written to apply only to what was found during testing. When reading the findings, others may extrapolate these results to other parts of the body. This sets up a follow-up study to see if the same results would be obtained in other areas of the body. As you can see, this can be an endless process. Every time more is learned it leads to additional questions.

Communicating the Findings

Designing a great study that meets the standards of the scientific method is very challenging. It is also important that published research is carefully checked to ensure that the study design is strong and the results are valid, accurate, reliable, and replicable.

The scientific community of researchers has a process to monitor themselves called *peer review*. Peer review is the process whereby research is scrutinized by a group of experts in the same or a similar field. These experts evaluate all aspects of the research design, execution, results, and conclusions and attempt to form an impartial opinion as to its quality. Peer review is used to determine which articles are published in scientific journals. Additionally, peer review is typically used by foundations and granting agencies to determine which grant proposals are funded. This process allows several experts to view the work from different perspectives, helping to ensure quality and avoid errors in the published literature. This is an essential part of the scientific process.

Scientific publications called *journals* distribute results of studies in specific fields, or areas of specialization called disciplines and subdisciplines. Because of this, journals that use the peer review process are referred to as *peer reviewed journals*. Articles go through a rigorous peer review process to ensure that only well designed, scientifically sound research is published. When you are looking for the best and most up-to-date information on a scientific topic, you will want to consult a peer-reviewed journal for information (see references for examples). Keep in mind that not all articles published are great articles, and you must read everything with a critical eye in an effort to determine the quality of the study.

ANATOMY OF A SCIENTIFIC ARTICLE

Scientific articles have a common structure. Although this may vary a bit from journal to journal or between fields of study, overall you can find the same type of information in specific locations in the article. This organization assists in the research process. If you are looking specifically for information on how to measure blood flow, you do not need to read the entire article, but you should look first to the methods section of an appropriate paper and read how the researchers completed their measurements. Scanning the abstract to get an idea of what was done and the results will tell you if you should spend the time reading the entire paper. This can be a great time saver. A good introduction can provide background information in an area that is new to you, and a great discussion section can help you decide whether you need a more in-depth understanding of the research and the findings.

Abstract. An abstract is a summary of the article and findings. It should allow for a quick review of all important aspects of the research: participants, methods, variables used, analysis completed, what was learned, and conclusions reached (see Box 5-1). The reader should be able to quickly scan the abstract to determine if he or she would like to read the entire article.

Introduction – The introduction provides an overview of the literature in the area related to the research. The introduction starts at a basic level and introduces the reader to the topic. It then proceeds to explain the deficits in the current research and builds a case for why this particular research study should be completed. It ends with the purpose of the study and the hypothesis.

Methods – The methods section is the recipe for conducting the study. This section includes details on the participants, equipment, protocols, and statistical analysis used. This section should be written so that the study could be replicated by following the methods step by step.

Results – The statistical analysis findings of the study are found in the results section. This is typically a brief section that reports what was found. Some publications or presentations will combine results with the discussion section. In this case a result is presented, then discussed; followed by the findings.

Discussion – The discussion section interprets the findings detailed in the results section. Here the author explains the results, the relevance to the literature, and any limitations inherent in the study. This is typically the longest section,

BOX 5-1

Sample Abstract

Massage accelerates brain development and the maturation of visual function.

J Neurosci. 2009 May 6;29(18):6042-6051.

Guzzetta A, Baldini S, Bancale A, Baroncelli L, Ciucci F, Ghirri P, Putignano E, Sale A, Viegi A, Berardi N, Boldrini A, Cioni G, Maffei L.

Department of Developmental Neuroscience, Istituto di Ricovero e Cura a Carattere Scientifico Stella Maris, I-56128 Calambrone, Pisa, Italy.

Abstract — Environmental enrichment (EE) was shown recently to accelerate brain development in rodents. Increased levels of maternal care, and particularly tactile stimulation through licking and grooming, may represent a key component in the early phases of EE. We hypothesized that enriching the environment in terms of body massage may thus accelerate brain development in infants. We explored the effects of body massage in preterm infants and found that massage accelerates the maturation of electroencephalographic activity and of visual function, in particular visual acuity. In massaged infants, we found higher levels of blood IGF-1. Massage accelerated the maturation of visual function also in rat pups and increased the level of IGF-1 in the cortex. Antagonizing IGF-1 action by means of systemic injections of the IGF-1 antagonist JB1 blocked the effects of massage in rat pups. These results demonstrate that massage has an influence on brain development and in particular on visual development and suggest that its effects are mediated by specific endogenous factors such as IGF-1.

and the author can elaborate and theorize as to the reason for the results.

Conclusion — The conclusion is a simple report of the findings as they relate to the study or study population. This is the shortest section. Some journals may include a "Clinical Applications" section at the end of the conclusions and provide specific ways in which the results can be applied clinically in the field.

References — The reference section is a detailed list of all literature used to justify and explain the study. This section is a great place to find more information regarding anything related to the article.

> *"It's time again. Tear up the violets and plant something more difficult to grow."*
> —James Schuyler

RESEARCH AND THE MASSAGE PROFESSION

Now that we know how researchers go about the process of gaining knowledge, the next question might be *What do we really know*, or *What is the current knowledge base for massage therapy*? How does this compare with other health care professions? The answers to these questions are important. Better knowledge will make us better therapists, enabling us to provide improved care for our clients. We must determine which of our methods are effective and which need to be replaced or modified because they do not produce the anticipated results. Moreover, as a profession, we have been striving to gain respect and improve our standing in both the medical community and society in general. To gain standing as a profession we must do several things:

1. Show that what we do is important and has a positive influence on society;
2. Show what we do is effective and based on research indicating massage therapy improves health and wellness;
3. Define the skills and abilities needed to participate in our profession;
4. Prove that we are a profession and not simply a trade. Professions and trades differ in several important ways, one of which is that someone in a profession completes research to improve their knowledge base; and
5. Conduct our own research rather than let those outside our profession do our research for us.

Research by the Profession for the Profession

Massage research conducted by the massage therapy profession is very important. While many research teams are comprised of individuals from different specialties and backgrounds, as a profession we must be involved in research in our own field. If we allow other professions (i.e. physical therapists) to do the vast amount of research in our field we lose the ability to define ourselves as a profession and allow others to control how we are perceived and the direction and progress of our profession. Thus as massage therapists it is incumbent upon us to support and advocate for massage therapy research, to read and implement new knowledge, and to support those massage therapists doing the research. This requires massage therapists to be involved at many levels; as clinicians, as researchers, and as academics; joining research teams, completing case studies and reports, and advocating for professional research support. This will help us all as a profession and will ensure that the treatments we provide for our clients will be constantly improving in efficacy and safety. Research by the profession for the profession also enables massage therapists to elevate our professional standing, increase physician referrals, and to fight for insurance reimbursement, all of which provides increased business opportunity and increases the access to treatment for those currently unable to afford it without insurance assistance.

How does the massage therapy research knowledge base stand up to other professions? We have learned a lot over the past decade. Massage therapy research is relatively new compared with the decades of quality research in other fields. While the first studies were important attempts to learn basic information, as with any new endeavor, there were some flaws and ways that the methods could be improved. Many of the first studies were small, lacked control groups, did not use certified massage therapists to do the treatments, or did not fully report the methods used.

Because of what we have learned from our past, research quality has improved dramatically. Each year the quality and quantity of the studies improves and massage therapy research is now receiving funding and support from major institutions such as the National Institutes of Health (NIH). Indeed, the establishment of the National Center for Complementary and Alternative Medicine (NCCAM) within the NIH, a subagency where massage research is most often funded, indicates a change in perspective of the massage by science and medicine. This agency only supplies funding for the top researchers in the country to answer the most pressing and well-defined research proposals. As we insist on quality research as a profession, more therapists will become involved in completing research, and the result will be a vast expansion of our knowledge base.

Research-Based Massage Effects

Our understanding of the massage therapy profession and the physiologic effects of massage change every time we learn something new. As such, it is important to become familiar with and stay current on the most up-to-date research literature. These broad conclusions are derived from numerous investigations and investigative approaches designed to study a specific topic. Different studies may have different results. Science is never simple, and knowledge is rarely black and white; unequivocal facts are very hard to come by.

Recent efforts have demonstrated that massage therapy is an effective treatment and support an ever-growing rationale for medically reimbursable massage therapy. Clinical studies and published reports of cases massage therapists see in practice (or *case reports*) helped to build our practic knowledge. More and more attention is turning to how massage therapy produces clinical effects, rather than if effects are produced. If we do not know the physiologic changes our therapy produces, effects themselves can still be held in question. Improving our evidence of clinical effects and finding how massage works (or the *mechanisms of action*) will be the focus of future research for a long time. In Chapter 6 we will take a close look at what we know and do not know about how massage therapy works.

RESEARCH LITERACY

Hopefully now you understand:
1. Research is important to the future of the profession;
2. Understanding research is an important part of being a massage therapy professional; and
3. The importance of actively supporting future research.

The next obvious question is how can you follow and keep up-to-date on what is going on in research? What are

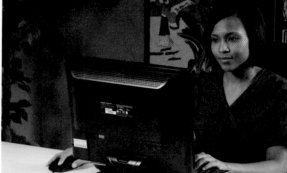

FIGURE 5-2 Therapist using the Internet to search for research literature.

the "new horizons" for massage therapy research, and how will that affect my practice in the years to come?

Ahh, I'm glad you asked.

Research literacy, or the ability to locate, read, and understand research literature, is an important part of being a professional, and is surprisingly easy to learn. (Remember, you still need to answer Sarah's question from the chapter introduction). If you are familiar with basic Internet search engines (e.g., Google), you have already mastered some of the techniques; now you just have to become familiar with a few new search engines and practice some easy techniques to help you to narrow search results to find your specific answers (Figure 5-2).

Internet Search Engines

Search engines are programs that use key words (e.g., subject, titles, authors) to help you search the Internet for information. These may direct you to databases of journals or the articles themselves. Key words are terms that the author identifies as important to help readers find information. The search engine will look for these words, as directed by you, within the title, abstract, or body of the published study. For example, a study assessing the effect of massage therapy on premature infant weight gain might include the key words *premature, infant, massage, cortisol, survivability,* or *obstetrics*. If the reader enters any of these words, or a word from the title, into a search engine this article would appear in the list of results. Learning and experimenting with determining the correct key words for your topic or using Boolean search methods is part of the art of database searching.

Some search engines are free to the public, others require subscriptions. Some valuable search engines are:
- Google Scholar (http://scholar.google.com)
- Web of Science (http://thomsonreuters.com/products_services/science/science_products/a-z/web_of_science)
- PubMed (http://www.ncbi.nlm.nih.gov/pubmed)

JACK MEAGHER, PT, MST

Born: July 6, 1923; died: March 6, 2005

"Massage is the study of anatomy in Braille."

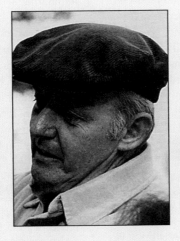

Jack Meagher was the father of sports massage. At age 74, with cancer at the time of this interview, he radiated the energy and demonstrated the quick wit rarely encountered in men half his age.

Before enlisting as a U.S. Army medic for 4 years, Meagher took a course in Swedish massage, hoping eventually to get into physical therapy. When he was in Epernay, France, he experienced a different type of massage from what he had learned back home. This massage, performed by a German prisoner of war, made Meagher move markedly better on the baseball field.

After his discharge, Meagher was signed by the Boston Braves as a pitcher, but a wartime shoulder injury threw him a curve that landed him in physical therapy, unable to continue a baseball career. The injury sent him looking for the same kind of massage that he had received in France. He found another German therapist, an instructor at the Viennese Massage School in Connecticut, who relieved his pain to the extent that Meagher was able to play semiprofessional baseball in his hometown of Gloucester, Massachusetts.

The success of his therapy did more than put Meagher's body into motion again; it got him thinking. The result was sports massage, the massage that can enhance athletic performance. Just as Swedish massage uses specific strokes, Meagher classified sports massage strokes as direct pressure, friction, compression, and percussion. He also recommended effleurage and kneading when necessary. "It took me 15 years of putting it together," says Meagher. "I was at a YMCA working on professional athletes and people for whom exercise was a way of life. The sports massage helped them do more before they faded. A loose body uses less energy."

Soon Meagher discovered that what made man go farther and faster might also help horses. That is when sports massage really took off. "In the 1976 Olympics, the horses I'd worked on took two golds and a silver," recalled Meagher. "I was written up and asked to do a book. Then the American Massage Therapy Association became interested, and I was invited to speak at one of their conferences."

The classic sports massage text he produced is *Sports Massage: A Complete Program for Increasing Performance and Endurance in Fifteen Popular Sports* (Doubleday, 1998). It more than introduces a specific massage technique to the reader; it provides a glimpse into the life of a warm, dedicated, and extremely results-oriented man with a sharp mind, who understands the intricate biomechanics of the body and is able to break it down into simple steps to make his life's work accessible to "weekend warriors" and professional athletes alike.

Meagher also had a wonderful sense of humor, exemplified in the title of his book *Never Goose an Appaloosa*. Ticklish himself, he does not even receive Swedish massage, but regarding the horses he massages, Meagher says, "I would not get on a horse, but I do get along with horses. I've never been kicked. Horses understand when you're trying to help them." He is still massaging 40 to 50 horses per week but not the workload he did in his prime. "I used to do 55 people and 30 horses a week," he says.

When asked what characteristics should be present in a successful massage therapist, Meagher says that the desire to help people and the ability to know how to use one's hands are of utmost importance. Additionally, a massage therapist should possess the education for putting it all together.

When asked if he would do it all over again, Meagher says, "I wouldn't do anything differently. It's taken years of hard work. One time a chief of orthopedics told me I had a real gift, and I had to disagree. Gifts come easily. What I do is not a gift. I work hard. I developed my instincts through my failures and my successes."

- Sports Discuss (http://www.ebscohost.com/thisTopic.php?topicID=585&marketID=1)
- Medline (http://www.nlm.nih.gov/medlineplus/)
- Biological Abstracts (http://thomsonreuters.com/products_services/science/science_products/a-z/biological_abstracts
- Academic Search Premiere (http://www.ebscohost.com/thisTopic.php?marketID=1&topicID=1)
- Journal Citation Reports (http://thomsonreuters.com/products_services/science/science_products/a-z/journal_citation_reports)

New search engines are developed daily and each researcher finds they have a favorite that seems to work for them. Finally, most libraries have reference librarians that are always willing to help.

MINI-LAB

Choose a disease or condition that you, a client, friend, or family member has experienced. Using the search engines listed previously, research this condition. (Example: arthritis; key words: *arthritis, massage, research, alternative therapy, pain, joint disease, range of motion*). Next, find any research that includes the use of massage therapy for this condition. What did you find? If you don't find any research involving massage therapy, look for investigations assessing another alternative or complementary treatment for this condition. If you cannot find research involving massage therapy and this condition, maybe it is time for you to get involved and help encourage massage research in this area.

Another way to stay current with research in a specific area of interest is to browse peer-reviewed journals that specialize in your field. This approach provides serendipitous discovery of unanticipated topics of relevance to your expertise and practice. Again, new journals appear frequently, but a few tried and true peer reviewed journals to investigate include:

Alternative Therapies (http://www.alternative-therapies.com/)

Medicine and Science in Sport and Exercise (http://journals.lww.com/acsm-msse/pages/default.aspx)

Journal of Preventative Medicine (http://www.elsevier.com/wps/find/journaldescription.cws_home/600644/description#description)

Journal of Bodywork and Movement Therapies (http://www.bodyworkmovementtherapies.com/)

Alternative and Complementary Therapies (http://www.liebertpub.com/products/product.aspx?pid=3)

Journal of Alternative and Complementary Medicine (http://www.liebertonline.com/loi/acm)

International Journal of Therapeutic Massage and Bodywork (http://www.ijtmb.org/index.php/ijtmb)

Alternative Medicine Review (http://www.ijtmb.org/index.php/ijtmb)

Complementary and Alternative Medicine (http://www.biomedcentral.com/bmccomplementalternmed)

Alternative Therapies in Health and Medicine (http://www.alternative-therapies.com)

If investigating a specific pathology (e.g., rheumatoid arthritis), go to a journal that specializes in medical conditions (e.g., *Journal of Rheumatology*). Use these same methods to look up client diseases or conditions you are unfamiliar with, or pharmaceuticals you have not encountered before. If you become overwhelmed when reading the research article, try reading the abstract.

Many journals also require the author to include a specific section on clinical applications that will be especially useful to you. The best authors can explain the most technical concepts and ideas simply for all to understand. Remember, you do not have to understand the full content of the article to learn from it. Use Box 5-2 to familiarize yourself with terms used in research studies and articles.

CHAT ROOM

Make it a habit to keep yourself up to date on new studies and discoveries in the field. This will help make you an outstanding massage therapy professional. But beware: a single study with exciting and often headline grabbing conclusions may not be supported over the course of time. Science generally advances in measured increments, so be sure to contrast new findings with foundational information. As you become a more seasoned consumer of scientific literature, you will hone your skill for understanding the evolving practice of massage therapy.

RESEARCH FUNDING

Research can be expensive. While some studies can be completed with little or no funding, most studies require significant funding. Where does this money come from? A creative researcher will learn to investigate government agencies and foundations, which are organizations with a mission to support research in specific areas. Business, corporations, local medical centers, doctors, universities or individuals will also support research efforts. Two important organizations that support massage therapy research are the Massage Therapy Foundation (MTF) (http://www.massagetherapyfoundation.org) and the National Center for Complementary and Alternative Medicine (NCCAM). (http://nccam.nih.gov).

The Massage Therapy Foundation is specifically designed to support small research studies investigating massage therapy. Grants are provided yearly to investigators who submit grants supporting their research efforts.

Grant writing is an art unto itself and is beyond the scope of this chapter. There are many websites devoted to this topic and interested individuals should start by visiting the website of the foundation or organization of interest.

NCCAM is a center within the National Institute of Health (http://www.nih.gov). The NIH is a government

BOX 5-2

Research Terminology

Accuracy. How close a result or measure is to the actual value. *For example, the temperature outside is 42.57° F. Due to limited accuracy of your thermometer, the temp reads 41° F.*

Bias. Prejudice, or tendency for preference; can be purposeful or accidental. *For example, if an investigator thinks massage improves range of motion, she may inadvertently record a larger angle when measuring movement at the shoulder.*

Blinding/Masking. A state where certain aspects of a study are kept from the participant and/or investigator to prevent bias. *For example, information on which treatment is the experimental treatment and which is the placebo treatment.*

Case report. A detailed report of the signs, symptoms, treatments, and results for an individual or case; typically an unusual case or condition.

Case study. A research study using an in-depth analysis of an individual or group over a long period of time to assess causation and factors involved in a condition.

Clinical trial. Biomedical or health-related research studies in human beings that follow a predefined protocol. ClinicalTrials.gov includes both interventional and observational types of studies. Interventional studies are those in which the research subjects are assigned by the investigator to a treatment or other intervention, and their outcomes are measured. Observational studies are those in which individuals are observed and their outcomes are measured by the investigators.[19]

Conceptual definition. A description of an idea that is measureable. *For example, defining how to measure a preference for massage therapy.*

Confounding variables. Any unanticipated or uncontrolled factor that might interfere with an experimental outcome. *For example, work associated stress may produce tightness in the trapezius that interferes with a massage study investigating the use of neck massage for increased range of motion in the cervical spine.*

Control group. A control is the standard by which experimental observations are evaluated. In many studies, one group of individuals will be given an experimental treatment, while the control group is given either a standard treatment for the condition or a placebo treatment.[19]

Data. (*sing.*, datum). Numerical or categorical information produced as part of a scientific study.

Data collection. The process of collecting data.

Dependant variable. What is measured in a study. *For example, heart rate or blood pressure.*

Double-blind. A study where both the investigators and the participants do not know treatment assignments (control or experimental) while data is collected and analyzed.

Extraneous variables. Any variable other than the independent variables that may affect the results and outcomes.

Exclusion criteria. A list of conditions, or reasons that a participant may not participate in a research study. *For example, neurological conditions, previous massage experience, or age limits.*

Experimental design. The organizational approach created to examine a scientific question free of bias and confounding variables in an effort to ensure accurate, reliable, and valid results.

Findings. Results of a study.

Hypothesis. A researcher's expected outcome of a study before data collection based on researching the literature and previous experience. The research hypothesis is the theory that is being tested in the study. A study tests the hypothesis, and accepts or rejects the hypothesis.

Independent variable. What the research manipulates or controls. *For example, group choice (experimental versus control), time of tests (5 minutes, 10 minutes after treatment), or sex (compare male and female groups).*

Institutional Review Board (IRB). An oversight committee within an organization where research is conducted whose charge is to protect research participants from undo harm caused by participation in research studies. The IRB evaluates and approves a study before the start of the research; monitors the study throughout the data collection; investigates any incidents that occur during the study; and evaluates a final report.

Investigator. A scientist or researcher.

Knowledge base. The sum total of what is known about a topic.

Limitations. Every study has drawbacks or inherent problems that cannot be overcome even by research design. A good design minimizes these drawbacks. A good researcher recognizes these drawbacks and lists them in an article to bring them to the attention of the reader. *For example, a narrow age range of participants.*

Mechanism of action. How a treatment produces an effect. *For example, increases in blood flow after a massage treatment would be a mechanism of action for massage therapy.*

Methods. The methods section of an article contains the procedures or protocols followed to complete a study. This can be thought of as the recipe for the study. It should be detailed enough that another research could repeat the study exactly.

Operational definition. Exact process by which a variable is measured.

Outcome variables. What you are measuring in a study. *For example, heart rate.*

Participant inclusion criteria. The criteria (often health or demographics related) used to define the subject population for a given study. *For example, people over the age of 55 might be excluded from a specific study for experimental reasons related to the aging process.*

Peer review. Process where subject matter experts assess the quality of a study, grant, or manuscript.

Peer review journal. Scientific magazine that publishes peer reviewed research.

Placebo. A sham treatment.

Placebo effect. A change in a participants' condition due to the thought that they are receiving a beneficial treatment.

Precision. Another term for accuracy of measurement.

(Continued)

BOX 5-2, cont'd

Qualitative research. Research that seeks to understand processes that underlie various behavioral patterns. Qualitative research revolves around words and themes in lieu of numbers and seeks answers to questions of how and why.

Quantitative research. Research that measures variables numerically. These values are analyzed statistically to examine relationships between variables. Quantitative research revolves around numbers rather than words.

Reliability. Ability of a test to yield the same results on repeated trials.

Results. Outcome of your assessment, measure, or study.

Research literacy. The ability to locate, read, and understand research literature.

Research question. The specific information to be determined by a study; specific question you want to answer.

Research studies. Experiments or investigations designed to learn new information about a particular topic or question.

Research team. A group of investigators or scientists working on a project.

Sample population. A group of individuals whose characteristics fit the experimental inclusion criteria.

Statistically significant outcome. A result that statistical analysis indicates is not the result of random chance.

Statistician. A person who uses statistics to assess outcomes and results of an investigation.

Scientific method. An accepted process or standards, which define the protocols used to create new knowledge through research.

Sham treatment. A placebo or fake treatment designed to mimic an experimental treatment for comparison purposes.

Subject/participant. Individual in a research study.

Treatment. An experimental intervention. *For example massage, heat pack, acupuncture.*

Validity. How well a test assesses what it is designed to measure. *For example, a valid test for range of motion should differentiate between joint laxity versus muscle tightness around the joint.*

---

agency designed to support the best research in the country. Funding from NIH is highly competitive and scientists often work for years to gain funding. NCCAM is a "center" that specializes in CAM. While the budget for NCCAM is small compared with other institutes within NIH, it specifically works to support CAM such as massage therapy. Massage therapy studies are not limited to applying to NCCAM; if a study assesses the effect of massage therapy on a specific disease (e.g., multiple sclerosis), the researcher may apply to the institute within NIH that specializes in neurological disorders. Obtaining funding is a long and often arduous process that requires a thick skin, hard work, and constant effort.

GET INVOLVED

How can massage therapists support research efforts? The easiest way is to become involved with an organization that supports research. You can become a member, donate money, or donate your time through volunteering. One easy way to support an organization financially is to donate the price of one massage each year to an organization that funds massage therapy research. Additionally, researchers are often looking for qualified massage therapists to assist with providing treatments for studies. That is, many studies collate data from multiple "sites" where massage therapists from across a region or country submit data from their practices. This research participation can be volunteer or paid work, and advances the profession.

Encouraging clients, family, or friends to participate is another way to support massage therapy research. Finally, supporting the continuing need for quality research through your professional organization, to other therapists and medical professionals, and to your political representatives

(NIH is funded through Congress so get in touch with your representatives and tell them how important NCCAM is to your profession. There are those in Congress who wish to eliminate NCCAM from the NIH[20]). Even seemingly small efforts when combined with those of other therapists can make a tremendous difference to the overall goal of establishing an outstanding research knowledge base for massage therapy.

So, back to Sarah. How *do* you answer her original question: how does massage work? Well, you can take several avenues depending on the client. You might want to try a short and specific answer: "massage works because human touch is a powerful and effective means of restoring balance to the muscles and soft tissues. There are a number of beneficial mechanical and chemical changes that take place when therapeutic touch is applied; here is a great article that references original research on the benefits of massage." If your client is a medical person or seeks a more in-depth answer, you can go into detail on the current knowledge base regarding massage and back pain. Never hesitate to offer to look deeper into a client's question and provide more information on their next visit. In doing this, you show a commitment to your client, a willingness to say "I don't know," a willingness to learn, and that you will put effort into helping them to more fully understand their condition and their treatment.

E-RESOURCES

©volve

http://evolve.elsevier.com/Salvo/MassageTherapy

- Chapter challenge
- Flash cards
- Additional information
- Weblinks

BIBLIOGRAPHY

1. Field T et al: Massage therapy reduces anxiety and enhances EEG pattern of alertness and math computations, *Int J Neurosci* 86(3-4):197-205, 1996.
2. Field T et al: Job stress reduction therapies, *Altern Ther Health Med* 3(4):54-56, 1997.
3. Burke C et al: The development of a massage service for cancer patients, *Clin Oncol (R Coll Radiol)* 6(6):381-384, 1994.
4. Corbin L: Safety and efficacy of massage therapy for patients with cancer, *Cancer Control* 12(3):158-164, 2005.
5. Moyer CA, Rounds J, Hannum JW: A meta-analysis of massage therapy research, *Psychol Bull* 130(1):3-18, 2004.
6. Collinge W, Wentworth R, Sabo S: Integrating complementary therapies into community mental health practice: an exploration, *J Altern Complement Med* 11(3):569-574, 2005.
7. Diego MA et al: Spinal cord patients benefit from massage therapy, *Int J Neurosci* 112(2):133-142, 2002.
8. Price C: Body-oriented therapy in recovery from child sexual abuse: an efficacy study, *Altern Ther Health Med* 11(5):46-57, 2005.
9. Danneskiold-Samsoe B, Bartels EM, Genefke I: Treatment of torture victims: a longitudinal clinical study, *Torture* 17(1):11-17, 2007.
10. Field T: Massage therapy, *Med Clin North Am* 86(1):163-171, 2002.
11. Field T et al: Massage therapy effects on depressed pregnant women, *J Psychosom Obstet Gynaecol* 25(2):115-122, 2004.
12. Field T et al: Massage and relaxation therapies' effects on depressed adolescent mothers, *Adolescence* 31(124):903-911, 1996.
13. Perlman AI et al: Massage therapy for osteoarthritis of the knee: a randomized controlled trial, *Arch Intern Med* 166(22):2533-2538, 2006.
14. Field T: Massage therapy for infants and children, *J Dev Behav Pediatr* 16(2):105-111, 1995.
15. Field T: Preterm infant massage therapy studies: an American approach, *Semin Neonatol* 7(6):487-494, 2002.
16. Field T et al: Children with asthma have improved pulmonary functions after massage therapy, *J Pediatr* 132(5):854-858, 1998.
17. Ouchia K et al: Changes in cerebral blood flow under the prone condition with and without massage, *Neurosci Lett* 407(2):131-135, 2006.
18. Guzzetta A et al: Massage accelerates brain development and the maturation of visual function, *J Neurosci* 29(18):6042-6051, 2009.
19. NIH: Understanding clinical trials, Clinical Trials (website): http://clinicaltrials.gov/ct2/info/understand#Q01. Accessed June 16, 2010.
20. Novella SM: President Obama—defund NCCAM, Science-Based Medicine (website): http://www.sciencebasedmedicine.org/?p=341. Accessed June 16, 2010.

FURTHER RESEARCH

Anderson PG, Cutshall SM: Massage therapy: a comfort intervention for cardiac surgery patients, *Clin Nurse Spec* 21(3):161-165; quiz 166-167, 2007.

Andrews L et al: The use of alternative therapies by children with asthma: a brief report, *J Paediatr Child Health* 34(2):131-134, 1998.
Arnold LE: Alternative treatments for adults with attention-deficit hyperactivity disorder (ADHD), *Ann N Y Acad Sci* 931:310-341, 2001.
Ayas S et al: The effect of abdominal massage on bowel function in patients with spinal cord injury, *Am J Phys Med Rehabil* 85(12):951-955, 2006.
Back C et al: The effects of employer-provided massage therapy on job satisfaction, workplace stress, and pain and discomfort, *Holist Nurs Pract* 23(1):19-31, 2009.
Billhult A et al: The effect of massage on cellular immunity, endocrine and psychological factors in women with breast cancer: a randomized controlled clinical trial, *Auton Neurosci* 140(1-2):88-95, 2008.
Billhult A, Dahlberg K: A meaningful relief from suffering experiences of massage in cancer care, *Cancer Nurs* 24(3):180-184, 2001.
Biondi DM: Physical treatments for headache: a structured review, *Headache* 45(6):738-746, 2005.
Braganza S, Ozuah PO, Sharif I: The use of complementary therapies in inner-city asthmatic children, *J Asthma* 40(7):823-827, 2003.
Brattberg G: Connective tissue massage in the treatment of fibromyalgia, *Eur J Pain* 3(3):235-244, 1999.
Bronfort G et al: Non-invasive physical treatments for chronic/recurrent headache, *Cochrane Database Syst Rev* (3):CD001878, 2004.
Brosseau L et al: Deep transverse friction massage for treating tendinitis, *Cochrane Database Syst Rev* (4):CD003528, 2002.
Ernst E: Complementary medicine, *Curr Opin Rheumatol* 15(2):151-155, 2003.
Fernandez-de-Las-Penas C et al: Are manual therapies effective in reducing pain from tension-type headache? A systematic review, *Clin J Pain* 22(3):278-285, 2006.
Field T et al: Bulimic adolescents benefit from massage therapy, *Adolescence* 33(131):555-563, 1998.
Field T et al: Burn injuries benefit from massage therapy, *J Burn Care Rehabil* 19(3):241-244, 1998.
Field T et al: Cortisol decreases and serotonin and dopamine increase following massage therapy, *Int J Neurosci* 115(10):1397-1413, 2005.
Field T et al: Labor pain is reduced by massage therapy, *J Psychosom Obstet Gynaecol* 18(4):286-291, 1997.
Field T et al: Moderate versus light pressure massage therapy leads to greater weight gain in preterm infants, *Infant Behav Dev* 29(4):574-578, 2006.
Field T, Delange J, Hernandez Reif M: Movement and massage therapy reduces fibromyalgia pain, *J Bodyw Mov Ther* 1:49-52, 2003.
Field T, Hernandez-Reif M, Diego M: Newborns of depressed mothers who received moderate versus light pressure massage during pregnancy, *Infant Behav Dev* 29(1):54-58, 2006.
Field T: Early interventions for infants of depressed mothers, *Pediatrics* 102(5 suppl E):1305-1310, 1998.
Field T: Maternal depression effects on infants and early interventions, *Prev Med* 27(2):200-203, 1998.
Field TM et al: Adolescents with attention deficit hyperactivity disorder benefit from massage therapy, *Adolescence* 33(129):103-108, 1998.

Gallagher G, Rae CP, Kinsella J: Treatment of pain in severe burns, *Am J Clin Dermatol* 1(6):329-335, 2000.

Gray RA: The use of massage therapy in palliative care, *Complement Ther Nurs Midwifery* 6(2):77-82, 2000.

Hernandez-Reif M et al: Breast cancer patients have improve immune and neuroendocrine function following massage therapy, *J Psychosom* 57:45-52, 2003.

Hernandez-Reif M et al: Low back pain is reduced and range of motion increased after massage therapy, *Int J Neurosci* 106:131-145, 2001.

Hernandez-Reif M et al: Migraine headaches were reduced by massage therapy, *Int J Neurosci* 96:1-11, 1998.

Ironson F et al: Massage therapy is associated with enhancement of the immune system's cytotoxic capacity, *Int J Neurosci* 84:205-217, 1996.

Ironson G et al: Massage therapy is associated with enhancement of the immune system's cytotoxic capacity, *Int J Neurosci* 84(1-4):205-217, 1996.

Khilnani S et al: Massage therapy improves mood and behavior of students with attention-deficit/hyperactivity disorder, *Adolescence* 38(152):623-638, 2003.

Lemstra M, Olszynski WP: The effectiveness of multidisciplinary rehabilitation in the treatment of fibromyalgia: a randomized controlled trial, *Clin J Pain* 21(2):166-174, 2005.

Reilly T, Ekblom B: The use of recovery methods post-exercise, *J Sports Sci* 23(6):619-627, 2005.

Sefton JM, Yarar C, Berry JW, Pasco DD: Effect of therapeutic massage on peripheral blood flow as assessed by skin temperature measures in the neck and shoulders, *J Altern Complement Med* 16(7):723-732, 2010.

Smith LL et al: The effects of athletic massage on delayed onset muscle soreness, creatine kinase, and neutrophil count: a preliminary report, *J Orthop Sports Phys Ther* 19(2):93-99, 1994.

Weerapong P, Hume PA, Kolt GS: The mechanisms of massage and effects on performance, muscle recovery and injury prevention, *Sports Med* 35(3):235-256, 2005.

MATCHING I

Place the letter of the answer next to the term or phrase that best describes it.

A. Analytical
B. Applied
C. Basic
D. Clinical trial

E. Confounding variables
F. Control group
G. Descriptive
H. Experimental

I. Placebo effect
J. Peer review
K. Scientific method
L. Validity

_____ 1. A controlled look at the safety and effectiveness of a treatment using human subjects

_____ 2. Steps taken to test the hypothesis of a research study; _____ design

_____ 3. Group of techniques used to investigate questions and develop new knowledge through gathering of evidence, experimentation, and testing theories

_____ 4. Uses investigations to examine questions on a functional level; _____ research

_____ 5. Includes surveys and interview studies; _____ research

_____ 6. How well a test assesses what it is designed to measure

_____ 7. Participants in a research study that do not receive treatment

_____ 8. Belief that a treatment or drug will be beneficial, whether or not it is actually administered; this effect can produce changes in the outcome measures of a research study

_____ 9. Includes in-depth investigations into complex issues and mechanisms; _____ research

_____ 10. Process whereby research is scrutinized by a group of experts in the same or a similar field

_____ 11. Influencing factors in research that cannot be controlled

_____ 12. Aims to find fundamental information at the molecular, cellular, or tissue level; research typically conducted in a laboratory; _____ research

MATCHING II

Place the letter of the answer next to the term or phrase that best describes it.

A. Abstract
B. Accuracy
C. Discussion
D. Findings

E. Hypothesis
F. Investigators
G. Journals
H. Methods

I. Reliability
J. Research literacy
K. Research question
L. Sample population

_____ 1. Ability of a test to yield the same results on repeated trials

_____ 2. Section of a research article that explains the results, the relevance to the literature, and any limitations inherent in the study

_____ 3. Specific information to be determined by the study

_____ 4. Scientific publications that distribute results of studies in specific fields, or areas of specialization

_____ 5. The participants in a research study

_____ 6. Summarizes a research article and findings

_____ 7. Expected result of a research study based on background research and knowledge

_____ 8. Ability to locate, read, and understand research literature

_____ 9. Those who are performing the research study; the scientists or researchers

_____ 10. Indicates how close the result is to the actual value of what is being measured

_____ 11. Section of a research article that contains the procedures or protocols followed to complete a study. This can be thought of as the recipe for the study.

_____ 12. The results of a research study

CASE STUDY

Form and Function

Sally is a massage therapist. Harold is an acupuncturist. Theresa is a medical doctor who recently decided to learn more about how to integrate less invasive, nonpharmaceutical treatments for her patients with chronic pain. Each made a good case for their approach, but Theresa asked Sally and Harold if they would be willing to give her one research study explaining the benefit of their clinical method on lower back pain.

Sally submitted a peer reviewed study titled "Reduction of anterior pelvic tilt using massage therapy reduces low back pain." The study included 5 subjects presenting with lower back pain and no history of disc pathology, nerve pathology, broken bones, or systemic pathology know to contribute to chronic pain. Each of the subjects presented with hyperlordosis, noted specifically by an increased anterior pelvic tilt of 5-10 degrees. Each subject was treated by the same massage therapist, using the same sequence of strokes. Subjects were instructed to refrain from using pharmaceuticals within 4 hours of each treatment, and to note each use of pharmaceuticals during the duration of the study. They were also instructed not to receive any other treatment for the condition. Each subject received five 40 minute treatments over the course of one month, 4 out of 5 of the subjects had significant relief of symptoms. One subject had moderate relief following the first two treatments, but no significant improvement subsequently. The study concluded that massage therapy reduces lower back pain resulting from anterior pelvic tilt. It was funded by Healing Hands Inc., a privately owned chain of clinical massage therapy clinics, and conducted on site at one of their facilities.

Harold submitted a peer reviewed study titled "Acupuncture significantly reduces lower back pain." The study was conducted over 24 months and included 121 subjects. 19 of the original subjects dropped because their health care provider disapproved. Subjects selected were evaluated for potential causes of lower back pain, and were accepted if cause of pain fell into one of 3 categories: herniated disc, lumbar ligament sprain, or strength imbalance between the hip flexors and lumbar extensors. Acupuncture treatment protocols differed depending on the cause of pain, and followed the traditional model of Chinese Medicine used for each condition. Each subject was consistently treated by one of 10 acupuncturists who received training from different institutions. 60% of subjects reported complete relief of symptoms. 20% reported moderate relief of symptoms. 10 reported moderate relief of back pain, but experienced new pain in another area of the body. 10% had no significant change in symptoms. The study was conducted at a respected university, and funded by the National Institutes of Health.

What are the pros and cons of each study design?

Are there any elements in either design that may affect the reliability of outcomes?

Are the study designs too narrow or too broad? Explain

Describe how you would improve each of the studies.

If you were to submit either of these studies for your client's consideration, would you explain the shortcomings even if you believe the outcome is reliable?

CRITICAL THINKING

If massage is beneficial for helping injuries to heal, why is massage contraindicated during the first few days after injury?

CHAPTER 6

Effects of Massage Therapy

JoEllen M. Sefton, PhD, ATC, CMT

LEARNING OBJECTIVES

After completing this chapter, the student should be able to:

- Describe how massage therapy works, including its mechanical, physiologic, and psychologic effects.
- Explain how massage therapy affects the cardiovascular system and blood circulation.
- Define massage therapy's effects on the lymphatic system and immunity.
- Describe effects of massage therapy on the musculoskeletal system and on connective tissues.
- Identify massage therapy's effects on the nervous and endocrine systems.
- State how massage therapy affects the skin, internal organs, and other body systems.
- List psychologic aspects of massage therapy.
- Describe whole body effects of massage therapy and indications for specific conditions and populations.
- Explain common misconceptions and false claims related to massage therapy treatment and effects.
- Describe the importance of keeping up to date on new massage therapy knowledge.

http://evolve.elsevier.com/Salvo/MassageTherapy

INTRODUCTION

As massage therapists, we believe that what we do makes a difference for our clients. You have probably already seen the beneficial results in those with whom you work or experienced the positive effects of massage in your own body. These effects can be as specific as the elimination of lower back pain, or as general as an overall feeling of well-being. The challenge to the profession is how to define and describe the effects of massage therapy.

It is very important, as a profession, to separate fact from myth. Like all medical and health care fields, much of what we thought we knew when we went to school has been brought into question as we improve our research into the effects of our therapies and treatments. Science is a constant process of discovery; we investigate, learn new things, replace old ideas, and investigate more. As discussed in Chapter 5, it is vital for all massage therapists to stay current on new knowledge being developed in our profession, and to share this knowledge with clients. As we learn more about how massage therapy affects the body's structures and systems, we may change how we apply our techniques to improve our clients' clinical outcomes. New knowledge can also elevate the overall standing of the field of massage therapy in the health, wellness, and medical communities.

The goal of this chapter is to discuss what we currently know about the effects of massage therapy. This chapter is not intended to be an in-depth assessment of the actual research, but rather a survey of what we know and do not know, and where our knowledge base stands. Perhaps this will lead you to further and continued investigation of the new research in these areas.

HOW MASSAGE THERAPY WORKS

If you are asked, "How does massage therapy work?", what would you say? Where would you even begin to answer this question? If you love spa massage you might immediately think about the wonderful relaxation massage therapy can produce and answer with a description of the importance of wellness and stress reduction. If you work with athletes you might answer with a detailed description about increases in blood flow, performance, and recovery. If you work in a hospital setting you might explain the benefits of touch in calming anxiety associated with cancer treatment or hospice care.

Massage therapy is an expansive profession encompassing a large variety of techniques and treatments. This incredible diversity makes this question even more challenging to answer. If we were to break this question down into type of effects, we might answer this question with more success. Let us begin by grouping effects into three basic categories: mechanical, physiologic, and psychologic. This grouping may help us to understand and investigate massage effects; however, it is important to understand that each category constantly interacts with and influences the others.

Mechanical Effects

The many benefits of massage therapy result from, quite literally, "hands on" manual manipulation of soft tissue, including squeezing, pushing, pulling, rubbing, stretching, and compressing. To most, these mechanical effects seem like the most logical consequences of massage therapy. However, these effects can be difficult to research and measure. It has long been thought that the mechanical forces used during massage treatment serve to push blood into and out of tissues, create changes in muscle fibers, and even move substances through the digestive tract. Current research is assessing the validity of these claims with mixed results. In the end, most massage effects can be related back to mechanical forces involving touch (or anticipated touch) during the massage therapy treatment (Figure 6-1).

Physiologic Effects

Changes in blood pressure, hormones, neurotransmitters, muscle fiber structure, and many other processes are the result of physiologic changes thought to result from massage therapy. Again, these are often the direct result of mechanical or psychologic effects. Physiologic changes are often easier to conceptualize and measure than other less quantifiable outcomes. As such, these physiologic alterations provided by massage are essential for scientifically verifying the myriad of benefits of massage therapy. For example, if mechanical pressure does help to move blood flow through muscle tissue, the resulting physiologic changes of improved tissue oxidation, nutrient exchange, and waste removal are the primary mechanisms resulting in the benefit of the therapy. Likewise, when a client relaxes and stress is reduced from a treatment, any resulting modulation in stress hormones or neurotransmitters would be considered a physiologic effect resulting in an overall benefit to the client.

Psychologic Effects

Tempered anxiety and stress levels, and improved well-being are some of the most well documented benefits resulting from massage therapy. Abstract psychologic concepts such as anxiety and stress can be easily measured through the use of questionnaires, surveys, and interviews. However, the difficulty of translating thoughts and feelings into numerical values suggests why psychologic factors are more challenging to quantify than the physiologic changes typically assessed in numerical values. Nonetheless, it is hard to deny that psychological effects influence physiologic outcomes. A client under a great deal of psychologic stress will produce increased cortisol and other hormones. This may affect the physiologic outcomes expected from massage therapy treatment.

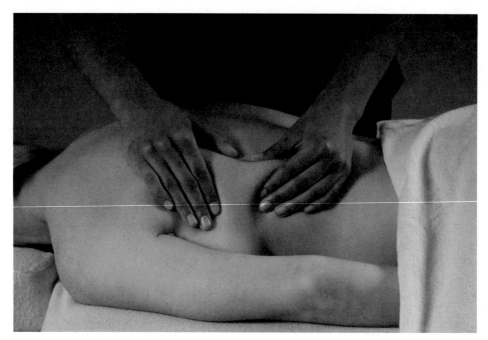

FIGURE 6-1 Many of the documented massage benefits are due to mechanical effects.

WHITNEY LOWE

Born: December 20, 1961

"Imagination is more important than knowledge."
—Albert Einstein

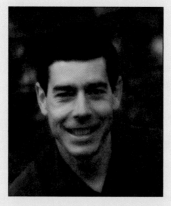

Whitney Lowe's earliest experiences laid a strong foundation for his vanguard contributions to the Massage Therapy profession. He was strongly influenced by his parents, both of whom encouraged his creativity and academic achievement. His mother Audrey was an audiologist who inspired Whitney's love of science and academic realization. She emphasized scholarly challenges, providing strong support for the achievement of her children's goals and dreams. His father Wade is a guitar and violin maker who cultivated Whitney's appreciation for the artistic elements found in nearly all facets of life. Lowe was captivated by the musicians who visited his father's store, absorbing as much as he could about what those musicians were contemplating and what they were creating.

As a young adult, Whitney attended Berklee College of Music in Boston, focusing his energy on becoming a musician himself. And though he chose not to continue that pursuit, the experience expanded his appreciation for the importance of being creative as he embarked upon his subsequent endeavors. But his curiosity led him toward the human mind and body, and he enrolled in the graduate program in psychology at Georgia State University. His professional objective was to become a counselor.

At the time, his wife was enrolled in massage school. Her stories about the body mind connection piqued his interest, and his ready access to massage therapy confirmed her reports. In the late 1980s, Whitney began to feel disillusioned by not being able to study the things he thought were important and valuable in his graduate studies, so he put psychology on hold and enrolled in massage therapy school with the intention of using his new skills to pay for the remainder of his degree in

If, at this point, you are thinking that this "effects stuff" seems like one big complex cycle, then you are getting the big picture! This is exactly why research into the mind-body interworking of massage therapy is such a difficult task. Let us proceed to what we do know about the effects of massage on different systems and structures. However, keep this complex cycle in mind while we are exploring the individual effects of massage therapy.

> *"He who feels it knows it more."*
> —Bob Marley

HOW MASSAGE THERAPY AFFECTS SPECIFIC STRUCTURES AND SYSTEMS

Cardiovascular System

Effects of massage therapy on the cardiovascular system naturally go along with changes in circulation. Massage therapy has been reported to decrease blood pressure, heart rate, and variations in heart rate.[1,2] These effects aid in cardiovascular health. Decreases in systolic, diastolic, and arterial pressure along with heart rate were found after 45-60 minutes of massage treatment in a study of 236 individuals.[3] These changes are thought to result from influences on parasympathetic nervous system activity. The autonomic nervous system controls involuntary nervous system function (see Chapters 23 and 29). While massage therapy has definitive influences on the cardiovascular system, research sufficiently indicates that massage therapy is safe for cardiovascular disease patients undergoing treatment, surgery, or rehabilitation.[4,5] Massage may reduce the workload on the heart by producing reductions in blood pressure. Thus, under normal scenarios, there is no reason to believe that massage would precipitate a pathological cardiac event.

Early studies[6,7] demonstrated increases in blood platelet count after massage. Recent studies[8] indicate increases in red and white blood cell counts in prostate cancer patients when massage was combined with other treatments. Similar

WHITNEY LOWE (*continued*)

counseling. But he got hooked on massage, fascinated by the exciting new insights developing in the field. There was so much to learn, and massage therapy became a passionate pursuit he had not anticipated.

Having worked in a wide variety of practice environments for several years, Whitney's keenness for science and research led him toward a more focused examination of the clinical applications of massage. Living in Atlanta, he found himself spending much of his spare time in the medical library at Emory University, scouring the wealth of resources relevant to improving his clinical practice of massage. During this time, he was also teaching at the Atlanta School of Massage Therapy, infusing his instruction with the clinical research he was discovering. He made it a goal to bring a bold and solid academic foundation to his courses in massage.

Whitney left Atlanta in mid-1990s and moved to Oregon where he developed OMERI—Orthopedic Massage Education & Research Institute. Recognizing a lack of resources that were useful for massage professionals in educational environments, his focus shifted away from clinical practice toward developing tools for clinical education and research. He began writing training materials related to the subjects he was teaching, including orthopedic assessment, pathology, kinesiology, and biomechanics. These original writings became the foundation for his first publication: *Functional Assessment in Massage Therapy*. He has since published two seminal resources for clinically oriented massage therapists: *Orthopedic Massage: Theory and Technique*, and *Orthopedic Assessment in Massage Therapy*. He has also written several peer reviewed articles and contributed to numerous texts on the subjects of orthopedic massage and teaching massage.

His parents taught him to do best in every endeavor, with integrity and honesty, and without getting caught up in the desire for fame, fortune or personal gain. "Integrity, honesty and critical thinking are some of the key principles that guide my personal and professional endeavors." Whitney names Albert Einstein among his mentors, not just because of his academic genius, but equally for his social stance and way of understanding the bigger picture. In his own focus on the transmission of information, a crucial guiding principle has been that encouraging creativity and open questioning is far more important that stuffing students' minds with data and details.

Whitney continues to bring innovative learning experiences to students and practitioners, advancing the appreciation and understanding for some of the more challenging scientific aspects of massage. He is currently spending much of his professional effort on developing high-quality online resources for teaching complex clinical reasoning skills, kinesiology, assessment and decision making in clinical treatment. And he's never abandoned his love of music and the arts.

increases were found in multiple immune system measures in a comparison between massage and aromatherapy massage.[9] Changes in cell counts reinforce the evidence supporting circulatory improvements as a mechanism of effect. This overall effect likely results from a combination of physiologic modulations such as increased blood vessel dilation; increases in acetylcholine and histamine, which increase and prolong blood vessel dilation; increased tissue temperature, which affects metabolic processes; and others. All of these modulate local circulation and improve exchange of nutrients and gases between the blood and cells.

Blood Circulation

One of the most commonly held beliefs in the profession is that massage therapy promotes healing and wellness through improved circulation. Improved blood flow to tissues would theoretically create enhanced delivery of metabolic fuels, removal of metabolic byproducts and improved gas exchange. These effects would promote tissue healing and help to maintain tissue viability and functionality. Improved circulation of lymph promotes enhanced immune system function (see section on Lymphatic System and Immunity). This theory of action seems intuitive as we consider the mechanical effects expected from adding rhythmic pressure, squeezing, lifting and shaking of tissue. As therapists, we can see hyperemia or red appearance of skin resulting from our work and feel the warming and change in tissue as treatment progresses.

The research, however, has been equivocal in this area, possibly due to the inherent difficulty in assessing changes in circulation from the treatment without interfering with these same treatment effects. An additional challenge in assessing changes in circulation comes from the fact that there are multiple types of circulation. When we discuss circulation, are we referring to changes in arterial volume, venous flow, capillary exchange, or lymph drainage? Even at the level of arterial flow, does massage affect change in flow in large supply arteries, or do we think this increase in flow occurs at small arteries supplying the tissue? A small change in flow in the femoral artery might not be detectable, but this same change in tiny arteries supplying tibialis anterior might produce important increases in blood supply. Finally, do these theoretical improvements occur just at the level of the skin where we feel the warmth, or does this increase in circulation occur in muscle tissue where it might create an improved healing environment for muscle injury? As you can see, these are complex issues, but progress is being made and a clearer picture is emerging.

One study[10] assessed the effect of mechanical pressure on capillary flow rate and blood viscosity after traditional Chinese medical massage. Measuring changes in massaged tissue compared with static tissue found increases resulting from enhanced hemodynamic mechanisms "promoting blood circulation and removing blood stasis." Other attempts to measure blood flow directly during massage have been hampered by technical constraints. Nonetheless, findings from several studies employing indirect blood flow assessment techniques suggest that massage increases circulation to the treated area.[1,11] For instance, assessment of intramuscular temperature demonstrated increased temperature after massage treatment.[12] A recent technical advancement in indirect flow assessment that has proved very useful for massage research is evaluation of noncontact surface temperature. This technique allows for a dynamic assessment of a specific point or changes across large areas. One study using this technique[13] indicated significant improvements in surface temperature not only in areas of treatment (neck and shoulders), but also down to the mid/lower back and down the arms along the treatment dermatomes. Naturally, the next question is does this represent simply a change in surface temperature or does this increase in circulation affect the deeper muscles and other structures? In a follow-up study,[14] changes in blood oxidation levels at the muscle were found in conjunction with changes in skin surface temperature after massage therapy. This work reinforces the theory that changes in blood flow occur at the muscle level as well and may be a primary mechanism of effect for the benefits of massage therapy (Figure 6-2).

Summary of Massage Effects on Cardiovascular Functions and Blood Circulation. Research to date suggests massage therapy provides the following physiologic improvements through a combination of mechanisms:

- Increases capillary flow rate, blood viscosity, and filtration rate
- Increases blood flow to the skin and muscular tissue
- Increases blood oxidation levels
- Increases surface tissue temperatures of the treated and adjacent areas
- Increases red and white blood cell and platelet counts
- Decreases heart rate, blood pressure, and variations in heart rate

Lymphatic System and Immunity

Continuing our discussion of circulation, there is both direct and indirect evidence that massage helps to promote lymphatic flow and drainage. Studies consistently show the effectiveness of massage for decreasing edema and lymphedema.[15-18]

Research to examine the physiologic effects of massage therapy on immunity is intriguing. Some introductory studies have indicated that massage promotes killer T cell levels and other measures of immune function in individuals with HIV infection and cancer.[19-21] Other studies suggest massage therapy combined with other treatments may increase white blood cell counts in cancer patients.[8,22] However, a randomized control trial (RCT) failed to find any effects of massage on many of these same measures.[23] RCTs are larger, more rigorous studies that, when well designed, can produce more reliable, accurate, and generalizable results. While smaller

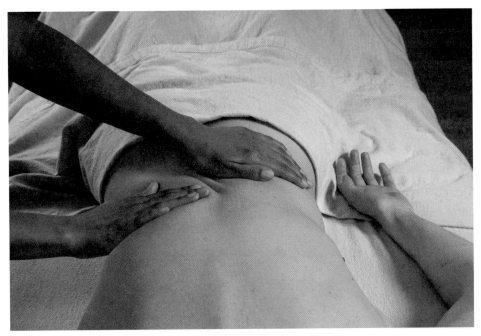

FIGURE 6-2 Massage increases blood flow to skin and muscular tissue.

studies are important to prove concepts, RCTs are an important step in proving the effects of massage therapy to the medical community. Collectively, cancer patients can benefit from massage due to increased lymph flow, and decreased anxiety, pain, and stress. New specialized training for massage therapists preparing to work in the field of oncology massage has been developed to teach safe and effective treatments in this rapidly expanding field of care.

Clearly, much remains to be done in this area. However, until definitive results on the physiologic mechanisms are determined, the positive physiologic effects suggest a clear rationale for the use of massage therapy for those with compromised immune function, cancer, other serious diseases, and for the general promotion of immune system function and overall health and well-being.

Summary of Massage Effects on the Lymphatic System and Immune Functions. Research to date suggests massage therapy may:
- Assist in lymphatic drainage
- Reduce edema and lymphedema
- Promote increases in lymphocyte levels
- Promote immune system health and function and overall well-being through combined mechanical, physiologic, and psychologic therapeutic effects

Musculoskeletal System

It may seem to even the newest massage student that massage must have significant effects on the musculoskeletal system. These are the tissues that we study, think about, and try to influence most often. The majority of massage therapy is prescribed or sought out for muscular aches and pains.

How then can there be any question that massage therapy directly affects musculoskeletal tissues? In reality, this is a very difficult area to study. How do you assess if a typical massage therapy session separates muscle fibers without cutting into the tissues themselves? (Most clients are opposed to that for obvious reasons). Much of what we know about massage and muscular tissues has been passed down over the years with little supporting evidence. That does not mean these ideas are incorrect or that massage is not beneficial. It simply means the research will validate some theories and invalidate others. As therapists we can see and feel changes. It is up to researchers to discover ways to assess and quantify these effects and enable us to move forward with the next generation of evidence-based massage therapy approaches.

So what *do* we know? Massage therapy improves range of motion (ROM) (Figure 6-3). Several studies have indicated an increased ability to move a joint through the entire range of motion after massage treatment.[24-27] This may be due to decreased pain or stiffness, decreased muscle tightness, or increased muscle length. The mechanism of action is not clear, but there are clear improved client outcomes. Clinically, improved ROM is an important treatment goal that may result in overall improvement in activities of daily living and general well-being. Flexibility is closely related to range of motion. The literature assessing flexibility is less clear, as most studies do not indicate improvement in flexibility after massage.[28-32] It is interesting to note that current research is questioning our understanding of flexibility and the value of stretching overall. It is likely that the massage therapy profession's thoughts in these areas will change in the future; a helpful way to track this is to watch research literature for the evolving knowledge on this topic.

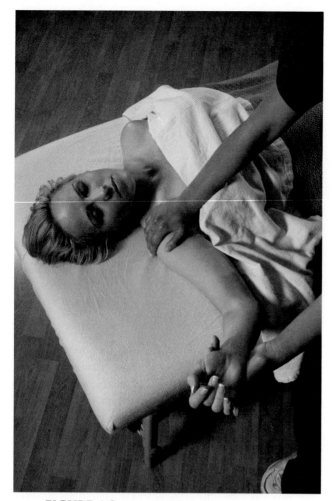

FIGURE 6-3 Massage improves range of motion.

There is little or no evidence to suggest that massage therapy actually lengthens muscle fibers as is commonly taught. There is, however, evidence that massage reduces tension in the muscle tendon unit,[1] which may have the effect of allowing the muscle to elongate. The aforementioned increase in blood flow and temperature may also lead to optimal muscle function and decreased spasm and tightness. Several studies[24,33-34] have assessed muscle electrical activity (electromyography or EMG) after massage. These studies have indicated a decrease in EMG activity after massage therapy. The difference in the findings comes from the variations in experimental design and interpretation. EMG can be used to assess multiple factors and its interpretation can be complex. A decreased EMG signal does not necessarily indicate a decrease in muscle strength or function; it may suggest a decrease in electrical activity. For example, a fatigued muscle recruits additional motor units to complete a task; this results in an increased EMG signal. Thus, the lower EMG signal can represent a more efficient muscular contraction.

While we are discussing muscle function, we must discuss muscle dysfunction. Trigger points are a common area of concentration for massage therapists. Working on these centers of myofascial dysfunction[35] has been shown clinically to relieve pain, increase range of motion, and restore function.[36] Pressure to trigger points has been shown to affect the parasympathetic nervous system, influencing heart rate and variability as well as other factors.[2,37] Trigger point work itself has been shown to reduce headaches,[38] as well as back and neck pain.[36,39-42] More research has been completed in this area than other areas of massage. While the positive results are encouraging, much remains to be learned regarding the cause and effect of trigger points and how to optimize protocols used to treat them.

Postevent massage has been thought to help "flush out toxins" and decrease postexercise soreness, called delayed onset muscle soreness (DOMS). Research investigating DOMS has been equivocal.[43,44] One study demonstrated a decrease in DOMS, edema, and creatine kinase levels (an indicator of muscle function and damage) after massage treatment.[45] Another study[46] found a possible improvement in perceived soreness, but not muscle swelling or range of motion. Other studies have failed to show a conclusive benefit.[1,47,48] It is important that we be careful about our claims in this area. Additional work is needed to further understand whether there is any effect in this area and any underlying mechanisms involved.

Another common claim for massage therapy is that it tones weak muscles. Massage does not make a muscle stronger. Massage may improve muscle health and function as discussed previously, especially when combined with active or passive movement and stretching. Improving circulation and neuromuscular activity in muscles in individuals with paralysis or on bed rest may help to delay muscle atrophy, reduce spasms, and improve overall wellness. Massage has also been reported to influence postural control, though little work has been completed in this area. As massage reduces spasms and assists in the restoration of symmetrical neuromuscular functioning, it is possible that postural control may be improved. Research is being conducted in this area and watching the literature for new developments is highly recommended.

Finally, can massage therapy have any effect on the skeletal system? Some research indicates that massage of preterm infants may assist in improved weight gain and bone development, while recent reviews bring this into question.[49-51] Restoration of joint motion, increases in circulation, decreases in muscle spasm, and other benefits of massage therapy may have an effect on bone health or healing. Use of massage on soft tissues surrounding healing fractures is common practice and has been shown clinically to assist in the restoration of motion and to decrease stiffness. This is an important area for future research.

Summary of Massage Effects on Muscles and Bones.
Research to date suggests massage therapy may:
- Directly affect both the muscular and skeletal systems through combined mechanical, physiologic, and psychologic effects
- Decrease tension within the muscle-tendon unit

- Increase range of motion (ROM)
- Decrease delayed onset muscle soreness (DOMS) and blood indicators of muscle damage
- Decrease electromyography (EMG) activity, suggesting increased muscle relaxation and decreased muscle fatigue
- Decrease pain and may activate the parasympathetic nervous system, causing relaxation through massage of trigger points

Connective Tissues

Several connective tissues are included in other sections of this chapter (i.e., blood, lymph, bone). In this section, we will focus on loose and dense connective tissues. What we understand about loose and dense connective tissues and their function may change dramatically over the next few years. Typically we are taught that these tissues simply fill in space, hold things together and help to form a scaffolding or structure for other tissues. As we learn about fascia and techniques to work with this tissue, the idea that connective tissue is an integral and important part of what we do may be a revelation. Newer studies suggest that different types of connective tissue respond as excitable tissue—more like muscle or nerve tissue. Watch the literature for dramatic changes in the way we view this important, responsive, ubiquitous, and complex substance.

One frequent use of massage therapy, especially techniques of transverse friction and cross fiber massage, is to reduce scar tissue and adhesion formation and to treat tendonitis. Does the current literature support these claims? One study[52] found massage minimized excessive scar formation and progressively increased tensile forces, enabling the scar tissue to serve the damaged tendon.

The use of massage for burn victims and to reduce scarring after burns has shown promise.[53,54] Important research continues in this area, and new research on adults and children should be published soon to assist us in optimizing these protocols to produce the best results. One study[55] found increased fibroblast activity after massage, with deeper pressure producing a greater effect than lighter pressure.[56] This increased fibroblast activity is thought to enhance healing in a way that promotes strong and mobile scar tissue.

Patients with fibromyalgia often seek relief from massage therapy treatments. Some research indicates that connective tissue massage may relieve pain and symptoms of this disorder[57-59]; however, strong randomized clinical trial evidence is still lacking.[60-65] There may be a strong psychological component to this work as well, and much remains to be done in this area to further understand the mechanisms of action and to optimize treatment protocols.[57,58]

Summary of Massage Effects of Connective Tissues.
Research to date suggests massage therapy may:
- Increase fibroblast activity, leading to improved healing
- Improve scar tissue formation

- Increase scar tissue strength to aid in tendon healing
- Assist in the treatment of tendonitis
- Be effective in the treatment of burns
- Be helpful in reducing pain and other symptoms of fibromyalgia

Nervous System

The nervous system is a vast and complex network involved in every aspect of the body's response to its environment. Naturally, it is an integral part of every aspect of massage therapy as well. From how the tissues respond to mechanical pressure to how the mind relaxes at just the thought of going to a massage appointment, the nervous system is involved. The nervous system is divided into the central nervous system and the peripheral nervous system. The peripheral nervous system is then subdivided into the autonomic and somatic systems, each playing a different role in orchestrating the body's response to the world around it (see Chapter 23).

Several studies have explored how spinal cord reflexes respond to different treatments and pressures.[66-74] These studies assessed the level of excitability of motor neurons in the spinal cord after different massage treatments. They found that massage influenced the level of spinal cord response. It is very exciting to think rather than just affecting the surface tissues our work is influencing the very heart of the nervous system. But what do these changes mean to our clients? The next step is connecting this spinal cord response to clinical changes. One study[24] found decreases in spinal reflexes, accompanied by decreases in EMG and increases in range of motion after massage to the neck and shoulders. This suggests the decreased excitability in the spinal cord may result in decreased tension and muscle firing, allowing for increased cervical spine ROM. More research is needed in this area, but the connection between spinal cord function and improved clinical outcomes is exciting.

Currently, most research is focused on assessing the effects of massage on relaxation and stress reduction,[75-77] and reduction of anxiety[78,79] and depression.[80-83] These studies examine the effects of massage on neurotransmitters. Neurotransmitters are chemicals that control neurologic functions. Examples of neurotransmitters are endorphins, dopamine, and serotonin (see Chapter 23 for more information). Endorphins reduce pain. Serotonin regulates mood, appetite, sleep, memory, learning, and even muscle contraction. Dopamine helps to regulate heart rate, blood pressure, and indirectly affects pituitary function and movement.

This is the process of research; newer studies will correct or contradict previous studies as we continue to learn new things. This is one reason why you must stay up to date, read research studies, and keep an open mind as our knowledge base changes. If massage has an effect on neurotransmitters, it stands to reason that massage has also been found to have direct effects on the parasympathetic nervous system,[1,2] lowering heart rate and blood pressure. Moreover, massage has been shown to directly affect brain wave activity[84-86] and assist in those with sleep disorders, whether from decreases in pain, depression, or anxiety, or from increased relaxation.[87] Finally, in a well-designed study using an animal model, massage was shown to directly influence brain development.[88] Together these responses comprise an important component of the body's response to massage therapy.

Summary of Massage Effects on the Nervous System.
Research to date suggests massage therapy may:
- Increase serotonin
- Increase dopamine
- Decrease motoneuron pool excitability
- Improve sleep
- Decrease stress, depression, and anxiety
- Increase relaxation
- Enhance brain wave activity
- Improve cognitive and memory functioning
- Activate parasympathetic response

Endocrine System

Like the nervous system, the endocrine system influences most other body systems. This makes assessing the influence of massage on the endocrine system independent of other systems difficult. It is thought that massage may have an influence on the levels of multiple hormones.[89] We have already touched on some influences of massage on the endocrine system in our discussions of cortisol alterations and the effects on labor, postpartum depression, and pregnancy massage.[90] This is a large area of study ripe for intense investigation.

The effect of massage therapy on cortisol levels is another area where we have gained substantial knowledge. Cortisol, an adrenal hormone, is integral to the body's stress response. A simple blood test can assess changes in cortisol after a treatment or change in a life situation. Any modulation in cortisol would produce important physiologic effects; and decreasing this stress hormone would have great benefits to health and wellness. These are areas in which a great deal of research has been done. There is substantial research assessing the effect of massage therapy on cortisol levels.[75,80,91-100] Most of these studies indicate a significant decrease in cortisol levels in various populations after massage therapy. One recent review of the literature in this area[101] suggests the evidence is lacking. As in any area of research, continued work only serves to improve what we know about our profession. The effect of massage on this important hormone will continue to be investigated and we will continue to learn more about how massage treatment influences the stress response. Stay tuned, and keep reading the literature to discover how this conversation develops.

We cannot discuss the endocrine system without a discussion of what is fast becoming an epidemic in this country—type 2 diabetes. Diabetes can have detrimental effects on the cardiovascular system, neurological system, tissue healing, vision and other sensory systems, and overall health and wellness. As the obesity problem grows to epidemic proportions, health conditions associated with obesity are fast becoming the primary health concerns for the medical community. In an effort to fight these trends federal research dollars are being funneled into ways to address this issue. These include the decreased activity levels in adults and children, poor nutrition, and drugs to fight the resulting health concerns that involves almost every system in the body. An exciting area of active research interest is the influence of massage on the secretion of insulin. Clinical evidence indicates improvement in diabetic symptoms with regular massage treatment. One animal study indicated improved insulin secretion after massage-like stroking in rats.[102] Studies indicate some changes in production or absorption of insulin after massage therapy.[103-107] Research in this area is promising and any positive effect massage therapy can have on patients with this devastating disease would be a wonderful result.

Summary of Massage Effects on the Endocrine System.
Research to date suggests massage therapy may:
- Influence levels of multiple hormones
- Influence production/absorption of insulin
- Produce changes in hormones related to pregnancy, labor, and postpartum depression
- Influence other massage outcomes and effects

Skin

It seems intuitive that massage therapy would influence the skin; all massage techniques featured in this text work through the skin. We often do not think of the skin itself as benefiting from the treatment unless we are specifically working to influence this organ (spa treatments, burn treatments, etc.). We have already said that massage increases skin temperature through changes in peripheral blood flow. Few articles assess the effect on the skin itself, but studies indicate improvements in eczema, including decreases in redness, lichenification (i.e., rough, thickened, dry skin), scaling, excoriation (i.e., crusting skin), and pruritus (i.e., itching).[108,109] Some research also suggests the use of massage to prevent pressure ulcers in bedridden patients.[110] Recent research indicates that the decrease in stress and anxiety after massage treatment may improve dermatological conditions, further supporting the interconnectedness between the various systems of the body.[111] The use of massage lubricant, the stimulation of blood flow, and the improvement of nutrient exchange may contribute synergistically to the overall health of the skin itself.

Summary of Massage Effects on Skin. Research to date suggests massage therapy may:

- Be effective in reducing scarring after burns
- Decrease symptoms of eczema and other skin conditions
- Be helpful in treating or preventing bed sores
- Reduce stress that may exacerbate dermatological conditions
- Increase skin temperature
- Contribute to the overall health of skin tissue

> *"A certain awkwardness marks the use of borrowed thoughts, but as soon as we have learned what to do with them, they become our own."*
> —Ralph Waldo Emerson

Internal Organs and Other Systems

As part of the general effect of massage, there is likely influence on individual internal organs and other body systems. Improved circulation, blood pressure, nutritional exchange, and other factors certainly affect tissues throughout the body. It has been suggested that massage therapy influences the urinary and digestive systems. Specific research in these areas is lacking. However, influences on the parasympathetic nervous system and on lymph circulation would necessarily have an influence on the functioning of these systems.

Massage therapy has been shown to assist respiratory function in individuals with chronic obstructive lung disease, although the exact mechanism of action is unknown.[112] There are also multiple studies indicating massage as an effective treatment for asthma symptoms, especially in children.[113-116] While more work needs to be done to confirm these results, a possible mechanism of action may be the decrease in stress and circulating cortisol in addition to alterations in serotonin and dopamine associated with the treatment.

Psychologic Aspects

The influence of massage therapy on the psychologic aspects of the client is a vast topic area well beyond the scope of this text. Areas of research have developed to investigate this mind-body connection and new fields of science are being created involving the neuropsychologic effects of massage.

We have already discussed changes caused by stress, depression, and anxiety and how these may occur. The improved mind-body connection often generates an overall feeling of health and wellness. This is an exciting new area of investigation,[117] and one that is difficult to quantify. Several studies have attempted to find ways to assess the effects of massage and other complementary and alternative medicine (CAM), or complementary and integrative medicines (CIM).[118-120]

One area of study is using massage in the treatment of hyperactivity disorders (ADHD, ADD, etc.) Several studies have found improved levels of focus, concentration, and overall functioning after massage therapy.[121-123] Other studies indicate massage as a useful treatment for victims of trauma and abuse.[124-126] Massage has also been successfully used with psychiatric patients for a variety of desired outcomes.[127] There are also studies that suggest massage influences communication, improves body image, improves mood, and helps us deal with strong emotions.[124,125,128-130] Clearly this is a vast field of study that will continue to evolve. It is important as massage therapists that we understand the effect of our work on psychologic aspects and the physical aspects of our clients. The psychologic changes inherent in massage will affect clinical outcomes. We must also ensure that we provide a safe and healthy environment for our clients, and that we do not attempt to treat psychologic aspects for which we are not specially trained. Scope of practice is discussed in Chapters 2 and 10.

Summary of the Psychologic Effects of Massage Therapy. Research to date suggests massage therapy may:

- Reduce anxiety, depression, and stress
- Promote well-being
- Promote a mind-body connection
- Be useful in treating hyperactivity disorders
- Be helpful in treating victims of violence and abuse (with proper training)

Whole Body Effects

Few of the changes brought about by massage therapy are isolated to one tissue type or system. Massage therapy may influence functioning of the nervous system, endocrine system, cardiovascular system, modulate circulation of blood and lymph, influence connective tissues, and influence psychologic factors that may influence multiple systems and tissues throughout the body. The effect of massage therapy on pain and fatigue are also whole-body effects that deserve special mention.

Massage therapy has long been used for pain resulting from multiple causes. Pain from muscle spasm and injury, tendonitis, bone fracture, skin conditions, trigger points, headaches, cancer treatments, osteoarthritis, orthopedic injury, fibromyalgia, labor and delivery, and other sources has already been addressed above. How massage influences pain in each case may vary depending on the type and source of the pain. Increased circulation, decreased spasm, modulation in neurotransmitters and hormones, or even the simple act of touch and comfort all likely influence the perception of pain in the patient[36,39,57,82,91,97,131-144] (Box 6-1 and Box 6-2).

Fatigue is another area that seems to respond to massage therapy. As discussed above, massage therapy influences multiple psychologic factors that may interfere with sleep and create fatigue. Massage treatment has been shown to

BOX 6-1

Massage and the Pain Cycle

The pain-cycle is initiated when painful stimuli result in muscle contraction and localized muscle splinting or guarding. The localized muscle guarding restricts movement and decreases local circulation, which restricts the amount of oxygen available to the tissues and the removal of metabolic wastes. Any subsequent swelling creates more pain as local nerves are compressed. Muscle splinting is then intensified and the cycle repeats itself. A more generalized secondary pain results that outlasts or exceeds the original discomfort. Massage may interrupt the pain cycle on all levels.

THE PAIN CYCLE

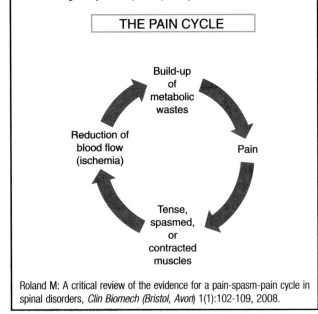

Build-up of metabolic wastes

Pain

Tense, spasmed, or contracted muscles

Reduction of blood flow (ischemia)

Roland M: A critical review of the evidence for a pain-spasm-pain cycle in spinal disorders, *Clin Biomech (Bristol, Avon)* 1(1):102-109, 2008.

BOX 6-2

The Gate Control Theory

In 1965, Ronald Melzack and Patricia Wall postulated the gate control theory of pain relief, which may explain a reason why massage, ice, and heat are effective in the treatment of pain. The gate control theory, or gate theory, states that transmission of impulses into the spinal cord is "gated" (can be open or shut). Gating is affected by the degree of activity, or transmission, in sensory nerves. Multiple signals may be competing for the same gate, or entrance into the spinal cord. The signal that hits the gate first wins. The gate then closes and prevents or inhibits other signals from entering.

Nerve transmission speed is affected by nerve diameter. Impulses traveling along larger nerve fibers are faster. Sensory nerves for pressure, temperature, and sharp acute pain lie close together in large concentrations near the body's surface. These sensory nerves are long, large-in-diameter, and transmit impulses quickly, protecting the body from harm. Strong stimuli to these receptors generate a quick sensory input to the spinal cord. A reflex is generated to move the affected body part out of harm's way. Touching the sharp point of a needle or a hot pan elicits this type of reflex response.

The sensory receptors for aching pain originate in the deeper tissues. These nerves are composed of short, thinner nerve fibers, which tend to transmit pain that has been present for some time (i.e., headache, dull pain) and requires no immediate protective action. These nerves transmit stimuli that are of lesser importance and lesser consequence to the body. The purpose of the deep, slower transmitting nerves is to make the conscious mind aware that a problem exists, which can be used to prevent overuse or dependence on an injured body part.

Suppose that a gymnast is having her performance compromised by soreness in her right calf. This pain originates from the deeper, slower nerves. When a pressure stimulus such as massage is applied to the calf, the new sensory input travels along the faster, larger nerve network, entering the spinal cord first. The gate closes, excluding pain information from entering the cord. The body experiences the pressure of the massage stroke as interruption of pain.

Massage therapists can use the gate mechanism when applying pressure, heat, and cold. All of these have the potential to interfere or interrupt pain signals.

Modified from Melzack R, Wall P: Pain mechanisms: a new theory, *Science* 150(699):971-979, 1965.

improve sleep[145-148]; decrease chronic pain, which often results in overwhelming fatigue[60,137,142,149-151]; treat fibromyalgia, which often is associated with fatigue[58-59,87,152]; and generally improves overall well-being that would reduce symptoms of fatigue.[153-155]

MASSAGE THERAPY: INDICATIONS FOR SPECIFIC CONDITIONS AND POPULATIONS

Massage therapy has been shown to be effective in working with many special populations. There are often special training requirements, contraindications, and treatment parameters associated with these groups. It is vital to ensure that you are properly trained, communicate with the client's health care provider, and conduct a thorough intake when working with these populations. When in doubt, refer your client to a qualified health care provider.

Research sufficiently indicates that massage therapy is safe for cardiovascular patients undergoing treatment or surgery.[4,5] It has been shown to decrease stress and anxiety, reduce blood pressure and heart rate, and improve overall well-being, which assists in the healing process.

Massage has been shown to decrease pain and symptoms in clients with fibromyalgia.[57,58] Suggestions are to use massage with moderate pressure and careful deactivation of tender points (see Chapter 14). Much work needs to be done in this area to optimize protocols.

Significant work has been done to develop safe and effective protocols for working with cancer patients. Research shows massage can be effective in reducing the stress associated with this disease.[82,91] Studies also indicate reductions in lymphedema associated with cancer and its treatment.[15-18]

Research is strong in advocating massage therapy for clients during pregnancy, labor, and postpartum, and with infants and preterm infants.[156]

Children and adult burn victims benefit from massage therapy treatment.[157]

Diabetic patients may benefit from massage therapy. As massage may influence production or absorption of insulin, it is important that clients monitor blood glucose levels before and after massage treatments and look for changes in the level of insulin dosage required. Be sure to know the signs of hypoglycemia and how to apply appropriate interventions. Patients should inform their health care providers that they are receiving massage therapy and work with them to monitor insulin dosage levels.[103-107]

Massage has also been found to be effective in working with children and adults with asthma.[113-116]

Research to date suggests massage therapy may be effective in working with the following special populations and individuals with specific disorders:

- Asthma
- COPD
- Fibromyalgia
- Hyperactivity disorders
- Multiple sclerosis
- Spinal cord injuries
- Alzheimer disease
- Accident victims
- Parkinson disease
- Cerebral palsy
- Chronic fatigue syndrome
- Hospice patients
- Postsurgical patients and other hospitalized populations

E-RESOURCES

@volve

http://evolve.elsevier.com/Salvo/MassageTherapy

- Chapter challenge
- Flash cards
- Additional information
- Weblinks

BIBLIOGRAPHY

1. Weerapong P, Hume PA, Kolt GS: The mechanisms of massage and effects on performance, muscle recovery and injury prevention, *Sports Med* 35(3):235-256, 2005.
2. Takamoto K et al: Compression on trigger points in the leg muscle increases parasympathetic nervous activity based on heart rate variability, *J Physiol Sci* 59(3):191-197, 2009.
3. Kaye AD et al: The effect of deep-tissue massage therapy on blood pressure and heart rate, *J Altern Complement Med* 14(2):125-128, 2008.
4. Kshettry VR et al: Complementary alternative medical therapies for heart surgery patients: feasibility, safety, and impact, *Ann Thorac Surg* 81(1):201-205, 2006.
5. Okvat HA et al: Massage therapy for patients undergoing cardiac catheterization, *Altern Ther Health Med* 8(3):68-70, 72, 74-65, 2002.
6. Aggeler PM, Lucia SP, Howard J: Platelet counts and platelet function, *Proc Am Fed Clin Res* 2:110, 1945.
7. Lucia SP, Richard JF: Effects of massage on blood platelet production, *Proc Soc Exp Biol Med* 31:87, 1933.
8. Hennenfent BR, Lazarte AR, Feliciano AE Jr: Repetitive prostatic massage and drug therapy as an alternative to transurethral resection of the prostate, *MedGenMed* 8(4):19, 2006.
9. Kuriyama H et al: Immunological and psychological benefits of aromatherapy massage, *Evid Based Complement Altern Med* 2(2):179-184, 2005.
10. Liu Y et al: Capillary blood flow with dynamical change of tissue pressure caused by exterior force, *Sheng Wu Yi Xue Gong Cheng Xue Za Zhi* 21(5):699-703, 2004.
11. Hovind H, Nielsen SL: Effect of massage on blood flow in skeletal muscle, *Scand J Rehabil Med* 6(2):74-77, 1974.
12. Drust B et al: The effects of massage on intra muscular temperature in the vastus lateralis in humans, *Int J Sports Med* 24(6):395-399, 2003.
13. Sefton JM, Yarar C, Pasco DD: Effect of therapeutic massage on peripheral blood flow as assessed by skin temperature measures in the neck and shoulders, *J Altern Complement Med* 2010 (in press).
14. Sefton JM et al: Assessment of blood flow changes to skin and muscle after massage therapy, 2010 (in press).
15. Jeffs E: Treating breast cancer-related lymphoedema at the London Haven: clinical audit results, *Eur J Oncol Nurs* 10(1):71-79, 2006.
16. Szuba A: Literature watch. The addition of manual lymph drainage to compression therapy for breast cancer related lymphedema: a randomized controlled trial, *Lymphat Res Biol* 3(1):36-41, 2005.
17. Bernas M et al: Massage therapy in the treatment of lymphedema. Rationale, results, and applications, *IEEE Eng Med Biol Mag* 24(2):58-68, 2005.
18. Cohen SR, Payne DK, Tunkel RS: Lymphedema: strategies for management, *Cancer* 92(suppl 4):980-987, 2001.
19. Hernandez-Reif M et al: Natural killer cells and lymphocytes increase in women with breast cancer following massage therapy, *Int J Neurosci* 115(4):495-510, 2005.
20. Shor-Posner G et al: Massage treatment in HIV-1 infected Dominican children: a preliminary report on the efficacy of massage therapy to preserve the immune system in children without antiretroviral medication, *J Altern Complement Med* 10(6):1093-1095, 2004.
21. Diego MA et al: HIV adolescents show improved immune function following massage therapy, *Int J Neurosci* 106(1-2):35-45, 2001.
22. Hennenfent BR, Feliciano AE: Changes in white blood cell counts in men undergoing thrice-weekly prostatic massage, microbial diagnosis and antimicrobial therapy for

genitourinary complaints, *Br J Urol* 81(3):370-376, 1998.

23. Billhult A et al: The effect of massage on cellular immunity, endocrine and psychological factors in women with breast cancer: a randomized controlled clinical trial, *Auton Neurosci* 140(1-2):88-95, 2008.

24. Sefton JM, Yarar C, Pasco DD: Physiological and clinical changes after therapeutic massage of the neck and shoulders, *J Bodyw Manual Ther* 2010 (in press).

25. James H et al: Rolfing structural integration treatment of cervical spine dysfunction, *J Bodyw Mov Ther* 13(3):229-238, 2009.

26. Perlman AI et al: Massage therapy for osteoarthritis of the knee: a randomized controlled trial, *Arch Intern Med* 166(22):2533-2538, 2006.

27. Hernandez-Reif M et al: Low back pain is reduced and range of motion increased after massage therapy, *Int J Neurosci* 106:131-145, 2001.

28. Boissonnault WG, Badke MB: Influence of acuity on physical therapy outcomes for patients with cervical disorders, *Arch Phys Med Rehabil* 89(1):81-86, 2008.

29. Badke MB, Boissonnault WG: Changes in disability following physical therapy intervention for patients with low back pain: dependence on symptom duration, *Arch Phys Med Rehabil* 87(6):749-756, 2006.

30. Losito JM, O'Neil J: Rehabilitation of foot and ankle injuries, *Clin Podiatr Med Surg* 14(3):533-557, 1997.

31. Wiktorsson-Moller M et al: Effects of warming up, massage, and stretching on range of motion and muscle strength in the lower extremity, *Am J Sports Med* 11(4):249-252, 1983.

32. McNicol K, Taunton JE, Clement DB: Iliotibial tract friction syndrome in athletes, *Can J Appl Sport Sci* 6(2):76-80, 1981.

33. Arroyo-Morales M et al: Psychophysiological effects of massage-myofascial release after exercise: a randomized sham-control study, *J Altern Complement Med* 14(10):1223-1229, 2008.

34. Barlow A et al: Effect of massage of the hamstring muscles on selected electromyographic characteristics of biceps femoris during sub-maximal isometric contraction, *Int J Sports Med* 28(3):253-256, 2007.

35. Lavelle ED, Lavelle W, Smith HS: Myofascial trigger points, *Anesthesiol Clin* 25(4):841-851, vii-iii, 2007.

36. Bell J: Massage therapy helps to increase range of motion, decrease pain and assist in healing a client with low back pain and sciatica symptoms, *J Bodyw Mov Ther* 12(3):281-289, 2008.

37. Delaney JP et al: The short-term effects of myofascial trigger point massage therapy on cardiac autonomic tone in healthy subjects, *J Adv Nurs* 37(4):364-371, 2002.

38. von Stulpnagel C et al: Myofascial trigger points in children with tension-type headache: a new diagnostic and therapeutic option, *J Child Neurol* 24(4):406-409, 2009.

39. Vernon H, Humphreys K, Hagino C: Chronic mechanical neck pain in adults treated by manual therapy: a systematic review of change scores in randomized clinical trials, *J Manipulative Physiol Ther* 30(3):215-227, 2007.

40. Hong CZ: New trends in myofascial pain syndrome, *Zhonghua Yi Xue Za Zhi (Taipei)* 65(11):501-512, 2002.

41. Offenbacher M, Stucki G: Physical therapy in the treatment of fibromyalgia, *Scand J Rheumatol Suppl* 113:78-85, 2000.

42. Trujillo L: Trigger point relief, *Nurse Pract* 23(2):119, 1998.

43. Cheung K, Hume P, Maxwell L: Delayed onset muscle soreness: treatment strategies and performance factors, *Sports Med* 33(2):145-164, 2003.

44. Ernst E: Does post-exercise massage treatment reduce delayed onset muscle soreness? A systematic review, *Br J Sports Med* 32(3):212-214, 1998.

45. Zainuddin Z et al: Effects of massage on delayed-onset muscle soreness, swelling, and recovery of muscle function, *J Athl Train* 40(3):174-180, 2005.

46. Bakowski P et al: Effects of massage on delayed-onset muscle soreness, *Chir Narzadow Ruchu Ortop Pol* 73(4):261-265, 2008.

47. Connolly DA, Sayers SP, McHugh MP: Treatment and prevention of delayed onset muscle soreness, *J Strength Cond Res* 17(1):197-208, 2003.

48. Moraska A: Sports massage. A comprehensive review, *J Sports Med Phys Fitness* 45(3):370-380, 2005.

49. Field T: Preterm infant massage therapy studies: an American approach, *Semin Neonatol* 7(6):487-494, 2002.

50. Vickers A et al: Massage for promoting growth and development of preterm and/or low birth-weight infants, *Cochrane Database Syst Rev* (2):CD000390, 2000.

51. Cassileth BR, Vickers AJ: Massage therapy for symptom control: outcome study at a major cancer center, *J Pain Symptom Manage* 28(3):244-249, 2004.

52. Rapp HJ et al: Management of acute tendinitis, *Tierarztl Prax* 20(6):615-620, 1992.

53. Field T et al: Postburn itching, pain, and psychological symptoms are reduced with massage therapy, *J Burn Care Rehabil* 21(3):189-193, 2000.

54. Patino O et al: Massage in hypertrophic scars, *J Burn Care Rehabil* 20(3):268-271; discussion 267, 1999.

55. Davidson CJ et al: Rat tendon morphologic and functional changes resulting from soft tissue mobilization, *Med Sci Sports Exerc* 29(3):313-319, 1997.

56. Gehlsen GM, Ganion LR, Helfst R: Fibroblast responses to variation in soft tissue mobilization pressure, *Med Sci Sports Exerc* 31(4):531-535, 1999.

57. Kalichman L: Massage therapy for fibromyalgia symptoms, *Rheumatol Int* 30(9):1151-1157, 2010.

58. Baranowsky J et al: Qualitative systemic review of randomized controlled trials on complementary and alternative medicine treatments in fibromyalgia, *Rheumatol Int* 30(1):1-21, 2009.

59. Brattberg G: Connective tissue massage in the treatment of fibromyalgia, *Eur J Pain* 3(3):235-244, 1999.

60. Tsao JC: Effectiveness of massage therapy for chronic, non-malignant pain: a review, *Evid Based Complement Altern Med* 4(2):165-179, 2007.

61. Morris CR, Bowen L, Morris AJ: Integrative therapy for fibromyalgia: possible strategies for an individualized treatment program, *South Med J* 98(2):177-184, 2005.

62. Melillo N et al: Fibromyalgic syndrome: new perspectives in rehabilitation and management. A review, *Minerva Med* 96(6):417-423. 2005.

63. Mease P: Fibromyalgia syndrome: review of clinical presentation, pathogenesis, outcome measures, and treatment, *J Rheumatol Suppl* 75:6-21, 2005.

64. Ernst E: Musculoskeletal conditions and complementary/alternative medicine, *Best Pract Res Clin Rheumatol* 18(4):539-556, 2004.

65. Field T, Delange J, Hernandez Reif M: Movement and massage therapy reduces fibromyalgia pain, *J Bodyw Mov Ther* 1:49-52, 2003.

66. Sefton JM, Yarar C: The effect of therapeutic neck and shoulder massage on flexor carpi radialis motor neuron pool excitability, Chicago, 2009, Society for Neuroscience Annual Meeting.

67. Morelli M, Chapman CE, Sullivan SJ: Do cutaneous receptors contribute to the changes in the amplitude of the H-reflex during massage? *Electromyogr Clin Neurophysiol* 39(7):441-447, 1999.

68. Morelli M, Sullivan SJ, Chapman CE: Inhibitory influence of soleus massage onto the medial gastrocnemius H-reflex, *Electromyogr Clin Neurophysiol* 38(2):87-93, 1998.

69. Goldberg J et al: The effect of therapeutic massage on H-reflex amplitude in persons with a spinal cord injury, *Phys Ther* 74(8):728-737, 1994.

70. Cramer GD et al: The Hmax/Mmax ratio as an outcome measure for acute low back pain, *J Manipulative Physiol Ther* 16(1):7-13, 1993.

71. Goldberg J, Sullivan SJ, Seaborne DE: The effect of two intensities of massage on H-reflex amplitude, *Phys Ther* 72(6):449-457, 1992.

72. Sullivan SJ et al: Effects of massage on alpha motoneuron excitability, *Phys Ther* 71(8):555-560, 1991.

73. Morelli M, Seaborne DE, Sullivan SJ: H-reflex modulation during manual muscle massage of human triceps surae, *Arch Phys Med Rehabil* 72(11):915-919, 1991.

74. Morelli M, Seaborne DE, Sullivan SJ: Changes in H-reflex amplitude during massage of the triceps surae in healthy subjects, *J Orthop Sports* 12:55-59, 1990.

75. Listing M et al: The efficacy of classical massage on stress perception and cortisol following primary treatment of breast cancer, *Arch Womens Ment Health* 13(2):165-173, 2010.

76. Lucini D et al: Complementary medicine for the management of chronic stress: superiority of active versus passive techniques, *J Hypertens* 27(12):2421-2428, 2009.

77. MacDonald G: Massage as a respite intervention for primary caregivers, *Am J Hosp Palliat Care* 15(1):43-47, 1998.

78. Hart S et al: Anorexia nervosa symptoms are reduced by massage therapy, *Eat Disord* 9(4):289-299, 2001.

79. Hadfield N: The role of aromatherapy massage in reducing anxiety in patients with malignant brain tumours, *Int J Palliat Nurs* 7(6):279-285, 2001.

80. Field T, Diego M, Hernandez-Reif M: Prenatal depression effects and interventions: a review, *Infant Behav Dev* 2010 (in press).

81. Field T et al: Pregnancy massage reduces prematurity, low birthweight and postpartum depression, *Infant Behav Dev* 2009;32(4):454-460.

82. Russell NC et al: Role of massage therapy in cancer care, *J Altern Complement Med* 14(2):209-214, 2008.

83. Field T et al: Massage therapy effects on depressed pregnant women, *J Psychosom Obstet Gynaecol* 25(2):115-122, 2004.

84. Diego MA et al: Massage therapy of moderate and light pressure and vibrator effects on EEG and heart rate, *Int J Neurosci* 114(1):31-44, 2004.

85. Field T et al: Massage therapy reduces anxiety and enhances EEG pattern of alertness and math computations, *Int J Neurosci* 86(3-4):197-205, 1996.

86. Jones NA, Field T: Massage and music therapies attenuate frontal EEG asymmetry in depressed adolescents, *Adolescence* 34(135):529-534, 1999.

87. Field T et al: Fibromyalgia pain and substance P decrease and sleep improves after massage therapy, *J Clin Rheumatol* 8(2):72-76, 2002.

88. Guzzetta A et al: Massage accelerates brain development and the maturation of visual function, *J Neurosci* 29(18):6042-6051, 2009.

89. Arkko PJ, Pakarinen AJ, Kari-Koskinen O: Effects of whole body massage on serum protein, electrolyte and hormone concentrations, enzyme activities, and hematological parameters, *Int J Sports Med* 4(4):265-267, 1983.

90. Field T et al: Pregnant women benefit from massage therapy, *J Psychosom Obstet Gynaecol* 20(1):31-38, 1999.

91. Post-White J et al: Massage therapy for children with cancer, *J Pediatr Oncol Nurs* 26(1):16-28, 2009.

92. Arroyo-Morales M et al: Massage after exercise: responses of immunologic and endocrine markers: a randomized single-blind placebo-controlled study, *J Strength Cond Res* 23(2):638-644, 2009.

93. Stringer J, Swindell R, Dennis M: Massage in patients undergoing intensive chemotherapy reduces serum cortisol and prolactin, *Psychooncology* 17(10):1024-1031, 2008.

94. Garner B et al: Pilot study evaluating the effect of massage therapy on stress, anxiety and aggression in a young adult psychiatric inpatient unit, *Aust N Z J Psychiatry* 42(5):414-422, 2008.

95. Field T, Diego M: Cortisol: the culprit prenatal stress variable, *Int J Neurosci* 8:1181-1205, 2008.

96. Bello D et al: An exploratory study of neurohormonal responses of healthy men to massage, *J Altern Complement Med* 14(4):387-394, 2008.

97. Beider S, Moyer CA: Randomized controlled trials of pediatric massage: a review, *Evid Based Complement Altern Med* 4(1):23-34, 2007.

98. Fujita M et al: Effect of massaging babies on mothers: pilot study on the changes in mood states and salivary cortisol level, *Complement Ther Clin Pract* 12(3):181-185, 2006.

99. Fogaca Mde C et al: Salivary cortisol as an indicator of adrenocortical function in healthy infants, using massage therapy, *Sao Paulo Med J* 123(5):215-218, 2005.

100. Field T et al: Cortisol decreases and serotonin and dopamine increase following massage therapy, *Int J Neurosci* 115(10):1397-1413, 2005.

101. Moyer CA, Rounds J, Hannum JW: A meta-analysis of massage therapy research, *Psychol Bull* 130(1):3-18, 2004.

102. Holst S et al: Massage-like stroking influences plasma levels of gastrointestinal hormones, including insulin, and increases weight gain in male rats, *Auton Neurosci* 120(1-2):73-79, 2005.

103. Field T et al: Insulin and insulin-like growth factor-1 increased in preterm neonates following massage therapy, *J Dev Behav Pediatr* 29(6):463-466, 2008.

104. Hildebrandt P: Subcutaneous absorption of insulin in insulin-dependent diabetic patients. Influence of species, physico-chemical properties of insulin and physiological factors, *Dan Med Bull* 38(4):337-346, 1991.

105. Ariza-Andraca CR et al: Delayed insulin absorption due to subcutaneous edema, *Arch Invest Med (Mex)* 22(2):229-233, 1991.

106. Linde B, Philip A: Massage-enhanced insulin absorption: increased distribution or dissociation of insulin? *Diabetes Res* 11(4):191-194, 1989.

107. Dillon RS: Improved serum insulin profiles in diabetic individuals who massaged their insulin injection sites, *Diabetes Care* 6(4):399-401, 1983.

108. Banner MA et al: Localized tufts of fibrils on *Staphylococcus epidermidis* NCTC 11047 are comprised of the accumulation-associated protein, *J Bacteriol* 189(7):2793-2804, 2007.

109. Field T: Massage therapy for skin conditions in young children, *Dermatol Clin* 23(4):717-721, 2005.

110. Duimel-Peeters IG et al: The effects of massage as a method to prevent pressure ulcers. A review of the literature, *Ostomy Wound Manage* 51(4):70-80, 2005.

111. Marshall M: Stress management in dermatology patients, *Nurs Stand* 5(24):29-31, 1991.

112. Beeken JE et al: The effectiveness of neuromuscular release massage therapy in five individuals with chronic obstructive lung disease, *Clin Nurs Res* 7(3):309-325, 1998.

113. Bielory L, Russin J, Zuckerman GB: Clinical efficacy, mechanisms of action, and adverse effects of complementary and alternative medicine therapies for asthma, *Allergy Asthma Proc* 25(5):283-291, 2004.

114. Field T: Massage therapy for infants and children, *J Dev Behav Pediatr* 16(2):105-111, 1995.

115. Field T et al: Children with asthma have improved pulmonary functions after massage therapy, *J Pediatr* 132(5):854-858, 1998.

116. Hondras MA, Linde K, Jones AP: Manual therapy for asthma, *Cochrane Database Syst Rev* (2):CD001002, 2005.

117. Dicker A: Using Bowen technique in a health service workplace to improve the physical and mental wellbeing of staff, *Aust J Holist Nurs* 12(2):35-42, 2005.

118. Wesa KM, Cassileth BR: Is there a role for complementary therapy in the management of leukemia? *Expert Rev Anticancer Ther* 9(9):1241-1249, 2009.

119. Mauboussin-Carlos S et al: Mind body therapy in palliative care, *Soins* 2009(737):43-44.

120. Wesa K, Gubili J, Cassileth B: Integrative oncology: complementary therapies for cancer survivors, *Hematol Oncol Clin North Am* 22(2):343-353, viii, 2008.

121. Sawni A: Attention-deficit/hyperactivity disorder and complementary/alternative medicine, *Adolesc Med State Art Rev* 19(2):313-326, xi, 2008.

122. Khilnani S et al: Massage therapy improves mood and behavior of students with attention-deficit/hyperactivity disorder, *Adolescence* 38(152):623-638, 2003.

123. Arnold LE: Alternative treatments for adults with attention-deficit hyperactivity disorder (ADHD), *Ann N Y Acad Sci* 931:310-341, 2001.

124. Price C: Dissociation reduction in body therapy during sexual abuse recovery, *Complement Ther Clin Pract* 13(2):116-128, 2007.

125. Price C: Body-oriented therapy in recovery from child sexual abuse: an efficacy study, *Altern Ther Health Med* 11(5):46-57, 2005.

126. Field T: Violence and touch deprivation in adolescents, *Adolescence* 37(148):735-749, 2002.

127. Elkins G, Rajab MH, Marcus J: Complementary and alternative medicine use by psychiatric inpatients, *Psychol Rep* 96(1):163-166, 2005.

128. Mackereth PA: Body, relationship and sacred space, *Complement Ther Nurs Midwifery* 4(5):125-127, 1998.

129. Kim HJ: Effect of aromatherapy massage on abdominal fat and body image in post-menopausal women, *Taehan Kanho Hakhoe Chi* 37(4):603-612, 2007.

130. Levine EG, Silver B: A pilot study: evaluation of a psychosocial program for women with gynecological cancers, *J Psychosoc Oncol* 25(3):75-98. 2007.

131. Field T: Pregnancy and labor massage, *Expert Rev Obstet Gynecol* 5(2):177-181, 2010.

132. Bauer BA et al: Effect of massage therapy on pain, anxiety, and tension after cardiac surgery: a randomized study, *Complement Ther Clin Pract* 16(2):70-75, 2010.

133. Sturgeon M et al: Effects of therapeutic massage on the quality of life among patients with breast cancer during treatment, *J Altern Complement Med* 15(4):373-380, 2009.

134. Livingston K et al: Touch and massage for medically fragile infants, *Evid Based Complement Altern Med* 6(4):473-482, 2009.

135. Cardenas DD, Felix ER: Pain after spinal cord injury: a review of classification, treatment approaches, and treatment assessment, *PM R* 1(12):1077-1090, 2009.

136. Vernon H, Humphreys BK: Chronic mechanical neck pain in adults treated by manual therapy: a systematic review of change scores in randomized controlled trials of a single session, *J Man Manip Ther* 16(2):E42-E52, 2008.

137. Suresh S et al: Massage therapy in outpatient pediatric chronic pain patients: do they facilitate significant reductions in levels of distress, pain, tension, discomfort, and mood alterations? *Paediatr Anaesth* 18(9):884-887, 2008.

138. Kutner JS et al: Massage therapy versus simple touch to improve pain and mood in patients with advanced cancer: a randomized trial, *Ann Intern Med* 149(6):369-379, 2008.

139. Field T et al: Massage therapy reduces pain in pregnant women, alleviates prenatal depression in both parents and improves their relationships, *J Bodyw Mov Ther* 12(2):146-150, 2008.

140. Sagar SM, Dryden T, Wong RK: Massage therapy for cancer patients: a reciprocal relationship between body and mind, *Curr Oncol* 14(2):45-56, 2007.

141. Gatlin CG, Schulmeister L: When medication is not enough: nonpharmacologic management of pain, *Clin J Oncol Nurs* 11(5):699-704, 2007.

142. Cassileth BR et al: Complementary therapies and integrative oncology in lung cancer: ACCP evidence-based clinical practice guidelines, ed 2, *Chest* 132(suppl 3):340S-354S, 2007.

143. Cassileth B, Trevisan C, Gubili J: Complementary therapies for cancer pain, *Curr Pain Headache Rep* 11(4):265-269, 2007.

144. Anderson PG, Cutshall SM: Massage therapy: a comfort intervention for cardiac surgery patients, *Clin Nurse Spec* 21(3):161-165; quiz 166-167, 2007.

145. Ejindu A: The effects of foot and facial massage on sleep induction, blood pressure, pulse and respiratory rate: crossover pilot study, *Complement Ther Clin Pract* 13(4):266-275, 2007.

146. Richards KC: Sleep promotion, *Crit Care Nurs Clin North Am* 8(1):39-52, 1996.

147. Zhou Y et al: The short-term therapeutic effect of the three-part massotherapy for insomnia due to deficiency of both the heart and the spleen: a report of 100 cases, *J Tradit Chin Med* 27(4):261-264, 2007.

148. Zhou YF et al: Multi-central controlled study on three-part massage therapy for treatment of insomnia of deficiency of both the heart and spleen, *Zhongguo Zhen Jiu* 26(6):385-388, 2006.

149. Cardenas DD, Jensen MP: Treatments for chronic pain in persons with spinal cord injury: a survey study, *J Spinal Cord Med* 29(2):109-117, 2006.

150. Walach H, Guthlin C, Konig M: Efficacy of massage therapy in chronic pain: a pragmatic randomized trial, *J Altern Complement Med* 9(6):837-846, 2003.

151. Harris RE, Clauw DJ: The use of complementary medical therapies in the management of myofascial pain disorders, *Curr Pain Headache Rep* 6(5):370-374, 2002.

152. Berman BM, Swyers JP: Complementary medicine treatments for fibromyalgia syndrome, *Baillieres Best Pract Res Clin Rheumatol* 13(3):487-492, 1999.

153. Afari N et al: Use of alternative treatments by chronic fatigue syndrome discordant twins, *Integr Med* 2(2):97-103, 2000.

154. Jones JF et al: Complementary and alternative medical therapy utilization by people with chronic fatiguing illnesses in the United States, *BMC Complement Altern Med* 7:12, 2007.

155. Yao F et al: Observation on therapeutic effect of point pressure combined with massage on chronic fatigue syndrome, *Zhongguo Zhen Jiu* 27(11):819-820, 2007.

156. Field T, Diego M, Hernandez-Reif M: Preterm infant massage therapy research: a review, *Infant Behav Dev* 33(2):115-124, 2010.

157. Hernandez-Reif M et al: Childrens' distress during burn treatment is reduced by massage therapy, *J Burn Care Rehabil* 22(2):191-195; discussion 190, 2001.

MATCHING I

Place the letter of the answer next to the term or phrase that best describes it.

A. Cortisol
B. Dopamine
C. EMG
D. Hyperemia
E. Increased fibroblast activity
F. Larger diameter nerves
G. Mechanic effects of massage
H. Physiologic effects of massage
I. Psychologic effects of massage
J. Serotonin
K. Smaller diameter nerves
L. Trigger point work

_____ 1. Red appearance of skin due to increased blood flow

_____ 2. Assesses electrical activity produced by muscles; acronym for electromyography

_____ 3. Clinically shown to relieve pain, increase range of motion, and restore function

_____ 4. Promotes healing for strong and mobile scar tissue

_____ 5. Neurotransmitter that helps regulate heart rate, blood pressure, and indirectly affects pituitary function

_____ 6. Effect of massage that result from squeezing, pushing, pulling, rubbing, stretching, and compressing soft tissues of the body

_____ 7. Neurotransmitter that regulates mood, appetite, sleep, memory, learning, and muscle contraction

_____ 8. Nerves that carry impulses for dull, aching pain that have been present for some time

_____ 9. Examples are changes in blood pressure, hormone and neurotransmitter levels, and muscle fiber structure

_____ 10. Hormone produced by the body in response to stress

_____ 11. Examples are decreased anxiety and stress levels, and improved well-being

_____ 12. Nerves that carry impulses for pressure, temperature, and sharp acute pain

MATCHING II

Place the letter of the answer next to the term or phrase that best describes it.

A. Application of pressure, heat and cold
B. Cardiovascular system
C. Connective tissues
D. Endocrine system
E. Gate control theory
F. Influence the perception of pain
G. Localized muscle guarding
H. Lymphatic system and immune functions
I. Muscles, bones, and joints
J. Nervous system
K. Pain-cycle
L. Skin

_____ 1. These may interfere or interrupt pain signals through the use of the gate mechanism

_____ 2. Massage effects on this body system include increased blood flow to the skin and muscular tissue, and an increase in the number of blood cells

_____ 3. Massage effects to this structure include treating or preventing bed sores and decreasing symptoms of eczema

_____ 4. When this occurs, there is a restriction of movement and a decrease in blood flow, which decreases the amount of oxygen available to tissues and the removal of metabolic wastes

_____ 5. Massage effects of these structures include increased range of motion and decrease in electromyography activity

_____ 6. Massage effects of these tissues include reduced pain and symptoms of fibromyalgia, and aiding in tendon injury healing

_____ 7. Initiated when painful stimuli result in muscle contraction and localized muscle splinting or guarding

_____ 8. Massage effects this symptom and its cycle in several ways including increased circulation, decreased spasm, modulation in neurotransmitters and hormones, and the simple act of touch and comfort

_____ 9. Massage effects of this system include improved sleep, and improved cognitive and memory functioning

_____ 10. Massage effects include decreased edema and increased level of white blood cells

_____ 11. Theory of pain relief where multiple nerve impulses compete for entrance into the spinal cord; the one that gets there first prevents other impulses from entering

_____ 12. Massage effects of this system include influencing the production and absorption of insulin, and producing changes in hormones related to pregnancy, labor and post partum depression

CASE STUDY

SOS Case

For the past few months, Adrienne has been having a variety of health problems. Her physician referred her to Jeremy in hopes massage would help her relax while waiting for test results. Adrienne explains to Jeremy that she has had pain in her neck and shoulders, and in her lower back. She sometimes feels a lightheaded. Her blood pressure is slightly elevated, but she is not taking medication. She has had digestive issues, ranging from pain in the upper abdomen after eating, to constipation and diarrhea. Sometimes after she eats, she feels short of breath. She also suspects plantar fasciitis because her feet hurt in the morning, and perhaps carpal tunnel syndrome because her wrist hurts and she feels tingling in her fingers.

During his assessment, Jeremy learns that Adrienne works as an administrative assistant, sitting at a desk for at 8 hours a day, plus an hour commute in either direction. Her hobby is sewing, so she spends a lot of time at a sewing machine. She gets regular exercise, but with her recent pain and digestive issues, she is less active. Jeremy also notes significant forward head posture. Adrienne's neck is rotated left and laterally flexed to the right. She has a considerable kyphotic curve.

Which techniques are best for Christine? Are there any cautions or contraindications to consider when formulating Adrienne's treatment plan? Should Jeremy wait for Adrienne's physician to make a diagnosis before proceeding? Why or why not?

CRITICAL THINKING

Does the Gate Control Theory address acute or chronic pain? Explain your answer.

Body Mechanics, Client Positioning, and Draping

"Hands are the heart's landscape."
—Pope John Paul II

LEARNING OBJECTIVES

After completing this chapter, the student should be able to:

- Define body mechanics.
- Discuss ways to prevent repetitive motion injuries.
- Identify basic foot stances.
- Explain principles of effective body mechanics.
- Discuss adaptive body mechanics used when the client is lying on the floor.
- Demonstrate effective uses of bolsters while the client is in various body positions.
- Using sheets and towels, demonstrate appropriate draping, and maintain draping while the client turns over.
- Assist the client off the massage table while maintaining appropriate draping.

 http://evolve.elsevier.com/Salvo/MassageTherapy

INTRODUCTION

A precursor to giving massage is learning and applying principles of effective body mechanics, client position, and draping. Each of these elements plays an essential role in the delivery of massage. The use of effective body mechanics can reduce or even eliminate the physical toll taken on the therapist's body, both on a daily basis and cumulatively over the span of a career. Additionally, the use of self-care techniques (see Chapter 4) helps to minimize the number of minor aches and pains. Assisting the client on and off the table is also addressed as it involves effective body mechanics.

BODY MECHANICS

Body mechanics is the use of postural techniques, foot stances, leverage techniques, and other elements to deliver massage therapy and related bodywork methods with efficiency and the least amount of trauma to the therapist. Body mechanics includes the principles of alignment, delivery of force, stamina, breathing, stability, and balance. Effective body mechanics positively influences the execution of the massage, decreases therapist fatigue and discomfort during and after the massage, and helps prevent repetitive motion injuries. See Box 7-1 for a discussion of these injuries. An essential aspect of a long, healthy career is the ability to provide treatment without incurring injury. Few health care occupations use upper body strength with the force or frequency required in massage (see Box 4-1).

A common perception is that Western cultures tend to focus on physical strength and stamina and Eastern cultures tend to focus on balance and the ability to become centered. Both viewpoints have merit in helping you explore your body's landscape and increase vigor.

Many elements of body mechanics used in massage and katas used in martial arts are similar in nature. To help us better understand these systems of movement, the ancient practices of kendo and aikido can be examined. Students of these martial arts are required to follow four basic principles: (1) *eyes first* (for focus and attention), (2) *footwork next* (foot position for weight transference), (3) *courage third* (assessing timing, space, your opponent, and how you are going to initiate your movements), and (4) *strength last* (body moves into action or weight effort). Notably, strength and weight effort come last in the list. If we apply these principles to massage therapy, then focus, foot stance, and self-assessment come before the massage strokes.

MINI-LAB

Using a full-length mirror, observe your body mechanics during a massage. Adjust your body position and foot stance when needed to feel stable, yet able to move into action.

BOX 7-1

Repetitive Motion Injuries

According to the American Massage Therapy Association, the second most common reason why therapists leave the profession is injury (first being inability to grow a business). Injuries can be sustained while giving massage. In most instances, these injuries result from poor body alignment and using muscular force rather than body leverage while applying pressure.

Repetitive strain injuries (RSIs), also called repetitive motion injuries, or cumulative trauma disorders, are most often caused by chronic misuse of the body (i.e., poor body mechanics). In many instances, repetitive motions are combined with compressive forces or joint hyperextension. RSIs may cause or contribute to neuropathy, paresthesias, subluxation, joint deterioration, or trauma, and related conditions such as bursitis and arthritis.

Symptoms of RSIs include pain and weakness in the arm, wrist, and/or hand. Symptoms and related damage can progress unless inefficient body mechanics or repetitive strain is altered. Examples of RSIs of the upper body include:

- Carpal tunnel syndrome
- Cubital tunnel syndrome
- Thoracic outlet syndrome
- De Quervain tenosynovitis
- Tennis elbow (lateral epicondylitis)
- Golfer's elbow (medial epicondylitis)

As therapists, our anterior forearm muscles (which, by design, are two-thirds stronger than our posterior forearm muscles) become overdeveloped from repeated finger flexing. Over time, this hypertrophy causes the flexor retinaculum to compress tendons and nerves supplying the hand. The digits most likely to be involved are the middle and ring fingers and the thumb such as seen in carpal tunnel syndrome.

If you have symptoms of RSI, visit your primary health care provider for medical evaluation and treatment.

Some prevention suggestions are:

- Massage anterior forearm muscles frequently.
- Learn to use your elbows and knuckles to deliver deep pressure.
- Strengthening posterior forearm muscles (e.g., 1 to 3 lb barbell)
- Prepare for the massage with movement (see Chapter 4).
- Adjust table height for best body mechanics.
- Use effective body mechanics.
- Avoid excessive wrist extension, flexion, abduction, and adduction during massage.
- Use a variety of strokes.
- Rest your hands by spacing appointments.
- Keep your body physically fit through a fitness program (see Chapter 4).

As you can see, RSIs will negatively affect your work as a therapist. Pain is the great equalizer. It eventually gets everyone's attention; therefore pay attention to your body when it is speaking to you and respond accordingly. But an ounce of prevention is worth a pound of cure.

ELEMENTS OF BODY MECHANICS

This section explores essential elements of body mechanics, which include (1) strength, (2) stamina, (3) stability, (4) breathing, (5) balance, and (6) centeredness.

Strength

Massage requires some physical strength. If you do not possess adequate strength through regular exercise and proper diet, you not only fatigue faster but are more prone to RSIs (see Box 7-1). You may be asked to assist your client onto and off the table or lift and move a client who is disabled or elderly. Activities that promote muscle strength are floor exercises (e.g., plank, side plank, bridge, sit-ups) and weight or strength training. Muscles become stronger when they are challenged (see Figure 4-3). Because massage involves the entire body, all major muscle groups should be addressed during strength training, with special focus on core muscles (abdominal muscles, back muscles, muscles of the shoulder and hip). Consult a personal or athletic trainer to help you develop a workout regime.

Stamina

Many massage sessions last at least 1 hour. The therapist must possess enough stamina and endurance throughout the day to provide every client a great massage. To gain or maintain stamina, include cardiovascular training in your fitness program. According to the American College of Sports Medicine and the American Heart Association, the current recommendation is *30 to 60 minutes of moderate physical activity daily*. Examples of moderate physical activity are walking, biking, swimming, and gardening.

Between massage sessions, you might want to try the 60-second energizer featured in Box 7-2. Additional complex carbohydrates added to a balanced diet are the best fuel food for keeping your energy level high. Be sure you get plenty of rest. Good body mechanics suffers when a therapist is tired. Fatigue can also be reduced by structured breathing techniques (see later section on breathing).

Stability

Massage movements are executed from a stable base. Your lower body is $2\frac{1}{2}$ times stronger and more stable than your upper body. With both feet firmly planted on the ground, stability is shared by both feet and legs. From a stable base, force is transmitted during massage from the lower body while the upper body becomes a flexible conduit. This helps you reduce stress, because your legs provide most of the force behind the movement.

Architecturally speaking, the triangle is the most structurally stable base. The structure of the foot produces three arches that resemble a geodesic dome. The three bony points of contact with the ground are the (1) calcaneal tuberosity,

---

BOX 7-2

60-Second Energizer

1. Slap the palms of your outstretched hands together, and rub them rapidly for 5 seconds (out of earshot of clients).
2. Hold your warmed palms over your cheeks and eyes for 5 seconds.
3. Make your hands into claws, and apply vigorous tapping tapotement to the scalp for 5 seconds.
4. Apply loose-fist tapotement up and down each arm for 10 seconds.
5. Gently grasp the hyoid bone, and mobilize it from side to side to stimulate the thyroid gland.
6. With your right hand, cup your palm around the back of your neck and squeeze firmly 10 times.
7. Repeat Step 6 with the left hand while nodding your head up and down at the same time.
8. Repeat Step 6 with the left hand while shaking your head side to side at the same time.
9. With the right hand, reach across the midline of your body, grasp the top of your left trapezius, and squeeze firmly 10 times.
10. Repeat Step 9 to the right trapezius with the left hand.
11. Perform three sets of shoulder rolls forward and three backward.
12. Pincer-grip the thumb web of each hand, and hold for 3 seconds.
13. Shake the hands several times.
14. Stomp the feet several times.
    You are now energized and ready to go.

---

(2) head of the first metatarsal, and (3) head of the fifth metatarsal. The three points of contact form the shape of a triangle (Figure 7-1). Both feet on the ground provide two stable bases, the foundation for movement.

Compare the relative stability of a pogo stick and a tripod. The tripod is stable, but the pogo stick is not. Techniques requiring the therapist to stand with most or all of his or her weight on one leg use poor body mechanics. Furthermore, the center of gravity is much higher, promoting instability. The therapist needs a stable base with both feet on the ground to initiate movement. In fact, when the therapist works from a stable body stance, he or she is more responsive to the client.

Breathing

Structured breathing will help you relax, pace massage movements, and fuel muscles with oxygen. Proper breathing technique enhances mental and physical health, thereby positively affecting the quality of massage. According to William Barry, author and instructor, structured breathing is the *foundation of massage*. Combine structured breathing and massage therapy. During the push of a gliding stroke,

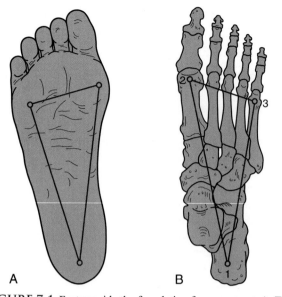

FIGURE 7-1 Feet provide the foundation for movement. **A,** Triangular base of support. **B,** Bony points of contact. *1,* calcaneal tuberosity; *2,* head of first metatarsal; *3,* head of fifth metatarsal.

exhale. Inhale while dragging your hands back. As you apply sustained pressure on a tender area, exhale. Inhale while releasing pressure. Encourage your clients to do the same.

Because the nose does a better job of warming and filtering the air over the mouth, nasal breathing is preferred over mouth breathing. Placing your tongue on the roof of your mouth as you breathe encourages nasal breathing.

Deep structured breathing is also a great way to release tension. Visualize all the tension and stress flowing out of your body as you exhale and vibrant energy entering your body as you inhale. Encourage your clients to take slow deliberate breaths before, during, and after the massage.

You may need to modify these techniques to minimize the excess noise produced by deep breathing, because some clients can find it distracting.

Aikido masters often use breathing to guide their students to shrink their focus to a space approximately the size of a quarter, 2 inches below and behind the navel. This ancient center of gravity is called the *hara* (Japanese term for lower abdomen) This area is a topographic *and* meditative point of reference known for thousands of years as the center of physical and spiritual balance. A simple way to experience the power of area is to allow your breath to move into and out of your hara. On expiration, contract your pelvic floor muscles to lower your center of gravity and tighten lower back muscles to help maintain a straight back.

While you breathe, be aware of facial expressions; keep your jaw unlocked and your face relaxed.

Balance

Effective body mechanics are a direct result of balanced posture that respects the laws of gravity. Gravity is the mutual attraction of two objects toward each other, such as

your body and the earth. When you are balanced, energy expended during the massage is reduced. The center of gravity, the point at which the body is balanced, is generally an inch or two below and behind your navel called the *dan tien* (Chinese term for this point). The principle of balance can be expanded to an emotional and spiritual awareness or energetic experience of ourselves in relation to our surroundings. Activites that encourage balance include yoga and martial arts such as tai chi, qi gong, and aikido, which can also be used for meditation or centering.

When teaching the concept of balance, aikido masters often tell students to place their weight underside and allow themselves to feel light on top. As mentioned earlier, abdominal breathing from the hara contributes to a sense of balance.

MINI-LAB

Choose a partner. Ask him or her to stand with both feet 24 inches apart. Next, ask your partner to concentrate on the head. After a moment, gently push against his or her shoulder. Question your partner about how his or her body responds to the change. Next, ask your partner to concentrate on the hara (lower abdomen). After allowing time for concentration, give another gentle push. Have your partner report on the difference he or she felt during each push. Which area of concentration felt more stable? Switch roles. Compare experiences, noting similarities or differences. The area that felt more stable is the area from which you initiate your massage movements.

Centeredness

Embedded in the art of massage is the concept of centeredness, which refers to the *mental, emotional,* and *physical* states of consciousness. The connection between the body and the mind is fundamental; the two are difficult, if not impossible, to separate. The best way to illustrate this relationship is to consider what happens and how your body feels when you are under considerable mental or emotional stress. The body mirrors your state of mind; headaches and insomnia are common. Conversely, when you are ill or experiencing chronic pain, you are affected mentally and emotionally. Mundane tasks become difficult, and you may express emotions easily or not at all. Thus taking time to center and prepare yourself not only physically, but also mentally and emotionally, helps you become a more compassionate and sensitive therapist.

When you are centered, you may feel the presence of God, nature, or a higher power (insert your personal preference) in addition to the company of your client. You become part of a larger whole and recognize that you are just a vessel for healing and positive influence. Surround yourself with the ubiquitous energy and power that bring peace and serenity. When stress, tension, and excess energy are released by your client, channel it to the ground rather than absorbing it. Being centered makes a difference in how you deliver the massage; it will help you stay focused and not become distracted by thoughts unrelated to the session. By clearing your mind and experiencing the moment, your body mechanics will be greatly enhanced.

CHAT ROOM

Can you pick up a client's negative energy or illness during a session? Some people think so. Pierre Pannetier (world's foremost authority on polarity therapy) says that when this phenomenon happens, "we try too hard to help our clients and in doing so are really using force instead of love. When we use force, we limit ourselves and create unnecessary difficulties."

*"You cannot solve problems with the same
level of thinking that existed when
the problems were created."*
—Albert Einstein

FOOT STANCES
7-1

We massage not only with our hands but with our whole body. This complete body involvement plays a role in how massage is delivered. Foot placement influences the depth of pressure and direction of the massage stroke. Remember, the lower body has $2\frac{1}{2}$ times more strength than the upper body; thus using the lower body to deliver massage makes sense. Foot placement has a profound effect on body mechanics and body alignment.

Massage therapists typically use two-foot stances when delivering massage strokes: the *bow stance* and the *horse stance*. Both stances provide a stable foundation and balanced body posture. Foot stance used depends on the style of massage you perform and the type of techniques used. Techniques that require excursion are done in the bow stance, whereas strokes that are performed with little or no excursion favor the horse stance. Each foot provides three points of contact with the earth (see Figure 7-1). Both feet represent six points of contact. While moving from one stance to the other, let movement be initiated from your feet up to the center of balance (hara or dan tien) and then

PAUL ST. JOHN

Born: July 27, 1945

*"Where all the growth is in this profession and in life is the line of most resistance. Oftentimes we
resist so much of what life wants to teach us and why we're here."*

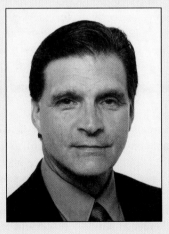

The St. John method of neuromuscular therapy is a comprehensive program of soft tissue manipulation techniques that balance the central nervous system with the structure and form of the musculoskeletal system. On a more basic level, it is the study of how form affects function. The St. John method can free the body to move, stand, and simply *be* the way it was created to be based on a structural and biochemical model.

Unlike some therapies that relax individuals and relieve minor pain, deep neuromuscular work zeroes in on both the problem and the effect. According to St. John, the five principles of neuromuscular therapy are (1) biomechanics, (2) postural distortion, (3) trigger points, (4) nerve entrapment–nerve compression, and (5) ischemia, all of which upset homeostasis.

Much of the charisma and commitment of Paul St. John, the man behind the method, was captured by Robert

Calvert in an interview for *Massage Magazine*. St. John was 3 years of age when his father, an illegal alien, was deported. Young St. John was a street kid and an average student who later discovered he had a learning disability. Playing high school football, he suffered a broken back, his first injury. This injury led him to take a U.S. Army recruiter's aptitude test. After doing exceptionally well, however, St. John still was not quite ready to join. Instead, his mother's battle with cancer motivated him into a career in radiology. While practicing radiology, he was drafted into military service during the Vietnam War. When his aircraft was shot down, two Chinese physicians accomplished in minutes what the hospital, which managed his earlier leg injury in high school, had not been able to do in weeks.

After he returned home, his family hounded him to get a job. He hitchhiked to Florida and worked as a
Continued

PAUL ST. JOHN (*continued*)

garbage collector until his third injury. With debilitating pain and mounting health bills, he experienced no improvement. A friend in chiropractic care then introduced St. John to the work of Dr. Raymond Nimmo, who was responsible for a technique known as *receptor tonus.* St. John studied this technique and soon began helping friends cope with pain. He then began a massage therapy school and is now a teacher and therapist who never wants to lose touch with clients. His own encounters with pain and other persons living with pain fuel his desire to do even more. He considers himself a perpetual student.

Today, St. John is changing the quality of lives with his methods, giving hope to people who have not found relief through conventional means. "Medicine has unconsciously become totally function oriented," explains St. John. "It ignores form, but if you have someone with a collapsed diaphragmatic posture, then peristaltic action and nutrient absorption are affected. The stomach collapses and loses tone. The medical community might suggest a laxative. You've got to treat the cause and not the effect. America spent over $4 billion for analgesics, medicines to suppress symptoms, this past year (1997)."

St. John shares the results of one of his latest cases: "A young woman who was about to have surgery to correct her scoliosis spent some time at my clinic. Doctors were going to put a rod in her back. We corrected her curvature 27%, and we have the x-rays to prove it."

St. John goes on to share other relationships between structure and disease. "Parkinson's patients almost all have a distortion in their cranium. In many stroke victims a forward-head posture of 6 to 8 inches is seen. This traps the arteries. Patients with cardiac problems usually have a slumping shoulder posture. An abdominal posture affects the diaphragm, aorta, vena cava, and esophagus. That's why so many of these people develop hiatal hernias.

"Neuromuscular therapy is the best value for the money. If your carburetor needs fixing, you get it fixed, right? But we let our bodies stay broken down."

After treatment, St. John's clients ask, "Why hasn't my doctor done this? It makes so much sense!" Nonetheless, skeptics abound. A man with a bad knee who had practically been dragged to the clinic told St. John, "I know what's wrong with my knee. I'm 72 years old." St. John then pointed to the patient's good knee and said, "Oh yeah, so how old is that knee?"

St. John has many success stories, but because of his commitment to his work, he has little time to recount them all. He has patients waiting. The interview is over with these words of advice for the beginning therapist: "Take personal responsibility. Specialize in a certain area if you really want to make a living. Techniques that work best conform to the laws of the universe. One third medicine is intellectual; two thirds is art."

In an earlier interview, St. John offered direction for anyone seeking success: "People who accomplish great things are ordinary people who have great dreams. It's not that they are more gifted and God has smiled upon them. People who become great have great work ethics and they put a lot of sweat equity into it. They aren't lucky people, you know; they work hard, and they're committed."

---

through the arms and hands. Massage movements feel smooth and rhythmic when initiated from a stable base.

Bow Stance

Also known as the *archer stance* or *lunge position,* the **bow stance** is used when applying massage techniques that proceed from one point to the next along the client's body (i.e., effleurage). Your feet are placed on the floor in a 30- to 50-degree angle, one pointing straight forward *(leading foot)* and the other pointing in the direction the therapist's body is moving *(trailing foot).* Your whole body follows the direction of the leading foot (Figure 7-2). Distance between the feet will vary from person to person.

When applying techniques that require excursion, begin the advancement by bringing your trailing foot to the leading foot; then move the leading foot forward, shifting your weight between the leading and trailing feet as you step forward to follow your hands. Without this weight shift, balance may be lost. If it is executed correctly, your client should not sense the step forward through your hands. Avoid balancing yourself by pushing on your client to move forward. Avoid movements that bring the knee beyond the placement of the leading foot.

With the bow stance, keep your spine straight from the cervical to the sacral region. Bend at the hips and knees, not at the waist, as you lunge forward.

Horse Stance

Also known as the *warrior stance,* the **horse stance** is used to perform massage techniques that traverse relatively short distances, such as pétrissage and most friction strokes. Place feet just beyond hip distance with toes pointing forward

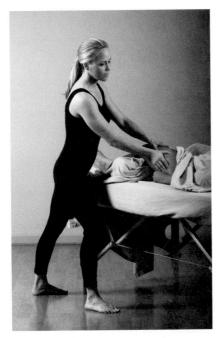

FIGURE 7-2 Therapist in the bow stance.

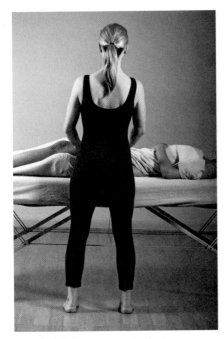

FIGURE 7-3 Therapist in the horse stance.

(Figure 7-3). Again, your knees are slightly flexed. Keep your back straight and your pelvis tilted posteriorly. This is aided with contraction of the abdominal muscles.

Your shoulders should be relaxed while your hands and arms are moving.

While moving side to side, shift your weight from one gluteal muscle group to the other as your hands move across the client's skin. If a lifting or lowering action is needed, raise or lower your body by extending and flexing your knees and keeping your back straight.

Evolve *Log on to the Evolve website for self-care suggestions for the therapist. Write down at least three more ways to reduce and relieve tension between sessions.* ■

▶ GUIDELINES FOR EFFECTIVE BODY MECHANICS
7-2

The following guidelines will assist you with effective body mechanics.

Use Proper Table Height

Proper table height allows you to use leverage to increase pressure without compromising body mechanics. Table height is determined by several factors: your height, the technique or method you are using, the position of the client, and the client's girth. For example, for performing side-lying massage, table height is often higher to accommodate the therapist's pushing his or her body weight across rather than downward.

Two generally accepted methods are used to determine table height. Take care to relax your shoulders fully to get an accurate measurement.

- Stand alongside the massage table with arms to your sides and make a fist with your hand. Table height is where the table touches your fist or first knuckles (Figure 7-4, *A*).
- Stand alongside the massage table, arms at your sides, with wrist and fingers extended. The height where your fingertips brush slightly against your table represents an appropriate table height (Figure 7-4, *B*).

Use a specific table height during a day when several clients are scheduled. Afterward, lie down and note how your body feels. If your arms or shoulders feel achy, the table is too high; you are overcompensating from not being able to use leverage. If your lower back feels stiff, your table is too low, or you might be bending your back instead of knees and hips. Raise or drop the tabletop until optimal table height is achieved (Box 7-3). After massage, the therapist should feel from relaxed to energized.

Additionally, take into account client girth, which can necessitate altering table height quite a bit. Clients with a large girth or torso thickness will require a lower table height. But remember to let the *comfort level of your body be your guide* when deciding appropriate table height.

Many therapists prefer to adjust their table heights lower than normal to take advantage of their body weight behind downward pressure. Table height may be set at just above the level of the therapist's patellas (or kneecaps). Conversely, many therapists who use methods such as Trager, craniosacral therapy, energetic practices such as Reiki, or polarity often prefer a higher-than-normal table because it is most comfortable for them.

Wear Comfortable Attire

Clothing should look professional, be comfortable, and allow freedom of movement. Cotton clothing is best because it absorbs perspiration, which helps keep you cool. Wear

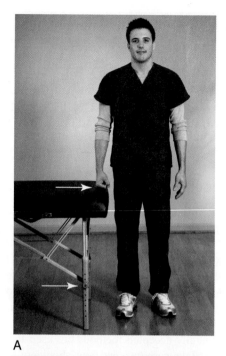

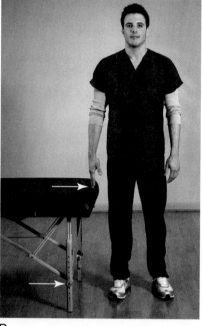

FIGURE 7-4 Methods of determining massage table height. **A,** Using fist; **B,** using fingertips.

sensible supportive shoes with low or no heels and good arch supports. Women should consider using a comfortably supportive sports bra.

Warm Up Before Massage

Before giving a massage, warm up first. Warm muscles are less susceptible to injury than cold muscles. The American College of Sports Medicine (ACSM) recommends that a person warm up by doing the movements he or she will

---

BOX 7-3

Listen to Your Pain

If you are in pain after giving a massage, your body is trying to tell you something. It *might* be saying that:

If your *neck* is sore, you are spending too much time looking down at your work.

If your *shoulders* are sore, your table is too high or you are using your upper body rather than your lower body when applying pressure.

If your *thumb pads* are sore, you are doing too much pétrissage (kneading) or sustained pressure with the thumbs.

If your *wrists* are sore, you are hyperextending them while applying pressure.

If your *lower back* is sore, your table is too low, you are not lunging, or your pelvis is neutral rather than posteriorly tilted.

If only *one side of your lower back* is sore, you are twisting your torso too much while applying pressure or your trailing foot is laterally rotated.

---

perform during activity, but with less intensity. Mild lunges, mild pressing of the hands against the massage table, and circling your foot using your ankles are excellent warm up activities for massage. See the Chapter 4 section entitled "Preparing for the Massage" for additional suggestions.

Stretch During Massage

Take stretch breaks while walking from one side of the table to the other. Use this time to shake out your arms, move your neck, and relax. Between massage sessions, spend time stretching your back, upper chest, and forearms (Figure 7-5). Your body mechanics will improve with regular stretching.

Use a Variety of Strokes

Most massage routines incorporate a variety of techniques. Changing from effleurage to pétrissage to tapotement to friction requires the therapist to change the position of both hands and feet, thus reducing fatigue and chances of repetitive motion injuries. Be sure to listen to your body. If the right hand is becoming fatigued, then use the left hand. If compressive movements are irritating wrists and knuckle joints, then change to a lifting technique such as pétrissage.

If you notice that the same body areas are fatiguing, consider appropriate exercise to strengthen those areas, rather than always relying on your "stronger" side.

Keep Wrists and Digits as Straight as Possible

Keep your wrists as straight as possible (Figure 7-6). Repeatedly applying pressure while wrists are out of alignment (flexion, extension, adduction, abduction) may cause injury.

At times, moving the wrist out of alignment will be necessary, but remember that the greater the pressure, the straighter the wrists. Do not let the digits become hyperextended while applying direct pressure. Use braced thumb techniques while working to prevent joint hyperextension. To brace your thumb, place your flexed index finger behind it (Figure 7-7).

Align Your Spine

Keep your spine straight, head erect, and eyes looking forward (as much as possible). This is more easily

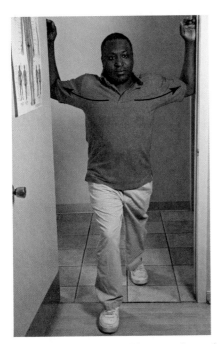

FIGURE 7-5 Therapist stretching his pectoral muscles between sessions.

accomplished with your shoulders back and rib cage lifted slightly. This posture also allows you ease of breathing so you can stay relaxed during the session. If you spend a great amount of time looking down, your neck may become stiff and sore. If you must observe your work, then lower yourself to the level of your hands by sitting on a stool or kneeling down on the floor. Look out a window or at the corners of the ceiling occasionally to stretch your neck while you move around the table (Box 7-4).

Check in With Lower Back, Hips, Knees, and Feet

Keep your back straight by tilting your pelvis posteriorly. This will reduce an exaggerated lumbar curve. Use the penny-pinching technique to tilt the pelvis (see the Mini-Lab on p. 117 for instructions). Hips should be level and knees slightly flexed. Keep your feet planted firmly on the ground while standing. Shift weight from one foot to another to reflect what your hands are doing. Freda Whalen, a fellow therapist and instructor, uses three phrases to remind students about effective body mechanics: *suck it* (pull abdomen in), *tuck it* (tilt pelvis posteriorly), and *drop it* (lower shoulders and flex knees).

Relax Shoulders

Place your shoulders comfortably on top of your rib cage, relaxed and dropped. Do not hunch over or round the shoulders while working, and try to keep your shoulders over your hips when possible. Keep your arms close to your upper body whenever possible. When your arms move away from your body, you lose leverage and fatigue more quickly. When gliding down the client's back or up the leg, follow your hands by taking a few steps rather than extending your shoulders.

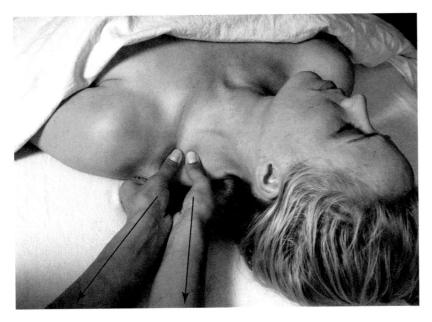

FIGURE 7-6 Therapist keeping wrists as straight as possible.

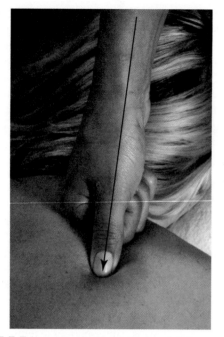

FIGURE 7-7 Use a braced thumb kept straight by support from the index fingers, while applying pressure.

BOX 7-4

Body Mechanics Quick Check

Answering the following questions will help you determine correct body mechanics during the massage and what areas might need improvement:

1. Is your massage table the correct height for you?
2. Are you warming up before your first massage of the day and stretching between massage sessions?
3. Are your knees slightly bent?
4. Are your feet firmly planted on the ground?
5. Are you shifting your weight as you move, working with your whole body?
6. Are your wrists straight?
7. Are your thumbs and fingers supported while applying direct pressure?
8. Is your back straight and your pelvis posteriorly tilted?
9. Is your head centered over your neck and shoulders?
10. Are you using a variety of techniques in your massage? Are you positioning yourself behind your strokes?
11. Is a stool nearby to be used during facial and foot massages?
12. Is your face relaxed and your jaw unlocked during the massage?
13. Are you using proper lifting techniques?

If you answered *no* to one or more of these questions, then you may be at risk for stress, strain, and injury resulting from poor body mechanics.

BOX 7-5

Body Mechanics While Working on the Floor

The same principles that are vital to massage therapy performed on a massage table apply to working on a mat or futon on the floor—strength, stamina, stability, breathing, balance, and centeredness.

Your center of gravity is your lower abdomen (hara). Keep your hara facing toward the area of the client's body you are working on. The hara can also be thought of as a pivot point for you to change your position. Keep your spine in proper alignment.

The strength for application of pressure, just like when working on a table, comes from the ground, up through your torso, then out through your arms and hands.

Several stances give you the most stability and proficient body mechanics when working on the floor.

One involves sitting with your gluteal muscles on your heels with your knees together. A variation of this is sitting in a wider position with your thighs open at least 45 degrees. From this position, you can rise up to apply more pressure.

Other stances include crawling, squatting, and lunging. *Crawling* is a natural way of moving around a client lying on a futon. *Squatting* provides a stable base from which to move into other positions easily. *Lunging* is modified squatting. Reaching certain parts of your client's body is easier when lunging.

A slight swaying motion can be included, then expanded on as you become more comfortable with the movements and the techniques being performed.

Never straddle a client. Keep in mind while working on the floor, avoid superfluous body contact.

Get Behind Your Work

Position yourself, as much as possible, directly behind your work. Both arms and legs should face the direction you are working or in which pressure is applied. When pushing an object, you would not stand beside it; you would stand directly behind. This is true while your client is on a table, in a chair, or on the floor (Box 7-5).

▌ MINI-LAB

Use a scale to learn how to lean into a client to increase pressure. Place a regular floor scale used for weighing people on your massage table. Press down with varying pressures and watch the scale reading. Try a palm, a thumb tip, elbow, etc. Have a classmate get on the massage table with the scale. Using the same pressure, press on the scale with one hand and on the person's back with the other. Ask your classmate for pressure feedback and compare the scale's readout. Come up with a number range for light, moderate, and deep pressure. What number is too painful?

Repeat the experiment, moving the scale both closer and farther away from your body as you lean. Repeat the experiment with the table lowered one to two notches.

Which position increases depth of pressure without additional excursion?

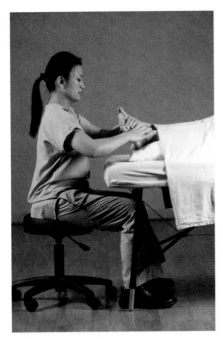

FIGURE 7-8 Therapist using a stool.

Sit Down Occasionally

It is okay to sit on a stool while working on your client's face, neck, shoulders, feet, or hands (Figure 7-8). Sitting will reduce fatigue and gives your back and feet a break. Keep both feet flat on the floor with the back straight. Lauriann Greene and Richard W. Goggins, authors of *Save Your Hands!*, suggest that about 25% of session time be spent in a seated position to avoid fatigue.

Use Effective Body Mechanics During Related Professional Activities

If you have to assist your client into a seated or standing position, use your legs, not your back, and keep your arms close to your body. Know and respect your own limits. Ask for assistance from other persons in your office when needed.

Adapt As You Age

It is no secret that a 20-year-old therapist is affected differently by giving massage than a 50-year-old therapist. So, as you age, adapt your body mechanics and your techniques accordingly. This may mean using a stool more often while you work or scheduling fewer clients per week. Monica Reno, a licensed and practicing massage therapist for more than 25 years, says that "the greatest likelihood of being able to practice massage as a 50-year-old is to practice the best body mechanics as a 20-year-old."

MINI-LAB

To experience a posterior-tilted pelvis, try the penny-pinching technique. While standing, imagine that you have a penny between your buttocks. To keep the penny from falling to the ground, contract your gluteal muscles and *pinch* the penny. This simple exercise straightens your back muscles, contracts your abdominal muscles, and tilts your pelvis posteriorly.

MINI-LAB

Stand in front of a full-length mirror. Place one foot 18 inches in front of the other, and place your hands on your hips. Lunge forward, shifting your weight from the back leg to the front leg. As you move forward and backward, keep your shoulders and hips level. Look in the mirror to check your progress. Maintaining a good posture while you are in motion promotes good working posture while performing massage.

"Close your hand. Do you feel absence or presence?"
—Brenda Hefty

 BOLSTERS

Bolsters, which include pillows and cushions, assist client comfort by supporting and enabling proper alignment of individual joints which, in turn, helps muscles relax. A small neck pillow maintains the normal anterior cervical curve, and a knee bolster reduces tension in the hips and lower back. An ankle bolster prevents excessive dorsiflexion and uncomfortable rotation of knees, which may cause leg or foot cramps in susceptible clients.

In the absence of commercially manufactured bolsters, a rolled-up towel, blanket, or pillow works great.

The most commonly bolstered areas are the face and ankles (see Figure 7-9) and the neck and knees (see Figure 7-11). The same bolster is often used for the knees and ankles. A cushion that rests on a frame extending from the table is used for the face. A soft smaller pillow is used for the neck. An additional soft pillow may be needed for female clients who are uncomfortable lying prone because of breast tenderness (see Chapter 11).

Always cover bolsters with a clean drape, such as a pillowcase or custom bolster cover. In the absence of a bolster cover, place the bolster beneath the bottom drape to avoid direct contact of the bolster fabric with the client's skin.

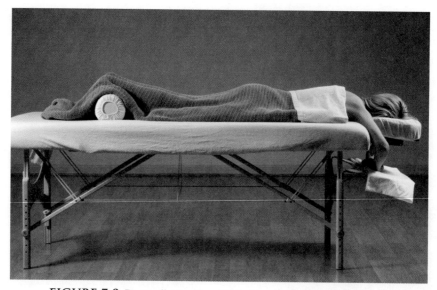

FIGURE 7-9 Prone client with ankle bolster, face rest, and arm shelf.

Be sure to remove any bolsters before the client gets up off the table. Otherwise, bolsters become obstacles for your client to maneuver around.

CLIENT POSITIONING

Certain client positions promote comfort and relaxation through proper body alignment. Client positioning also addresses medical and health issues that often necessitate the client to be positioned on the table in a particular way. The client intake and interview will help you decide what positions to use and which to avoid (if any). For example, a client in advanced pregnancy requires a different set of positions from those used for an athlete. A client with physical limitations might require a lower table height or additional bolstering. A client with severe lordosis may need a higher-than-normal knee bolster while in the supine position.

Regardless of which positions you and the client decide, a good question to ask your client is, "How can you become even more comfortable?" This process allows you to fine-tune the client's position and address directly his or her comfort needs.

The four main client positions are prone, supine, side-lying, and seated. Supine clients may also be placed in a semireclining position.

Prone Position

7-4 In the prone position, the person is lying face down. The most commonly supported areas when the client is prone are the ankles and face (Figure 7-9). Occasionally, female clients may be more comfortable with additional bolstering to reduce pressure on breast tissue.

A vinyl-covered 3-, 6-, or 8-inch-diameter bolster under the ankles of a prone client helps the hips, legs, and ankles

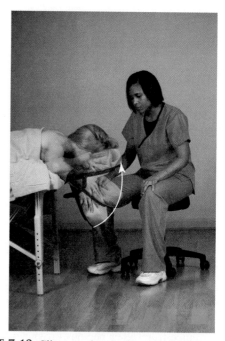

FIGURE 7-10 Client moving the face rest frame into a comfortable position before the therapist locks it into place.

to relax during the massage. Try different bolster heights to see which one works best for your client (See Mini-Lab on page 121 in Chapter 3 for a related activity). If your client complains of lower back pain while prone, try a pillow under the abdomen or hips.

If you have an adjustable face rest, let the client decide the angle of the frame to maximize personal comfort (Figure 7-10). Larger-breasted women may require the face rest frame to be adjusted above the level of the table (see Figure 11-9). Unlock all the cams and ask your client to pull the

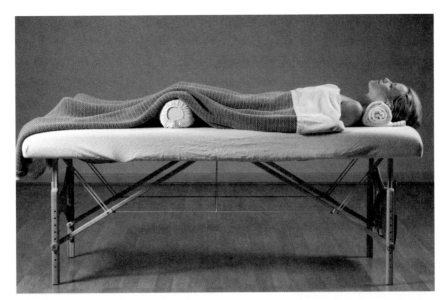

FIGURE 7-11 Supine client with knee bolster and rolled-up towel for a cervical pillow.

face rest and frame up to the face while flexing the neck forward slightly until a comfortable position is found. Next, lock the cams in place to maintain the position of the face rest.

Some tables possess a wide slit for the face, allowing the client to lie prone without a face rest. Because of the slit built into the table top, specially made sheets must be used. If a face rest is not available, use one or two standard-size pillows. Place them either horizontally or diagonally under the forehead and/or the shoulders.

As mentioned previously, many women may experience breast discomfort when lying prone. Breast tenderness may be due to a variety of reasons including menopause, menstruation, pregnancy, lactation, fibrocystic breast disease, or surgeries such as augmentation or mastectomy. Be sure to offer additional support with a small soft pillow or rolled-up plush towel when needed. These may be placed lengthwise along the sternum, below the breasts, across the clavicles, or in any combination of these arrangements.

For added client comfort while prone, use an arm shelf or linen-draped stool placed under the face rest.

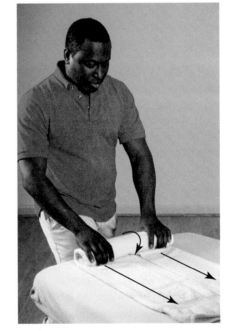

FIGURE 7-12 Rolling up bath-size towel for a cervical pillow.

▶ Supine Position

7-5 In the supine position, the person is lying on his or her back. The most commonly supported areas are the neck and the knees (Figure 7-11).

A soft cloth-covered pillow is best placed under the neck. In the absence of a pillow, a rolled-up bath-size towel can be substituted. There is a trick to rolling up the towel for use as a cervical pillow. Lay it flat on the table and bring the two opposing edges toward the center, leaving a 1-inch gap down the middle. Roll up the towel so that the gap is in the center (Figure 7-12). This will create a space for the cervical

spinous processes while adding additional padding for muscles located on either side of the cervical spine. The thickness of the towel can be adjusted by unrolling to accommodate the normal cervical curve. Avoid hyperextending the client's neck with a cervical pillow that is too thick.

A knee bolster helps relax the lower back and hips while the client is supine. In fact, it is recommended to use a knee bolster to flex the knees before performing abdominal massage. If your client complains of lower back pain while using a knee bolster, try a higher knee bolster (i.e., 8-inch

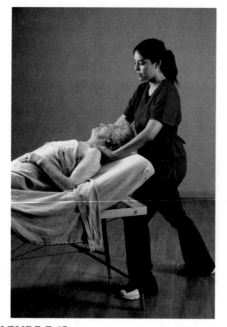

FIGURE 7-13 Client in a semireclining position.

height) to further flex the knees. If the additional knee bolster height does not provide adequate relief, place the client's feet on a pillow. This same client positioning is ideal for when you massage the client's feet in the supine position by providing easier access to the feet by raising them at or above the level of the flexed knees and facilitating effective body mechanics (see Figure 7-8). You may sit on the table or on a stool while massaging the feet.

Semireclining

In some instances, the client's upper body needs to be elevated while supine to create a semireclining or semisitting position. This can be accomplished in several ways: (1) your table may be designed so that a portion of the tabletop can be elevated (Figure 7-13); (2) use a special wedge-shaped bolster; or (3) several pillows may be stacked to create the incline. For the last choice, use two pillows to create a wide base, with a single pillow on top to create an inclined plane. Be sure that the pyramid of pillows or table elevation begins at your client's hip joints and not the midback.

For your pregnant clients, use a semireclining supine position. As her uterus expands, also include a wedge pillow or rolled towel tucked under her right side to reduce compression of abdominal blood vessels (see Figure 11-3).

Side-Lying Position

7-6   The side-lying position is just that: the client lies on his or her left or right side. The side-lying position offers a number of advantages for both the client and the therapist. Overweight, frail, and elderly clients can more readily relax

in this position and it encourages easier breathing over that in the prone position. Those with back and neck issues usually find side-lying to be a more comfortable option than the prone or supine position. It offers unparalleled access to the hip and shoulder girdle, and neck. The side-lying position is best for clients in advanced pregnancy.

The side-lying position may also be used when working on clients with catheters, colostomy bags, drain ports, or other surgical appliances. Although massage may be safely administered to clients with surgical appliances, in some cases, you may need to obtain physician clearance to perform massage on the client.

Effective positioning helps the side-lying client feel comfortable and provides accessibility for the therapist. The client's head, torso, and upper leg should be in a neutral position and properly supported so that the client feels stable and not apt to roll when pressure is applied to the neck, back, or hip area. The pregnant client may need additional support under her belly.

Be sure to ask your client to lie on the side he or she feels most comfortable in, because he or she will likely spend most of the treatment time on this side (i.e., most of the body can be accessed from one side).

Once your client is on one side, place your hands approximately 4 inches from the table edge. Next, ask your client to scoot backward until the back touches your hands. Having your client scoot back accomplishes two things. First, it is easier to massage the back when it is closer to the table's edge, because you are leaning over the table less. Second, it provides ample room on the table top to place pillows under your client's arms and legs.

Using three or four pillows, place the first pillow underneath the head and place your client's lower wrist on this pillow. The next pillows are placed in front of your client's chest with the upper arm (i.e., on the side of the body not lying against the table) resting on it. The next pillow(s) are needed to rest your client's leg. Be sure that the ankle and hips, as well as the arms and shoulders, are at or near the same height (Figure 7-14). An additional, smaller pillow may be used to support the lower ankle.

While massaging a client in the side-lying position, adjust your body for the best leverage, which may include using a stool, squatting, or kneeling down on the floor (see Figure 7-20B). When using a stool for side-lying massage work, avoid rolling stools, because the lateral pressure applied may push the therapist away from the client, increasing strain on the therapist's body.

Before you roll the client over, remove all the pillows except for the one supporting the head. Ask your client to scoot toward the center of the table *before* you ask them to roll over (remember that the client is close to the edge of the table). After your client has rolled over to the opposite side and has scooted back, place the pillows in their proper positions.

Be sure to remove all pillows before asking your client to get up and get dressed (Box 7-6).

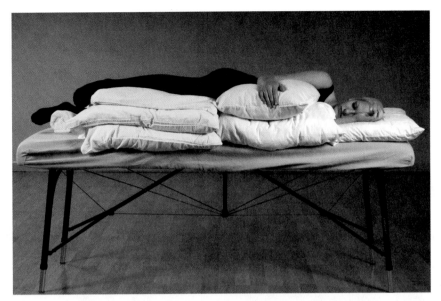

FIGURE 7-14 Pillow placement for side-lying positioning.

BOX 7-6

How to Begin: Prone? Supine?

Read this section, weigh the pros and cons, and decide which position sequence you and your client prefer.

Beginning Prone, Ending Supine

Most clients complain of back-related pain. Beginning with the client in the prone position allows you to massage this essential area first. Ending supine allows your client's sinuses to drain; otherwise, client may leave with a nasal congestion from lying prone last. Beginning prone also allows the genital region to be underneath the client's body (a physically and emotionally vulnerable area) and allows time for trust between client and therapist to develop. Even with the best face rest, the client's neck may become stiff while lying prone. Beginning prone and ending supine allows the neck to be worked easily during the last part of the session to reduce or eliminate any neck stiffness that may have occurred from lying prone. Many therapists wrap their clients up in the bottom sheet (like a cocoon). Ending supine allows this type of session conclusion.

Beginning Supine, Ending Prone

Starting a client in the supine position allows him or her to observe what you are doing, which may put the client at ease. Clients often enjoy conversing with their therapists but also enjoy silence during the massage. When you begin with the client in the supine position, eye contact between client and therapist is easy. Conversation flows effortlessly. The client who rolls onto his or her abdomen often signals a time of quiet rest. Ending prone also allows the back to be worked last, which is often a primary area of complaint.

No matter how you begin, you may decide to finish the massage with the client in the side-lying position, allowing him or her to rest before getting up off the table. The side-lying position also facilitates stretching of the client's back, especially if you ask him or her to pull both knees to the chest into a fetal position.

MINI-LAB

Acquire approximately six pillows of various sizes, a massage table, and a partner. Ask your partner to lie on the massage table in the supine position, and use the pillows to create a variety of comfortable positions. Once all possibilities are explored, remove the pillows from the massage table and ask your partner to turn over and lie on his or her side. Use the pillows again to position your partner's arms, legs, and so on. Repeat the activity with the person in the prone position. This method will help you discover new and creative ways to work with pillows as positioning equipment.

Seated Position

7-7   The seated position is used to give massage while the client is seated in a regular chair, stool, massage chair (Figure 7-15, *A*), or even a wheelchair (see Figure 11-14). Learning how to massage a client while he or she is seated is important because you will have a diverse clientele and, although a massage chair is the current standard, it does pose problems for the physically challenged, some individuals with musculoskeletal or neurological diseases, women in advanced pregnancy, and clients who are elderly or who have a debilitating illness.

A seated position is preferred if a massage table is not available or there is not adequate space for a massage table. It is also ideal when a full massage might not be appropriate or if the client has reservations about removing clothing.

When a regular chair is used, the client may lean forward while sitting up and relaxing (Figure 7-15, *B*) or lean forward onto a pile of pillows atop a table (Figure 7-15, *C*). Avoid having the client straddle the chair. Devices are also

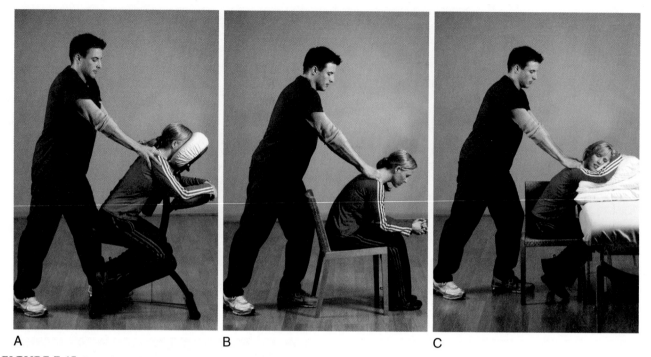

A   B   C

FIGURE 7-15 Seated position. **A,** Client in a massage chair. **B,** Client in a regular chair. **C,** Client in a chair leaning forward on a mountain of pillows.

available that sit or clip onto a tabletop that accommodate the client leaning forward. If using a rolling stool or wheelchair, make sure the wheels are locked before proceeding with the massage.

DRAPING

Draping is essentially covering the body with cloth and allows the client to be undressed while receiving massage. The purposes of using a drape are to (1) provide a professional atmosphere, (2) support the client's need for emotional privacy (modesty) and sense of security, and (3) provide warmth. As the massage progresses and the client becomes more relaxed, basal body temperature drops. When this occurs, the client may feel cold. It is more difficult to relax while you are cold. For this reason, ask whether the client is comfortably warm at least twice during the session—once as you start the massage and again halfway through. If the client indicates that he or she is cold, place a blanket over the top drape. If the opposite occurs and your client becomes too warm (e.g., advanced pregnancy, perimenopausal women), uncover the arms and legs.

Be sure that all reusable draping material is freshly laundered for each client. A clean drape is placed over the table or mat before the massage begins. A second clean drape is placed over the client (clothed or unclothed). Even if your client elects to wear a swimsuit or shorts and a loose shirt, cover him or her with a clean drape during massage. Disposable linens must be disposed of properly after each use.

Comply with state or local laws regarding draping. In most instances, the genital area, the gluteal cleft, and female breast are never undraped.

Only the area massaged is undraped. For example, if you are massaging the back, then both legs should be draped. If you are working on the posterior aspect of the left leg, then the back *and* the right leg should be draped.

Avoid lifting or fluffing the drape when uncovering or covering body areas or when your client is turning over. A draft may disturb your client's feelings of warmth, security, relaxation, and privacy. Use the anchor method (described next) to help keep the drape in contact with your client's body while he or she is turning. Turning a client is the most challenging draping experience for students because this is when most accidental exposures occur. However, the danger of exposure is greater in the classroom setting than in a massage room. The vantage point of surrounding classmates is better than that of the therapist who makes a draping mistake, so extra caution should be taken with draping in classroom settings.

If you accidentally expose your client, look away while redraping the exposed area. Looking away is a gesture of respect because your client will look at your face first if accidental exposure occurs. Generally, the best thing to do is to acknowledge your error with a simple pardoning of yourself while remaining composed. A look of horror on your face only makes the uncomfortable situation worse.

The two main types of drapes are sheets and towels. Become proficient at using *both* types of drapes. Be patient while learning draping techniques; time and practice are required. Proper draping is an art in itself.

MINI-LAB

One way to practice draping is to put on a pair of bright undergarments over your regular attire. Lie on a table with the drape over you. Have a classmate practice turning you over while *not* exposing your bright undergarments. Then trade roles with the classmate.

▶ Towel Draping

7-8 Towels are thicker, heavier than sheets, and are used to cover female breasts while accessing the abdomen (even when sheet draping is used). Typically, one towel is used for draping male clients, and two towels are used to drape female clients. However, provide additional draping if your client requests it or feels cold. A flat or fitted sheet is used to drape over the table and one or more towels are used to drape your client. Avoid using a towel to drape over the table or the face rest cushion because terry material often leaves pits on a client's skin and face as a result of compression.

When using towel draping, fold the towel back or under to reveal the area to be massaged. In most circumstances, the towel stays where it is folded, but it may be secured by tucking underneath the body.

Towel Draping Male Clients. Instruct the client to undress, lie supine on the table, and drape himself with one towel horizontally across the hips. After you reenter the room, rotate the towel 90 degrees so that it drapes from his waist down his legs to the ankles. To do this, grasp the bottom corner of the towel closest to you with your lower hand and the top corner of the towel (opposite side of the table) with your upper hand. Pull these corners apart until slight traction is felt. While maintaining traction and keeping the center of the towel over the hips, rotate the towel 90 degrees, with the top hand pulling the far corner of the towel across the midline of the client's body to the hip nearest the therapist. At the same time, with the same speed, move the lower hand away until the corner held is on the opposite side of the client's body (see Figure 7-18). The towel is now draped down the legs. The towel will be turned back to its original position before the client is turned over.

Towel Draping Female Clients. Instruct the client to undress, lie supine on the table, and drape herself with the two towels: one across her torso covering her breasts and the other across her hips. The two towels should be parallel to each other like an equal sign (=). After you reenter the room, use the technique detailed previously to rotate the bottom towel 90 degrees. When towel rotation is complete, the bottom towel will be parallel to the body, creating a T where it meets the top towel (Figure 7-16). The towels will be returned to the equal sign formation before the client is turned over.

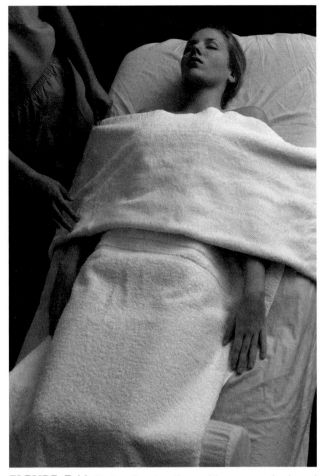

FIGURE 7-16 Supine female client with two towels draped across chest and down hips and legs.

Accessing the Abdomen on Female Clients. Towel draping is used for accessing the abdomen in the supine position. The bottom edge of the towel is lifted and fanfolded on itself across the breasts to act as a bikini top (Figure 7-17, *A*). Be sure to use a covered bolster to keep the knees flexed when working the abdomen. To redrape the client's abdomen, simply anchor the top edge of the towel with one hand and pull bottom edge of the towel downward with the other hand, unfolding the fanfolds as you go (Figure 7-17, *B*).

Turning Your Client Over. This discussion assumes that the therapist is using two towels. Modify the instructions for use with a single towel.

Remove all bolsters from the table. If your client is prone and is using a face rest, give instructions to scoot down until the head is resting on the table and off the face rest. Be sure to guide the towels down for proper draping. Then, rotate the lower towel back to the equal sign position (Figure 7-18).

Anchor the towel edges nearest you by leaning on them, thus securing them to the table. Reach across the table and grasp the top corner of the top towel with your upper hand

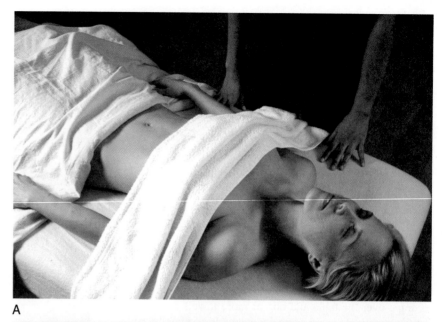

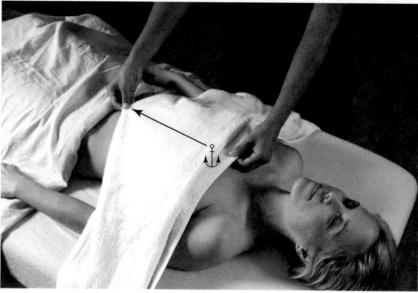

FIGURE 7-17 **A,** Supine female client with towel draping, abdomen exposed. **B,** Therapist redraping the abdomen by holding top of towel while unfolding fanfolds with the other hand.

and the lower corner of the top towel and upper corner of the bottom towel with your lower hand. Lift them up to form a tent. Instruct the client to turn over. Be sure the drape remains in contact with the client as he or she is turning over to prevent the feeling of air space. Return the bottom towel to the T formation (see Figure 7-16). If your client is now supine, place bolsters under the client's neck and behind the knees. If your client is prone, instruct him or her to scoot up to take advantage of the face rest and then place a bolster under the ankles (see Figure 7-9).

 Sheet Draping

7-9 Two sheets are required for each client: one sheet draped over the client and one sheet covering the massage

table. Twin-size sheet sets are preferred (fitted sheet for the table drape and flat sheet for the client drape), but a twin flat or a double-size flat sheet folded in half may be used as the table drape. Arrange the top flat sheet neatly on the bottom sheet, folding down the top edge to reveal the bottom sheet. This arrangement gives the draped massage table an inviting appearance. As you undrape specific areas of the body for massage, edges of the fabric may be tucked underneath the client's body. Untuck the sheet, and redrape when moving to a different area for massage.

Accessing the Abdomen on Female Clients. The easiest method of accessing the abdomen requires the use of a towel or king-size pillowcase. A towel is draped on top of the sheet, across the breasts, and perpendicular to the body. The bottom edge of the towel is lifted and fanfolded on itself across the breasts to act as a bikini top (Figure 7-17, *A*). Be sure to use a covered bolster to keep the client's knees flexed when working the abdomen. To redrape the client's abdomen, simply anchor the top edge of the towel with one hand and

pull bottom edge of the towel downward with the other hand, unfolding the fanfolds as you go (Figure 7-17, *B*). You can remove the towel after redraping the breasts with the sheet drape.

Turning Your Client Over. Remove all bolsters from the table. If your client is prone and is using a face rest, give instructions to scoot down until the head is resting on the table and off the face rest. Be sure to guide the sheet down for proper coverage. Ask the client to place their arms under the sheet. Uncover the feet, because they may become entangled in the sheet while the client is turning over.

Slightly elevate the sheet along the opposite edge of the table to form a tent and pull it taut. Anchor the sheet with your thighs on the side of the table closer to you (Figure 7-19). Instruct the client to turn over. Be sure the drape remains in contact with the client as he or she is turning over to prevent the feeling of air space. If your client is now supine, place bolsters under the client's neck and behind the knees. If your client is prone, instruct him or her to scoot up to take advantage of the face rest and then place a bolster under the ankles.

Side-Lying Using Sheet Draping. Drape the side-lying client with a sheet. Be sure to use the suggestions for bolstering side-lying clients in the previous section entitled "Client Positioning." Proceed with the massage as usual, exposing one area at a time. When the back and neck are uncovered, use a towel folded in half lengthwise, draping it over the client's side to help secure the sheet drape (Figure 7-20, *A*). The back can be worked while the therapist is seated in a stool or chair (Figure 7-20, *B*). The arm is worked from the

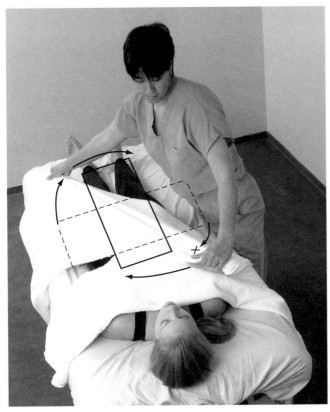

FIGURE 7-18 Therapist rotating the lower towel.

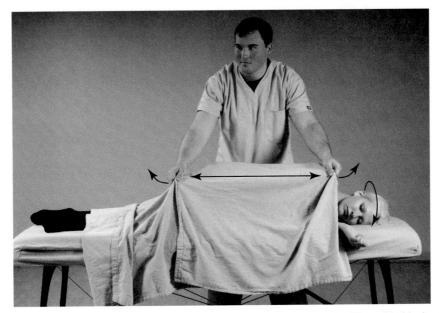

FIGURE 7-19 Client with feet uncovered, turning over to prone while her therapist lifts and holds the sheet in place.

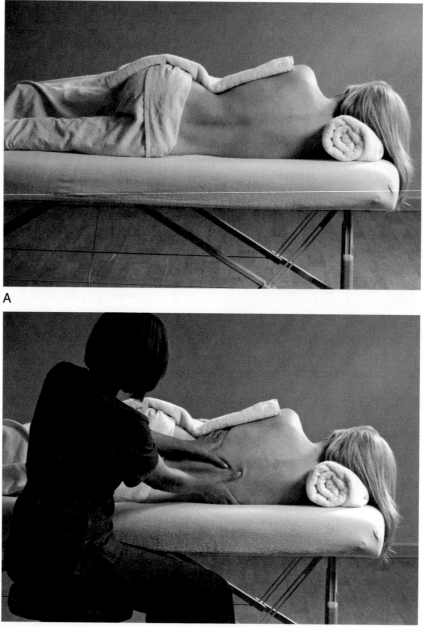

A

B

FIGURE 7-20 Sheet draping for the side-lying client. **A,** Side-lying female client with back exposed while towel holds sheet in place. **B,** Therapist massaging client's back while sitting on a stool.

front while the client is draped from the chest down (Figure 7-20, *C*). For the bottom leg, drape as you would if the client were lying prone or supine (Figure 7-20, *D*). A rolled towel can be placed under the ankle. For the top leg, undrape and tuck the sheet back around under the leg (Figure 7-20, *E*).

 ## ASSISTING CLIENTS ONTO
7-10 ## AND OFF THE MASSAGE TABLE

From time to time, a client may need assistance getting on the massage table or sitting up and getting off the table once

the massage is complete. Geriatric clients may use a low, stationary stool when getting on the table. The therapist may offer a forearm as support when the client is maneuvering onto or off of the table.

Practice is needed to prevent strain or injury resulting from assisting your client onto or off of the massage table. Also, it is prudent to check your liability insurance policy to be sure it covers any injuries resulting from this type of professional activity.

Assistance is most often requested by clients when getting *off* the table. A variety of methods are used to assist the client

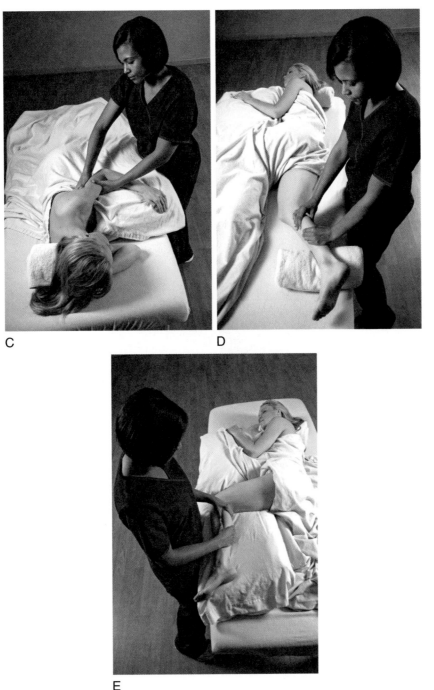

FIGURE 7-20, cont'd **C,** Therapist massaging client's arm. **D,** Therapist massaging client's calf. **E,** Therapist massaging client's upper calf.

getting off the table while keeping the client comfortably draped and protecting the therapist's back against injury. This method assumes the therapist is using sheets as the drape.

The client needs to be in the supine position. Remove all positioning equipment and undrape the feet. Next, explain the procedure to the client. Follow these steps:

1. Face the client while standing with the side of your hip or thigh against the massage table at the client's waist level.

2. Place your closer arm under the client's closer arm, slide your arm under the axilla and grasp the shoulder blade and the head of the humerus. Ask the client to reach under your arm and grasp your closer arm or shoulder (Figure 7-21, *A*).

3. Slide your other arm under the client's back until you are supporting the opposite shoulder from behind. Bend your knees. Grasp the edge of the top drape while supporting the shoulder with your arm (Figure 7-21, *B*).

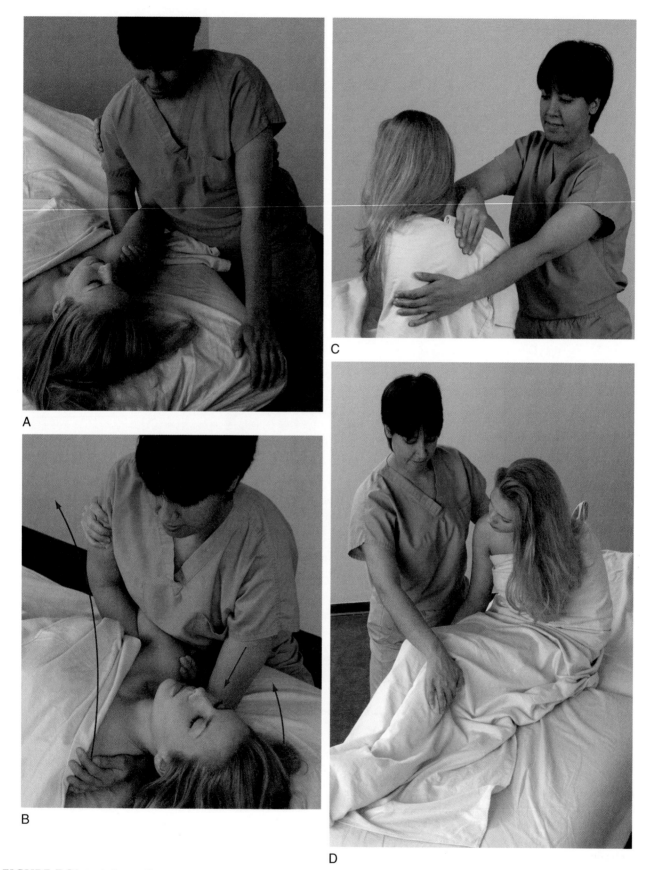

FIGURE 7-21 Assisting a client off of the table. **A,** Therapist grasping behind client's shoulder and client grasping behind therapist's shoulder. **B,** Therapist sliding other hand under client to opposite shoulder. **C,** Therapist adjusting and securing drape once client is in seated position. **D,** Therapist reaching over both client's knees.

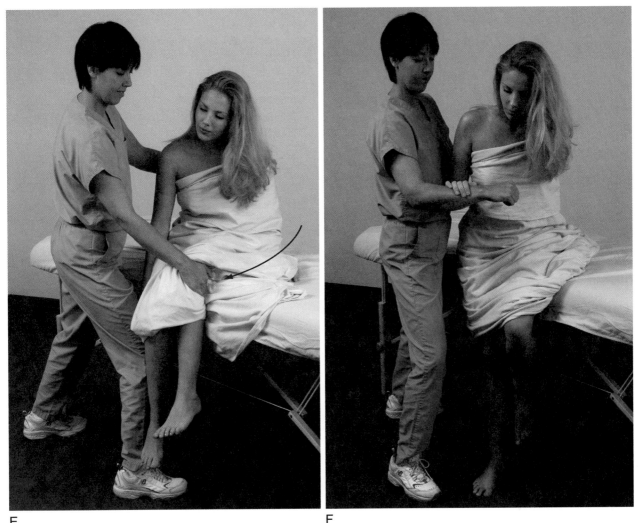

E   F

FIGURE 7-21, cont'd **E,** Therapist rotating client until feet dangle off table edge. **F,** Therapist maintaining drape while client gets off table, using therapist's other arm as support.

4. Using your legs, not your back, to assist in lifting, and with the client assisting, raise him or her to a seated position. Some clients will still need back support in this sitting position.
5. Pull the sheet loosely about the client's neck and shoulders while continuing to secure the top edge of the drape (Figure 7-21, *C*).
6. Reach over the client's knees, and cup your palm around and over the side of his or her opposite knee (Figure 7-21, *D*).
7. While supporting the client's back with your upper arm, pull his or her knees toward you in a swivel so that the client's legs dangle off the table edge (Figure 7-21, *E*).
8. Maintaining your upper arm around the client's shoulders, use your other arm to support the client into a standing position (Figure 7-21, *F*). Do not let go of the top edge of the drape until your client has it

securely in his or her hand and drapes him or herself appropriately.

It is important to note that clients who use mobility devices such as a wheelchair may also require assistance. Proper training and practice are needed to prevent strain or injury resulting from assisting in the transfer of wheelchair-bound clients. If providing massage in a health care facility, ask a qualified person for assistance with transfer if needed.

ⓔvolve   *How to assist a client off the table is featured on the Evolve website that accompanies this text. Log on and access your student account, then locate resources for Chapter 7. Click on "How to Assist a Client Off the Table."* ∎

E-RESOURCES

⊜volve

http://evolve.elsevier.com/Salvo/MassageTherapy
- Chapter challenge
- Flash cards
- Photo gallery
- Technique videos
- Additional information
- Weblinks

▶ DVD

- 7-1: Foot stances
- 7-2: Body mechanics
- 7-3: Bolstering
- 7-4: Prone position
- 7-5: Supine position
- 7-6: Side-lying position
- 7-7: Seated position
- 7-8: Towel draping
- 7-9: Sheet draping
- 7-10: Assisting client off of the massage table

These videos can also be viewed on the Evolve website.

BIBLIOGRAPHY

AMTA: http://www.llcc.edu/LinkClick.aspx?fileticket=IC0ot%2FcU4dc%3D&tabid=5196. Accessed May 19, 2010.

AMTA Council of Schools 2008 Leadership Conference and Annual Meeting, Savannah, Ga, Jan 24, 2008.

Barry W: Massage body mechanics, *Massage Mag* 60:72-75, 1996.

Barry W: Personal communication, 2010.

Beck MF: *Theory and practice of therapeutic massage*, ed 4, Albany, NY, 2005, Thomson Delmar Learning.

Coughlin P: *Principles and practice of manual therapeutics*, New York, 2002, Churchill Livingstone.

Foster MA: *Somatic patterning: how to improve posture and movement and ease pain*, Longmont, Colo, 2004, Educational Movement Systems Press.

Foster MA: Your birthright: a case for the human stance, *Massage Bodyw* 20(2):72, 2005.

Fritz S: *Essential sciences for therapeutic massage*, ed 3, St Louis, 2009, Mosby.

Fritz S: *Fundamentals of therapeutic massage*, ed 4, St Louis, 2009, Mosby.

Frye B: *Body mechanics for manual therapists: a functional approach to self-care*, ed 3, Philadelphia, 2010, Lippincott Williams & Wilkins.

Grafelman T: *Graf's anatomy and physiology guide for the massage therapist*, Aurora, Colo, 1998, DG Publishing.

Greene L, Goggins RW: *Prevention tips*, Save Your Hands (website): http://www.saveyourhands.com. Accessed May 20, 2010.

Greene L, Goggins RW: *Save your hands! the complete guide to injury prevention and ergonomics for manual therapists*, ed 2, Coconut Creek, Fla, 2008, Body of Work Books.

Prudden B: *Pain erasure*, New York, 1980, M Evans.

Rose MK: *Comfort touch: massage for the elderly and the ill*, Philadelphia, 2010, Lippincott Williams & Wilkins.

Stillerman E: *Prenatal massage: a textbook of pregnancy, labor, and postpartum bodywork*, St Louis, 2008, Mosby.

Torres LS: *Basic medical techniques and patient care for radiologic technologies*, Philadelphia, 1993, JB Lippincott.

MATCHING I

Place the letter of the answer next to the term or phrase that best describes it.

A. Aligned spine
B. Body mechanics
C. Bolsters
D. Bow
E. Being balanced
F. Dan tien
G. Fists or fingertips
H. Hara
I. Horse
J. Knees
K. Mild lunges
L. Triangle

_____ 1. A major contributor to the reduction of energy expended while performing massage

_____ 2. These joints should be flexed and extended if a lifting or lowering action is needed while in the horse stance

_____ 3. Japanese term for lower abdomen

_____ 4. Architecturally speaking, the most structurally stable base

_____ 5. Accomplished by having a straight spine, erect head, and eyes looking forward, shoulders back and rib cage lifted slightly

_____ 6. Chinese term for the point located an inch or two below and behind the navel

_____ 7. This accessory is to be removed before the client gets up off the table or it becomes an obstacle for the client to maneuver around

_____ 8. Stance characterized by placing the feet just beyond hip distance with toes pointing forward

_____ 9. Stance recommended during strokes that require excursion

_____ 10. One activity that can be performed to warm up the therapist's body before massage

_____ 11. Appropriate table height can be determined where the table top touches these structures

while the therapist stands next to the massage table

_____ 12. Use of postural techniques, foot stances, and leverage techniques to deliver massage therapy and related bodywork methods with maximum efficiency and least amount of trauma to the therapist

MATCHING II

Place the letter of the answer next to the term or phrase that best describes it.

A. Balance and centering
B. Client's body
C. Breathing
D. Centeredness

E. Draping
F. Moderate physical activities
G. Prone
H. Seated

I. Semireclining
J. Strength and stamina
K. Supine
L. Towel

_____ 1. Term used to describe the connection between the body and mind; refers also to mental, emotional and physical states of consciousness

_____ 2. Term used to describe lying face down

_____ 3. Position in which the upper body is elevated while supine

_____ 4. Covering the client's body with cloth in a manner that allows him or her to be undressed while receiving massage

_____ 5. Western cultures tend to focus on these two aspects of physical activity

_____ 6. Avoid balancing yourself or pushing off the _____ _____ while shifting your weight to move forward in the bow stance

_____ 7. Included in essential elements of body mechanics along with strength, stamina, stability, balance, and centeredness

_____ 8. Client position used if a massage table is not available, if there is inadequate space for a massage table, or if the client has reservations about removing clothing

_____ 9. Term used to describe lying on the back

_____ 10. Eastern cultures tend to focus on these two aspects of physical activity

_____ 11. Drape that can be used to access the abdomen of female clients in the supine position

_____ 12. Examples are walking, biking, swimming, and gardening

CASE STUDY

The Bachelorette

For the most part, Nikki sees clients with sports-related injuries, so she spends most of her treatment time working on a specific structure or area of the body. She spends most of a session seated. Not only does this spare her a bit of energy, but she's found that sitting sharpens her focus.

Today is a very busy day for Nikki. In addition to five half-hour sessions with athletes, Nikki's sister hired her to provide Swedish massage for her three bridesmaids. Nikki, her sister's maid of honor, was given a gift certificate to receive a massage from her preferred therapist at a later date. After the massages today, the bachelorette party begins! The bridal party will meet their other girlfriends for dinner and then dancing. The wedding is next weekend and Nikki and her sister have both taken the week off to prepare for the event.

The wedding party arrived at the designated time and the women spent a little while talking and laughing before starting the treatments. About 15 minutes into the first Swedish massage, Nikki noticed that she was having a difficult time controlling her pressure. The client didn't complain, but Nikki realized that she was using her whole body to try to keep herself from using too much strength, and it was causing discomfort in her upper back and neck. By the middle of the second session she began feeling discomfort in her low back as well. She remembered to adjust her posture to a lunge, but found that she'd fall out of that posture without even noticing until she felt pain in her back again. Nikki realized how long it had been since she'd practiced Swedish massage.

CASE STUDY—cont'd

Discuss how the table height that Nikki uses when sitting while working might be different from the table height that is more appropriate for Swedish massage.

Discuss the importance of the proper table height for maintaining control of your strength and pressure.

Does performing shorter sessions impact the choices a therapist might make about table height and other aspects of proper body mechanics?

What suggestions for proper body mechanics might Nikki have used during these sessions to minimize the stress she was feeling?

Should she interrupt the massage to make adjustments, or just wait for the next session?

What can Nikki do after the sessions to keep the aches she's feeling now from affecting her sister's party? Keep in mind that she will be sitting in a car and then at a dinner table, followed by dancing.

Discuss how Nikki's preference for the seated posture when doing focused work might be beneficial for both herself and her clients.

CRITICAL THINKING

Why are bolsters needed for client comfort during a massage, when most people sleep each night without any cushion but a head pillow?

CHAPTER 8

"When the only tool you have is a hammer, every problem looks like a nail."
—Albert Einstein

Massage Techniques, Joint Mobilizations, and Stretches

LEARNING OBJECTIVES

After completing this chapter, the student should be able to:

- Define massage therapy.
- Describe qualities of massage application, which include intention, touch, depth and direction of pressure, excursion, speed, rhythm, continuity, frequency, duration, and sequence.
- Explain and perform basic massage techniques such as effleurage, pétrissage, friction, compression, tapotement, and vibration, as well as their variations.
- Identify cautionary sites and general massage contraindications.
- Explain and perform joint mobilizations and stretches on the neck, wrists and hands, arms and shoulders, spine, hips and knees, and feet and ankles.

http://evolve.elsevier.com/Salvo/MassageTherapy

INTRODUCTION

Massage has been around for millennia, probably since early man hit his head on the roof of a cave and instinctively began to rub the area to reduce the pain. Massage in Asian countries developed according to Eastern philosophy, spirituality, theories of energy movement, and clinical practice. Massage in Western society took its roots from the East, blending it with their religious and medical ideas. It continued to evolve under the influence of research, modern medicine, biology, and sports models.

This chapter features *Swedish massage.* The practice of Swedish massage includes the combined use of joint mobilizations and stretches to help clients restore and maintain pain-free movement. Collectively, these movements are historically called *Swedish gymnastics.* According to a 2007 survey conducted by the Federation of State Massage Therapy Boards, Swedish massage is the most popular massage method practiced in the United States. This survey is the largest of its kind conducted in history.

Massage therapy is known by many different terms. For purposes of clarity and consistency in this text, Swedish massage, massage therapy, therapeutic massage, and classic massage all fall under the umbrella term *massage therapy*, or simply *massage.*

Massage therapy is the manual and scientific manipulation of the soft tissues of the body for the purpose of establishing and maintaining good health and promoting wellness. The practice of massage revolves around a client, and using sessions and a wide variety of techniques to fulfill the client's goals (see Chapter 6). These goals are established through treatment planning, which includes an intake process (see Chapter 10). The therapist employs body mechanics to deliver massage therapy with efficiency and to reduce trauma on his or her own body (see Chapter 7). Techniques, procedures, and client positions may be modified during treatment depending on the client's current health status and level of comfort (see Chapters 3 and 11). Standard precautions are employed to protect the client and the therapist by reducing disease transmission (see Chapter 9).

As health care providers, massage therapists demonstrate respect to clients, client advocates, and colleagues, acknowledging their wholeness. This includes appreciation of and tolerance for a client's mental, physical, emotional, spiritual, environmental, social, and occupational aspects. The therapist is also aware of and maintains professional boundaries and respects the boundaries of others (see Chapter 2).

The era of modern massage began in the early nineteenth century, when a wide variety of practitioners were advocating massage and developing their own systems. The most important of these was Pehr Henrik Ling (1776-1839), a Swedish physiologist and gymnastics instructor. Because of his nationality, Ling's system became commonly known as *Swedish massage,* and he became known as the father of Swedish massage.

Basic massage techniques include (1) effleurage, (2) pétrissage, (3) friction, (4) compression, (5) tapotement, and (6) vibration. Dutch physician Johann Mezger promoted Swedish massage using the Western medical model and is given credit for introducing and popularizing the use of French terminology into the profession. Also, French was considered the international language in the nineteenth century. See Chapter 1 for more information about Ling and Mezger.

Your massage session can be compared to a blank canvas on which you paint, using your techniques. Primary colors are the basic techniques used in Swedish massage. Once you are comfortable and proficient with these techniques, you can mix them to create your own unique variations. You may find yourself using one hand to massage the sole of the foot and your other hand to massage the calf at the same time. You might try massaging around the scapula and up the neck simultaneously, thereby creating a new and distinctive massage variation. You can even combine joint mobilizations and stretching techniques with massage. For example, you can be performing a deep effleurage up the hamstring while flexing and extending the knee simultaneously. Your session will indeed be unique as long as you keep your client's therapeutic goals as the central focus of the massage.

As you progress through your career, learning never stops. As you explore a variety of continuing education classes, you will add many different shades of color to your artist's palette. But all these new techniques can still find their origins in the "primary colors" of Swedish massage.

> *"It is not enough to do your best; you must know what to do, and THEN do your best."*
> —W. Edwards Deming

QUALITIES OF MASSAGE APPLICATION

During your study of massage therapy, you will quickly discover that applying massage techniques is much more than placing your hands on the body and manipulating skin, muscle, and fascia. Skillful application of massage is largely a blend of hand holds, hand movements, and your own body mechanics (see Chapter 7). Basic massage techniques possess unique qualities and characteristics. Several qualities are common to all techniques, such as depth of pressure and direction, excursion, speed, rhythm and continuity, frequency, duration, and sequence. These affect not only the body's response to massage therapy but also the intensity of that response. An understanding of these qualities is necessary for the skillful application of massage.

Your massage techniques will be more effective if your client is relaxed. Use Box 8-1 to evaluate your massage environment and application of techniques to ensure client relaxation. Be sure to make any adjustments as needed. Let us examine the qualities of massage to deepen your understanding, and use them as you evaluate your own progress and digest the assessments of others.

BOX 8-1

Factors That May Inhibit Client Relaxation

- Strange or new surroundings
- Fear of unknown treatments
- Unpleasant odors
- Excessive noise
- Bright lights or total darkness
- Cold, drafty rooms
- Fear of undressing
- Shortness of breath or other breathing difficulties
- Inadequate or uncomfortable support, draping, or positioning

Adapted from DeDomenico G: *Beards massage: principles and practice of soft tissue manipulation*, ed 5, Philadelphia, 2007, Saunders.

Intention

Intention, in massage, is a consciously sought goal and defines the purpose of the session. All qualities of massage rest on intention. This intention is stated by the client during treatment planning during each visit. Sometimes the desire to help our clients interferes with our ability to listen and observe subtle messages. It is important to suspend your own agendas, both personal and therapeutic, as they may interfere with your ability to listen and respond to what the client is saying verbally or with his or her body. If your own agenda is in the forefront, it is like having a one-sided conversation with someone; when you do all the talking, all you hear is yourself. Approach the session as a *tabula rasa*, or blank slate, and let your client's story unfold. This attitude sets the stage for a session that is client focused and experience-led. In this time of being both full and empty, you will choose the best technique and apply it with purpose to serve the client's intention or goal of the session.

MINI-LAB

Touching With Intent

1. Work with a partner.
2. Assign one person to be the giver and one person to be the receiver. Sit facing each other.
3. The receiver extends his or her hands, palms up. The giver places his or her hands on the receiver's hands, palm down. Both the giver and the receiver then close their eyes.
4. The giver becomes unfocused, disinterested, and mentally distracted as the receiver is relaxed and receptive for 2 minutes.
5. After that time, the giver becomes very aware, interested, and concerned about the receiver. This attitude is maintained for 2 minutes.
6. Reverse roles and repeat.
7. Share your experiences with each other. Did you notice any differences when the attitudes changed? Do intent and focus alter how touch is received? How can you use this information during a massage therapy session?

Touch

Touching, holding, or resting the weight of your hands on the client is not only a powerful therapeutic tool but the medium of massage itself. In a therapeutic setting, touch is not casual but is full of meaning and intention. Touch may be the only technique used during a session such as seen in methods such as Therapeutic Touch and Healing Touch. Touching the client on the head, feet, or back is a wonderful way to begin and end the massage session (Figure 8-1). In many instances, a brief period of stillness accompanies initial contact with your client, giving him or her the opportunity to relax and to become accustomed to your touch without distracting conversation.

MINI-LAB

Enhancing Awareness and Sensitivity

The following exercise is designed to increase your level of awareness and sensitivity as a therapist and to strengthen proprioception. Select a partner, and decide who will be the giver and who will be the receiver for the first round. Sit facing each other, and raise your hands just below shoulder level. Gently flex your fingers; allow your fingertips to touch your partner's fingertips. Both the giver and the receiver then close their eyes.

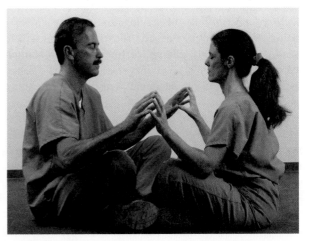

Demonstration of the position needed for push hands.

The designated "giver" slowly begins to move his or her hands in space, allowing the "receiver" to follow his or her hands while remaining connected only by fingertips. This movement may feel awkward at first, but as the receiver expands his or her awareness, it begins to feel as though the two are dancing. After a minute of following your partner's movements, reverse roles.

After the exercise, answer the following questions. How confident were you as the giver? How did you feel as the receiver? When you were the giver, did your receiver relax or become tense and uncomfortable? Sometimes people try to anticipate the moves rather than relaxing and following. The more relaxed you are, the more sensitive and responsive you become. How does this type of sensitivity apply to massage therapy?

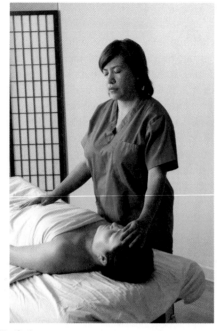

FIGURE 8-1 Therapist touching client in a quiet, focused manner.

Depth and Direction of Pressure

Depth of pressure is the application of manual forces applied to the body's surface. The therapist most often uses his or her hands, elbows, or forearms when applying pressure, but knees or feet may also be used. Pressure may be applied using handheld tools or other external apparatus.

Pressure varies from light to deep; this is accomplished by using more (or less) of the therapist's body weight and proper leverage. Initially the pressure should be light to moderate, gradually increasing until the desired effect is achieved. In general, the deeper the pressure, the broader the base of contact required on the body's surface (heel of hand versus fingertip). Raising or lowering the massage table will assist you in achieving the desired amount of pressure. Be sure to reduce pressure over bony areas such as the knee and shin.

Pressure depends on several factors, such as:
- Purpose or intent of the technique
- General health of the client (healthy clients can take more pressure)
- Area on the body where the pressure is applied (more pressure is needed to address thick, dense tissues than delicate, thin tissues)
- Client tolerance to pressure (avoid applying pressure past the client's pain threshold)
- Client preference

Whether on different clients or on the same client within the session, the therapist must be able to vary the pressure exerted with each technique. There is a significant difference in the amount of stroke pressure exerted when treating a young man who is fit and that used for an 80-year-old female who weighs 100 pounds and has osteoporosis. The pressure used with any technique must be appropriate for the individual.

Because pain experienced by the client when pressure is applied is subjective, consider using a 1- to 10-point pain scale with 1 being no pain and 10 quite painful. This will indicate how your depth of pressure is being experienced. Do not exceed 7 on a 10-point scale. If pressure goes beyond your client's tolerance, he or she may state this aloud or respond nonverbally by tensing up, changing facial expression and breathing pattern, or lifting a limb or the head off the table. When you notice these messages, reduce the pressure without breaking contact. Ask for feedback regarding pressure. Adjust pressure until it is appropriate.

Too much pressure, especially combined with extended treatment times, can cause soreness and/or bruising. With training, practice, and common sense, you will make good pressure judgments.

Direction of pressure is usually related to some anatomic structure or physiologic event. For example, deep effleurage is usually applied centripetally because effleurage promotes venous and lymphatic flow (and circulation in veins and lymph flow toward the chest). In contrast, deep frictions are usually performed at right angles to target fibers (e.g., muscles, tendons, ligaments) to mobilize them. Direction of pressure must be considered for the technique to be effective.

Direction of pressure can make the difference in locating a trigger or tender point. After applying depth of pressure, slide the skin over the underling tissue while moving back and forth, tracing the number "8," or by moving in the directions of a compass; north, northeast, east, southeast, south, southwest, west, northwest, and north, until the spot of the greatest tenderness is located (see Figure 14-3). When possible, pressure is applied against an underlying bone, using the bone as if it were a backboard. Be sure to release pressure before repeating the stroke, transitioning to a new stroke, or breaking contact.

CHAT ROOM

When I get to a spot that is really tender and the client says, "Oh, that hurts!", I ask them to clarify this response by asking, "Are you saying, 'Oh that hurts, keep going' or 'Oh that hurts, stop'?"

Excursion

Excursion is the distance traveled during the length of a massage stroke. After you have made a decision on the depth and direction of pressure, the next decision is how far across the tissues the movement will go. Will it cover the length of the muscle, just the area of tissue dysfunction, or a topographical region such as the back or lateral border of the scapula? Excursion has a relationship with body mechanics in that longer strokes are performed while in the bow stance and shorter strokes are performed in the horse stance. Proper foot stance is vital to ensure a smooth excursion without a change in depth of pressure or a break in continuity. See Chapter 7 for a discussion of foot stances.

Speed

Speed is the rate at which massage movements are applied (how rapidly or slowly your hands are moving). The following general rules apply:
- Slower and rhythmic movements are more calming and relaxing.
- Rapid and arrhythmic massage movements are more stimulatory and energizing.
- Quick delivery of massage movements may alarm the client, causing a tensing reaction.
- Fast massage movements may be tiring to a fatigued client.
- If hand speed is too fast or too slow, it is difficult to palpate and assess tissues.

Rhythm and Continuity

Rhythm refers to the regularity of technique application and often depends on its purpose. If massage movements are applied at regular intervals, they are considered even or rhythmic. If they are applied in a disjointed or irregular fashion, they are considered uneven or arrhythmic.

Alter the rhythm of the massage to fit the intent of the session; rhythmic strokes are ideal for stress reduction, whereas arrhythmic strokes are more energizing and stimulatory.

Continuity in massage refers to the uninterrupted flow of strokes and to the unbroken transition from one stroke to the next. The massage is more relaxing when strokes are delivered with continuity and fluid transitions. To accomplish this, keep your hands relaxed and flexible, which allows them to be lifted, without losing contact, around the bony regions and contours of the body.

Rhythm and continuity come not only from what the hands are doing but also from what the rest of the therapist's body is doing (e.g., foot placement, distance between the client and the therapist) and the height of the table.

A skilled therapist can renew massage lubricant without the client's ever being aware of any hesitation or interruption in the rhythm and continuity of the strokes.

Frequency

Frequency is the rate at which massage strokes are repeated in a given time frame. In general, a stroke is repeated in multiples of three (3, 6, 9, 12, etc.) until the desired effect is achieved. The therapist may then switch to a different stroke and may move to another area of the client's body. The first strokes (which are usually effleurage) are used for assessment, the second (or more) set of strokes is used for treatment, and the third set is for reassessment (again, usually effleurage). If tissue dysfunction is still noted during reassessment, the strokes are repeated, which may include an increase in stroke frequency during retreatment of the area.

Duration

Duration, in massage therapy, has two aspects: (1) length of the massage session or the (2) length of time massage is performed on a given area. The purpose of the massage determines how long the treatment is to be given and for how many sessions. The duration of the treatment varies according to the size of the area to be treated and the technique chosen. Even if the treatment area is confined to a small location, there will be physiologic changes in adjacent areas. Therefore, the treatment may not be limited to the area of complaint. This will affect treatment duration.

If your client is in significant pain, he or she may not be able to remain still for long periods of time. It is best to decrease duration of the session to 15-30 minutes. Be sure your client is comfortable by using well-supported positions.

Keep in mind that, unless the client is accustomed to receiving massage, working too long in one area is rarely a good idea. And yes, the desire to help may be overwhelming because you really want to help and, well, more massage is better, right? Wrong. More massage, especially deep pressure massage, often creates a localized inflammatory response that may leave your client sore. Learn to work effectively by using a variety of strokes, and use ice packs after treatment if you suspect your client may become sore. Massage soreness is similar to exercise soreness or even overexposure to sunlight. You really do not know you have overdone it until later and often not until the next day.

Sequence

Sequence is the arrangement or order of massage strokes. The therapist combines strokes to achieve a desired result. Typically, effleurage is applied initially to evaluate and warm up the tissues and used as a transition stroke. Pétrissage often follows effleurage to treat tissues more deeply. Friction is used to address specific areas. Vibration and percussion may be used when the therapist deems them necessary. A series of ending effleurages often soothes the area and assists in tissue re-evaluation. Using a sequence also helps prevent repetitive motion injury to the therapist.

When applying a sequence of strokes, work the area most proximal first; then proceed distally. For example, while the direction of the stroke is typically toward the heart, the thigh is massaged before the calf. Doing so clears the fluids from the thigh back to the trunk, giving the fluids from the more distal area a clear path as the therapist moves to address the calf.

The union of these aforementioned qualities applied to massage techniques results in a routine. In the classroom and under the supervision of a caring and experienced instructor, you will learn several routines. By their very nature, routines are dynamic. Each time you begin a massage, your routine will vary. And as you evolve as a therapist, so will your routines. With each postgraduate seminar you attend, and with each massage you receive, your routines will evolve. Stay in tune with the client during the routine. A conscientious therapist continually listens to the client and the client's body, modifying his or her sequence to meet the needs of the client.

> *"You can map out a fight plan or a life plan, but when the action starts, it may not go the way you planned, and you're down to your reflexes—which means your training."*
> —Joe Frazier

MASSAGE TECHNIQUES

Basic massage techniques, or strokes, have been categorized into groups according to their application characteristics. These categories are *effleurage, pétrissage, friction, compression, tapotement,* and *vibration.* Each stroke is described, technically discussed, and photographically represented. Also included are technique variations. Sometimes the description of these moves may seem abstract, as though they are describing a kitten; you have a better chance of understanding them through sight and touch. Hence learning these strokes takes more than a book. Rely on your experienced instructor or instructors to demonstrate properly each stroke, to model technique as you go, and to guide your practice. Use the self-assessment guide to help you evaluate your progress (Box 8-2).

Effleurage and pétrissage are usually done on lubricated skin. Friction, compression, tapotement, and vibration are performed on skin with little or no lubricant.

Hybrid strokes exist, as they do in most methods. Some pétrissage variations such as ocean waves combine lifting and squeezing followed by a downward compression often seen in effleurage strokes. Pincement tapotement is a hybrid of pétrissage and tapotement because it has elements of both. The classifications presented here are based on tradition, observation, innovation, and experience (Table 8-1).

▶ Effleurage (Gliding Strokes)

8-1

Effleurage is the application of gliding movements that are repeated and follow the contours of the body. These

---

BOX 8-2

Self-Assessment Guide

- Are the movements smooth and easy for you to perform? Are the movements jarring, rough, or abrupt?
- Are your transitions smooth?
- Is your own body as fluid, easy, and open as the movement qualities you want to give to the client?
- Do you leave time for the client to respond?
- Do you know how far a stroke needs to go? Are your excursions long enough, or are they too long?
- Is the depth sufficient without invasion or intrusion?
- Are you using a variety of strokes?
- Do you know when to stop so as not to overwork part of the body?
- Do you use your body well (positioning, foot stance, leverage, and wrist angle)? Are your body mechanics complementing your massage movements?
- Are you working within an appropriate amount of time?
- Is the session feeling whole and integrated?

TABLE 8-1 Massage Techniques and Their Variations

TECHNIQUE	VARIATIONS
Effleurage *(gliding)*	One-handed *(ironing, circular)*
	Two-handed *(heart, circular)*
	Alternate hand *(raking, circular [sun-moon])*
	Nerve stroke *(feathering)*
Pétrissage *(kneading)*	One-handed
	Two-handed *(praying hands, ocean waves, fulling [broadening])*
	Alternate hand
	Skin rolling
Friction	Superficial warming *(heat rub, sawing, towel friction)*
	Rolling
	Wringing
	Cross-fiber *(deep transverse friction)*
	Chucking *(parallel friction)*
	Circular
Compression	One-handed
	Two-handed
Tapotement *(percussion)*	Tapping *(raindrops)*
	Pincement *(plucking)*
	Hacking *(quacking)*
	Cupping
	Pounding *(loose fist beating, rapping)*
	Clapping *(slapping, splatting)*
	Diffused
Vibration *(shaking)*	Fine
	Jostling *(course vibration, fluffing)*
	Rocking

movements may be linear or circular. Pressure may be superficial (light) or deep. Variations include *one-handed, two-handed, alternate hand,* and *nerve stroke.*

The term *effleurage* (ef-flur-ahzh) originates from the French verb *effleurer,* meaning "to flow" and "to glide." This is the most versatile massage stroke; you can perform an entire session with effleurage by simply changing depth of pressure, direction of pressure, excursion, speed, and rhythm. Effleurage can be used on virtually every type of body surface.

Effleurage is used to apply lubricant and is excellent for assessing, treating, and reassessing tissues. It is also the stroke used to begin and end a massage, as well as the preferred transition stroke to use between other strokes. Effleurage is the most commonly used stroke.

Technique. Effleurage is delivered using a *lean-and-drag* technique. Lean and push your body weight downward to achieve depth of pressure and then begin the excursion. Once the excursion is complete, drag your hands back using only the weight of your hands. Maintain contact with the skin during each repetition. Remember, the deeper the pressure, the slower the stroke, and the broader the base of contact (heel of hand versus fingertip).

When working on the extremities, apply pressure *centripetally,* or toward the heart (or center). This action promotes venous blood and lymphatic flow. When applying effleurage on the back, centripetal direction is not an issue because the heart is centrally located. There are some exceptions to the centripetal direction rule (e.g., nerve stroke).

Keep your wrists as straight as possible and avoid hyperextending the wrist (see Figure 7-6). The therapist's hands, arms, shoulders, back, and legs should all be aligned along the path of movement. This alignment will increase the ease of stroke application and help prevent self-inflicted injuries of repetitive motion.

Variations

One-Handed Effleurage – One hand (finger, thumb, fist, forearm, elbow, knee, foot) is used to apply pressure (Figure 8-2). It may be helpful to anchor the client's wrist or ankle with traction so that the limb will remain in place as pressure is applied upward (Figure 8-3).

The hands may be stacked to increase depth of pressure; this is still considered one-handed effleurage because only the bottom hand makes contact with the client's body (Figure 8-4). A deep one-handed (fist, heel of hand, ulnar side of the forearm) effleurage is called *ironing effleurage* (Figure 8-5). Combine deep ironing effleurage with joint mobilizations. For example, perform deep effleurage up the hamstring while flexing and/or extending the knee (Figure 8-6). Joint mobilizations are discussed in a later section.

Two-Handed Effleurage – Two-handed effleurage is done using both hands gliding on the skin simultaneously. The hands may glide together in the same direction or move apart. Two-handed effleurage is used to perform *heart*

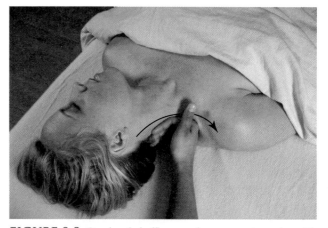

FIGURE 8-2 One-handed effleurage down upper trapezius with client supine.

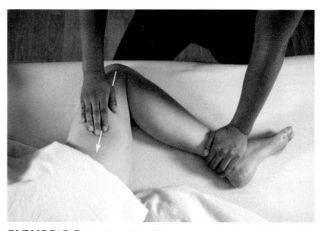

FIGURE 8-3 One-handed effleurage on the lateral thigh with the opposite hand holding the limb still.

effleurage, which covers the back, neck, and shoulders in one continuous stroke (Figure 8-7, p. 141). Two-handed effleurage can be used up the leg (Figure 8-8, p. 142), or up the arm.

Alternate Hand Effleurage – To perform alternate hand effleurage, glide one hand or digit (finger or thumb) across the skin, lifting it up as the other hand or digit follows behind in succession (Figure 8-9, p. 142). Done properly, the sequence resembles a paddlewheel (Figure 8-10, p. 143). Alternate hand effleurage can be applied in a circular direction with one hand moving in a circle while the other hand moves behind the first hand in a half circle or crescent shape (Figure 8-11, p. 143). This variation is also known as *sun-moon.*

Nerve Stroke – Considered a light effleurage, nerve stroke or *feathering* is light finger tracing over the skin. Avoid pressure that is too light, because it may be ticklish or produce goose bumps. The direction of nerve strokes is always *down* the body (as in petting a dog or cat), because downward movements are more relaxing (Figure 8-12, p. 143). Many therapists regard nerve stroke as "icing on the

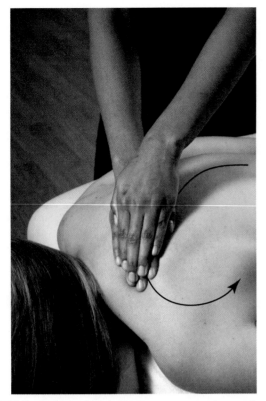

FIGURE 8-4 One-handed effleurage around scapula with stacked hands to increase pressure.

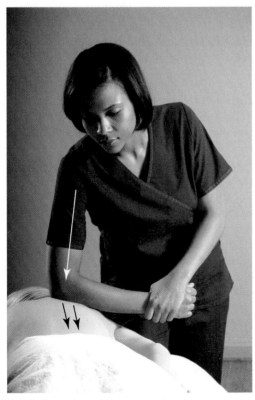

FIGURE 8-5 One-handed effleurage (ironing) on the back with client prone.

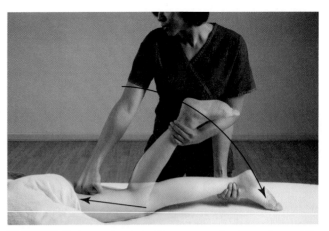

FIGURE 8-6 One-handed effleurage up the hamstrings while the therapist extends the knee with the opposite hand.

cake", and it is typically done at the end of massaging a body segment and at the completion of the massage. The stroke may be applied to bare skin or clothed clients (sports or seated massage) or over the massage drape.

Therapeutic Effects and Uses
- Relaxing effect when done slowly, which may help relieve pain and muscle spasm
- Stimulating and invigorating effect when performed rapidly
- Increases skin temperature
- Increases blood flow
- Stimulates lymph flow
- Increases mobility of the skin and subcutaneous tissues, which helps to increase range of motion in joints
- Helps both the client and the therapist become accustomed to the feel of each other's tissues. For the client, it is the feel of the therapist's hands. For the therapist, it is the feel of the client's body contours, tissue quality, and other palpatory assessments
- Provides transition between other massage techniques to achieve smoother sequence and continuity
- May promote movement of intestinal contents
- Promotes absorption of inflammatory byproducts (exudates) in subacute and chronic stages of soft tissue injury

⊖volve   *Log on to your student account from the Evolve website and view the basic strokes demonstration and their variations from this chapter. Use this as you practice at home.* ∎

▶ Pétrissage (Kneading Strokes)

8-2   **Pétrissage** consists of lifting soft tissues vertically, and then compressing and releasing them. The compression is accomplished by either squeezing or rolling the tissues before releasing, using rhythmic alternating pressures. Several variations of pétrissage are *one-handed, two-handed, alternate hand,* and *skin rolling.*

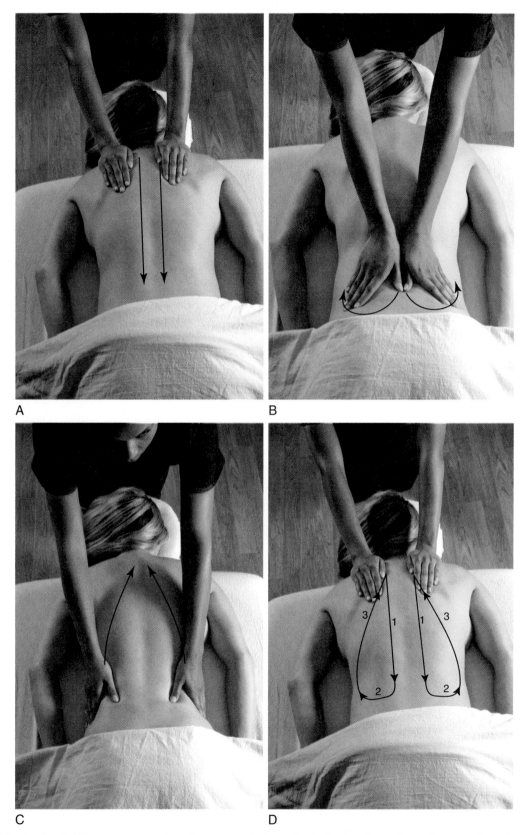

FIGURE 8-7 Two-handed heart effleurage with client prone. **A,** Down back. **B,** Stopping at base of spine and moving toward sides. **C,** Moving up the sides of the back. **D,** Back to original position.

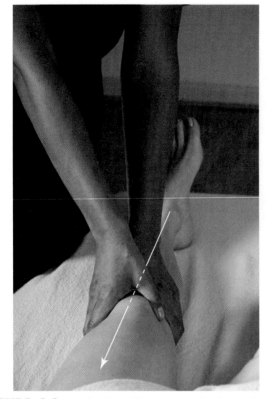

FIGURE 8-8 Two-handed effleurage up the leg with client supine. Notice how pressure is reduced while moving across the patella or kneecap.

The term *pétrissage* (peh-tre-sahzh) comes from the French verb *petrir*, meaning "to mash" or "to knead." Pétrissage is the stroke of choice to *milk* the tissue of metabolic wastes and draw new blood and oxygen into the tissues.

Technique. Grasp the skin or muscle firmly and lift. Done properly, this action should raise the skin or muscle from its usual position. Next, compress the lifted tissue by kneading, squeezing, wringing, or rolling. Then relax your grip enough to release the tissue while still remaining in contact with the skin and repeat the grasping and squeezing movement with the same or the opposite hand. Do not lose contact with the skin while switching hands. When using both hands, they may move simultaneously or alternately. Repeat the movements until the tissues feel warm and elastic.

As much as the entire hand or as little as the pads of the fingers and thumb can be used to lift the tissue, depending upon the area of treatment.

If your client has a lot of body hair, avoid small, circular moves, as they may mat and pull the hair. As an alternative, use the back-and-forth pattern (as with ocean waves, described later), or perform the pétrissage movement over the drape.

Variations

One-Handed Pétrissage – Use one hand (fingers or thumb) to perform the lifting, compressing, and releasing sequence.

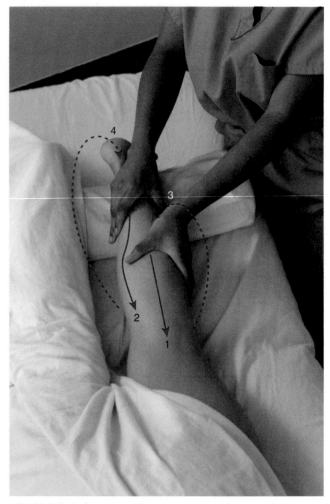

FIGURE 8-9 Alternate hand effleurage on prone client's leg.

(Figure 8-13, p. 144). This variation is well suited for smaller muscular areas such as the arms, forearms, or shoulders (Figure 8-14, p. 144).

Two-Handed Pétrissage – Both hands are performing the lift, compress, and release sequence simultaneously. Interlace the fingers and use the heels of both hands moving simultaneously for a new twist on this variation (called *praying hands*) (Figure 8-15, p. 144). Alternatively, the hands can move in opposite directions simultaneously (called *ocean waves*) (Figure 8-16, p. 144).

Tissue can be compressed with both hands or fists; lift it up and away from the bone while compressing and then spreading it out laterally before releasing (called *fulling*) (Figure 8-17, p. 145). It should feel as though you are kneading the muscles around the bone. This technique is effective for broadening muscles and their related tissues and mimics the movement of a muscle when it contracts. Because of this effect, fulling is also referred to as *broadening*.

Alternate Hand Pétrissage – In alternate hand pétrissage, both hands are performing the lift, compress, and release sequence alternately, rather than simultaneously (Figure 8-18, p. 145).

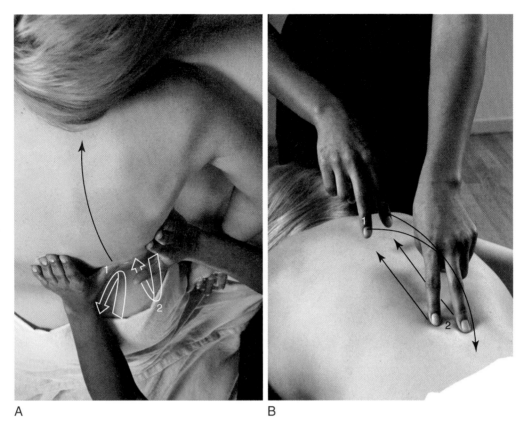

A   B

FIGURE 8-10 Alternate thumb effleurage. **A,** Up one side of the paraspinals. **B,** Up both sides of the paraspinals (raking).

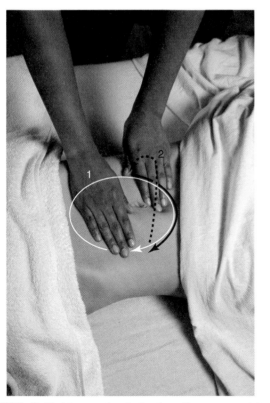

FIGURE 8-11 Alternate hand circular effleurage on abdomen with client supine.

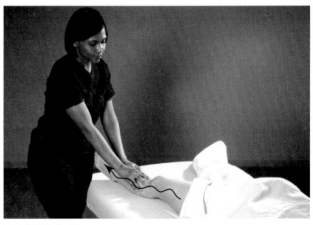

FIGURE 8-12 Nerve stroke down the leg while client is supine.

Skin Rolling – Grasp and lift the skin between the fingers and thumbs, compressing the tissue. Roll the skin as though you were rolling a pencil, using your fingers to scoop up the skin as you move across the treatment area before releasing the tissue (Figure 8-19, p. 145). Because the superficial fascia lies in several planes, lift and roll the skin in several directions. If the skin is not lifting, then do not force the tissue into position. It may feel uncomfortable initially for the client; therefore move gently and avoid going past your client's pain threshold; otherwise your client may be bruised and sore from treatment.

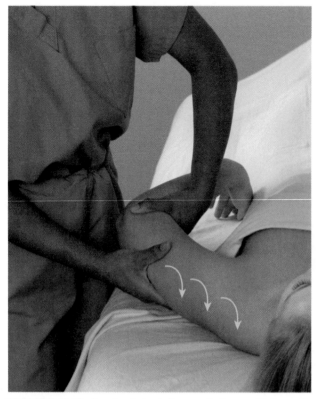

FIGURE 8-13 One-handed pétrissage of triceps with inwardly rotated shoulder and flexed elbow on supine client.

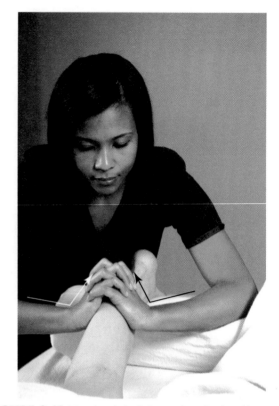

FIGURE 8-15 Two-handed pétrissage (praying hands) on prone client's calf.

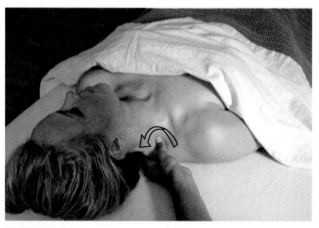

FIGURE 8-14 One-handed pétrissage using fingers and thumb on upper trapezius with client supine.

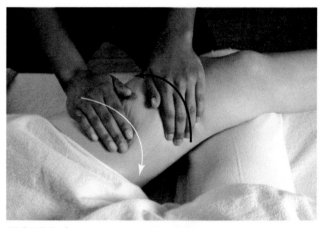

FIGURE 8-16 Two-handed petrissage (ocean waves) across the anterior thigh.

Tissue may be lifted using the sides of two hands (Figure 8-20, p. 145) or between the thumb web of one hand and the fingers of the other hand (Figure 8-21, p. 146). Although most variations of pétrissage lift muscle from the underlying bone, skin rolling lifts the skin from the underlying muscle.

Skin rolling is applied best on dry skin with little or no lubricant. Hot packs may be used to prepare the area before technique application.

Skin rolling is a technique essential to *Bindegewebsmassage* and other methods of connective tissue and myofascial release. Because no downward force is used, skin rolling is one of the few massage techniques that may be applied over bony areas.

Therapeutic Effects and Uses
- Relaxing effect, which may help relieve pain and muscle spasm

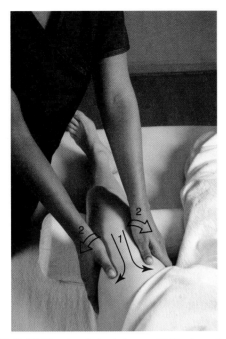

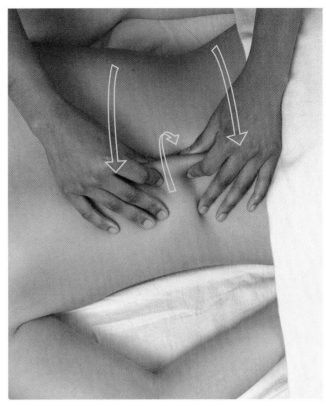

FIGURE 8-17 Two-handed pétrissage (fulling) on the anterior thigh.

FIGURE 8-19 Skin rolling by lifting it between fingers and thumb.

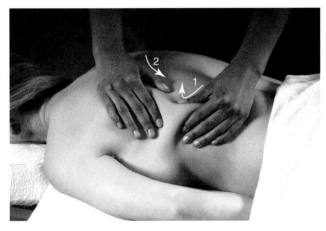

FIGURE 8-18 Alternate hand pétrissage on latissimus dorsi muscle with client prone.

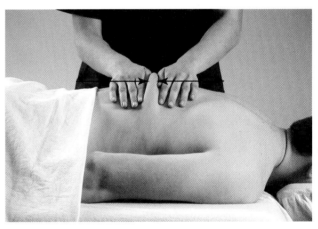

FIGURE 8-20 Skin rolling by lifting it between two hands.

- Stimulating and invigorating effect (when performed rapidly)
- Increases skin temperature
- Increases blood flow
- Improves range of motion
- Reduces muscle soreness and stiffness
- Promotes absorption of inflammatory byproducts (exudates) in subacute and chronic stages of injury

 Friction

Friction massage is performed by rubbing one surface over another in several directions. Friction can be applied superficially with hands gliding over the skin or deeply while moving skin across underlying tissue layers. Varieties of superficial friction are *superficial warming, rolling,* and *wringing.* Deep friction variations include *cross-fiber, chucking,* and *circular.*

The term *friction* (frik-shon) comes from the Latin word *frictio,* meaning "to rub." Friction movements are performed dry, or using little or no lubricant. When applied correctly, friction generates a shearing force.

Technique. For superficial friction, slide your hands, palms, fingers, or knuckles back and forth over the client's

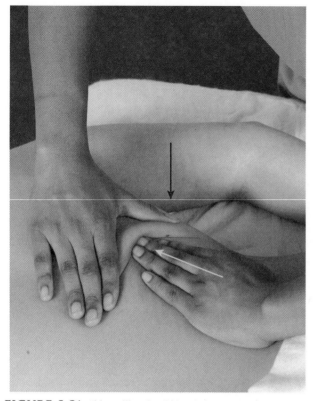

FIGURE 8-21 Skin rolling by lifting it between fingers of one hand and thumb web of the other.

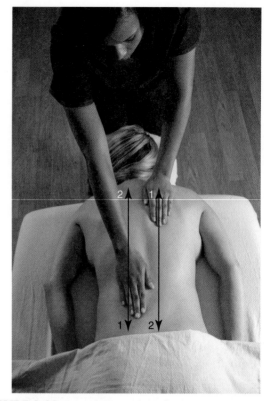

FIGURE 8-22 Superficial warming friction on the back of prone client. Shorter strokes can be used while moving up and down the back.

skin briskly. Use quick strokes. For deep friction, the therapist first engages and then moves the skin (and superficial fascia) over the underlying tissue layers. The direction can be circular (pressing down and then around) or linear (pressing down and then up and down or back and forth).

Variations

Superficial Warming Friction – Also known as a *heat rub,* superficial warming friction generates heat by creating resistance to motion. Place one or both hands on lightly lubricated skin. Fingers are held together firmly. Move the hand(s) briskly up and down or back and forth. If both hands are used, they will move in opposing directions (Figure 8-22). Use your shoulder and upper arms to propel your hands. The fingertips, knuckles, or ulnar surface of one or both hands may be used (Figure 8-23). The latter variation is called *sawing* (Figure 8-24, p. 148). Superficial warming friction may also be done with a towel, rubbing it quickly across the client's skin. This is called *towel friction.*

Rolling Friction – Compress the tissues firmly using both hands, fingers extended. Move the hands back and forth first, in a clockwise motion, changing quickly to a counter-clockwise motion. This action rolls the tissues back and forth around the underlying bone(s) (Figure 8-25, p. 148). Begin these movements distally, sliding your hands proximally to complete the stroke. This variation is best suited

for the extremities with the client assisting by holding the limb up. See "Wringing Friction," next.

Wringing Friction – Compress lightly lubricated skin with your hands and fingers and begin moving them in opposing directions. One hand moves in a clockwise direction while the other moves in a counter-clockwise direction simultaneously, changing directions of both hands quickly (Figure 8-26, p. 148). As in rolling friction, movements begin distally, sliding your hands proximally to complete the stroke. Also as in rolling friction, this variation is best suited for the extremities with the client assisting by holding the limb up.

Both wringing and rolling friction are performed vigorously, as though you were squeezing water from a cloth. To wring or roll fingers or toes, modify your technique; compress the tissue using only your fingers rather than your entire hand.

Cross-Fiber Friction – Also known as *deep transverse friction,* cross-fiber friction is a precise and penetrating friction popularized by Dr. James Cyriax of London (see p. 158), who called it the "most rehabilitative massage stroke." The direction of movement should be perpendicular to the fibers of the body part being treated (muscle, tendon, ligament).

One or more fingers are placed on the skin at the site of pain or tissue dysfunction. Move the skin back and forth perpendicular to the fibers of the treated structure (Figure 8-27, p. 149). Apply enough pressure to meet (and not

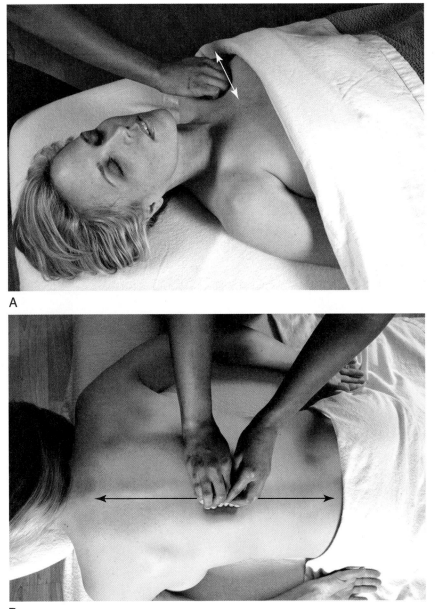

FIGURE 8-23 Superficial warming friction **A,** Using knuckles of one hand on pectoralis major below clavicle with client supine. **B,** Using fingertips up and down the paraspinals with client prone. Shorter strokes may be used while moving up or down the back.

exceed) the client's pain tolerance. Continue the movements for up to 10 seconds (Figure 8-28, p. 149). Repeat if needed.

Being a rehabilitative stroke, cross-fiber friction is remarkably effective in treating most muscular, tendinous, or ligamentous injuries, especially when adhesions and fibrosis are involved.

***Chucking Friction* –** Chucking friction, or *parallel friction,* refers to deep linear friction applied parallel to fiber direction of the treated structures (muscle, tendon, ligament). Using one or more fingers, apply enough pressure to meet (and not exceed) the client's pain tolerance. Continue the movements for up to 10 seconds (Figure 8-29, p. 150). Repeat if needed.

These movements are often applied between bony areas (e.g., metacarpals, metatarsals, forearms, legs). Chucking is often performed using one hand while the other hand is supporting the limb that is being massaged.

***Circular Friction* –** The fingertips or the palm of the hand is placed on the skin at the site of pain or tissue dysfunction. Move the skin over the underlying tissue layers in a circular direction (Figure 8-30, p. 150). Apply enough pressure to meet (and not exceed) the client's pain tolerance. Continue the movements for up to 10 seconds. Repeat if needed.

This movement is particularly useful around joints and on bony areas. Circular friction is also great to use before skin rolling and myofascial release techniques.

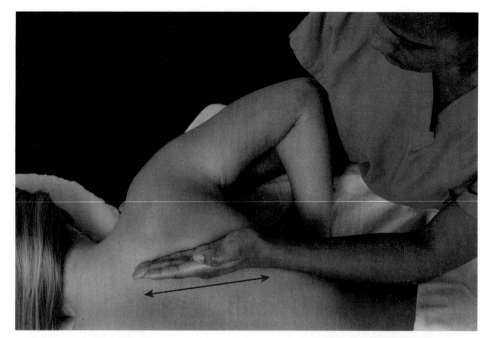

FIGURE 8-24 Superficial warming friction (sawing) using the ulnar sides of the hands on medial border of the scapula.

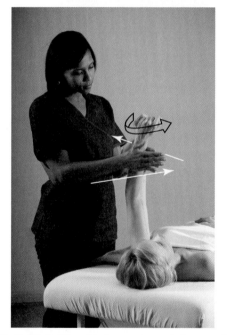

FIGURE 8-25 Rolling friction on extended arm with client supine.

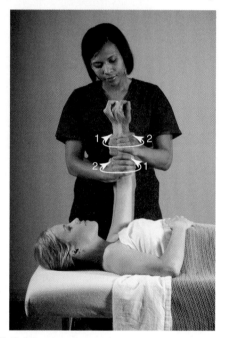

FIGURE 8-26 Wringing friction on extended arm with client supine.

Therapeutic Effects and Uses

- Increases blood flow
- Stimulates lymph flow
- Promotes absorption of inflammatory byproducts (exudates) in subacute and chronic stages of injury
- May reduce posttraumatic scar tissue and adhesions in skin, muscle, tendons, tendon sheaths, ligaments, and joint capsules
- Relieves pain and muscle spasm, thereby promoting relaxation and healing
- Produces localized vasodilation

MINI-LAB

To illustrate how cross-fiber friction can have an effect on scar tissue and repatterning, perform the following activity. Place a box of toothpicks in a haphazard formation under a thick towel. Lay your hand, palm down, on the towel and begin moving your hand using a back and forth motion. Continue moving your hand for several seconds and notice what happens to the toothpick arrangement. Do they remain haphazard, or do they line up straight? How does this activity relate to applying cross-fiber friction on restricted tissue? Write down your conclusion and share it with your class.

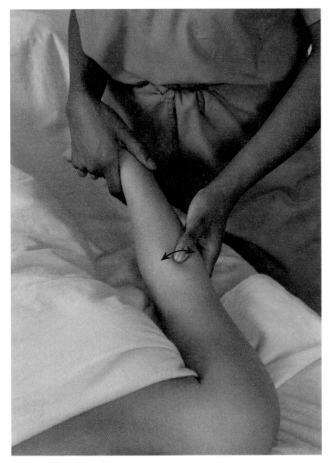

FIGURE 8-27 Cross-fiber friction using a one-thumb technique on the forearm musculature.

Compression

Compression is a non-gliding technique of sustained pressure or a sequence of rhythmic alternating pressures. Variations include *one-handed* and *two-handed compressions*.

The term *compression* comes from the Latin *compressare,* which means "to press together" or "to squeeze." This technique commonly uses sustained pressure or a pumping action over muscle and other tissues. Compressed tissue blanches during pressure application, and then becomes hyperemic when pressure is released. This mechanism enhances fluid exchange. Compression can be performed directly on bare skin, as well as over a clothed or draped client.

Technique. Press the muscle(s) into the underlying bone(s) using your finger, thumb, knuckle, palm, fist, forearm, or elbow. Force is commonly applied at a 90-degree angle or perpendicular to the muscle belly. A 45-degree angle is often needed to address muscles along the spine or anterior leg. Direct pressure can be sustained for 8 to 10 seconds. Repeat if needed. Compression may be applied using rhythmic alternating pressures and may resemble a rocking motion. An outward rotation of the shoulder or forearm can be added before the downward pressure, causing a twist or torquing at the end.

Variations

One-Handed Compression – Use one hand (finger, palm, fist, or forearm, knee, foot) is used to apply the press-release

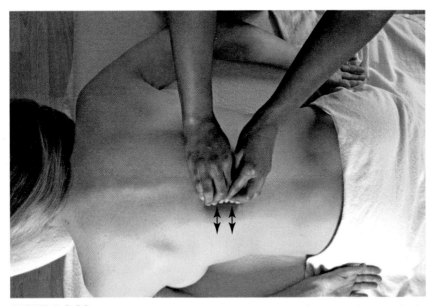

FIGURE 8-28 Cross-fiber friction using the tips of several fingers on the paraspinals.

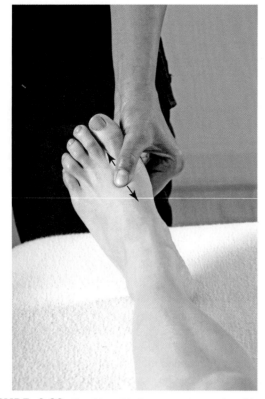

FIGURE 8-29 Chucking friction on metatarsals with client supine.

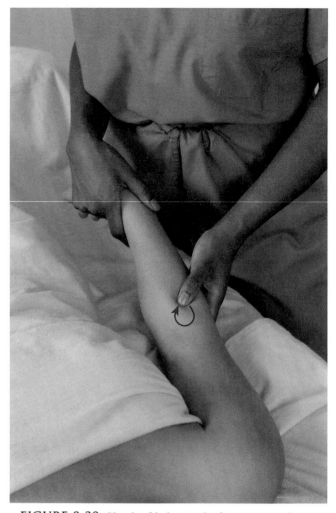

FIGURE 8-30 Circular friction on the forearm musculature.

action (Figure 8-31). Pressure may be sustained for 8 to 10 seconds or rhythmically pressed and released. The hands may be stacked to help increase pressure (Figure 8-32, p. 151). One hand can also be used to maintain pressure while the other hand mobilizes nearby joint(s).

Two-Handed Compresssion – During two-handed compression, both hands are performing the press-release action simultaneously, usually with the hands positioned side by side.

Therapeutic Effects and Uses
- Relaxing effect, which may help relieve pain and muscle spasm
- Stimulating and invigorating effect (when performed rapidly)
- Increases localized blood flow
- Improves range of motion

> *"Often the hands will solve a mystery that the intellect has struggled with in vain."*
> —C. G. Jung

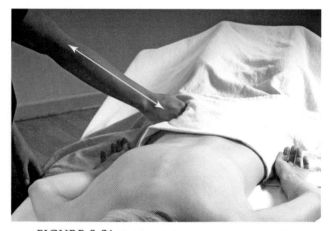

FIGURE 8-31 One-handed compression using a fist.

Tapotement (Percussion)

Tapotement involves repetitive staccato striking movements of the hands, moving either simultaneously or alternately. Movements can be rhythmic or arrhythmic. This

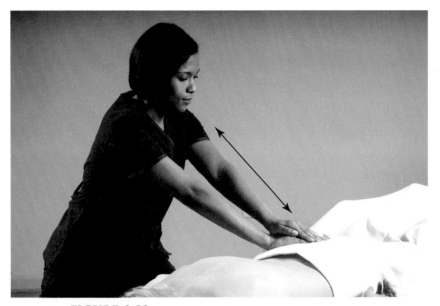

FIGURE 8-32 One-handed compression with hands stacked.

stroke can be delivered with the ulnar surface of the hand or loosely closed fist, tips or flats of the fingers, open or cupped palm, or the knuckles.

Different variations, which include *tapping, pincement, hacking, cupping, pounding,* and *clapping,* require the therapist to use different parts of his or her hands. The variation used often depends on the location where it is employed and the therapist's intention (relaxing versus stimulating). Muscular areas such as legs and hips can withstand a more energetic, vigorous strike whereas thin-tissued or delicate areas such as the face require a lighter tap.

The term *tapotement* (tap-ot-mon) is a derivation of an Old French term, *taper,* that means "a light blow," which, in turn, was derived from the Anglo-Saxon term *taeppa,* meaning "to tap," in the sense of draining fluid from a cavity. At first, this word origin may seem strange, but interestingly, cupping is still used by respiratory therapists and nurses to loosen phlegm congestion in the lungs. The synonym *percussion* comes from *percussio,* which means "a striking."

Tapotement can be performed directly on bare skin or over a clothed or draped client. When performed over bare skin, you may want to warn the client about the possibility of the loud noises that often accompany some varieties (e.g., cupping, clapping). Most therapists use tapotement to finish treatment of an area or end the massage, along with nerve stroking.

Avoid the application of tapotement immediately after exercise, because this stroke can activate muscle spindles, causing spasm. Vigorously applied tapotement over the kidneys in the lower back area is avoided, because these organs are not adequately protected by the rib cage or the abdominal peritoneum.

Technique. Move your hands either alternately or simultaneously to strike the body's surface. Allow your hands to spring back after contact to control the impact (as if your hands are bouncing off the client). The client should feel the onset and removal of pressure. Begin with lighter pressure and moderate strike speed and gradually increase pressure and speed according to the desired effect, tapering off toward the end. Practice will improve your application of qualities such as rhythm and speed.

Variations

Tapping – Using your fingertips on one or both hands, strike the body's surface. Fingers can be held together (Figure 8-33) or apart. Use just the flats of your fingers, tapping lightly on the face or scalp to produce a variation called *raindrops* (Figure 8-34).

Pincement – Strike, grasp, lift, and release the skin quickly using several fingers and thumb of one or both hands (Figure 8-35). Pincement, or *plucking,* lifts the skin much the same way as for skin rolling mentioned previously, but strikes the skin before lifting and releasing it. It's similar to the action used when quickly plucking tissue from a tissue box.

Hacking – Using the ulnar edge of one hand or both hands moving alternatively or simultaneously, strike the skin's surface and release. The wrists should be flexible and the fingers slightly spread apart (Figure 8-36). On skin contact, the momentum of the stroke causes each finger to contact the one above it. This produces a vibratory effect.

Hacking *along* muscle fibers (fingers parallel) produces muscular relaxation. Hacking *across* muscle fibers (fingers perpendicular) stimulates muscle spindles and produces contraction. See Chapter 23 for information about muscle

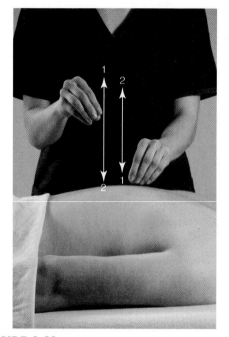

FIGURE 8-33 Tapping tapotement applied to the back.

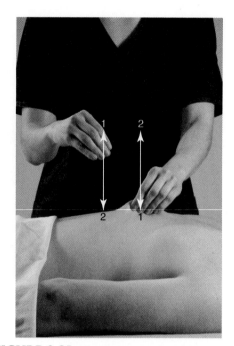

FIGURE 8-35 Pincement tapotement on the back.

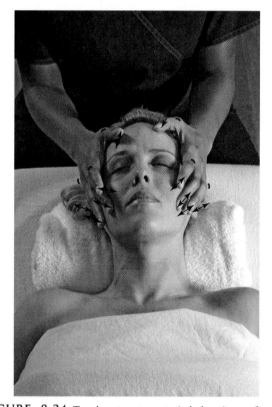

FIGURE 8-34 Tapping tapotement (raindrops) on face of supine client.

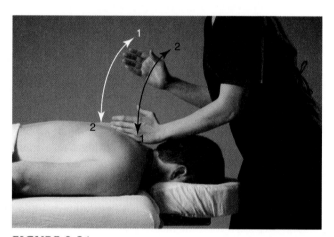

FIGURE 8-36 One-hand hacking along the back parallel to the paraspinals with client prone.

8-37). Air moving out of the hands during the strike makes the quacking sound.

⊖volve *To see alternate hands hacking perpendicular to the hamstrings on a prone client, log on to the Evolve website and go to the course materials for Chapter 8.* ■

---

spindles. Avoid the latter variation on already fatigued muscles (e.g., after athletic events).

A variation of hacking, called *quacking*, places the palms of both hands facing each other (but not touching). The skin is struck using only the sides of the last three fingers (Figure

Cupping – Strike the client's skin with the edges of a cupped hand (Figure 8-38). The strike makes a muffled horse-hoof sound. Done properly, it produces a vibratory effect. Cupping over the posterior and lateral thorax is the stroke of choice for loosening mucus and phlegm and may

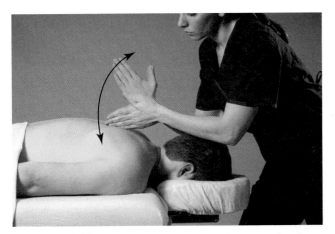

FIGURE 8-37 Hacking tapotement (quacking) on the rhomboids with client prone.

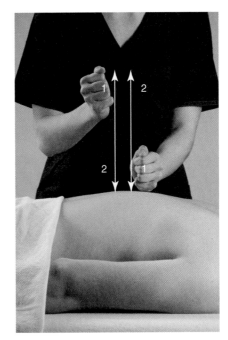

FIGURE 8-39 Pounding tapotement on prone client's back.

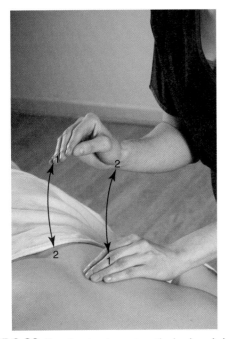

FIGURE 8-38 Cupping tapotement on the back and sides while client is prone.

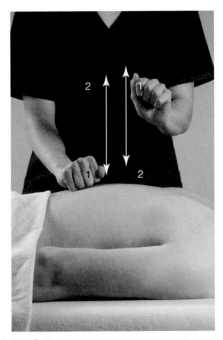

FIGURE 8-40 Pounding tapotement (rapping) on prone client's back.

induce coughing. Have tissues handy. Consider lowering your client's head and torso by using pillows under the abdomen to help with gravity-dependent drainage.

Pounding – Using the sides of one or both loose fists, strike the skin simultaneously or alternately (Figure 8-39). Pounding, or *loose fist beating,* is used on large, muscular areas such as the back, thighs, and hips.

Knuckles of a loose fist can be used to strike the skin as if knocking on a door (Figure 8-40). This variation is called *rapping.*

Clapping – Clapping, *slapping,* or *splatting* is performed by striking the skin with the palmar surface of one or both hands moving simultaneously or alternately (Figure 8-41).

Hands and fingers are held together firmly. A loud smacking sound is heard if clapping is done correctly. If it is done on the face, lighter pressure is used and the force is directed upward.

Diffused – Lay the palmar surface of your relaxed hand on the client's skin. Strike this hand using the other held in

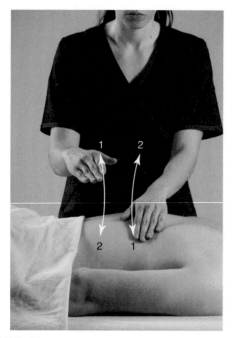

FIGURE 8-41 Clapping tapotement (slapping) on prone client's back.

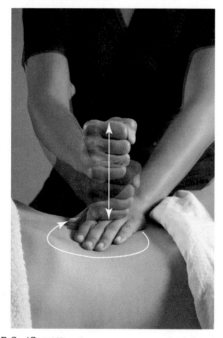

FIGURE 8-42 Diffused tapotement on supine client's abdomen.

a loose fist (Figure 8-42). If your bottom hand is not relaxed, it will not be able to transmit the force of the strike into the treatment area. Drag rather than lift the bottom hand when moving across the skin's surface. This variation is most commonly applied over the abdomen.

BOX 8-3

Ultrasound

Ultrasound is acoustic mechanical vibration of high frequency that produces thermal and nonthermal effects. Therapeutic ultrasound is unique because it falls within the acoustic spectrum and not within the electromagnetic spectrum. Physical and physiotherapists use an ultrasound machine to project microwaves beyond human hearing. Although ultrasound therapy is outside the scope of massage therapy, sonic (sound) energy can be transmitted into the body during tapotement. Therapeutic ultrasound is known for its thermal effects, but its acoustic pressure changes are also important. Therapeutic ultrasound is referred to as *micromassage*. It is also interesting that lower frequencies of sound penetrate farther into the tissue than higher frequencies.

Therapeutic Effects and Uses
- Stimulates mechanoreceptors in skin, muscle, and tendons
- Reduces pain
- Increases skin temperature
- Produces localized vasodilation
- Loosens and mobilizes phlegm in the lungs, thereby assisting with expectoration
- Provides relief of neuralgic pain after amputation, trauma, or another pathology

▶ Vibration

8-5 **Vibration** refers to shaking, quivering, trembling, or rocking movements applied with the fingers, full hand, or an appliance. Variations include *fine, jostling,* and *rocking.* Some vibration involves a back-and-forth or up-and-down motion, whereas other types such as rocking, involve a slower, rhythmic, swinging motion. The speed of vibration varies from rapid to slow.

The term *vibration* comes from the Latin *vibrationem,* which means "a shaker." Vibration can be performed directly on bare skin as well as over a clothed or draped client. Most varieties take coordination and practice to master (Box 8-3). Vibration is the key stroke used in Trager techniques (see page 208 for biography of Milton Trager).

Technique. Use your fingers or full hand to apply the vibrational or rocking movements. Vibration differs from tapotement in that, during vibration, the hands do not break contact with the client's skin. The therapist will notice that each body has its own type of movement pattern, depending on the size of the body, density of the tissues, and health of the joints. Avoid imposing an unnatural rhythm on the body.

Variations

***Fine Vibration* –** Place your hands and/or the fingers of one or both hands on the skin and begin the trembling movements (Figure 8-43). The tissue can be compressed, or

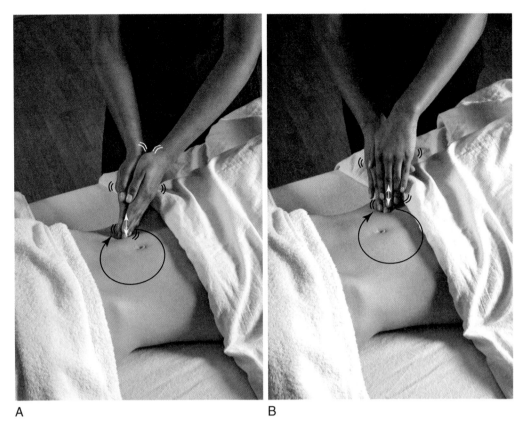

A   B

FIGURE 8-43 Fine vibration on abdomen with client supine. **A,** Praying hands. **B,** Stacked hands.

compressed and lifted, before vibration begins. Movements can be side to side or up and down, or a combination of the two. The therapist's hand may remain in one location or glide down or around an area (Figure 8-44).

Jostling – Jostling is essentially fine vibration applied more vigorously. Grasp the muscle or joint in one or both hands. Shake it vigorously up and down or back and forth (Figure 8-45, p. 156). Movement can be rhythmic or arrhythmic. Your hands can move in the same or different directions. During jostling, or *coarse vibration,* the therapist may lean back and pull to apply traction in joints while delivering the shaking movements (Figure 8-46, *A*). A slight variation of jostling, called *fluffing,* is done while lifting and shaking the tissues from underneath (Figure 8-47, p. 157). A bouncing motion enhances the vibratory effect.

Rocking – Rocking involves pushing the body with one or both hands and either tossing the body back toward you (Figure 8-48, p. 157) or allowing momentum to carry it back. As you pitch and catch your client (which is not unlike the feeling of pushing someone on a swing), you will find your client's unique rhythm. Some bodies have a quicker rattle, whereas others have a slower, fuller cadence. Gentle rocking in a mother's womb or in a parent's arms is probably the first motion the body experiences. Even as adults, we still find this movement comforting.

Vibration Using an Appliance – Be sure your client is draped or clothed and inform the client before using the unit.

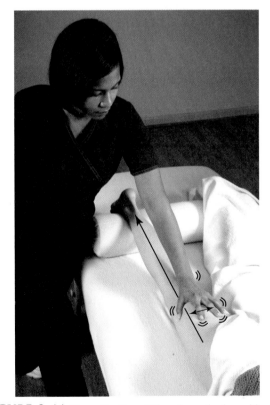

FIGURE 8-44 Fine vibration sliding down the leg with client prone.

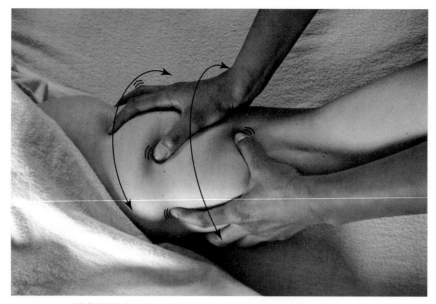

FIGURE 8-45 Jostling on the hamstrings with client prone.

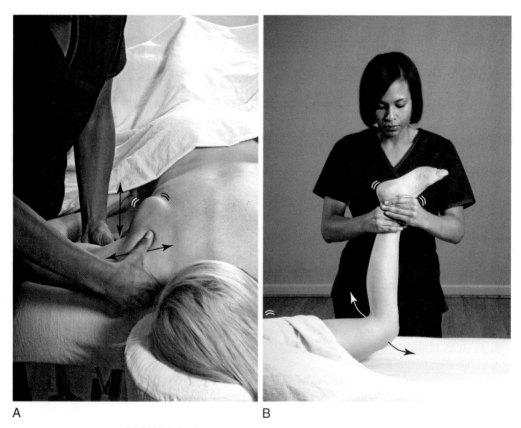

A   B

FIGURE 8-46 Jostling. **A,** Shoulder joint **B,** Hip joint.

Place the unit on the client before turning it on. Move the unit around slowly and avoid bony prominences. Limit its use to no more than 5 minutes, because longer periods of application may cause irritation, numbness, or a feeling of itchiness.

If the unit is corded, be sure the cord does not touch the client. While the corded unit is not being used, be sure it is unplugged and stowed securely so that it will not become a tripping hazard. Check cords often for wear; replace immediately when frayed.

Therapeutic Effects and Uses

- Promotes relaxation, which may help relieve pain and muscle spasm
- Stimulates and invigorates when performed rapidly
- Loosens and mobilizes phlegm in the lungs, thereby assisting with expectoration
- May promote movement of intestinal contents
- May facilitate muscle contraction

Properly applied strokes used in massage therapy go a long way toward addressing pain reduction and stress reduction, as well as a host of other effects included in Chapter

5. Box 8-4 features guidelines to help you integrate massage therapy principles into your practice.

MINI-LAB

To demonstrate the ability to relax the body during vibration, perform the following activity. With a partner, decide who will be the giver and who will be the receiver. Stand approximately 18 to 24 inches apart. The giver grasps the receiver's wrist and pulls, using moderate force. Note the response of the receiver's body. Let go and again grasp the receiver's wrist, keeping it stable. Pull, using moderate force; only this time, rock or shake the arm as you do so. Note the response of the receiver's body. Ask the receiver to share his or her experience with both techniques. Perform the exercise again, reversing roles. Is tensing up and resisting the forward movement more difficult while your body is being rocked? Might the rocking movement also be providing a distracting element, interfering with the body's tendency to become tense during massage?

"The humble improve."
—Wynton Marsalis

CHAT ROOM

Some textbooks group tapotement and vibration under the umbrella of *oscillation*, which encompasses any stroke that involves the up-and-down or springy movements of tapotement/percussion or the back-and-forth or swinging movements of vibration.

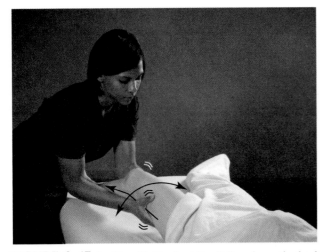

FIGURE 8-47 Jostling (fluffing) while sliding down the back of the thigh with client supine.

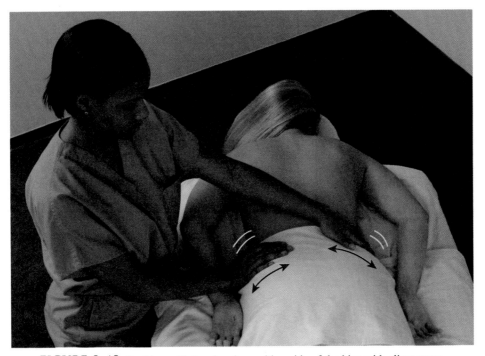

FIGURE 8-48 Rocking with two hands on either side of the hips with client prone.

JAMES HENRY CYRIAX, MD, MRCP

Born: 1904; died: June 17, 1985. Physician. Father of orthopedic medicine.

"He could often be seen walking backwards along Lambeth Palace Road round to the bus stop on Westminster Bridge so as to keep an eye on the oncoming buses."

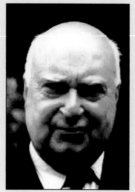

James Cyriax was born in London to Edgar and Annyuta (Kellgren) Cyriax, both of whom studied medicine. His mother's family used exercise and manipulation in the treatment of musculoskeletal disorders, something that was not a common practice at the time and that became very influential in Cyriax's medical career.

Young James was educated at University College School (Gonville) and Caius College (Cambridge) before finally graduating from St. Thomas's Hospital Medical School (London). Soon after passing his qualifying medical examinations, Cyriax became affiliated with St. Thomas's Hospital in the department of orthopedic surgery. He is generally given credit for coining the term *orthopedic medicine* and was probably one of Great Britain's most noted orthopedic practitioners of this time. In 1938 Cyriax transformed the massage department at St. Thomas's into the first department of orthopedic medicine. His new department did much to help transform the art of manipulation into a science that was practiced by trained medical physicians and physical therapists.

Especially important among Cyriax's contributions was his system of soft tissue diagnosis. According to his book *Textbook of Orthopedic Medicine* (1982 edition), Cyriax had a four-step process for determining problems of soft tissues: (1) active motion (to assess the patient's range of motion, strength, and willingness to move the affected area); (2) passive motion (to assess the degree of motion available and the direction of limitation, the use of palpable sensation at the end of passive motion that Cyriax called *end-feel,* and the determination of resistance felt by the practitioner during the end-feel testing); (3) resisted contractions (to determine the reaction of the muscle, tendon, and bony attachments to contraction); and (4) palpation (to confirm involvement of the structures suggested by the preceding three steps in the diagnostic procedure) (Hayes et al, 1994).

In an effort to determine the exact location of a soft tissue lesion, Cyriax's work is extremely important (although not without numerous critics) in that it helps therapists identify the tissues causing the pain and, consequently, select the best methods of treatment to diminish the pain. In general, Cyriax advocated the use of manipulation, deep friction massage (without the use of creams or oils), and the injection of selected drugs in the treatment of soft tissue lesions. Even though Cyriax's ideas were (and remain) controversial, he provided the first systematic diagnostic approach to determine the cause of a patient's soft tissue pain and dysfunction .

An important point to note is that Cyriax was a firm believer in deep massage (cross-fiber or deep transverse friction), either alone or in conjunction with passive or active movements, for the treatment of muscular, ligamentous, and tendinous lesions. In *Textbook of Orthopedic Medicine* (1982 edition), he wrote, "Deep transverse friction restores mobility to muscle in the same way a manipulation frees a joint. Indeed, the action of deep transverse friction may be summed up as affording a mobilization that passive stretching or active exercises cannot achieve."

According to Cyriax's obituary in the *British Medical Journal* (July 1, 1985), he was apparently *persona non grata* within the British medical establishment because of his nontraditional views and consequently was never elected a fellow of the British Royal College of Physicians. His work continues to be scrutinized, as an examination of the various journals within the physical medicine profession will attest. He was an individual who brought out the extremes in individuals, with both his supporters and his critics being adamant about their views. Regardless, Cyriax was instrumental in advancing the concepts of manipulation and massage in the medical profession, making incalculable contributions to those professions.

A key indicator of the importance of James H. Cyriax's contributions is the fact that his book, *Textbook of Orthopedic Medicine,* is presently in its ninth edition.

BOX 8-4

General Guidelines for Massage Therapy

- Practice hand hygiene before and after each massage.
- Protect yourself by using good body mechanics.
- Promote client comfort through providing a restful environment and bolstering devices.
- Screen your client for contraindications.
- Address the client's therapeutic goals.
- Work deeply enough to contact and release tension but not so deep that you cause tension and pain.
- Stroke lightly over bony prominences and pulse points.
- Stay relaxed and present; be focused and respect the client.

MINI-LAB

Once you have learned a basic massage routine, perform a massage while blindfolded. The recipient on the table may have to assist with the draping and turning aspects of the massage because these activities may be too difficult for you without your sense of sight. This exercise will help you get out of your head and intellect and into your hands and feeling skills.

CAUTIONARY SITES AND MASSAGE CONTRAINDICATIONS

During professional practice, you will be making decisions regarding treatment planning and implementation including when to reduce pressure over an area, to avoid an area, or to postpone massage on a certain day. The prudent therapist looks, listens, inquires, palpates, and evaluates constantly. Decisions regarding the safe administration of techniques, and all other treatment modifications, are made on the basis of information gathered about the client as well as knowledge of anatomy, physiology, pathology, and current scientific research.

Certain areas of the body contain structures that, when massaged, may negatively impact the client's health. These areas are called **cautionary sites** or **endangerment sites**.

In many parts of the body, major arteries, veins, and nerves are bundled and wrapped by fascia. Consideration should be given to location and pressure. Pressure over nerve structures can easily create paresthesias (i.e., tingling, numbness) of a spinal nerve. Usually, this effect stops as soon as the pressure is relieved. Peripheral neuropathies can be aggravated by sustained pressure. Peripheral neuropathies are inflammation or degeneration of peripheral nerves leading to loss of sensations and/or motor function. This may occur with use of sustained pressure on the *facial nerve*, *brachial plexus*, and *sciatic nerve* (Figure 8-49) when peripheral neuropathies are present, caution is warranted.

In some people, plaque is located along the walls of arteries and can be dislodged with rigorous movement and create emboli (floating masses). The *carotid arteries* in the throat are the primary vessels of concern (see Figure 26-13). In addition, rubbing over the area of the carotid arteries can create changes in heart rhythm, which may lead to the feeling of dizziness in some people. Avoid any area in the throat that has a pulse.

Deep pressure massage may compromise an abdominal aortic aneurysm. Because this condition may be undiagnosed, avoid using deep pressure on the *abdominal aorta*. This artery lies near the psoas major muscle. A strong pulse arises from this artery; so any area where a strong pulse is felt in the abdomen should be avoided.

Veins are much more fragile structures than arteries, especially in elderly or diabetic clients, or when visible varicosity is evident. Limit your technique to gentle effleurage gliding strokes over these damaged vessels. See Chapter 26 for more information about varicose veins.

Avoid vigorous percussion to the *lower back* just below the floating ribs, as the kidneys are located here (see Figure 30-1). These organs are not as protected as other visceral organs. The kidneys are located behind the protective peritoneum, or retroperitoneally. Limit treatment with electrical massager over this area to a minute.

Also be mindful of local and absolute contraindications. A *local contraindication* is one in which massage can be administered safely while avoiding an area of the body. Examples of local contraindications are areas that have been recently injured, inflamed, or contain a lump, lesion, suspicious mole, or localized skin rash.

Absolute contraindications are factors or conditions for which receiving massage would put you or your client at serious health risk or the client's condition could be made worse. Examples of absolute contraindications are if your client has a highly contagious disease, widespread or systemic infection or inflammation, a fever, a chronic disease that is in exacerbation, or if they are in a state of medical emergency (e.g., hypoglycemia, or low blood sugar). When a client has an absolute contraindication, massage is not advised. When the client's disease resolves, is in a state of remission, or is cleared by the physician who managed the client's medical emergency, the client can then receive massage.

Superficial lymph nodes are found in great numbers in the *groin* (inguinal nodes), in the *armpit* (axillary nodes), and in the *neck* (cervical nodes). When palpated, lymph nodes feel dense, and are similar in size and shape to a raw black-eyed pea. The location of enlarged palpable lymph nodes is just under the skin and superficial to muscle (see Figure 27-1). Enlarged lymph nodes are local contraindications. If enlarged lymph nodes are accompanied by systemic infection, treat as an absolute contraindication until your client is symptom free for 48 hours. If you possess advanced certification in manual lymphatic drainage or lymphatic massage, your education has made you familiar with workable and unworkable conditions.

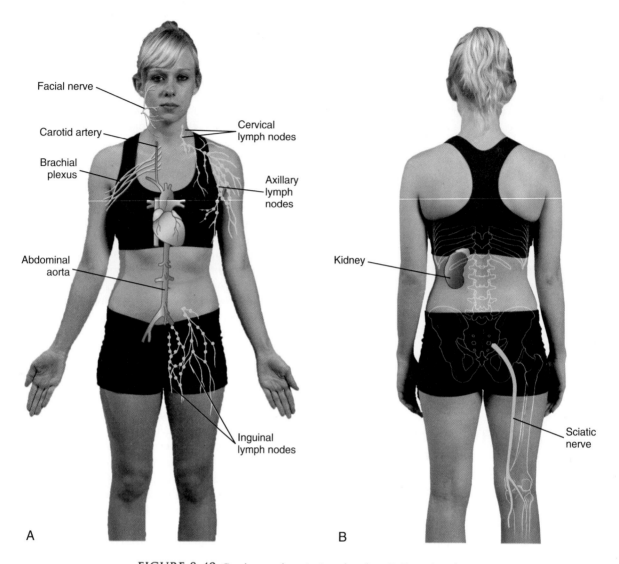

FIGURE 8-49 Cautionary sites. **A,** Anterior view. **B,** Posterior view.

Discussions of local and absolute contraindication are found in Chapter 9. Specific modifications for clients with various diseases and conditions are found in Chapters 19 through 30.

JOINT MOBILIZATIONS AND STRETCHES

Joints, muscles, and other soft tissues that benefit from massage will also benefit from joint mobilizations and stretching techniques to improve function, restore mobility, and increase range of motion. These techniques provide additional treatment options and can easily be applied before, during, or after the massage, or they may be used as the primary technique. Furthermore, these techniques can be administered passively or actively.

Most joint mobilization and stretching techniques are best administered on unlubricated skin; you may need to wipe off any excess lubricant if massage was previously

administered before you begin these movements. If the entire session is devoted to joint mobilizations and stretching, the client may remain clothed, although the routine is best performed on a client wearing flexible clothing such as sweats, tights, or leggings.

Tell your client about the movements you will be performing beforehand. You may need to demonstrate any movements, especially if they are to be done by the client (actively).

Description

Joint mobilizations involve moving a joint through its full normal range of motion (Box 8-5). It is helpful to apply a little traction to the joint before mobilizing it. Use three repetitions (reps) in one direction before reversing direction and repeating three more reps. Repeat this sequence if needed. Be familiar with the type of joint with which you are working and its range of motion capabilities (see Chapter 21). **Range of motion** (ROM) is the range, usually expressed

BOX 8-5

Joint Mobilizations and Stretches

Neck
  Neck circles
  Neck lateral flexion
  Neck lateral flexion with rotation
  Neck forward flexion
Wrist and Hand
  Flip wrist
  Interlace fingers and mobilize wrist
  Metacarpal scissors
  Pull and circumduct fingers
Arm and Shoulder
  Arm pull
  Shoulder circles
Spine
  Spinal twist I
  Spinal twist II
  Spinal twist III
  Spinal twist IV
Hip and Knee
  Leg pull
  Leg rock
  Hip clock stretch
  Hip circles
  Hip flexion
  Groin stretch
  Heel to hip
  Hip hyperextension
Foot and Ankle
  Plantar flexion
  Dorsiflexion
  Metatarsal scissors
  Pull and circumduct toes

in degrees of a circle, through which bones of a joint can move or be moved.

Stretching is a method that lengthens and elongates soft tissues. When deciding how to stretch a particular muscle, just perform the opposite action of the target muscle(s). For example, to stretch the psoas, medially rotate and extend the hip.

Have your client demonstrate actively a baseline range of motion before use of these techniques. This will help you evaluate the effectiveness of the technique.

Technique

Use jostling, rocking, or superficial warming friction to prepare the area. The principle is simple; similar to clay, warm tissues are pliable and can move and stretch more easily. Cold tissues tend to be rigid and less malleable, making them more susceptible to injury.

During application of both joint mobilizations and stretches, ask your client to relax and inhale at the beginning of the movement and exhale during the movement. You can hold a stretch for up to 30 seconds and can repeat the stretch for up to three times.

Stretching should be performed slowly and rhythmically and not cause pain. This application method is called *static stretching*. *Ballistic stretching* uses a bouncing motion and is not preferred because it stimulates muscle spindles rather than Golgi tendon organs (see Chapter 23 for more information).

How far a muscle can stretch or a joint can be mobilized depends on numerous factors, including the client's flexibility, genetic limitations, the health of the involved joint, fascial restrictions, muscle tension, muscle guarding, past injuries, and past surgeries.

Furthermore, it is essential to use proper body mechanics when applying these movements because they can be physically demanding on the therapist, particularly when the client is large.

Variations: Active and Passive

Two primary variations of joint mobilizations and stretching techniques are (1) *passive* and (2) *active.* Two additional variations of active mobilizations are: *active assisted* and *active resisted.*

- *Passive movements*: Client relaxes or is passive while the therapist performs the movement
- *Active movements*: Client actively performs the movement after the therapist describes or demonstrates it
- *Active-assisted movements*: Client actively performs the movement while the therapist assists
- *Active-resisted movements*: Client actively performs the movement while the therapist resists it

When active-assisted or active-resisted movements are performed at home, the client may use a wall, towel, or other object to provide the assistance or resistance.

MINI-LAB

Place your hand, palm down, on your anterior thigh. Keeping your hand flat, raise your index finger and notice how high it can go. Now raise your index finger again, but this time, use your other hand to lift your finger to its fullest extent. Notice how much farther your index finger can go with active assistance.

Therapeutic Effects and Uses

- Helps to maintain or increase range of motion and improves functional ability
- Stimulates production of synovial fluid
- Reduces pain
- Increases blood and lymph flow in area mobilized or stretched because of the mechanical pumping effect produced as tissues are alternately squeezed and released
- Increases kinesthetic awareness

- Aids in rehabilitation
- May improve body alignment and posture
- Assists in assessing tissues

Caution

Use caution if the client has any disease process or abnormality present (i.e., surgical replacement, pins or wires, osteoporosis, osteoarthritis, scoliosis, etc).

Inflamed or swollen joints are best avoided.

Avoid fast, bouncy, or *ballistic* movements because they can cause the muscle to contract, thereby limiting the effectiveness of the movement. A succession of ballistic movements can cause irritation or even tear the muscle, fascia, tendons, and ligaments. Rather, use a slow *static* stretch.

The techniques presented in the following sections are passive movements. A brief description of the movement is presented with pictorial representation. Both mobilization and stretches are addressed in the prone and supine positions. Perform the movements on both sides of the body when applicable.

Additionally, be sure and check your state's definition of scope of practice for the inclusion or exclusion of these techniques.

MEMO: Because this section contains movement terminology not yet discussed, it is highly recommended that you refer to Chapter 21 when you encounter a term you do not understand (e.g., flexion, rotation).

 Neck

Joint mobilizations and stretches of the neck, which are performed while the client is in the supine position, include *neck circles, neck lateral flexion with and without rotation,* and *neck forward flexion.* Movements of the neck include flexion, extension, lateral flexion, and rotation.

Neck Circles. Place one hand on the client's forehead, rocking the head side to side while your other hand intermittently compresses the tissue in the lamina groove on the opposite side up and toward you (Figure 8-50). Done correctly, it will feel as if your hands are pushing and pulling alternately.

Neck Lateral Flexion. With one hand, pull the client's head toward the near shoulder while your hand stabilizes the client's far shoulder (Figure 8-51). Do not lift the head while pulling.

Neck Lateral Flexion with Rotation. With one hand, pull the client's rotated head toward the near shoulder; the client's head is rotated away from you or toward the far shoulder. Use your other hand to stabilize the client's far shoulder (Figure 8-52). Do not lift the head while pulling. Repeat on the opposite side.

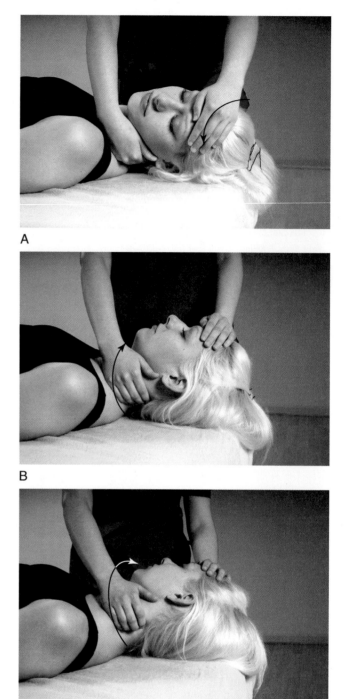

A

B

C

FIGURE 8-50 Neck circles. **A,** Begin by moving the head away from you. **B,** Then to the center. **C,** Move the head toward you. .

Neck Forward Flexion. Support the base of the skull with one or both hands or forearm while you lift the head toward the chest (Figure 8-53). If both forearms are used, they can be crisscrossed at the base of the client's skull before the lift.

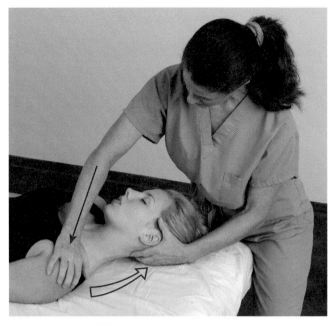

FIGURE 8-51 Neck lateral flexion.

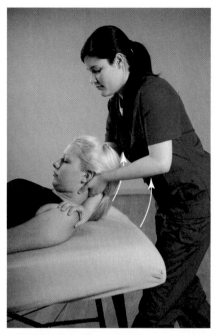

FIGURE 8-53 Neck forward flexion.

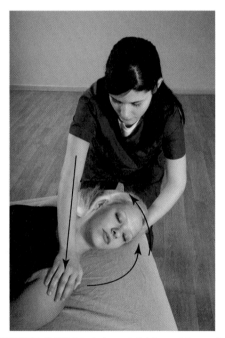

FIGURE 8-52 Neck lateral flexion with rotation.

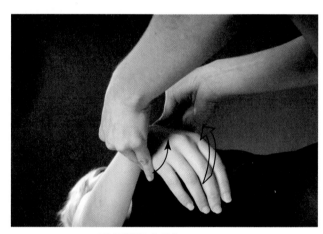

FIGURE 8-54 Flip wrist.

Wrist and Hand

Joint mobilizations and stretches of the wrist and hand are *flip wrist*, *interlace fingers and mobilize wrist*, *metacarpal scissors*, and *pull and circumduct fingers*. Do not apply excessive force while moving the wrist and hand. The four movements of the wrist are abduction, adduction, flexion, and extension.

Flip Wrist. Lightly pincer grip just above wrist with your thumbs and index fingers of both hands. Use your remaining

fingers to flip your client's hand up and down while you stabilizing the wrist (Figure 8-54). This action will move the wrist into flexion and extension.

Interlace Fingers and Mobilize Wrist. Holding the client's forearm vertically, interlace your fingers with the client's fingers, then move the wrist into flexion, extension, abduction, and adduction as your other hand stabilizes the client's forearm just above the wrist (Figure 8-55).

Metacarpal Scissors. Lightly pincer grip two of the metacarpal bones with the thumbs and index fingers of both your hands. Alternately move them up and down; then move to the next pair of bones and repeat (Figure 8-56). Be sure to mobilize the tissues between each pair of metacarpals.

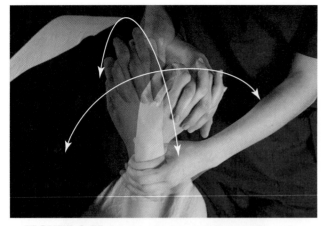

FIGURE 8-55 Interlace the fingers before moving wrist.

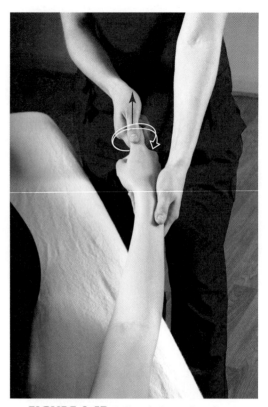

FIGURE 8-57 Pull and circumduct finger.

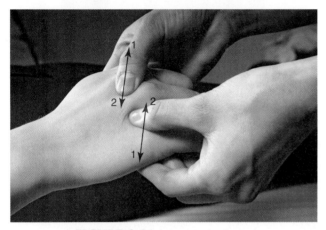

FIGURE 8-56 Metacarpal scissors.

Pull and Circumduct Fingers. Support the client's wrist with one of your hands while you pull and circumduct each finger with the other hand (Figure 8-57). Move in both directions (i.e., clockwise and counterclockwise).

Arm and Shoulder

8-9 Joint mobilizations and stretches of the arm and shoulders are *arm pulls* and *shoulder circles*. These movements are best applied while the client is supine but can be adapted for the prone or side-lying client. The movements of the shoulder are flexion, extension, adduction, abduction, rotation, and circumduction. The elbow permits flexion, extension, and rotation (the latter movement permits pronation and supination of the forearm).

Arm Pull. This technique has four parts:
1. While standing tableside near your client's hip, grasp just above the wrist. Pull and release the arm several times (Figure 8-58). The arm can be tapped or gently bounced on the massage table while you pull or traction it.
2. Grasp just above the wrist and stand several feet away from the table's side. The shoulder will be abducted

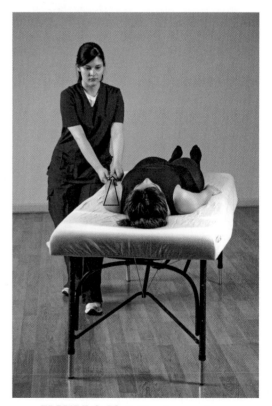

FIGURE 8-58 Pulling the arm down.

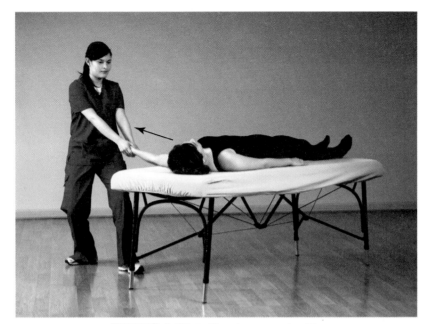

FIGURE 8-59 Pulling the arm to the side.

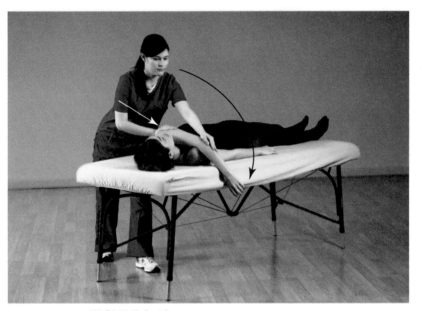

FIGURE 8-60 Pulling the arm across the chest.

90 degrees. Pull and release the arm several times (Figure 8-59).

3. Adduct the client's shoulder by draping his or her arm across the chest. Push the arm horizontally across the table using one hand over the shoulder and the other hand over or under the elbow (Figure 8-60).

4. Grasp just above the wrist and position yourself several feet away from the top of the table. Pull and release the arms several times (Figure 8-61).

Shoulder Circles. Beginning with the client's arm at his or her side, create an arc by pulling the arm up toward the

ceiling until it is vertical; continue pulling the arm until it is over the client's head (Figure 8-62, *A*, p. 166). With your other hand, bend the client's elbow and bring the arm laterally to the client's side (Figure 8-62, *B*). Maintain traction during the entire movement sequence. Repeat three times.

Spine

8-10 Techniques for the spine that use a lengthening and rotational motion on the supine-lying client and fall under the umbrella term *spinal twist*. These movements are repeated on each side of the client.

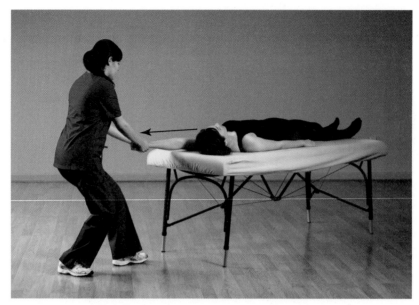

FIGURE 8-61 Pulling the arm overhead.

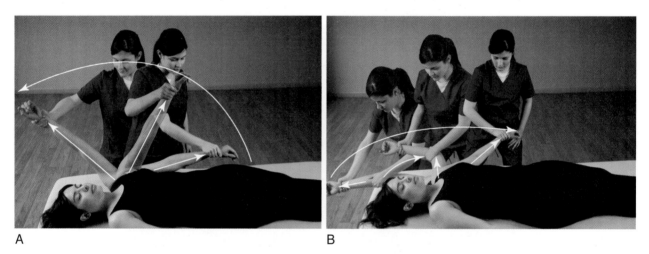

A   B

FIGURE 8-62 Shoulder circles. **A,** Pull arm over the client's head. **B,** Pull arm down to the client's side.

Spinal Twist I. Anchor the client's far hip with your lower hand while you pull the far shoulder up and toward you with your upper hand. The client's arms can be relaxed or placed with hands behind the head (Figure 8-63).

Spinal Twist II. With the client's near leg bent and the foot placed on the lateral side of the far knee, push the bent knee away from you while pulling the far shoulder up and toward you (Figure 8-64).

Spinal Twist III. Anchor the client's far shoulder while you pull the bent far knee toward you and down (Figure 8-65).

Spinal Twist IV. Anchor the client's near shoulder while you push the bent near knee away from you (Figure 8-66).

 ### Hip and Knee

Joint mobilizations and stretches of the hip and knee areas are *leg pull*, *leg rock*, *hip clock stretch* and *circles*, *hip flexion* and *hyperextension*, *groin stretch*, and *heel to hip*. Hip movements are flexion, extension, adduction, abduction, rotation, and circumduction. Knee movements are essentially flexion and extension.

Leg Pull. While standing at the foot of the table, grasp just above the client's ankle. Pull and release several times (Figure 8-67). The leg can be tapped or gently bounced on the massage table while you are pulling or tractioning it.

Leg Rock. While standing tableside, place your hands above and below the client's knee. Rock the leg back and forth to rotate the hip (Figure 8-68).

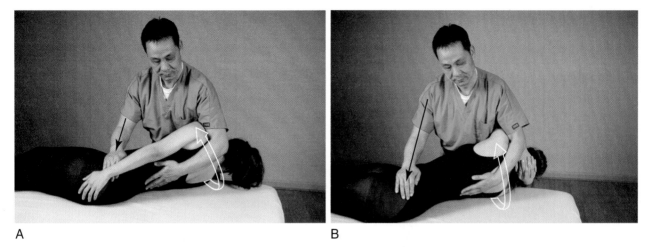

A

B

FIGURE 8-63 Spinal twist I. **A,** Client's arms relaxed. **B,** Client's hands behind her head.

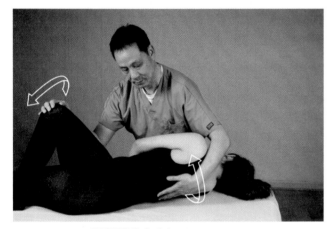

FIGURE 8-64 Spinal twist II.

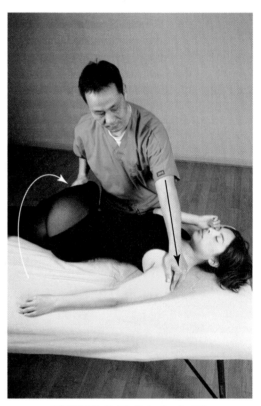

FIGURE 8-65 Spinal twist III.

Hip Clock Stretch. Flex the client's hip and knee while supporting both the knee and heel; while imagining that the client's leg is the hour hand of a clock, push and stretch the hip in a 10 o'clock, 12 o'clock, and 2 o'clock stretch (Figure 8-69). Repeat in the opposite direction.

Hip Circles. After performing the hip clock stretch, move the client's flexed hip and knee in a circle three times (Figure 8-70). Reverse direction and repeat.

Hip Flexion. Flex the client's hip by placing one hand just above and behind the ankle and raise the leg. Be sure to place your other hand above the knee to maintain knee extension during the movement (Figure 8-71). To stretch the calf after hip flexion, dorsiflex the ankle (Figure 8-72).

Groin Stretch. Flex and laterally rotate the client's near hip and flex the near knee. Place the near foot by the far knee. Stretch the hip adductors by gently pressing down on the iliac crest of the far hip with one hand and just above the near flexed knee with the other hand (Figure 8-73).

Heel to Hip. Flex the client's near knee by moving the heel toward the near hip (Figure 8-74). A dorsiflexion of the ankle can be added during the stretch (Figure 8-75).

Hip Hyperextension. Flex the client's knee and lift the thigh until the hip is hyperextended. The hand lifting the thigh should be above the flexed knee while the other hand anchors the sacrum (Figure 8-76). Release and repeat two more times.

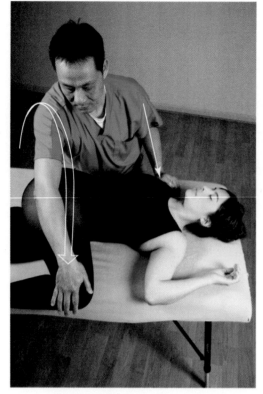

FIGURE 8-66 Spinal twist IV.

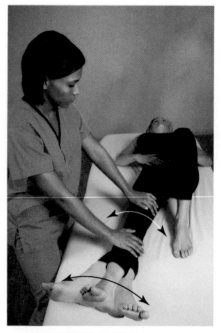

FIGURE 8-68 Leg rock.

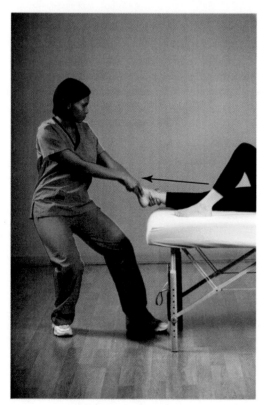

FIGURE 8-67 Leg pull.

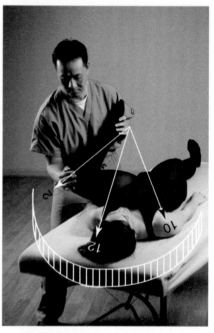

FIGURE 8-69 Hip clock stretch.

Ankle and Foot

8-12 Joint mobilizations and stretches of the ankle and foot are *plantar flexion* and *dorsiflexion*, *metatarsal scissors*, and *pull and circumduct toes*. The ankle and foot movements, which include dorsiflexion, plantar flexion, inversion, and eversion, can be applied while the client is prone or supine.

Plantar Flexion. While holding the client's heel with one hand, push down on the top of the foot with the other hand to move the ankle into plantar flexion (Figure 8-77).

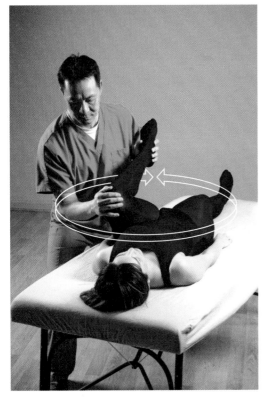

FIGURE 8-70 Hip circles.

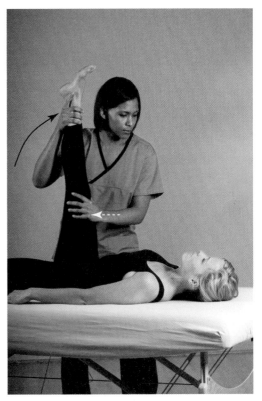

FIGURE 8-71 Hip flexion.

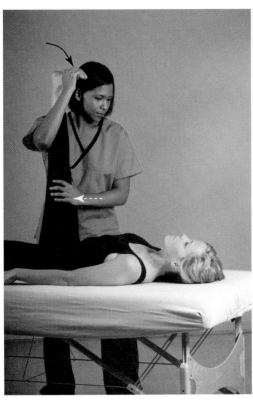

FIGURE 8-72 Hip flexion with ankle dorsiflexion.

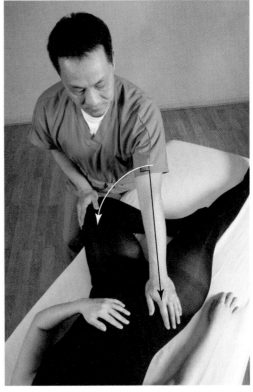

FIGURE 8-73 Groin stretch.

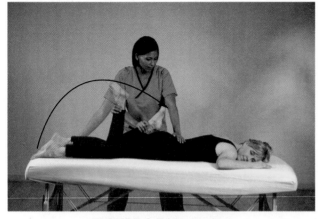

FIGURE 8-74 Heel to hip.

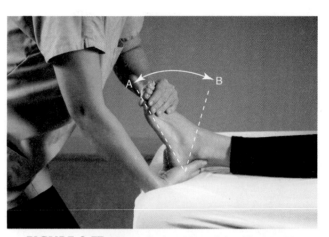

FIGURE 8-77 Plantar flexion (**A**) and dorsiflexion (**B**).

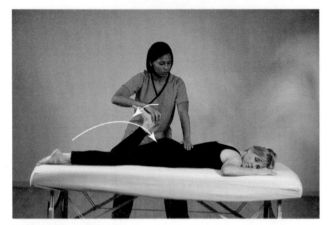

FIGURE 8-75 Heel to hip with the additional ankle dorsiflexion.

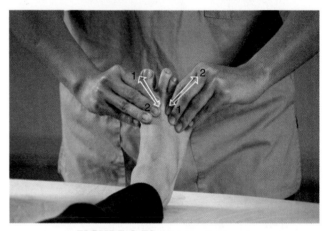

FIGURE 8-78 Metatarsal scissors.

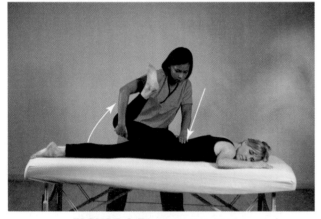

FIGURE 8-76 Hip hyperextension.

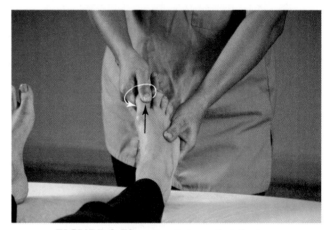

FIGURE 8-79 Pull and circumduct the toes.

Dorsiflexion. Hold the client's heel with one hand while pushing the ball of the foot toward the knee with the other hand to move the ankle into dorsiflexion (see Figure 8-77).

Metatarsal Scissors. Lightly pincer grip two of the metatarsal bones with the thumbs and index fingers of both your hands. Alternately move them up and down, then move to the next pair of bones and repeat (Figure 8-78). Be sure to mobilize the tissues between each pair of metatarsals.

Pull and Circumduct Toes. Support the client's foot with one hand while you pull and circumduct the each toe with the other hand (Figure 8-79). Move in both directions (i.e., clockwise and counterclockwise).

E-RESOURCES

⊜volve

http://evolve.elsevier.com/Salvo/MassageTherapy

- Chapter challenge
- Flash cards
- Photo gallery
- Technique videos
- Additional information
- Weblinks

▶ **DVD**

- 8-1: Effleurage
- 8-2: Pétrissage
- 8-3: Friction
- 8-4: Tapotement
- 8-5: Vibration
- 8-6: Joint mobilizations and stretches
- 8-7: Neck
- 8-8: Wrist and hand
- 8-9: Arm and shoulder
- 8-10: Spine
- 8-11: Hip and knee
- 8-12: Ankle and foot

These videos can also be viewed on the Evolve website.

BIBLIOGRAPHY

Anderson B: *Stretching*, Bolinas, Calif, 1980, Shelter Publications.

Beck MF: *Theory and practice of therapeutic massage*, ed 4, Albany, NY, 2005, Thomson Delmar Learning.

Benjamin PJ: *Tappan's handbook of healing massage technique*, ed 5, Upper Saddle River, NJ, 2004, Prentice-Hall.

Buckwalter JA: Effects of early motion on healing of musculoskeletal tissues, *Hand Clin* 12(1):13-24, 1996.

Chaitow L: *Modern neuromuscular techniques*, ed 2, New York, 2003, Churchill Livingstone.

Chamberlain G: Cyriax's friction massage: a review, *J Orthop Sports Phys Ther* 4:16-22, 1982.

Coughlin P: *Principles and practice of manual therapeutics*, New York, 2002, Churchill Livingstone.

DeDomenico G: *Beards massage: principles and practice of soft tissue manipulation*, ed 5, 2007, Saunders.

Drez D: *Therapeutic modalities for sports injuries*, St Louis, 1989, Mosby.

Evans P: The healing process at cellular level, a review, *Physiotherapy* 66:256-259, 1980.

Fritz S: *Mosby's fundamentals of therapeutic massage*, ed 4, St Louis, 2009, Mosby.

FSMTB: 2007 job task analysis survey report (website): http://www.fsmtb.org/downloads/jtaDemo.pdf. Accessed June 11, 2010.

Greene L: *Save your hands! the complete guide to injury prevention and ergonomics for manual therapists*, ed 2, Coconut Creek, Fla, 2008, Gilded Age Press.

Hayes KW, et al: An examination of Cyriax's passive motion tests with patients having osteoarthritis of the knee, *Phys Ther* 74(8):697-708, 1994.

Juhan D: *Job's body, a handbook for bodyworkers*, ed 3, Barrington, NY, 2003, Station Hill Press.

Kendall FP, McCreary EK, Provance PG: *Muscles: testing and function*, Baltimore, 1993, Lippincott Williams & Wilkins.

Krieger D: Therapeutic touch: the imprimatur of nursing, *Am J Nurs* 75(5):784-787, 1975.

Mackey B: Massage therapy and reflexology awareness, *Nurs Clin North Am* 36(1):159-170, 2001.

Massage Therapy Body of Knowledge: Version 1, 2010 (website): http://www.mtbok.org/index.html. Accessed June 11, 2010.

Mennell JB: *Physical treatment*, ed 5, Philadelphia, 1945, Blakiston.

Moore KL: *Clinically oriented anatomy*, ed 5, Baltimore, 2005, Lippincott Williams & Wilkins.

Muscolino J: *The muscle and bone palpation manual*, St Louis, 2009, Mosby.

Platzer W: *Color atlas and textbook of human anatomy: locomotor system*, vol 1, ed 3, New York, 1984, Thieme.

Prudden B: *Pain erasure*, New York, 1980, M Evans.

Reed B, Held JM: Effects of sequential connective tissue massage on autonomic nervous system of middle-aged and elderly adults, *Phys Ther* 68(8):1231-1234, 1988.

St. John P: *St. John neuromuscular therapy seminars: manual I*, Largo, Fla, 1995, self-published.

Thompson C: Oil on troubled waters? *Nurs Times* 97(15):74-77, 2001.

Travell JG, Simons D: *Myofascial pain and dysfunction, the trigger point manual*, Baltimore, 1992, Lippincott Williams & Wilkins.

Venes D, Thomas CL, Taber CW: *Taber's cyclopedic medical dictionary*, ed 20, Philadelphia, 2005, FA Davis.

Voss DE, Ionta MK, Myers BJ: *Proprioceptive neuromuscular facilitation*, Philadelphia, 1985, Harper & Row.

Walker H: Deep transverse frictions in ligament healing, *J Orthop Sports Phys Ther* 6(2):89-94, 1984.

Williams RE: *The road to radiant health*, College Place, Wash, 1977, Color Press.

MATCHING I

Place the letter of the answer next to the term or phrase that best describes it.

A. Compression
B. Continuity
C. Cross-fiber friction
D. Effleurage

E. Friction
F. Joint mobilization
G. Nerve stroke
H. Pétrissage

I. Rhythm
J. Swedish gymnastics
K. Tapotement
L. Vibration

_____ 1. Regularity of applied massage techniques

_____ 2. Uninterrupted flow of massage strokes, and unbroken transition from one stroke to the next

_____ 3. Gliding movements that are repeated and follow the contour of the client's body

_____ 4. Considered a light effleurage, the massage technique that consists of light finger tracing over the skin

_____ 5. Shaking, quivering, trembling, or rocking massage movements applied with fingers, full hand, or an appliance

_____ 6. Lifting soft tissues vertically and then compressing by either squeezing or rolling the tissues before releasing them, using rhythmic alternating pressures

_____ 7. Rubbing one surface over another in several directions; can be applied superficially with hands gliding over the skin or deeply while moving skin across underlying tissue layers

_____ 8. Precise and penetrating massage technique, popularized by Dr. James Cyriax of London, in which the direction of movement is perpendicular to the fibers being treated

_____ 9. Repetitive staccato striking movements of the therapist's hands, moving either simultaneously or alternately

_____ 10. Historical collective term for stretches and joint mobilizations designed to restore and maintain pain-free movements

_____ 11. Moving a joint through its full normal range of motion

_____ 12. Non-gliding technique of sustained pressure or a sequence of rhythmic alternating pressures

MATCHING II

Place the letter of the answer next to the term or phrase that best describes it.

A. Absolute contraindication
B. Active-assisted movements
C. Active movements
D. Active-resisted movements

E. Cautionary sites
F. Excursion
G. Local contraindication
H. Massage therapy

I. Passive movements
J. Range of motion
K. Sequence
L. Stretching

_____ 1. Movements described or demonstrated by the therapist while the client performs the movements

_____ 2. Manual and scientific manipulation of the soft tissues of the body for the purpose of establishing and maintaining good health and promoting wellness

_____ 3. Condition in which massage can be administered safely while avoiding a certain area of the body

_____ 4. Distance traveled during the length of a massage stroke

_____ 5. Movements performed by therapist on the client while he or she remains relaxed

_____ 6. Technique that lengthens and elongates soft tissues

_____ 7. Situation in which receiving massage would put the therapist or the client at serious health risk or the client's condition could be made worse with massage

_____ 8. Arrangement or order of massage strokes

_____ 9. Areas of the body containing structures that, when massaged, may negatively impact the client's health

_____ 10. Movements performed by client with therapist assisting

_____ 11. Therapist gently opposes movement while client is performing it

_____ 12. The extent to which bones of a joint can move or be moved; usually expressed in degrees of a circle

CASE STUDY

More than Just an Accident

Margaret was a recent graduate from the Gulf Coast School of Massage. She acquired her state license and began her practice at a well-established chiropractic clinic. Margaret massaged the physicians' patients before their spinal adjustments. The patients loved the massage, and the physicians loved that the patients reported improving more quickly with the addition of the massage before the spinal adjustments.

Mark was Margaret's next client. It was Mark's first massage at the clinic. He was a car sales associate uptown and was recently involved in a minor car accident. Mark's chiropractor gave clearance for him to begin receiving massages. Because Margaret was asked to address his back, neck, and shoulder only, Mark left on his trousers.

When Margaret reentered the massage room, Mark was lying prone with the sheet draped across his back and legs. Margaret lowered the sheet and observed a large portion of his back covered with red circles. The edges of the circles were slightly elevated, and she noticed a slight odor to his skin.

Should Margaret continue with the massage?

Should Margaret ask the client or his physician about the circles?

When should she make the inquiry?

Should she consult the physician before, after, or during the massage?

CRITICAL THINKING

Why is the order of the application of techniques important for massage therapy? Give examples.

CHAPTER 9

Infection Control and Emergency Preparedness

"In the End, we will conserve only what we love, we will love only what we understand, we will understand only what we are taught."

—Baba Dioum (Senegalese conservationist)

LEARNING OBJECTIVES

After completing this chapter, the student should be able to:

- Contrast and compare types of disease.
- State types of pathogens and examples of infections they can cause.
- Discuss how disease can be transmitted.
- Outline several host defenses against infection.
- Contrast and compare local and absolute contraindications.
- List suggestions for good personal hygiene.
- Name the recommended guidelines for standard precautions.
- Demonstrate the recommended hand hygiene procedures.
- Discuss glove use in a massage practice, and determine when gloves might be necessary.
- State what to do in medical emergency situations that the therapist may encounter in professional practice.

http://evolve.elsevier.com/Salvo/MassageTherapy

INTRODUCTION

Massage therapy is one of the safest, least intrusive, and most effective treatments for pain and discomfort in the health care field today. However, the client is still susceptible to infection as well as injury. For example, contagious diseases may be transferred to clients by unclean hands or by unsanitary equipment and supplies.

A system of infection control is needed to protect clients and minimize disease transmission. These measures include hand hygiene and sanitary lubricant dispensing. Part of client safety includes good personal hygiene on the part of the therapist. Infection control and good hygiene are some of the best ways to prevent the spread of disease. These standards are part of professional massage practice across the country.

Hippocrates, the father of Western medicine, is frequently quoted as saying that physicians should "do no harm." The therapist must adopt a policy of impeccable cleanliness before coming into contact with a client. This chapter examines procedures regarding infection control and standard precautions, including hand hygiene, glove use, and the disinfecting of equipment. This chapter goes beyond infection control to include strategies for a safe work environment and procedures for medical emergency situations.

DISEASE AWARENESS

As health care professionals, massage therapists seek to improve the health and well-being of their clients through massage therapy. Regardless of your work setting or treatment style, you will encounter clients who have diseases or medical conditions and who are under medical supervision. You need to be aware of disease and infectious agents to control their transmission. To build understanding, a fundamental overview of disease is needed.

Diseases can be grouped according to similar characteristics or how they were acquired. The major types of diseases are autoimmune, cancer, deficiency, degenerative, genetic, infectious, and metabolic. Table 9-1 summarizes types of diseases, their description, and examples of each.

Disease awareness also means that we will be discussing infections and how they occur. For example, the mere presence of a virus does not mean infection will take place. Infection is the invasion of pathogens occurring in a series of events termed a *chain of infection* (Figure 9-1). Infection

TABLE 9-1 Types of Diseases

DISEASES	DESCRIPTION	EXAMPLES
Autoimmune	Caused by an overactive immune system. The immune system mistakes body tissue for something foreign. It then launches an attack, destroying normal tissue.	Rheumatoid arthritis (synovial membranes of joints are affected), systemic lupus erythematosus (connective tissues are affected), multiple sclerosis (brain and spinal cord nerve sheaths are affected)
Cancer	Characterized by abnormal cells that possess uncontrollable cell division, lack programmed cell death, and can accumulate into masses called tumors. Tumors can be localized or spread to distant sites. This spreading is called metastasis.	Lung cancer (cancerous cells in the lungs), colon cancer (cancerous cells in the colon), malignant melanoma (cancerous cells in pigmented tissue [usually the skin])
Deficiency	Caused by a lack of dietary vitamins, minerals, or nutrients. Deficiency can also result from inability to properly digest or absorb a particular nutrient. Lack of the nutrient interferes with the affected individual's growth, development, or metabolism.	Scurvy (lack of vitamin C), rickets (lack of vitamin D), beriberi (lack of vitamin B_1), pernicious anemia (vitamin B_{12} malabsorption)
Degenerative	Occur when an organ or its function deteriorates over time. This is caused by overuse or results from the aging process seen in senescence.	Osteoporosis (bone degeneration), Alzheimer and Parkinson diseases (brain degeneration), osteoarthritis (joint degeneration)
Genetic	Caused by abnormalities in genetic material. Genes are the cell's hereditary units found in cell nuclei; they are arranged in single file along chromosomes. Genetic diseases are passed from one generation to the next, which means they are inherited. Some result from mutation (either natural or induced).	Turner syndrome (1 of the 2 X chromosomes are absent or incomplete), Down syndrome (3 rather than the normal 2 copies of chromosome 21), hemophilia (mutation in a clotting factor gene), albinism (defect in the skin pigment gene)
Metabolic	Caused by abnormal metabolic processes and disruption of homeostasis. Can be congenital due to an inherited abnormality acquired from a preexisting disease, or failure of a metabolically important organ (i.e., pancreas, adrenals, liver)	Cushing disease (cortisol overproduction by the adrenals affecting protein, carbohydrate, and fat metabolism), diabetes mellitus (inability to produce and/or use insulin)
Infectious	Caused by disease-causing agents called pathogens. The most common pathogens are bacteria, fungi, protozoa, and viruses. Pathogenic animals such as parasites and prions can also cause disease.	Impetigo (bacterial infection), ringworm (fungal infection), malaria (protozoal infection), influenza (viral infection), lice (infestation), mad cow disease (prionic infection)

TABLE 9-2 Disease Causing Agents

PATHOGEN	DESCRIPTION	EXAMPLES OF INFECTIONS
Virus	Nonliving entities that can only replicate themselves within the cell of a living host. After viral replication, the host cell bursts. Each virus then travels and infects a new host cell.	Common cold, influenza, AIDS, herpes simplex, and viral hepatitis
Bacteria	Bacteria are unicellular microorganisms. Most are not pathogenic.	Boils, tuberculosis, Lyme disease, and strep throat
Fungi	Fungal agents include molds and yeast. Only a few varieties are pathogenic (*Candida albicans,* dermatophytes). Warm, moist environments promote their growth.	Ringworm, athlete's foot, jock itch, and thrush
Protozoa	Protozoa can only survive in a host organism.	Trichomoniasis, amoebic dysentery, African sleeping sickness, and malaria
Prions	Prions, or proteinaceous infectious particles, are involved in central nervous system diseases. Prion diseases are rare, currently untreatable, and fatal.	Bovine spongiform encephalopathy (mad cow disease) and Creutzfeldt-Jakob disease
Pathogenic animals	Pathogenic animals include parasites, which live in or on a host organism and rely on that host for nourishment.	Tapeworms, hookworms, lice, and scabies

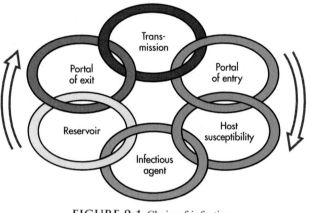

FIGURE 9-1 Chain of infection.

control includes breaking this chain and is discussed later in the chapter.

Pathogens

A *pathogen* is an infectious agent capable of causing disease. Bacteria and viruses are examples of pathogens. One way to acquire disease or infection is to be exposed to a pathogen.

As stated in Table 9-2, the pathogens are bacteria, fungi, protozoa, viruses, prions, and pathogenic animals. The last-named group causes infestation rather than infection. Toxic agents and plant resins may also cause disease such as in the case of poison oak, causing contact dermatitis. The resultant disease caused by pathogens is also called a communicable disease because it is contagious, some more so than others.

DISEASE TRANSMISSION

Disease transmission occurs when pathogens travel from a *reservoir* (source) to a *host* (destination). There are several modes of transmission. These include direct contact, vehicle and vector transmission, and inhalation of infected respiratory droplets. Effective exposure and successful transfer of pathogens result in a condition called *contamination*. The time between pathogen exposure to onset of signs and symptoms is the *incubation period*.

Direct Contact

The most common route of disease transmission is by direct contact. Spread can occur:
- **Person to person**. Pathogens pass from an infected person to an uninfected person by physical contact (including sexual contact) and through blood transfusions.
- **Animal to person**. This includes touching and a bite or scratch from an infected animal.
- **Mother to fetus**. Pathogens cross the placenta and can infect an unborn child.

Examples of diseases spread by direct contact are sexually transmitted infections, ringworm, herpes simplex, hepatitis B, and chickenpox.

Vehicle and Vector Transmission

Vehicle transmission occurs when infectious organisms are transmitted in or on a common vehicle or source such as food and water or objects such as computer keyboards or doorknobs. Such vehicles may include undercooked meats or food that has not been properly prepared or stored. Another example is not washing the hands after handling raw meat or after using the toilet while preparing or serving meals. Examples of diseases spread by vehicle transmission are *Salmonella*, gastroenteritis, and some cases of influenza.

Vector transmission involves stings or bites from insects and/or animals that act as intermediaries of disease exchange between two or more hosts. Examples of vector-borne diseases are malaria, Lyme disease, and Rocky Mountain spotted fever.

Respiratory Droplets

Infections can also spread through the air by infected respiratory droplets propelled by coughing or sneezing. The droplets are inhaled through the nose or mouth into the upper respiratory tract, where they can cause infections such as influenza or colds. They may also be absorbed into the lower respiratory tract, where they can cause infections such as pneumonia. Most respiratory diseases are spread by this method.

Infection

Infection is the period after disease transmission. During infection, pathogens use host resources to multiply (usually at the expense of the host). These processes, which include pathogenic growth and replication, interfere with the normal functioning of the host.

The ability of pathogens to cause disease depends on several factors, which include (1) number of pathogens that gain access; (2) areas of the body attacked; (3) the pathogen's ability to spread and replicate itself; and (4) the pathogen's resistance to host defenses. Thus a weak host with a strong pathogen results in disease; a strong host with a weak pathogen will overcome the infection and the introduction of disease.

HOST DEFENSES

A host has numerous ways to keep infection from progressing to disease. Collectively, these are referred to as *host defenses*. These defenses can be natural or acquired (see Chapter 27).

Natural defenses include barriers (e.g., intact skin and mucosa), chemicals (e.g., digestive enzymes, vaginal secretions), and reflexes (e.g., coughing, sneezing).

Infection also triggers an immune response, which stimulates production of specialized cells (e.g., lymphocytes, antibodies). These cells serve to immobilize and destroy pathogens. White blood cells, the body's mobile army, begin to multiply. Body temperate may elevate, resulting in fever. Another host defense is inflammation.

In most instances, these defenses are successful in keeping infection from either entering the body or invading into deeper tissues. However, if chronic stress, malnutrition, radiation, certain medications, or a preexisting illness (e.g., diabetes, AIDS) suppresses the person's immune system, then the person is increasingly susceptible to diseases.

Inflammation

Inflammation may occur during infection, but it also is part of the body's response to tissue damage after injury. The purpose of inflammation is to stabilize the injured area, contain infection, and initiate the healing process for damaged tissue. Inflammation can be localized or systemic; the latter often results in fever. Cardinal signs of inflammation are:

- Heat
- Redness
- Swelling
- Pain
- Loss of function (rarely seen unless inflammation is severe)

Inflammation is also discussed in Chapters 16 and 18.

CHAT ROOM

It is important to note that inflammation is not synonymous with infection.

Infection occurs when pathogens reside in or on the body. Inflammation is the body's response to a pathogen or tissue damage, such as a wound, burn, or from attack by the body's immune system as occurs in certain autoimmune diseases.

In cases of local infection or inflammation, avoid the affected area during massage. When infection or inflammation is more widespread or systemic, postpone massage until the condition has resolved.

CONTRAINDICATIONS

A **contraindication** is the presence of a disease or condition that makes it unsafe to treat a particular client in the usual manner. When you determine that a client has a contraindication (usually during the intake process, but this determination can also occur during the session), usually one of three things will happen:

1. Your client can receive massage, but an area of the body will be avoided.
2. Your client cannot receive massage that day.
3. Your client can receive massage with a few treatment modifications.

The first example represents a *local contraindication*, and the second example represents an *absolute contraindication*. Remember, when making treatment decisions, use the adages "Do no harm" and "When in doubt, don't." The third example, which involves treatment modifications, is discussed in detail later.

Local Contraindication

A **local contraindication** is one in which massage can be administered safely while avoiding an area of the body. Areas of local contraindication can be:

- Recently injured
- Inflamed
- Excessively tender when pressure is applied
- A lump, lesion, suspicious mole, or localized skin rash

Be sure to avoid enlarged lymph nodes. However, if you possess advanced certification in manual lymphatic drainage or lymphatic massage, your education has made you familiar with workable and non-workable conditions. Superficial lymph nodes are located in the groin (inguinal nodes), in the armpits (axillary nodes), and in the neck (cervical nodes). When palpated, enlarged lymph nodes feel hard, similar to a raw black-eyed pea under the skin.

Absolute Contraindication

Absolute contraindications occur when receiving massage might put you or your client at serious health risk or the client's condition could be made worse with massage. Examples are a:

- Reported disease that is highly contagious
- Client who has widespread infection or inflammation
- Client who has fever
- Chronic disease that is in exacerbation
- Client who is in a state of medical emergency

When a client presents with an absolute contraindication, massage is not advised. When the client's disease resolves, is in a state of remission, or is cleared by the physician who managed the medical emergency, the client can then receive massage.

Treatment Modifications

In many cases, all that is needed are a few adaptive measures or treatment modifications. The type and extent of disease, as well as the client's health status, determine modifications to treatment. More on treatment planning and medication use (e.g., pain killers, hypoglycemics) can be found in Chapter 10. Chapter 11 is devoted to treatment modification for special populations (e.g., elderly or pregnant client).

Most treatment modifications are either positional or procedural. Examples of *positional modifications* are (1) use of a seated or semireclining position, (2) avoidance of the prone position, and (3) placement of a supportive cushion under the right pelvis and trunk to tilt the lower body to the left in cases of advanced pregnancy.

Examples of *procedural* or *modifications of technique* are (1) use of lighter-than-normal pressure, (2) avoiding percussion or joint mobilizations, and (3) assisting the client off the massage table. The last modification may be needed if your client is taking blood pressure medication, is pregnant, or is elderly and frail.

CHAT ROOM

Chronic diseases often have stages of remission and exacerbation. During *remission*, signs and symptoms subside or disappear. Also called flare-ups or relapses, *exacerbation* ushers in an increase in sign and symptom severity. Example of diseases with remission and exacerbation are multiple sclerosis and rheumatoid arthritis. Be sure to postpone massage in cases of disease exacerbation.

"A musician must make music, an artist must paint, a poet must write, if he is to be ultimately at peace with himself."
—Abraham Maslow

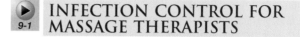

INFECTION CONTROL FOR MASSAGE THERAPISTS

As a massage therapist, you are at a slightly higher risk for contracting infection by direct contact or inhalation of infected respiratory droplets. Massage therapists who are hospital-based or who work with individuals who are sick or injured are at increased risk for contracting and spreading disease. Infection control decreases the risk of disease transmission in all settings.

So what are some ways infection can spread? You may unknowingly massage over an infectious rash in a treatment room with low lighting and spread the infection from one part of the client's body to another. Fluid from a boil may seep and enter broken skin. A client with a cold sore may touch the lip; then, after massaging your client's now infected hand, you may touch your own face. Additionally, infection can be spread through contact with contaminated linens, massage tools, and open containers of massage lubricant.

In December 1991, the Occupational Safety and Health Administration (OSHA) supported and helped pass federal legislation that requires all health care providers to adhere to a plan that helps prevent transmission of pathogens, namely human immunodeficiency virus (HIV), hepatitis B virus (HBV), and other blood-borne pathogens.

From this legislation, the Centers for Disease Control and Prevention (CDC) established *universal precautions*. Under universal precautions, blood and certain body fluids of all patients are considered potentially infectious.

In 1996, CDC published new guidelines for health care providers called *standard precautions*. These new guidelines expounded on original universal precautions, which dealt mainly with blood-borne pathogens. Standard precautions represent a wider range of infection control measures such as glove use when touching mucous membranes and guidelines for hand sanitation. Standard precautions for massage therapists include:

- Hand hygiene
- Using disposable gloves
- Laundering contaminated linens appropriately
- Disinfecting contaminated massage equipment and tools
- Dispensing uncontaminated massage lubricant
- Personal hygiene
- Maintaining a clean and sanitary office and treatment environment

In some circumstances, state law or employers require massage therapists to be immunized against diseases such as rubella, rubeola, diphtheria, tuberculosis, and hepatitis B. Some employers of massage therapists, such as hospitals, may highly recommend vaccinations but not require them.

The chain of infection can be broken by implementing procedures of sanitation. These practices aim to (1) remove the infectious agent (by hand hygiene, laundering of contaminated linens, and disinfecting contaminated surfaces); (2) create a barrier against entry (with glove use); and (3) prevent disease transmission (dispensing uncontaminated massage lubricant). Standard precautions also prevent *cross-contamination*, which is passing of pathogens from one source to another. In states where massage therapy is a licensed profession, infection control is mandatory.

Infection control, which protects both you and your client, starts with a little self-assessment and personal hygiene.

Hygiene

Hygiene is defined as collective principles of health preservation. Personal hygiene not only preserves health but also is part of infection control because it helps protect the public by reducing disease transmission. A list of tips has been compiled to aid you in practicing good hygiene. As you observe these hygiene tips, develop and maintain a respect for the diversity of different cultures found throughout the globe. Hygienic practices that are commonplace to some may be offensive to others. Apply these tips to your own situation, common sense, and knowledge of local customs. Good hygiene includes:

- Keep hair clean and off your face. Secure long hair so it does not accidentally touch your client while you are leaning over the table.
- Fingernails should be clean, short, and without colored polish. Be sure the polish is not chipped. The area between the chip and the nail can be a reservoir for infectious agents.
- Wear a clean garment each day. Clothing should not fit too loosely because it may brush against your client as you lean over the table. Sleeves should be short (midarm or higher).
- Avoid wearing wristwatches or ornate jewelry while massaging, especially rings. Ornate rings can harbor germs, potentially injure your client, or break the protective barrier of gloves.
- Bathe or shower daily. Use an antiperspirant or deodorant if necessary.
- Brush your teeth at least twice a day, and floss daily. Because massage requires close contact with clients, you may elect to use a mouthwash or avoid food that can cause an offensive odor.
- Shave or keep facial hair trimmed and groomed.
- If you perspire heavily while performing a massage, then wear sweatbands at the wrists and forehead to ensure that perspiration does not drip onto your client's skin. (Yes, this has happened to me when I was the client.)

 ## Standard Precautions

This section discusses guidelines and procedures of standard precautions. It includes how to disinfect contaminated linens and equipment surfaces, as well as massage tools. It also discusses ways to dispense uncontaminated lubricant. This list also contains a brief discussion on glove use and hand hygiene as aspects of standard precautions, then, later in the chapter, an entire section will be devoted to these important topics.

Use Clean Linens for Each Massage. This not only demonstrates your commitment to professionalism but also helps prevent the transfer of disease. Cover or drape everything that touches your client with clean linens. After the massage, launder linens before they are reused.

Massage linens include (1) top and bottom sheets, (2) bolster covers, (3) face rest covers, and (4) pillowcases.

If Massage Linens Become Contaminated. Be sure to follow the recommended procedure to disinfect linens when they become contaminated. Linens are contaminated if they contain any body fluid (e.g., blood, fluid from skin lesions, respiratory fluids, breast milk) or if they were in contact with a known or suspected infection source. Examples are cold sores, athlete's foot, and genital warts (even though the genitals remained draped during massage, if the client indicates there are lesions present and undergarments are not worn, treat linens as contaminated). The following is a recommended protocol. Note that the massage table fabric and accessory fabric are disinfected as well.

- Don a pair of disposable gloves.
- Remove linens with gloved hands.
- Wash linens in hot water; use laundry detergent and $\frac{1}{4}$ cup of household bleach. Dry linens using hot air.
- Discard the gloves and don a new pair of disposable gloves.
- Clean the massage table fabric and accessory fabric with soap and water, and then disinfect it with a 1 : 10 solution of household bleach and water.
- Discard the gloves and paper towels.
- Finally, wash and dry your hands.

If you are unable to immediately wash contaminated linens, place them in a container away from other linens. Wash these linens as soon as you can and be sure to wear gloves while handling before washing them. If you have to carry your linens back to your home or office to launder them, be sure you bag contaminated linens separately.

And remember to treat any substance that cannot be identified as unsafe.

If Massage Tools Become Contaminated. Contaminated massage tools, including massage stones, can be immersed for at least 10 minutes in a 1 : 10 solution of household bleach and water or a 1 : 7 solution of isopropyl alcohol and water. Some therapists surround their massage tools with plastic wrap before using and then discard the wrap afterward. Be sure to wash your hands after placing the massage tool in the solution or after discarding the plastic wrap.

CHAT ROOM

I have always been leery of massage tools made of porous materials such as wood and stone. After I made this comment in class, a student (who was a glass blower) later presented me with a glass massage tool she had made. It has three sides and fits in my hand nicely. And it is easy to disinfect. Thank you, Simone.

Avoid Using Open Containers of Lubricant. Dispensing massage lubricant from an open container contaminates the lubricant if the same container is used for multiple clients. This is an example of cross-contamination. To avoid this, use containers with a flip top or pump mechanism. If your lubricant is too thick to pump (e.g., butters), use a clean spatula or tongue depressor to remove enough lubricant for single-client use, and place it on a sanitary dish (I use the cleaned top of the lubricant jar). Also, placing your lubricant container on a dirty counter or floor or in an unclean holster may contaminate the container. As an extra safety measure, wash the lubricant container after each massage. Discard disposable single-use items properly.

Use Standard Hand Hygiene Procedures. Either wash and dry hands thoroughly or use an alcohol-based hand sanitizer before and after performing massage. Guidelines for hand hygiene are provided in the next section.

Use Disposable Gloves When Appropriate. Disposable gloves are to be worn (1) during the massage when you have an open wound on the hands, (2) when handling contaminated linens, (3) when in contact with mucous membranes such as in the mouth or nose. Disposable gloves are to be removed promptly after use and discarded, with hands resanitized. Guidelines for glove removal are found later in the chapter.

Do Not Perform Massage When Ill or When Experiencing Coldlike Symptoms. You may be the reservoir in the chain of infection (see Figure 9-1). Symptoms include sneezing, coughing, fever, or a runny nose. In these cases, canceling appointments or arranging for an associate to take your place is preferred.

Avoid Massaging Clients Who Are Ill. Your client may be the reservoir in the chain of infection. Postponing massage while your client is ill helps prevent disease transmission.

Maintain a Clean and Sanitary Office and Treatment Environment. This includes removing the trash from your office daily. Be sure all trash receptacles are lined with a disposable bag. Also, exterminate (and then dispose of) any insects or rodents on the premises because they can be a source of disease.

Avoid Working Under the Influence of Alcohol or Recreational Drugs. Making good judgments regarding infection control is difficult while under the influence of mood-altering substances.

Follow a Personal Health Plan and Get Regular Physical Examinations. As seen in the chain of infection, host susceptibility plays a part in infection control. The healthier you are, the more you will be able to overcome disease when exposed to infectious agents. Chapter 4 is devoted to self-care, which includes regular physical activity, proper nutrition, adequate rest, and stress reduction.

CHAT ROOM

If you happen to sneeze or cough while giving a massage, be sure do so into the crook of your elbow or sleeve if tissue is not readily available. Then excuse yourself and disinfect your hands with soap and water or with an alcohol-based hand sanitizer before resuming the massage. Be sure and tell your client what you are doing and why.

HAND HYGIENE

The number one source of disease transmission is contact with human hands. Cleaning your hands with soap and water or an alcohol-based hand sanitizer is the best measure to prevent infection. You must sanitize your hands before and after each massage, as well as during the session if deemed necessary.

So when, besides before and after massage, should hand hygiene occur? Hands should be sanitized:

- After using the toilet
- Before, during, and after food preparation
- Before eating
- Before inserting or removing contact lenses
- After touching animals or handling animal waste
- Before and after caring for or visiting someone who is ill
- Treating wounds
- Handling something that could be contaminated, such as a cleaning cloth or massage linens
- After sneezing or coughing

Next, let us look at two procedures for hand hygiene. Both are used by health care providers to ensure that appropriate steps have been taken to protect themselves and their clients.

Hand Washing

9-3 Washing hands with soap and water is one way to sanitize them. Liquid soap is preferred over bar soap because

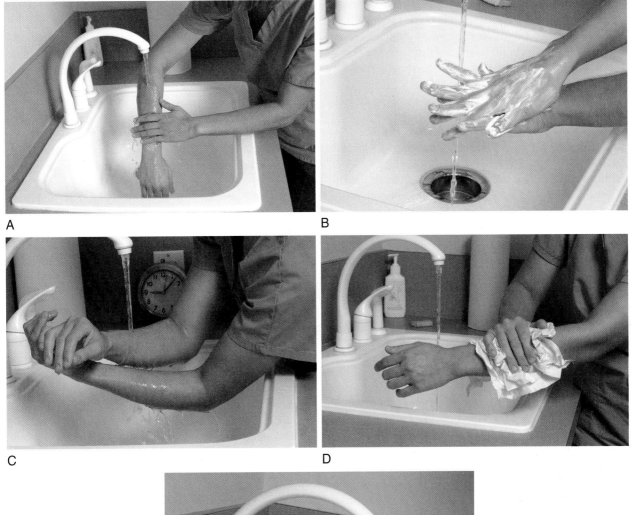

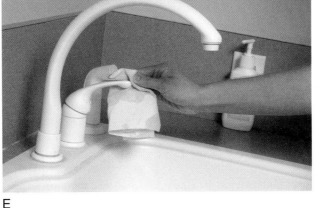

FIGURE 9-2 **Hand washing. A,** Wetting hands, forearms, and elbows. **B,** Soaping the hands. **C,** Rinsing. **D,** Drying the hands. **E,** Turning off the water.

the latter can be contaminated by vehicle transmission. Liquid dishwashing soap or baby wash can be used as an alternative to liquid hand soap. Also, antibacterial soap is no more effective at killing germs than regular soap. Using antibacterial soap may even lead to the development of bacteria resistant to the product's antimicrobial agents, making it more difficult for the product to kill germs on your skin in the future.

Six-Step Procedure

1. Wet hands, forearms, and elbows with warm, running water. Keep your hands lower than your elbows (Figure 9-2, *A*). This will prevent water, soil, and germs from running up the arms and onto garments.
2. Apply soap and generate lather. Then, using firm circular motions, rub the soap to lather your hands, forearms, and elbows briskly (Figure 9-2, *B*). Be sure to include the

backs of hands, wrists, between fingers, tips of fingers, and under fingernails (a nailbrush is best). Do this for at least 15 seconds.* Friction created by rubbing hands together is essential to lift germs and dirt from the skin's surface. These unwanted impurities become suspended in the lather, which will be rinsed away.

3. Rinse thoroughly until all lather is removed (Figure 9-2, *C*). Allow water to run from fingers to the elbows.
4. Using clean paper towels, pat dry the hands and forearms well (Figure 9-2, *D*). Rubbing can chap or irritate the skin.
5. Using the same paper towels, turn off the water valves (Figure 9-2, *E*). If washing hands before massage, then continue to use the same paper towels when touching door handles.
6. Discard the paper towels.

CHAT ROOM

Instead of counting to 15 while generating lather during hand washing, many therapists mentally sing the "Happy Birthday" song.

 ### Hand Sanitizer

Using foam or gel alcohol-based hand sanitizer is more effective and takes less time than hand washing with soap and water. Furthermore, hand sanitizer does not promote antimicrobial resistance if antibacterial soap is used, is less irritating to skin, and can be used when there is no access to running water. If your hands are visibly soiled, wash them with soap and water before applying hand sanitizer. To work effectively, alcohol content of the product should be between 60% and 70%.

Three-Step Procedure

1. Apply product to palm of one hand (exact amount will depend on type of product).
2. Rub hands together, covering all surfaces of hands, forearms, and elbows.
3. Continue rubbing until the product is absorbed (about 15 seconds).

You can also use a waterless hand sanitizer wipe. Be sure to follow the directions on the container.

⊖volve *Hand washing is an important aspect of the health care profession. Log on to the Evolve website and view the segment on proper hand washing. While you are there, watch the section on sanitation to review important guidelines for the massage therapist.* ■

---

*Increase the time from 15 seconds to 2 minutes if you have touched any known or suspected contaminate.

 # GLOVE USE

As stated previously, disposable gloves are to be worn (1) when handling contaminated linens; (2) when in contact with mucous membranes, such as in the mouth or nose; or (3) during the massage when you have an open wound on the hands. If the open wound is small and contained to one finger, a finger cot may be used over a bandage to keep the edges smooth.

When your are using gloves, your palpatory skills may be reduced until you become proficient at palpating through them.

Be sure to remove gloves promptly after use and discard, and to resanitize your hands before touching noncontaminated items and surfaces and before providing care to the same or another client.

The three most popular gloves used in the health care industry are latex, nitrile, and vinyl.

Latex Gloves

Latex material is thin and strong and conforms to your hands well when the correct size is selected. There are two possible disadvantages to latex: (1) Most massage lubricants are oil based and break down latex. If latex gloves are used, a water-based lubricant is needed. (2) Latex should be avoided if you or your client has latex allergies. Allergy symptoms can include rashes, itching, or, more seriously, respiratory difficulties.

Nitrile Gloves

Nitrile gloves are the most popular nonlatex glove used in the health care profession. These gloves can be used with oil-based lubricants and are almost as flexible as latex.

Vinyl Gloves

Vinyl is thicker than latex and nitrile, and does not have the same stretch capability; therefore vinyl gloves do not conform as well to your hands. But like nitrile glvoes, vinyl gloves can be used with oil-based lubricants. Vinyl gloves tend to be the most expensive.

Glove Removal

Care must be taken when removing and disposing of gloves to restrict contamination from the glove surface. One safe method of glove removal is as follows:

1. Peel the first glove from the cuff to fingers so that it is inside out (Figure 9-3, *A*).
2. Place the removed glove into the palm of the other hand (Figure 9-3, *B*).
3. Peel off the second glove from cuff to fingers so that the first glove is contained inside (Figure 9-3, *C*).
4. Discard the gloves (Figure 9-3, *D*).

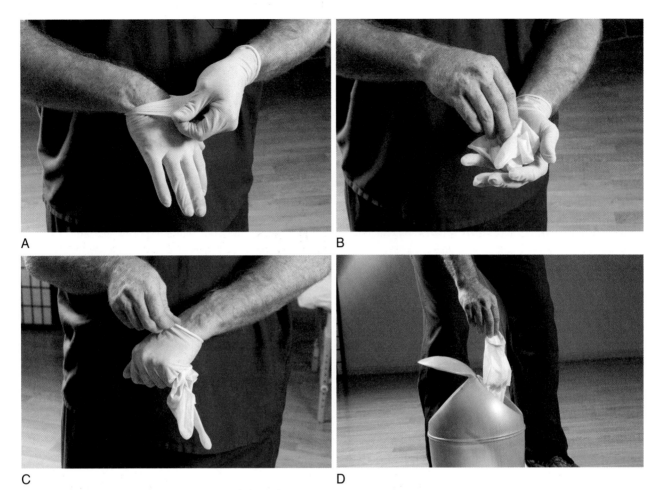

FIGURE 9-3 Glove removal. A, Pulling off one glove. **B,** Putting the removed glove in the palm of the gloved hand. **C,** Removing the other glove with the first removed glove inside. **D,** Disposal of the used gloves.

5. Wash and dry your hands immediately after glove removal.

"I happen to feel that the degree of a person's intelligence is directly reflected by the number of conflicting attitudes she can bring to bear on the same topic."
—Lisa Alter

EMERGENCY PREPAREDNESS

Not exactly infection control but an important aspect of being a health care provider is to know what to do in the event of medical emergency. Every therapist should obtain training in basic first aid and cardiopulmonary resuscitation (CPR). Agencies such as the American Red Cross and the American Heart Association offer training and certification programs in these areas. Also, keep a first aid kit on hand. These kits are inexpensive or can be assembled easily (Box 9-1). Be sure everyone in your office knows its location.

If you encounter an unconscious adult, try to rouse the person to consciousness before you call 911 because he may be just resting.

If you need to contact emergency services, use 911 emergency telephone systems. When the emergency dispatcher answers, begin with the following:
• What the emergency is
• Where the emergency happened

When stating where the emergency is happening, street addresses are preferred over name of an office building. If you are calling about a medical emergency, include the condition of the victim.

In this section, we will look at first aid measures for clients who are choking, who may be in insulin shock, experiencing a stroke or heart attack, or having a seizure. After the emergency has ended and your client has received proper medical care, be sure to take the time to write an incident report of the event. Look on Evolve for this and other important forms (see Chapter 2 Resources).

CHAT ROOM

Emergency preparedness also means having a fire evacuation plan and a designated safe area in which to retreat during events such as tornados or earthquakes.

DAVID LAUTERSTEIN

Born: December 4, 1947

"It is not the educational intention but the meeting which is educationally fruitful."
—Martin Buber

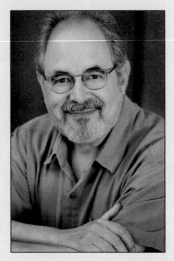

David Lauterstein entered the world surrounded by art, science, and a commitment to social justice. His father was a dentist, writer, and visual artist; his mother a homemaker and pianist. Both parents were social activists in Chicago, paving the way for David's involvement in the peace movement and his work to end segregation. With great enthusiasm for music and poetry, David began playing guitar at 13, meeting and learning from many of the great folk and rock talents of the 1960s: Michael Bloomfield, Fleming Brown, Big Joe Williams, Muddy Waters, Otis Spann, and Bob Dylan.

But it was while studying with the German composer Wolf Rosenberg that David began to question the absence of body awareness, emotion, and spirit in his exclusively intellectual education. He turned to Gestalt psychotherapy and yoga to reconnect his mind and body. Following a series of Rolfing and other forms of bodywork, David began to truly understand that the body is a source of profound wisdom, deep feeling, and heightened energy. In the mid-1970s he began a study group with Rolfers, massage therapists, martial artists, and psychotherapists to explore the frontiers of body, mind, and spirit.

Shortly thereafter he began to practice massage therapy and found that he was being as creative as he had been as a composer, but in a much more profound medium and with an incredible instrument—the human body, mind, and spirit. In 1979 David entered the training course at the Bodymind Center, which later became the Chicago School of Massage Therapy. In 1983 he completed advanced studies with Daniel Blake, one of the first Rolfers to look beyond fascial binding to include postural kinesiology and the role of chronically contracted muscles in postural and movement distortions.

BOX 9-1

First Aid Kit

It is advisable for the therapist to have a first aid kit available for minor emergencies. A preassembled one can be purchased or you can assemble your own. A simple kit could include adhesive bandages and antiseptic solution such as isopropyl alcohol. More complex kits could include some or all of the following:

- A first aid manual
- Sterile gauze
- Adhesive tape
- Adhesive bandages in several sizes
- Elastic bandage
- Antiseptic wipes
- Liquid soap
- Antibiotic cream
- Hydrocortisone cream (1%)
- Antiseptic solution (such as isopropyl alcohol or hydrogen peroxide) or alcohol wipes
- Acetaminophen and ibuprofen
- Tweezers
- Sharp scissors
- Safety pins
- Disposable instant cold packs
- Calamine lotion
- Disposable gloves (at least two pairs)

Additionally, it is highly recommended that massage therapists become trained or certified in first aid and CPR, and to maintain certification. In some municipalities, this may be a requirement for licensure.

Adapted from Holland PM, Anderson SK: *Chair massage*, St Louis, 2010, Mosby.

DAVID LAUTERSTEIN (*continued*)

David became an instructor at the Chicago School of Massage Therapy, and began presenting his signature workshops entitled "Deep Massage: The Lauterstein Method." In 1984 he wrote the book, *Putting the Soul Back in the Body: A Manual of Imaginative Anatomy for Massage Therapists*. While studying Zero Balancing with its founder Dr. Fritz Smith, he developed the vocabulary to best articulate in his teaching, and a methodology to best demonstrate in his touch, the way to simultaneously and consciously optimize one's contact with both energy and structure. He refers to his subject of instruction as "deep massage" rather than "deep tissue" to underscore the holistic practice of treating more than just the injured tissues.

David met John Conway while serving as the Dean of Faculty at the Texas School of Massage Studies. The two later partnered to open The Lauterstein-Conway Massage School. Believing strongly in the holistic art and science of massage, they embarked upon the mission "to run the school in a manner as healing as the subjects we teach."

In his series "The Seven Dimensions of Touch," David outlines core aspects of powerful healing: contact, movement, breath, graceful verticality, heart, mind, and alchemy. The modalities we practice do not embody healing power. That power is found in the body, mind,

and spirit of the practitioner and the receiver. When love is present, the body is more likely to heal. The techniques of the massage therapist create meaning in the human body—"every stroke sends a message."

The fourth dimension of touch, graceful verticality, is created by the structural and energetic aspect of posture, while the heart mediates our healthy movement between our protection and intimacy. With the mind we understand the health history, the postural deviations, and their potential causes, although this understanding is never attained in the mind alone. And alchemy is the positive transformation that the client experiences through the therapist's truly meeting the client with their whole self.

Music never stopped being an integral part of David's life. When scheduling teaching engagements, David requests that the host provide an acoustic guitar. "Playing the guitar softens the heart, quiets the mind, and very quickly puts the students in a place where learning is easier and goes quickly to a greater depth, therefore it is more memorable." In 2009 he recorded his first CD in an innovative context. David arranged to have three therapists perform massage in the recording studio while he played acoustic guitar in accompaniment to their sessions. This resulted in "Roots and Branches," his first CD recorded live to massage.

Choking

Choking occurs when the trachea is blocked and the affected person cannot breathe. Choking may occur when a person is talking while eating and inhales at the same time as swallowing. In massage, choking is more likely when your client has a mint or piece of gum in the mouth while he or she is lying supine and tries to speak.

First Aid Measures

If your client is choking, he or she appears distressed, grasps the throat, and cannot inhale or exhale. When this occurs, help him or her to sit upright and encourage coughing.

If the person cannot cough or speak, use the Heimlich maneuver, also called abdominal thrusts, to open an suddenly obstructed trachea (Figure 9-4).

1. From behind, wrap your arms around the victim's waist.
2. If the person is standing, put your leg between the victim's legs to prevent the victim from falling should he or she become unconscious.

3. Make a fist and place the thumb side of your fist against the victim's upper abdomen, below the rib cage and above the navel.
4. Grasp your fist with your other hand and press into victim's upper abdomen with a quick upward thrust. Do not squeeze the rib cage; confine the force of the thrust to your hands.
5. Repeat until object is expelled.

If you cannot reach around the victim:
1. Place the victim on back.
2. Facing the victim, kneel astride the victim's hips.
3. With one of your hands on top of the other, place the heel of your bottom hand on the upper abdomen below the rib cage and above the navel.
4. Use your body weight to press into the victim's upper abdomen with a quick upward thrust.
5. Repeat until object is expelled.

If the victim becomes unconscious, call 911 immediately.

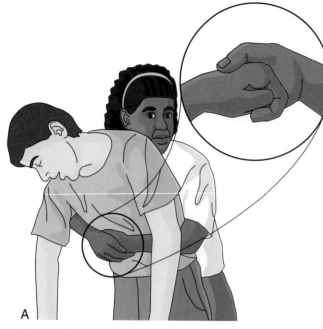

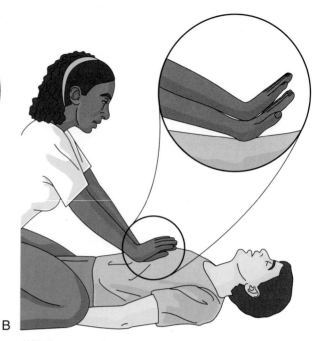

A

With the conscious victim standing or sitting, place your fist between the victim's lower rib cage and navel. Wrap the palm of your hand around your fist. A quick inward, upward thrust expels the air remaining in the victim's lungs, and with it the foreign body. If the first thrust is unsuccessful, repeat several thrusts in rapid succession until the foreign body is expelled or until the victim loses consciousness.

B

With the unconscious victim lying supine, straddle the victim's thighs. Place one hand on top of the other as shown, with the heel of the bottom hand just above the victim's navel. Quickly thrust inward and upward, toward the victim's head.

FIGURE 9-4 Heimlich maneuver performed while choking victim is standing or sitting (**A**) or is lying supine (**B**).

Hypoglycemia and Insulin Shock

Hypoglycemia is low blood sugar. This condition may occur in clients who have diabetes mellitus. Hypoglycemia is more common in diabetes mellitus type 1 but can also occur in type 2.

Your diabetic client may become hypoglycemic by consuming a smaller-than-usual meal, or by delaying or missing meals. It can also be from an increase in physical activity over the client's norm or by taking too much medicine (i.e., insulin or certain diabetes pills). Some signs and symptoms of hypoglycemia are:

- Mental confusion, disorientation, and slurred speech; the person may appear intoxicated
- Visual disturbances
- Sweaty, cool, pale skin
- Tremors or shaking
- Irritability or fatigue
- Seizures and loss of consciousness, though uncommon

If left untreated, hypoglycemia can develop into a medical emergency called *insulin shock* (insulin reaction), which may lead to coma and death.

First Aid Measures

What do you do if suspect that your diabetic client has hypoglycemia? If he or she is conscious and coherent:

1. Give sweet food or beverage such as sugar cubes, cake frosting dispensed in a tube, 4 oz of orange juice, or 6 oz of regular, not diet, soda.
2. Repeat this step after 10 minutes if your client does not claim to feel better
3. When the client feels better, offer a snack that includes carbohydrates and protein, such as about six crackers with cheese or peanut butter.

If the client becomes unconscious or if giving anything by mouth is unsafe, call 911.

Stroke

A *stroke*, also called a *cerebrovascular accident* or *brain attack*, is a sudden disruption in blood flow to the brain caused from blood clot or hemorrhage from a broken blood vessel. The sequelae depend on the location and extent of ischemia.

The acute care principle is *time is brain*. Because strokes require immediate medical attention, it is important to know the signs of stroke, which are:

- Sudden or transient weakness, numbness, or tingling in the face, an arm or leg, or on one side of the body
- Temporary loss of speech, failure to comprehend, or confusion
- Sudden loss of vision

- Sudden severe headache
- Unusual dizziness or loss of balance

First Aid Measures

Call emergency medical services (EMS) by dialing 911.

Heart Attack

Heart attack, also called a *myocardial infarction* (MI), is death of heart muscle from interrupted blood supply. MIs are usually caused by occluded coronary arteries as a result of (1) blood clots that have developed in coronary arteries from a disease process, such as atherosclerosis or (2) floating blood clots (emboli) that become lodged in coronary arteries. The tissue supplied by the occluded artery is often destroyed by infarction.

The acute care principle is *time is muscle* —heart muscle, in this case. Some signs of heart attack are:

- Chest pain, which may be described as crushing, burning, viselike, heaviness, or fullness (this pain is not relieved by rest or nitroglycerin)
- Discomfort in other areas of the upper body such as the left arm, shoulder, neck, or jaw
- Shortness of breath, profuse sweating, fatigue, or dizziness
- Nausea and indigestion (more common in women)
- Anxiety or fear

First Aid Measures

If your client complains of chest pain that lasts more than a few minutes, especially with the other signs listed above:

1. Call EMS by dialing 911.
2. If the client becomes unresponsive before emergency medical services (EMS) arrives, he or she may be in cardiac arrest, which means the heart has stopped beating.
3. Begin CPR if you are qualified to do so.

When EMS arrives, give any information regarding the incident, including any medications, such as nitroglycerin, that your client took before EMS arrival.

Seizures

Seizure disorders are characterized by explosive episodes of uncontrolled and excessive electrical activity in the brain. This activity results in a sudden change in behavior called a *seizure*. A seizure may be subtle and consist of abnormal sensations, or it may produce overt involuntary repetitive movements and loss of consciousness. Once a seizure begins, it cannot be stopped. Seizures can be triggered by physical stimuli, loud noises, bright lights, or stress.

The two main types of seizures are partial and generalized. One type of generalized seizure is called tonic-clonic (previously called a grand mal seizure). These are the most intense type of seizures and produce an intermittent contract-relax pattern in muscles called a convulsion. These are often preceded by peculiar visual or auditory sensations, called auras, minutes before a convulsion. There are often two phases of a tonic-clonic seizure, the tonic phase and the clonic phase.

- During the tonic phase, general tone increases and muscular contraction begins. A cry may be heard as abdominal and thoracic muscles contract, forcing air out of the lungs. This phase lasts approximately 10 seconds.
- The clonic phase is the classic presentation of alternating contraction and relaxation of muscles. These contractions gradually subside in several minutes; the person is then confused, weak, and drowsy, and has no memory of the event.

Your client with a seizure disorder is more likely to have a seizure if he or she has stopped taking his or her prescribed medications.

First Aid Measures

If your client appears to be having a seizure, follow these basic first aid measures. Every situation will be different.

1. Remain calm and begin to time the seizure.
2. Clear the area of objects (if possible).
3. Gently place the person on the floor (if possible).
4. Place a cushion or soft material, like a jacket, under the person's head. Lift the chin slightly to open the airway.
5. If the person is choking or vomiting, roll him or her onto the side.
6. Remain with the person until the seizure has ended.

After a seizure, several things can be expected to happen. The person may be groggy or feel very tired. The person could be confused, disoriented, or even embarrassed. The person may also complain of a headache or general soreness.

If the seizure lasts more than 5 minutes or immediately repeats, call EMS by dailing 911, and then:

1. Roll the person onto his or her side and speak calmly until EMS arrives.
2. Inform EMS how long the seizure has lasted and the symptoms exhibited.

E-RESOURCES

⊕volve

http://evolve.elsevier.com/Salvo/MassageTherapy

- Chapter challenge
- Flash cards
- Photo gallery
- Educational animations
- Technique videos
- Additional information
- Webquest
- Weblinks

▶ **DVD**

- 9-1: Infection control for massage therapists
- 9-2: Standard precautions

- 9-3: Hand washing
- 9-4: Hand sanitizers
- 9-5: Glove use

These videos can also be viewed on the Evolve website.

BIBLIOGRAPHY

Applegate EJ: *The anatomy and physiology learning system*, ed 4, Philadelphia, 2010, WB Saunders.

Damjanov I: *Pathophysiology for the health-related professions*, ed 3, Philadelphia, 2006, WB Saunders.

Frazier MS, Drzymkowski JW: *Essentials of human diseases and conditions*, ed 3, Philadelphia, 2004, Saunders.

Fritz S: *Essential sciences for therapeutic massage*, ed 3, St Louis, 2009, Mosby.

Fritz S: *Massage online for essential sciences for therapeutic massage*, ed 3, St Louis, 2011, Mosby.

Gould BE: *Pathophysiology for the health professions*, ed 3, Philadelphia, 2006, Saunders.

The Heimlich Institute: *How to do the Heimlich maneuver* (website): http://www.heimlichinstitute.org/page.php?id=34. Accessed March 12, 2010.

Holland PM, Anderson SK: *Chair massage*, St Louis, 2010, Mosby.

Jacob S, Francone C: *Elements of anatomy and physiology*, Philadelphia, 1989, Saunders.

Jones NL: *The Americans with Disabilities Act: overview, regulations, and interpretations*, Hauppauge, NY, 2003, Novinka Books.

Larson E, Mayur T, Laughon BA: Influence of two hand washing frequencies on reduction in colonizing flora with three products used by health care personnel, *Am J Infect Control* 23:17, 1989.

Louisiana State Department of Social Services: *Uniform federal accessibility standards accessibility checklist*, Baton Rouge, LA, 1995, United States Architectural and Transportation Barriers Compliance Board.

Ogg S: Personal communication, 1997.

Perry AG: *Clinical nursing skills & techniques*, ed 6, St Louis, 2009, Mosby.

Pliszka M: The truth about antibacterial soaps, *Twins Mag*, Jan/Feb:38-39, 2006.

Salvo SG: *Mosby's pathology for massage therapists*, ed 2, St Louis, 2009, Mosby.

Smith DG: *The challenge of diversity: involvement or alienation in the academy. Report No. 5*, Washington, DC, 1989, School of Education and Human Development, George Washington University.

Thibodeau G, Patton K: *Anatomy and physiology*, ed 6, St Louis, 2006, Mosby.

Thibodeau G, Patton K: *Structure and function of the body*, ed 12, St Louis, 2004, Mosby.

Torres LS: *Basic medical techniques and patient care for radiologic technologies*, Philadelphia, 1993, JB Lippincott.

Tortora GJ: *Introduction to the human body: the essentials of anatomy and physiology*, ed 5, Hoboken, NJ, 2000, John Wiley & Sons.

U.S. Department of Justice. *Americans with Disabilities Act* (website): http://www.usdoj.gov/crt/ada/adahom1.htm. Accessed October 21, 2009.

U.S. Department of Labor. Office of Disability Employment Policy (website): http://www.dol.gov/odep/. Accessed October 21, 2009.

Williams A, editor: *Teaching massage: foundation principles in adult education for massage program instructors*, Philadelphia, 2008, Lippincott Williams & Wilkins.

MATCHING I

Place the letter of the answer next to the term or phrase that best describes it.

A. Absolute
B. Chemical
C. Contamination
D. Contraindication
E. Exacerbation
F. Incubation period
G. Inflammation
H. Local
I. Pathogen
J. Reservoir
K. Standard precautions
L. Virus

_____ 1. Nonliving entity that requires a living host cell for replication

_____ 2. Digestive enzymes are examples of this type of barrier against disease

_____ 3. Type of contraindication in which massage can be administered safely while avoiding a certain area of the body

_____ 4. Infectious agent capable of causing disease

_____ 5. Type of contraindication in which massage is postponed because receiving massage might put the therapist or client at serious health risk or the client's condition could be made worse with massage

_____ 6. Wide range of infection control measures such as hand hygiene, use of disposable gloves, and correct laundering of contaminated linens

_____ 7. Term for successful transfer of pathogens

_____ 8. Characterized by heat, redness, swelling, and pain

_____ 9. State of a chronic disease in which massage is an absolute contraindication

_____ 10. In disease transmission, the term used to describe the source of infection

_____ 11. Presence of a disease or condition that makes it unsafe to treat a particular client in the usual manner

_____ 12. Time between exposure to a pathogen and onset of signs and symptoms

MATCHING II

Place the letter of the answer next to the term or phrase that best describes it.

A. Bleach
B. Disposable gloves
C. Fifteen
D. Five

E. Heart attack
F. Heimlich
G. Human hands
H. Hypoglycemia

I. Open
J. Stroke
K. Ten
L. Visibly soiled

_____ 1. Dispensing massage lubricant from this type of container contaminates the lubricant if the same container is used for multiple clients.

_____ 2. Number one source of disease transmission is contact with this structure

_____ 3. Number of seconds soap lather should be rubbed into your hands, forearms, and elbows during hand washing

_____ 4. Number of minutes to immerse contaminated massage tools in a 1:10 solution of household bleach and water or a 1:7 solution of isopropyl alcohol to disinfect them

_____ 5. Condition for which a diabetic client would need sweet food or beverage

_____ 6. 1/4 cup of this substance should be included in the wash water when washing contaminated linens

_____ 7. A seizure lasting more than this number of minutes means you should call 911

_____ 8. Maneuver that may serve to open an obstructed trachea if your client is choking and cannot cough or speak

_____ 9. Acute care principle for persons experiencing this medical emergency is _time is muscle_

_____ 10. Waterless hand sanitizer alone should be avoided if hands have this appearance

_____ 11. Worn while cleaning contaminated massage table fabric or handling contaminated linens

_____ 12. Acute care principle for persons experiencing this medical emergency is _time is brain_

CASE STUDY

Seize the Day

Moxie is a middle-aged African-American female who recently had her second child. While in her early twenties, she began having anxiety attacks with occasional mild seizures. Her physician prescribed medication to control her seizures. While she was pregnant, she discontinued the medication as directed by her obstetrician. Her doctor told her to remain off the medication until she stopped nursing as the medication is excreted in her milk.

Many of Moxie's pregnancy-related discomforts were alleviated with massage. Her loving husband frequently bought her massage gift certificates to a local therapist, Chantell. Moxie received a massage at least twice a month. She had a standing appointment with Chantell: 2 PM every other Tuesday. A neighbor cared for Moxie's 2-month-old infant so she could get away and relax. The demands of a new infant on top of caring for a 2-year-old child and a new home were beginning to take their toll on Moxie. She tried hard to get the nourishment her body needed, but it was not easy.

Moxie was on time for her 2:00 appointment. She entered the massage room and began to prepare herself for the session. She felt unusually

CASE STUDY—cont'd

tired and thought, "Timing for this massage is perfect! I really need a break." She pulled the sheet over as she lay down on her back and closed her eyes.

Chantell entered the room and asked Moxie a few health-related questions. Moxie replied in single syllables. After about 5 minutes, Chantell asked Moxie to comment on the pressure. Moxie did not answer. Chantell asked again. She looked down at Moxie and saw that her eyes were moving rapidly under her closed lids. Because Chantell had done an in-depth client intake, she knew about Moxie's history of seizures. Not ever seeing one in the past, Chantell assumed that Moxie was experiencing a seizure.

Chantell immediately discontinued the massage, anchored her leg to the tableside nearest her, and waited for the seizure to pass. While in school, Chantell was taught to place pillows around the massage table, but doing that meant she had to leave Moxie's side. What if Moxie fell onto the floor while Chantell was gathering pillows? There were only two pillows in the massage room; two pillows are not enough. Where should they be placed on the floor? The reality of the situation was very different from what she expected.

If you were Chantell, how would you handle the seizure incident?

Once the seizure has passed, how would Chantell explain the incident to Moxie?

If you were Moxie, how might you feel coming out of the seizure?

If Moxie's seizure had been physical, how might Chantell respond?

If Chantell had called emergency services and an ambulance had been dispatched, what would have happened if Moxie did not want to be treated once they arrived?

CRITICAL THINKING

Why is it important for massage therapists to understand how diseases can be transmitted?

CHAPTER 10

"You know the rule: If you are falling, dive. Do the thing that has to be done."
—Joseph Campbell

Treatment Planning: Intake, Assessment, and Documentation

LEARNING OBJECTIVES

After completing this chapter, the student should be able to:

- Define and state the value of documentation.
- Outline aspects of the Health Insurance Portability and Accountability Act that are significant in a massage therapy practice.
- Compare and contrast different documentation formats.
- Contrast and compare subjective and objective information.
- Define scope of practice, outlining what is commonly in and what is commonly out of a massage therapist's scope.
- Discuss informed consent, identifying important elements of the process and the document.
- Define treatment planning, identifying important elements of the process and the plan document.
- Outline important features of a client intake.
- State the importance of client communication.
- Give examples of nonverbal communication.
- List important skills used during the client interview.
- Compare and contrast open- and closed-ended questions.
- Describe and give examples of information gathered using PPALM assessment domains.
- Compare and contrast medical referral and medical clearance.
- Discuss the importance of palpation as an assessment tool.
- Formulate a plan of care.
- List protocols used after the massage and during subsequent sessions.
- Discuss networking with health care providers, including the role of prescriptions, referral forms, and medical release forms.

http://evolve.elsevier.com/Salvo/MassageTherapy

INTRODUCTION

Time spent with each client is limited and structured. Within this time frame, you decide which activities will occur for the massage to have a safe and satisfactory outcome for the client. Before the massage begins, decisions are made about how time will be spent, which may based upon:

- Information gathered on a completed client intake form or furnished by the client's primary health care provider and primary caregivers (if applicable)
- Goals stated by the client during an interview
- The client's personal time and financial restraints, or parameters set by third party payers such as insurance companies
- Relevant assessments performed by the therapist
- The therapist's training and experience
- The scope of practice as defined by the state or municipality where services are provided

This chapter examines the process of collecting client information, performing basic client assessments, and developing an individualized treatment plan. This plan serves as an organizational framework of care for a particular client on a particular day. Because this process includes dialogue that takes place in an interview, treatment planning also enhances rapport and trust between the client and the therapist, forming the foundation of a positive and cooperative therapeutic relationship (see Chapter 2). This process is documented, which reflects our quality of care and professionalism.

Documentation is the process of providing written information regarding client care. A massage therapist needs to collect and document client information for many reasons (as described in the next section on documentation). Proper documentation helps the therapist ascertain the client's therapeutic goals and to create a holistic picture of the client's health, both past and present. This information forms the basis for planning individual sessions and future sessions, also known as the *treatment plan* or *plan of care*. So the treatment plan is essentially the therapist's strategy used to help the client achieve his or her therapeutic goals. The plan also takes into account any precautions or contraindications based on the client's health. A treatment plan is formulated before each massage begins.

One of the most valuable skills a therapist can acquire is effective communication, which includes verbal and nonverbal forms. Through effective communication, you will be able to properly gather and synthesize all client information (Figure 10-1). This is a cooperative process revolving around the client's needs and is demonstrated during formation, evaluation, and modification of the treatment plan.

The chapter also features methods to organize your client interview using assessment domains. This information is essential when developing a treatment plan. **Assessment** is the process involved in evaluating or appraising a client's condition based on subjective reporting and objective findings.

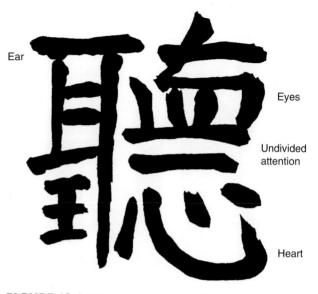

FIGURE 10-1 Chinese calligraphy depicting communication.

Experience is the best teacher. By palpating, questioning, listening, and treating, the massage therapist develops a sense of what is familiar. This, in turn, breeds knowledge, enhances skill, and promotes confidence. With practice, the intake, assessment, and documentation will flow effortlessly.

 ## DOCUMENTATION

As stated in the introduction, **documentation** is the process of providing written information regarding client care. The primary reason is to gather information and then develop a treatment plan that seeks to fulfill client therapeutic goals. There are many other reasons why documentation is part of our professional activities.

Documentation is a vital tool for communicating with other health care providers about client care. The written word is the communication of choice in all professional arenas. Guidelines for sharing this information between your office and another health care provider as outlined in the Health Insurance Portability and Accountability Act (HIPAA) are provided in Box 10-1. Consult with your state board to find if massage therapists in your state must be HIPAA-compliant.

Next, systematically collecting and documenting client information sharpens the therapist's critical thinking skills. Through the written record, the therapist can confirm his or her educated assessments, choice of methods or techniques, decisions to avoid or focus on an area, and pressure judgments. Alterations are made on the basis of client preference and response.

Another reason for documentation is that client records are legal evidence, which serves to protect the therapist by establishing professional accountability. Written communication decreases liability risks by verifying the information your client has shared with you and supports the treatment that the client received. Adequate and accurate

BOX 10-1

Health Insurance Portability and Accountability Act (HIPAA): Guidelines for Massage Therapist

- Obtain a signed consent form from each client.
- Obtain a signed medical release form from the client before any information about your client is disclosed to a third party.
- Do not disclose any information regarding clients to individuals in your office.
- Protect electronic client files by assigning passwords to anyone who has access to them. Computers that are connected electronically to the Internet must be fitted with a firewall to protect information from hackers.
- Obtain client authorization before dispensing any marketing material such as newsletters, facsimile referrals, greeting cards, or e-mail.
- Place confidentiality notices on all facsimiles and e-mails.
- Store client files in a locked fireproof cabinet and restrict access.
- Create a client information sheet outlining how you intend to use the information obtained from the client, how this information will be maintained and stored, and under what circumstances this information will be disclosed, as well as how the therapist will obtain permission for such incidents, how copies can be obtained by the client of his or her files, how long these files will be kept once the client is released, and how these records will be destroyed. Give a copy of this document to each client. Go over each item with the client, asking him or her to sign and date a separate statement that he or she received the *Notice of Privacy Policies*.
- Keep the appointment book and all client files out of view.
- When talking on the telephone, do not use the caller's name if others who might overhear are in the room.
- If you have a computer in your office, make sure the screen is out of view or shows a screen saver when clients or unauthorized individuals are nearby.

BOX 10-2

Tips for Documenting

Here are some suggestions for documenting client information on the intake form, treatment plan, and other client documents. Most suggestions apply to handwritten rather than electronic documentation.

- Use blue ink color. Currently, blue is the preferred ink color for documentation of client records because it differentiates an original from a facsimile or a photocopy. More important is that the color ink be consistent from initial treatment until release. Changing from blue to black then back to blue may cause a record to be thrown out of a court proceeding because it might appear as though the other colors were added as an afterthought instead of as part of the original treatment documentation.
- Write legibly. Documentation that cannot be read is worthless.
- Correct errors with a single line through the writing and your initials, avoiding correction fluid and tape.
- Use precise and correct medical terminology. Be careful of intangible words such as *energy* or *energy work*. For a medical record or a chart that will be read by someone working for an insurance company, using words that describe exact anatomy, physiologic response, or specific technique is best.
- Use sentence fragments to highlight the information gained from the client, as well as objective assessments, but be sure the fragment makes sense to the reader.
- Use direct quotes stated by the client when applicable.
- Be careful with abbreviations and use of symbols. Remember, one reason to document is that this information may be shared with others. *SOB* might offend someone, even though it often means *shortness of breath*.
- If a client misses an appointment, document this event with an entry indicating *no show* or *canceled, no reschedule*.
- Keep in mind the scope of practice. You can make observations of a client, but you cannot diagnose a condition. For example, *anxiety* is a medical diagnosis. You can, however, report when the client says, "I feel stressed out."

documentation also helps in supporting payment reimbursement, improving the quality of client care, and it demonstrates to the public that the therapist followed accepted standards of care. In all professional arenas, "If it isn't documented, it didn't happen" (Box 10-2).

Furthermore, many state licensing boards are mandating systematic collection and ongoing documentation, which may be used in peer review, licensing determinations, and other legal proceedings.

Finally, relying on memory is poor record keeping. Written or electronic records serve to jog memory and to outline particular details for review; the more detailed and specific client notes are, the more accurate the assessment and planning will be (Box 10-3). If written information is recorded, or documented, the therapist can reread it when needed.

CHAT ROOM

Minimum paperwork most often consists of a (1) health history or an intake form, a (2) consent form, and a (3) treatment plan using a method of data collection (PPALM, SOAP, CARE, APIE).

Documentation Formats

Client information must be organized. Currently, the two most popular formats are the SOAP note and the APIE note. Two other formats are CARE and PPALM notes. The notation form used will depend on which system is in place where you are employed or on your personal preference.

SOAP notes are the probably the most widely used and most complex documentation format. They are used chiefly by the medical community, perhaps because their complexity makes them a good fit for a large team of health care providers to keep track of orders, procedures, surgeries, prescriptions, and allergies. Massage therapy is often a more simple form of health care with considerably fewer variables than physical or occupational therapy. Thus it is easy to see that a less complex form of documentation is a better fit for our needs. This chapter emphasizes PPALM as a documentation format because its assessment domains are relevant to massage treatment planning.

Let us take a brief look at other formats.

SOAP. SOAP stands for:
S: subjective
O: objective
A: assessment
P: plan

In the initial SOAP note, the *subjective* section contains the client's experience of his or her condition, including symptoms, when and how the condition started, what makes it better or worse, what has been done about it until now, and the results. In future sessions, the *S* section will state the client's updated, current experience of his or her condition, including impressions or responses to the previous session.

The *objective* section contains the therapist's visual and palpatory findings, as well as the results of any examinations or tests.

If you are working under prescriptive directives or billing insurance, all subjective and objective data must directly correspond to the physician's diagnosis.

In the initial SOAP note, the *assessment* section outlines the physician's diagnosis of the client's condition. In future sessions, the *A* section will contain therapist notes of what was done for that session.

The *plan* portion in the initial SOAP note contains the treatment plan as directed by the physician, including the type, duration, and expected outcome or results. In future sessions, the *P* section will outline methods and techniques used and any suggested home activites such as stretching or stress reduction.

One criticism of this format is that it lacks flexibility and often focuses on one problem only. In addition, within massage journals and textbooks, no consistency exists as to what *A* or *P* means or what information is placed in the *A* or the *P* section of the format. For example, *A* might mean application, activity, or even analysis; *P* might mean procedure (past or present) or planning (future tense). For this reason, always include a legend on the documentation form.

Another variation of the SOAP note is the SOAPIER note. This abbreviation stands for subjective, objective, assessment plan, implementation, evaluation, and review. SOAP notes are discussed in the Appendix.

APIE. APIE stands for:
A: assessment
P: plan
I: implementation
E: evaluation

The *assessment* section contains subjective data and objective data, as well as the physician's diagnosis. Assessment addresses pretreatment conclusions.

The *plan* (treatment plan) portion states what should be done today and in the near future. This section is written before the massage.

The *implementation* section contains the methods and techniques used during that day's session. This section is written after the massage.

Finally, the *evaluation* section is the therapist's determination of treatment outcome to date. Evaluation addresses posttreatment conclusions.

CARE. CARE stands for:
C: condition of client
A: action taken
R: response of client
E: evaluation

CARE notes are completed after the session and document what was done (therapist *action*), why it was done (client *condition*), and how the client *responded* to the session. The fourth element, E or *evaluation*, is optional and is used to document observations, recommendations, or questions that arise from the session.

Subjective Versus Objective

During the assessment process, the massage therapist collects subjective and objective information and combines these findings to formulate the treatment plan. In SOAP notes, this information is separated. In all other documenting formats, this information is combined.

Subjective data consist of any information learned from the client or the client's family and friends; this information includes most written information obtained on the intake form and information gathered during conversation. The information is referred to as *subjective* because the client cannot present the information without personal bias; it is his or her perception or point of view. Of special interest are the client's chief concerns or complaints and explanations of various symptoms. Important symptoms such as pain, headache, fatigue or depression, or *paresthesia* (sensations of tingling, prickling, pins-and-needles, or numbness) will affect the treatment plan and subsequent sessions. Listening, which is focused on the client, is the primary skill used when gathering subjective information. This information, when documented, may include direct client quotes, such as "My head is killing me!"

Objective data are measurable and quantitative and obtained by the therapist through *empirical* means (measurable and verifiable via the senses). Objective findings include the size and shape of a mole, whether the right shoulder is higher than the left shoulder, and whether the left knee is more swollen (larger) than the right knee and by how much. The data may be obtained by comparing of range of motion in one hip joint with the other. The main skills used for gathering objective information are observation and palpation, even though all senses participate in the process.

To understand the difference between objective and subjective information, consider the following example: If a client comes into a massage therapist's office and enters his or her height and weight on the intake form, this information is subjective. If the therapist uses a tape measure and a scale to determine the client's height and weight, the information is objective.

> *"If you communicate with clients in terms of what he/she needs, they will begin to show you where to look."*
> —Stanley Smith

SCOPE OF PRACTICE

Scope of practice outlines the activities and procedures that can be performed by members of a licensed profession. Scope of practice is derived from the profession's legal definition. Even if you possess training in a particular technique or method (e.g., ear candling, herbalism), unless your scope of practice permits its use, it cannot legally be part of your professional activities.

What's In

Be sure you know the scope of practice pertaining to massage therapy in the state you are licensed (or intend to be licensed). The scope of practice for massage therapists in your state often includes:

- Client assessment by health history and intake, interview, observation of posture and movement such as joint range of motion, palpation, and, with client permission, consultation with the other health care providers participating in a client's care
- Formulation of an individualized treatment plan based on client assessment
- Determination of whether massage therapy is indicated or contraindicated
- Informing client regarding treatment and obtaining consent before initiating treatment
- Documenting a client's health history, intake interview, assessment findings, treatment protocols, and treatment outcomes
- Use of touch with or without pressure includes effleurage (gliding), pétrissage (kneading), tapotement (percussion) lifting, compression, holding, vibration, friction, and pulling by use of the digits, hands, forearms, elbows, knees, or feet, and mechanical appliances that enhance massage therapy techniques
- Use of lubricants such as oils, gels, lotions, and creams, as well as powders, liniments, ointments, antiseptics, rubbing alcohol, and similar preparations
- Application of therapeutic modalities and agents, which include hot and cold applications (such as compresses, ice or hot packs, stones, and heat lamps), hydrotherapy, topical herbal agents (e.g., poultices, muds, clays), body wraps (for therapeutic musculoskeletal or constitutional intentions), topical application of sugars or salts for exfoliation and detoxification purposes, tools, electric massagers, essential oils, and application of tape for the purpose of therapeutic benefit that does not restrict joint movement
- Use of joint mobilizations and stretching
- Energetic methods through the use of touch contact or noncontact techniques
- Offering suggestions and recommendations of self-care and health maintenance activities, including but not limited to self-massage, self-administered hydrotherapy applications, movement and stretching activities, and stress reduction and stress-management such as structured breathing techniques, progressive relaxation, and meditation
- The determination of whether referral to another health care provider is appropriate or necessary to address the client's condition when the care needed is beyond the therapist's scope of practice and training

What's Out

Massage therapists cannot provide any other service or therapy that would require a separate license to practice, such as psychotherapy, chiropractic, acupuncture, physical therapy, or any other branch of medicine, unless they have a required license to do so. The following is a partial list of what is commonly outside of a massage therapist's scope of practice, but *may be included with special training, certification, and/or additional licensure*:

- Acupuncture
- High-velocity/low-amplitude thrust force to any articulation of the human body as performed in chiropractic, osteopathic, or naturopathic procedures
- Application of ultrasound, electrotherapy, laser and microwave therapy, injection therapy, diathermy, or transdermal electronic nerve stimulation
- Dietary and nutritional counseling, which includes recommending nutritional supplements, herbal preparations, and other nutraceuticals
- Cosmetology or specific practices to beautify the skin
- Depilation, waxing, hair extractions, and electrolysis
- Colonic irrigation and other methods of internal hydrotherapy
- Ear candling
- Herbalism
- Homeopathy, which includes recommending Bach flower remedies
- Naturopathy
- Diagnosis of medical or orthopedic conditions or illnesses
- Performing surgery, psychotherapy, hypnotherapy, or counseling, or other practices or procedures
- Prescribing, dispensing, or administering legend and over-the-counter drugs

CHAT ROOM

Recently a massage therapist with advanced certification in pregnancy massage shared a situation where a client's OB/GYN suggested that she not receive massage during her pregnancy. The therapist was incensed that the doctor was trying to limit her clientele. However, when a client is being seen by an MD, DO, or other higher-level medical practitioner, that person is the primary health care provider and every other provider is secondary. The best approach for the massage therapist might be to contact the OB/GYN and identify his or her credentials and then, with the utmost professionalism, educate and encourage the inclusion of massage therapy. If that conversation goes well, perhaps suggest a lecture campaign for all of the doctor's expectant moms.

INFORMED CONSENT

Informed consent is permission for treatment given by a client after he or she has been informed of the risks, benefits, and consequences of the techniques and procedure(s). The consent form may be part of the client intake form or a separate document. Contents of the consent form are discussed with the client during the initial appointment. Be sure to go over each item and check for understanding before obtaining client signature. Keep the original signed form for your files; give one copy to your client for his or her records.

---

evolve *The Evolve website that is linked to this textbook contains a sample consent form.* ∎

To give consent, the client/patient must be a legal adult, have adequate reasoning faculties, and be in possession of all relevant facts. Persons who are minors or who have mental impairments must have a legal guardian consent to therapy on his or her behalf.

To fulfill mandatory requirements for informed consent, it must include a detailed explanation of the treatment plan, treatment costs and client financial obligations, therapist's scope of practice, and products used during treatment.

Along with the aforementioned required content, your consent form may include, but is not limited to:

- *Therapist's credentials:* This information includes the massage school the therapist attended, the year graduated, college degrees, postgraduate training and certifications held, and professional affiliations. If the therapist is in an office where a single consent form is shared by several therapists, this information needs to be verbalized to the client. Discussing your educational and professional background with your client helps establish a foundation of confidence and trust in the emerging therapeutic relationship.
- *Description of techniques, methods, and modalities:* This information will depend on the therapist's education, skills, and abilities and will vary among therapists.
- *Expected benefits:* Outline the benefits of treatment and how it can positively affect the client's condition and level of stress.
- *Potential risks and possible undesirable effects:* Discuss any known risks of treatment. For example, someone who has just been discharged from a week-long hospital stay and is taking medications may be at risk for bruising, soreness, or blood clot dislodgement. Be sure to mention that clients are screened before every massage and modifications are made when indicated (such as avoiding the lower extremities of persons who are prone to blood clots). Unless both benefits and risks are listed, the consent is not a valid, legally sound document.
- *Statement of scope of practice:* This statement should include that you do not have the authority to diagnose or prescribe and that services you provide are not a substitute for medical treatment.
- *Fees for services:* Inform your client about your fee schedule so he or she can make treatment decisions. This includes when fees are assessed and consequences, such as additional fees, for checks or charges made against accounts with insufficient funds.
- *Office policies:* Include your office procedures and policies of your practice, such as how to cancel appointments and how missed appointments, or "no shows," are handled. Be sure to also explain your policy regarding when the session officially begins (e.g., when massage begins versus when treatment planning begins).
- *Right of refusal:* This includes both the client's and therapist's rights. (1) Right of refusal by the *client* means that he or she has the right to terminate the session at any time

or for any reason and that the therapist will comply immediately. (2) The right of refusal by the *therapist* means that, when a contraindication is suggested or presented, the therapist has a right, responsibility, and obligation to refuse to treat the client or the local area involved. The therapist right of refusal also means that we have the right to refuse a client who makes us feel unsafe or who makes continued sexual advances once warned.

- *Information use:* Include information on how the client's records will be used and stored, as well as the circumstances for its disclosure such as obtaining a signed medical release form. You might also discuss exceptions to this rule including by subpoena or by statute to protect public health or the welfare of a third party.
- *Filing complaints:* Provide the client with written information on how to report professional misconduct to national, state, or other regulatory boards or agencies.

The following are samples of items to include in a consent form:

- The therapist's credentials are (list credentials)

Or

- The therapist has told me of his or her credentials.
- The information contained on the intake form is true to the best of my knowledge.
- I freely give my permission to receive massage therapy treatments.
- I understand that massage is contraindicated for some medical conditions and that obtaining a medical clearance or prescription may be necessary before beginning treatment.
- The primary methods used will be (list methods). Secondary methods will be (list methods).
- Using these methods, the client can expect (list documented effects of massage; see Chapter 6 for suggestions).
- Potential risks and undesirable effects of massage are (list risks and undesirable effects such as soreness, bruising, and exacerbation of symptoms).
- I agree to inform the therapist of any experience of pain during initial and subsequent sessions.
- I understand that I have the right to refuse any treatment or ask that it be modified in regard to pressure or technique.
- I understand that I will be draped during treatment in accordance with state laws and that I may request additional draping if desired.
- During future sessions, I agree to update the therapist on changes in my health status and understand that no liability on the therapist's part shall exist if I should neglect to do so.
- I understand that massage therapy should not be construed as a substitute for medical examination, diagnosis, and treatment and that I should see a medical physician, chiropractor physician, or other health care provider to address concerns that are outside the scope of a massage therapist's practice.

- I have been asked to report any professional misconduct to (list agencies or other resources).
- I understand that information obtained from me will be used only to provide a safe professional treatment and will not be disclosed. If an outside party requests this information, it will be released only after written permission is obtained from me or through a court order.
- Client printed name
- Client signature
- Therapist signature
- Date of signatures

"The question is not what you look at, but what you see."
—Henry David Thoreau

▶ TREATMENT PLANNING

10-2

From the moment a client enters the massage therapist's office until the time he or she leaves, the massage experience is literally and figuratively in the therapist's hands. Client experience depends on the therapist's communication skills, critical thinking skills, and hands-on skills. During the client's initial session, time is spent gathering client information, obtaining consent for therapy, performing assessments, and devising a treatment plan.

Treatment planning is the documented process of planning a client's treatment or course of treatment. This process takes into account (1) the client's therapeutic goals or reasons for seeking massage therapy, (2) his or her current health status, (3) information gathered on a completed intake form, (4) answers to questions asked by the therapist, (5) palpation of tissues, and (6) assessment procedures such as for range of motion, gait, and posture.

The resultant treatment plan, or plan of care, consists of strategies the therapist will use to resolve issues and address goals identified by the client. The plan also takes into account the therapist's training and experience, his or her scope of practice, and clinical reasoning skills. The treatment plan also documents, but is not limited to, the date and length of the session, techniques used, and parts of body treated or avoided. A well-designed treatment plan will be individualized for every session with client safety the first priority.

Treatment planning may involve working with a health care team to ensure that all health care providers for a particular client understand each other's treatment goals, and that these goals are complementary.

Let us look at steps taken to create the treatment plan.

CLIENT INTAKE

As stated previously, the primary reason for collecting and documenting client information is to develop a plan of care that seeks to fulfill your client's therapeutic goals. We find out this information through an intake process. Even though a formal protocol if followed, each client intake is unique. Each session is planned according to a particular client's needs and expectations with respect to his or her current health and abilities. The fact that some therapists are successful and some are not is not happenstance. Massage therapists who develop a large clientele are masters at finding and meeting, or exceeding, client's expectations while providing care that is both safe and effective.

Intake Location

Provide an environment conducive to the exchange of information. The area should be:
- Private and free of distractions
- Safe, well lit, and provides unobstructed passage
- Comfortable for you and your client
- Seating of relatively close proximity

Intake Form

A completed intake form, or health questionnaire, is the first element in the treatment planning process. A well-designed client intake form should encompass a variety of entries, such as the client's personal and contact information, as well as health and medical histories (Box 10-4). Please note that third party payers, such as insurance companies, may have their own particular forms for use if you are a part of their provider network. Questions to ask while you design an intake form are:
- Are the font style (serif versus sans serif) and point size (8 versus 12) easy to read?
- Is it brief and confined to a single page?
- Is it organized logically?
- Can the client check off or circle applicable items quickly?
- Is the information requested relevant and important for you to know?
- Is the information on the form understandable to all clients (called *health literacy*)?

According to the U.S. Department of Education, the average adult American reading level is between eighth and ninth grade.

A well-designed intake form includes the client's:
- Personal and contact information
- Date of birth
- Emergency contact information
- Name and contact information of the primary health care provider
- Health and medical data
- Date on which the information is recorded

Conditions (both past and present) or situations that have relevance to a massage and may need to be included in a checklist format:
- Allergies (especially to topical agents)
- Arthritis
- Blood clots
- Bulging or herniated disk

- Easily bruised
- Cancer
- Diabetes
- Infection
- Inflammation
- Pregnancy
- Recent motor vehicle accidents or trauma
- Seizure disorders
- Stroke or heart attack survivor
- Recent surgeries (including cosmetic surgeries)
- Vascular disorders such as varicose veins
- Medications and supplements

MINI-LAB

Collect a variety of intake forms from other professionals, including massage therapists, physicians (e.g., medical, chiropractic, dental), hospitals, physical therapists, and mental health counselors. Use these forms to create your own *health intake form*. Ask your teacher or a massage therapist to critique your form for design, flow, and relevance. Edit the form until it is complete and precise.

Filling Out the Form

After greeting your client, escort him or her to a private area with adequate lighting for reading and writing. Offer a writing utensil and the health intake form on a clipboard to complete. While your client is filling out the form, be available for questions.

If the client is unable or unwilling to fill out the form, ask your client for the information. Some therapists prefer to ask the client all queries on the intake form and write down the information instead of asking the client to do so. For one thing, they can read their own handwriting. It also provides the perfect opportunity to ask any questions needed to clarify information immediately. In such instances, write down the client's responses legibly on the form. Be sure to place your initials next to the entry when the writing on the form is your own and not your client's, or insert a handwritten statement at the bothom of the form.

Once the form is filled out, you are ready to begin the interview.

CHAT ROOM

Be sure to keep the intake form with you and the client at all times. Demonstrate that the information will be kept confidential, and will not be viewed by anyone other than you.

THE INTERVIEW

The interview is an essential component to a customized, client-centered treatment plan. The purpose of the interview is twofold. First, it gives you a greater insight into your client's overall health. You have the opportunity to review

---

BOX 10-4

Client Intake Form

Name: _____

Address: _____

Telephone (__) _____ Telephone (__) _____

Email _____

Date of birth: _____ Occupation: _____

Emergency contact: _____ Telephone (__) _____

Previous massage experience: _____

Are you under medical supervision? _____

Regular physician: _____ Telephone (__) _____

Referring by: _____

Check all that apply:

☐ Allergies	☐ Heart condition	☐ Previous MVA/trauma
☐ Arthritis	☐ Infection	☐ Ruptured/bulging disk
☐ Blood clots	☐ Inflammation	☐ Seizure disorders
☐ Bruise easily	☐ Kidney disorder	☐ Stroke
☐ Cancer	☐ Medications affecting blood clotting	☐ Recent surgery
☐ Diabetes	☐ Pregnancy	☐ Varicose veins/thrombophlebitus

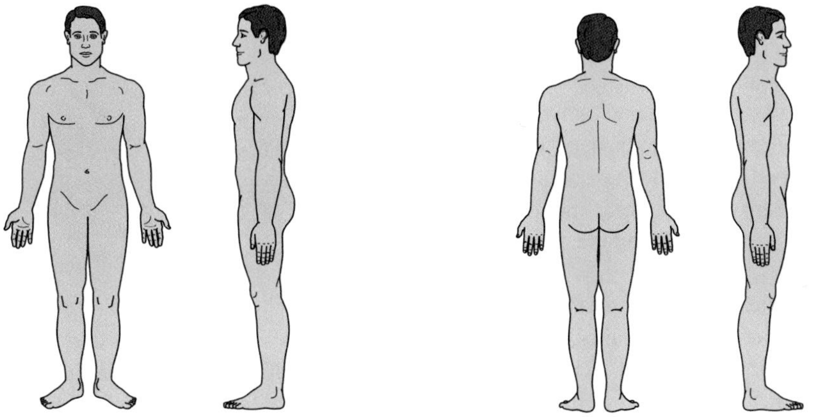

Identify your painful areas on these drawings using an X

Please briefly explain all checked items: _____

_____

_____

Signature: _____ Date: _____

---

the intake form, clarify information, and ask specific questions. This will help you screen for contraindications, realize the need for hypoallergenic lubricant, or when adaptive measures are needed, such as a side-lying position. An interview gives you more pieces of the puzzle.

Second, collaboration helps you devise a treatment plan that best suits your client's needs and wishes. An interview gives you a chance to find out your client's (1) primary purpose of the session and (2) his or her personal likes and dislikes. This information goes a long way toward establishing a positive therapeutic relationship, which often results in client satisfaction and continued patronage.

If your client speaks a foreign language that you do not understand, ask him or her about the possibility of bringing a support person to act as an interpreter.

Length of the Interview

Reasons for your client's visit will determine how much time is spent during the interview. A healthy client with no specific complaints does not require a lengthy interview—about 4 minutes on average. In contrast, a client with a lengthy medical history, recent injury, painful symptoms, or a physician's prescription may need a lengthier discussion and a focused evaluation of posture, gait, or joint range of motion (see Chapter 14). So a prudent therapist should set aside approximately 15 minutes for a new client interview, just in case. Keep in mind that most clients, new or established, want to spend most of the appointment time receiving a massage.

Building Rapport

Skills can be learned to help you build rapport while obtaining the information needed for the treatment plan. This rapport will also enhance the therapeutic relationship. For these and many other reasons, the person conducting the interview needs to be the attending therapist.

Begin by greeting your client by name, making eye contact, shaking hands firmly, and smiling. If you are not sure about the pronunciation of your client's name, ask how to say it correctly. Then introduce yourself and state your title. Reiterate why the interview is needed and how long it should take.

During the interview, sit facing your client at eye level (Figure 10-2). This creates an atmosphere of interaction, a sense of trust and goodwill, and facilitates conversation. If your client is bedridden, elevate his or her head with either the use of pillows or by bed setting. If there is a guardrail or rolling bed table between you and your client, move it during the interview and replace it after the interview or conclusion of the massage.

Once you and your client are comfortable, the next task is to review information on the intake form. Ensure that it is complete, dated, and signed. Then, verbally highlight health and medical issues, as well as personal preferences that will affect the massage. Use a systematic approach to avoid overlooking important information. In the next section, an organizational framework called PPALM will be featured, which contains five assessment domains.

While speaking, be sure to consider the background or education of your client. Anatomic names and medical terms may be inappropriate for clients who do not have background or training in these areas. If you do use anatomic terminology, you may want to give the common synonym (e.g., collarbone for clavicle); or you may want to touch the area on your body to show the client the anatomical location.

By the conclusion of the interview, you should know why your client is seeking massage services, areas to be addressed or avoided, any allergies or skin conditions, details about daily activities, medical history, and past trauma-producing events.

End the interview with a question that encourages discussion of any additional issues such as, "Is there anything else

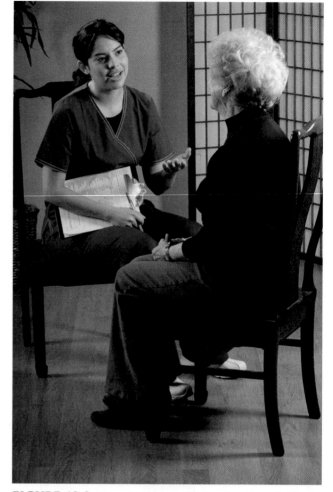

FIGURE 10-2 Therapist is seated facing the client during the interview.

you would like to tell me that I have not already asked?" This gives the client the final say.

Importance of Communication

Communication is the act of exchanging information through words, actions, behaviors, body language, and feelings. Communication skills are used in initiating, developing, and maintaining the therapeutic relationship; greeting the client; explaining and informing the client of services and procedures; collecting and reviewing client information; gaining consent; assessing needs of the client; developing a treatment plan; and room orientation. When the client reveals honesty and openly personal knowledge as well as his or her thoughts and feelings, this is known as **disclosure**. This information is needed to make decisions regarding therapy. Successful communication leads to a satisfied client, one who believes that he or she has been heard.

Nonverbal Communication

Communication occurs using five main methods: (1) words, (2) tones, (3) gestures, (4) posture, and (5) facial expressions. Because four out of five methods of communicating are nonverbal, body language often gives more complete information than the spoken word. Nonverbal cues indicate how the client is feeling and his or her internal state. Body language includes the following:

- Facial expressions such as grimaces, frowns, puckers, rapid blinking, and eye contact
- Gestures such as making a fist, gripping the table, fidgeting, looking down, and nodding
- Sudden movements such as the toes coming up off the table, buttocks tightening, change in breathing, and lifting the head
- Sounds such as sighs, grunts, groans, "hmm," and "uh-huh"
- Posture in relation to others (when a person is seated higher than another, or one is standing and one is sitting, usually implying that the higher person is more important or has more power)

In many instances, the client may not tell you that a certain massage technique or pressure is painful. Body language will communicate his or her unspoken discomfort. Look for congruency between what your client says and his or her body language.

Report your observations. Telling the client what you observe often improves the communication process because what you are observing can be affirmed or denied. Direct inquiry is preferred over assumptions.

Remember that, whether consciously or unconsciously, the client is also reading your body language. The information you project with your body language may affect therapeutic relationships. You may be considered insincere if you speak in a way that says your client is important but are also glancing at the clock or cell phone or are ruffling through papers as if in a hurry. How will you be perceived if your body language says you are tired when you greet your client? Generally, the strongest message is the unspoken message, because it is perceived to be the most honest. What is seen by the client, what is felt, and what is heard must all match to deliver a congruent, consistent message.

CHAT ROOM

What do our words really mean?

Research provided by Dr. Albert Mehrabian, Professor of Psychology at the University of California, Los Angeles, offers his classic statistic on the effectiveness of spoken communication.

Words we say: 7%
How we say them: 38%
Body language: 55%

This model is important to consider factors other than words when conveying a message.

"No man ever listened himself out of a job."
—Calvin Coolidge

Interview Skills

10-3 Skills can be developed to increase your success of obtaining client information while setting the stage for an enjoyable experience for both you and your client. These skills include:

Stay focused. Conversation is centered on your client's health and issues related to massage therapy. Guide the conversation back if it strays to other topics.

Look at your client more than the clipboard. During the interview, take notes sparingly by jotting down key words. Excessive note taking is distracting and interferes with listening and observing.

Listen intently and signal your interests. Active listening is conveyed by eye contact and occasional nodding or using facial expressions that coincide with the tone of the message. Neutral phrases or sounds, such as "uh-huh," "hmm," "I see," and "okay" show interest and encourage conversation.

Use both open-ended and closed-ended questions. Open-ended questions are broader in scope; close-ended questions are narrower. These questions are discussed next.

Open- and Closed-Ended Questions

Open-ended questions offer little restriction in answering and allow your client to reflect and clarify thoughts and feelings. Asking these kinds of questions helps you to explore topics with your client. Examples of open-ended questions are:

- "What brings you to the clinic?"
- "Tell me about your headache."
- "How can I help you be more comfortable?"
- "Anything else?"

Closed-ended questions are more direct, usually requesting a factual or denial statement such as "yes," "no," or "the right shoulder." These questions are used to gain specific information about a topic or the client. They are also useful to keep the client focused on the interview. Examples of closed-ended questions are:

- "Does it hurt to raise your right arm?"
- "Does pain radiate down your left leg?"
- "Can you take more pressure on this tender area?"
- "Do you want me to spend more time on your right shoulder or your left?"

Organizing the Interview

To ensure all necessary client information is obtained during the interview, an organizational framework is needed. A structured interview also helps prevent errors of omission. The next section features five assessment domains to help you systematically collect the information needed to formulate an appropriate treatment plan for your client.

Since massage therapists have a broad practice spectrum ranging from wellness to rehabilitation, information within each assessment domain will vary from general and nonspecific to detailed and precise.

MINI-LAB

Pair up with another student. Decide who will be the therapist and who will be the client. Ask the client to complete an intake form. Afterward, the therapist looks over the form, examines it for accuracy, fills in any omitted information, and makes certain that the form has been signed and dated. Next, interview the client and formulate his or her treatment plan. Reverse roles and repeat.

PPALM: ASSESSMENT DOMAINS

PPALM is a method of obtaining and recording data relevant to client assessment and treatment planning. It features five assessment domains that encompass observable and palpable data, as well as information from direct client inquiry. PPALM is an acronym for the first letter of the five assessment domains, which are:

- **P**urpose of Session
- **P**ain
- **A**llergies and Skin Conditions
- **L**ifestyle and Vocation
- **M**edical Information

During the interview, each assessment domain is discussed with your client. Information gathered is jotted down on a treatment planning diagram (Figure 10-3), which can be the backside of the client intake form. Even though some information requested is listed on the client intake form, revisit the information, even if the comment is "Mrs. Brown, are there any health conditions that would affect your massage today?" Then pause for a reply. If there is nothing to report in a particular domain, place a null symbol, or "Ø," instead of leaving it blank to indicate that it was discussed during the interview.

The duration and depth of the interview are determined by the session's purpose, which is one of the first questions answered by the client.

Purpose

The first domain identifies your client's reason for wanting massage. Find out what motivated today's visit. Is it pain reduction? Relaxation? A combination of the two perhaps? Begin with an open-ended question such as "What is your primary goal for today's session?" Then pause.

If this question does not bring a satisfactory answer, perhaps offer a more direct, closed-ended question such as "Do you need pain relief or stress relief today?" These questions go a long way in determining your client's primary concern or problem that is regarded as paramount.

This is also a good time to discuss any past experiences your client has had with massage therapy.

Pain

The second assessment domain addresses your client's pain. Use questions related to the acronym OPPQRST to gain further insight (Figure 10-4). This acronym stands for:

- **O**nset
- **P**rovocative
- **P**alliative
- **Q**uality
- **R**adiation
- **S**ite
- **T**iming

Answers to these questions will help you decide where to massage, if the area needs to be avoided, or to postpone massage.

Timing may be further explored by asking, "Does it hurt more first thing in the morning or at the end of your day?" "What makes it better or worse?" These types of questions will give the therapist clues to discover whether the pain is more related to postures such as sleeping position or to physical or mental stress from the client's job.

When describing the quality of pain, a 1- to 10-point pain scale can be used, with 10 being the worst (Figure 10-5). Note that severe pain is an absolute contraindication. Clients who report severe pain should be referred to a physician for evaluation before massage can safely be administered.

Pain may be either acute or chronic. Acute pain begins abruptly. It usually has a recognizable cause (e.g., auto accident, slipping or falling) and is characterized by swelling, localized heat, redness, tissue damage, and loss of function. Chronic pain usually develops slowly and persists for longer periods of time. This type of pain may be associated with multiple episodes of illness or injury or it may recur because of incomplete recovery from previous illness or injury. Because of the length of time, the original cause of chronic pain may or may not be known. See Table 10-1 for a comparison of chronic and acute pain.

Allergies and Skin Conditions

Next, inquire about any allergies your client may have to latex (used to make latex disposable gloves), ingredients in massage lubricants, or plants from which essential oils are derived.

Keep an alternate glove type or hypoallergenic lubricant on hand in case your client has allergies or has skin that is hypersensitive. The term *hypoallergenic* does not mean that the product will not cause allergic reactions; it means that the product underwent lengthy testing and that a majority of the subjects in the study were unaffected. Scented lubricants are more likely to cause allergic reactions.

Ask your client about skin conditions. These may be overlooked on the intake form as not all skin conditions are bothersome (some cases of psoriasis and eczema). Most skin conditions are avoided during massage. Some, such as oral herpes simplex, constitute an absolute contraindication.

Be sure to assess your client's skin by looking and feeling. Note any swelling, redness, bruising, lacerations, and other abnormalities.

Treatment Plan for _____

P	_____ _____ _____
P	_____ _____ _____
A	_____ _____ _____
L	_____ _____ _____
M	_____ _____ _____

Treatment Plan:

_____
_____
_____
_____
_____
_____
_____
_____
_____
_____

Client signature: _____

Therapist signature: _____

Date/s: _____

Legend	**P** = Purpose **P** = Pain **A** = Allergies/skin conditions **L** = Lifestyle **M** = Medical history/meds

FIGURE 10-3 PPALM form.

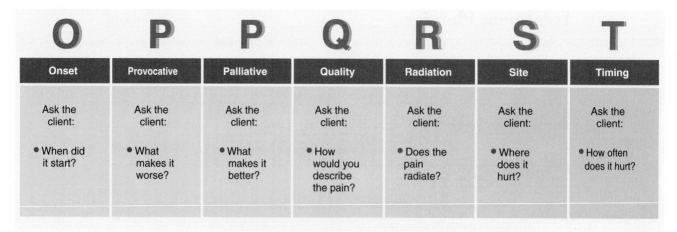

O	P	P	Q	R	S	T
Onset	**Provocative**	**Palliative**	**Quality**	**Radiation**	**Site**	**Timing**
Ask the client: • When did it start?	Ask the client: • What makes it worse?	Ask the client: • What makes it better?	Ask the client: • How would you describe the pain?	Ask the client: • Does the pain radiate?	Ask the client: • Where does it hurt?	Ask the client: • How often does it hurt?

FIGURE 10-4 Pain assessment using OPPQRST.

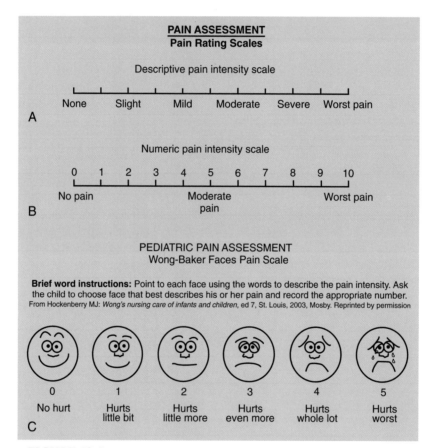

FIGURE 10-5 Pain scales. **A,** Descriptive; **B,** numeric; **C,** Wong-Baker Faces.

"Pay attention to your patient's allergies or you will have to pay attention to his lawyer."
—Rebecca Swanson, MD

Lifestyle and Vocation

This domain explores how your client uses his or her body throughout the day. Find out about your client's occupation, avocation (hobby or pastime), regular leisure or sports activities, and routine physical exercise. Investigate frequent activities at work and home such as sitting, standing, chasing small children, or carrying heavy books. These are also called activities of daily living (ADL), and are essential to quality of life.

If a client indicates a high level of stress, your treatment plan might include relaxation massage, which may mean a longer session if your client originally scheduled a half-hour massage for lower back pain.

TABLE 10-1 Acute and Chronic Pain: A Comparison

CHARACTERISTIC	ACUTE PAIN	CHRONIC PAIN
Experience	An event	A situation: state of existence
Source	External agent or internal disease	Unknown; if known, treatment is prolonged or may be ineffective
Onset	Usually sudden	May be sudden or develop insidiously
Duration	Transient (≤6 months)	Prolonged (≥6 months or years)
Pain identification	Painful and nonpainful areas generally well identified	Painful and nonpainful areas less easily differentiated; change in sensations becomes more difficult to evaluate
Clinical signs	Typical response pattern with more visible signs	Response patterns vary; fewer overt signs (adaptation)
Significance	Significant (affected person perceives something is wrong)	Affected person looks for significance
Pattern	Self-limiting or readily corrected	Continuous or intermittent; intensity may vary or remain constant
Course	Suffering usually decreases over time	Suffering usually increases over time
Actions	Leads to actions to relieve pain	Leads to actions to modify pain experience
Prognosis	Likelihood of eventual complete relief	Complete relief may not be possible

From Black RG: The chronic pain syndrome. *Surg Clin North Am* 55(4):999, 1975.

Ask about nutrition and personal habits. Insufficient fluid intake, inadequate sleep, or use of tobacco, alcohol, or prescription drugs often affects tissue health. Answers to these questions will uncover potential areas of muscle tension trigger points, as well as expected tissue response and recovery time after the massage. The answers will also help you decide which self-help activities to suggest after the massage.

Medical History

The last assessment domain addresses your client's medical history. Note any medical conditions on the intake form. Ask how long your client has had the disease (or condition) and how it is managed, as well as about any limitations on activities. Ask about signs and symptoms; find out your client's experience with the disease. As about medical treatment or other forms of therapy the client is undergoing and any related adverse effects.

Many medical conditions and diseases are managed with medications. Ask about medication use and any side effects related to medication use. Table 10-2 includes medication examples (ibuprofen [Advil, Motrin, Nuprin]) for your convenience.

If the client has a comorbid disease, be sure it is addressed along with the primary disease in the treatment plan. An example of someone with comorbid disease is a client who is diabetic and suffers from chronic bronchitis. If the client reports the presence of a disease or medical condition with which you are unfamiliar, look it up in a current pathology textbook or other reliable source.

Interview Conclusion

10-5 The treatment plan outlines the best approach to address your client's goals by synthesizing all client information. After you have formulated the plan, discuss it briefly with your client and make any appropriate revisions. Once you both have come to a mutual agreement, ask your client to sign and date the document.

Medical Referral and Medical Clearance

A therapist who is competent and accountable acts in the client's best interest. This also includes recognizing when your client needs a medical evaluation or services outside your scope of practice. If this occurs, refer your client to an appropriate health care provider.

Additionally, medical clearance may be needed before treatment is initiated (Box 10-5). For example, if your client reports a recent worsening of symptoms or if you note any symptom instability, medical clearance should be obtained before initiating treatment. Here is an example of symptom instability: Your client has been taking drugs to manage high blood pressure and reports that it has been higher than normal the last 3 days even though the client has not missed any medications. This change indicates symptom instability, and massage should be postponed until medical clearance is obtained.

PALPATION AS AN ASSESSMENT TOOL

Palpation is touching with purpose and intent and is part of the premassage assessment, as well as ongoing during the session. In massage, the primary purpose of palpation is to locate treatment areas such as taut bands, spasms, and trigger points. However, palpation can also reveal other aspects of the client's health (e.g., swollen lymph nodes), which affect treatment (i.e., local or absolute contraindications). Palpation requires you to touch the client with different parts of

TABLE 10-2 Prescribed Medication Types and Massage Considerations

TYPE	SIDE EFFECTS AND MASSAGE CONSIDERATIONS

MEDICATIONS FOR PAIN AND INFLAMMATION

Nonsteroidal antiinflammatory drugs (NSAIDs)	GI distress? Avoid abdomen or use semireclining position.
	Easy bruising or reduced sensation? Use caution with deep pressure and aggressive techniques.
	Dizzy or drowsy? End session with stimulating strokes and instruct client to move slowly and carefully; be ready to assist.
	Acetaminophen does not produce any side effects that would affect massage.
Corticosteroids	Avoid areas of dermatitis.
	Caution with deep pressure and aggressive techniques because of reduced tissue integrity (long-term use).
	No massage considerations for short-term use (30 days or less) of corticosteroids.
Skeletal Muscle Relaxants	Constipation? Use abdominal massage.
	Dizzy or drowsy? End session with stimulating strokes and instruct client to move slowly and carefully; be ready to assist.
Narcotics	Reduced sensation? Caution with deep pressure and aggressive techniques.
	GI distress? Avoid abdomen or use semireclining position.
	Constipation? Use abdominal massage.
	Dizzy or drowsy? End session with stimulating strokes and instruct client to move slowly and carefully; be ready to assist.

DIABETIC MEDICATIONS

Antidiabetic Agents and Hypoglycemics	GI distress? Avoid abdomen or use semireclining position.
	Injectable insulin? Avoid vigorous massage over recent injection sites for 24 hours.
	Insulin pump? Avoid massage over the patch where insulin is administered up to a 4-inch radius around the patch. Do not get lubricant on the sensor, transmitter, pump, or its tubing.
	Watch for signs of hypoglycemia (see Chapter 9).

MEDICATIONS FOR CARDIOVASCULAR DISEASE

Anticoagulants and Antithrombotics	GI distress? Avoid abdomen or use semireclining position.
	Easy bruising? Use caution with deep pressure and aggressive techniques.
	Dizzy? Instruct client to move slowly and carefully; be ready to assist.
Vasodilators	Severe or pitting edema? Seek medical clearance before massage begins.
	Mild edema? Elevate and use gentle centrifugal stroking.
	Dizzy? Instruct client to move slowly and carefully; be ready to assist.
Antiarrhythmic drugs	If antiarrhythmics are given because of a medical emergency, postpone massage until the condition has resolved.
	Dizzy? Instruct client to move slowly and carefully; be ready to assist.
Angiotensin-converting enzyme inhibitors (ACE inhibitors)	Dizzy or weakened? Instruct client to move slowly and carefully; be ready to assist.
Angiotension II receptor blockers (ARBs)	Dizzy or weakened? Instruct client to move slowly and carefully; be ready to assist.
Alpha receptor drugs	Dizzy or drowsy? End session with stimulating strokes and instruct to move slowly and carefully; be ready to assist.
Beta blockers	Dizzy or drowsy? End session with stimulating strokes and instruct to move slowly and carefully; be ready to assist.
Calcium channel blockers	Severe or pitting edema? Seek medical clearance before massage begins.
	Mild edema? Elevate and use gentle stroking.
	Dizzy? Instruct client to move slowly and carefully; be ready to assist.
	Constipation? Use abdominal massage.
Diuretics	GI distress? Avoid abdomen or use semireclining position.
	Dizzy or weakened? Instruct client to move slowly and carefully; be ready to assist.
	Suggest use of toilet before the session begins.
Lipid-lowering drugs	GI distress? Avoid abdomen or use semireclining position.
	Refer back to physician if severe or persistent muscle weakness, muscle pain, or joint pain (may indicate medication problem).

MEDICATIONS FOR RESPIRATORY DISORDERS

Antihistamine	Dizzy or drowsy? End session with stimulating strokes and instruct to move slowly and carefully; be ready to assist.
Antitussives (cough suppressants)	Dizzy or drowsy? End session with stimulating strokes and instruct to move slowly and carefully; be ready to assist.
Bronchodilators	Shortness of breath? Regardless if this is related to a symptom of disease or medication side effect, avoid prone position and use semireclining position while the client is supine.
Decongestants	Restless? A relaxing massage with long, gliding strokes is beneficial.
Expectorants	GI distress? Avoid abdomen or use semireclining position.

TABLE 10-2 Prescribed Medication Types and Massage Considerations—cont'd

TYPE	SIDE EFFECTS AND MASSAGE CONSIDERATIONS
FEMALE GONADAL HORMONES	
Estrogens	Breast tenderness? Prop soft pillows under the chest and shoulders when prone or avoid the prone position.
	A serious side effect is an increased risk of blood clots and phlebitis, most often in the legs. S/S* includes redness, heat, swelling, and leg pain. If these are present, refer her back to her physician for immediate evaluation with massage postponed until medical clearance is given.
Progesterone	See massage consideration under estrogens.
MEDICATIONS FOR DEPRESSION AND ANXIETY	
Antianxiety, sedative, and hypnotic drugs	Reduced sensation? Caution with deep pressure and aggressive techniques.
	Dizzy or drowsy? End session with stimulating strokes and instruct to move slowly and carefully; be ready to assist.
Antidepressant drugs	Postpone massage and refer client back to physician if the client is experiencing severe tremors or muscle weakness (may indicate medication problem).
	Dizzy or drowsy? End session with stimulating strokes and instruct client to move slowly and carefully; be ready to assist.
	Restless? A relaxing massage with long, gliding strokes is beneficial.
Antipsychotics	GI distress? Avoid abdomen or use semireclining position.
	Dizzy or drowsy? End session with stimulating strokes and instruct client to move slowly and carefully; be ready to assist.
Anticonvulsants	Dizzy or drowsy? End session with stimulating strokes and instruct client to move slowly and carefully; be ready to assist.

*S/S = signs/symptoms.

BOX 10-5

Medical Clearance Form

Client: _____   DOB: _____

Massage therapist: _____

Address: _____

Telephone number: _____   Fax: _____

Type of massage therapy: _____

☐ Cleared

☐ Cleared after completing evaluation/rehabilitation for: _____

_____

_____

_____

☐ Not cleared for: _____   Reason: _____

Recommendations/Restrictions: _____

_____

_____

_____

Name of physician (print/type): _____   Date: _____

Address: _____

Telephone number: _____   Fax: _____

Signature of physician: _____

Signature of client: _____   Date: _____

---

your hands using varying degrees of pressure. Through palpation, the therapist may detect:

- **Anomalies**. Do any superficial or deep masses exist, such as lipomas or swollen lymph nodes? These masses often represent a local contraindication. Swollen lymph nodes accompanied by fever represent an absolute contraindication.

- **Client reaction**. Does pressing the area produce pain or discomfort? Is the pain localized, or does it refer to other areas? These areas often represent a massage indication.

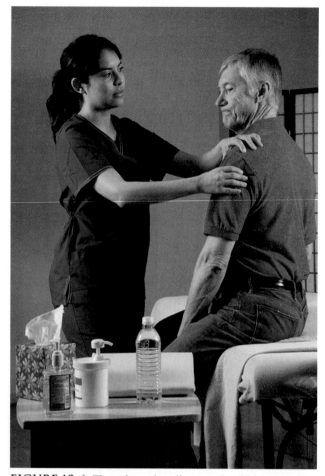

FIGURE 10-6 Therapist noting client reaction during palpation.

Does the client report lack of sensation? This circumstance necessitates lighter-than-normal pressure during massage (Figure 10-6).

- **Edema**. Does the area feel swollen, mushy, or congested? Does any pitting edema exist (i.e., dents produced by applying pressure)? The cause needs to be ascertained because edema from heart or kidney conditions will affect treatment.
- **Twitching**. Is a muscle firing involuntarily or twitching when pressure is applied, indicating a trigger point? This circumstance often represents a massage indication.
- **Temperature**. Is the skin overly warm, suggesting inflammation, or cool, indicating ischemia? Localized heat represents a local contraindication, and fever (systemic heat) represents an absolute contraindication. Or is the room temperature adversely affecting the client?
- **Superficial fascia**. Does the skin glide easily or with difficulty when moved over the underlying structures? Most fascial restrictions can be addressed with massage.

In massage, touch is not a monologue but rather a dialogue. The client's body leads you in a certain direction, and you follow. Your hands, in turn, communicate with the client's tissue, and it responds accordingly. Spoken communication and the tissue response you feel in the client's skin give you the information you need to create therapeutic impact. During palpation, your hands become sensitive miniature microphones sensing restrictions in the tissue. With this information, you can verify or discard your original therapeutic assessment and offer the client the fullness of your therapeutic abilities.

MINI-LAB

Without using your sense of sight, work in pairs and use palpation to find and note the differences among bone, muscle, tendons, lymph nodes, veins, arteries, and hair. This activity will help sharpen your palpatory skills.

FORMULATING THE PLAN

10-6

During the planning process, the therapist uses the information gathered to set the course of action for the massage session. The treatment plan itself represents the culmination of all of the information gathered: the client's intake form, the interview, and other assessments such as palpation. It is also based on the therapist's critical thinking skills; knowledge of anatomy, physiology, and pathology; massage therapy skills; and understanding the effectiveness of techniques. It embodies the approach you will use to address your client's goals. The plan also takes into account your scope of practice and your client's financial and time constraints. With practice, the planning process will flow naturally.

If unsure how best to design a treatment plan, begin with shorter sessions using moderate pressure. This approach gives you an opportunity to see how your client responds to massage.

While collecting and synthesizing information, the therapist is also screening each client for contraindications. A **contraindication** is the presence of a disease or physical condition that makes treating a particular client in the usual manner impossible or undesirable (see Chapters 8 and 9). If a local or absolute contraindication is determined through assessment, then it influences how massage will be applied, or it may rule out massage therapy entirely.

Elements of a Treatment Plan

Your client's treatment plan may include:

- Techniques and areas to include or avoid
- Duration, frequency, and length of sessions
- Goals related to improved function
- Method of reassessment to measure improvement (or lack of improvement)
- Whether your client needed assistance
- Use of any adjunctive therapies, such as aromatherapy or hydrotherapy

- Client education and self-help techniques suggested after the session
- Referrals made to persons who provide a service that can help clients achieve their goals, such as a chiropractor, nutritionist, personal trainer, or yoga or tai chi instructor
- Referrals made to other health care providers
- Use of support or bolstering devices that are out of the ordinary
- Your client's general demeanor

> *"The body never lies."*
> —Martha Graham

AFTER THE MASSAGE AND SUBSEQUENT SESSIONS

After the session, make appropriate suggestions for self-help techniques or home care activities that will help the client achieve better results with massage. Offer your client water, perhaps suggest another appointment, and ask if he or she has any questions. Be sure to say goodbye and express your hope that the client enjoyed the massage today or is feeling better (find a closure that fits you and your work).

Client Education

Suggest ways your clients can help achieve their therapeutic goals. For stress management, recommend light exercise (going for a walk around the block), deep breathing, meditation, and taking time out for enjoyable activities. Approach stress management as a health care issue by pointing out all the benefits the body receives from lowered stress levels: increased stamina, better concentration, and enhanced immune functions. If the client is not an avid water drinker, explain the benefits of water intake, how it improves the body's metabolism and slows the aging process. Think of creative ways to increase water consumption.

Unless restricted by scope of practice, you can teach clients self-care techniques to help them achieve their goals. Teaching clients health-building skills is an important part of the treatment plan and empowers them to take control of their own health. These activities are to be done between scheduled appointments. Suggest an activity that would fit easily into the day and that would tie into something your client does daily. For example, suggest sleeping with the cervical spine in a neutral position. Other suggestions are:

- Stretching
- Joint mobilizations
- Self-massage
- Applications of ice and heat

Use of stretching helps to lengthen tight muscles. Joint mobilizations help improve range of motion and facilitate pain-free movements (see Chapter 8). When teaching self-help techniques, explain and demonstrate how to do them properly and not cause injury. Have your client mirror the activity back to you. Be sure the client is doing it correctly. If stretches or joint mobilizations are performed bilaterally, ask the client to complete the movement on both the left and the right sides of the body.

Updating the Plan During Subsequent Sessions

Prepare for your client's subsequent sessions by briefly reviewing your past treatment plan or PPALM notes. Begin the interview by asking about the prior massage. If your client sought pain reduction, ask about any changes (better or worse) in the frequency, intensity, or duration of pain. If your client needed stress reduction, ask if an increase in relaxation and a decrease in anxiety were achieved.

Next, ask if there were any adverse effects such as soreness or bruising. Update your PPALM notes by asking if there are any changes in health status since the last session. Finally, inquire about goals for today's session. Answers to these questions will help you decide if the last session was well received and whether the treatment plan should be repeated or if modifications are needed (Box 10-6).

Helping Clients Achieve Their Goals

Keep your client's desired results and goals clearly in mind. It is difficult to know, given the variable of client response, how often and how many massages may be needed to achieve your client's desired results or goals. In general, the initial period consists of frequent sessions, tapering off as symptoms subside and goals are achieved. Goals expressed in functional terms (e.g., massage needed to increase ROM in right shoulder) is easier to demonstrate progress.

Ideally you hope to see a decrease in the frequency and severity of symptoms, most notably pain, and an increase in flexibility and range of motion. Be sure to remind your client about self-care measures, such as ice packs, stretching, and self-massage, so that the client takes responsibility for maintenance of therapeutic progress.

Realize that a 100% return of function and complete freedom from pain are not possible in all cases. Sometimes

---

BOX 10-6

Treatment Planning: Basic Steps

Collect. Gather client information from a completed intake form and a structured interview.
Formulate. The treatment plan is formulated to address client goals.
Implement. The treatment plan is implemented.
Revise. The treatment plan is revised as needed.

MILTON TRAGER

Born: April 20, 1908; died: January 20, 1997

"Not until we experience it is it more than just words. After we experience it, there is no need for words."

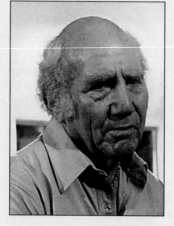

It is the roaring '20s in sunny Miami. However, for a high school dropout who lied about his age to get a job at the post office, it is all work and no play. He barely has time to breathe—until today. Today the posted health tip instructs him to do so and to sign his name indicating that he had done so.

Milton Trager slowly inhaled, then exhaled. He had no idea that he possessed a talent that would develop—without outside influence—into a revolutionary method of bodywork. That one deep breath put Trager in touch with his body for the very first time. "It was the beginning of me," he recalls. Soon he started working out at the beach, doing acrobatics, developing his muscles, and listening to the waves as he swayed to their ebb and flow. Fascinated by the movements of boxers in the ring, he took up the sport. One day he offered to turn the tables and massage his trainer. His trainer was stunned at his ability. From there he went home to massage his father, who had severe sciatic pain. After four treatments, the pain was gone, never to return.

At 19, Trager helped a child walk who had not walked in 4 years. The proverbial 90-lb weakling had grown into a strong, agile young man whose acrobatic antics along his mail route captured the attention of the Hollywood studios. However, his unique mode of hands-on therapy went virtually unnoticed.

He enlisted with the Navy medical corps. After his release, he decided it was time to get the credentials that would make physicians take notice of his work. However, the only medical school that would accept a 42-year-old person was in Guadalajara, Mexico, so he headed south with his wife and embarked on the arduous task of earning a medical degree in a completely Spanish-speaking environment.

Establishing a medical practice was difficult for someone with his background, but the Tragers finally settled in Honolulu. Sadly, the medical community remained deaf and blind to his work. However, Trager did not need the medical community's blessing to know what he was doing was right. His method of holding,

---

50% improvement represents tremendous progress. The purpose of massage treatments is to benefit the client and to meet his or her needs, not to meet the expectations of the therapist. A therapist who is mindful of this is truly a professional.

CHAT ROOM

Functional goals possess certain characteristics. When formulating these goals, therapist Mirra Greenway uses the acronym **F-A-R-M-S**, which stands for *F*unctional, *A*chievable, *R*elevant, *M*easurable, and *S*pecific.

ⓔvolve　*Try your hand at creating treatment plans by viewing the sample client interviews provided in the course materials for Chapter 10. Share them with your instructor for additional suggestions on how best to proceed with a particular client.* ∎

NETWORKING WITH OTHER HEALTH CARE PROVIDERS

In some instances, the massage therapist part of a team of health care professionals assembled by the client. Members are selected according to the client's needs, as well as the skill and expertise of the health care providers. Your professional experience and opinion may be needed to further develop an overall treatment plan for the mutual client. Health care team members may include:

- Doctors and surgeons
- Nurse practitioners
- Osteopaths and chiropractors
- Physical and occupational therapists
- Mental health counselors
- Nutritionists

Be sure to obtain written permission from the client before releasing confidential records or before discussing your client with team members. Respect professional boundaries of other health care providers involved in your client's

MILTON TRAGER (*continued*)

listening to, rocking, and freeing the body continued to evolve.

By chance, a well-known psychologist experienced Trager's methods and convinced Trager to demonstrate at Esalen, a workshop and meeting place for developing human potential. Jack Liskin, Trager's biographer, writes: "And so it was that an aging and unusual doctor with an unusual talent, unattached to any movement, New Age or conventional, came face-to-face with the California counterculture."

The Trager Approach uses nonintrusive movements to lull the body into a better, more mobile, lighter state of being by releasing deep-seated physical and mental patterns.

Essential to Trager's work is a state that has been termed *hook-up*, which means that the practitioner becomes so totally focused that he or she achieves a hypersensitivity to body cues. "It's as though the practitioner's mind and body communicates, without using words. And what is being said to the receiver is, though you may have hidden them from your consciousness, you hold the keys to unlock patterns that are holding you physically and mentally hostage. I'm just here to give your body the cues to gently remind you of your own potential—nothing more."

A Trager session does not end with table work. Mentastics reinforces the results. *Mentastics* is Trager's term for mental gymnastics, the gentle, mindful movement exercises that help the body recall positive physical or mental changes that occurred on the table and reinforce these changes.

Though Trager never cared for explaining his work, people who experienced, practiced, and witnessed its results have filled in the gaps.

"The practitioner uses the vast sensory capacities of the skin and deeper tissue to transmit messages. Using wavelike, moving rhythms that are at the core of all forms and matter of life, it communicates its messages thousands of times during a session to break habitual patterns," writes Jack Liskin in *Moving Medicine: The Life and Work of Milton Trager, M.D.*

Trager never cared to be referred to as a genius, guru, or healer, claiming instead to have a talent. However, his talent touched lives and changed minds about what was possible.

For instance, Betty Fuller, a frequent seminar leader at Esalen, was prepared to live the rest of her days in chronic pain. When Trager reached out to examine her, she practically shrieked, "No one touches my neck." Nonetheless, Trager persisted in his gentle but unyielding manner. Soon she was pain-free and became Trager's first instructor. In Trager she saw the same deep reverence for the mind's ability to heal the body that she had experienced as a student of Moshe Feldenkrais. Trager turned to Fuller to protect his name and his work, and in April of 1980 the Trager Institute was founded. Today practitioners all around the world are using the Trager Approach and Mentastics Movement Education techniques to ease headaches, back pain, and the debilitating effects of Parkinson's disease, cerebral palsy, polio, and multiple sclerosis.

---

care (see Chapter 2). For example, if a physical therapist has assigned activities such as exercise, it might be inappropriate for you to add more or different activities.

Massage therapists have direct access to the public, meaning that no prescription or referral is needed to receive treatment. However, most insurance companies require documentation of referral or prescription when insurance is billed for massage services (see Chapter 17 for information regarding insurance reimbursements). In these cases, a medical physician, chiropractor, physician assistant, or nurse practitioner must complete one of two forms: (1) prescription and (2) referral.

Prescriptions

A **prescription** is a physician's order for medication, medical treatments (physical or massage therapy), or medical devices

(hearing aids, eyeglasses). If a therapist accepts a prescription for therapy, the prescription must specify massage therapy, not physical or occupational therapy. A prescription may include the following:

- Patient's name
- Age of patient (if significant, such as child)
- Date written
- Diagnosis or diagnostic code
- Treatment order
- Frequency of treatments
- Duration of treatments
- Prescriber's information (name, address, and identification) and signature

If a prescription is for medications, it indicates the drug name and amount, dosage, route of administration, and permission for additional quantities.

BOX 10-7

Ownership of Client Records

In most states, therapists are required to maintain documentation for each client session. However, client records are considered the property of the facility where they were created. For example, a therapist in private practice owns his or her clients' records; client records acquired in a spa or clinic are the facility's property.

For example, if you had a medical procedure done in a local clinic and, a year later, needed copies of your documents, you would contact the clinic where the procedure was performed rather than the person who provided the service.

As a protection in the event of litigation, records should be kept until the applicable statute of limitations period has elapsed, which is generally 4 to 5 years after the last date of client service. This procedure is also the recommendation of the National Certification Board for Therapeutic Massage and Bodyworkers (NCBTMB), but requirements may vary from state to state.

Massage client records are not protected under the law because they are subject to subpoena by a court of law. However, treat client records with the same care for confidentiality that a physician's office would use.

The prescription may instruct the therapist to *evaluate and treat* at the discretion of the therapist, or it may state a specific method such as soft tissue mobilization or massage therapy. The prescription may also state how the massage is to be *taken* or *administered*. Massage is *taken* in increments known as sessions, with a specific time frame such as 60 minutes *(strength)*. The prescription may also specify frequency, such as once a week, and duration, such as 6 weeks *(dosage)*. Prescriptions must be followed exactly or they may be challenged by an insurance company or court of law.

If you have any problem understanding the order, or believe you need to amend the treatment, contact the physician's nurse or assistant.

At the end of the prescriptive period, the client returns to the referring health care provider for follow-up and re-evaluation. The original prescription becomes a permanent part of the client's file (Box 10-7). The client may request a copy, and some insurance companies may require a copy as well, but the therapist retains the original.

Referral Forms

A referral form is produced by the therapist (you) and filled out by a health care provider authorizing massage therapy treatment. These forms may be personalized with the massage therapist's logo, name, regular and e-mail addresses, telephone number, fax number, and other contact information. The form should have room for the patient's name, diagnosis, treatment choices (preferably with check boxes), and blank spaces for frequency and duration. At the bottom is a space for the health care provider's signature and office stamp.

A referral form can be given to a specific patient who is seeking your services. Instruct the person to bring the referral form to his or her health care provider for completion and signature. Or you can provide these forms to health care providers to be given to patients who need your services. Keep in mind that the patient can bring the form filled out by a health care provider to any licensed massage therapist for services. Just as people have their choice of pharmacy for medication, they also have their choice of therapist for massage.

Medical Release Forms

Because of its confidential nature, the client must authorize, in writing, release of any medical or personal information to a third party. The release of information encompasses all possible methods of communication such as paper or electronic documents or discussing your client's treatment with other individuals involved in his or her care.

The medical release form includes the client's name, the name of address of the institution who maintains client information, and the name and address of the institution receiving the information.

The release of client information should have an expiration period. Only the information requested should be released. If the client is a minor or has mental impairment, then a parent or legal guardian must sign. An example of a medical release form is presented in Box 10-8.

Do not release client information without his or her consent. Exceptions include legally required disclosures, such as those ordered by subpoena or by statute to protect public health or the welfare of a third party.

> *"I am different from [George] Washington; I have a higher, grander standard of principle. Washington could not lie. I can lie, but I won't."*
> —Mark Twain

▌ MINI-LAB

Using a medical dictionary, such as *Dorland's Illustrated Medical Dictionary,* or a reference book, such as Travell and Simons' *Myofascial Pain and Dysfunction,* find definitions of words that might be used to describe a knot or ropiness, tonus or tension, thickening or swelling, tenderness or discomfort, and numbness. Use these appropriately in your treatment record.

E-RESOURCES

⊜volve

http://evolve.elsevier.com/Salvo/MassageTherapy

- Chapter challenge
- Flash cards
- Photo gallery
- Technique videos

BOX 10-8

Release of Medical Information

I authorize: Name of person or institution: _____
                                                        (Provider of information)

   Street address: _____
   City, state, ZIP code: _____
To release client information to: _____

_____

   Name of person or institution: _____
                                                        (Recipient of information)

   Street address: _____
   City, state, ZIP code: _____
   Attention: _____

_____

Client's name: _____   Date: _____
Signature of client or legal guardian: _____
Complete address: _____
Relationship, if not the client: _____   Client's date of birth: _____

_____

The authorization will automatically expire one year from the date of signature, unless specified otherwise.

- Additional information
- Downloadable forms
- Weblinks

▶ **DVD**

- 10-1: Documentation tips
- 10-2: Treatment planning
- 10-3: Interview skills
- 10-4: PPALM: Assessment domains
- 10-5: Sample interviews
- 10-6: Formulating the plan

BIBLIOGRAPHY

Abdenour J: *TN magazine: the professional magazine with the personal touch*, Montvale, NJ, 1999, Medical Economics.

NALS: *Adult literacy in America.* Washington DC, 2002, National Center for Education Statistics, U.S. Dept of Education, Office of Educational Research and Improvement (NCES 1993-275).

American Health Information Management Association: *Time for a HIPAA tuneup?* 2006, AHIMA (website): http://library.ahima.org/xpedio/groups/public/documents/ahima/bok1_031356.hcsp?dDocName=bok1_031356. Accessed June 5, 2010.

American Massage Therapy Association: *Code of ethics*, Evanston, Ill, 1994, The Association.

Black HC: *Black's law dictionary*, ed 9, St Paul, 2009, ThomsonWest Publishing.

Bolton R: *People skills*, New York, 1979, Simon & Schuster.

Bucci C: *Condition specific massage therapy*, Baltimore, Lippincott Williams & Wilkins (in press).

Burley-Allen M: *Listening: the forgotten skill*, New York, 1995, John Wiley & Sons.

Chaitow L: *Palpation skills: assessment and diagnosis through touch*, New York, 1998, Churchill Livingstone.

Charting made incredibly easy, Springhouse, Pa, 1998, Springhouse.

D'Ambrogio KJ, Roth GB: *Positional release therapy – assessment & treatment of musculoskeletal dysfunction*, St Louis, 1997, Mosby.

Davis NM: *Medical abbreviations: 7000 conveniences at the expense of communications and safety*, ed 5, Huntington Valley, Pa, 1990, Neil M Davis Associates.

Dilks T: Personal communication, 2010.

Diamond B: *The legal aspects of complementary therapy practice: a guide for health care professionals*, New York, 1998, Churchill Livingstone.

Dolan DW: *Objective structural findings in massage therapy: key to insurance reimbursement & specialty physician referrals*, Jacksonville, Fla, 1995, Advanced Therapeutics America.

e-university: Documentation (website): http://www.childbirths.com/euniversity/documentation.htm. Accessed June 8, 2010.

Expert 10-minute physical examination, St Louis, 1997, Mosby.

Fritz S: *Mosby's fundamentals of therapeutic massage*, ed 4, St Louis, 2009, Mosby.

Health Privacy Project: *Welcome to health privacy 101*, Health Privacy (website): http://www.healthprivacy.org. Accessed June 12, 2010.

Henry MC: *EMT prehospital care*, ed 4, St Louis, 2009, Mosby.

Ignatiavicius DD, Bayne MV: *Medical-surgical nursing: a nursing process approach*, ed 2, Philadelphia, 1995, Saunders.

Jusdon K, Hicks S: *Law and ethics for medical careers*, ed 3, New York, 2003, Glencoe McGraw-Hill.

Liskin J: *Moving medicine: the life and work of Milton Trager, M.D.*, Barrytown, NY, 1996, Station Hill Press.

Loving J: *Massage therapy: theory and practice*, Stanford, Conn, 1998, Appleton & Lange.

Lowe WW: *Functional assessment in massage therapy*, Corvallis, Ore, 1995, Pacific Orthopedic Massage.

Lowe WW: *Orthopedic massage,* ed 2, St Louis, 2009, Mosby.

Mackey B: Massage therapy and reflexology awareness, *Nurs Clin North Am* 36(1):159-169, 2001.

Massage Therapy Body of Knowledge Project, 2010 (website): http://www.mtbok.org/index.html. Accessed June 10, 2010.

McKay M, Davis M, Fanning P: *Messages: the communication skills book,* ed 2, Oakland, Calif, 1995, New Harbinger Publications-Mosby.

National Association for Nurse Massage Therapists: *Standards of practice,* West Milton, Ohio, 2006, National Association for Nurse Massage Therapists.

National Certification Board of Massage Therapy: *Code of ethics,* McLean, Va, 2006, National Certification Board of Massage Therapy.

Institute for Integrative Health Care Studies. *Ethics: therapeutic relationship.* Montgomery, NY, 2004, self-published.

Potter PA: *Basic nursing: essentials for practice,* ed 6, St Louis, 2006, Mosby.

Reese-Berryman N: *Muscle and sensory testing,* ed 2, Philadelphia, 2005, WB Saunders.

Rose MK: *The art of the chart: documenting massage therapy with CARE notes,* http://www.massageandbodywork.com/Articles/AprilMay2003/CAREnotes.html Accessed May 23, 2010.

Rubino J: *Been there done that,* Charlottesville, Va, 1997, Upline Press.

Salvo SG: *Mosby's pathology for massage therapists,* ed 2 St Louis, 2009, Mosby.

Shealy NC: *Alternative medicine – the complete family guide,* Versailles, Ky, 1996, Rand McNally.

Sohen-Moe C: Taking care of business: the ultimate client interview, *Mass Ther J* Fall:133-136, 1996.

St. John P: *St. John neuromuscular therapy seminars manual I,* Largo, Fla, 1995, self-published.

Starlanyl D, Copeland ME: *Fibromyalgia and chronic myofascial pain—a survival manual,* ed 2, Oakland, Calif, 2001, New Harbinger Publications.

Strong J et al: *Pain: a textbook for therapists,* New York, 2002, Churchill Livingstone.

Successful business handbook, Evergreen, Colo, 2001, Associated Bodywork & Massage Professionals.

Thibodeau G, Patton K: *Anatomy and physiology,* ed 6, St Louis, 2006, Mosby.

Thompson DL: *Hands heal,* ed 3, Baltimore, 2005, Lippincott Williams & Wilkins.

Torres LS: *Basic medical techniques and patient care for radiologic technologies,* Philadelphia, 1993, JB Lippincott.

U.S. Department of Health and Human Services: *Guidance on compliance with HIPAA transactions and code sets* (website): http://aspe.hhs.gov/admnsimp/HIPAACP.pdf. Accessed June 9, 2010.

MATCHING I

Place the letter of the answer next to the term or phrase that best describes it.

A. Assessment
B. Documentation
C. Informed consent
D. Intake form

E. Medical release
F. Null
G. Objective
H. Plan of care

I. Scope of practice
J. Subjective
K. Treatment plan
L. Written word

_____ 1. Data that is essentially a client's perception or point of view

_____ 2. If there is nothing to report in an assessment domain, place a _____ symbol or "∅" rather than leaving it blank

_____ 3. Best mode of communication in all professional arenas

_____ 4. Process of providing written information regarding client care

_____ 5. Strategies used by the therapist to resolve issues and address goals identified during the client intake

_____ 6. Form signed by the client authorizing the release of his or her records to a third party

_____ 7. Permission for treatment given by a client after he or she has been informed of the risks,

benefits, and consequences of the techniques and procedure(s)

_____ 8. The treatment plan is also referred to as the

_____

_____ 9. Client data that are measurable and quantitative

_____ 10. Health questionnaire that is the first element in the treatment planning process

_____ 11. Process involving appraisal of a client's condition based on subjective reporting and objective findings

_____ 12. Outlines activities and procedures that can be performed by members of a licensed profession

MATCHING II

Place the letter of the answer next to the term or phrase that best describes it.

A.   Activities of daily living
B.   Acute
C.   Chiropractic, acupuncture
D.   Chronic

E.   Client interview
F.   Closed-ended
G.   Disclosure
H.   Nonverbal

I.   Open-ended
J.   Palpation
K.   Paresthesia
L.   Part of informed consent

_____ 1.   Sensations of tingling, prickling, pins-and-needles, or numbness

_____ 2.   Commonly outside scope of practice for massage therapy (unless additional licensure is obtained)

_____ 3.   Descriptions of methods and modalities, potential risks and possible undesirable side effects, and right of refusal

_____ 4.   Communication using tones, gestures, posture, and facial expressions

_____ 5.   Types of questions that offer little restriction when answering and allow the client to reflect and clarify his or her thoughts and feelings

_____ 6.   Frequent movements or behaviors done at work and home such as sitting, standing, or chasing small children

_____ 7.   Provides the opportunity to review the client intake form, clarify information, and ask specific questions

_____ 8.   Pain that begins abruptly, has a recognizable cause, and is characterized by swelling, localized heat, redness, tissue damage, and loss of function

_____ 9.   Pain that usually develops slowly and persists for longer periods of time; original cause may not be known

_____ 10.   Assessment through touching with purpose and intent

_____ 11.   Type of question that is direct, usually requesting a factual or denial statement

_____ 12.   Honest and open revealing of personal knowledge as well as by the client thoughts and feelings

CASE STUDY

Scar Tactics

Rebecca, 28-year-old Caucasian female, is your next client. She just had her third child and her mother bought her a gift certificate for a 90-minute massage. Rebecca mainly wants to relax. On her intake form, she indicated that about 7 years ago, she had surgery on her left knee with no residual effects. You noticed the surgical scar is hypertrophic (elevated).

You read an article recently about the effects of massage on hypertrophic scars and how it improves their appearance. Rebecca wants to give the scar tissue massage a try today.

After placing a little Shea butter on your fingers, you mobilize the scar and the adjacent area with deep cross-fiber friction. As you massage the area, you focus on Rebecca's face, watching for signs of discomfort. After a few minutes, you glance back at the scar. The scar itself looks paler than it did before the application of pressure and the surrounding skin, in contrast, looks quite reddened. Additionally, the scar looks swollen and more hypertrophic than it did previously.

What do you think happened to the scar?
How would you explain this tissue reaction to Rebecca?
Is this type of massage out of your scope of practice?
What should you do next?

CRITICAL THINKING

When is it important to pay attention to nonverbal clues from a client? Give some examples.

CHAPTER 11

Special Populations and Pregnancy

"It is only with the heart that one can see rightly. What is essential is invisible to the eye."

—Antoine de Saint-Exupéry

LEARNING OBJECTIVES

After completing this chapter, the student should be able to:

- Implement individualized strategies for clients in special populations.
- Modify massage techniques and positions for expectant mothers during all stages of normal pregnancy.
- Customize or postpone treatments for clients who have a high-risk pregnancy.
- Provide a comfortable position for clients experiencing breast tenderness.
- Help provide massage to infants by instructing their parents and caregivers.
- Provide massage tailored to children and adolescents.
- Modify massage techniques to suit the needs of elderly clients.
- Provide massage that is appropriate for persons nearing the end of life.
- Explain modifications that are appropriate when working with obese clients.
- List ways massage can benefit clients who have substance abuse or addiction issues.
- Define ways massage can be modified for survivors of sexual abuse.
- Outline an appropriate strategy for clients who experience an emotional release during massage.
- Adjust massage techniques to accommodate clients with orthopedic disabilities.
- Compare and contrast disability and handicap.
- List ways to accommodate clients who have speech, hearing, or visual impairments.

http://evolve.elsevier.com/Salvo/MassageTherapy

INTRODUCTION

Therapists will encounter unique individuals with special needs and some with physical, emotional, and health-related challenges. Massage is safe during all stages of life if tailored to the client's health and particular situation and circumstance. Modifications might involve placing a client in advanced pregnancy on her side or massaging an elderly client while he or she sits in a comfortable chair. It may also entail using touch-based methods, working around catheters and intravenous lines connected to a client nearing the end of life, or being totally present while a client becomes emotionally overwhelmed during a session and begins to cry. As a therapist, you must be willing and able to accommodate the needs of all clients, no matter where they are on this journey called life.

Massage modifications for special populations and persons with disabilities and impairments are not difficult to provide. It usually involves reduced pressure over an area, positioning your client for comfort, or limiting sessions to 20 to 30 minutes. This chapter offers treatment guidelines as well as guidance regarding appropriate etiquette for behavior. However, no one can predict every possibility; be creative and innovative when needed, keeping safety and your client's best interests in the forefront.

Just as you do with all clients, approach these individuals with attitudes of loving kindness, reverence, and acceptance. It is important that you view these individuals as people first and their special need(s) as a secondary consideration. Furthermore, it is helpful to regard persons with special needs and disabilities as having a different ability or exceptionality. These terms bring to mind a positive connotation, focusing on the individual's strengths. As stated by Henry Holden, *attitudes are the real disabilities*. Fear may arise as you contemplate working on a client with disabilities or one who is elderly, but rest assured that knowledge combined with loving kindness, reverence, and acceptance will overcome fear.

GENERAL SUGGESTIONS

When your client mentions his or her special need or disability when making an appointment, spend time preparing for the session. This may include reviewing applicable information in this textbook or a pathology book written for massage therapists, or authoritative websites on the Internet. However, the best source of information comes from the client. Each situation will be different, and you must be willing to be open-minded, patient, tolerant, and flexible. Each client will teach you, if you are willing to listen and learn.

Keep your facilities as barrier-free as possible; the floor in your office, hallway, bathroom, and massage room should be free from clutter and from items such as throw rugs and wires from appliances.

Your client may be dealing with emotions and physical discomforts. It is a good idea to have tissues and drinking water handy.

The chapter on treatment planning (Chapter 10) discusses strategies used during the interview portion of the client intake. The information presented in the following list builds on those strategies, while modifying some to better fit the needs of your client with special needs.

- Sit near the client at eye level during the intake, if possible, not more than 5 feet away. This not only displays respect but also assists the exchange of information.
- Sit in a well-lighted place but avoid sitting with your back to a light source (i.e., lamp, window) as this will create a shadow over your face, making lip reading difficult.
- Speak naturally (not more slowly or more loudly) and enunciate clearly.
- Use your client's name as you speak to him or her.
- Be sure your client understands what is being said, and allow time for asking and answering questions.
- Rephrase any sentence that your client does not understand; do not just repeat the same words over again in the same sequence.
- Inquire about accommodations that can be made on your client's behalf.
- Not all health problems are written on an intake form. Take extra time each visit to look at and listen to your client. Do you see or hear something that was not disclosed previously? Before each subsequent session, update your client's health status to set goals for that day's treatment.
- When explaining procedures, tell your client which parts of the body you will be massaging or avoiding, using simple, nonanatomic terms. Reinforce verbal information with hand gestures such as touching the body area as you discuss it.

Additionally, be familiar with how to respond during medical emergencies (see Chapter 9).

PREGNANT CLIENTS

Pregnancy massage has many benefits for the expectant mother. Massage has been found to reduce stress, decrease swelling in the arms and legs, and relieve aches and pains in muscles and joints. Massage therapy has been found to reduce anxiety and depression. "Pregnant women are becoming more aware of what massage can offer them. I haven't met a pregnant woman who didn't like massage. They savor the moment, because they know that at the end of nine months, moments of free time and quiet are few and far between," says Sallie Mowles, LMT, who specializes in prenatal massage at Urban Oasis in Chicago.

The therapist can provide much-needed compassion and support. Pregnancy is often a time for reflection and introspection. Frequently, unresolved childhood issues come to the forefront. Active listening and massage will help your client better cope with the stress surrounding her pregnancy; caring, nurturing touch can bring comfort and solace.

There are many different responses to discovering one is pregnant. Some women are shocked, stunned, or confused, whereas others are elated. Some women may be struggling with new responsibilities facing them as parents, how the new family member will affect the relationship between themselves and their partner, and how the new baby will affect family finances, including concerns about the baby's health or resentments about discomforts surrounding the pregnancy. All of these feelings are normal and understandable.

Massage benefits can extend to the expectant mother's relationship with the co-parent. Offer the co-parent the opportunity to attend massage sessions. Teach loved ones massage strokes they can do at home to bring the pregnant woman much-needed relief. This activity will also facilitate the bond between co-parents and baby. Invite the co-parent to make loving remarks to both the pregnant woman and the new life within her. In this way, family bonding can be enhanced and nurtured through touch. Family bonding helps strengthen the shared love and responsibility of this new life.

Pregnancy is divided into three trimesters. The first trimester is the first 14 weeks of pregnancy (from the first day of the last period). The second trimester is week 14 to week 28. The third trimester spans from the 28th week to birth, which is around week 40. Pregnancy is discussed in Chapter 25.

Some discomforts of pregnancy are more prevalent in the first trimester (i.e., morning sickness, breast changes) and others are more common in the third trimester (i.e., backaches, edema, frequent urination).

Massage in the First Trimester. Massage is safe during the first trimester, which lasts till week 14. Massage should be postponed if your pregnant client is experiencing symptoms of miscarriage such as severe abdominopelvic pain, cramping, and spotting or vaginal bleeding. Advise her instead to seek immediate medical attention. In these cases, medical clearance is needed with subsequent massage. *This is true not only with pregnant clients in the first trimesters, but ALL trimesters as well.*

Additionally, postpone massage if your client is nauseated.

Massage in the Second Trimester. Many discomforts of the first trimester have resolved by the second trimester. The mother-to-be usually begins to feel energetic. She will begin to experience her baby moving between 18 and 22 weeks for first-time mothers and earlier for women who have had subsequent advanced pregnancies.

The pregnancy, with her changing body, begins to *show.* As the uterus grows, it crowds the intestines, and the mother may experience heartburn or constipation. Pressure on blood vessels occurs when she is lying supine. A small wedge or pillow tucked under her right hip tilts her abdomen

just enough to move the baby off the abdominal blood vessels. *These techniques should also be used in the third trimester.*

Massage in the Third Trimester. During the last trimester, the baby's growth is greater and postural changes in the mother are evident. Follow the applicable massage suggestions for position and technique modifications listed under the section "Preferred Positions." The mother may notice occasional, preparatory, or Braxton Hicks contractions in which the uterus tenses and then relaxes. Colostrum, the early form of breast milk, may leak from the breasts. Because of this, many women leave on their bras during the massage.

Massage and Common Discomforts of Pregnancy

A pregnant woman's body is challenged, changed, and stressed in many ways. Yes, the sweet burden of motherhood begins long before the baby is born. Throughout her pregnancy, the expectant mother watches her body change and she may have pregnancy-related discomforts with each passing month. Understanding these discomforts and implementing simple massage modifications will help your pregnant client get the most from her session.

Fatigue. Pregnancy puts a strain on the body (e.g., eating, breathing, eliminating for two) and requires a great deal of energy. Pregnancy-induced anemia and hormonal changes often cause the pregnant woman to feel unusually tired and fatigued, especially in the first and third trimesters. Getting a full night's rest is difficult if frequent urination is a problem. Nausea certainly costs the expectant mother energy, and feelings of depression or anxiety can be draining.

Massage Modifications – If she is overly fatigued, reduce treatment time to 30 minutes and use lighter-than-normal pressure to avoid further fatiguing the client. If she feels dizzy when getting up from the massage table, have her sit up slowly and remain seated for at least 30 seconds before standing. Be ready to assist.

Breast Changes. Blood supply to breasts increases and they become enlarged and tender, usually by the eighth week. Breasts may swell, tingle, throb, or hurt. Nipples enlarge and may become sensitive and sore. The areolae (pigmented areas around the nipple) darken and become broader. Stretch marks may also appear. During later pregnancy, colostrum may leak from her breasts in preparation for their job of infant nourishment.

Massage Modifications – Make her comfortable with a combination of client positions and soft but supportive cushions. Suggestions can be found in the section on breast comfort. If she elects to wear a bra during the massage, modify your technique to work around the bra. If breast secretions (colostrum) stain your sheets, treat them as contaminated (see Chapter 9).

Nausea and Vomiting of Pregnancy (NVP). Approximately 75% of pregnant women experience nausea and sometimes vomiting during their first trimester. Also known as *morning sickness*, NVP can begin as early as 10 days after fertilization and normally fades by the end of the third month. Some women feel nauseated off and on throughout pregnancy.

Massage Modifications – Massage is contraindicated while the woman is experiencing nausea. When she feels better and massage can be provided, avoid movements that cause rocking of the body. In some instances, she might be more comfortable receiving massage in a semireclining position. Have lemon drops, peppermints, or ginger candy nearby if she suddenly becomes nauseated during massage.

Heartburn. Heartburn is experienced as a burning sensation in the chest and is common during the third trimester. The sensation may extend to the lower throat. Heartburn may be caused by an expanded uterus, causing overcrowding of internal organs. Progesterone, a hormone that relaxes the smooth muscles of the uterus, also has an effect on the gastrointestinal tract. The valve between the esophagus and the stomach relaxes, allowing gastric juice to enter the lower esophagus. Progesterone also slows down motility, making digestion sluggish.

Massage Modifications – Avoid the prone position and, while she is supine, use a semireclining position by elevating her upper body. As her uterus expands, also include a wedge pillow or rolled towel tucked under her right side to avoid compression of abdominal blood vessels (more under "Preferred Positions").

Nasal Congestion. Approximately 30% of pregnant women have congestion without any other cold symptoms. Congestion usually starts in the third month of pregnancy and can last until the baby is delivered. Elevated and sustained levels of estrogen and progesterone cause increased blood flow to nasal mucosa, which results in mucosal swelling and increased mucus production. Pregnancy can also make allergies worse or cause hypersensitivity to allergens and other irritants.

Massage Modifications – Avoid the prone position and, while she is supine, use a semireclining position by elevating her upper body. As in cases of NVP, avoid scented lotions and aromatherapy, as many pregnant women are hypersensitive to odors. Box 11-1 includes a list of essential oils that are safe during pregnancy.

CHAT ROOM

To help create a more hypoallergenic space for your pregnant clients (or clients with hay fever), avoid plants, candles, dried leaves or flowers, and fabric drapes because they attract dust.

BOX 11-1

Essential Oils Safe for Pregnancy*

Grapefruit	Orange
Lavender	Petigrain
Lemon	Rose
Mandarin	Rosewood
Neroli	Frankincense

*Be sure they are used in dilutions appropriate for a child (diluted by one half).

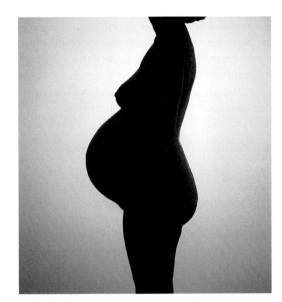

FIGURE 11-1 Silhouetted side view of a pregnant woman showing an exaggerated lumbar curve.

Lower Back Pain. Lower back pain is a common complaint as her uterus expands and she leans backward to compensate. This changes her center of gravity and she may rotate her pelvis forward, which places stress on the sacroiliac joints and lumbar spine (Figure 11-1). Another contributing factor is referred pain from overstretched uterine ligaments (see Figure 25-4).

Relaxin and other hormones increase the flexibility of the pelvic girdle and help the cervix relax and dilate during childbirth. Relaxin may have a slight effect on all joints in pregnant women by making them hypermobile. The effects of relaxin remain in the new mother's body for 4 to 6 months after childbirth.

Massage Modifications – Extra time can be spent on her lumbosacral area and buttocks; this may offer her temporary relief from pain. If she experiences pain while repositioning herself or getting off the massage table, suggest that she lie back down slowly and remain there until the pain subsides. After a few moments, suggest that she try again, moving more slowly this time. This type of abdominopelvic pain is often related to stretching and pulling of uterine ligaments.

Leg Cramps. Leg cramps (or Charley horses) are caused by the extra weight of a heavy uterus pressing against blood vessels and compromising blood flow to the legs. Other causes are muscle fatigue and electrolyte imbalances. Leg cramps can be painful and alarming, especially at night when they cause a sleeping pregnant woman to wake suddenly. Cramps can also occur in the foot.

Massage Modifications – Plantar flexion can stimulate leg cramps, so undrape her feet while she is supine or use a light drape to prevent the drape from creating this foot position. If a leg cramp occurs during the massage, place the ankle into dorsiflexion to stretch the calf muscles. If this does not stop the cramp, slide your fingers on the top of her foot and ask her to resist this movement by moving her toes toward her shin. Hold this position for about 5 seconds. Repeat if needed for a maximum of two more times. *Note: if pain occurs during dorsiflexion, it may be sign of deep vein thrombosis (DVT). If so, treat legs as a local contraindications.* See next section for more information.

Deep Vein Thrombosis and Blood Clots. Because of the decreased clot-dissolving property of blood during pregnancy and the increased clot-producing factor, she is at a higher risk for blood clots (5 to 6 times greater). This may lead to DVT, or blood clots in deep leg veins. Blood clotting factors typically normalize 8 to 10 weeks after childbirth.

To assess for DVT and possible blood clots, lightly palpate the entire leg, feeling for areas of localized heat or "hot spots." Hot spots may indicate the presence of DVT and/or blood clots.

Massage Modifications – If your pregnant client has hot spots on her leg, treat her entire legs as a local contraindication until the condition has resolved.

Varicose Veins. Many women develop varicose veins or find that they worsen during pregnancy. A heavy uterus pressing on blood vessels also increases the pressure in leg veins. Blood volume increases during pregnancy, which adds to the burden on the compromised venous system. Progesterone relaxes smooth muscles, dilates peripheral blood vessels, and contributes further to varicose veins and even hemorrhoids (varicose veins in the rectum).

Massage Modifications – Avoid the affected area if pressure causes pain. Less severe varicosities may benefit from massage. During massage, place the client's legs on bolsters or pillows to raise them above the level of the heart. Alternating gliding strokes toward the heart helps milk superficial veins and aids circulation.

Edema. Fluid volume increases during the third trimester and the growing uterus puts pressure on abdominal blood vessels. This often leads to swollen feet and ankles. Edema, or swelling, is more prevalent at the end of the day and is worse during the summer months. While some edema, or swelling, is normal in pregnancy, edema that increases all over the body, particularly in the legs, arms, lower back, and face, or a type of edema called pitting edema is cause for alarm. *Pitting edema* is a term used to describe the pit or dent left in the edematous skin when compressed for a few seconds and released.

Massage Modifications – Both widespread edema and pitting edema may indicate a serious problem requiring immediate referral to her physician. Postpone the massage until after she has received medical evaluation and clearance.

For mild edema, elevate the affected area using bolsters or pillows. This will help facilitate lymphatic and venous flow. Next, use gentle superficial gliding strokes applied centripetally. Massage proximal to the affected area first and then proceed distally (e.g., massage the thigh, then the leg, then the ankle, and then the feet). This will help clear the path for lymph and venous blood from distal areas. It is recommended to use 30 g of pressure or less to move the lymph.

Frequent Urination. As the uterus enlarges and presses on the urinary bladder, she may have to urinate more frequently. Hormonal changes also cause the retention of and the release of fluids.

Massage Modifications – Suggest that she void before massage as a comfort measure and be prepared for toilet breaks during the session. Avoid any sound of running water (e.g., rain, waterfalls, bubbling brooks). This sound may intensify the already frequent urge to urinate.

Stretch Marks. As the scales show weight gain in the later stages of pregnancy, stretch marks may appear on the abdomen, buttocks, thighs, hips, or breasts. At least one half of all pregnant women acquire stretch marks related to pregnancy weight gain. Stretch marks start out pink, reddish brown, or very dark brown, depending on the color of her skin, and later fade although they never totally disappear.

CHAT ROOM

The first trimester is an excellent time to recommend pubococcygeus exercises (formerly called Kegels). These are a regimen of isometric exercises involving voluntary contractions of the muscles of her pelvic diaphragm and perineum (in women, this is the area between the vaginal orifice and the anus) in an effort to increase the tone of the pelvic floor. Laxity and weakness of the pelvic floor muscles, often a result of childbirth, may predispose certain women to looseness of the vaginal wall and to urinary incontinence (loss of voluntary bladder control). Kegels involve the familiar muscular squeezing action that is required to stop the flow of urine while voiding. Instruct the pregnant client in how to duplicate the squeezing, pulling-up action. Hold the contraction for 10 seconds, allowing the muscles to relax between contractions. Perform four to six repetitions of the contraction in a series, and repeat the series three to four times each day.

Massage Modifications – Light pressure is indicated over stretch marks. Massage will not reduce stretch marks, because they are areas of overstretched, thinned skin rather than scar tissue.

Additional Suggestions

The following are some other suggestions to help make the massage safe and enjoyable for your pregnant clients.

Technique Restriction. Avoid connective tissue and deep myofascial release techniques because of the presence of the hormone relaxin. Also, avoid techniques that require manual traction of the lower extremities as this may cause separation of the pubic symphysis and produce pain over the area. As pregnancy progresses, joint mobilizations must be adjusted to protect and support all of the woman's increasingly lax joints.

Body Temperature. Avoid hot packs or any heating elements (including hot stones). If she states that she is feeling uncomfortable warm during the massage, help keep her cool by covering her with just a sheet or by uncovering the arms and legs. A cool washcloth may be placed over the forehead or across the base of the neck. An oscillating fan may also be used.

Belly. Use only light pressure over her abdomen after obtaining permission to massage this area.

Comfort. Also be willing to make adjustments in techniques, pressure, or her position on the table or chair. Be responsive to the pregnant woman's mood, both in conversation and body language. If your client is experiencing sadness or is grieving, be accepting and support of emotional expressions such as crying.

"The moment a child is born, the mother is also born. She never existed before. The woman existed, but the mother, never. A mother is something absolutely new."
—Bhagwan Shree Rajneesh

Preferred Positions

Traditional prone and supine positions are not appropriate and may be unsafe during most of her pregnancy without the appropriate use of supportive cushions. Positions recommended for a pregnant client who is no longer able to lie comfortably prone or who is past her first trimester include:

Supine. While she is supine, be sure her upper body is elevated and that she is tilted slightly toward the left by placing a small pillow, rolled towel, or wedge-shaped cushion under her right hip (Figure 11-2). This will prevent **supine hypotensive syndrome**. This syndome is dizziness

experienced when her blood pressure drops suddenly because her uterus is compressing major abdominal blood vessels and reducing circulation (Figure 11-3).

Side-Lying. Side-lying is a safe position for pregnancy massage. While she is lying on her side, place a pillow underneath her head. Place another pillow under the upper arm. A third pillow props her knee and ankle. Three additional smaller pillows may be added under the wrist of the lower arm, under the lower ankle, and under the abdomen, respectively (Figure 11-4). To avoid overstretching the sacroiliac joint, be sure her hip, knee, and ankle are aligned on the same horizontal plane. See Chapter 7 for more information regarding side-lying positions.

Prone. The prone position is not recommended once the client begins to "show" unless the therapist has, and is skilled in using, specialized body cushion systems. These are designed to properly support the pregnant woman's body. Pregnancy tables are not safe alternatives, because they may cause overstretching of uterine ligaments and may cause or aggravate lower back pain.

High-Risk Pregnancies

High risk pregnancies are ones that put the mother, the developing fetus, or both at higher-than-normal risk for complications during or after the pregnancy and birth. Factors that contribute to a high risk pregnancy are:
- Twins, triplets, or higher-order multiples
- History of preterm labor or delivery
- Maternal age (<15 and 35>)
- Vaginal bleeding
- Complications caused by pregnancy itself, such as gestational diabetes or preeclampsia
- Abnormalities or infections of the urogenital tract
- History of miscarriage
- More than five previous pregnancies
- Prepregnant weight is less than 100 lb or the woman is obese (a body mass index [BMI] of 30 is considered obese)
- When prenatal tests indicate fetal abnormalities
  Pregnancy massage expert Elaine Stillerman divides high-risk pregnancies into low, mid-, and high levels.

Low-Level Risk Factors. These include maternal age, multiples, use of ARTs (artificial reproductive technologies), complications from previous pregnancies, multiple past miscarriages, and fetal genetic abnormalities.
Massage Modifications – No treatment modifications needed other than those recommended for normal pregnancy featured previously in the chapter.

Midlevel Risk Factors. These are maternal illness or preexisting conditions, anemia, low weight gain or obesity, smoking, and substance abuse.

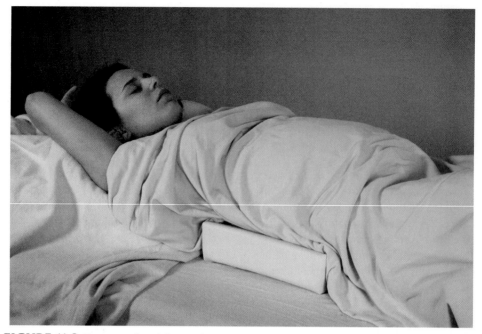

FIGURE 11-2 Pregnant client lying supine with cushion under her right side, tilting her to the left.

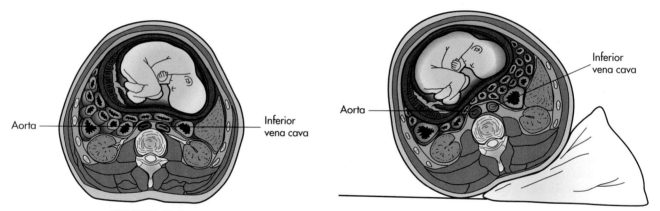

FIGURE 11-3 Cushion under the right side decreases abdominal blood vessel compression.

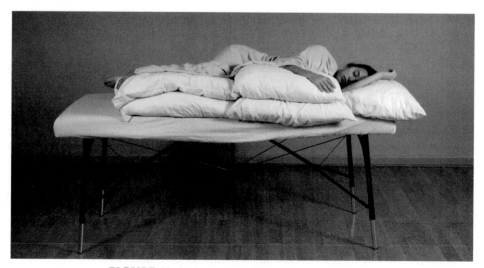

FIGURE 11-4 Pregnant client in a side-lying position.

Massage Modifications – Minimize treatment time to see how your pregnant client tolerates massage and then make modifications during subsequent sessions.

High-Level Risk Factors. These include vaginal bleeding, gestational diabetes, placenta previa or abruption (placement of the placenta over the cervical os or its premature detachment), premature labor, pitting edema, and lack of fetal movement in 8 to 10 hours.

Massage Modifications – Postpone massage until medical clearance is given (and may be denied).

Massage Post Partum

Once the baby is born, the mother's body begins its journey back to a prepregnant state. Some texts refer to this time as the fourth trimester. Postpartum massage can help the mother by reducing tension and soreness in muscles and enhancing relaxation. Vaginal bleeding (lochia) is normal and not a contraindication. This bleeding may occur for about the first 2 to 6 weeks after a vaginal birth or cesarean section (C-section).

Vaginal Births. Position your client for comfort. There are no restrictions for prone and supine positions, although her breast might need extra support in the prone position. The uterus will return to normal size relatively quickly with fundal massage done every 4 hours for 10 days to 2 weeks post partum. Teach and encourage the new mother to massage her own abdomen. Additionally, the rectus abdominis heals and returns to normal relatively quickly with massage and can begin as early as 3 days post partum. You may draw muscles together toward the midline and manually vibrate them or knead the two sides of the rectus abdominis as they are moved toward the midline (see Figure 21-159).

C-Section. Position her for comfort, which may include avoiding the prone position since the incision is located on her abdomen. Because surgery involves cutting into the body, blood clots form as part of the healing process. Blood clots can also form in the veins of the pelvis and lower extremities as a result of reduced blood flow. Reduced blood flow can also occur because of inactivity and bed rest, both common after surgery.

Because of these risks, deep pressure and vigorous massage should be avoided on the lower extremities. These restrictions should apply for 10 days after she is ambulatory. Scar mobilization can begin once the incision is fully healed (6 to 8 weeks).

Breastfeeding. Offer the nursing mother water before and after the massage because her fluid needs increase during this time. She may elect to wear her nursing bra during the massage because she may leak milk. Her breasts may be sore and tender, and she may feel more comfortable in a side-lying position during the massage. Be sure to address tension in her back, neck, shoulders, and arms, which may be tight from holding the baby during feedings. If mother's milk accidentally spills on the linens, treat them as contaminated (see Chapter 9).

> *"A baby is born with a need to be loved—and never outgrows it."*
> —Frank A. Clark

BREAST COMFORT

Finding comfort in the prone position can be a challenge for clients who have large breasts or breast tenderness regardless of size. Breast tenderness may be due to a variety of conditions including menopause, menstruation, nursing, pregnancy, breast surgery, biopsy, and fibrocystic breast change. See Chapter 25 for further information.

There are several options you can use to help make your female client more comfortable while she is lying prone. You may offer her a rolled-up towel or cylindrical pillow placed under, above, or between her breasts, whichever is most comfortable. Many clients prefer a supportive device both above *and* below the breasts (Figure 11-5). Use a face rest that can be adjusted above the level of the table. Several massage table manufacturers now carry tables fitted with recessed channels that allow the client to lie prone comfortably (see Figure 3-2) or have specially designed bolstering systems.

With the client in the supine position, addressing muscles in the pectoral region may be difficult. It is appropriate to ask her to use the back of her hand to retract the breast medially (Figure 11-6). This technique establishes a safe physical boundary between client and therapist. You may decide to work on this area with the client in a side-lying position, holding her top arm above the elbow with her bottom hand (Figure 11-7). These modifications are also useful to a postpartum or nursing mother.

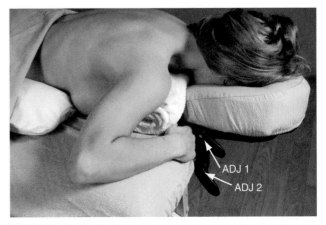

FIGURE 11-5 Cushions placed above and below the breasts. Face rest frame is adjusted above the level of the table.

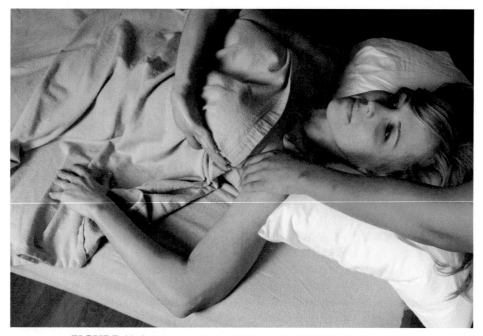

FIGURE 11-6 Woman retracting her breast with the back of her hand.

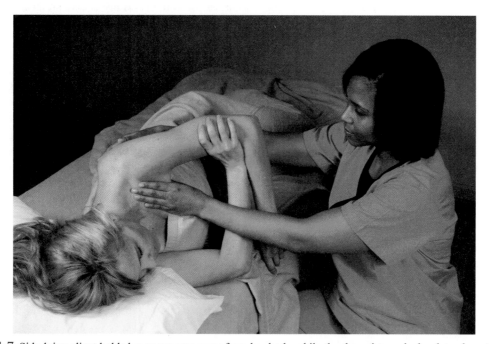

FIGURE 11-7 Side-lying client holds her upper arm away from her body while the therapist works her lateral pectoral muscles.

INFANTS

Infant massage has many benefits for both the giver (parents or caregivers) and the receiver (baby). Infant massage may foster parent-infant bonding; relieve discomfort from teething, congestion, gas, and colic; and promote deeper and longer sleep for the baby. In infant massage, the massage therapist does not massage the baby, but rather instructs and encourages the parents and caregivers to provide massage and loving touch to the baby. The infant massage instructor often uses a doll to demonstrate strokes while the mother or caregiver mimics what is seen (Figure 11-8).

According to Drs. Marshall Klaus and John Kennell, **bonding** is a "solid connection between the parent and child that nourishes the child on a core level." Bonding occurs when certain elements are in place soon after the baby's birth. These elements include skin-to-skin contact, odor or scent, high-pitched voice, prolonged eye contact, warmth, and the reestablishment of biorhythmic activity that existed between the mother and the baby in utero. Infant

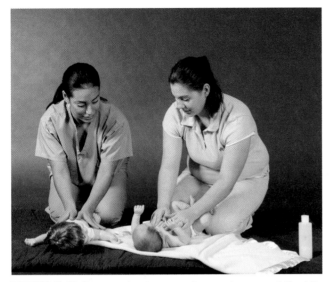

FIGURE 11-8 Therapist demonstrating strokes on a doll while the mother mimics her moves.

massage is especially suitable as a vehicle for all of the necessary elements for parent-infant bonding, a process that builds trust and intimacy, calls forth the innate protective and nurturing instincts in parents, and sets the tone for a quality, long-term parent-child relationship.

Massaging the Baby

Depending on the age and developmental stage of the baby (e.g., 4 months, 8 months) the positioning of the infant ranges from lying beside the baby, holding the baby, placing the baby between your knees, or having the baby draped across your lap.

Do not massage the baby for 30 minutes after bottle feeding. However, breast-fed babies can be massaged shortly after feeding because breast milk is predigested.

When massaging the baby, the most commonly used strokes are touch-holds, thumb-over-thumb gliding, and thumb spreading, as well as full-hand gliding. Rather than applying strokes as a routine, use massage to enjoy the time with the baby. Strokes can be modified, refined, or even created according to the baby's response and tolerance. Remember, never leave the baby unattended.

▌MINI-LAB

Without judgment, observe parent-infant interaction and notice how the parents calm their baby. Do they use movement, voice, touch, or visual engagement? What else do you observe?

Additional Suggestions

The following are suggestions to help the parent or caregiver and baby get the most from the experience.

Warmth. The room should be warm and without drafts. Keep areas that are not being massaged covered with a blanket, especially for newborn or very young babies.

Lighting. Natural light or low light is best. Babies can become overstimulated with fluorescent lighting.

Music. Soft background music can assist the parent in creating the rhythm for the massage and promote the relaxation response. The favorite music for the baby is the parent's voice singing a lullaby or just talking or humming.

Lubricant. Use food-grade oils such as almond, safflower, and olive because oil will inevitability end up in the baby's mouth. Avoid mineral oils because they clog the skin's pores and are not digestible. Also avoid scents; they may cause an allergic reaction in a sensitive baby. Keep all supplies handy, but keep oil bottles closed because they are easily knocked over during the massage.

CHILDREN AND ADOLESCENTS

Children and adolescents, or pediatric clients, are defined as young people between 3 and 18 years of age. Working on this age group is not much different than working on adults. Because most children have a small stature and short attention span, the massage session may only last 30 to 45 minutes. Extra time can be used to establish a rapport.

Because children are not of legal age, they must have a parent or legal guardian consent to therapy on their behalf. Be sure this person is present during treatment planning and during discussions of policies and procedures. Any documents requiring a legal signature (such as the intake form and consent form) must be signed by the attending parent or legal guardian (e.g., John Doe Salvo, minor, by Susan G. Salvo).

During the intake, be sure the child or adolescent understands all of the procedures and willingly gives consent. Even with consent from the parent or guardian, massage is inappropriate on a child who does not want it. Touch is a powerful experience, one that cannot be undone. The potential for influencing the attitude and acceptance of touch cannot be underestimated. How touch is given, and how the child receives it, will determine whether the child becomes a person who views touch, especially during massage treatments, as nurturing, positive and beneficial or as something to be avoided.

Because reflexes that stimulate neurologic responses such as erections are often overly sensitive in adolescent boys, keep the top drape bunched up in the groin area and use a blanket over the top drape. This helps disguise any sexual response to the massage that is innocent, but often embarrassing to the client. If an erection does occur, ask a few questions about a mundane topic such as school or sports. This often reduces the "tent-effect."

"I'm not 70, I'm eighteen with 52 years experience."
—Anonymous

Elderly

The elderly, or geriatric, clients represent the fastest-growing segment in the massage client population. **Geriatric** refers to someone who is 70 years of age or older. However, just as there are no typical 30 year olds, there are no typical 70 year olds. An elderly person can be quite active and independent, living without assistance. Some older adults require some assistance with various daily activities and may live at home or in an assisted-living facility. Others may be frail and cannot function without skilled help. Most persons in the latter group are in long-term care facilities or at home with family or caregivers.

The elderly present massage therapists with some unique challenges. There are physical changes ranging from thinning skin, reduced muscle mass, and vision and hearing impairments. Ninety percent of the elderly reported having at least one chronic medical condition, most often managed with medications. It is also necessary for the therapist to implement a thorough intake procedure and have an understanding of medication side effects that affect massage (see Table 10-2).

This age group faces many lifestyle and emotional changes such as retirement, reduced income, and the loss of loved ones. To meet the needs of this population segment, the therapist needs to cultivate understanding, patience, thoroughness, kindness, caring, and caution.

Sensorineural deficits and the effects of illness predispose the elderly to accidental injury. Reported disability increases with age. Over 50% of older persons stated that they had some type of disability (sensory, physical, or mental). Some disabilities were minor, whereas others required assistance; 57% of persons over 80 years of age reported severe disabilities.

Diseases such as heart disease and high blood pressure (hypertension) occur more frequently in the elderly; both are seen in more than 50% of the elderly. The therapist must be aware of the possibility and frequency of *orthostatic hypotension* (dizzy spells) related to medication use. Many elderly women, and even some elderly men, have osteoporosis (decreased bone density). Cerebral changes increase the likelihood of Alzheimer disease, the most common form of dementia. Roughly 9% of seniors report having problems with balance and coordination. Cataracts, glaucoma, macular degeneration, and diabetic retinopathy are the most common problems of aging eyes and contribute to visual impairments. Hearing impairment increases with age: 1 in 3 people older than 60, and half of all people older than 85, have significant hearing loss.

How does all this relate to massage? Sixty-five years is the age at which massage therapists begin to take into account the aging process and how it may have affected a client's body. Although each client is assessed individually, physical changes might affect massage treatment in persons 65 and older. A table on the Evolve website lists many physical changes seen in the elderly.

Assess the client's vitality and vigor during the intake interview (Figure 11-9). Decide, based on the client's health status and activity level, which category of aging he or she falls into (robust or frail). Active, robust seniors still experience body changes that accompany the aging process, but can benefit from a more vigorous massage. If the client is frail, he or she would benefit from a shorter and gentler massage with techniques using a broader, perpendicular, more even pressure.

The attitude with which a therapist approaches the elderly client is often different. Respect your client's slower pace rather than maximizing massage time. Schedule time in the appointment to allow for the client to undress (sometimes layers of clothes have to come off); you may have to help him or her onto the table and off the table, perhaps with the use of a stepstool (see Figure 11-10). The client may need a time of transition after the massage or would like to share a personal story with you.

Additional Suggestions

The following suggestions will help you provide the best care possible for your elderly clients. Keep in mind that a robust senior may not require any accommodations, whereas a frail person may require a combination of several. Tailor sessions to the needs of the individual client.

Reduce Pressure. Aging skin is more easily injured owing to reduced skin elasticity and decreased subcutaneous fat. Because of this risk, reduce downward pressure and sliding (or shearing) force. However, reduced pressure does not

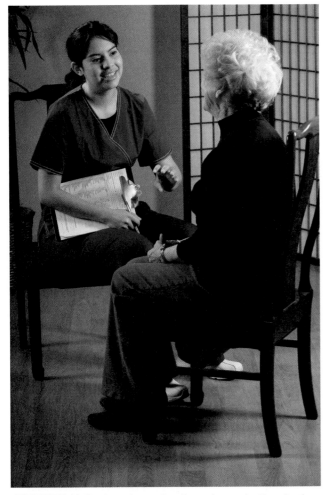

FIGURE 11-9 Therapist performing a thorough client intake.

translate into a light massage. Maria Mathias, massage instructor and author, uses the phrase "gentle strength" when describing the reduced pressure. Even with reduced pressure, strokes are still firm and broad; use the entire palm surface of the hand.

Avoid Stretches and Limit Joint Movements. It is vital to perform only gentle joint mobilizations such as rocking on elderly clients, especially if they are sedentary or bedridden. Be sure to constantly monitor the client, because these movements can be tiring.

Extreme stretches are avoided owing to the possibility of damaging fragile bones, ligaments, and tendons.

Shorter Sessions

If your client is frail or chronically ill, treatment time is shorter, about 30 minutes, to reduce the possibility of fatiguing the client. Sharon Puszko, PhD, LMT, owner and director of Day-Break Geriatric Massage Institute, recommends:

- 5 minutes of unhurried effleurage, deep breathing, and gentle rocking
- 20 minutes of focused work on feet, legs, back, shoulder, or neck (client determined)
- 5 minutes of closure work

Avoid Prone Position. Many frail elderly clients are uncomfortable or have difficulty breathing while lying prone or have problems turning from supine to prone (or vice versa). Supine, side-lying, and seated positions are best. Note that medical facilities such as hospitals also avoid the prone position for this age group.

Inspect Feet. Physical limitations and visual impairments make it difficult for the elderly to inspect their feet. Because foot problems are common, it's a good idea to inspect your client's feet. If the client is wearing socks or slippers, obtain permission to remove them. Explain that you will inspect the feet before massage. Avoid any areas in the feet that look or feel unhealthy including swollen or inflamed joints. Bring these areas to the attention of the client (or caregiver). If socks or slippers were removed, replace them before moving to another area of the client's body.

Warmth. Because of reduced metabolism and decreased subcutaneous fat, many elderly persons tend to feel uncomfortably cold. Use lightweight blankets over the client's draped naked or clothed body. You can use a heated table pad during cooler weather, but turn off the pad when the client gets on the table as heated pads can potentially damage fragile skin.

Session Location and Time. Most visits to your office should be scheduled during daylight hours because many elderly people do not like to drive after dark. Sometimes, it is better if the massage is performed at the client's residence rather than the therapist's office. Be flexible; if your client feels unsafe getting onto and off your massage table, be willing to massage him or her in a chair or on a sofa or bed. The floor is not an option because it may be difficult for the elderly to get up from the floor.

Safety Issues. Falling is the most common safety issue for the elderly. There are several contributing factors:

- Many elderly people have sensorineural or musculoskeletal conditions or commonly use medications. These can alter balance, coordination, and response time.
- Orthostatic hypotension is common, which causes dizziness.
- Visual impairments are common.

To reduce the risk of falling, provide unobstructed passage to and from the massage table. Be sure to assist in the removal of any eyeglasses, hearing aids, or placement of walkers. At the conclusion of the session, replace these items. Additional information is located in the sections on visual and hearing impairment.

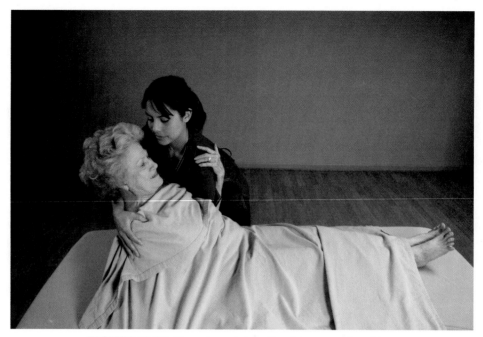

FIGURE 11-10 Therapist assisting client into a seated position.

Remove excess lubricant from the client's feet with a plush towel. Remind your client to sit up for a moment before standing and to move slowly rather than quickly when moving upright. If needed, assist the client (Figure 11-10).

"Tell them that death is absolutely safe.
It's like taking off a tight shoe"
—Pat Rodegast, in contact with a
disembodied being named Emmanuel

Hospice: Persons Nearing the End of Life

Massage during the final stage of life can bring comfort and is an important method of relating when communicating verbally is difficult or impossible. Hospice is often an integral part of this life stage. The goal of hospice is provide caring, compassionate, and high-quality care to clients and their family members during the final stage of life. These services include pain management, as well as emotional support.

Because the goal of massage is palliative, some of the standard rules of contraindications do not apply. For example,

if your client has a fever or pitting edema, gentle massage is still appropriate. **Palliative care**, also called comfort care, seeks to improve the quality of life by relieving symptoms and reducing suffering. You are not trying to fix or correct anything; you are there to offer comfort.

As your client moves closer to death, body systems begin to slow and shut down. When this occurs, certain changes can be noted; some are listed below. These changes do not cause your client pain or discomfort, nor are they contraindications to gentle massage strokes. Not all are seen in every dying person; just as every life is unique, so is every death.

- Skin becomes cool to the touch and becomes mottled.
- The feet, hands, lips, and nose often appear grayish-blue.
- The underside of the body may darken in color.
- Body temperature varies, causing the affected person to feel unusually cold or warm.
- Breathing can be irregular and shallow with periods of apnea (temporary cessation of breathing) that increase in length.
- A gurgling sound may be heard during breathing as air moves across saliva and mucous pools in the back of the throat.
- At the moment of death, laryngeal spasm may produce a gasp or a cry. This is normal reflex and does not mean your client is in pain or distress.

Be sure to teach loved ones and caregivers to perform gentle massage strokes. This makes massage accessible to everyone. Also, encourage frequent expressions of affection, such as holding the client's hand (Figure 11-11).

When massaging someone who is near the end of life, addressing your own feelings about death and dying is helpful. You might attend workshops that are part of a local

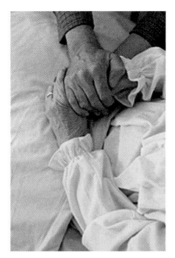

FIGURE 11-11 Therapist holding a client's hand.

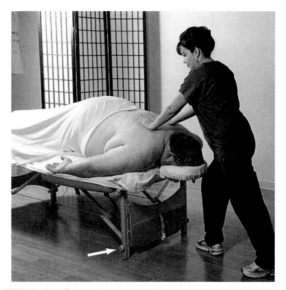

FIGURE 11-12 Lower your table height to ensure proper body mechanics.

hospice program and read books on the subject. Several authors who have written books on the subject are Elisabeth Kübler-Ross, Stephen Levine, and Bernie Siegel. These resources may be helpful in working with people near the end of life, because they and their loved ones face grief issues.

Before you decide to work with a client who is dying or terminally ill, make a personal commitment to stay with him or her until death, because abandonment is often difficult for your client to face at this time. Additionally, take care of yourself. Find something that will serve as an outlet for the energy you spend around sickness, sadness, fear, and grieving. Know that you will probably become attached to the client, cry when death comes, mourn the loss, grieve with his or her family, and grow from the experience.

Additional Suggestions

The following guidelines may be used to help you provide a safe, nurturing massage.

Positioning. Side lying and semireclining are often the most comfortable positions. Avoid the prone position.

Technique and Duration. Use only light compression or gentle gliding strokes. The massage rarely exceeds 30 minutes.

OBESE INDIVIDUALS

Incidence rate of obesity has increased significantly over the past 2 decades. A person is regarded as obese when his or her BMI is 30 or over. A desirable BMI for most middle aged adults is 22 to 27.

The three leading causes of death in the United States are associated with obesity (cardiovascular disease, type 2 diabetes, and cancer). Obesity is also a risk factor for hypertension, stroke, gallstones, osteoarthritis, and sleep apnea.

Many obese individuals have suffered criticism and prejudice; they often feel vulnerable and sensitive. When the obese client encounters a therapist who expresses loving kindness and is nonjudgmental, it can be a healing and transforming experience.

Some obese clients may feel uncomfortable within their bodies and may elect not to disrobe for the massage. In these cases, be willing to work through clothing.

Additional Suggestions

The following suggestions will help you provide a comfortable, safe, and nurturing environment for your obese clients.

Positioning. Because most obese clients have a wider-than-normal girth, consider lowering your massage table height or have a small platform on which you can stand. This will provide better leverage and improve your body mechanics (Figure 11-12). A lower table also assists the client, as he or she may feel awkward or unsafe getting onto and off the table. Have a foot stool available for client use, and be willing to offer assistance.

Because many obese clients suffer from sleep apnea and other breathing problems, elevate their upper body while they are supine and limit the time spent in the prone position.

Draping. Use a large flat sheet as a top drape during the massage. Drape your client even if he or she is fully clothed.

Pressure. Avoid deep pressure in areas that contain excessive amounts of fat because this tissue is extremely vascular and is susceptible to bruising. Also reduce pressure in edematous areas.

PERSONS WITH ADDICTION ISSUES

Addiction is a persistent, compulsive dependence on a behavior or substance. Addiction may develop when a person becomes overwhelmed with life's stressful events or as a temporary escape from uncomfortable feelings. Examples of these feelings are pain, inadequacy, sadness, loneliness, anger, and fear. The person becomes trapped in a cycle of pain and escape. The addictive behavior continues to escalate until the consequences of addiction exceed the pain of the emotions. Examples of additive substances are nicotine, alcohol, and narcotics. Acts of overeating, sex, or gambling can be regarded as an addiction if the act is used continually to escape painful feelings.

When a client enters recovery and during episodes of relapse, massage can be used to relieve stress and promote body awareness.

Although massage can assist the recovering addict by increasing relaxation, the combination of education, support, and counseling by a qualified mental health care provider is the best tool for overcoming this disorder. Most massage therapists are not licensed to provide counseling services, but they can offer these special clients acceptance and moral support as a part of their recovery.

SURVIVORS OF SEXUAL ABUSE

You will likely encounter clients who are survivors of sexual abuse. Sexual abuse crosses all population barriers, with a majority of incidents perpetrated by family members, extended family members, friends of family members, or personal friends (as in date rape). Massage can help heal the wound of abuse by making touch an emotionally and physically safe experience.

One of the reasons that sexual abuse is so traumatic is that sex is such a powerful experience. Sex has the potential of being the ultimate expression of intimacy or one of the worst bodily assaults possible. Many survivors become people of extremes, often developing compulsive habits. They may overeat to a point of obesity, cocooning themselves physically and emotionally by hiding inside excess body weight. Or they may relate to their bodies as a source of self-esteem and become compulsive about exercise and diet.

Extreme behaviors may also involve sexual inappropriateness (more common with long-term childhood molestation). Survivors may have difficulty understanding proper sexual boundaries and either fear or encourage sexual interactions. It is imperative that the therapist become a role model by possessing and enforcing appropriate boundaries while avoiding the slippery slope of sexual misconduct (see Chapter 2).

To anesthetize the pain of sexual abuse, many survivors develop addiction (see previous section). In fact, mental disorders involving anxiety, depression, or addiction are often what propel survivors of sexual abuse into counseling.

Then, as different layers of various issues begin to reveal themselves, he or she may come to discover incidents of sexual abuse, or he or she may have always been aware of the abuse.

Massage can be a wonderful adjunct to therapy and help your client heal the wounds of sexual abuse. It is best to begin with shorter sessions to see how your client responds to massage. Because much of sexual and physical abuse is more about power and control than the physical act, let your client have a lot of control over the massage environment.

Additional Suggestions

Body Boundaries. Because the body is the medium for the wound, and massage is performed on the body, take extra precautions to ensure a nurturing, emotionally safe, and healing environment. Remind your client that he or she controls the session. If your client indicates she would rather you not touch a certain area of her body, honor this request even if prior consent was given. For example, if your client initially requests deep massage on her lower back, but suddenly becomes uncomfortable and asks you to move on to another area, do so without asking for an explanation.

Draping. Emphasize that he or she can disrobe down to a personal comfort level and that draping will be used at all times. Heavier draping material may help your client feel more safe and secure.

> *"Seek not, forbid not."*
> —A.W. Tozer

Emotional Release

Occasionally, clients release emotions during a massage session. These releases can be expressed as deep sighs, laughter, shaking, and/or tears (the most common expression). Clients release emotions for a lot of reasons. Emotional tension may be stored as muscle tension and when one is released, so is the other. Clients may feel a high level of safety with their therapists, safe enough to let down defenses and release emotional tension. Although we are not counselors, we can support the client during the process. Here are some tips on handling your client's emotional release.

- Approach the situation with the attitude of total acceptance. Do not interfere with probing questions.
- Discontinue massage and make touch contact in an area that is neutral (examples are shoulders, arms, and feet). Your client has another task now—releasing emotions (Figure 11-13).
- Remain in the room unless instructed to leave by your client. Abruptly leaving the room without client directive may be interpreted as abandonment.
- When appropriate, remind your client that tears and feelings are normal and that he or she is in a safe place. Ask

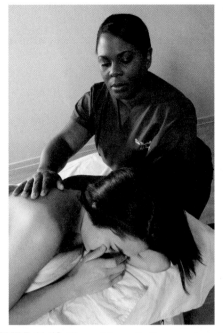

FIGURE 11-13 Therapist comforting a crying client.

if he or she would like to take a short break and then continue with the massage or end the massage for that day. Regardless of which option is chosen, be calm and accepting, and avoid encouraging or discouraging a particular response.

If the client asks for an explanation of what happened, mirror back what you observed. Do not offer your personal interpretation or analysis.

Clients in counseling or psychotherapy are more likely to experience emotional releases. Also, clients who suffer from chronic pain or who have a debilitating illness are also more likely to experience emotional releases. In these cases, it is appropriate to discuss how you will handle the situation if and when it occurs. In fact, the neutral area being touched during the emotional release can be determined by the client at this time.

CHAT ROOM

Do not be quick to offer facial tissues to a client experiencing emotional release. Drying someone's tears or offering the tissue too fast can be taken as disapproval of crying and of the feelings beneath it. But have tissues within client reach so there is an option.

After an emotional release, clients may feel fractured, confused, or in an emotional void. Some clients will feel self-conscious. Provide a safe, private space for your client to wind down and collect his or her thoughts after the session. Avoid asking your client to leave your office while he or she is in a raw, wounded, or disassociated state.

Note that the client may feel embarrassment or shame connected to the release, and may (sadly) choose not to return to your office. This decision must be respected.

As professionals, it is important that we get in touch with our own feelings about others who express emotions. You must be willing to witness another person's pain without interruption. If you are truly uncomfortable with emotional release, be honest with yourself. Support the client through the experience the best way you can. It is inappropriate to discuss your discomfort with emotional release while he or she is on the massage table or immediately after the emotional release when he or she may feel vulnerable. Later, share your feelings of apprehension with a counselor, preceptor, fellow therapist, or a peer support group. If you choose not to work with clients prone to emotional release, discuss your limitations with your client during the intake of the next session. Perhaps you both can come up with a mutually satisfying resolution. If this is not possible, refer your client to a massage therapist who is trained and comfortable in dealing with these issues.

More detailed discussions on boundaries and the therapeutic relationship are in Chapter 2.

CHAT ROOM

Legal statutes do a good job of outlining our scope of practice. However, situations can arise in everyday practice that can create confusion and "muddying the waters" of scope of practice. Massage therapists need to have solid and impeccable boundaries regarding the type of care they offer a client. Although the mind, body and spirit cannot be separated in their physiologic functioning, massage therapists must be absolutely sure that their treatments, advice, and focus remain on the soft tissue of the body. We can recognize the imprint that the emotions make on the fascial structures of the body, but we should avoid engaging the client in conversations or exercises that address the human psyche directly.

PERSONS WITH ORTHOPEDIC DISABILITIES

People with orthopedic disabilities experience a decreased range of physical movements, causing difficulties with tasks such as sitting or walking. These individuals often use mobility aids such as wheelchairs, canes, or walkers. Causes of these disabilities include spinal cord injury, stroke, arthritis, heart disease, emphysema, diabetes, obesity, inactivity, and amputation. Some disabilities are temporary, such as those incurred while healing from surgery or injury.

The first consideration in working with clients using mobility devices is how they will enter your massage establishment. Most municipalities require businesses to be barrier-free as well as wheelchair-accessible, but if yours is not, then schedule a home visit and perform the massage off site.

During the intake, ask your client to describe the impairment and the degree of limitation. Do not overlook limitations caused by the disability indirectly. For example, it is not uncommon for a person with an orthopedic disability to be physically fatigued from moving. Your client may need

VIMALA SCHNEIDER McCLURE

Born: June 7, 1952

"Do all the good you can in all the ways you can, for all the people you can for long as ever you can."
—P. R. Sarkar

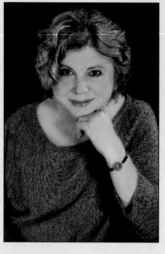

Vimala Schneider McClure, the pioneer of infant massage in the United States, always had the feeling that she was put on earth to fulfill a specific purpose. At age 21, the starry-eyed humanitarian sold everything she had and took off for India. "I was terrified," she confided, "but my sense of purpose was so strong it was worth putting myself in harm's way."

In India, McClure studied with yogi master P. R. Sarkar until a bout with malaria cut her trip short and landed her in a New York hospital for a couple of weeks. Somewhat recovered from the malaria, McClure returned to India and worked in an orphanage. The nun who ran the orphanage spent much of her time begging for money for its support; thus McClure was left to care for the children along with two Indian girls. "They couldn't speak my language, and I couldn't speak theirs," she remembers. It was here that she learned traditional Indian baby massage.

"They've done it in India for 10,000 years or more," she explains. Mothers massage their infants and pass along the skill to their daughters. "I began to see how relaxed these children were ... how different [they were]

from American children. They were easier with each other and less aggressive. Boys and girls alike walk around with their arms around each other. Then it began to click. I began to see massage as something that could change lives. A good analogy is that we're like a cup, and the more love that goes into that cup, until it is overflowing, the more you can give. If your cup didn't get filled as a child, then you're always looking for someone to fill it up."

McClure returned to the United States in 1976 and became pregnant with her first of two children. In addition to everything she had learned in India, she asked friends to teach her some Swedish massage techniques for her newborn. She writes: "This joyful blend provided my son with a wonderful balance of outgoing and incoming energy, of tension release, and stimulation. Additionally, it seemed to relieve the painful gas he had been experiencing that first month."

McClure began to keep copious notes. Eventually, she invited mothers over to show them what she was doing. During these sessions, she distributed a small hand-made flyer. One of these flyers fell into the right

to rest a bit when he or she first arrives. Furthermore, the client may be taking prescribed medications with accompanying side effects such as headaches, drowsiness, disorientation, and reduced sensation (the last is often a therapeutic effect rather than a side effect). Information provided by your client will determine any modifications.

In addition, be sure to check for any compensatory patterns that develop as the result of the disability itself, from treatments, or from the use of assistive devices. Many of these areas of muscle tension can be reduced with massage.

Wheelchairs

Your client can be massaged in a wheelchair. Place pillows atop a massage table onto which your client can lean forward. If a table is unavailable, place a cushion in the client's lap

and have the person lean onto it (Figure 11-14). Be sure that the chair wheels are locked.

Because of the degree of upper body strength needed to propel a wheelchair, trigger points may be located in the shoulders and chest area. Locate and deactivate them using pressure within the client's tolerance.

Clients with greater mobility usually elect to use the table. The person in the wheelchair knows how to transfer, or move, him or herself into and out of the chair.

Additional Suggestions

Suggestions for clients with orthopedic disabilities include:

Wheelchair Etiquette. When speaking to a person in a wheelchair, sit down so both of you will be at eye level. A wheelchair is part of the body space of the occupying

VIMALA SCHNEIDER McCLURE (*continued*)

hands, and she was invited to speak at a childbirth education conference. There, she met the owner of a baby products company who asked, "Have you ever thought about writing a book? Write one, and I'll publish it."

And so, McClure's notes became *Infant Massage: A Handbook for Loving Parents,* which was then published by Bantam Books, then Random House, and is still the definitive work on infant massage today. Pressed by others to begin an organization, she founded the International Association of Infant Massage, now a worldwide operation.

McClure's advice is to start with a different mindset because what happens between parent and child is different from what happens during a therapeutic massage. McClure says, "It's the act of bonding and impacting a lifetime. That's why I trained instructors to teach parents rather than training massage therapists to massage infants. As an instructor, you have to allow parents to develop their own style. Even if they don't apply strokes in an expert manner, the message comes through. You have to empower parents and not allow them to turn over their power to the instructor as the expert."

McClure is quick to share her philosophies of infant massage:

- Teach the parents to ask permission before they massage their baby. Initially a show of thoughtfulness, this action becomes an authentic sign of respect as the baby grows. If the baby indicates no, then the massage is postponed.
- Teach them slowly. Parents are often sleep-deprived, overwhelmed with new responsibilities, and cannot

process a lot of new strokes. Just give them a few massage movements. Parents can practice and keep building their skills each week while the baby's tolerance increases. In this way the massage is effective both for parents and baby.

- Give them credit for their successes. Given that the parent is the one who is massaging the baby, success is attributed to parental competence rather than to the skills of either a massage therapist or an infant massage instructor.
- Take your cues from the baby. Parents want to know that they are doing the strokes correctly. Teach them that they need to look to the baby for confirmation rather than to the instructor. A baby is a person; connect to this person to determine what works best.

Discovering what works best is a process. Infants cannot tolerate massage as long as adults; parents need to be prepared to be finished when the baby is finished. The length of time varies with each child and each session. Babies also do not do well with unconscious touch. You know how a massage feels when a therapist is hurrying or not paying attention. The same applies with infant massage: if the parent is hurried or unfocused, then the massage will not feel good to the baby.

Students are often amazed to hear that massage is not always so great for a baby. Remember that less is more. Infant massage is not about the volume of strokes; it is about sharing a moment of time and going deeper into it together.

---

person. Avoid leaning on it and push it only when asked. If it appears the client needs assistance, offer it. Respond to a "no thank you" graciously if your help is declined.

Pressure. Use lighter pressure over areas of *paresthesias* (sensations of tingling, prickling, pins-and-needles, or numbness) or over the legs, where there is an increased risk of blood clot formation. On other areas, use only moderate pressure.

Technique Restriction. Generally speaking, the longer your client has been inactive, the weaker the bones will be, so limit all stretching and joint mobilizations, especially on the spinal column and hip joints.

Skin Inspection. Inspect the skin before massage begins. Skin ulcers are local contraindications; avoid up to 4 inches

around the ulcer's edge. Bring these to the client's and caregiver's attention. Decubitis ulcers are discussed in Chapter 22 under the "Dermatologic Pathologies" section.

Body Temperature. Many clients with orthopedic disabilities have poor thermal regulation; check in with your client periodically and make appropriate adjustments such as a fan or warm blanket.

MINI-LAB

Obtain a wheelchair and use it to move about your home or neighborhood for at least 20 minutes. Next, lie on the floor and see if any part of your body feels strained or fatigued. Use this information as you look for compensatory patterns on your wheelchair-bound clients.

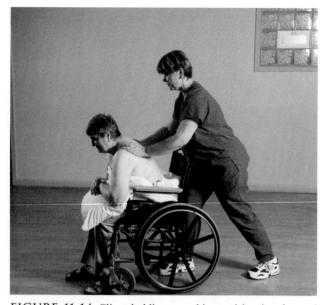

FIGURE 11-14 Client holding a cushion and leaning forward during the massage.

Persons With Speech and Hearing Impairments

Speech impairments create limited speech patterns or ones difficult to understand. Speech impairments, which include stuttering, stammering, and hoarseness, can be caused neurologically, or by drug abuse, vocal abuse, or hearing loss.

Hearing impairments create partial to total loss of hearing; the latter condition is referred to as *deafness*. These types of impairments can be due to genetic or hereditary factors or result from childhood disease. Most persons who are deaf use one or more visual methods of communication, such as American Sign Language (ASL) or lipreading.

Speech and hearing impairments often coexist, especially if a hearing impairment was acquired when the person was very young.

When communicating with your speech or hearing impaired client before the massage begins, consider note writing or typing on a computer using an Arial or Comic Sans font and the zoom view feature set at 200%.

Older persons often develop a hearing impairment as a result of the aging process. The affected person may correct some hearing loss by wearing a hearing aid. If your client is wearing a hearing aid during the massage, avoid moving your hands close to the client's ears. Proximity to the hearing aid generates feedback, producing an uncomfortable squeak in the wearer's ear.

If your client has removed a hearing aid for the massage or has severe hearing loss, be sure to gain your client's attention before you begin to speak. Eye contact is considered a sign of attention. Waving a hand in the person's direction or tapping a person lightly on the shoulder or arm is acceptable; the latter method can be used when your client is lying face down in the face cradle and cannot see you.

Additional Suggestions

Communication Etiquette. Enunciate clearly and normally, but do not exaggerate your lip movement, because this makes lipreading difficult. Keep your language simple and to the point. Do not eat, smoke, chew gum, or hold your hands in front of your mouth while you talk. Stand close and do not let any object obstruct the person's view of you. Use facial expressions and body language to clarify your message. Do not be embarrassed to be expressive.

Interpreter. If your client has a sign language interpreter, direct your conversation to your client rather than to the interpreter.

PERSONS WITH VISUAL IMPAIRMENTS

Visual impairment is the consequence of loss of vision and can range from partially sighted to total blindness. This can be the result of disease (cataracts, glaucoma, diabetic retinopathy), trauma (sports, chemicals), brain and nerve disorders (lazy eye, crossed eyes), or a congenital or degenerative condition (albinism, macular degeneration).

As a reminder, keep your facilities barrier-free. Bright, ambient lighting is best. For client safety, it is a good idea that your table linen color contrast with the color of the floor. Some therapists also have contrasting top and bottom sheets.

When you step into the room where your client awaits, announce your presence while speaking in a normal tone of voice. Begin by addressing your client by name, and then state your name. When transferring your client from one area to another, stand just in front of the person or to his or her left. He or she may choose to touch your right elbow and follow you. Be sure to announce ahead of time any changes in direction, such as when you turn to enter the massage room.

Describing surroundings, using the face of a clock as a reference, may be helpful. Instead of saying, "There is a table in front of you," say, "There is a table at 2 o'clock." Next, tactually familiarize your client with the massage room and placement of equipment (such as a massage table) before the session begins.

Next, go into detail about what you are going to do and what you would like the client to do. Use descriptive words such as straight, forward, left, and right. Avoid vague terms such as *over there*, *here*, *this*, and *that*. When handing your client an object (such as bottled water), touch it to the hand so he or she does not have to grope for it.

When you exit the room, let the client know you are leaving. Never begin a massage unless he or she knows that you have reentered the room and maintain physical contact throughout the massage as much as possible. If room lights were dimmed before the massage, be sure and raise the lighting level back up before you exit the room. This is true for any client, not just those who are visually impaired.

Keep equipment and supplies in the same place and explain to the client about any changes during subsequent sessions.

Additional Suggestions

Suggestions to accommodate students who have visual impairments include:

Printed Materials. For printed materials, choose Arial or Comic Sans in 16 to 18 point or larger font and use white or yellow paper with black ink. When enlarging printed materials using a copy machine, use a 160% to 175% setting. This will enlarge an 8.5 × 11-inch page to an 11 × 17-inch page. It might be helpful to use a dark sheet of paper placed behind the printed paper to make a window for reading.

Support Persons and Animals. If your client has an assistant, acknowledge that person, but direct all conversation to the client, not the assistant. Do not pet or touch a guide dog, because this may distract the dog from his task of assisting the client. Be sure to provide a comfortable place for the assistant or animal during your client's session.

MINI-LAB

Working with a partner, take turns blindfolding each other and allow approximately 20 minutes each to explore your environment. How can this experience be used to better understand and provide appropriate care to your clients who are visually impaired? Share your experiences with your classmates. This activity can also be done with earplugs to simulate hearing impairments.

E-RESOURCES

⊜volve

http://evolve.elsevier.com/Salvo/MassageTherapy
- Chapter challenge
- Flash cards
- Photo gallery
- Educational animation
- Additional information
- Weblinks

BIBLIOGRAPHY

Applegate EJ: *The anatomy and physiology learning system*, ed 3, Philadelphia, 2006, Saunders.

Artal R, Friedman MJ, McNitt-Gray JL: Orthopedic problems in pregnancy, *Phys Sports Med* 18:93-105, 1990.

Avery MD, Van Arsdale L: Perineal massage: effect on the incidence of episiotomy and laceration in a nulliparous population, *J Nurse Midwifery* 32(3):181-184, 1987.

Barnett K: A survey of the current utilization of touch by health team personnel with hospitalized patients, *Int J Nurs Stud* 9:195, 1972.

Barstow C: *Tending body and spirit: massage and counseling with elders*, Boulder, Colo, 1985, Cedar Barstow.

Bass E, Davis L: *The courage to heal*, Philadelphia, 1994, HarperCollins.

Beera MH, Berfow R: *Merck manual of geriatrics*, ed 3, Whitehouse Station, NJ, 2000, Merck Research Laboratories.

Bernard K: *Keys to caregiving. Nursing child assessment satellite training (NCAST) manual*, ed 2, Seattle, 1995, University of Washington School of Nursing.

Curties D: *Massage therapy and cancer*, Moncton, New Brunswick, Canada, 1999, Curties-Overzet.

Damjanov I: *Pathology for the health professions*, ed 3, Philadelphia, 2006, Saunders.

Diego MA et al: Massage therapy of moderate and light pressure and vibrator effects on EEG and heart rate, *Int J Neurosci* 114:31-44, 2004.

Dychtwald K: *Age power: how the 21st century will be ruled by the new old*, New York, 1999, Jeremy P Tarcher/Putnam.

Dychtward K, Flower J: *Age wave: the challenges and opportunities of an aging America*, Los Angeles, 1989, Jeremy P Tarcher.

Ebersole P et al: *Gerontological nursing and healthy aging*, ed 2, St Louis, 2005, Mosby.

Ebersole P, Hess P, Schmidt Luggen A: *Toward healthy aging, human needs & nursing response*, ed 6, St Louis, 2004, Mosby.

Eisenberg A, Murkoff HE, Hathaway SE: *What to expect when you're expecting*, New York, 1991, Workman.

Eliopoulos C: *Manual of gerontologic nursing*, ed 2, St Louis, 1999, Mosby.

Engelmann GJ: Massage and expression or external manipulation in the obstetric practice of primitive people, *Massage Ther J* 33(3):34-40, 92-110, 1994.

Evans M: Complementary therapies: reflex zone therapy for mothers, *Nurs Times* 86(4):29-31, 1990.

Falconer J: Being of service, *Massage Bodyw* Feb/Mar: 132-137, 2002.

Feldman W: *Learning disorders: a guide for parents and teachers*, Buffalo NY, 2000, Firefly Books.

Feldt KS: *Increasing physical activity in frail, older adults: guidance for clinicians.* Presented at American Geriatrics Society Annual Scientific Meeting, Washington, DC, 2002.

Field T, et al: Elder retired volunteers benefit from giving massage therapy to infants, *J Appl Gerontol* 17:229-239, 1998.

Fordyce M: *Geriatric pearls*, Philadelphia, 1999, FA Davis.

Fritz S: *Fundamentals of therapeutic massage*, ed 4, St Louis, 2009, Mosby.

Gorsuch R, Key M: Abnormalities of pregnancy as a function of anxiety and life stress, *Psychosom Med* 36:353, 1974.

Gould BE: *Pathophysiology for the health professions*, ed 3, Philadelphia, 2006, Saunders.

Guthrie RA: Lumbar inhibitory pressure for lumbar myalgia during contractions of the gravid uterus at term, *J Am Osteopath Assoc* 80:264-266, 1980.

Heath H, Schofield I: *Healthy ageing—nursing older people*, St Louis, 2000, Mosby.

Heller S: *The vital touch*, New York, 1997, Henry Holt and Company.

Hernandez-Reif M et al: Parkinson's disease symptoms are differentially affected by massage therapy versus progressive muscle relaxation: a pilot study, *J Bodyw Mov Ther* 6:177-182, 2002.

Hiniker PK, Moreno LA: *Developmentally supportive care, theory and application*, Norwell, Mass, 1994, Children's Medical Ventures.

Ignatiavicius DD, Varner Bayne M: *Medical-surgical nursing: a nursing process approach*, ed 2, Philadelphia, 1995, WB Saunders.

Inkeles G: *Massage and peaceful pregnancy*, New York, 1983, Putnam.

Jones NL: *The Americans with Disabilities Act: overview, regulations, and interpretations*, Hauppauge, NY, 2003, Novinka Books.

Kahn RL, Rowe JW: *Successful aging*, New York, 1998, Pantheon Books.

Klaus MH, Kennell JH, Klaus PH: *Bonding: building the foundations of secure attachment and independence*, San Francisco, 1983, Addison-Wesley.

Knaster M: Researching massage as real therapy: an interview with Dr. Tiffany Field, *Massage Ther J* 33(3):45-53, 1994.

Leboyer F: *Loving hands: the traditional art of baby massage*, New York, 1997, Newmarket Press.

Leigh S: Aromatherapy: making good scents, *Mothering* 59:77-79, 1991.

Linton AD, Lach HW: *Matteson & McConnell's gerontological nursing: concepts and practice*, ed 3, Philadelphia, 2007, Saunders.

Liu BA et al: Falls among older people: relationship to medication use and orthostatic hypotension, *J Am Geriatr Soc* 43(10):1141-1145, 1995.

Lohman JS: Massage for elders: an ever-growing opportunity, *Massage Ther J* 40(3):60-79, 2001.

MacDonald G: Easing the chemotherapy experience with massage, *Massage Mag* 84:85-91, 2000.

MacDonald G: *Medicine hands: massage therapy for people with cancer*, Tallahassee, Fla, 1999, Findhorn Press.

Mathias M, Mathias W: *Infant touch and massage instructor manual*, Albuquerque, NM, 2002, Self-published manuscript.

Mathias M: *Instructor training for infant massage*, Presented at workshops in Dallas, Tex, 1986 and Lake Charles, LA, 1992.

Mathias M: Personal communication, 2006.

McCance KJ, Huether SE: *Pathophysiology: the biologic basis for disease in adults and children*, ed 5, St Louis, 2006, Mosby.

McConnellogue K: The courage to touch: massage and cancer, *Massage Bodyw* Dec/Jan: 12-20, 2000.

McKay M, Davis M, Fanning P: *Messages: the communication skills book*, Oakland, Calif, 1987, New Harbinger.

Meek S: Effects of slow stroke back massage on relaxation in hospice clients, *Image J Nurs Sch* 25(1):17-21, 1993.

Meiner SE, Lueckenotte AG: *Gerontologic nursing*, ed 3, St Louis, 2006, Mosby.

Miesler DW. *Readings in geriatrics: topics for bodyworkers*, ed 3, Sunrise, Fla, 2001, Massage Review.

Milinare C: *Birth*, New York, 1990, Random House.

Monohan FD et al: *Phipps' medical-surgical nursing: health illness perspectives*, ed 8, St Louis, 2007, Mosby.

Montagu A: *Touching: the human significance of the skin*, ed 3, New York, 1986, HarperCollins.

Napolitano R: *Loving pregnancy massage: a manual for practitioners and educators*, Pine Bush, NY, 2000, Natural Wellness.

Nelson D: *Compassionate touch: hands-on caregiving for the elderly, the ill and the dying*, Barrytown, NY, 1994, Station Hill Press.

Nelson D: *From the heart through the hands: the power of touch in caregiving*, Findhorn, Scotland, 2001, Findhorn Press.

Nelson D: Growing old with massage, *Facility Care, Massage Bodyw Mag* Feb/Mar, 2001.

Nelson D, Allen B: *Therapeutic massage in facility care: benefits, effects, and implementation*, Sunrise, Fla, 1996, Massage Review.

Osborne-Sheets C: Massage and the pregnant pelvis, *Mass Ther J* 37(2):88-96, 1998.

Osborne-Sheets C: *Pre- and perinatal massage therapy*, San Diego, 1998, Body Therapy Associates.

Ostgaard HC et al: Prevalence of back pain in pregnancy, *Spine* 17(1):53-55, 1992.

Puszko S: Personal communication, 2007, 2010.

Rich GJ: *Massage therapy: the evidence for practice*, St Louis, 2002, Mosby.

Rich P: *Practical aromatherapy*, Bath, UK, 1994, Parragon Book Service.

Rockwood K, et al: A global clinical measure of fitness and frailty in elderly people. *Can Med Assoc J* 173(5):489-495, 2005.

Rose MK: *Comfort touch: massage for the elderly and the ill*, Philadelphia, 2010, Lippincott Williams & Wilkins.

Rose MK: *Comfort touch massage for the elderly and the ill, DVD*, Boulder, CO, 2004, Wild Rose.

Rose MK: *Comfort touch: nurturing acupressure massage for the elderly and the ill* (website): http://www.massagetherapy.com/articles/index.php?article_id=566. Accessed June 18, 2010.

Rounseville C: Phantom limb pain: the ghost that haunts the amputee, *Orthop Nurs* 11(2):67-71, 1992.

Salvo SG: *Mosby's pathology for massage therapists*, ed 2, St Louis, 2009, Mosby.

Salvo S: *Massage therapy: principles and practice*, ed 1, Philadelphia, 1999, WB Saunders.

Schneider McClure V: *Infant massage: a handbook for loving parents*, New York, 2000, Bantam Books.

Schrag K: Maintenance of pelvic floor integrity during childbirth, *J Nurse Midwifery* 24(6):26-30, 1979.

Scott D et al: The antiemetic effect of clinical relaxation: report of an exploratory pilot study, *J Psychosoc Oncol* 1(1):71-83, 1983.

Sloane PD: *Normal aging, primary care geriatrics: a case-based approach*, ed 3, St Louis, 1992, Mosby.

Smith DG: *The challenge of diversity: involvement or alienation in the academy. Report No. 5*, Washington, DC, 1989, School of Education and Human Development, George Washington University.

Smith S, Gove J: *Physical changes of aging*, EDIS (website): http://edis.ifas.ufl.edu/HE019. Accessed June 20, 2010.

Stillerman E: *Mothermassage: a handbook for relieving the discomforts of pregnancy*, New York, 1992, Dell.

Stillerman E: *Prenatal massage: a textbook of pregnancy, labor, and postpartum bodywork*, St Louis, 2008, Mosby.

Thibodeau G, Patton K: *Anatomy and physiology*, ed 6, St Louis, 2006, Mosby.

Thibodeau G, Patton K: *Structure and function of the body*, ed 12, St Louis, 2004, Mosby.

Tortora GJ: *Introduction to the human body: the essentials of anatomy and physiology*, ed 5, Hoboken, NJ, 2000, John Wiley & Sons.

Tortora GJ, Grabowksi SR: *Principles of anatomy and physiology*, ed 11, New York, 2005, John Wiley & Sons.

Trenter ME: *From test tube to patient*, Food and Drug Administration (website): http://www.fda.gov/oc/seniors/. Accessed January 14, 2010.

Turner Bernhardt R: Massage therapist as doula, *Massage Ther J* 33(3):46-48, 1994.

United States Department of Justice: *Americans with Disabilities Act* (website): http://www.usdoj.gov/crt/ada/adahom1.htm. Accessed January 10, 2010.

United States Department of Labor: *Office of Disability Employment Policy* (website): http://www.dol.gov/odep/. Accessed January 10, 2010.

Waters B: *Massage during pregnancy*, ed 3, Saint Augustine, Fla, 2003, Bluewaters Press.

Weidner N: Personal communication, 2002.

Williams A, editor: *Teaching massage: foundation principles in adult education for massage program instructors*, Philadelphia, 2008, Lippincott Williams & Wilkins

Williams D: Touching cancer patients, *Massage Mag* 84:74-79, 2000.

Wold GH: *Basic geriatric nursing*, ed 3, St Louis, 2004, Mosby.

Worfolk JB: Keep frail elders warm! *Geriatr Nurs* 18(1):7-11, 1997.

MATCHING I

Place the letter of the answer next to the term or phrase that best describes it.

A. Blood clots
B. First trimester
C. Food-grade
D. Hip, knee, and ankle
E. Medical clearance
F. Pitting
G. Relaxin
H. Right hip
I. Supine hypotensive syndrome
J. Third trimester
K. Weeks 14 to 28
L. Weeks 18 to 22

_____ 1. Needed before massaging a pregnant client who complains of cramping or vaginal bleeding (and it may be denied)

_____ 2. Trimester in which backaches, edema, and frequent urination are more prevalent

_____ 3. Usually the time in pregnancy when the mother begins to experience her baby moving

_____ 4. Where to place a rolled up towel or small cushion under a supine pregnant client to prevent abdominal blood vessel compression

_____ 5. Type of edema in a pregnant client may indicate a serious problem requiring immediate medical referral

_____ 6. Week range indicating the second trimester of pregnancy

_____ 7. Dizziness experienced in pregnant women when blood pressure drops suddenly because the uterus is compressing major abdominal blood vessels

_____ 8. Presence of this hormone requires avoiding connective tissue and deep myofascial release techniques on a pregnant client

_____ 9. Joints aligned in the same horizontal plane to avoid overstretching the lower back sacroiliac joints in a side-lying pregnant client

_____ 10. Type of oil such as almond, safflower, and olive that is recommended for use during infant massage

_____ 11. Trimester in which discomforts such morning sickness and breast changes are more prevalent

_____ 12. These may be present in a pregnant woman's deep leg veins when pain is felt with dorsiflexion of her relaxed feet

MATCHING II

Place the letter of the answer next to the term or phrase that best describes it.

A. 65
B. Acceptance
C. Barrier-free
D. Consent

E. Dizzy spells
F. Education, support, counseling
G. Geriatric
H. Hospice

I. Orthopedic
J. Over 50 percent
K. Palliative
L. Stretching

_____ 1. Technique avoided on the elderly because of the possibility of damaging fragile bones, ligaments, and tendons

_____ 2. Phrase synonymous with orthostatic hypotension

_____ 3. Type of care that seeks to improve the quality of life by relieving symptoms and reducing suffering

_____ 4. Percentage of older persons stating they have some type of disability

_____ 5. Someone who is 70 years of age or older

_____ 6. Attitude with which the therapist approaches his or her client who is experiencing an emotional release

_____ 7. Type of care that offers pain management as well as emotional support to a client and client's family during the final stage of life

_____ 8. Best tools for overcoming any type of addiction

_____ 9. Must be provided by a parent or legal guardian before a child who is not of legal age can be treated

_____ 10. Condition in which the office floor, hallway, bathroom, and massage room are free from clutter and items that can be tripped over

_____ 11. Client age when massage therapists should begin to take into account effects of the aging process

_____ 12. These types of disabilities include decreased range of physical movement, which cause difficulties with tasks such as sitting or walking

CASE STUDY

Up in Smoke

Susan was the mother of four children and the wife of a loving husband. For their fifteenth wedding anniversary, Susan's husband bought her a massage with her therapist, Delilah. He had been laid off work recently and saved up to give this anniversary gift to his wife. She had been stressed because of a recent diagnosis of a chronic illness. He would stay home with the children while she relaxed.

Susan was diagnosed with chronic obstructive pulmonary disease, specifically, chronic bronchitis. She had smoked for 20 years and it had taken its toll on her lungs. Susan's doctor instructed her to avoid cigarette smoke. She was currently on a drug regimen to quit smoking and it was successful.

When Susan arrived for her appointment, she was ready for tranquil moments. The receptionist greeted her and asked her to have a seat and that Delilah would be with her shortly.

When Delilah called Susan to the massage room, she was anticipating the smell of clean linens, soothing music, and an inviting atmosphere. To her surprise, there was an overwhelming stench of cigarette smoke in the room and on Delilah's clothes. Delilah greeted her with a welcoming smile and asked Susan about her health since her last visit. Susan informed her of the recent diagnosis. She told Delilah about the avoidance of cigarette smoke. Delilah, who was a cigarette smoker, thought nothing of this as she did not smoke in the building.

CASE STUDY—cont'd

About 10 minutes into the massage, Susan started to fill nauseated and began to cough. Delilah asked her if she would like a glass of water. Susan nodded. Delilah left the room. When she returned, Susan was still coughing and nearly dressed. Susan drank the water and told Delilah that she could not continue with the massage, stating that she had a headache and felt queasy. Delilah felt that Susan was upset as well.

How should Delilah respond to Susan's sudden illness? Should Delilah address that Susan seemed upset? If so, how might she do this? If Delilah was told the truth, how might she respond to the criticism? Once told, should Delilah assume responsibility and refund the charges? Since this was a gift, how should Delilah involve the gift giver? Should Susan be referred to a nonsmoking therapist for future sessions?

How should Susan tell Delilah about the offensive odor? Susan does not want to change therapist, because she loves Delilah's work, so how might she address the situation for future sessions? How might Susan tell her husband that the massage was an awful experience?

CRITICAL THINKING

What points are helpful to remember when working with any client with a special need? In particular, what should the therapist do if he or she is presented with an unfamiliar condition?

CHAPTER 12

Hydrotherapy and Spa

"Nothing on earth is as weak and yielding as water, but for breaking down the firm and strong, it has no equal."

—Lao Tzu

LEARNING OBJECTIVES

After completing this chapter, the student should be able to:

- Define hydrotherapy and discuss its history.
- Define spa; then compare and contrast types of spas.
- Describe the factors that contribute to the effects of water on the body.
- Describe benefits of heat and cold, contraindications, and application methods.
- Name several bath and shower techniques and application methods.
- Identify methods of exfoliation.
- Demonstrate how to apply a wet and a dry body wrap.
- Discuss the specialized hydrotherapy methods listed in this chapter.
- Discuss how aromatherapy works.
- Define essential oils and give several examples.
- Describe proper storage and handling of essential oils.
- Identify characteristics of and rationales for the use of essential oil carriers.
- Discuss essential oil safety.
- Name ways aromatherapy and essential oils are used in massage and spa services.

http://evolve.elsevier.com/Salvo/MassageTherapy

INTRODUCTION

Water, transformational by its very nature, has always been used to obtain and maintain health, manage pain, and treat physical and emotional ailments. The Babylonians, Egyptians, Indians, Cretans, Chinese, Japanese, and Mesopotamians have all advocated and used water's healing effects in the form of various baths and other treatment methods. Water also has been an essential component in religious rituals and healing rites of these various cultures (e.g., rites of passage such as baptism). Hippocrates, the father of Western medicine, advised both hot and cold bathing. He was the first to record the use of contrast baths.

Although both ancient Greece and Rome had adopted the beliefs that water had healing properties, the Romans were the first to integrate hydrotherapy into their social and political life, building temples and baths near natural springs. Ancient Greek societies built public baths in conjunction with gymnasiums to facilitate sound bodies and sound minds (Figure 12-1). Bath temperatures were adjusted to the needs of each individual bather and to achieve the intended therapeutic outcome. In Sparta, laws were passed that made frequent bathing mandatory.

Hydrotherapy is the internal and external therapeutic use of water and complementary agents. Agents added to the water to enhance its therapeutic value are soaps, essences, aromatics, minerals, seaweed, salt, carbon dioxide, and oxygen. The word *hydrotherapy* finds its roots in the Greek word *hydro*, meaning "water." Hydro as a prefix is defined as fluid or liquid.

Water is often heated, cooled, or pressurized for use in specific applications. Water, in its various forms, continues to be used to enhance the health and well-being of individuals and can be used to add therapeutic value to massage therapy.

Father Sebastian Kneipp (1821-1897), from Worshofen, Bavaria, in western Germany, is regarded as the father of hydrotherapy. Father Kneipp possessed exceptional knowledge and skill in using water to heal the ailments that afflicted his community. These treatments, known collectively as Kneipp therapy, are still used today and are found on menus of services at world class spas. Key components of this therapy are herbal and mineral baths, as well as cold or alternating hot and cold treatments administered by water, stones, or pebbles. Kneipp published his only book on hydrotherapy, *My Water Cure,* in 1886.

In the nineteenth and early twentieth centuries, sanitariums were established as a type of health resort where individuals could go to regain health after a long-term illness such as tuberculosis. Water treatments and massage were central components. The most famous sanitariums were located in Hot Springs, Arkansas; Saratoga Springs, New York; and White Sulphur Springs, West Virginia. John Harvey Kellogg (see Chapter 1) opened his sanatorium in Battle Creek, Michigan. These began to close after the arrival of antibiotic therapy.

SPA

The term **spa** is used to describe a place where water therapies are administered. The common denominator for both massage and water therapies, according to international spa expert Robin Zill, is that the "skin is the portal of entry" for both. *Spa therapies* include a variety of body treatments administered in spas that may or may not incorporate massage, but water is the heart of the spa experience.

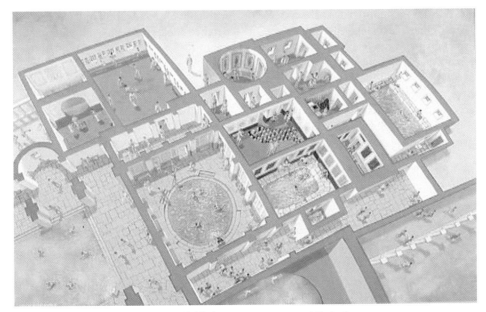

FIGURE 12-1 Ancient Roman public bath.

The origin of the word *spa* is uncertain. Some scholars believe the term is derived from the Walloon (Wallonia, Belgium) phrase *espa,* meaning "fountain." Other scholars, however, believe that the word comes from the letters *S-P-A* that were scribbled on the marble walls of ancient public baths of Rome. This is translated from the Latin term *sanus per aqua,* meaning "healing through water" or "cure of water." In those times, the spa was more than just a place to relax; it was considered a sacred space—a place to experience nurturing, transformation, and healing on both spiritual and physical levels.

In the sixteenth century, people traveled to the town of Spa, Belgium, to "take the waters" as a way to rest, retreat, find lost health, preserve vitality, and rejuvenate.

Massage therapists have begun to add spa services to their repertoire, which can range from hot towels to scrubs to steam baths to body wraps. Clients enjoy these additional ways to relax and revive themselves. This chapter offers exposure and training in several hydrotherapy and spa applications.

Spa esthetics and ambience play an important role because beauty and art go hand in hand with the spa experience. Spas have evolved to include four basic types of facilities: day spas, hotel or resort spas, destination spas, and medical spas. Most spas offer their own signature treatments.

- **Day spa.** Day spas provide beauty, health, and therapeutic treatments, with services varying by provider. Most are combined with a hair salon. As the name suggests, day spas offer their services on a day-use basis where clients remain for a few hours or the day. Overnight accommodations are not available.
- **Hotel or resort spa.** These spas are owned by and located within a resort or hotel. These facilities provide professionally administered spa services, fitness and wellness components, and spa cuisine menu choices.
- **Destination spa.** These facilities offer overnight accommodations, professionally administered spa services, physical fitness and wellness elements, educational programming, and spa cuisine to provide their guests with lifestyle improvement and health enhancement.
- **Medical spa.** Medical spas provide both medical and wellness care in an environment that integrates spa services. These services are supervised under a medical doctor and may include modalities such as Botox injections and aggressive chemical peels.

CHAT ROOM

In 1785, Antoine Lavoisier proved that water is composed of two parts hydrogen and one part oxygen. (Author C. S. Lewis added "one part magic.")

WATER AS A HEALING AGENT

Water turns into a solid called *ice* at 32° F and into a vapor called *steam* at 212° F. Heat can be added to or removed from water to change its physical state. Adding heat to ice excites the molecules and causes them to move farther apart, changing a block of ice into a puddle of water and a puddle of water into a cloud of water vapor. Removing heat from water turns vapor into liquid and liquid into solid. Chemically, water remains unchanged; it is always H_2O even though its state has changed.

The four major factors that contribute to the effects of water on the body are its *temperature,* its *moisture and mineral content,* and its *mechanical effect.*

Temperature

Temperature variation is the most common method of influencing hydrotherapy treatments. The body's ability to maintain homeostasis in a changing environment is the key that unlocks one of hydrotherapy's primary benefits. As the nervous system perceives the difference between the body temperature and the temperature of the water, it responds to warm or cool the body by altering the diameter of blood vessels and, therefore, alters blood flow (Box 12-1). Lymph flow is also affected. The greater the difference between the body temperature and water temperature, the greater the effect will be; this may be harmful.

By increasing and decreasing blood and lymph flow, hydrotherapy can assist the body in detoxifying. Water is the universal solvent; the flow of water parallels the movement of electrolytes. By using water externally, the internal flow of water (blood and lymph) is altered to move oxygen and nutrients to a desired location and remove metabolic wastes. Both cold and hot applications reduce pain and discomfort through the gate control theory (see Box 6-2), by competing with pain for recognition in the nervous system. For a more detailed look at the physiologic effect of temperature, see Table 12-1.

BOX 12-1

Temperature Conversion

Fahrenheit to Celsius
Subtract 32, then multiply by $\frac{5}{9}$:
$(° F − 32) \times \frac{5}{9} = ° C$
EXAMPLE: $(212° F − 32) \times \frac{5}{9} = 100° C$

Celsius to Fahrenheit
Multiply by $\frac{9}{5}$, then add 32:
$(° C \times \frac{9}{5}) + 32 = ° F$
EXAMPLE: $(0° C \times \frac{9}{5}) + 32 = 32° F$

HAROLD DULL, MA

Born: December 18, 1935

"The body is movement. Breath is life. And the base of our being is the support of others."

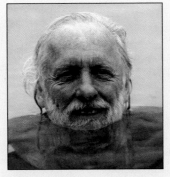

No direct path to a career in facilitating health is evident; thus it is no surprise that a physics major who decided to become a beatnik poet is the man behind one of the latest forms of hands-on therapy. *Watsu* is the combination of water and shiatsu. The name was coined by wordsmith and bodyworker Harold Dull. Developed 15 years ago, it is a hybrid of Zen shiatsu, flotation, joint mobilization, and stretching.

The oldest of four boys, Harold Dull was born in Seattle to parents in real estate. He attended the University of Washington with the intention of studying physics, prelaw, or philosophy. He wound up studying poetry instead, became a writer, and was part of the Poetry Renaissance. "At age 40 I had never had a massage," Dull says, "but I decided to begin studying Zen shiatsu in San Francisco with Wataru Ohashi and Reuho Yamada." Dull finally traveled to Japan to complete studies with world-renowned master Shizuto Masunaga. When he returned home, Dull began teaching others the ancient Japanese art and later emphasized how to combine shiatsu with the hot spring therapy he had enjoyed at Harbin Hot Springs Resort in California. In its earlier incarnation, Watsu was dubbed Wassage. Dull used a board set up in a hot tub. In time, however, he began doing his unique form of bodywork in Harbin's hot springs.

In Watsu, the water is the medium as is the massage. Its buoyancy helps practitioners and clients by supporting body weight so that small practitioners are able to handle large clients. The water also helps the therapist see, feel, and listen to what is going on with the client's body. As the body rises and falls with each breath, the water helps the practitioner identify areas that need work. The water, maintained at body temperature, also soothes the client, releasing tense muscles, taking the load off joint articulations, and helping increase flexibility and range of motion.

Step into a conventional massage room and you may not feel the result of your massage until after the therapist begins, but immerse yourself in water and you immediately feel different—lighter. As you relax into your breathing pattern, supported by your therapist, you gradually let go as the tickle of the water filling your ears silences a chaotic world and lulls you into a heightened state of relaxation.

One writer describes her experience with Watsu as follows:

"The surprise, for me, was just how profound this was. It has become a cliché to say that a therapy works 'on many different levels,' but that is actually an excellent description of Watsu. Deeply rooted physical tensions and ailments are worked on more easily, while the experience of being safely held and moved through the water also touches profound emotional and spiritual levels."
—Diana Brueton: "Watsu, Flowing Free in Water," *Kindred Spirit Quarterly.*

Dull notes that it is "the unconditional acceptance that is so powerful. So many injured people are treated as less than what they once were." In addition to its emotional impact, Watsu has reportedly helped headache pain. Muscle spasms disappear, and chronic lower back pain and spine misalignment have been corrected.

Dull's vision is to make the therapeutic value of his work, especially the added benefit of the sense of unconditional acceptance it brings, available to everyone. "From an equipment standpoint, you need a 10-foot diameter pool with about 4 feet of water, which should be maintained at body temperature," he explains, adding that new ways will be discovered to heat water at a lower cost.

TABLE 12-1 Water Temperatures and Effects on the Body

FAHRENHEIT	CELSIUS	DESCRIPTION	EFFECTS ON THE BODY
212	100	Boiling point of water	Burn
111+	43+	Painfully hot	Possibly injurious
102-110	40-43	Very hot	Tolerable for short periods
98-102	38-40	Hot	Tolerable, may redden the skin
92-98	33-38	Warm-neutral	Comfortable
80-92	27-33	Tepid	Slightly below skin temperature
65-80	18-27	Cool	Produces goose flesh
55-65	13-18	Cold	Tolerable, but uncomfortable
32-55	0-13	Very cold	Painfully cold
32	0	Freezing point of water	Burn

Moisture

Moisture content in hydrotherapy is the amount of humidity or dampness in the air. The moisture content of a steam bath is about 100%. This much moisture will help moisten the nasal passages and throat and help keep skin supple. However, high-humid air feels heavier than low-humid air and may cause breathing difficulties in susceptible persons.

In contrast, the moisture content of a sauna ranges from 10% to 20%. Breathing is often easier as the air feels lighter, but low-humid air, lacking moisture, can be drying and irritating to skin and mucous membranes.

Mineral Content

The mineral or chemical content of water is another factor that influences its therapeutic effect. Water, being a wonderful solvent, can readily dissolve minerals to form therapeutic solutions. Three kinds of mineral waters most often used in spas are:

- *Saline:* Used for its purgative effects. Saline water appears milky white.
- *Iron oxide:* Used for its restorative and healing effects. Iron oxide water is a brownish, rust color.
- *Sulfur:* Used for its cleansing and purifying effects. Sulfur water is a light lime green color.

Adding minerals to water may duplicate the effects of natural springs. The most commonly used substances are sea salt (sodium chloride), Epsom salt (magnesium sulfate), and baking soda (sodium bicarbonate). Historically, these minerals are thought to draw out toxins as the body attempts to balance the percentages of saline content between the water and skin.

CHAT ROOM

A common practice in massage is to recommend that a client soak in a tub with salt and baking soda after the massage to enhance the detoxification process and reduce postmassage soreness. The recipe for the bath is one part salt and one part baking soda (e.g., 1 cup of each) in a tub of warm water and a soaking for 20 minutes. Rinse off after the tub soak.

CHAT ROOM

Thalassotherapy is the therapeutic use of sea and marine products, primarily seaweed. The term *thalassotherapy* comes from the Greek word for sea. Seawater and blood plasma are chemically similar. Proponents of thalassotherapy often cite this fact. Spa treatments that use thalassotherapy are seawater baths and body wrap treatments using seaweed paste.

Mechanical Effect

Water, weighing 8.33 lb per gallon, is often used for its mechanical effect. Water may be pressurized as in a whirlpool or in a shower. The mechanical effect of water intensifies with increased pressure. The two important mechanical effects of water are *density* and *hydrostatic pressure*.

Density. The most important mechanical effect in water immersion is the *principle of relative density,* discovered by Archimedes (c. 287-212 BC). This famous discovery, made during a bath, prompted him to run down the street naked shouting, "Eureka!" meaning "I found it!" He realized that when a body is immersed in water, it experiences an upward force equal to the weight of water. The relative density of water is set at 1.0. Objects with a density less than 1.0 will float, and objects that have a density greater than 1.0 will sink. The adult human body has a relative density of 0.97.

Because the density of water is near that of the human body, it produces a buoyant effect on immersion equal to the weight of the water displaced. The water pressure exerted against the body when in water offsets some or all of the effect of gravity and allows it to bob or float. This property is particularly useful for clients who are unable to move freely on land; the body weighs less in water and is therefore easier to move. Similarly, water therapies are highly recommended for clients with chronic pain. Although these individuals may be in pain during weight-bearing activities while on land, if they are placed in a pool of warm water, the water buoys up some of their weight and takes pressure off the spine and faulty disks, reducing pain.

Density is also influenced by water's mineral content. The more mineral in the water, the denser it becomes and the greater the upward force. Water in flotation tanks often contains about 100 lb of salt, so the client in the tank will always float.

CHAT ROOM

The Dead Sea has a salt concentration of 33%, whereas the ocean has a salt concentration of 3%. For thousands of years, individuals have been drawn to the Dead Sea for bathing and for using its salts and mud.

Hydrostatic Pressure. The *law of Pascal* (1623-1662) states that when a body is immersed in water, the pressure exerted on it is equal everywhere at a constant depth and is exerted equally in a horizontal direction at any level. In other words, the sideways pressure is equal on all surfaces at certain depths. Hydrostatic pressure increases with depth and fluid density.

When you place an edematous leg in water, hydrostatic pressure will gently compress the tissues. This pressure acts as a compressive bandage and thus will reduce swelling. These now-displaced fluids will find their way to the kidneys. This will in turn increase urine output. In fact, research indicates that when a body is immersed for 1 hour, urination increases by 50%.

"Everything flows."
—Heraclitus

HEAT AND COLD

The therapeutic use of heat and cold in massage is very common. The external therapeutic application of heat is called **thermotherapy** and the external therapeutic application of cold is called **cryotherapy**. Heat moves from an area of greater concentration to an area of lesser concentration (Box 12-2). So when the temperature of the application method, such as a hot pack or bath water, exceeds body temperature, heat moves from that source into the body. Likewise, when temperature of the application method, such as an ice pack or cold towel friction, is less than that of the body, heat moves out of the body. This movement will continue until the temperatures of the two sources are roughly equal or until the application method is removed (Table 12-2).

CHAT ROOM

Heat is energy resulting from the motion of molecules, atoms, and other subatomic matter. *Temperature* is a measure of this atomic activity.

Effects of Heat and Cold

In general, heat and cold have four main effects:
- Pain relief
- Muscle relaxation
- Blood flow alterations
- Connective tissue effects

Pain Relief. Both heat and cold decrease pain. It is not well known how heat application reduces pain; perhaps by increasing pain nerve fiber conduction rates, which would raise pain thresholds and reduce the current level of pain experienced. Cold, on the other hand, reduces nerve fiber conduction rates, which inhibits pain. This effect occurs when temperature reaches 50°F to 59°F (10° to 15°C).

Muscle Relaxation. Both heat and cold reduce muscle spasm. Heat promotes muscle relaxation by softening and lengthening collagen within muscles and tendons. It is also suspected that heat relaxes muscle by decreasing muscle spindle activity. Client experience indicates that heat induces general relaxation. Cold reduces nerve fiber conduction rates, which helps muscles relax.

Blood Flow Alterations. Heat applications cause an initial increase in localized blood flow by reflexive vasodilation, mainly in the skin. Skin in contact with the heat source often appears hyperemic or reddened. This in turn raises tissue temperature, brings nutrients to the area, increases the rate of clearing metabolic wastes, and increases capillary permeability and fluid exchange. After a few minutes, blood vessels constrict in an attempt to reduce heat. The client often begins to perspire to help cool the body. Prolonged application depresses localized blood flow. It should be noted that superficial heat application does not increase blood flow to the underlying muscle.

Cold applications cause an initial decrease in localized blood flow by reflexive vasoconstriction; the skin may initially appear blanched or pale. If cold application is maintained for longer than approximately 15 minutes (and tissues reach 50° F or 10° C), vasodilation occurs as the body tries to increase the local temperature and restore homeostasis. This lasts for 4 to 6 minutes. If cold application continues, vasoconstriction resumes, and the cycle continues. This cycle of vasoconstriction and vasodilation is known as the **hunting response**. Even though the goal is homeostasis, these cycles of vasoconstriction and vasodilation bring blood into and then pushes it out of the area, flushing out tissue debris and bringing in oxygen. This vascular action is one of the most important effects of cold application. This effect has not been noted consistently and typically occurs in superficial rather than deeper tissues.

Benefits related to blood flow alterations include decreased hemorrhage and swelling within injured tissues, although some animal studies have shown a paradoxical increase in swelling with cold application.

BOX 12-2

How Heat Transfers

Heat is transferred by several delivery methods:
- **Conduction** involves the exchange of thermal energy while the body's surface is in direct contact with the thermal agent or conductor (e.g., hot packs, hot stones). Water has 27 times greater capacity for conducting heat than air.
- **Convection** involves transferring heat energy through movement of air or liquid (e.g., sauna, steam bath).
- **Radiation** is the transfer of heat energy in rays (e.g., infrared lamps). Heat transfer occurs without direct contact.

- **Evaporation** is the transfer of heat through the process of changing a liquid into a vapor, such as sweating.
- **Conversion** involves one energy source changing (or converting) into a heat energy source as it passes into the body (e.g., diathermy, ultrasound). This method generally is not used by massage therapists but is within the scope of practice for chiropractic, physical, and occupational therapy.

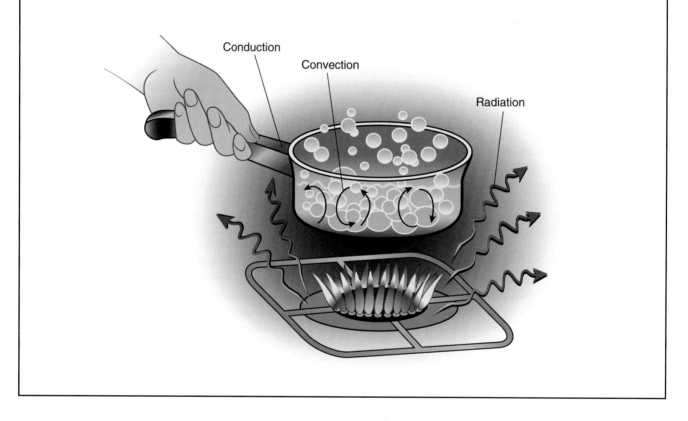

TABLE 12-2 Comparative Effects of Heat and Cold

PHYSIOLOGIC RESPONSE	INITIAL EFFECTS OF HEAT	PROLONGED EFFECTS OF HEAT	INITIAL EFFECTS OF COLD	PROLONGED EFFECTS OF COLD
Heart rate	Decreases	Increases	Increases	Decreases
Vascular response	Vasodilation	Vasoconstriction	Vasoconstriction	Vasodilation
Depth of action	Superficial	Superficial	Superficial	Deep
Effect on pain	Reduces	Reduces	Reduces	Reduces
Fascial response	Softens	Softens	Unchanged	Softens
Tissue damage	Nonapplicable	Nonapplicable	Decreases	Decreases
Analgesic	Yes	Yes	No	Yes
Anesthetic	No	No	No	Yes
Inflammatory response	Increases	Increases	Decreases	Decreases
Renal response	Nonapplicable	Nonapplicable	Stimulates	Inhibits
Digestive response	Inhibits	Inhibits	Stimulates	Inhibits
General response	Stimulates	Depresses	Stimulates	Depresses

Connective Tissue Effects. Heat increases extensibility of collagen and decreases joint stiffness and is often used to soften and distend superficial fascia. So heat therapy promotes relaxation of muscle through lengthening of the collagen within these and related structures. Cold, on the other hand, decreases collagen extensibility.

CHAT ROOM

Heat alters the viscoelastic state of fascia, just as the heat created by handling modeling clay makes it pliable. Massage manipulations are much more effective after the tissues have been prepared by heat.

Contraindications to Heat and Cold

Avoid the use of heat with the following clients or situations:
- Women who are pregnant (with the exception of limited local heat applications [avoid the abdomen])
- Very old or young individuals
- Poor or compromised circulation
- Cardiac insufficiency (i.e., congestive heart failure)
- Metal in the treatment area such as for some joint replacements and surgical implants (rods and pins)
- Over areas where chemical topical agents (i.e., liniments) have recently been applied
- Acute injury
- Inflammation (local or systemic)
- Edema or lymphedema
- Recent or potential hemorrhage
- Fever
- Recent burns, including sunburn
- Any skin lesions or rashes
- Thrombophlebitis
- Impaired sensation and paresthesias (e.g., Raynaud, cryoglobulinemia, Buerger disease)
- Impaired mental state of mind or cognition

Avoid the use of cold with the following clients or situations:
- Hypertension (i.e., high blood pressure)
- Very young or old
- Cold hypersensitivity
- Cold intolerance
- Cold allergies
- Rheumatoid conditions
- Pectoralis angina
- Previous cold injury (frostnip and frostbite)
- Any skin lesions or rashes
- Impaired sensation and paresthesias (e.g., Raynaud, cryoglobulinemia, Buerger disease)
- Impaired mental state or cognition
- Poor or compromised circulation

HEAT AND COLD APPLICATIONS

In general, heat is better to use before massage to help prepare the area. Cold is better after a massage to minimize any swelling and inflammation resulting from deep prolonged pressure. Cold can also be used over areas of acute injuries while massaging nonaffected areas.

Avoid heat therapy during the acute phase of an injury (usually 72 hours). Heat applied during this phase can actually increase pain and swelling because of the effects of heat on the blood vessels.

Heat therapy is best when injury enters the subacute phase (3 to 7 days) because heat has the beneficial effects of increased blood flow to help purge the area of debris and by-products of tissue injury.

Caution

Temperatures above 113°F (45°C) can cause tissue damage. Recommendations for water temperature to heat stones to be used during massage ranges from 110° to 140°F. *Hot stones can burn the skin.* Also, bear in mind when using hot water from a faucet, hot water heaters are set between 120° to 140°F (48° to 60°C).

Be sure to use a thermometer, such as infrared, to ascertain water temperature.

Cold therapy can be applied at any stage of injury. However, applications should not exceed 20 minutes because this increases the risk of skin injury.

Discussed next is descriptive and procedural information on hot and cold packs, contrast packs, hot and cold compresses, ice immersion, ice massage, and cold mitten friction (Table 12-3).

Be sure to use safe practice procedure for these and any other hydrotherapy techniques (Box 12-3).

Hot and Cold Packs

Both hot and cold packs are used in professional settings are commercially manufactured and available in a variety of styles. The liability for either is that they block access to and observation of the treatment area, but massage to adjacent areas may be performed.

Hot Pack. Hot packs, or *fomentation packs,* range from electric devices, to ones heated in the microwave oven, to ones filled with hot water. The most common hot pack is heated in a *hydrocollator,* a stainless steel kettle that keeps water temperature at approximately 165°F (73°C) (Figure 12-2, *A,* p. 250). Submerged in the hot water are canvas pouches containing channels filled with silicon granules; these retain heat. To prevent burning yourself, remove the hot packs from the unit using a pair of tongs or by grasping the cloth tabs that extend above the water's surface. To prevent burning the client's skin, wrap the pack in a towel or terrycloth pouch before placing it on the client's skin (Figure 12-2, *B*). Avoid placing the pack beneath the client's body or over an area containing liniment. Hot packs can remain on the client for up to 30 minutes.

TABLE 12-3 Hydrotherapeutic Applications at a Glance

HEAT AND COLD APPLICATIONS	BATH AND SHOWER TECHNIQUES	EXFOLIATIONS	BODY WRAPS	SPECIALIZED METHODS
Hot and cold packs	Immersion baths: whirlpool, spa tub, hot tub	Scrubs	Wet sheet wrap: Herbal wrap	Stone massage
Contrast pack: alternate and simultaneous	Pool plunge	Glows	Dry sheet wrap	Watsu
Hot and cold compresses	Contrast bath	Polishes		Thermal mittens and booties
Ice immersion	Sauna	Dry brush massage		Shirodhara
Ice massage	Steam bath: steam canopy, steam cabinet			
Cryokinetics	Paraffin bath			
Cold-towel friction	Vichy shower			
	Swiss shower			
	Scotch hose			
	Shampoo: Swedish, Turkish			
	Underwater massage			

Cold Pack. Professional cold packs are strong vinyl bags filled with a special gel that does not freeze to a solid block mass. They retain cold for approximately 20 minutes (Figure 12-3, p. 250). Other packs are filled with ice or icy water before use (see Figure 12-4). Some therapists prepare their own cold packs by mixing a solution of two-thirds water and one-third alcohol placed in a vinyl pouch, which is then placed in the freezer. The alcohol will prevent the water from freezing-solid so that the pack remains somewhat pliable.

During cold application of 20 minutes, your client will most likely experience (1) coldness or cooling, (2) burning, (3) stinging or aching, and then (4) numbness. The pack should remain on the treatment area until the fourth stage.

Procedure
1. Prepare the hot or cold pack.
2. Place the wrapped pack on the client's skin.
   a. If using a hydrocollator, wrap the hot pack in up to three layers of terrycloth.
   b. If using a cold pack, wrap the pack in a single paper towel or thin cloth such as a pillowcase (if the cloth is too thick, then treatment effectiveness is reduced).
3. Every 5 minutes, lift the pack and observe the skin underneath. If the skin appears puffy or raised, then remove the pack immediately; if not, then continue treatment.
4. If the client begins to shiver or perspire, then place a cold or hot compress, respectively, near the pack. You can also cover the client with a blanket or uncover the client's back and feet, whichever makes the client more comfortable. If the client still complains, remove the pack.
5. Hot pack can remain on the treatment area for up to 30 minutes. Cold pack can remain for 20 minutes.

Contrast Packs

One of the most potent techniques in hydrotherapy is to combine heat and cold during the same treatment. This technique is known as the **contrast method**. By alternating between hot and cold, the tissue vasculature experiences a vigorous pumping of fluids into and out of the tissue. Two variations of contrast packs are alternate and simultaneous.

Alternate Contrast Pack. This involves alternating hot and cold packs, which is thought to intensify the circulatory effects of each.

Procedure
1. Place the cold pack over the treatment area for 10 to 15 minutes.
2. Remove the cold pack and apply a hot pack for 10 minutes.
3. Remove the heat pack.
4. Repeat this sequence two more times, for a total of three times.
5. End with a cold pack application of 10 minutes.

Simultaneous Contrast Pack. This involves placing a cold pack over the treatment area and a hot pack near the cold pack at the same time (Figure 12-4). Not only do the heat impulses interfere with the cold impulses, but the sensation of heat also comforts the client and helps induce relaxation.

Procedure
1. Place a cold pack on the affected area and a hot pack on the affected area's opposite side or juxtaposed to the cold pack.
2. After 15 to 20 minutes, remove both packs.

Hot and Cold Compresses

A **compress** is a wet cloth, generally a washcloth or towel, that has had water wrung from it and is applied to the skin's surface, most often across the forehead or back. The most common types are hot and cold compresses. Both lose their desired temperature quickly, so refresh often.

BOX 12-3

General Hydrotherapy Treatment Guidelines

Before

- Follow all safety recommendations outlined in Chapter 9.
- Explain to the client any critical safety points such as emergency buttons.
- Maintain hot tubs, spas, steam cabinets, and whirlpools in compliance with public and multiple-use standards.
- Require that spa guests wear waterproof shoes or sandals.
- Require that spa guests take a shower before entering pool to prevent waterborne infections.
- Be sure individuals with long hair have it either tied up or secured beneath a cap. Long hair might also become trapped in water outlets.
- If hydrotherapy equipment is kept in the massage room, then be sure it is not in a high-traffic region of the room. For example, electrical cords can create a tripping hazard, and a hydrocollator and units for heating stones can burn if touched.
- Plan ahead and assemble all necessary articles.
- Be sure the treatment room is warm.
- Ask the client not to eat at least 1 hour before scheduled appointment.
- As with massage, perform a client intake, obtain consent, and conduct a premassage interview.
- Wash or sanitize your hands.
- Drape stools or tables used by the client with linens.
- Use nonslip floor mats.
- Avoid using liniments before treatment.
- Offer water or juice before, during, and after treatment.

Questions Relevant to Spa and Hydrotherapy Clients Before Treatment

Along with a thorough intake, the following questions may be added to the premassage interview to provide the client with comfort and safety:

- *Do you have any allergies?* Have an ingredient list that the client can review. Have an alternate product or treatment to substitute if the client is allergic to any ingredients in the products.
- *Do you suffer from claustrophobia?* If the answer is *yes*, then treatments such as body wraps, steam cabinets or canopies, or other spa therapies may be inappropriate or may require creative modifications.

During

- Check and monitor water temperature. For an accurate reading, use a thermometer, which can be purchased at a pool supply or spa supply store. Although testing the water temperature using your fingertips is helpful, use caution when placing a hand or foot into water of unknown temperature.
- Use a timer to monitor treatment duration. Do not overtreat.
- Ask for client feedback regarding comfort level of water temperature. Adjust temperature as needed.
- Remain with the client or within easy calling distance during treatment.
- If water collects on the wet room or bathroom floor, wipe it up immediately to prevent accidents (floor drains are helpful).
- In the event of body fluid seepage, glove up and use paper towels to absorb the spill, and then clean the area with mild soap and water. Next, disinfect equipment with a solution of water and chlorine bleach in a 10:1 solution. Discard the contaminated gloves and paper towels in a safe manner (determined by the local department of health). Finally, wash and dry your hands.
- Implements used during the massage such as stones that become contaminated should be immersed in a 10% bleach solution or a 70% alcohol solution for 10 minutes.

After

- Make certain the client's skin is dry.
- Assist the client to an upright position because hydrotherapy treatments may cause the client to feel light-headed.
- After treatment, allow the client to rest for at least 10 minutes so that body temperature can return to normal.
- Document the type of treatment, products used, duration of treatment, and the client's reactions.
- Clean all surfaces that come in direct contact with clients and all reservoirs that collect perspiration or exfoliated skin cells.
- Items such as brushes, sponges, or loofahs can be disinfected by placing them in a dishwasher's top basket and run through a cleaning and heated dry cycle.

Poultices and dressings are other types of compresses but are used as home treatments and not part of spa or massage treatments. *Poultices* are packs in which products, such as mustard, are spread between layers of cloth and applied hot to provide heat or counterirritation. Poultices are the forerunners of today's body wraps. A *dressing* is a cloth applied to a clean area for protection and absorption of secretions.

Hot Compress. Hot compresses are used primarily to soothe, relax, or warm clients during or after massage or

during local cold application. An infrared light can be used to keep compresses hot longer. Many therapists have compresses, such as washcloths and towels, warmed in electric towel cabinets so they are readily available.

Cold Compress. Cold compresses are frequently used to help keep clients comfortable during hot baths, steam or sauna baths, or during body wraps. They can also be used to soothe an area after a deep pressure or aggressively applied massage techniques.

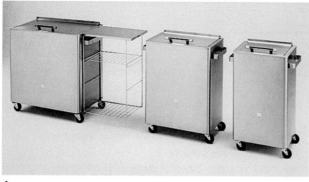

A

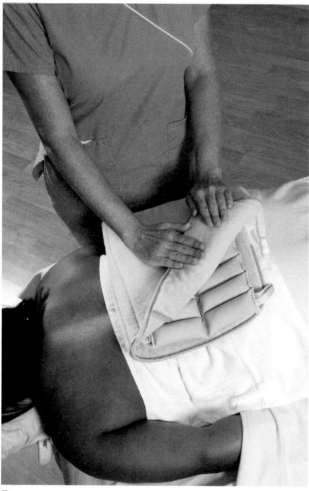

B

FIGURE 12-2 Hot packs. **A,** Hydrocollator units. **B,** Hydrocollator pack in a terrycloth pouch.

Procedure
1. For a hot compress, dip a washcloth in hot water. For a cold compress, dip a washcloth in icy water.
2. Squeeze out excess water.
3. For a small area such as the forehead, layer the cloth by folding.

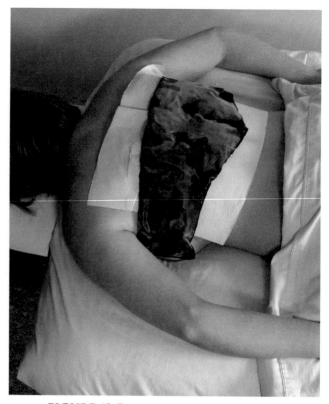

FIGURE 12-3 Cold gel pack on a prone client.

4. Apply to the desired area.
5. Allow it to remain on the skin until it reaches near body temperature.
6. Remove or replace with a fresh compress (therapist's discretion).

Ice Immersion

Ice immersion baths involve soaking the affected area, usually hand or foot, in icy water. Because this treatment is often uncomfortable, clients may elect to leave the tips of their fingers or toes out of the icy water.

Procedure
1. Immerse the affected area in a container of tepid water.
2. Add plenty of ice to the water, enough to chill it quickly.
3. Keep the area immersed for 5 minutes.
4. Remove and dry immediately.

To include **cryokinetics** (cold therapy combined with joint movement):

1. After the treatment area is numb, ask your client to draw pictures or trace the alphabet with his or her fingers or toes in the icy water for approximately 3 minutes. The additional movements will assist in the transport of fluids through the treatment area.
2. Remove the treatment area from the water and dry immediately.

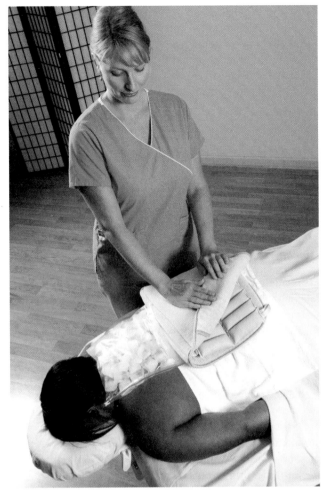

FIGURE 12-4 Simultaneous contrast method using ice pack (*on upper back*) and hot pack (*on lower back*).

> ⊖volve *Mostly used as a rehabilitative tool, ice immersion combines the therapeutic effects of ice with movement. An image of this technique is located on the Evolve website under Chapter 12's course materials.* ■

Ice Massage

Ice massage combines the use of ice with friction massage. To begin, either (1) partially fill a 6-oz foam or paper cup with water and place in the freezer until water turns to solid ice; then tear the top edges or bottom of the cup to expose the ice and use the cup to insulate the ice as you hold it, or (2) insert a tongue depressor into a paper or foam cup filled partially with water before freezing; the tongue depressor can be used as a handle.

Procedure

1. Place a towel under the treatment area or a rolled-up towel around the treatment area to absorb the water from the melting ice.
2. Using circular friction, rub the ice on the client's skin (Figure 12-5).
3. Continue until the area is numb. This may take up to 10 minutes.
4. Remove the ice and dry the treatment area.

To include *cryokinetics (*cold therapy combined with joint movement*)*:

1. After the treatment area is numb, remove the ice and ask your client to actively and slowly move the joint by mirroring back to you demonstrated movements.

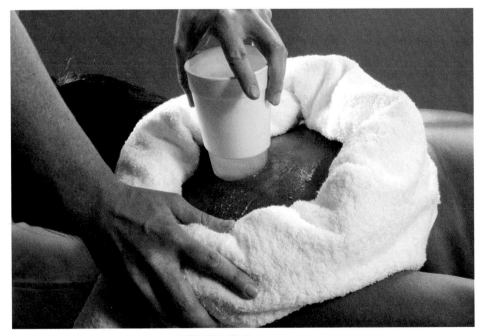

FIGURE 12-5 Ice massage.

Active-assisted, resisted, or passive movements can be used. These movements will assist in the transport of fluids through the treatment area.

2. Continue movements until feeling is restored (approximately 1 to 2 minutes).
3. Reapply ice and move in a circular direction until the area is renumbed.
4. Continue two more cycles of ice and movement, for a total of three cycles.

Cold-Towel Friction

Cold-towel friction, also called *cold mitten friction,* combines ice application through towels dipped in icy water and friction massage. This application method is regarded as a tonic treatment because it is thought to increase vigor and endurance while improving circulation (Figure 12-6). The client may stand, sit on a water-resistant stool, or lie on a wet table.

Procedure
1. Dip two hand towels into icy water. Do not wring out the excess water.

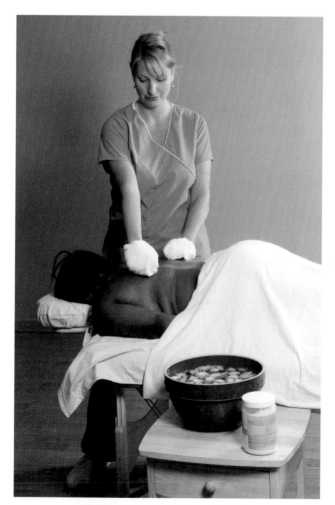

FIGURE 12-6 Cold-towel friction.

2. Apply the towels to client's skin using vigorous back-and-forth friction movements.
3. Dip the towels again, and repeat the process.
4. Cover the treated area with a dry towel, and rub vigorously until dry.
5. Repeat on another area until the client's back and extremities are treated.

MINI-LAB

Arrange a meeting with a local physical or occupational therapist. Ask how and why he or she uses hot and cold therapy in rehabilitation. Prepare a summary and present it to the class.

BATH AND SHOWER TECHNIQUES

For centuries, people from all cultures have enjoyed the relaxing pleasures and therapeutic benefits of soaking in warm water. **Balneology** is the art and science of bathing for therapeutic and relaxation purposes. The broad category of baths and showers encompasses submerging all or part of the body in water, wax, light, heated air, or steam.

A range of shower techniques, which is a type of bath, is included in this section. The two most popular varieties of spa showers are Swiss and Vichy showers. The client stands in a Swiss shower and lies down in a Vichy shower. Showers are often used to remove body masks and exfoliants. A type of shower, called a *spray* or a *hose,* is a single fine jet of pressurized warm or cool water.

Combining applications of hot water with cold is called a *contrast bath.* Cool pool plunges or tepid showers after hot immersion baths, a sauna, or steam baths are a great way to have the best of both worlds.

Immersion Baths

Immersion baths include whirlpools, spas, hot tubs, footbaths, and underwater massage. Immersion baths are best used before a massage session, or they can revolve around the massage itself, as in underwater massage.

Additives such as minerals, milk, whey, or herbs are added to bath water to suit the client's need. Epsom salts (named for the mineral springs in Epsom, England) or preparations such as Batherapy create a *mineral bath.* Blended herbs, herb extracts, or essential oils create a *herbal bath.* Goat or cow milk creates a *milk bath,* a luxurious bath choice. The hot water disperses the healing qualities of these additives and opens the pores to facilitate absorption.

A general rule about bath treatment times is that the greater the difference is between body and water temperatures, the shorter the treatment time will be. Most people find that 100°F to 102°F is a comfortable temperature. If the client becomes too warm during treatment but is not ready to leave the tub, then he or she may lift the arms out of the water, exposing a greater surface area of the skin to allow

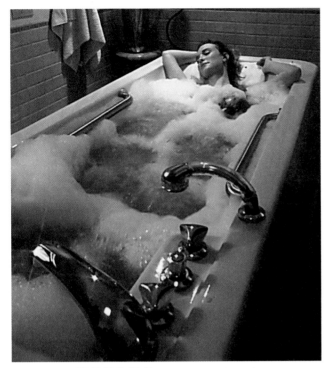

FIGURE 12-7 Client in a whirlpool.

for evaporative cooling. If the client feels weak or dizzy, then immediately discontinue bathing and assist him or her out of the tub.

Whirlpool. A whirlpool is a tub with jets positioned along the sides. It is filled with hot water just before use and drained after each use (Figure 12-7). After it is filled, the jets can be activated, which agitate and circulate the water.

Spa Tub. A spa tub uses high-pressure jets to agitate and circulate the water. These jets are positioned on the sides and sometimes the bottom of the tub. The water temperature is maintained at a preset temperature. Water remains in the tub, so it is chemically treated to remain clean and sanitary for multiple uses. Ozonators may also be used, which use ozone to sanitize the water.

Hot Tub. A hot tub is essentially an immersion bath that uses a wooden barrel filled with water. The barrel does not contain jets. Water can be heated using an electrical heating device or heat from a fire. Like a spa tub, the water is chemically treated to remain clean and sanitary for multiple uses.

Procedure
1. Because the tub is a soaking rather than a cleaning vessel, ask clients to shower before entering the tub. A body shampoo can be performed rather than a shower (see later discussion).
2. Instruct the client on how to enter and exit the tub safely. Assistance may be required.

3. While the client is in the tub, offer a cup of water in a nonbreakable cup and a cool compress for the face and neck.
4. Soaking time ranges from 5 to 20 minutes, depending on the water temperature and client's comfort level.
5. If desired, the client can take a 2- to 3-minute tepid shower after bathing.
6. When the client is dry and wrapped in a warm towel or robe, escort him or her to a warm, quiet place, to rest and drink water or tea for 10 to 20 minutes.

CHAT ROOM

The age-old tradition of barrel making (cooperage) dates back thousands of years, and such barrels have long been used to hold liquids such as wines and spirits. Cedar and oak are the most popular woods as they have a natural resilience to decay. This led to the early development of wooden barrels used as tubs for bathing.

When water immersion is combined with light exercise, a *Hubbard tank* is used. Named after its inventor, Carl Hubbard, this large tub is used in rehabilitation clinics.

Pool Plunge

A **pool plunge** consists of a brief dip in a cold, deep water pool (usually a chilly 50°F to 60°F). The cold plunge is invigorating following a sauna, steam, or immersion bath.

Procedure
1. Follow the procedure for a sauna, steam, or immersion bath.
2. Direct the client to quickly submerse himself or herself in the pool water. Thirty seconds is recommended.
3. Once out of the pool, dry off immediately.

Sauna

The **sauna** is a dry heat bath where the client sits or stands in a wood-lined room. Humidity is set between 10% and 20% with temperatures ranging from 160° to 210°F; 185° is ideal. A Finnish sauna is the type on which most modern saunas are based. In a Finnish sauna, a fire (preferably using birch wood) heats a pile of stones until they are red hot. The radiant heat warms the air. Water may be thrown on the stones to create steam. After the initial sweat, the person's skin is gently slapped with leafy birch twigs to stimulate circulation.

Procedure
1. Ask the client to shower before treatment.
2. Assist the client into the room.
3. Offer a cup of cool water in a nonbreakable cup and a cool compress for the face. Because of water lost during sweating, clients must be well hydrated before, during, and after treatment.
4. After the initial sweat, which may take from 5 to 15 minutes, have the client take a tepid shower or cool pool plunge.

5. If desired, the client may reenter the sauna for a second sweat.
6. After the session, allow the client to take a brief tepid shower or cool pool plunge.
7. When the client is dry and wrapped in a warm towel or robe, escort him or her to a warm, quiet place, to rest and drink water or tea for 10 to 20 minutes.

Steam Bath

A **steam bath** is conducted in a ceramic-tiled room filled with water vapor. Temperatures are maintained between 105° and 120° F. Essential oils may be added to the water before vaporizing to create an aromatherapy steam bath.

A *steam canopy* fits over a wet table and is an inexpensive way to offer clients the benefits of a steam bath. It not only can be used in the privacy of a massage room but also keeps the head exposed while the client remains supine.

Similar to the canopy, the *steam cabinet,* or *Russian bath,* allows the head to be exposed while the client remains seated.

Procedure
1. Ask the client to shower before treatment.
2. Assist the client into the room, instructing him or her to sit on a towel placed there for comfort and sanitation. It is also a good idea to show your client where the steam pipe is and avoid it.
3. Offer a cup of cool water in a nonbreakable cup and a cool compress for the face. Because of the water lost during sweating, clients must be well hydrated before, during, and after treatment.
4. Allow the client to remain in the steam room, canopy, or cabinet for up to 20 minutes.
5. After the steam bath, suggest that the client take a brief tepid shower or cool pool plunge.
6. When the client is dry and wrapped in a warm towel or robe, escort him or her to a warm, quiet place, to rest and drink water or tea for 10 to 20 minutes.

⊖volve *My first experience in a steam cabinet was in a Japanese spa in San Francisco. This, along with a massage, was my way of unwinding after taking the National Certification Exam in the mid-1990s. Shortly thereafter, I purchased one for my practice. To see an illustration of a steam cabinet, access your student account from the Evolve website.* ■

Paraffin Bath

Paraffin baths are dips in a heated waxy mixture. Paraffin wax treatments are used to apply heat and are particularly useful on angular bony areas such as the hands, wrists, elbows, knees, ankles, and feet. The paraffin wax is kept in a thermostatically controlled vat. The molten wax can be painted on the affected part instead of dipped. Lotion or cream can be applied to the treatment area to assist in hardened wax removal. These treatments soften the skin and are used for pain relief.

Procedure
1. Clean and dry the treatment area thoroughly.
2. Dip the client's hand or foot into the vat for 1 to 3 seconds.
3. Remove the hand/foot and let any excess drip into the vat.
4. Wait 5 to 10 seconds and repeat the sequence four more times (for a total of five times). This will help build up a thick layer of wax (at least $\frac{1}{4}$ inch thick). The thicker the layer, the longer the heat will be retained.
5. Place the hand/foot in a special mitten/bootie or wrap with a plastic wrap and then with a towel.
6. Repeat on the other hand/foot.
7. Allow the client to rest for up to 15 minutes or until the client reports that he or she can no longer feel heat. During this time, perhaps perform a scalp massage.
8. Remove the wax covering.
9. Discard the wax; do not reuse because this wax is now unclean.

CHAT ROOM

More of a physical therapy modality than spa application, a *sitz bath* is a sitting bath with the water covering the hips and often coming up to the navel. This type of treatment requires a tub shaped as a chair designed so that the legs remain out of the water. Water temperature ranges from 90° to 102°F. If the water is cool for a tonic effect, then the bath lasts only 3 to 8 minutes. Warm water creates a sedating, calming effect, with treatment times ranging from 20 to 30 minutes. Healing agents such as salt or alum usually accompany the bath water. A sitz bath is often indicated for relief of menstruation pain or postchildbirth pain; however, it is contraindicated in cases of pelvic inflammation.

Another type of sitz bath uses a small pan designed to be placed over the toilet seat or bowl. A hose from a nearby faucet provides a constant flow of controlled temperature water to the front of the pan while the client sits (or sitz). The excess water spills out an overflow notch in the back falling into the toilet bowl. This treatment is generally used following pelvic surgeries such as episiotomy or hemorrhoidectomy.

And for the etymology fans, *sitz* is the German word for "sit."

Vichy Shower

The **Vichy shower** is taken while a client reclines on a special table as jets of water spray from a horizontal bar with multiple down-facing showerheads along its length. This bar is suspended above a table. Some Vichy shower are equipped with a separate hand-held shower hose. The temperature and pressure of the water can be adjusted as needed. Treatment time is usually 10 to 20 minutes.

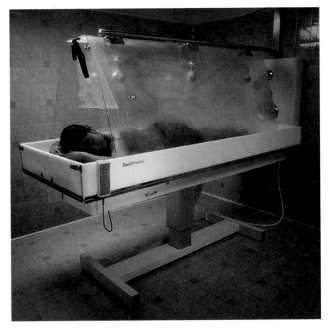

FIGURE 12-8 Vichy shower.

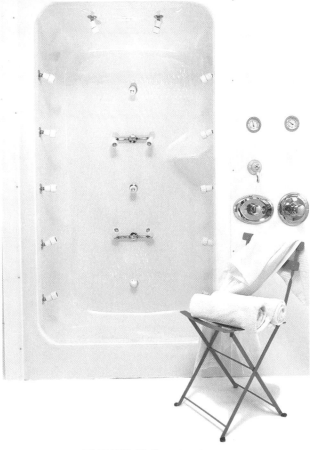

FIGURE 12-9 Swiss shower.

The Vichy shower gets its name from its city of origin, the renowned spa town of Vichy, France. This type of shower is typically incorporated into body wrap and exfoliation procedures to rinse off products from the body (Figure 12-8).

Procedure
1. Instruct the client how to lie on the table.
2. Assist your client with draping (i.e., genitals and female breast are draped at all times).
3. Turn on the shower and adjust the temperature and water pressure according to the desired result.
4. After treatment, assist the client upright while maintaining the drape.
5. When the client is dry and wrapped in a warm towel or robe, escort him or her to a warm, quiet place, to rest and drink water or tea for 10 to 20 minutes.

Swiss Shower

During a **Swiss shower**, the client is standing in a shower stall rather than lying down on a table . Typically, the Swiss shower has one large showerhead on the ceiling of the shower and several showerheads positioned vertically on each of the three walls. Water pressure and temperature vary to create stimulating and invigorating effects (Figure 12-9). Treatment time is usually 5 to 10 minutes.

Swiss showers get their name from its country of origin, Switzerland. Swiss showers can be used as part of a contrast bath or used to remove products after body wrap and exfoliation procedures.

Procedure
1. Instruct the client how to enter the shower stall and turn on the shower.
2. Adjust the temperature and water pressure according to the desired result.
3. For a traditional Swiss shower, begin with water temperature at about 100°F. Increase the temperature to 110°F within 30 seconds. This is maintained for a full minute, then switched to 70°F for 30 seconds, then back again to 100°F. This cycle is repeated two more times, for a total of three times.
4. When the client is dry and wrapped in a warm towel or robe, escort him or her to a warm, quiet place, to rest and drink water or tea for 10 to 20 minutes.

Scotch Hose

This shower type is received while the client stands about 9 to 10 feet from the therapist. The therapist uses a large hand-held hose (resembling a fire hose) to spray strong jets of water over the client's body. The water temperature alternates from hot to cold at regular intervals to create a contrast effect.

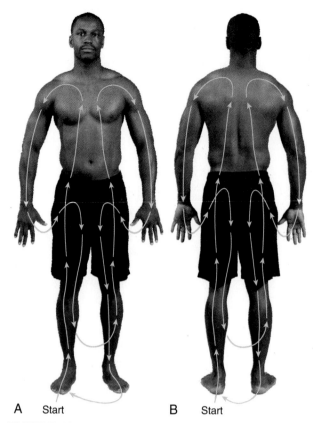

A Start   B Start

FIGURE 12-10 Scotch hose technique. Arrows indicate direction of water stream. **A,** Anterior view. **B,** Posterior view.

This treatment combines the benefits of alternating water temperatures (see contrast method) with that of massage (caused by water pressure).

This treatment is also known as a *Scotch douche, Scotch shower, jet blitz,* or a *blitz gus. Douche* is a French word meaning *shower*.

Procedure

1. Turn on the valve and begin with water temperature at 90° F. Begin at the feet and direct the water stream up the client's leg, thigh, back, and shoulder; then down the arm, and switch to the opposite side of the body (Figure 12-10). Be sure the water stream is moving constantly.
2. While you are moving the stream over the client,* increase the temperature to 110° F and maintain this for 1 minute. Turn the water temperature down to 60°F for 30 seconds. This cycle is repeated two more times, for a total of three times. End with the water temperature on 90° F.
3. When the client is dry and wrapped in a warm towel or robe, escort him or her to a warm, quiet place, to rest and drink water or tea for 10 to 20 minutes.

---

*The therapist can place a thumb partially over the nozzle to widen the column of water. This technique is called *fanning*.

Shampoos

Body shampoos involve gently scrubbing the client's skin using a cloth or brush dipped in warm, soapy water. The client may stand, sit on a water-resistant stool, or lie on a wet table. Body shampoos may be administered indoors or outdoors. The final rinse temperature determines if the procedure is a Swedish or a Turkish shampoo.

Swedish Shampoo. A Swedish shampoo includes pouring a pail of hot water (105° F) over the client's skin as the final rinse.

Turkish Shampoo. Follow the hot pail pour (105° F) with a tepid pail pour (90° F) for a Turkish shampoo.

The procedures for a Swedish and a Turkish shampoo follow.

Procedure

1. Dampen the client's skin.
2. Using a mild liquid soap, generate a thick lather.
3. Gently scrub the client's skin. Use circular strokes around joints and linear strokes over larger body areas.
4. Remove the lather with a shower, hose, or a pail of water poured over the client's skin. Water temperature varies according to whether you are providing a Swedish (105° F) or Turkish (90° F) shampoo.
5. Dry the client's skin immediately.

Underwater Massage

This method combines an immersion bath with massage. Water temperature is a comfortable 97°F to 101°F. The massage is provided by a stream of water under pressure from a hand-held hose.

Procedure

1. Ask the client to shower before entering the tub. A body shampoo can be performed rather than a shower (see previous section on shampoos).
2. Instruct the client on how to enter and exit the tub safely. Assistance may be required.
3. While the client is in the tub, offer a cup of water in a nonbreakable cup and a cool compress for the face and neck.
4. Soaking time ranges from 5 to 20 minutes, depending on the water temperature and the client's comfort level.
5. Using a hand-held hose, massage the base of the neck, shoulders, back, hips and thighs, legs and feet with a moderate-pressure stream of water. The client is supine and occasionally rolls onto the left or right sides to access the back of the body. Both linear and circular movements of the hose can be used. The hose can be operated by the client for self-massage or by a therapist.
6. The water massage typically lasts 20 to 30 minutes.
7. If desired, the client can take a 2- to 3-minute tepid shower.

8. Provide a warm, quiet place for the client to rest for 10 to 20 minutes.

"The cure for anything is salt water—sweat, tears, or the sea."
—Isak Dinesen

EXFOLIATIONS

Exfoliation procedures are any treatment in which the client's skin is stimulated by abrasion. It includes use of a textured cloth, sponge, loofah, brush, or grainy product. The procedure can be performed on a wet or dry table with the client lying down, standing, or sitting on a stool.

One of the most popular exfoliants is salt (noniodized); the granule size ranges from fine to course. Other exfoliants are sugar, corn, or oatmeal; coffee; and ground herbs (the last type is popular in ayurvedic treatments). Nut and seed meals, which include ground almond, walnut, and other nut shells, as well as fruit seeds, such as apricot and peach, are also used. Liquid soap can be added to the exfoliant to provide a cleansing effect.

The primary strokes used during procedure are linear and circular superficial friction, both done with a relaxed hand and open palm. Pressure used during frictioning must be monitored, because some areas may become easily irritated. If a burning sensation occurs, then reduce the pressure or speed or discontinue treatment altogether. Avoid using salt on skin that has been freshly shaved or waxed or has a rash, because it can feel uncomfortable and irritating.

Scrubs, Glows, or Polishes

A body *scrub* is procedure that uses a coarse grainy substance as the exfoliant. The word *glow* is often used to describe a scrub because of the way skin "glows" during and immediately after the procedure (it's really just hyperemia).

A body *polish* uses a fine, grainy substance as the exfoliant. These products are not as coarse or abrasive as scrubs and glows. Clients who have fair, ruddy, thin, or fragile skin should use a polish instead of a scrub. Some polishes use a *gommage*, which is a cream-based polishing agent.

Procedure
1. Dampen the client's skin.
2. Use about a tablespoon of exfoliant and apply it to the skin using both hands. Replenish when you begin a new area or when needed.
3. Use short, brisk back-and-forth friction strokes to apply the compound over the client's body. Use circular friction around joints. Do not apply exfoliant to the neck or face.
4. Rinse off the product with a warm shower, hand-held nozzle, pail pour, or damp washcloth. Dry the skin

immediately. Some products can be brushed off with a towel rather than rinsed off with water.
5. Apply a skin moisturizer.

Dry Brush Massage

Highly stimulating to skin glands and lymph circulation, dry brush massage uses a natural bristle brush or loofah to friction massage the skin. In most cases, this procedure precedes another spa service or as a stand-alone treatment.

Garshana, an ayurvedic dry brush treatment, is performed with textured cotton gloves, loofah, and wool or raw silk gloves.

Procedure
1. Use strokes that are short and brisk and directed upward toward the primary lymph nodes to assist lymphatic drainage.
   a. Circular brush strokes can be used on the soles of the feet, palms, and hands, and on joints.
   b. Linear brush strokes are used on limbs, back, abdomen, and upper chest (Figure 12-11).
   c. Avoid the face and head.
2. Be sure to use mild to moderate pressure within the client's tolerance level. If a burning sensation occurs, reduce pressure or speed.
3. Session time can range from 10 to 20 minutes.

CHAT ROOM

If a client feels nauseated during a spa treatment, a cup of peppermint tea should help ease the queasiness.

"Give me the power to create a fever, and I shall cure any disease."
—Hippocrates

BODY WRAPS

A body wrap uses large wet or dry sheets or bandages to wrap most of the body. For a *wet sheet wrap*, the sheets are soaked in a therapeutic agent and wrung out before wrapping the body. For a *dry sheet wrap*, the therapeutic agent is applied to the skin before wrapping. These two methods can be combined in which a therapeutic agent is applied to the skin and then wrapped in damp sheets that have been soaked in a therapeutic agent. Total treatment time for either type of wrap is approximately 50 minutes.

The body is wrapped to create a uniform snug fit around the body (except for the head). This technique is often referred to as *cocooning*. After cocooning, if the client begins to experience anxiety from claustrophobia, loosen up the wrap around the neck and shoulders. If this does not bring immediate relief of anxiety, remove the arms from the

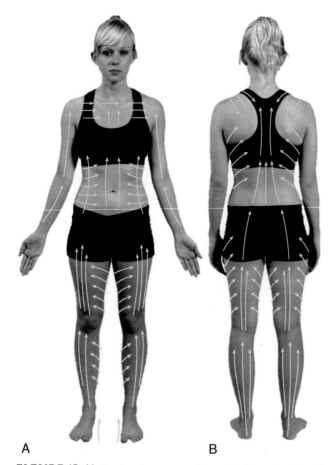

FIGURE 12-11 Dry brush massage. Arrows indicate direction of strokes. **A,** Anterior view. **B,** Posterior view.

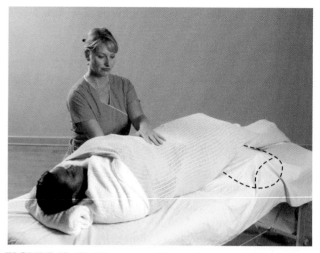

FIGURE 12-12 Client encased in a body wrap lying supine with a bolster under knees.

temporary. Avoid misleading the client into thinking that compression wraps are a method of weight reduction.

Wet Sheet Wrap

As stated previously, sheets used for a wet sheet wrap are soaked in a therapeutic agent and wrung out before wrapping the body. The most popular wet sheet wrap is the herbal wrap. Sheets are soaked in herbal tea. Select herbs are used to make a tea decoction or infusion. A *decoction* is a tea made from boiling parts of the plant (e.g., bark, roots, seeds). An *infusion* is a tea made from steeping the parts of the plant (e.g., stems, leaves). Instead of herbal teas, sheets may also be soaked in coffee, milk, cider, or juice.

Ideally, the client must be warmed before being wrapped. This can be done by immersion bath, or steam or sauna bath.

Procedure

1. Prepare the table. Be sure sheets, blankets, other layers are lined up at the head of the table (see Figure 12-13).
2. Place a towel at the head of the table. Fold the towel lengthwise, tucking the sheet and blankets in between. This towel will surround the client's head and neck when the body is wrapped.
3. Lay the wrung-out sheet over the thermal blanket.
4. Ask the client to lie supine on the table quickly.
5. Wrap the sheet tightly around the client. Then wrap the remaining layers around the client. Keep the face exposed.
6. Place a bolster behind the knees.
7. Allow the client to stay wrapped for up to 20 minutes. Remain nearby. If the client becomes overheated, place a cool compress across the forehead. Refresh when needed. If the client becomes thirsty, offer cool water in a cup with a bendy straw from which the client can sip.
8. Unwrap the client and then cover him or her with a warm towel or robe. Allow the therapeutic agents to dry on the

wrap. These methods work in most cases. However, if the client is still experiencing anxiety, it is best to unwrap the client and discontinue the procedure.

If the client becomes too warm, loosen the sheet or uncover the feet and ankles. A cool compress across the forehead offers quick relief.

It is important to use a bolster behind the knees while your client is supine because the weight of the wrap may cause hyperextension of the lower back (Figure 12-12).

One principle behind use of body wraps is to raise body temperature. With the body covered in sheets, blankets, and other insulating material, the body temperature rises and the body registers a fever. This rise triggers a sweat response, cools the body, and helps eliminate the toxins the body *thinks* is causing the fever. During this process, circulation and metabolism are increased, as is the opening of skin pores. This response encourages absorption of the therapeutic agent.

A *slimming wrap* or *compression wrap* is a type of body wrap that encases the body in plastic wrap or elastic bandages that have been soaked in a special solution. Therapeutic agents can also be applied to the skin. The objective is to contour the body and reduce fluids. The effects are

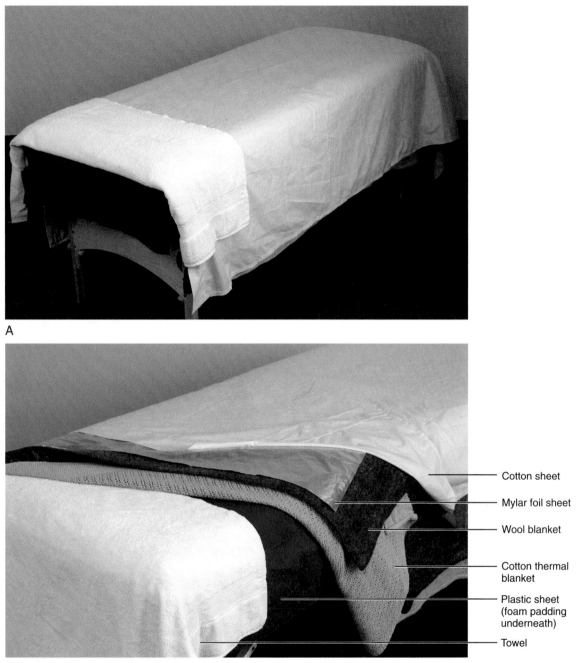

A

B

Cotton sheet

Mylar foil sheet

Wool blanket

Cotton thermal blanket

Plastic sheet (foam padding underneath)

Towel

FIGURE 12-13 Body wrap. **A,** Table set up for body wrap. **B,** Bottom edge pulled back to reveal layering.

skin. Allow him or her to rest for 10 to 20 minutes. Showering is optional after a wet sheet wrap.

Dry Sheet Wrap

For a dry sheet wrap, therapeutic agents are applied to the client's skin before he or she is wrapped in a dry sheet. A number of substances can be used as therapeutic agents, including muds, clays, fango (Italian for "mud" but can include peat and clays), paraffin, parafango (fango and paraffin), volcanic ash, charcoal, seaweed, algae, and honey.

These products can be applied to the skin with a clean brush or with gloved hands.

Ideally, the client's skin is stimulated with a dry brush massage before application of the therapeutic agent (see prior section on dry brush massage).

Procedure

1. Prepare the table. Be sure sheets, blankets, and other layers are lined up at the head of the table (see Figure 12-13).
2. Place a towel at the head of the table. Fold the towel lengthwise, tucking the sheet and blankets in between.

This towel will surround the client's head and neck when the body is wrapped.

3. Ask the client to lie supine on the table and drape him or her with a towel.

4. Apply product to the client's skin using long gliding strokes.
   a. Apply product to the fronts of the legs. To apply product to the backs of the legs, flex the hip and knee.
   b. To apply product to the buttocks, flex the hip and knee, then rotate the hip medially to expose the buttocks.
   c. To apply product to the back, help the client into a seated position while maintaining the drape.

5. Wrap the sheet tightly around the client. Then wrap the remaining layers around the client. Place a bolster behind the knees.

6. Allow the client to stay wrapped for up to 20 minutes. Remain nearby. If the client becomes overheated, place a cool compress across the forehead. Refresh when needed. If the client becomes thirsty, offer cool water in a cup with a bendy straw from which the client can sip.

7. Unwrap the client.

8. Remove the product with warm, wet towels; a Vichy, Swiss, or regular shower; or a hand-held hose.

9. Apply moisturizer to hydrate the skin.

CHAT ROOM

Massage therapists can apply exfoliants to improve the condition of soft tissues and to help the client relax or feel invigorated (i.e., help the client achieve his or her therapeutic goals), but not to beautify skin because this is the scope of practice for cosmetologists and estheticians.

SPECIALIZED METHODS

This section deals with hydrotherapy methods that do not quite fit within the previous treatment categories. These specialized methods are either ancient methods used in different cultures, such as Shirodhara, or they consist of new interpretations and presentations of hydrotherapy principles such as Stone Massage and Watsu.

It is highly recommended that therapists who wish to include these specialized methods as part of their repertory undergo specialized training and practice before offering them to clients.

Stone Massage

Stone Massage uses smooth stones as a massage tool or as a method of heat and cold application. Native Americans have been using hot and cold stones for centuries. Teaching application of hot and cold stones to massage therapists began in Arizona by Mary Nelson, and she called it *LaStone therapy*. Hot stone massage is a popular spa technique, especially in ayurvedic treatments.

Stones of various sizes are used. For example, large stones are needed for large areas of the body, such as the back, and small stones are needed for between the toes. Basalt is recommended for the *hot stones*, and marble is recommended for the *cold stones*. Exercise caution when using hot stones because if too hot, they can burn the skin.

According to the Associated Bodywork and Massage Professionals, the greatest number of lawsuits filed against massage therapists are due to skin injuries from hot stones. Be careful when using the method.

Stones used during treatment should be cleaned with antibacterial soap and water after each use. Some therapists add a little salt to the soapy lather. If stones contain any massage lubricant, an additional step of rubbing isopropyl alcohol over them is recommended. Water in the unit where stones are heated should be replaced each day. At the end of each week, stones should be washed, rinsed, and placed on a towel to dry. The heating unit should then be emptied, cleaned and sanitized, and then dried.

Procedure

1. Heat basalt stones in water 110° to 140° F, or chill marble stones in a refrigerator or freezer.

2. For treatment with hot stones, remove and dry the stones you wish to use.

3. Stone arrangement suggestions are:
   a. Ask your client to sit up for a moment while you arrange approximately 10 large stones on the table; place 6 stones on either side of the spine, base of the neck, backs of the shoulders, and on the sacrum.
   b. Place four large stones on the top drape over chakra areas (lower belly, belly, solar plexus, upper chest). Place two additional large stones over the shoulders (Figure 12-14).
   c. Place two middle-sized stones on the sides of the neck.
   d. Place two middle-sized stones in the palm of each hand.
   e. Place four small flat stones between the toes.

4. Massage the client using the stones until the desired effect is achieved or until the stones reach body temperature. Massage can be performed using the stones in long, gliding strokes and for more specific point work on tender areas.

5. Replace with warmer stones as needed.

CHAT ROOM

A value-added service is a treatment offered in addition to performed spa procedure to increase its value to the client. The most popular value-added services are reflexology and neck, face, and scalp massage.

Watsu

Watsu is a type of massage that takes place in a warm water pool. Water temperature of 95°F is suggested. During Watsu (a term derived from "water shiatsu"), the therapist stands

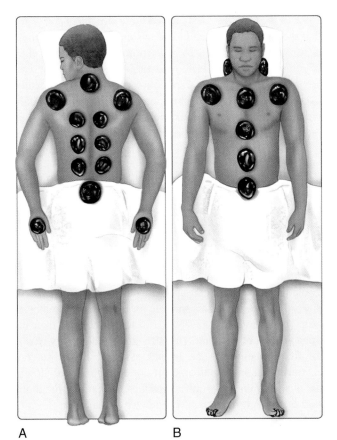

A   B

FIGURE 12-14   Stone placement. **A,** Posterior view, **B,** Anterior view.

in chest-deep water helping the client to float, sometimes with the aid of flotation devices. The therapist uses techniques of compression, body movements, and stretching to achieve deep relaxation.

Therapists who wish to offer Watsu to their clients must undergo specialized training and months of practice. See the biography box to learn more about Watsu and its founder, Harold Dull.

Thermal Mittens and Booties

Thermal mittens and booties are a value-added service and rarely used as a stand alone treatment. Two types of thermal mittens or booties are available for use. The first type is filled with buckwheat or a similar material and warmed in a microwave oven. The second type consists of small, electrically warmed sleeves for the hands and feet.

In most cases, a moisturizing agent such as Shea or cocoa butter, jojoba oil, or paraffin wax is applied to the skin before the warmed mittens or booties are slipped on.

Procedure
1. Preheat the mitts or boots.
2. Apply a moisturizing agent to the hands or feet (if desired). Wrap the hands or feet in plastic wrap.
3. Slide the heated mitts or boots on the hands or feet.

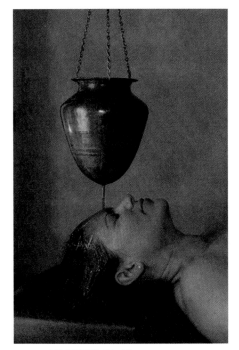

FIGURE 12-15   Shirodhara.

4. Slip off after 15 minutes.
5. Remove any excess product (if applicable).

> ⊖volve *I use heated mittens and booties as a free special treat during massage for a client who are also be celebrating a birthday or another special event. See a picture of how these therapy aids are used on the Evolve website that accompanies this text.* ■

Shirodhara

Shirodhara is an ayurvedic treatment that delivers a steady stream of oil over the client's forehead to achieve deep relaxation. The term shirodhara comes from *shiro*, which means head and *dhara* which means the flow of liquid. This treatment is usually combined with other spa treatments, such as body wraps, or massage, but is suitable as a standalone service.

During the procedure, the client lies on a massage table with the upper portion of the head over the edge. Warm oil (usually sesame) flows from a vessel in a steady stream over the client's forehead, particularly the brow and in the region between the eyes (Figure 12-15). This vessel is held in place by a support stand. Essential oils are added to the oil to enhance doshic balance (see Chapter 16 for more information about doshas).

Procedure
1. Cover the client with a drape, and place a bolster under the client's knees.
2. Assist the client in lying on the table properly.
3. Position a large basin on the floor under the client's head to catch the oil as it runs off the forehead.

4. With a copper vessel positioned approximately 6 inches above the client's forehead, begin the oil stream.
5. Allow the stream to run for approximately 30 minutes. The treatment may last for a shorter time, if needed.
6. Dispose of the used oil in the catch basin.

MINI-LAB

Choose one or all of the hydrotherapy and spa treatments listed in this chapter and administer to a classmate or willing volunteer. Afterward, write a narrative report.

AROMATHERAPY

The use of aromatherapy and essential oils dates back more than 10,000 years to India. The Indians have used essential oils in their practice of ayurvedic medicine. The Egyptians, dating back to 4500 BC, were experts in the art of aromatherapy, especially with their embalming process.

Aromatherapy, also called *essential oil therapy,* is the use of plant-derived essential oils for therapeutic purposes. Rene'-Maurice Gattefosse' was the first to coin the phrase *aromatherapie,* from which the English *aromatherapy* is derived. The French physician Dr. Jean Valnet contributed a great deal to the medical acceptance of aromatherapy, and his book *The Practice of Aromatherapy* has become a classic for aromatherapists. Essential oils can be used in baths, candles, massage lubricants, incense, and specially designed aromatherapy diffusing units. In spa treatments, essential oils are widely used in water to make a steam bath in products used for body masks or body scrubs.

Why then should a massage therapist use aromatherapy?
- **Enhances treatment effectiveness.** Many spas and massage therapists use aromatherapy as a way of enhancing the effectiveness of their treatments.
- **Creates an inviting atmosphere.** A pleasant aroma will help clients relax and feel welcome the moment they walk into the room.

Aromatherapy and Olfaction

We do not smell with the nose; we smell with the brain. With the sense of smell (olfaction), aromatherapy can be used to relax or stimulate the nervous system. The olfactory bulb, located on the superior surface of the nasal cavity, is the only place in the body where the central nervous system is exposed and in direct contact with the environment. When olfactory receptors are stimulated, impulses travel along olfactory nerves toward the brain.

The olfactory bulb is part of the limbic system, which is regarded as the neurological seat of the emotions. Other parts of the limbic system are the hypothalamus, hippocampus, amygdala, thalamus, and a marginal section of the cerebral hemispheres close to the thalamus. Research indicates that these structures work as a system to regulate emotional behaviors.

In 1937, J. W. Papez identified these structures and stated that the structures of the limbic system responded to smell, taste, sound, sight, and painful stimuli, all of which elicit emotional responses. He found that when these structures are damaged, emotional experience decreases significantly. Conversely, when these structures are stimulated, individuals experience emotions such as anger, aggression, fear, sadness, pleasure, happiness, and sexual arousal. Structures of the limbic system are also associated with memory and hunger.

The easiest way to stimulate the limbic system is through the sense of smell.

Essential Oils

Concentrated essences of aromatic plants are known as **essential oils.** There are approximately 300 essential oils available for commercial use. However, only 50 to 100 of these oils have properties suitable for use by the aromatherapist. These essences are 75 to 100 times stronger than the dried version of the plant. This strength is the primary reason for dilution before its use. In fact, essential oils are so concentrated that only small amounts, or drops, are used. Essential oils enter the body either through absorption through the skin or through mucous membranes by inhalation.

Essential oils are extracted from botanicals by several methods, most commonly steam distillation. Many aromatherapists regard essential oils as the soul of the plant. Essential oils can be obtained from many parts of the plants (Figure 12-16). Examples are:
- Flowers (e.g., lavender, jasmine)
- Fruits (e.g., bergamot, lemon)
- Grasses (e.g., citronella)
- Leaves (e.g., eucalyptus, peppermint)
- Roots (e.g., ginger, vetiver)
- Seeds (e.g., black pepper, fennel)
- Tree blossoms (e.g., ylang-ylang, clary sage)
- Woods and resins (e.g., sandalwood, frankincense)

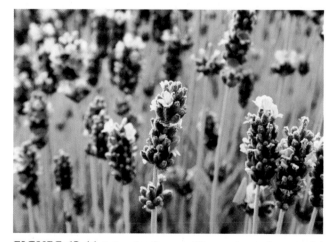

FIGURE 12-16 Lavender flowers. The most popular essential oil is derived from these.

Storage of Essential Oils. Store essential oils in a dark, airtight container, and place in a cool, dry place away from direct sunlight. Be sure the container does not have a rubber cap or rubber squeeze bulbs because these oils will deteriorate the rubber; and dissolved rubber will contaminate the oil.

If properly cared for, essential oils can have a shelf life of up to 7 years. However, when mixed with carrier oils, their shelf life is only as good as that of the carrier oils.

Although they are technically classified as oils, their consistency is similar to that of water. As with water, essential oils are *volatile* (French, "to fly") and will easily evaporate without a trace when exposed to open air. So be sure to replace the bottle top after use.

Keep them out of children's reach.

Carrier Oils. As stated earlier, essential oils must be diluted before use because of their concentration. Not just any substance will do. Essential oils, being *lipophilic* (Greek, "fat loving"), require a fatty material not only to dilute, but also to suspend them. This material is referred to as *carrier oil* because it helps to carry the essential oil. Carrier and essential oils also complement one another's effects; the skin easily absorbs them.

Most fatty substances are appropriate as carriers. These include vegetable and nut oils, such as olive oil or almond oil. Other fatty products that work well are jojoba oil and Shea butter. Whole milk is also an appropriate carrier because it contains fat. Other carriers are creams, lotions, shampoo, conditioner, and liquid soap.

Generally, the higher the fat content, the more stable the carrier oil will be. Stability refers to its shelf life and resistance to oxidation and resultant rancidity. Jojoba is very stable. Safflower oil is not very stable and will go rancid quickly. Vitamin E, which helps stabilize carrier oils, can be added to lengthen shelf life.

Even though essential oils are not soluble in water, they can be added to water if they are properly dispersed, as in shaking a mist bottle before spraying, water used in a steam bath, or water moved through a pump in an immersion bath. If not dispersed, the essential oil will then float, concentrated, on top of the still water.

Essential Oil Safety

- Use only the oils that you are familiar with and that you can use on yourself (you are inhaling and absorbing them too).
- Avoid using on infants.
- Cut the dose for children in half.
- Avoid using essential oils on or near the eyes.
- Ensure that you have adequate ventilation when working with or using essential oils, and take frequent breaks.
- Always use a carrier oil. (There are some exceptions, such as lavender and tea tree.)
- For the therapist, vary the essential oils worked with or diffused on a daily basis to prevent overdose. For example,

daily use of black pepper essential oil can cause allergies.
- Therapists using relaxing essential oils on their clients for prolonged periods risk lowering their own immune system function. Use stimulating oils at least twice on yourself between treatments during the day to lower this risk.
- Predetermine possible contraindications such as those for pregnancy or nursing women (see Chapter 11 for more information). Some essential oils are not recommended for certain neurologic conditions such as seizure disorders, especially birch, cedar, clary sage, jasmine, juniper, marjoram, peppermint, and rosemary. Research and know your essential oils before use.
- Do not apply angelica, lavender, lemon, orange, tangerine, mandarin, and especially bergamot before direct sun exposure. These essential oils are photosensitive and may cause hypersensitivity in ultraviolet light or sunlight.
- Many essential oils carry a high level of toxicity, such as juniper, cinnamon, pennyroyal, fennel, hyssop, and wintergreen. This concern is primarily for the therapist; if he or she is using the aforementioned oils regularly throughout the day, toxicity through frequent exposure may then develop.

Aromatherapy in Massage and Spa

According to Robert Tisserand and Tony Balacs, the following are important to remember in using essential oils as part of a massage therapy experience:

- Use on clean skin (clean skin absorbs better than dirty skin).
- Warmth and massage both enhance absorption.
- Covering the skin after a massage aids in the absorption of the essential oils.
- The stratum corneum (layer in the skin's epidermis) acts as a reservoir; some components of essential oils can remain here for hours.
- The amount of essential oil absorbed through inhalation will be greatly increased by deep or rapid breathing.
- Absorption of substances through the nasal mucosa have easier access to the central nervous system than absorption through the skin.

The following are suggested uses in massage and spa settings. It is recommended that you not blend more than three or four oils at a time until you gain considerable training and experience in aromatherapy, because the blend can become overpowering and even nauseating.

- **Inhalation:** For inhalation, place 5 to 10 drops of essential oil on the center flap of a face rest cover, on a corner of a pillowcase, or on a tissue placed on the arm shelf while the client is prone.
- **Diffusion:** A diffuser is used to disperse essential oils into the air. Add 10 to 15 drops of essential oils to a diffuser. Add more drops as needed.

- **Room mister:** Add 2 to 10 drops per 1 oz of water in spray bottle. Shake before use.
- **Baths:** For immersion bath, add 5 to 10 drops of essential oil in a tub for a single user. Be sure the water is moving while the client is in the water. For steam bath, add 5 to 10 drops in the water well.
- **Compress:** Add 2 to 5 drops of essential oil to a small dish of water. Drench washcloth in scented water. Wring out excess water and apply to client.
- **Massage lubricant:** Add 15 to 20 drops of essential oil to 1 oz of a fat-based lubricant for a full-body massage. This gives a 2.5% to 3% dilution. For massaging a localized area (e.g., muscle spasm in the shoulder), a slightly stronger dilution can be used. Add 12 to 15 drops of essential oil to ½ oz of carrier oil or lubricant for this purpose.
- **Body treatment product:** When using essential oils in body masks or body scrubs, mix the essential oil in a carrier, and then add it to the body treatment product.

Essential Oil Starter Kit

The following oils are recommended to begin building a supply of oils. They are chosen for versatility and economic value.

1. **Eucalyptus.** Widely used for respiratory congestion, eucalyptus helps bring comfort when experiencing loss and grief. This oil is also used during periods of physical and mental fatigue and exhaustion.
2. **Lavender.** The most widely used essential oil, it combats insomnia, calms and balances the mind and emotions, and helps ease irritability.
3. **Lemon.** Lemon is used for added energy to the mind and body and a sense of clarity, which makes it useful during times of indecisiveness. Lemon essential oil may irritate the skin.
4. **Peppermint.** Peppermint adds a sense of excitement and enthusiasm. It is great for a pick-me-up or after a long period of depression. This oil is used for headaches, nausea, and motion sickness. Do not use during pregnancy. If your client is taking homeopathic remedies, then avoid using peppermint because it can act as an antidote.
5. **Rose geranium.** Relaxing and soothing, rose geranium also can enhance sensuality and assist in confidence building.
6. **Rosemary.** Aiding in stimulating mental clarity, concentration, and memory, rosemary promotes cerebral activity (and is used by some students during exams). Rosemary also brings balance by helping detoxify the mind and body. Do not use during pregnancy or for clients with seizure disorders.
7. **Sandalwood.** Sandalwood promotes deep relaxation, abates depression, and quiets the mind and emotions.
8. **Tangerine.** Tangerine is said to clear away negativity and opens up the heart by inspiring sensitivity and empathy. It also helps calm an overactive nervous system.
9. **Tea tree.** Tea tree acts as an antiseptic, so it can be used to disinfect contaminated items. It also helps strengthen the immune system.
10. **Ylang-ylang.** This oil can calm the nervous system, ease depression, and reduce frustration. Used topically, ylang-ylang can irritate the skin.

E-RESOURCES

@volve

http://evolve.elsevier.com/Salvo/MassageTherapy
- Chapter challenge
- Flash cards
- Photo gallery
- Additional information
- Weblinks

BIBLIOGRAPHY

Associated Bodywork & Massage Professionals (ABMP): *Touch training manual*, Evergreen, Colo, 1998, ABMP.

Arnheim DD: *Modern principles of athletic training*, ed 8, St Louis, 1992, Mosby.

Barnes L: Cryotherapy: putting injury on ice, *Phys Sportsmed* 7(6):130-136, 1979.

Cameron MH: *Physical agents in rehabilitation: from research to practice*, ed 3, St Louis, 2008, Elsevier Health Sciences.

Capellini S: *The complete spa book for massage therapists*, Florence, KY, 2010, Cengage Learning.

Clark S: *Essential chemistry for safe aromatherapy*, New York, 2002, Churchill Livingstone.

Corio C: *Aromatherapy educational package for the retailer and health practitioner: part one*, 1996, self-published manual.

Crebbin-Bailey J, Haracup J, Harrington J: *The spa book: the official guide to spa therapy*, London, 2005, Thomson.

De Vierville JP: Taking the waters: a historical look at water therapy and spa culture over the ages, *Massage Bodyw* Feb/Mar: 12-20, 2000.

Drez D: *Therapeutic modalities for sports injuries*, St Louis, 1986, Mosby.

Eidson R: *Hydrotherapy for health and wellness: theory, programs, and treatments*, Florence, KY, 2009, Cengage Learning.

Hannigan MD: *LaStone therapy: the original hot stone massage*, Tucson, 1999.

Hecox B, Mohrotoab T Weiberg J: *Physical agents: a comprehensive text for physical therapists*, Upper Saddle River, NJ, 1993, Prentice-Hall.

Herriott E: Steam and sauna therapy applications with massage, *Massage Mag* May/June: 32-35, 1997.

Knight K: *Cryotherapy: theory, technique and physiology*, Chattanooga, Tenn, 1985, Chattanooga Corp.

Lavabre M: *Aromatherapy workbook*, Rochester, Vt, 1990, Healing Arts Press.

Lawrence DB: *Waterworks*, New York, 1989, Putnam.

Leibold G: *Practical hydrotherapy*, Wellingborough, UK, 1980, Thomson.

Lepak V: *Heat & cold*, University of Oklahoma Health Science Center (website): http://moon.ouhsc.edu/llepak/7223/lecture/hotcold.pdf. Accessed February 9, 2010.

Marx L: An odyssey through spa therapies, *Massage Mag* May/June: 45-48, 1997.

Mellion MB: *Sportsmedicine secrets*, Philadelphia, 1994, Hanley and Belfus.

Minton M: Body and spa, *Massage Mag* Sept/Oct: 89-99, 2001.

Nikola RJ: *Creatures of water*, Salt Lake City, 1997, Europa Therapeutic.

Northern Lights Cedar Hot Tubs: *Cedar tub history* (website): http://www.cedartubs.com/index.html. Accessed June 3, 2010.

Osborn K: Liquid therapy: pouring water on your routine, *Body Sense: Massage, Bodyw, and Healthy Living Mag* Autumn/Winter: 34-42, 2004.

Price S, Price L: *Aromatherapy for health professionals*, ed 2, New York, 1999, Churchill Livingstone.

Rose J: *The aromatherapy book: applications and inhalations*, Berkley, Calif, 1992, North Atlantic Books.

Salvo SG: *Mosby's pathology for massage therapists*, ed 2, St Louis, 2009, Mosby.

Schnaubelt K: *Advanced aromatherapy: the science of essential oil therapy*, Rochester, Vt, 1999, Healing Arts Press.

Tepperman PS, Devilin M: Therapeutic heat and cold: a practitioner's guide, *Postgrad Med* 73(1):69-76, 1983.

Thomas DV: Aromatherapy: mythical, magical, or medicinal? *Hol Nurs Pract* 17(8):8-16, 2002.

Thrash A, Thrash C: *Home remedies: hydrotherapy, massage, charcoal and other simple treatments*, Seale, Ala, 1981, Yuchi Pines Institute.

Tisserard R: *The art of aromatherapy handbook*, Boulder, Colo, 1977, Healing Arts Press.

Tuckerman B: How to add body wraps to your practice, *Massage Mag* Nov/Dec: 92-96, 1999.

Williams A: *Spa bodywork: a guide for massage therapists*, Philadelphia, 2007, Lippincott Williams & Wilkins.

Wissell S: *Aromatherapy educational package for the retailer and health practitioner: part two*, 1996, self-published manual.

Wnorowski D: *Heat and cold therapy*, Runner's Corner (website): http://www.genufix.com/heat_and_cold_therapy.htm. Accessed February 9, 2010,

MATCHING I

Place the letter of the answer next to the term or phrase that best describes it.

A. Body temperature
B. Contrast
C. Cryotherapy
D. Father Sebastian Kneipp

E. Friction
F. Hippocrates
G. Hunting response
H. Hydrotherapy

I. Sauna
J. Spa
K. Steam
L. Vichy

_____ 1. Technique used for administering ice massage

_____ 2. Regarded as the father of hydrotherapy

_____ 3. Dry heat bath in which the client sits or stands in a wood-lined room

_____ 4. Type of shower in which the client reclines on a special table with overhead multiple down-facing showerheads

_____ 5. Early physician who advised both hot and cold bathing; father of western medicine

_____ 6. External therapeutic application of cold

_____ 7. Place where water therapies are administered

_____ 8. Type of bath taken in a ceramic-tiled room filled with water vapor

_____ 9. Type of hydrotherapy treatment in which heat and cold are combined

_____ 10. Cycles of vasoconstriction and vasodilation experienced during cold applications

_____ 11. The greater the difference between this and water temperature, the greater the effect of hydrotherapy

_____ 12. Internal and external therapeutic use of water and complementary agents

MATCHING II

Place the letter of the answer next to the term or phrase that best describes it.

A. 50-59°F (10-15°C)
B. 113°F (45°C)
C. Aromatherapy
D. Balneology

E. Destination
F. Dry brush massage
G. Eucalyptus
H. Heat therapy

I. Lavender
J. Medical
K. Paraffin
L. Thalassotherapy

_____ 1. Art and science of bathing for therapeutic and relaxation purposes

_____ 2. Method used to stimulate skin glands and lymph circulation.

_____ 3. Type of spa where services are supervised under a medical doctor; services may include measures such as Botox injections and aggressive chemical peels

_____ 4. Therapeutic use of sea and marine products, primarily seaweed

_____ 5. Temperature range at which cold reduces nerve fiber conduction rates

_____ 6. Type of spa that offers overnight accommodations, traditional spa services, wellness elements, and spa cuisine

_____ 7. Therapeutic use of plant-derived essential oils

_____ 8. Therapy that promotes relaxation of muscle through lengthening of the collagen within these and related structures

_____ 9. Most widely used essential oil; obtained from flowers

_____ 10. Application of this heated product may be used for pain relief and to soften skin; commonly applied on angular bony areas of the body such as the hands, wrists, elbows, knees, ankles, and feet

_____ 11. Essential oil obtained from leaves

_____ 12. Temperature above this range can cause tissue damage

CASE STUDY

At Your Service

The Transformation Station is a full-service spa in an active convention center. Services include massage therapy, stone massage, shiatsu, sauna, steam bath, whirlpool, contrast pool plunge, Vichy shower, saline bath, and a variety of body wraps, scrubs, and exfoliations.

Therapists are trained in all spa treatments. This versatility allows each therapist to accommodate each client's needs. And the average client is a one-time user of services, scheduling when the convention permits free time. Appointment cancellation is not likely to result in rescheduling, so management makes every effort to be sure that each scheduled client keeps his or her appointment.

Tara has been working at the spa for 2 years. Her ratings are very high and she hopes to be chosen to replace the spa manager, who is moving to another location this fall.

On a Wednesday evening in January, Brett has scheduled a Swedish massage with Tara. She greets Brett and brings him into the massage room to do an initial intake. Brett tells Tara that he scheduled the massage because he feels congested and is afraid he has caught a cold. He needs to be in tip-top shape for an important presentation at his conference. He was told that massage therapy might make the cold go away faster.

Tara is not sure massage is the best option. Tara also knows that a cancellation will not result in rescheduling, and that management frowns upon turning a client away. She is concerned that discouraging Brett from having treatment will hurt her chances of being promoted.

What is the best way for Tara to proceed with this client?

Does she have an ethical obligation to discuss this with Brett, even if he is not certain that he has a cold?

Are there offerings at the spa that may improve his symptoms? If so, what might be the best option for a client with congestion who needs to be in the best shape possible 12 hours later?

What self-care recommendations, within her scope of practice, might Tara offer to Brett?

How can Tara turn this situation into a positive way to elevate her chances of being promoted to manager?

CRITICAL THINKING

Spa applications are not always considered massage therapy per se. Why would a massage therapist want to know how to apply these treatments?

Foot Reflexology

LEARNING OBJECTIVES

After completing this chapter, the student should be able to:

- Discuss the theories of foot reflexology.
- Identify the 10 zones and the horizontal landmarks on the feet.
- Locate all of the reflex points on the feet and ankles.
- Describe basic techniques used in foot reflexology.
- Explain the treatment guidelines, contraindications, and precautions used in foot reflexology.
- State what a client might experience during a foot reflexology session.
- Using techniques provided in this chapter, perform a foot reflexology treatment session.

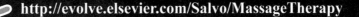

INTRODUCTION

While foot reflexology itself is a relatively new method, various forms of foot massage originated over 5000 years ago. The roots of modern reflexology can be traced back to many countries, including India, Egypt, China, and Japan. Early statues from India of the Hindu god Vishnu depict Sanskrit symbols placed on his feet at the same location where modern reflexologists locate reflex points. One of the earliest pieces of evidence depicting reflexology is an Egyptian tomb that dates back to approximately 2500 BC. It features a physician performing foot reflexology to ease his patient's pain. Underneath the pictograph is carved the words "Do not hurt me." To this statement, the physician replies, "I will act only to help you."

Feet have been revered and considered sacred in many cultures. Jesus washed the feet of his disciples, and Asian students traditionally kissed the feet of their spiritual teacher. Native Americans believed the feet were sacred because they are in contact with the earth's energy; therefore feet should be uncovered to receive life force.

Modern reflexology developed out of zone therapy and the research and writings of Dr. William Fitzgerald in the early 1900s. It was popularized in North America by **Eunice Ingham,** a physiotherapist, who is affectionately referred to as the "mother of reflexology" (Figure 13-1). She spent most of her life mapping the exact location of reflex points on the feet. Ingham spread her love and knowledge of reflexology through teaching, writing, and demonstrating reflexology on as many people as possible. Her work is still carried on by the International Institute of Reflexology through seminars held worldwide.

To receive reflexology, disrobing is not necessary and lubricants are not needed. Furthermore, reflexology can be practiced practically anywhere that is comfortable for both the therapist and the client. For these and many more reasons, reflexology is a very popular form of massage and bodywork. According to a 2007 survey conducted by the Federation of State Massage Therapy Boards, reflexology is the fifth most popular massage method in the United States. In order, the top five methods are:

1. Swedish massage
2. Deep tissue
3. Trigger point therapy
4. Myofascial
5. Reflexology.

This survey is the largest one conducted thus far in the history of massage therapy.

⊜volve *An Egyptian tomb carving that dates back to around 2500 BC can be seen on the Evolve website that accompanies this text. According to the carving, the patient is saying, "Do not hurt me." In hearing this, the physician replies, "I will act only to help you."* ∎

▌MINI-LAB

Use a golf ball or tennis ball to stimulate your feet when you are tired and your feet ache. Simply roll the bottom of your foot over a ball placed on the floor, pressing down on areas that are tender. Maintain a comfortable pressure for approximately 10 seconds. Return to these areas for additional work as needed.

THEORY OF REFLEXOLOGY

According to ancient Eastern principles, all living things are enmeshed in a life force. This life force is called several things such as Chi, Qi, Ki, and Prana. In our polarized world, Chi flows between North and South poles. Just as iron filings form a specific configuration when a magnet is held over them, this energy travels through the body in a distinct pattern.

In reflexology, this energy travels through the body through 1 of 10 zones (Figure 13-2). When the body is in a state of health, energy flows freely. Disease or pain impedes the flow of energy and represents an imbalance in the life force. Congestion or tension in any part of the zone will affect the entire zone. Direct pressure stimulates and directs the life force through its respective zone. This reduces stress by inducing relaxation.

Reflexology, which was originally called *zone therapy*, is a method of stimulating life force through applied pressures on reflex points located on the hands, ears, face, and feet. These reflex points correspond to the body's organs and structures, as they are *reflections* of the body. Pressure is typically applied with the fingers and thumbs. Knuckles

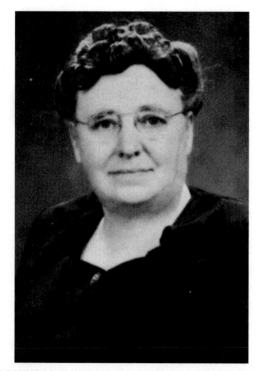

FIGURE 13-1 Eunice Ingham: The mother of reflexology.

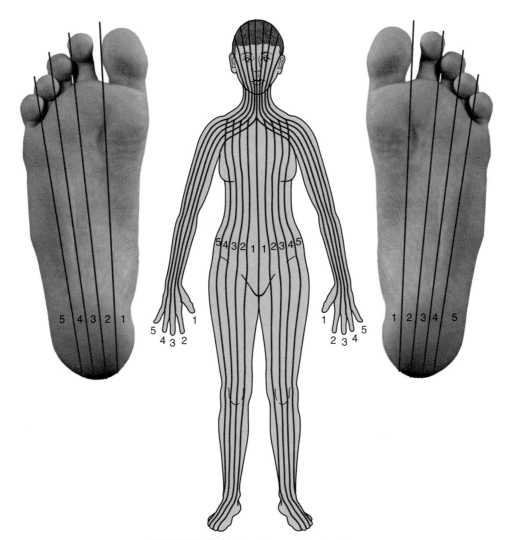

FIGURE 13-2 The 10 zones in reflexology.

or hand-held tools may be used when working on the client's heels. This chapter focuses on the feet, or on foot reflexology.

Reflexology should not be confused with a reflex action, which is an involuntary muscular response to a nerve stimulus, such as when the knee extends when the quadriceps tendon is tapped with a physician's rubber hammer. However, many reflexologists agree that applying specific techniques to the reflex areas and points produces a calming and relaxing effect.

Aside from the energetic (energy-based) theory of reflexology, other theories suggest that by pressing on reflex points, toxins and impurities are released by improving local circulation. The feet are the most distal region of the body. Venous and lymphatic circulation may not be adequate to push these wastes back toward the heart. Reflexology can act to release and return these wastes back into the circulation.

> *"Always do right. This will gratify some people and astonish the rest."*
> —Mark Twain

MAP OF THE BODY: ZONES, LANDMARKS, AND REFLEXES

The feet can be mapped in several ways such as by zone, landmarks, and reflex points.

Zones

According to the theory of reflexology, 10 zones exist in the body through which energy travels. Five zones are located in each foot (see Figure 13-2). These zones are used for mapping the reflex points. Imagine a line passing from the area between each toe and then continuing straight up to the head. Everything in this area, including glands, organs, and body parts, is found in that particular zone located on the foot. If you follow zone 2 from the center of the second toes up through the body, you will pass through the kidneys and eventually the iris of the eyes. Zone 1 passes through the great toe, zone 2 passes through the second toe, and so on, until you reach the smallest toe, which is zone 5. Life force stimulated on a zone located on the foot affects the entire zone within the body.

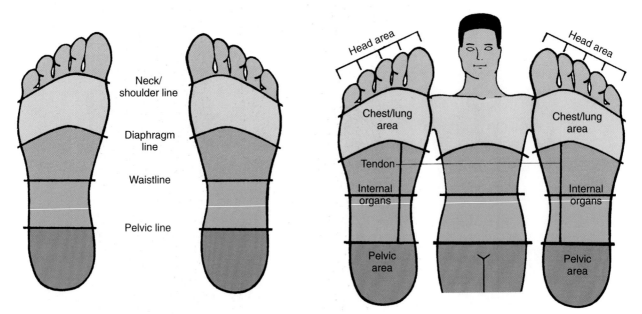

FIGURE 13-3 The four horizontal landmarks in reflexology. (Norman L: *Feet first: a guide to foot reflexology*, New York, 1998 Simon & Schuster)

Landmarks

Four horizontal landmarks traverse the bottom (or plantar surface) of each foot and provide assistance in locating reflex points (Figure 13-3).

- **Neck/shoulder line:** The first landmark is the neck/shoulder line. Above this line are the toes, which reflect the head area in reflexology; below is the ball of the foot, which corresponds to the chest/lung area.
- **Diaphragm line:** The next landmark is the diaphragm line located where the ball of the foot meets the lateral arch.
- **Waistline:** The waistline is the third horizontal landmark. To locate this line, find the base of the fifth metatarsal and trace an imaginary line across to the foot's medial edge. Internal abdominal organs are located above and below the waistline (between the diaphragm line [discussed previously] and the pelvic line [discussed next]).
- **Pelvic line:** The fourth and final landmark is located in front of the heel. The area below the pelvic line contains reflex areas and points for the abdominopelvic organs.

Reflex Points

Once you have an understanding of the zones and how to use horizontal landmarks, you are ready to locate the foot reflexes or reflex points. Reflex locations and their positional relationships to each other follow a logical anatomic pattern that closely resembles that of the body itself. Glancing at a reflexology chart, imagine that you are laying the feet alongside the body, with the toes next to the head (Figure 13-4). During a reflexology session, pressure will be applied along the zones and on reflex points.

BASIC TECHNIQUES

Several techniques are used in foot reflexology; two important techniques are (1) finger and thumb *walking* and (2) *pointwork*.

Walking

The walking technique is used for working an entire area or zone. This technique, which is usually applied with the thumb on the bottom of the foot or with the finger on the top of the foot, allows the therapist to stimulate many reflexes located along its path.

To create the *walking* action, bend and straighten the thumb's (or finger's) interphalangeal joint. As you move your thumb up in small increments, press and release over reflex points. This strategy ensures that all of the reflexes within the zone are stimulated.

While the thumb of one hand is walking, the fingers of that hand are supporting the foot receiving treatment. The other hand is also providing support (Figure 13-5).

Pointwork

Pointwork is used to stimulate specific reflex points. Two pointwork methods are used to isolate a specific point and to increase pressure on the point. The first is *direct pressure*; pressure can be increased by rotating, pivoting, or flexing the foot onto the thumb (or finger) as it remains stationary. Hence, the client's foot moves rather than your thumb.

The second method is called the *hook-in and backup*; it requires the therapist to apply pressure to the reflex point, then flex and extend the distal joint of the working thumb (or finger). This technique can be broken down into three

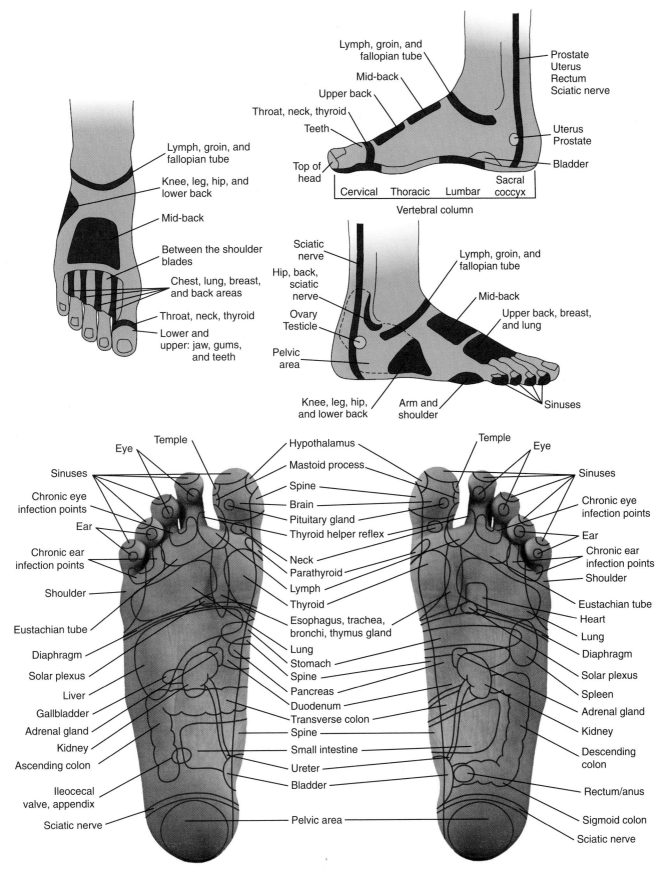

FIGURE 13-4 Reflexology foot map.

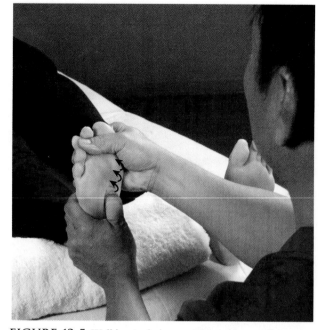

FIGURE 13-5 Walking technique used to address reflex points in an area or zone.

parts. First, locate the desired reflex and apply pressure. Next, bend the distal joint while maintaining contact with the reflex point. Last, straighten the distal joint while maintaining contact. It is as though you are applying the walking technique, only you are not walking to other reflexes (essentially *walking* in place). Pressure is concentrated on one spot, and the movement of the thumb pushes the tissue aside so pressure feels more intense without the therapist's actually applying more pressure. This technique is used for deeper reflex points, including the pituitary, the ileocecal valve, and the sigmoid colon.

CHAT ROOM

Many therapists also use hand-held tools for pointwork. Refer to Chapter 9 to learn more about disinfection of hand-held tools used during treatment.

Relaxation Techniques

Relaxation techniques, also called *desserts,* are used for relaxing the feet before, during, and after a reflexology session. These techniques include shaking the feet (the foot flop) and ankles from side to side (the ankle flop) (Figure 13-6) and taking the foot through its range of motion such as dorsiflexion, plantar flexion, inversion, and eversion (Figures 13-7 and 13-8). If you do whatever feels good to you while you are receiving a reflexology session, it will also feel good to the client. Clients enjoy having their feet kneaded and stroked. Do not be afraid to invent moves. You will discover that your hands and your client's feet work well together.

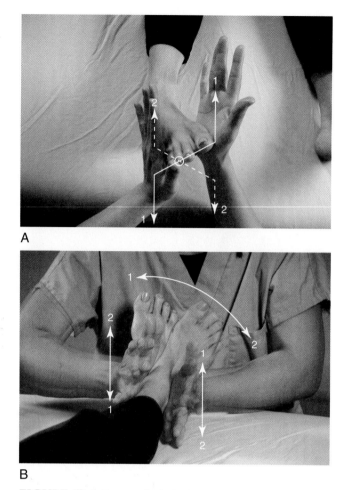

FIGURE 13-6 Desserts include the foot flop **(A)** and the ankle flop **(B)**.

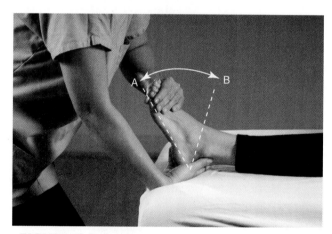

FIGURE 13-7 Foot plantar flexion **(A)** and dorsiflexion **(B).**

TREATMENT GUIDELINES

Reflexology can be practiced almost anywhere. Your client may be seated or lying down during the session. Presented next are guidelines and suggestions for the session.

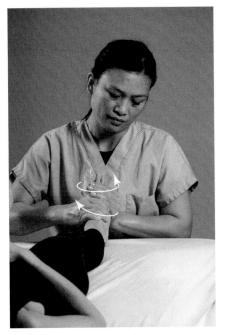

FIGURE 13-8 Inversion and eversion or *wringing out the foot.*

- Conduct a client intake to rule out any contraindications and to establish therapeutic goals (see Chapter 10).
- Escort the client to the area where the reflexology session will take place, and discuss the procedure, answering all questions to the best of your ability.
- Ideally, the client should remove socks or stockings and his or her feet should be resting on a clean drape.
- Sanitize your hands before and after each session.
- Use efficient body mechanics (see Chapter 7).
- Avoid the use of massage lubricants because the therapist's fingers and thumbs may slide off reflex points. If lubricant is used, check for possible allergies to topical agents. Have a hypoallergenic lubricant available in case it is needed (see Chapter 3).
- Warm up the area well with relaxation techniques. Use pressures within the client's pain tolerance and avoid inducing pain. Watch for signs indicating discomfort such as tension in the client's face, hand clenching, or body rigidity.
- Avoid overtreating; limit the time spent working on one area. Work a reflex point for 10 to 15 seconds. Revisit tender areas up to three times during a session.
- For pressure on the top of the foot, use the fingertips because of the close proximity of the tendons and because there is less padding located here. Thumb pressure may be too strong. Thumbs can be used on the bottom of the foot. On the thick skin of the heel, you can use your knuckle.
- If your hands tire, interject relaxation techniques.
- After the session be sure to wipe off any excess lubricant (including between toes); this will help prevent

accidental slips and falls. You may remove any lubricant, help your client put on shoes and socks or stockings, if appropriate. Suggest that the client to drink plenty of fluid, namely pure water, for a day or two following the session is helpful.

---

evolve *Watch a therapist performing reflexology by accessing your student account through the Evolve website. Note how the therapist applies direct pressure to the adrenal reflex point while he flexes the client's foot. Included are two photos of how the therapist works on a reflexology client while in supine and prone positions, with the feet placed on a support in the latter position.* ■

Contraindications and Precautions

Reflexology is safe to use with most clients. Precautions and contraindications are the same as with massage clients. Information about infection control and standard precautions are found in Chapter 9.

General precautions include:

- Clients with diabetes or neurologic conditions such as multiple sclerosis and paralysis often have various degrees of neuropathy (reduced or lack of sensation); a lighter-than-normal pressure should be used over affected areas.
- Avoid pressing on tendons that become prominent when the toes are extended.
- If the client is in a weakened state caused by illness, age, or disability, then treatment time is shorter than normal (10 minutes per foot); pressure should be lighter than usual and sessions can be more frequent.

Local contraindications include:

- Localized cysts
- Corns, calluses, and bunions
- Bone spurs
- Ulcerations, fissures, and other skin lesions
- Warts
- Fungal infection of the toenails
- Ingrown toenails

Absolute contraindications include:

- Gout
- Pitting edema (unless the therapist is trained in advanced protocols of lymphatic massage)
- Athlete's foot
- Recent injury of the foot or ankle (avoid the affected area for 72 hours)
- Recent surgery (postpone treatment until after the 10th day from when the client became ambulatory)

DWIGHT BYERS

Born: February 11, 1929

"You may be walking on the solution to many of your health problems."

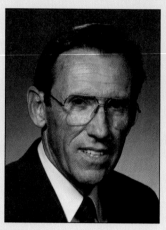

Dwight Byers claims he was one of the guinea pigs for his aunt's early work in reflexology. His aunt, Eunice Ingham, a physical therapist and member of the New York Medical Massage Therapist Association, worked during the early 1930s for a physician who had a passing interest in the art of zone therapy. Zone therapy was a predecessor of reflexology and was introduced in the early 1900s by Dr. William H. Fitzgerald, who successfully used different devices to place pressure on certain points on the hands to relieve pain.

Eunice Ingham took this work a step further and put her own mark on this ancient healing art, which was practiced as far back as 2330 BC. According to Byers, his aunt was strong-willed, extremely intuitive, and totally dedicated to easing suffering in her fellow man.

Along with a compassionate heart, Ingham had a keen mind. Her time-honored techniques are the result of experiment, research, and copious notes. She threw out what did not work and perfected what did. Her books, *Stories the Feet Can Tell Through Reflexology* (Ingham Publishing, 1984) and *Stories the Feet Have Told Through Reflexology* (Ingham Publishing, 1984) provide more details on this subject.

Ingham's dedication to helping relieve suffering proved inspirational to her young nephew, who was at first skeptical. His skepticism, along with his hay fever and asthma, vanished after experiencing his aunt's healing touch firsthand.

"At first we kind of laughed at her," remembers Byers, as he shares the stories of traveling with his aunt as she conducted seminars on reflexology across the United States. "I helped her carry her bags and set up. But soon I became fascinated, and eventually my sister and I began helping her teach."

Byers's background as a medic in the U.S. Army and his later experience in mortuary science helped hone some of his anatomy skills as he began practicing reflexology part time. When his aunt died in 1974, Byers formed the International Institute of Reflexology to help preserve the original Ingham method. In 1983, he published his book, *Better Health with Foot Reflexology* (Ingham Publishing, 2001), for the same reason.

In the foreword of Byers's text, Dr. Ray C. Wunderlich, Jr., offers some compelling theories to account for reflexology's success:

"Quite probably, it will eventually be shown that foot reflexology alters energy flow in the body… There are 7200 nerve endings in each foot. Perhaps this fact, more than any other, explains why we feel so much better when our feet are treated. Nerve endings in the feet have extensive interconnections through the spinal cord and brain with all areas of the body." (from Byers D: *Better health with foot reflexology,* 1983)

Byers, whose favorite adage is *"experience is the father of all knowledge,"* claims that the best results are obtained by those who practice, practice, practice. "You've got to work on thousands of feet," he says. "My advice for beginning massage therapists is to master your art. Don't be a jack-of-all-trades and master of none."

Byers believes that the therapist must be the type of person who wants to help people, not someone who thinks of money first. "You've got to give a lot," he says. This statement is not idle lip service from Byers. He has done his share of throwing in an extra free visit for clients and has helped senior citizen clients by providing them with discounted sessions.

Byers is a man who understands people. He is down to earth and pragmatic, and so are his seminars. The final is hands-on, and his feet are up for grabs after a 200-hour program. His criterion for grading: "Would I pay to have this treatment done?"

Massage therapists who become certified in reflexology use it to enhance their business. Beginning the session with reflexology can induce relaxation and increase circulation, which benefits muscles, glands, and internal organs from the inside out.

WHAT THE CLIENT MAY EXPERIENCE

Most clients experience deep relaxation during and after the reflexology session. He or she may fall asleep. After the session, your client may feel light-headed or dizzy when sitting or standing up suddenly after lying down. This is due to a sudden drop in blood pressure (orthostatic hypotension). In these cases, suggest that the person sit back down, wait a few moments, and try again, moving more slowly this time. Be ready to assist. Some therapists offer their clients pure water after the session.

Other clients may experience a headache or an increase of elimination through the skin, bowels, or urination. He or she may even experience a flare-up of a current or past illness that had never healed fully. All of these scenarios can be classified as a *healing response* or *healing crisis*; it is the body's way of throwing off excess toxins or impurities. More than likely, most of these symptoms will go away in a few days. However, of course, if the client has any questions or concerns, refer the client to his or her physician.

What Tenderness May Mean

Generally speaking, if the client feels only pressure and not pain, then the reflexes are healthy and the person has a good general constitution. When the client feels tenderness, sensitivity, discomfort, or pain during the application of pressure, it may then mean that there is a localized condition such as a bunion or plantar wart (for which you avoid the area). Tenderness may mean that the client is under stress or may simply not be accustomed to having the feet massaged. With ongoing sessions, tenderness often diminishes. It is important that you do not imply that tenderness indicates a health problem.

As reflexes are palpated, the therapist may feel a lumpy or grainy deposit. Some therapists believe that these areas are crystal deposits of uric and lactic acid that accumulate in the feet. These deposits create congestion and blockage around vital nerve functions, and interfering with blood circulation to the feet. Also believed is that pressure applied to these areas breaks them down so that the body can more easily reabsorb them into the bloodstream or lymph system, where they can be eliminated.

"Grow in any dimension and the pain, as well as the joy, will be your reward. The only alternative is not to live fully or not to live at all."
—M. Scott Peck

A FOOT REFLEXOLOGY TREATMENT SESSION

The foot can be divided into six treatment areas: the head, the chest, the abdomen, the pelvic area, the reproductive organs, and the spinal area. The four horizontal landmarks mentioned previously (neck and shoulder, diaphragm, waistline, and pelvic lines) are used to delineate five of the six treatment areas; the last area is located on the medial side of the foot from the base of the heel to the base of the toenail of the great toe.

Begin by establishing physical contact with the client. Locate the solar plexus reflexes with your thumbs (just under the ball of the foot between the second and third toes). The solar plexus is often referred to as the *abdominal brain* because it contains a large number of nerves. In reflexology, the solar plexus reflex is also referred to as the *key to relaxation*. The client will often reward you with a generous sigh of relief once you locate this spot. Apply pressure while your client inhales; release pressure while the client exhales. Follow the client's breath with your own. Do this three to six times.

Next, locate the diaphragm line. Use the walking technique along this line, moving across the foot. This will help your client relax and set the stage for a more effective reflexology session.

As the session progresses, return to the solar plexus reflex because pressing it returns the client to a place of relaxation, especially after deep pointwork.

> *evolve* For a sample foot reflexology routine, log on to the Evolve website and choose materials for Chapter 13. ∎

Head Area

The great toe is the reflex area for the head, containing the pituitary gland. Locate the pituitary reflex by looking for the center of the swirl on the great toe and hook into that point with your thumb. It will often feel similar to a small pea. This reflex is effective to work if a boost of energy is needed or for any glandular problems because of its importance in the endocrine system.

Next, gently squeeze the pads of each toe to stimulate the sinus reflexes. Use the walking technique along the bottom and sides of each toe, pressing from the tip to the base.

CHAT ROOM

Some schools of thought on reflexology state that the great toe contains all five zones.

Chest Area

The ball of the foot is the reflex area for the chest, which contains the heart and lungs. In our bodies, the heart is located two thirds to the left of the midline and one third to the right. This area is represented on the feet: The heart reflex is located primarily on the left foot, with a small portion on the right foot.

Abdominal Area

The area housing the abdominal reflexes is located between the diaphragm and the pelvic lines. The spleen and stomach reflexes are located on the left foot, and the liver and gallbladder reflexes are on the right foot. Another important reflex to stimulate is the pancreas area, located on the left foot just behind the stomach reflex. The pancreas is involved in regulating glucose levels, which is the body's main source of energy. Avoid overworking the reflexes of the abdominal area during the first few sessions because it may leave the client feeling overwhelmed and exhausted.

Pelvic Area

Between the pelvic line and the heel is the area containing pelvic reflexes, which houses the organs of the lower abdomen and pelvis. The right foot contains the reflexes for the ascending colon and part of the transverse colon. The left foot contains reflexes for the rest of the transverse colon and the descending colon.

The reflexes for most of the urinary structures are located here. The urinary bladder area is located where the pelvic line meets the arch of the foot. The kidneys' reflexes are located along the waistline demarcation, between the second and third toes.

Reproductive Area

One of the last areas worked in reflexology is the area containing the reproductive reflexes, which are located on the heel and the ankle. The uterus or prostate reflex is on the medial ankle, and the ovaries or testes reflex is on the lateral ankle. To locate the reflex for the uterus or prostate, imagine a diagonal line from the high point of the medial ankle (malleolus) to the base of the heel; in the middle of the line is the uterus/prostate reflex point. Use the same measuring procedure to find the ovaries or testes on the lateral ankle.

Working on the uterus point during pregnancy is controversial, although no documented evidence indicates that this would stimulate labor via uterine contractions.

The next set of foot reflexes worked is the sciatic nerve. To locate it, imagine a stirrup running from beneath the heel, behind the ankle, and on both sides of the Achilles tendon.

Spinal Area

The last sets of reflexes to be addressed, and one of the most important, are the spinal reflexes, which are located along the medial aspect of the feet. As you look at the arch of the foot, notice how the medial edge possesses four distinct curves, just as does a vertebral column. Because of the importance of these reflexes, they are to be worked in every session. Walk your thumb along the spinal reflexes, pressing continuously from the base of the heel to the base of the nail of the great toe.

E-RESOURCES

ⓔvolve

http://evolve.elsevier.com/Salvo/MassageTherapy
- Chapter challenge
- Flash cards
- Photo gallery
- Weblinks

BIBLIOGRAPHY

Berkson D: *The foot book*, New York, 1977, HarperCollins.
Byers DC: *Better health with foot reflexology: the original Ingham method*, St Petersburg, Fla, 1996, Ingham.
Dougans I: *The complete illustrated guide to foot reflexology*, Boston, 1996, Element Books.
FSMTB: 2007 job task analysis survey report (website): http://www.fsmtb.org/downloads/jtaDemo.pdf. Accessed May 28, 2010.
Ingham E: *Stories the feet can tell through reflexology*, St Petersburg, Fla, 1984, Ingham.
Kunz K, Kunz B: *The complete guide to reflexology (revised)*, Upper Saddle River, NJ, 1986, Prentice Hall.
Micozzi MS: *Fundamentals of complementary and alternative medicine*, Philadelphia, 2011, Saunders.
Monohan FD et al: *Phipps' medical-surgical nursing: health illness perspectives*, ed 8, St Louis, 2007, Mosby.
Norman L: *Feet first: a guide to foot reflexology*, New York, 1988, Simon & Schuster.
Salvo SG: *Mosby's pathology for massage therapists*, ed 2, St Louis, 2009, Mosby.
Stillerman E: *Modalities for massage and bodywork*, St Louis, 2009, Mosby.

MATCHING I

Place the letter of the answer next to the term or phrase that best describes it.

A. Chi
B. Desserts
C. Eunice Ingham
D. Landmarks

E. Lubricant
F. Mother of reflexology
G. Reflex action
H. Reflexology

I. Roots of modern reflexology
J. Ten
K. William Fitzgerald
L. Zone therapy

_____ 1. Individual whose research and writings helped develop modern reflexology

_____ 2. Involuntary muscular response to a nerve stimulus

_____ 3. Can be traced back to countries including India, Egypt, China, and Japan

_____ 4. What reflexology was called originally

_____ 5. Title by which Eunice Ingham is referred

_____ 6. Method of stimulating life force through applied pressures on reflex points located on the hands, ears, face, and feet

_____ 7. Total number of zones the body possesses, which run vertically from the toes up to the head

_____ 8. Physiotherapist who popularized modern reflexology in North America

_____ 9. Horizontal areas that traverse the bottom of each foot and provide assistance in locating reflexes

_____ 10. Term to denote techniques used specifically to relax the feet before, during, and after a reflexology session

_____ 11. A term used in Eastern principles to denote life force

_____ 12. Product not required in reflexology treatments

MATCHING II

Place the letter of the answer next to the term or phrase that best describes it.

A. Bone spur
B. Diaphragm line
C. Direct pressure
D. Knuckles, hand-held tools

E. Neuropathy
F. Pelvic line
G. Pointwork
H. Reflex points

I. Walking
J. Zone 1
K. Zone 5
L. Zones

_____ 1. Term used in reflexology to describe the body's energy pathways

_____ 2. Landmark located where the ball of the foot meets the arch of the foot

_____ 3. Client with this condition requires lighter-than-normal pressure when receiving reflexology

_____ 4. Zone that passes through the smallest toe

_____ 5. Points located on the hands, ears, face, and feet where pressure is applied in reflexology; these points correspond to the body's organs and structures

_____ 6. This reflexology technique can be used to work an entire area rather than a specific reflex point

_____ 7. Landmark located in front of the heel of the foot

_____ 8. The therapist may use these instead of the tops and sides of the fingers when performing reflexology on the client's heels

_____ 9. Zone that passes through the great toe

_____ 10. Primary method used to stimulate and direct life force through its respective zone

_____ 11. An example of a local contraindication in foot reflexology

_____ 12. This reflexology technique can be used to stimulate a specific reflex point rather than an entire area

CASE STUDY

Be Cautious of Labels

Delores has been practicing massage therapy for 10 years. She has a small practice in a local business area. Most of her clients are professional men and women, who typically have standing appointments. On rare occasions, Delores can work with a new client.

Natalie, the wife of a prominent bank owner, telephoned Delores late one afternoon and requested a massage for 9 AM the next day. Delores had a cancellation and was able to work in this new client on short notice. When Natalie arrived, Delores noted that Natalie was a tall, middle-aged, well-dressed woman adorned with furs and elaborate jewelry. As Delores ushered her to the massage room, Natalie became louder and even more expressive as she talked about her pet poodle, Phoebe. As they sat down to discuss Natalie's health, the stench of whiskey filled the air. Delores realized that her client may be intoxicated.

How should Delores address the situation, if at all?

What risks are involved if Delores decides to massage Natalie in her current state? What modifications should Delores make during the session? Is alchohol a stimulant or a depressant?

How might Natalie feel if confronted with her alcohol consumption?

What if Delores made an incorrect assumption and Natalie was on prescription medication, had Parkinson disease, or diabetes mellitus?

What issues might be discussed if the roles are reversed and the therapist showed signs of intoxication?

CRITICAL THINKING

Why is it important for a massage therapist to receive regular massages and foot reflexology?

CHAPTER 14

Clinical Massage

Susan G. Salvo, BEd, LMT, NTS, CI, NCTMB,
Judith DeLany, LMT, and Monica J. Reno, LMT

"If a pickpocket meets a holy man, he will see only his pockets."

—Hari Dass Baba

LEARNING OBJECTIVES

After completing this chapter, the student should be able to:

- Define and explain the importance of clinical massage.
- Discuss fascia, muscle, and muscle spasm.
- State the definition of a trigger point, how they are formed, types of trigger points, and their characteristics.
- List ways of locating and deactivating trigger points.
- Define muscle soreness, listing prevalent theories.
- Contrast and compare acute, subacute, and chronic pain.
- List the stages of rehabilitation and related activities.
- Discuss and perform a postural assessment.
- Explain gait assessment.
- Define and demonstrate techniques used in clinical massage.
- Explain how to avoid common mistakes of clinical massage.
- List aftercare recommendations.
- Discuss sports massage, types, and causes of sports injury.
- List muscles to be addressed when the client is experiencing pain or limited function in the neck and head, shoulder area, and lower back and hip areas.

INTRODUCTION

Massage therapists are part of a health care team serving clients, many of whom exhibit various injuries and conditions. Research has documented the effectiveness of massage. The need for massage in clinical and athletic settings has never been greater. **Clinical massage** involves the use of specific focused techniques that, when applied properly, reduce reported signs and symptoms and improve function.

Regardless of work setting, clinical massage can be used. For example, you may have a client who has requested a massage focused on relaxation because he or she lacks the terminology to ask for what is needed, which may be to feel better and to not be hurt by techniques that are too deep. A well-trained, skilled massage therapist conducts an intake interview and, during this process, may reveal not only the client's definition of "relaxation" massage, but also his or her actual needs, which may include focused techniques.

In this chapter, for purposes of clarity and consistency, clinical massage will be the umbrella term for all of the following: *medical massage, orthopedic massage, treatment massage, neuromuscular therapy, trigger point work, deep tissue massage, deep tissue work,* and *deep pressure massage.*

The goal of this chapter is to provide general information on trigger points, injuries, rehabilitation, basic postural and gait assessments, clinical massage techniques, and recommendations for a few area-specific treatments. These treatment protocols can be used as (1) a stand-alone treatment in a clinical setting (e.g., 15- to 30-minute rotator cuff treatment), (2) a rehabilitative approach within a sports massage session, or (3) a focused segment with a relaxation massage.

To accomplish these tasks, this chapter reviews and develops information that has been covered in other chapters, including assessment, planning (see Chapter 10), and technique (see Chapter 8). It also introduces sports massage and describes how the needs of athletes differ from those of the general public. An *athlete* is someone who possesses natural or acquired abilities, such as strength, endurance, or agility, required for participating in physical exercise or sports, especially competitive sports. Different types of sports massage and their goals are also presented.

Several reasons exist for using clinical massage techniques. The first reason is *time.* Whether dealing with prescribed treatments and third-party payers, a client who is self pay, or an athlete who is near an event, time is often the limiting factor. In these cases, techniques designed to rehabilitate the client in a timely manner is important. Recovery time is swifter when targeting specific tissues.

The second reason is *effectiveness.* Studies show that subjects who received massage using deeper pressure healed faster than those who received massage using lighter, less specific pressure. This was evidenced by an increased number of fibroblasts in injured tissue. These cells, present in connective tissue, are important for tissue healing.

The third reason to learn clinical massage techniques is *need.* Many clients who seek massage have aches and pains and need techniques that focus on tissue repair and recovery, rather than on general relaxation. Therapists who possess knowledge and skills in both relaxation and clinical massage can address their clients' multiple needs. If you work in clinical settings or if you want more information than is presented in this chapter, pursue specialization through well-designed continuing education programs or schools offering augmented education in these areas.

Developing precision with your massage techniques begins with a solid understanding of anatomy (see Chapters 18 to 30). Being knowledgeable about the effects of massage is mandatory (see Chapter 6). Repeated opportunities to palpate and compare structures strengthen hands-on skills and increase the practical knowledge of anatomy immensely. Most abnormalities that you encounter will be muscle spasms, trigger points, myofascial restrictions, and adhesions.

Let us first review information on fascia, muscles, spasms, trigger points, and muscle soreness. This will provide a solid foundation for the clinical massage therapist.

FASCIA

The most abundant tissue type in the body is connective tissue. The eight families of connective tissues include loose and dense fibrous connective tissues and their subsets. And like all types of connective tissue, it contains a ground substance in which its various cells and fibers are embedded. According to Juhan, the ground substance of fascia possesses two physical states:

- *Sol state.* Fascia is relatively thin and more pliant and elastic, and offers less restriction during movement.
- *Gel state.* Fascia is thicker, more gelatinous, tougher, more inflexible, and can restrict movement.

Fascial states can be altered to some degree because fascia's ground substance possesses a property called **thixotropism,** the ability to change from one state to the other. With use of massage techniques such as friction, torquing, skin rolling, or applied heat, fascia can change from a gel to a sol state. When fascia softens, it becomes flexible and elastic, allowing muscles, and trigger points to be manipulated more easily. Thixotropism also occurs during exercise (blood flow increases, and muscle activity generates heat).

CHAT ROOM

Effective conversion of fascia, from a gel state to a solid state, will occur more easily if the body is well hydrated. Suggest to clients to consume water on a daily basis (i.e., 0.5 oz for every 1 lb of body weight). A healthy 140-lb person should consume 70 oz of pure water each day.

MUSCLE

As you move into the realm of clinical massage, it is beneficial to review kinesiology and basic musculoskeletal anatomy such as attachments, actions, fiber direction, synergist, antagonists, and types of contraction from Chapters 20 and 21. Muscle produces body movements, stabilizes body position such as standing or sitting (posture), and produces heat via contractions. Muscles receive and respond to signals from the nervous system for movement to occur; skeletal muscle contractions are mostly voluntary.

Spasm

A muscle **spasm** is an abnormal sustained muscle contraction. Spasms usually result from overuse or overstimulation. This lowers the threshold stimulus (strength of stimuli required to generate a nerve impulse), producing localized spasm. Spasms may or may not cause pain and tenderness. The environment that created the spasm is one of hyperirritability; the muscle's motor units generate contraction with reduced stimuli and the electrophysiologic properties surrounding the sarcomere fail to allow the muscle to relax after contraction (see Chapter 20). Spasms are essentially a neuromuscular event.

Muscle Soreness

Muscle soreness is subjective discomfort felt after physical activity and is a frequent complaint of clients. Two kinds of muscle soreness are immediate and delayed.

Immediate Muscle Soreness. Soreness is experienced during or shortly after exercise or activity, disappearing when the person has rested (see Mini-Lab).

Delayed-Onset Muscle Soreness (DOMS). Here, discomfort is not felt until 8 to 14 hours after the activity, often reaching a peak after 48 hours. Clients often report that they feel stiff the morning after the activity. Even though DOMS has been under scientific scrutiny since 1902, at present the actual biologic process behind it remains a mystery.

The following discussion does not include all theories of DOMS, such as lactic acid. However, the lactic acid theory was once so prevalent, it deserves a mention. Within 1 hour after exercise, most, if not all, lactic acid produced is removed by the circulatory system.

CHAT ROOM

Muscle Fatigue

In contrast with muscle soreness, *muscle fatigue* is the loss of muscle strength or endurance felt after strenuous physical activity. It is believed that muscle fatigue occurs when muscles burn glucose without adequate amounts of oxygen. Muscle fatigue occurs with prolonged contraction; the muscle becomes temporarily weak, unable to generate force. A resultant buildup of lactic acid may cause a burning sensation in the affected muscles.

Prevalent Theories

The two prevailing theories of delayed-onset muscle soreness are inflammation and connective tissue damage. Please note that these theories are related physiologically.

Inflammation Theory. Muscles subjected to prolonged periods of activity can be injured, causing microscopic tears. Pain felt during DOMS is simply part of the inflammatory process as the body attempts to repair microscopic damage caused by prolonged physical activity. DOMS and related inflammation does not result in long-term tissue damage. This theory may also explain why deep-pressure massage may cause soreness in some clients.

Connective Tissue Damage Theory. A relationship has been established between DOMS and connective tissue damage. A substance called hydroxyproline is produced and released into the blood as a result of connective tissue damage and is later excreted by the kidneys. The highest levels of this substance were found in urine of individuals claimed to be the most sore. Interestingly, hydroxyproline is one of the chemical markers associated with the inflammatory response.

DOMS is not felt at rest. If someone with DOMS were sitting watching television, he or she would not experience DOMS until he or she began to move.

Additionally, DOMS usually follows excessive or difficult exercise, and appears to fit into the idea of sports specificity, meaning DOMS occurs commonly after the person performs an activity to which they are unaccustomed. For example, if a person worked out in the gym performing exercise at every station for 4 days a week for the past year, he or she would rarely be sore. However, if this same person decides to rake leaves for 4 hours one fall afternoon, he or she might experience DOMS if no exercise in the gym mimics raking leaves.

Studies show that the vast majority of pain and discomfort associated with DOMS is caused by eccentric muscle contraction. Eccentric contractions (or *negatives*, as they are sometimes called in the gym) occur when muscles experience resistance as they lengthen working against gravity (i.e., descending phase of a biceps curl).

▮ MINI-LAB

Stand with your arms extended in front of you. With your back straight, slowly lower yourself into a deep knee bend. Stop when your thighs are parallel to the floor. Hold this position, noting where you begin to feel a burning discomfort (it is usually felt in the thigh or the shoulder or both). Maintain this position for a few more moments. Stand up again. Notice how long it takes for this burning sensation to disappear. Normally, when the stress on your muscle ceases, the discomfort should subside. This discomfort is an example of immediate muscle soreness.

Discontinue this activity immediately if you experience pain.

TRIGGER POINTS

Similar to spasms, **trigger points** are localized areas of hyperirritability. Unlike spasm, trigger points, when pressed, may refer sensations (usually pain) to other areas of the body. Even though trigger points can be found in tendons, ligaments, and periosteum, most are found in skeletal muscles and their related fascia. Another term used to describe this type of trigger point is a myofascial trigger point. *When the term trigger point is used during the remainder of this chapter, it refers to myofascial trigger points.*

Trigger points are a *neurochemical* event. Muscle spasms are a *neuromuscular* event.

CHAT ROOM

Tender points are specific spots on the body that elicit pain and discomfort where compressed. These points do not refer pain. In some cases, tender points may be caused by muscle spasm, which may be addressed during massage. Presence of tender points is used in the diagnosis of fibromyalgia, a chronic noninflammatory condition characterized by widespread pain, fatigue, and other symptoms.

Review of Contraction and Relaxation

Let us review briefly muscular contraction and relaxation before we look at trigger point formation.

Normal Muscular Contraction. When a muscle is at rest, actin and myosin (myofilaments) lie side by side. When activated by a motor neuron, calcium ions are released from the sarcoplasmic reticulum (membrane surrounding the myofilaments). The presence of calcium ions expose binding sites located on actin; myosin heads can now attach. The myosin heads then toggle (like a light switch). If adenosine triphosphate (ATP) is present, myosin heads then detach themselves, bind to the next exposed site, and pull again. This repetitive pulling causes the ends of the sarcomere to move toward its center. If the force of contraction is great enough to overcome whatever resistance force there is, the muscle will shorten concentrically and muscle attachments will move toward each other.

Normal Muscular Relaxation. Almost immediately after the sarcoplasmic reticulum releases calcium ions into the sarcoplasm, it begins to actively pump calcium back into its sacs. Within a few milliseconds, much of calcium is recovered. The lack of calcium causes the binding sites to be restored. This action, along with the required ATP, releases the myosin heads and returns them to their precontraction state. The muscle is now at rest.

Trigger Point Formation

According to Chaitow and DeLany, trigger points accur from excessive neurotransmitter release in axon terminals. This effect leads to shortening of muscle fibers and localized ischemia. The resulting oxygen and nutrient deficiency leads to reduced energy production in the cell. Energy is needed to release myosin heads and stop myofascial tissue shortening. In the area of the trigger point, energy is not available, so localized contraction is sustained. Trigger points are often caused by sustained muscular contraction and the resultant ischemia. Without blood glucose, cells cannot generate the ATP needed to release the contraction.

Once a trigger point forms, the pulling action causes a taut band to form. Trigger points may be found at the center of the taut band, at musculotendinous junctures, or at the muscle attachment sites.

Causes of Trigger Points

Some activities that generate both trigger points and spasms are:

- *Repetition of any activity.* Examples are sitting long hours at a computer, working out at a gym, yard work, or participating in sports.
- *Direct trauma.* Tissues can be traumatized or injured as seen in motor vehicle accidents, slips and falls, surgical procedures, or sports injuries (Box 14-1).
- *Disease and disorders.* Trigger points can develop in conditions such as myofascial pain syndrome, arthritis, and temporomandibular joint dysfunction.
- *Stress and fatigue.* This includes feelings of anxiety and depression.
- *Miscellaneous factors.* These include structural asymmetry, insufficient strength, lack of flexibility, inadequate hydration and/or electrolytes, or emotional trauma.

Most skeletal muscle contractions are voluntary and stimulated by nerve impulses. *Spasms* are due to a lowering of the threshold, which produces shortening of muscle fibers. *Trigger points* are thought to be due to localized ischemia, the presence of abundant calcium, and inadequate adenosine triphosphate or ATP, resulting in localized contractures. Ischemia is reduced blood supply. We cannot shut off the mechanisms of spasm or a trigger point voluntarily. In most instances, it requires some form of intervention such as massage, stretches, nutritional interventions, medications, or joint mobilizations, and, in some cases, the tincture of time.

Types of Trigger Points

Trigger points can be classified as latent or active.

Active Trigger Points. While all trigger points cause discomfort when pressed, active trigger points cause symptoms such as pain, even at rest. Other symptoms include

BOX 14-1

Causes of Sports Injury

Improper warm-up. Soft tissues are more likely to achieve optimal elasticity if they are warm. Most studies show that a warm-up reduces the risk of muscular tears and fascial restrictions that limit or prevent performance. Aerobic activity such as running in place should be used to raise the heart rate and move oxygen-rich blood through muscle groups associated with the activity. The warm-up should continue until the client feels "mildly breathless." Additionally, for competing outdoors, a good rule of thumb is that the cooler the weather is, the longer the warm-up should be.

Lack of flexibility. Muscles that are flexible stretch easily and are injured less. Studies show that stretching increases flexibility in muscle tissue when compared with subjects that did not stretch. The question is what type of stretching is more beneficial: static or dynamic? On this subject different studies show different results. Even though the jury is still out on which type of stretch is more beneficial, most coaches, trainers, and athletes will tell you that performance benefits from warm-up followed by some form of stretching. For this reason many people have a stretching schedule in their training routine. Remind the athlete that muscles and fascia are similar to clay; they tend to stretch when warm and remain stiff when cold, so warm up first.

Unsuitable equipment. These items include braces, helmets, or pads that do not fit; worn-out shoes; a bow that is not the right size for the archer; and handlebars and bicycle seats that are not positioned correctly. Unsuitable equipment can contribute to injury or reduce athletic performance.

Overtraining. Working too hard or not getting enough recovery between sessions can negatively affect health and performance. Look for overtraining symptoms: lack of enthusiasm for the sport, irritability, fatigue, depression, sleeplessness, and weakening of the immune system. The older the athlete and the closer in time to the competitive event, the more recovery time will be required.

Miscellaneous factors. These factors include improper diet and dehydration; competing in abnormal weather conditions such as rain, snow, or extreme temperature and humidity; structural factors such as fallen arches, spinal curvatures, and pelvic distortions; and emotional distractions.

sensations of tingling, prickling, pins-and-needles, itching, burning and/or numbness, collectively called *paresthesias*.

Latent Trigger Points. Latent trigger points have the same characteristics as active trigger points, but they do not cause referred pain or other sensations until direct pressure is applied. When latent trigger points are found during palpation, the client may comment, "I didn't even realize it hurt there."

Characteristics of Trigger Points

Besides producing pain and paresthesias, trigger points can possess other interesting characteristics during palpation.

Local Twitch Response. A local twitch response is a reflexive impulse causing the affected muscle or adjacent muscles to twitch spontaneously.

Jump Sign. The jump sign is the spontaneous reaction of pain or discomfort that causes a client to wince, jump, or verbalize on application of pressure.

Referred Pain Phenomena. During palpation, some trigger points refer pain to a target area associated with the particular point. These sensations include not only pain but paresthesias.

According to Simons et al (1999), the trigger point is located within its referral pattern (target zone) only 27% of the time. This means that if you are working only where your client reports pain (or other sensation), you are in the wrong spot nearly 75% of the time.

Active trigger points refer to a pattern that the person recognizes or reports is familiar. It refers even when it is not being provoked. Latent trigger points also refer when provoked, but the person will report it as not a common pattern.

Trigger point location and the corresponding target zones of referred pain are fairly constant from one person to the next. Drs. Janet Travell and David Simons charted the target zones over the course of decades of research on myofascial pain syndromes. Because the locations of trigger points and their pain referral patterns are moderately consistent, they are somewhat predictable (Figure 14-1).

Locating and Deactivating Trigger Points

Locating taut bands and trigger points is done mainly by palpation and client inquiry. The identification of possible trigger point (or spasm, for that matter) is most likely to occur during effleurage and friction; as you are sliding your hands over tissues. Direction of pressure is important during palpation (Figure 14-2, *A* and *B*).

Palpation strategies solely for trigger point evaluation include sliding skin over underlying tissue while moving back and forth, tracing the number "8," or by moving in the direction of a compass; north, northeast, east, southeast, south, southwest, west, northwest, north, until an area of localized tenderness is reported (Figure 14-3).

You may also notice a change in the "feel" of the tissues over and around the area; the client will report tenderness. The area can be described as cordlike, nodular, or *crepitant* (pertaining to sounds of crackling, grating, or rattling).

When locating and palpating trigger points, you may also note:
- Changes in thickness of tissue, resistance to pressure
- Muscle shortening with weakness

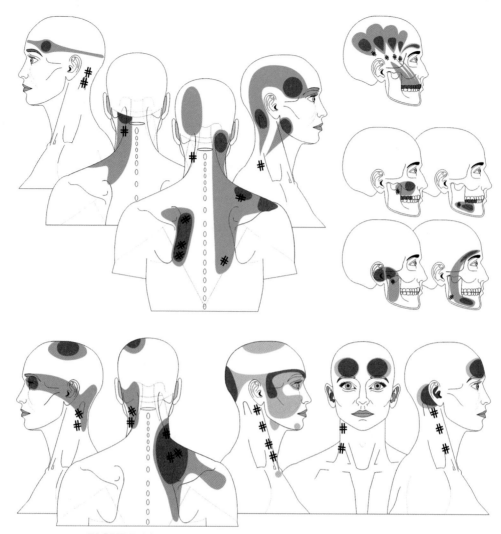

FIGURE 14-1 Common trigger points and their referral patterns (#).

- Temperature changes (area is usually colder, but may be warmer)
- Edema

When the point is located, use a series of 30 to 60 firm gliding strokes. The depth of pressure will depend on the depth of the trigger point you are trying to release. Apply pressure to the client's tolerance just above the taut band and maintain the pressure over the band, releasing pressure just beyond it (see Figure 14-2, *A*). Use of deep gliding strokes accomplishes (1) an increase local circulation and (2) a slight stretch of the tissues. These combined actions help release the cross-bridges.

On a scale of 1 to 10, with 1 being barely felt and 10 being the most pain imaginable, the goal is to apply pressure that registers as a 5, 6, or 7 (preferably). It should not be painful, but, instead, will be moderately uncomfortable. Pressure that produces distorted facial expressions, feet leaving the bolster, fist tightening, and other gestures of painful reaction are entirely too heavy and should be avoided. When these painful reactions occur, reduce pressure and verbally check in with the client. Be sure to encourage

relaxation through deep breathing. Chapter 8 contains additional suggestions regarding working within a client's pain tolerance.

Afterward, stretching techniques should be applied to affected muscles to increase their resting length.

Other techniques to address myofascial trigger points are discussed later in the chapter.

When Not to Deactivate Trigger Points. When deciding whether or not to deactivate and release trigger points, consider their purpose and usefulness. If trigger points are from an activity such as raking leaves and the client used inefficient body mechanics, he or she would benefit from trigger point deactivation. However, if trigger points are in tight lower back muscles that might also limit range of motion (ROM) because of a bulging or herniated intervertebral disk, they might be serving a useful purpose. This type of muscle tightening is often called muscle splinting. In this and similar cases, the underlying problem needs to be assessed and corrected before deactivation of trigger points begins.

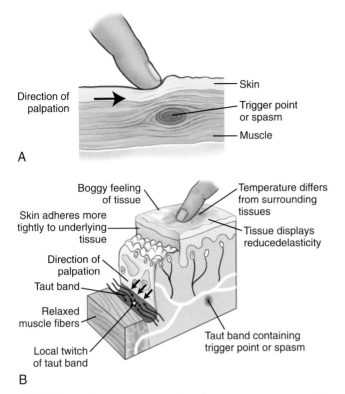

FIGURE 14-2 Trigger points (A) and direction of pressure (B).

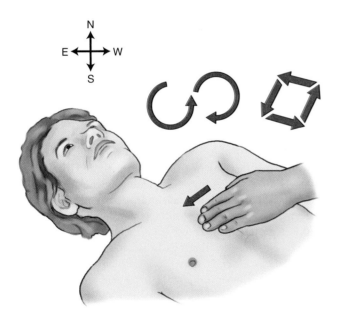

FIGURE 14-3 Compass and "figure 8" method for locating trigger points.

In general, if massage increases the client's pain or produces other adverse reactions, the problem may not be myofascial and may need medical evaluation.

"Pain is inevitable. Suffering is optional."
—Kathleen Casey Theisen

PAIN

Acute Pain

Acute pain is the normal and predictable physiologic response to an adverse stimulus. The adverse stimulus is often tissue damage caused by trauma such as from auto accidents, slipping, falling, or surgical procedures. The duration of acute pain will vary depending upon the condition. For example, if tissue damage was involved, the affected area may be inflamed, with swelling, localized heat, redness, and loss of function. Management of inflamed areas may involve protection, rest, ice, compression, and elevation (PRICE). Many cases also involve the use of pharmacotherapy (drugs recommended or prescribed by qualified health care providers [this is outside the massage therapist's scope of practice]).

Subacute Pain

Subacute pain lies between acute and chronic pain. In these cases, the client appears to be clinically well (there are no presenting signs such as swelling and localized heat), but he or she is still experiencing symptoms such as pain and discomfort. Several studies indicate that massage is beneficial for clients in this stage of pain (e.g., *effectiveness of massage therapy for subacute low-back pain: a randomized controlled trial* by Preyde released in 2000).

Signs are clinical findings that can be observed and measured, so they are objective. Examples of signs are edema, fever and localized heat. *Symptoms* cannot be measured and only the person experiencing them is aware of them, which means they are subjective. Examples of symptoms are headaches, pain, and anxiety.

Chronic Pain

Chronic pain persists for a longer period of time than expected for the condition. Many individuals with chronic pain are unable to identify a cause because it may stem from a situation such as years of sitting improperly at a work desk. This type of pain may be associated with multiple episodes of, or incomplete recovery from, illness or injury. See Table 11-1 for a comparison of chronic and acute pain.

"A muscle can never be neutral—if it doesn't work for you, it works against you."
—Jack Meagher

REHABILITATION

Physical rehabilitation is the process used after illness, injury, or surgery to help the affected individual regain as much function and self-sufficiency as possible. Many clients seek out massage therapy to rehabilitate injuries and address painful symptoms. Rehabilitation begins on day four, after the acute phase when inflammation has reduced significantly. Actual time depends of the severity of the trauma. Moving trauma out of the acute phase promptly is imperative because a prolonged acute state may slow total healing time.

Rehabilitation occurs in three stages; evaluation, conditioning, and maintenance. The objective of each stage should be met before progressing to the next. Disregard of this strategy or omitting one of the stages may hinder the rehabilitation process or exacerbate symptoms. For example, stretching and strengthening activities used before eliminating spasm may interfere with treatment progress and meeting treatment goals.

These stages of rehabilitation are discussed next, highlighting the role of the massage therapist. Be sure to review the neurological laws (see Box 23-2).

Your client's treatment team may include the client's physician, chiropractor, physical or occupational therapist, personal or athletic trainer, and dietitian or nutritionist.

NOTE: Some activities listed may be outside the massage therapist's scope of practice.

First Stage: Evaluation

This stage of rehabilitation begins approximately 72 hours after the injury (day 4) and lasts approximately a week.

First, determine if your client has recovered enough to exhibit the stamina needed to participate in any evaluations you will conduct. Observe your client's skin color, ease of movements, and nonverbal signs of pain. Finally palpate affected areas for spasms and trigger points and use deep stroking to deactivate them (see "Locating and Deactivating Trigger Points" in the Trigger Points section). Palpation and client inquiry are the best methods for locating these tender areas. Furthermore, the location of these tender areas may lead the therapist to speculate about the client's posture and gait, given that muscle tightness is often related to their dysfunction. Massage reduces spasms, trigger-point activity, and ischemia. Massage relieves neurovascular entrapment by relaxing taut muscles and fascia.

Address faulty body mechanics by evaluating shoe wear, dysfunctional postures, and inefficient movement habits (see Assessments section). Positive changes seen during rehabilitation is enhanced by teaching your client alternative postures for sleeping, sitting, or working, or referring them to other specialists for braces, orthoses, or therapeutic exercise.

This stage also includes encouraging your client to begin or to maintain a balanced diet and drink plenty of fluids because these measures will positively influence rehabilitation. This may include a diet high in protein and reduced alcohol consumption (the latter may slow metabolism and therefore slow the healing process).

Second Stage: Conditioning

Once spasms have been located and reduced with massage, and after dysfunctional posture and gait patterns have been identified and addressed, a period of postinjury conditioning begins. This period includes a regime of stretching, weight training, and aerobic exercise. Notify the client's physician of the treatment plan you have devised, and obtain approval and further recommendations before beginning this stage of rehabilitation.

The first activity is aerobic movements. The appropriate treatment team member may suggest activities such as walking, water walking, stationary bike cycling, jump rope, or slow jogging. Classes taught by certified instructors are excellent choices. The purpose of aerobic movements is to increase circulation and deliver oxygen to stiff muscle and thickened fascia.

The next activity is stretching. In most cases, the injured area is stretched using active isolated stretching techniques until an increased range of motion is observed. The client increases his or her activity level slowly, adding more repetitions and time each week but never more than a 10% increase until a maximum goal is reached (physician or trainer determined). The injury may become irritated as the workload gradually increases, but this irritation is often a necessary step toward improvement. The addition of any new therapy (e.g., massage, chiropractic, stretching, exercise) may cause a temporary inflammatory response in the tissue. The client may experience subsequent soreness. Be sure to convey this to your client. The body normally acclimates to the newer treatment by the fourth to sixth session.

Remind the client to listen to his or her pain. Soreness is acceptable, but sharp pain is not. If you feel your client is overdoing it, refer him or her back to the person who devised the exercise plan for coaching and possible reevaluation.

As regular stretching becomes a daily habit, the next step is to increase activity with weight training. This usually occurs 1 to 2 weeks after your client began a stretching program. These and the aforementioned activities are usually done under the supervision of the client's physician or other qualified professional. To prevent repeated injury, involved muscles and muscles that cross over affect joints must be strengthened. Strength or weight training can be accomplished with rubber tubing, free weights (dumbbells or canned goods), or exercise machines.

Your role is to support and encourage your client to follow the prescribed program, along with keeping him or her as pain free as possible with massage. This process will reduce the likelihood of future problems while allowing the client to lead a lifestyle compatible with his or her wishes and desires.

Third Stage: Maintenance

The third stage is essentially maintenance, with the continuation of conditioning activities tailored to the client's lifestyle. This stage also includes suggesting stress reduction and a massage therapy maintenance plan. Be sure to continue supporting and encouraging your client in his or her quest for health and wellness.

To review the stages of rehabilitation:

- **First stage.** Eliminate spasm and trigger-point activity and address faulty body mechanics.
- **Second stage.** Restore flexibility and strength to muscles and joints and rebuild endurance.
- **Third stage.** Address diet, stress, and emotional well-being.

CHAT ROOM

Maximum Medical Improvement

Maximum medical improvement (MMI) refers to the state reached by the client where his or her condition cannot be improved any further or when a treatment plateau has been reached. The two main types of MMI are clinical and statutory.

Clinical MMI is based on clinical findings and no further recovery from or lasting improvement to an injury can reasonably be expected. The client's physician determines MMI and it is an important area of concern for insurance providers.

Statutory MMI is based on the elapsed time since the injury and is partially based on the nature and the extent of the injury (e.g., ankle versus spinal injury) and methods used to repair the injury (e.g., physical therapy, surgery). The time frame of statutory MMI varies from state to state.

ASSESSMENTS

Performing assessments is an important component of clinical massage as it gives direction and purpose to the session and ample use of the therapist's critical thinking skills. Assessments are performed during the intake process (see Chapter 10) and may be indicated during treatment. The client's treatment goals determine if assessments of posture, gait, and range of motions are needed, as well as the extent of the assessment.

Before these assessments begin, explain briefly what you are planning to do, why you are doing it, how long it will take, what changes in position it will require, and what equipment you will use. Eliminate as many distractions and disruptions as possible during the assessment process. Sanitize your hands before and after the assessment, preferably in your client's presence. Warm your hands and any equipment before touching your client, and be aware of your nonverbal communication and reactions from your client.

POSTURE

How the body distributes itself in relation to gravity over a base(s) of support is referred to as **posture**. To maintain postures such as sitting, standing, or lying down, the body must overcome the forces of gravity.

The efficiency with which the body overcomes gravity is individual and depends on many factors, including muscle strength, length and tone of muscles, movement habits, the health of ligaments, and emotional components. The body is constantly making adaptations and compensations to maintain its sense of balance and posture.

Unrelenting gravitational forces may make musculoskeletal overload inevitable. Structural misalignment and postural decline and are commonly observed as the battle against gravity is slowly lost over a lifetime. Although we will rarely encounter *picture-perfect posture*, many adaptations and compensations allow the body to function as close to optimal as possible. Aiming for well-compensated function should be a principal clinical goal. To help a client achieve this goal, we must recognize that a multitude of local and global (whole body) interactions are occurring.

Observations and actual postural assessments are simply a snapshot of your client in a particular moment in time. Many factors influence posture such as a client's emotional state, proprioceptive and other types of neural input, congenital or posttraumatic characteristics such as leg length discrepancy, as well as patterns of habitual movements. While we can observe characteristics of a client's posture, understanding why distortions are present involves a detailed evaluation and may remain a mystery.

One significant influence on posture is the response of muscles to stress (i.e., physical, emotional, structural). Types of muscles include postural and phasic. **Postural muscles** help to maintain the body's vertical position and **phasic muscles** primarily provide movement. In response to stress, postural muscles have a tendency to shorten and strengthen while phasic muscles tend to lengthen and weaken. These responses may produce dysfunctional postural patterns, such as forward head, slumping shoulders, and upper or lower crossed syndrome.

Other possible observations may include muscular atrophy (shrinking) and hypertrophy (enlargement).

Postural changes can have a profound influence on other muscles, joints, breathing patterns, blood and lymphatic flow, neural health, and numerous biochemical, biomechanical, and psychological processes. Abnormal posture is often caused by, but may also be the source of, spasms and trigger points, which can produce chronic pain. Improved posture often reduces spasms and triggers points, alleviates pain, and significantly improves function.

⊖volve An anterior and a posterior view of the human body featuring major postural muscles are located on the Evolve website. Access your student account and choose Additional Resources for this chapter. ■

Although perfect posture is rarely observed in a clinical setting, an understanding of standard or ideal alignment is necessary to recognize abnormalities.

In observing standard posture, the:

- Spine has four normal anterior/posterior curves, which include cervical, thoracic, lumbar, and sacral (see Figure 21-21)
- Pelvis is in a neutral position (anterior superior iliac spine is approximately level with the posterior superior iliac spine bilaterally, and the iliac crests are level with each other)
- Bones of the lower extremities are in an ideal alignment for bearing weight
- Chest and upper back are in a position that favors optimal function of the respiratory organs
- Head is erect in a well-balanced position that minimizes stress on the muscles of the neck

As stated previously, the presence of poor posture does not always explain why it exists or how well the client is adapting to changes in alignment. Nonetheless, it is still important to ask "Why is this happening?"

- *Is it due to overuse?* Question this possibility during the client's intake.
- *Could there be a reaction to joint problems or other influences (such as a diseased organ or systemic illness)?* Careful evaluation of symptom history, along with palpation and other assessments, may provide clues.
- *Are trigger points present?* Evaluation and palpation will confirm their presence or absence.
- *Are neurological factors involved?* Referral to an appropriate health care provider may be necessary to assess these factors.
- *Are there structural asymmetries, such as short leg or pelvic rotations for which soft tissues are compensating?* Careful observation, palpation, and assessments may provide clues.
- *Are adaptations the result of "tight" or "weak" musculature?* If so, the treatment plan should address these factors.

Regardless as to whether you have answers to these and other questions, the following static postural assessment will assist you in developing an appropriate treatment plan for your client. Static assessment is an important part of postural evaluation and will help you refine your observational skills. Findings can be recorded on a postural assessment form and compared with future postural assessments to indicate if the current plan is effective in obtaining client treatment goals or if the plan needs modification. Postural assessment forms can be downloaded from the Evolve website under Course Materials for Chapter 14.

Static Postural Assessment

While dynamic, moving postural assessment such as gait analysis has tremendous value, static postural assessment offers important information on a client's structural alignment and balance. Deformities, such as leg length difference, pelvic distortion, and scoliosis, may be verified by observation and palpation. Assessment will point toward the use of a particular modality, or suggest need for further testing or referral to another therapist.

Keep in mind that, while you may note postural distortions, clients who present with these findings should be referred to a qualified health care provider for definitive diagnosis.

Evaluate posture by noting baseline measurements in several anatomical planes, including midsagittal, coronal, and horizontal. A plumb line or posture grid may be used, and often deviations can be determined by observational skill alone, but findings should be quantified by measurement to assist in subsequent assessments.

Advanced training in postural assessment will assist the therapist in becoming more proficient. While postural assessments are not diagnostic, they often reveal conditions that require attention. Also note asymmetry in major bilateral muscle groups. Look for imbalances between anterior and posterior musculature. Survey for other signs of dysfunction such as:

- Anterior pelvic tilt, which spills abdominal contents forward (see Figure 21-38)
- Knees locked back, which may also contribute to anterior pelvic tilt
- Slumped shoulders that are rolled forward and inward
- Forward head posture
- Abnormal spinal curvatures such as scoliosis, kyphosis, or lordosis (see Chapter 19)
- Differences in leg length, creating pelvic obliquity
- Collapsed arches, which contribute to a faulty base of support

A more precise assessment can also be performed using a number of postural landmarks. The vertical and horizontal axes are assessed in all three planes mentioned previously. Landmarks should appear relatively symmetrical when comparing left and right. Document any abnormal findings.

Anterior Landmarks (Figure 14-4). A vertical line, or plumb line, lying within the midsagittal plane should bisect the:

- Nasal septum
- Manubrium of the sternum
- Umbilicus
- Pubic symphysis

It should also be equidistant between the knees and ankles.

Horizontal symmetry should (ideally) be observed between the:

- Acromioclavicular joints
- Iliac crests
- Anterior superior iliac spines
- Greater trochanters
- Tips of the fingers
- Patellae
- Fibular heads
- Medial malleoli
- Height of the medial arches of the feet

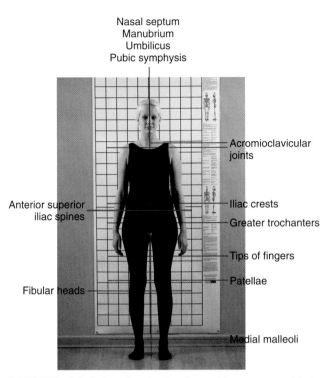

FIGURE 14-4 Anterior landmarks, with posture grid in background.

Memo: the ASIS may be slightly lower in women owing to natural elongation of this protuberance.

Posterior Landmarks (Figure 14-5). A vertical line, or plumb line, lying within the midsagittal plane should bisect the:
- Occipital protuberance
- Vertebral spinous processes
- Sacral tubercles
- Coccyx
  Horizontal symmetry should be observed between the:
- Mastoid processes
- Scapulae
- Posterior superior iliac spines
- Tops of the greater trochanters
- Calcanei (*singular,* calcaneus)

Coronal Plane Landmarks (Figure 14-6). A vertical line, or plumb line, lying within the coronal plane on the left and the right side should bisect the:
- External auditory meatus
- Humeral head
- Femoral head
- Lateral epicondyle of the femur
- Lateral malleolus

ⓔvolve *Images of anterior and posterior pelvic tilts, as well as how a difference in leg length can affect pelvic alignment, are found in the Additional Resources for Chapter 14. Log on to the Evolve website to access these important images.* ▪

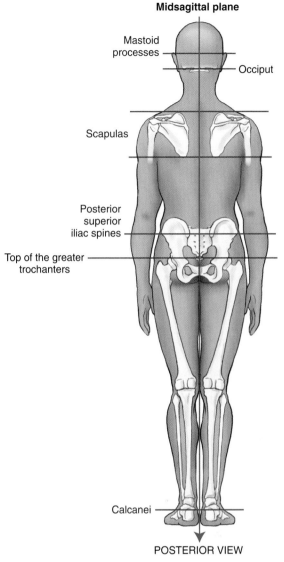

FIGURE 14-5 Posterior landmarks.

GAIT

While static postural analysis offers clinical value, a different perspective is gained with dynamic assessments. These might include walking forward or backward, hopping, jumping, running, and a variety of functional movements, such as swinging a racquet or club or bending at the waist in various directions. Observation of the person while walking reveals his or her unique gait, and includes movements of the arms, pelvis, knees, and feet, head motions and undulations of the torso. The quality and efficiency of each movement is dependent upon factors ranging literally from head to toes. By definition, **gait** is the manner in which a person moves on foot; it includes activities such as walking or running.

In order for an individual to walk or run, muscular action combined with gravity is required to propel a musculoskeletal frame through a series of complex and (ideally) highly efficient stages. Gait *analysis* is a complex skill that requires significant training and advanced levels of understanding, and may include computerized methods with pressure-sensitive equipment. However, basic gait *observation* and resultant evaluation offer clues to dysfunctional patterns. These patterns can be the result of, or are produced by, compensations made by the body. For the purpose of remaining brief, only the components of forward walking are included in this discussion. This is not to be confused with gait analysis, which remains a vastly complex and intriguing concept for advanced therapists.

Walking is a progressive *falling forward*, which is checked by alternating legs being thrust forward to stop the fall. Two functional units are considered: the *passenger unit* (or HAT, for head, arms, and torso, including pelvis), which is being carried, and the *locomotor unit* (pelvis and lower extremities), which is responsible for weight bearing and propulsion. Note that the pelvis serves as a transitional segment in both units.

The locomotor unit provides structural stability and mobility simultaneously. These factors must be maintained while transferring weight from one leg to the other and back again repeatedly. This *gait cycle* is repeated at varying speeds, on numerous terrains, and often while the passenger unit is carrying a variety of items (purses, luggage, children, etc.), all of which can alter the body's center of gravity.

Each lower limb has three basic tasks during the gait cycle:

1. Accept the transfer of the weight
2. Support the weight of the entire body
3. After unloading the weight, move the limb forward.

A normal gait cycle, or stride, contains two steps; one step by each foot. In normal gait, each step begins with a heel strike.

Each gait cycle is divided into two periods or phases (Figure 14-7):

1. **Stance period.** The foot is in contact with a surface; approximately 60% of gait cycle.
2. **Swing period.** The foot is moving forward and usually not in contact with the surface; approximately 40% of gait cycle.

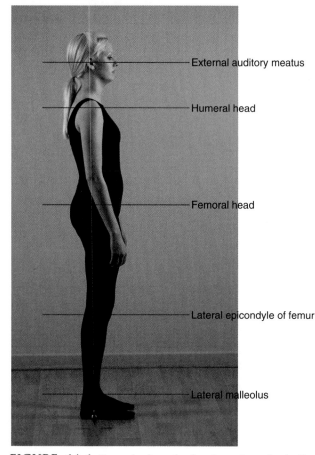

- External auditory meatus
- Humeral head
- Femoral head
- Lateral epicondyle of femur
- Lateral malleolus

FIGURE 14-6 Coronal plane landmarks using plumb line (lateral view).

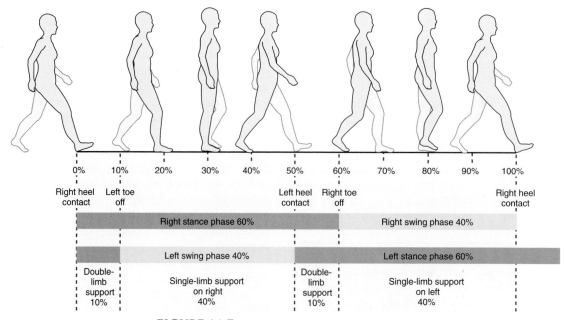

FIGURE 14-7 Gait cycle: Stance and swing phases.

Approximately 25% of the gait cycle involves double limb support, that is, when both feet are touching the ground at the same time.

Abnormalities are more easily seen during the stance period rather than the swing period. This is due to its weight-bearing duty and the greater length of time spent in the stance period. However, the swing period also places high demands on the body as it strives to maintain balance during lifting and positioning of the airborne limb. This highly orchestrated chain of events includes hip flexion, knee flexion, eventual knee extension, and foot positioning in preparation of its task to bear weight. Gait also includes pelvic movements including rotation, tilt, and shift.

A more detailed look at gait can be found in Chaitow and DeLany's *Clinical Application of Neuromuscular Techniques, Vol. 2,* "The Lower Body."

Observing Gait

Greenman (1996) suggests using a multidirectional approach when observing gait. Be sure to observe the client:
1. Walking toward you
2. Walking away from you
3. Walking viewed from the side
4. Length of stride, swing of arm, heel strike, toe off, and adaptation of the shoulders
5. Functional capacity of gait such as cross-patterning and symmetry of stride

For evaluating the functional capacity of the gait as just described, Kuchera et al (1997) suggest including the following key elements of normal gait:
1. Weight transferring in a continuous manner from initial contact to push-off
2. No sign of limp
3. Correct foot orientation, without toeing in or toeing out
4. No evidence of excessive inversion or eversion
5. Symmetric motion throughout the pelvis, lumbar and thoracic regions, and shoulders
6. Arm swinging bilaterally equal

These elements can be observed in both normal and abnormal gait. The person may compensate to avoid painful weight-bearing positions or a painful range of motion. Additionally, tight muscles or those housing trigger points may not contract normally and movements may appear jerky or misaligned, or they may cause synergists or antagonists to overcompensate.

Other factors that affect normal gait are a reduced stance period compared with the other foot and limping caused by painful arthritic changes or stiffness in weight-bearing joints, such as the hip, knee, or ankle, and leg length discrepancy. Other factors include foot problems such as bunions, ingrown toenails, Morton toe, fallen arches, bone spurs, and gout.

Neurologic conditions can also affect gait, such as foot drop, diabetic neuropathy, hemiplegic gait (associated with stroke), a shuffling gait (associated with Parkinson disease), an unsteady gait (associated with multiple sclerosis), or a waddling gait (associated with muscular dystrophy).

While assessments of posture and gait do not provide all the answers, they may point to issues that may be addressed by massage. Students and therapists are encouraged to begin observing posture and gait, not only in classroom and clinical settings but also in day-to-day life, where people are just being themselves and using their bodies without regard to those who may be observing them.

CHAT ROOM

How you handle cases in your own practice is built upon an ongoing accumulation of skills, including your base knowledge obtained in formal training, deeper understanding through self-imposed study, continuing education, information acquired from the patient/client, medical tests, and other health care providers; experience with your own body; and experience gained in clinical practice. The acquisition of these skills takes patience and commitment; they will deepen with time and professional experience.

MINI-LAB

Divide the class into two groups: One group will observe while the other classmates walk. The observers will assess posture and gait. Hold a group discussion to identify structures and the muscle groups used. Have the two groups trade roles and repeat.

"When my daughter was about seven years old, she asked me one day what I did at work. I told her I worked at the college—that my job was to teach people how to draw. She stared back at me, incredulous, and said, 'You mean they forget?'"
—Howard Ikemoto

TECHNIQUES

During clinical massage, the therapist uses the same techniques featured in Chapter 8, but treatment is focused on reducing reported signs and symptoms, and to improve function. For example, if your client states that a treatment goal is to reduce lower back discomfort, you might select the most appropriate massage techniques and apply them to lower back muscles.

Several techniques used in clinical massage are a variation of basic massage techniques and include *compression*, *pin and glide,* and *torquing.* Compression is included in our discussion because sustained pressures are frequently used by clinical massage therapists. These techniques, which use little or no lubricant, target fascia and use mild to moderate stretching pressure in specific directions. This attempts to release fascial restrictions from surrounding tissue to which fascia may have become adhered.

Compression

Compression is a nongliding technique of sustained pressure or a sequence of rhythmic, alternating pressures.

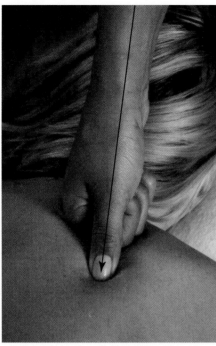

A

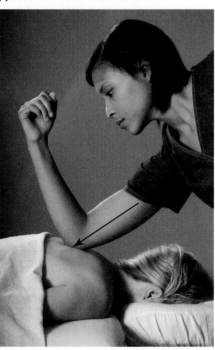

B

FIGURE 14-8 Compression: **A,** Using a braced thumb; **B,** using an elbow.

Compression over spasms and trigger points is applied using a finger, knuckle, thumb, fist, forearm, or elbow (Figure 14-8). Hand-held tools can also be used. Be sure to vary the direction of pressure until you locate the spot that is most *exquisitely* sore. Pressure can be maintained for various lengths of time, but you can usually elicit a therapeutic

response in 8 to 10 seconds (Figure 14-9, pp. 293-294). Repeat as needed.

Some tender areas, such as those found in the sterno-cleidomastoid, require the tender area to be compressed between the thumb and finger(s) in a pincer grip approach. Some muscles have a tendency to roll under pressure, such as the biceps brachii or muscles of the erector spinae. You may need to stabilize the muscle with one hand while treating it with the opposite hand to prevent rolling.

Pin and Glide

Pin and glide (or anchor and glide) uses slow, deep gliding pressure. While one hand is gliding, the other anchors the tissue where the glide began (Figure 14-10, p. 295). Deep gliding pressure creates a wave effect, stretching and separating muscle and fascial layers.

Torquing

Torquing, or applied shearing force, is used for extremities and involves grasping skin with both hands and rotating tissues in one direction around the bone's axis (Figure 14-11, p. 295). Pressure is maintained for 90 seconds. As fascia and muscular layers release, tissues begin to loosen and unwind.

Skin Rolling

Skin rolling and tissue lifting techniques are used to soften fascia. Skin rolling involves lifting and compressing skin and superficial fascia; no downward force is used. Tissue can be rolled between the fingers and thumb (see Figure 8-19) or just lifted and maintained (see Figure 8-20). Both thumbs may be used moving in opposite directions, creating an S-curve in the skin's surface (Figure 14-12). Because superficial fascia lies in several planes, lift and roll the skin in several directions. If the skin is not lifting, do not force it into position. Be sure to address the area two or three times in a session.

CHAT ROOM

Lymphatic Drainage

Lymphatic drainage techniques enhance fluid movement in the treatment area, thereby improving oxygenation, nutrient supply, and waste removal. Therapists trained in lymphatic techniques often use lighter pressure (i.e., less than an ounce per 2 cm^2—barely the weight of a nickel or a dime), usually directed toward the lymph node cluster draining a particular area. Lighter pressure is needed to encourage lymph flow without increasing blood filtration. Deep pressure, which often creates a shearing force, and can temporarily inhibit lymph flow.

Therapists not trained in lymphatic techniques may prepare and flush the treatment area using light effleurage applied centripetally (toward the heart) before and after treatment.

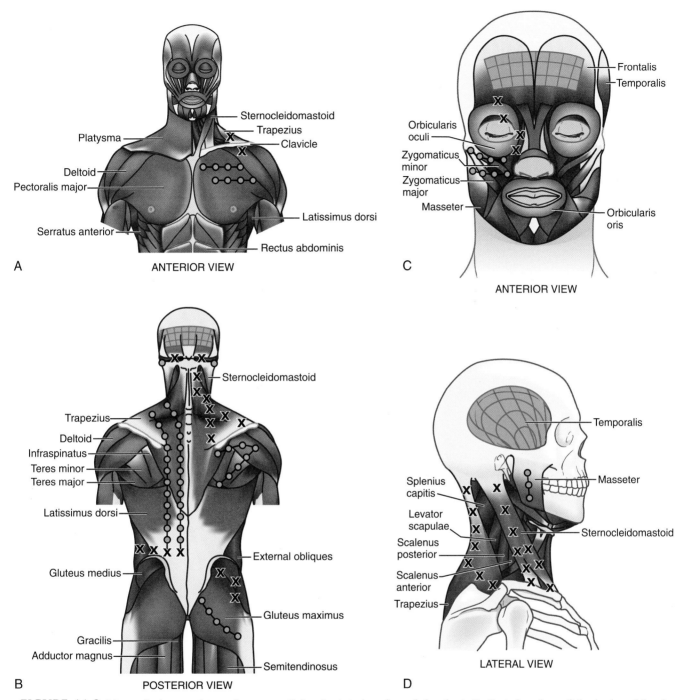

FIGURE 14-9 Maps of trigger points and spasm activity. **A,** Anterior view of the chest. **B,** Posterior view of the back and head. **C,** Anterior view of the head. **D,** Lateral view of the head.

COMMON MISTAKES: OVERWORKING THE AREA

Reviewed next are common mistakes novice therapists make when applying clinical massage techniques.

Overworking tissue, especially injured tissue, is the most common mistake of a novice therapist. The two types of overworking mistakes are (1) working too deep and (2) working too long. Experience is the best teacher. Until you

progress to a point at which you are comfortable judging pressure, tissue density, and tissue resistance, limit your pressure and duration of treatment. For the beginning therapist, the general rule for deep pressure is no more than 2 minutes of treatment to any given region. The best course of action is to treat the area for a short time and then move to another muscle for a while before returning to the original treatment site. In other words, three 2-minute treatments to the rhomboids are better than one 5-minute treatment.

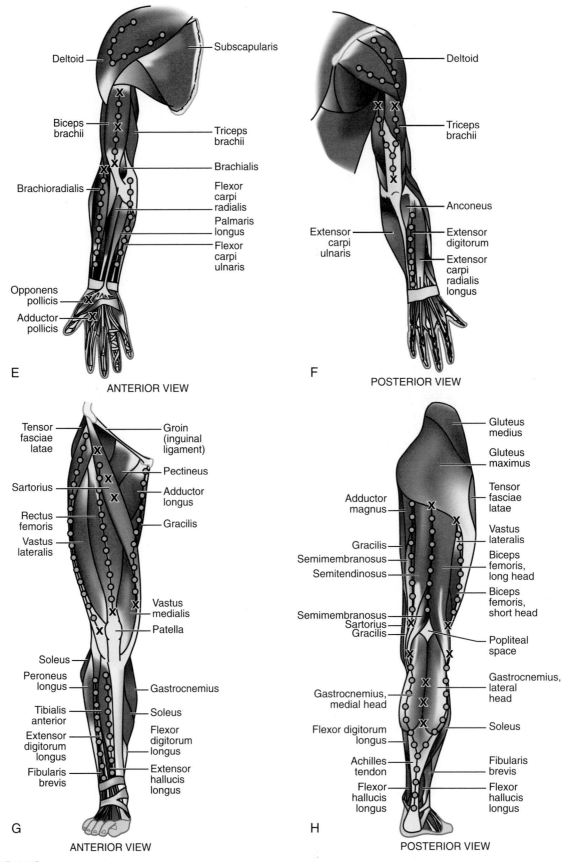

FIGURE 14-9, cont'd E, Anterior view of the right upper extremity. **F,** Posterior view of right upper extremity. **G,** Anterior view of right lower extremity. **H,** Posterior view of right lower extremity.

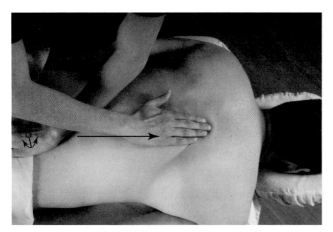

FIGURE 14-10 Pin and glide.

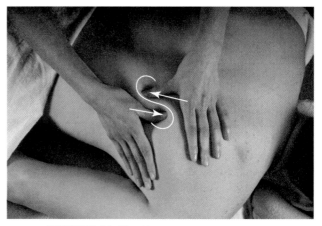

FIGURE 14-12 Skin rolling with an S-Curve.

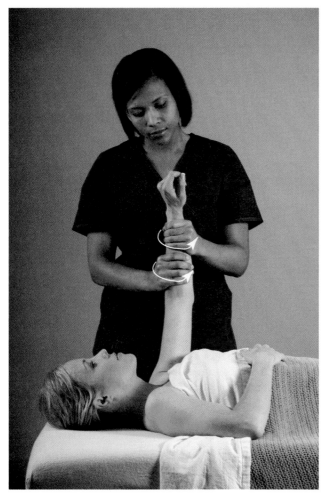

FIGURE 14-11 Torquing.

CHAT ROOM

Treatment Tools

Hand-held tools are commonly used and may help prevent overuse injuries to the thumb, as well as treat hard-to-reach areas such as between ribs or spinous vertebral processes.

Be sure all tools used are washed with soap and water or sanitized in the top tray of a dishwasher run on a hot water cycle. A plastic bag or sheet of plastic can be used to wrap the treatment tool and discarded after use. See Chapter 9 for other sanitation guidelines.

CHAT ROOM

Question of Pressure

Pressure applied in clinical application of massage is more varied and specific than in relaxation massage. Sometimes your touch will be nothing more than a static hold; other times you will apply firm pressure to overcome resistance in tissue. Mild discomfort is often a sensation associated with clinical massage. This is easily governed by presenting an analog scale to be used by the client when expressing level of pressure tolerance. On a 1 to 10 scale, with 1 being barely felt and 10 being the most pain imaginable, the goal is to apply pressure that registers between 5 and 7. It should be moderately uncomfortable, not painful.

With experience, the therapist gains skill and confidence. Using the following factors, the clinical therapist can properly judge pressure and treatment times.

Client's Massage Experience

Someone who has had weekly massages for the last 5 years is going to be more comfortable receiving deep pressure than a client who has never received a massage or who has had few massages. An experienced client will be better able to give direction and feedback to the therapist, even if it is their first session with the therapist. You can increase treatment pressure and time at the request of an experienced massage receiver.

Experience of the Therapist

An experienced therapist with 4+ years of experience can better use his or her judgment when determining what is best for a particular client in regards to techniques used and how they are applied. Time on the job does not count unless you are seeing clients.

Level of Familiarity Between Client and Therapist

If you are just starting clinical massage applications but have done 20 to 50 massages on one certain client, then the established rapport and familiarity with the client's body are reason enough to exceed the treatment protocol for that client.

Physical Condition of the Client

Clients who are robust and physically fit are more conditioned and more body-aware and can handle deeper pressure and longer treatment times than clients who are weak and debilitated.

AFTERCARE

When working with injuries, treatment may increase the local discomfort and the referred pain patterns initially. Educating clients about expectations regarding their pain level following injury and treatment will be necessary.

First of all, clients should be made aware that some increase in soreness is common and to be expected. This circumstance is true for almost any new therapeutic method or modality (chiropractic adjustments, electrostimulation, acupuncture, exercise, stretching, yoga movements), but is especially applicable when the client has been injured. The body perceives the treatment as increased sensory input. While the occasional miracle client will feel better after just one session, in most instances, three sessions per week, 30 minutes in duration for 2 to 4 weeks, is recommended before a client becomes acclimated to the new treatment and begins to respond.

Some recommended aftercare activities are:
- Regular physical activity
- Stretching
- Self-massage with or without tennis balls
- Stress reduction techniques such as meditation, guided imagery, structured breathing, and strolling outdoors
- Sleeping in a neutral position with proper support
- Good nutrition such as increasing intake of dietary fiber and water
- Ergonomics, such as computer monitor height, keyboarding, or telephone headset
- Ice and heat

Before making aftercare recommendations, take into account important variables such as the client's age and physical condition, treatment progress, and time and financial restraints. And be sure to know your scope of practice and limitations on professional activities.

Ⓔvolve *Log onto your student account on Evolve for a detailed list of injury management techniques.* ▪

"Success is not found in what you have achieved, but rather in who you have become."
—Anonymous

SPORTS MASSAGE

The goals of sports massage are similar to those of clinical massage, with one big difference: Athletes want increased performance, and fast—whether massage is used for recovery after an event, restoring range of motion, or increasing oxygen to an area of injury to speed repair. Performance is the bottom line for the athlete. Sports massage is divided into three categories: event, maintenance, and rehabilitative massage.

Event Massage

Event sports massage is administered during sports events and can be further divided into preevent, interevent, and postevent massage.

Pre-event Massage. Preevent sports massage focuses on increasing circulation to muscles and increasing flexibility. Massage is given from 2 hours before to immediately before the event. Techniques are delivered using brisk movements and moderate pressure, leaving the athlete relaxed, yet ready for action. The most effective techniques to accomplish this are compression, fulling, tapotement, jostling, and nonspecific friction. These techniques are often applied without lubricant because it can reduce sweating during the event, thereby causing the athlete to overheat. Sports massage can also enhance performance potential by reducing precompetition apprehension. Because time is also a consideration, avoid the use of headrests or bolsters because their use increases treatment time. Begin with the client prone, shoes left on with toes off the end of the table. The time frame is usually 10 to 15 minutes.

Interevent Massage. Interevent massage is given between games or events and within a 1- or 2-day period. The massage is brief with use of moderate pressure; problem areas are addressed generally, and receive attention later. The goal here is to assist the return of the body to homeostasis. Apply the same techniques used in preevent massage, minus tapotement.

Postevent Massage. Postevent massage occurs 30 minutes to 6 hours after the event. Techniques focus on reducing soreness and spreading muscle fibers while promoting rest and recovery. Faster recovery time means that athletes can return to activity promptly. Avoid tapotement or deep, specific techniques because the athlete's muscles may spasm

MONICA J. RENO

Born: April 18, 1957

"Leadership is the art of accomplishing more than the science of management says is possible."
—Colin Powell

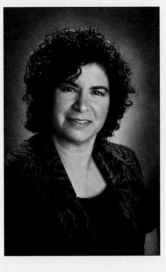

Monica Reno, the second of five children, grew up on Long Island during what she fondly remembers as the greatest time for kids in America. "The 60s saw endless bike rides, baseball games, and sleigh riding. Every family had 4 to 6 children, so every block had its own baseball team."

When Monica was a young child, her mother began to suffer from chronic heart disease, the long-term effect of the rheumatic fever she endured as a teenager, undergoing her first aortic valve replacement in 1961. Taking over household duties became a priority, and the need to cope with her mother's long hospitalizations forced Monica to mature at a young age. "It was not an issue then, just what needed to be done." Her escape became schoolwork, with science as a favorite subject. She wanted to know the human body and understand her mother's illness.

In 1984, Monica graduated from the Swedish Institute in Manhattan. She purchased a failing massage business and turned it around and was on her way to a successful career before she even graduated. In 1985, she teamed up with Dr. George Rizos, DC, to create an unofficial relationship with the New York Jets. After a changing of the guard in the training room in 1986, they began working under contract with the NFL's New York Jets.

"I practiced Swedish massage. It was more or less all that was taught in those days. Benny Vaughn (see Chapter 17) was just beginning to write on the subject, so I did whatever seemed to work, applying what I knew about kinesiology and muscle physiology."

Monica moved to Florida in 1998 and switched from a clientele of anaerobic athletes (football) to more aerobic athletes (triathletes and marathon runners). She discovered that her mainstay of techniques wasn't ideal for endurance athletes. "...Once I *became* the athlete and started training for triathlon, the intimate relationship between sports physiology, the cycles of training, and the clinical effects of massage merged to create protocols so useful and accurate that it changed my entire approach to massage after 17 years in practice."

Exertion sports, such as field events, football, and fencing, are anaerobic exercises. These activities focus on strength, explosive actions, and, in some cases, flexibility to achieve the ultimate performance. The physiologic considerations for the anaerobic athlete stresses maximum exertion during a single action. Here, maximal effort is the key. For this athlete, Monica has found circulatory massage to be more beneficial.

Endurance sports such as running, swimming, and cycling are aerobic exercises. The physiologic consideration for this athlete is submaximal exertion maintained at a steady state for long periods of time. In the case of some triathletes during certain races, this could be 14 hours or more. The training goal is to delay the lactate threshold—the state at which the athlete enters an oxygen debt and goes anaerobic. She realized that the lactate threshold is poorly influenced by the use of circulatory massage and, after taking a workshop with Thomas Myers, began focusing more on myofascial treatment for endurance athletes.

Her treatment plans are designed with Tudor Bompa's theory of periodization in mind—training divided into cycles with specific goals and performance measurements leading to an individual competitive event.

For each cycle, the treatment plan is adjusted for the time in training, the stresses and loads on the body during that cycle, the frequency and duration of each training session, and the specific activities during each session, phase, and cycle. Knowing just what changes will occur in the body during these phases allows Monica to determine the most effective treatment plan.

"This may seem more complicated than choosing pre/post-event protocols over rehabilitation protocols but the outcomes are so much more accurate."

easily in their hypersensitive state. Be sure the athlete has cooled down before the massage begins.

Maintenance Massage

Maintenance massage addresses any of the athlete's treatment goals and emphasizes prevention. During massage, spasm and trigger points are located and reduced by alternating gliding strokes (see Trigger Points section). This is also the time to implement self-care programs that facilitate independence and support the athlete's goals.

Rehabilitative Massage

Rehabilitative massage takes into consideration presentation of soft-tissue injuries. Enhanced recovery after injury is another benefit of sports massage. When the question arises concerning which type of sports massage is most appropriate, the answer is simple: The physiologic effect of the technique must always match the physiology of the soft tissue complaint (see Chapters 6 and 8).

> *"This is not a time in which to complete anything.*
> *It is a time for fragments."*
> —Marcel Duchamp

COMMON TREATMENT AREAS

The following are common treatment areas for a variety of conditions. Each includes a list of muscles that should be on the therapist's "must treat" list for a given area. Use the trigger points map (see Figure 14-8) to locate important trigger points and spasms. Be sure to review Chapter 21 for information on specific muscles.

Neck and Head

Suboccipitalis (rectus capitis major and minor, capitis oblique superior and inferior)
Temporalis
Sternocleidomastoid
Frontalis
Trapezius
Levator scapulae
Paraspinals (transversospinalis and erector spinae)
Splenii (capitis and cervicis)
Scalenes (anterior, medius, posterior)
   Figure 14-13 shows a great technique for deactivating trigger points and spasms at the cranial base. Be sure to sustain pressure for 8 to 10 seconds. Release and repeat.

Shoulders

Rotator cuff (supraspinatus, infraspinatus, teres minor, subscapularis)

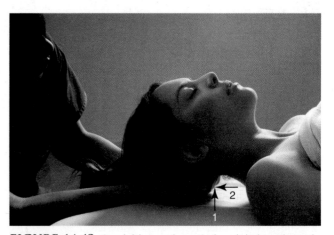

FIGURE 14-13 Cranial base release (suboccipitals and attachment sites of neck and shoulder muscles).

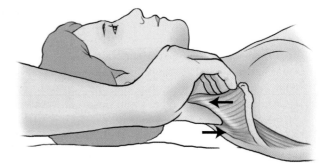

FIGURE 14-14 Unrolling the upper trapezius.

Deltoid
Trapezius
Pectoralis (major and minor)
Rhomboids (major and minor)
Serratus anterior
   Figure 14-14 shows a great technique for deactivating trigger points and spasms in the upper trapezius. Grasp the tissues between fingers and thumb. Move in opposite directions using equal pressure. Release and repeat.

Lower Back and Hip

Quadratus lumborum
Paraspinals (transversospinalis and erector spinae)
Iliopsoas (iliacus and psoas major)
Gluteus maximus, medius, and minimus
Piriformis
Quadriceps femoris (rectus femoris and vastus intermedius, medialis, and lateralis)
Hamstrings (semitendinosus, semimembranosus, biceps femoris)

E-RESOURCES

evolve

http://evolve.elsevier.com/Salvo/MassageTherapy

- Chapter challenge
- Flash cards
- Photo gallery
- Educational animations
- Additional information
- Weblinks

BIBLIOGRAPHY

Abraham WM: Exercise-induced muscle soreness, *Physician Sports Med* 7:57-60, 1979.

Applegate EJ: *The anatomy and physiology learning system*, ed 3, Philadelphia, 2006, Saunders.

Beers MH, Berkow R: *The Merck manual of diagnosis and therapy*, Whitehouse Station, NJ, 2006, Merck Research Laboratories.

Biel A: *Trail guide to the body: how to locate muscles, bones, and more*, ed 3, Boulder, Colo, 2005, Books of Discovery.

Bompa TO: *Periodization: theory and methodology of training*, ed 5, Champaign, Ill, 2009, Human Kinetics.

Chaitow L: *Modern neuromuscular techniques*, ed 2, St Louis, 2003, Churchill Livingstone.

Chaitow L, DeLany J: *Clinical application of neuromuscular techniques*, vol I, ed 2, Edinburgh, 2008, Churchill Livingstone.

Chaitow L, DeLany J: *Clinical application of neuromuscular techniques*, vol II, Edinburgh, 2002, Churchill Livingstone.

Como D, editor: *Mosby's medical, nursing, and allied health dictionary*, ed 6, St Louis, 2002, Mosby.

Crawley J, Van De Graaff KM: *A photographic atlas for anatomy and physiology*, Englewood, Colo, 2002, Morton.

Damjanov I: *Pathophysiology for the health-related professions*, ed 3, Philadelphia, 2006, Saunders.

Davies C: *The trigger point therapy workbook: your self-treatment guide for pain relief*, Oakland, Calif, 2001, New Harbinger.

Dominguez R, Gajda R: *Total body training*, New York, 1984, Warner Books.

Fernandez F: *Deep-tissue massage treatment: a handbook of neuromuscular therapy*, St Louis, 2006, Mosby.

Foldi M, StroBenreuther R: *Foundations of manual lymph drainage*, ed 3, St Louis, 2005, Mosby.

Frazier MS, Drzymkowski JW: *Essentials of human diseases and conditions*, ed 3, Philadelphia, 2004, Saunders.

Fritz S: *Sports and exercise massage: comprehensive care in athletics, fitness, and rehabilitation*, St Louis, 2005, Mosby.

Gehlsen GM, Ganion LR, Helfst R: Fibroblast responses to variation in soft tissue mobilization pressure, *Med Sci Sports Exerc* 31(4):531-535, 1999.

Gould BE: *Pathophysiology for the health professions*, ed 3, Philadelphia, 2006, Saunders.

Gray H, Pick TP, Howden R: *Gray's anatomy*, ed 29, Philadelphia, 1974, Running Press.

Greenman PE: *Principles of manual medicine*, Baltimore, 1996, Williams & Wilkins.

Haubrich WS: *Medical meanings: a glossary of word origins*, New York, 1984, Harcourt Brace Jovanovich.

Hendrickson T: *Massage for orthopedic conditions*, Baltimore, 2004, Lippincott Williams & Wilkins.

Jacob S, Francone C: *Elements of anatomy and physiology*, Philadelphia, 1989, Saunders.

Juhan D: *Job's body, a handbook for bodyworkers*, ed 3, Barrington, NY, 2003, Station Hill Press.

Kalat JW: *Biological psychology*, ed 8, Belmont, Calif, 2003, Wadsworth.

Kapit W, Elson LM: *The anatomy coloring book*, ed 3, New York, 2002, Benjamin Cummings.

Klafs D, Arnheim DD: *Modern principles of athletic training*, ed 8, St Louis, 1992, Mosby.

Kordish M, Dickson S: *Introduction to basic human anatomy*, Lake Charles, La, 1995, McNeese State University.

Kuchera W, et al: Musculoskeletal examination for somatic dysfunction. In Ward R, editor: *Foundations of osteopathic medicine*, Baltimore, 1997, Williams & Wilkins.

Lowe WW: *Orthopedic massage: theory and technique*, ed 2, St Louis, 2009, Mosby.

Marieb EN: *Essentials of human anatomy and physiology*, ed 8, New York, 2005, Benjamin Cummings.

Mattes AL: *Flexibility: active and assisted stretching*, Sarasota, Fla, 1995, self-published.

McAleer N: *The body almanac*, Garden City, NY, 1985, Doubleday.

McAtee R: *Facilitated stretching*, ed 2, Colorado Springs, Colo, 1999, Human Kinetics.

Merck manual, ed 17, Whitehouse Station, NJ, 1998, Merck and Company.

Moore KL: *Clinically oriented anatomy*, ed 5, Baltimore, 2005, Lippincott Williams & Wilkins.

Muscolino JE: *Kinesiology: the skeletal system and muscle function*, ed 2, St Louis, 2011, Mosby.

Muscolino JE: *The muscle and bone palpation manual: with trigger points, referral patterns, and stretching*, St Louis, 2009, Mosby.

Muscolino JE: Understanding and working with myofascial trigger points, *Massage Ther J* Fall: 159-162, 2008.

Newton D: *Pathology for massage therapists*, ed 2, Portland, Ore, 1995, Simran.

Perry J: *Gait analysis: normal and pathological function*, New York, 1992, McGraw-Hill.

Platzer W: *Color atlas and textbook of human anatomy: locomotor system*, vol I, ed 5, New York, 2003, Thieme.

Premkumar K: *Pathology A to Z, a handbook for massage therapists*, Baltimore, 1999, Lippincott Williams & Wilkins.

Salvo S: *Massage therapy: principles and practice*, Philadelphia, 1999, Saunders.

Salvo SG: *Mosby's pathology for massage therapists*, ed 2, St Louis, 2009, Mosby.

Simons DG, Travell JG, Simons LS: *Myofascial pain and dysfunction: the trigger point manual*, vol 1, ed 2, Baltimore, 1999, Lippincott Williams & Wilkins.

Solomon EP, Phillips GA: *Understanding human anatomy and physiology*, Philadelphia, 1987, Saunders.

Stanton P, Purdam C: Hamstring injuries in sprinting: the role of eccentric exercise, *J Orthop Sports Phys Ther* 10:343-348, 1989.

Synder GE: Fascia—applied anatomy and physiology, *J Am Osteopath Assoc* 68:675-685, 1969.

Thibodeau G, Patton K: *Anatomy and physiology*, ed 6, St Louis, 2006, Mosby.

Thibodeau G, Patton K: *Structure and function of the body,* ed 12, St Louis, 2004, Mosby.

Tortora GJ: *Introduction to the human body: the essentials of anatomy and physiology,* ed 5, Hoboken, NJ, 2000, John Wiley & Sons.

Tortora GJ, Grabowksi SR: *Principles of anatomy and physiology,* ed 11, New York, 2005, John Wiley & Sons.

Venes D, Thomas CL, Taber CW: *Taber's cyclopedic medical dictionary,* ed 20, Philadelphia, 2005, FA Davis.

Walter JB, Israel MS: *General pathology,* ed 4, New York, 1974, Churchill Livingstone.

Weineck J: *Functional anatomy in sports,* Chicago, 1986, Year Book Medical.

Wilmore JH, Costill DL: *Physiology of sport and exercise,* Leeds, UK, 2006, Human Kinetics.

Wilmore JH, Costill DL: Cardiovascular regulation. In *Training for sport and activity: the physiological basis of the conditioning process,* ed 3, Dubuque, Iowa, 1988, William C Brown.

MATCHING I

Place the letter of the answer next to the term or phrase that best describes it.

A. Acute
B. Athlete
C. Chronic
D. Clinical massage
E. Crepitant

F. Delayed-onset muscle soreness
G. Gel state
H. Muscle fatigue
I. Physical rehabilitation
J. Sol state

K. Thixotropism
L. Trigger points or myofascial trigger points

_____ 1. Loss of muscle strength or endurance felt after strenuous physical activity

_____ 2. Injuries that begin abruptly, usually have a recognizable cause, and are characterized by severe symptoms such as pain, swelling, and loss of function

_____ 3. Type of soreness and discomfort felt 8 to 14 hours after the activity, often reaching a peak after 48 hours

_____ 4. Ability of fascia to change from a sol state to a gel state and back

_____ 5. Physical state which fascia is relatively thin, more pliant and elastic, and offers less restriction during movement

_____ 6. Someone who possesses natural or acquired abilities such as strength, endurance, or agility required for participating in sports, especially competitive sports

_____ 7. Process used after illness, injury, or surgery to help the affected individual regain as much

function and self-sufficiency as possible; this process includes stages of evaluation, conditioning and maintenance

_____ 8. Localized area of hyperirritability found in skeletal muscles and their related fascia and, when pressed, may refer sensations (usually pain) to other areas of the body

_____ 9. Term used to describe sounds of crackling, grating, or rattling

_____ 10. Physical state in which fascia is thicker, more gelatinous, tougher, more inflexible, and can restrict movement

_____ 11. Injuries that develop slowly and persist for long periods, sometimes for the remainder of the individual's lifetime

_____ 12. Term used to describe the use of specific focused techniques that, when applied properly, reduce reported signs and symptoms as well as improve function

MATCHING II

Place the letter of the answer next to the term or phrase that best describes it.

A. Active
B. Causes of trigger point formation
C. Connective tissue damage theory

D. Eccentric muscle contractions
E. Inflammation theory
F. Jump sign
G. Latent
H. Local twitch response

I. Referred pain
J. Spasm
K. Splinting
L. Tender point

_____ 1. Phenomena that may occur when a trigger point produces pain to an associated target area during palpation

_____ 2. Specific spots on the body that elicit pain and discomfort where compressed but do not refer pain

_____ 3. Reflexive impulse that may occur a when an affected muscle or an adjacent muscle twitches spontaneously during trigger point palpation

_____ 4. Type of trigger points that cause pain even at rest

_____ 5. Examples are strain, overuse, and direct trauma leading to shortened muscle fibers and localized ischemia

_____ 6. Spontaneous reaction of pain or discomfort that may occur during trigger point palpation that causes a client to wince, jump, or verbalize

_____ 7. Term used to describe an abnormal sustained muscle contraction

_____ 8. Type of trigger points that go unnoticed by client until pressure is applied

_____ 9. Term used to describe muscle tightening that serves a useful purpose by protecting an area

_____ 10. Theory that states muscle soreness is part of an inflammatory process as our bodies attempt to repair microscopic damage caused by activity such as a workout.

_____ 11. Theory that states muscle soreness is due to hydroxyproline produced and released in the bloodstream as a result of connective tissue damage

_____ 12. Type of muscle contraction associated with the vast majority of cases of delayed-onset muscle soreness, pain, and discomfort

CASE STUDY

Do No Harm

Garrett was in a bicycle accident about 10 days ago. He was wearing his helmet, but as he fell, the left side of his head struck and slid down the side of a mailbox, stretching the left side of his neck as he slid down. He did not feel any pain right after the accident, but the next day his head, neck, and especially his right shoulder were in pain. Garrett saw his doctor, who recommended rest and analgesic medications to manage the pain. These helped temporarily, but each morning when he woke, Garrett felt the pain as intensely as he had the day after the accident.

Audrey, one of Garrett's colleagues, referred him to Baila, a massage therapist who had helped relieve her pain related to a whiplash injury from an automobile accident. Garrett was ready to try anything, and made an appointment for that day. He told Baila that he felt a pain in his right shoulder and neck most of the time, and that 2 days ago he began to feel tingling in his right arm and hand.

During postural assessments, Baila noticed right lateral flexion of the neck and an elevated right shoulder. When she asked him to laterally flex his neck to the left, he immediately felt sharp pain in the left side of the neck. During palpation, Baila felt dense, hypertonic tissues on the right side of the neck, and overstretched weak tissue on the left. She suspected that the tingling in his right arm might be the result of hypertonic tissues

compressing a nerve, but the sharp pain on the left made her concerned about the possibility that vertebrae may also have moved out of alignment.

Baila has many years of training and experience in neuromuscular therapy and clinical massage. She feels confident that she can release the spasm that may be causing the nerve compression on the right side, and can aid in the healing of any strain that may be present in the over-stretched, weakened muscles on the left side. But she is concerned about the possibility of damage to the vertebrae.

At the time that Garret visited Baila, was his pain acute, subacute, or chronic?

Should Baila offer to discuss her findings and concerns with Garrett's doctor before initiating massage therapy?

Should Baila recommend that Garrett return to his doctor for a more thorough medical assessment before initiating massage treatments?

If she does believe that further medical testing is necessary to determine whether any vertebral malalignment, is it OK for Baila to rely on her training and experience to treat the spasms and overstretched tissues today?

If Baila performs massage today, should she treat trigger points if she finds them?

CRITICAL THINKING

What does it mean to say that body structure governs function?

CHAPTER 15

Seated Massage

Ralph R. Stephens

> *"We can be knowledgeable with another man's knowledge, but we cannot be wise with another man's wisdom."*
> —Michel De Montaigne

LEARNING OBJECTIVES

After completing this chapter, the student should be able to:

- List major considerations when purchasing a massage chair.
- Describe types of seated massage equipment.
- State reasons that a massage therapist might choose to massage a client in the seated position.
- Explain and demonstrate procedures of sanitation and hygiene unique to seated massage.
- Properly adjust the massage chair for the client.
- Describe effective body mechanics and safety considerations for the massage therapist who uses a massage chair.
- Use adaptive professional communication to communicate effectively with the client before and during the seated massage.
- Perform a basic seated massage routine.

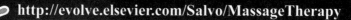

http://evolve.elsevier.com/Salvo/MassageTherapy

INTRODUCTION

Rubbing a person's shoulders while he or she is sitting in a chair is often instinctive. It is a natural and therapeutic urge. Seated massage is often referred to as *chair massage* and came to prominence through the efforts of David Palmer, whose vision was to make massage therapy safe, convenient, and affordable for anyone, anywhere, anytime. He introduced seated massage in the workplace in the early 1980s. Working at corporations such as Apple Inc. and Pacific Bell, he developed a chair to complement the massage. In 1986 Palmer introduced the first massage chair and coined the term *onsite massage*. Palmer adapted the traditional Japanese system of massage, called amma, to create massage routines performed on the client in the chair (see Chapter 1 for more information about amma). Amma routines use acupressure techniques, stretching, and percussion (tapotement). Today, seated massage routines incorporate a variety of other massage methods such as Swedish massage and myofascial release techniques.

Seated techniques have made massage more accessible to the mainstream public by making it convenient and affordable. Enterprising therapists have expanded this concept to every imaginable venue. Some of the opportunities to use seated massage are airports, beauty salons, large and small businesses, concerts (public and backstage), chiropractic offices, day spas, numerous events such as fairs and festivals, golf courses, health food stores, hospitals, hospices, locker rooms, offices, private practices, retail stores, schools, shopping malls, sporting events, and even street corners. The massage emergency response team (MERT) also uses seated massage.

A MERT, sponsored by the American Massage Therapy Association, was deployed during the rescue efforts after the September 11, 2001, terrorist attacks on the World Trade Center, and the Pentagon. MERT teams primarily used massage chairs and appropriate techniques to treat rescue workers and others at the disaster sites.

Seated massage sessions are typically short (5 to 15 minutes), although they can last as long as 30 minutes. The cost is usually $10 to $20, currently averaging $1 per minute. Some individuals who are not familiar with massage find seated massage more acceptable than table massage. Disrobing is unnecessary. Lubricants are not used. People generally feel less vulnerable seated in a chair than lying on a table, and the time commitment is considerably less, especially when the therapist goes to the client's place of business or on site.

HOW TO SELECT A MASSAGE CHAIR

Many different massage chairs are available today. Just as with a massage table, different features appeal to different people. The following factors should be kept in mind when purchasing a massage chair:

- The chair should be lightweight because you may be moving it from location to location.
- It should be quick and simple to set up and take down.
- It should have enough adjustments to fit a variety of body styles but not so many that you spend a lot of time adjusting the chair. Avoid massage chairs requiring a series of smaller adjustments after making a major adjustment. Simple is better; simple and quick is best.
- It should be sturdy and strong. A creaky or wobbly chair makes the person sitting in it feel insecure and unsafe.
- Be sure that the armrest is strong enough to withstand deep compression and deep frictioning techniques performed on the client's arm. The arm rest's positioning should be high enough off the floor that the therapist can maintain good body mechanics when massaging the forearm and hand.
- The chair manufacturer should offer a trial period during which the chair can be returned for a full refund if the therapist is not completely satisfied. The chair should come with a 5-year or longer warranty.
- Buying from a manufacturer that is well established is generally best. Such a manufacturer usually provides better customer service, and recognized brands typically have a better resale value should you decide to sell your chair.

Professional-grade massage chairs sell for $300 and up. There are less expensive chairs from $150. If you perform seated massage only occasionally (a few times a year) a cheaper chair may suffice so long as it is structurally sound and not poorly constructed because client safety is the most important determining factor when purchasing a chair. Cheaper chairs are also typically less comfortable for the client and will not last long if used regularly. If you plan to include seated massage as part of your massage practice, it is well worth the price to buy a professional-grade chair.

Massage chairs are offered by most massage table companies (Figure 15-1). Some companies offer a desktop face support, which is typically the face support designed to be clamped to or balanced on the edge of a counter, table, or desk. Many of these items have chest pads that hang vertically over the edge. A system of specially designed cushions can hang over the back of an armless chair. If none of the previously mentioned options are available to you, then you can use a stack of pillows on a massage table, a regular table, desk, counter, or chair (see Figure 7-15, *C*) As a last resort, the therapist may use a stool or chair, but this option provides no support for the head, upper body, or arms (see Figure 7-15, *B*).

REASONS FOR OFFERING SEATED MASSAGE

Reasons for offering seated massage are:

- Massage therapists may use seated massage techniques as their primary modality and source of revenue.

DAVID PALMER

Born: November 27, 1948

"My vision is to make touch a positive social value in our culture."

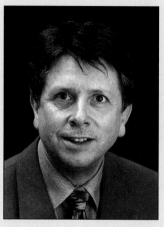

The topic of chair massage can hardly be discussed without the name David Palmer surfacing at least once. Read any article on the subject, and you will soon discover that he is the father of contemporary chair massage.

His career in massage began in 1980. Considering his previous profession of 10 years as an administrator of social service programs for nonprofit agencies in Chicago and San Francisco, it seemed only natural that he would focus on a field in which he could have a great effect on the mental well-being of people through the art of touch. He first encountered massage in his late 20s during a Rolfing session. He had been experiencing chronic neck pain, and the Rolfing combined with tai chi and stretching gave him a feeling of being back inside his body. It was this experience that led him to explore massage.

After he received a massage in a spa in San Francisco, a series of events over a 3-year period led to his position as director of a massage institute specializing in the Japanese art of *amma*. After only a short period of teaching, he realized that a serious gap existed between people who wanted to give and those who wanted receive professional massage. After a little investigating, he came to the conclusion that a significant packaging problem existed in the massage industry.

"The package that the mainstream massage community was selling to the general public was a package that the general public was not interested in buying," he says. It was hard to convince most people to accept an idea that required going into a private room, removing clothing, lying on a table, and being rubbed with oils by a stranger for a costly fee on a regular basis. The whole idea was just too frightening for the average individual. It was then that he gave massage a hard look from a marketing point of view. He says, "They [mainstream massage community] were selling a graduate-level understanding of the field of touch to a population who had not even begun kindergarten regarding touch."

Palmer's solution to this problem was to make massage less frightening and more affordable. The result was his legacy of the seated chair massage.

Although this type of massage had been done for thousands of years, as can been seen in ancient Japanese and Chinese woodcuts, Palmer's contribution was to revive its visibility and identity. It would be more difficult to perceive as strange if the massage is given with the client fully clothed on an open sidewalk in a chair.

Initially Palmer's chair massage was being done on a drummer's stool, but in 1983, he decided to create a special chair. He had seen one of the Scandinavian computer chairs called *Balance* with slanted leg rests and thought it would be perfect, if only it had some sort of head rest and chest support. He enlisted a French cabinetmaker named Serge Bouyssou to be his design partner, and after 2 years the chair was introduced to the national market. The year was 1986, and chair massage was now viewed as being significant enough to have its own physical product.

Vision has clearly been an important factor in David Palmer's career. From the beginning, he saw a challenge and immediately acted on it. Chair massage has given so many people the opportunity to experience the wonderful benefits of massage. It allows the client to safely experience the much-needed sense of touch. "We're so touch phobic that you can't grow up in this culture without having some serious issues about touch," says Palmer. "Parents are afraid to touch their kids; teachers can't touch their students; it's crazy out there. My feeling is that we need to shift that around, and massage is a vehicle for doing that because it provides structured touch." Although he fully appreciates the many wonderful benefits of massage, it is not his main interest. He states, "My vision is to make touch a positive social value in our culture." He admits that this is what primarily motivates his professional life.

The most important thing he feels that students can do in their massage therapy program is first learn how to touch and how to be touched. He confesses, "I'm one of those unreformed 1960s brats who thinks it's still possible to change the world." If his previous record is any reflection on his future, he just might succeed.

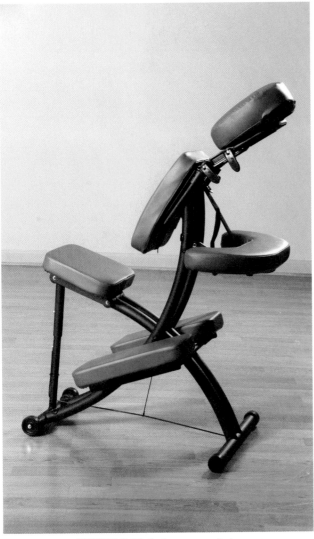

FIGURE 15-1 A massage chair.

• Massage therapists may use seated massage as their secondary modality and supplemental source of revenue.
• Seated massage can be used as a promotional tool to introduce the public to massage in a safe, nonthreatening way.
• Seated massage may be done on site or in the therapist's office.
• Seated massage is often used at sporting events.
• Other opportunities include fundraisers, concerts, conventions, airports, beauty salons, and spas.
• Onsite massage services may be used at professional offices and other work places for stress reduction, pain relief, and injury prevention.
• Seated massage is used by therapists in their offices for short treatments.
• The massage chair is ideal for clients who have difficulty getting onto and off a massage table.
• The chair is as versatile as your imagination.

Seated massage is often used for stress reduction and relaxation, as a *stress-buster break;* however, routines can be designed to address specific complaints such as lower back pain, headaches, and neck and shoulder tension. Adapting massage techniques to the seated position gives the therapist the option of doing clinical massage in either an onsite or a private office setting.

A massage chair takes up less room than a table, making it more adaptable to space limitations. This and the through-clothes technique have brought the chair into therapy areas, athletic training rooms, chiropractic offices, and many massage therapists' treatment rooms as an adjunct to their tables for specific work. Acquiring a massage chair and learning how to use it effectively are well worth the massage therapist's financial investment and time.

CHAT ROOM

In research published in 1996, Dr. Tiffany Field of the Touch Research Institute in Miami found that individuals who received a 15-minute seated massage twice a week showed increased cognitive ability, performed better on math tests, and completed problems with increased accuracy and speed. These individuals also experienced a significant decrease in tension compared with individuals who practiced traditional relaxation techniques while seated in a chair without receiving massage. Hence massage does not cost an employer; it pays.

SANITIZATION AND HYGIENE CONSIDERATIONS

The need for infection control and hand hygiene cannot be overemphasized. The public is aware of the importance of cleanliness, and your clients will notice and appreciate that your equipment is sanitary and your work environment clean. However, when working on site, washroom facilities may not be readily accessible. Seated massage therapy procedures must be self-contained, including hygiene. Hand hygiene is discussed in Chapter 9.

Seated massage therapists can purchase antimicrobial disposable towelettes. These sanitize the massage chair fabric between client sessions. These cleansers help protect the therapist and the client by preventing the spread of disease.

Use a cover on the face rest cushion to make your clients feel more comfortable and to facilitate keeping it clean. These covers help keep makeup off the fabric. One type of cover is a *nurse bouffant cap,* which is available through medical or massage supply businesses. Other types of covers are paper towels and specially designed paper covers, with the latter available through massage supply sources.

A list of items you might wish to bring to on-site massage events can be found in Box 15-1.

BOX 15-1

On-site Massage Events: What to Bring

- Massage chair (or other seated system)
- Face cradle covers
- Antimicrobial wipes*
- Waterless hand sanitizer
- Facial tissue
- Business cards
- Appointment calendar (paper or digital)
- Receipt book
- Bank bag and small bills for change
- Pure drinking water
- Pad for kneeling
- Stool for sitting
- Sunscreen, sunglasses, cap or hat (if working outdoors)
- First aid kit†

*Antimicrobial wipes may be used to sanitize both your equipment fabric and your hands.
†See Box 9-1 for first aid kit suggestions if you are creating your own kit.

SAFETY CONSIDERATIONS AND BODY MECHANICS

Before you set up your massage chair, select an area that allows you to move completely around the chair during the massage. If you use a massage chair carrying case, then place it out of the way. Provide a clear, unobstructed pathway for your clients to and from the chair.

Use effective body mechanics to prevent repetitive motion injuries. When in the lunge (bow) stance, keep your feet and body pointed in the direction of force. Keep your back straight and your head erect. Your movement and pressure will be generated from the pelvis; move your pelvis to shift your weight from back leg to front leg. Be sure to flex your knees. For the greater part of the massage session, your wrists should not be flexed more than 45 degrees.

When using the thumbs, maintain proper alignment by *stacking the bones*. This method means that the bones of the thumb are in relatively straight alignment with the bones of the wrist and arm. If you look straight down your arm, the thumb is then pointing straight ahead. As you use your thumb, the fingers of the working hand may be open or loosely closed. You may also use your fingertips, palm of the hand, loosely clenched fist, or elbow to apply massage techniques (see Figure 15-5). Use of these alternative methods gives your thumbs a needed break and varies the quality of touch for the client. However, be sure to maintain effective body mechanics at all times. Spread your feet farther apart as you work closer to the floor. Avoid bending the back and neck.

> *"Ultimately, your only source of funding is satisfied clients."*
> —Tim Mullen

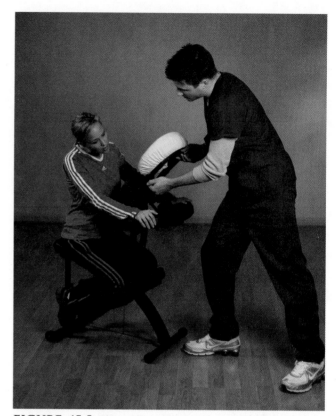

FIGURE 15-2 Therapist making adjustments on chair while client is seated.

Before Seated Massage Begins

If this session is your client's first time to sit in the massage chair, physically demonstrate how to do it properly. As you are sitting in the chair, explain what you are doing. For example, "I am sitting in the chair placing my knees and legs on these cushions while my forearms rest on this shelf and my face is supported by this crescent-shaped pillow." Be specific with your directions and actions. If your client tries to climb on the chair as if it were a motorbike, he or she might upset the chair and become injured. Stand by the chair and offer additional guidance if needed.

Make any chair adjustments before the massage begins (Figure 15-2). The primary adjustments are the seat height, chest pad height, face support height and angle (tilt), and armrest height. A client will typically arch the back or slump if the chair is improperly adjusted to the person's body. *Be sure the client's back is straight and that the armrest is low enough so that the client's shoulders are not raised.* For most clients, the most comfortable position of the face cradle is when the neck is slightly flexed forward. Once the chair is completely adjusted to the client, ask if any additional adjustments should be made. This simple question takes a few seconds and has a significant impact on the session.

Chair Adjustments

- The client's back is straight and his or her chest is relatively flat against the chest pad.
- The face cradle is positioned around the face and tilted to allow the therapist access to the posterior cervical muscles, without subjecting the client's neck to excessive flexion (see Figure 15-4).
- The armrest is at a height that does not elevate the client's shoulders; the shoulders should be at a natural height with the elbows lightly touching or just a few millimeters above the armrest.

TECHNIQUES USED FOR SEATED MASSAGE

Seated massage routines consist of techniques found in East Asian and basic Swedish massage (without lubricant). Techniques most frequently used are featured next.

Compression

Rhythmic compression is effective on the muscles of the forearm and back. Apply firm pressure primarily from the heel of the hand or loosely clenched fists. During rhythmic compression of the forearm, face the client with your fingers relaxed and pointed toward the client's elbow. Apply pressure straight down while maintaining contact.

Compression using sustained pressure is usually applied with a finger or thumb, elbow, or a hand-held tool. This technique displaces fluids in the tissues being compressed, spreads muscle fibers, and relieves muscle spasms. It is primarily used to relieve trigger and tender points. In East Asian techniques, pressure is applied to points in a pattern to improve or balance energy flow in the meridians.

Deep Friction

Deep friction is applied with the thumb, finger, elbow, loosely clenched fist, palm, or heel of the hand. During friction, engage the skin through the client's clothes and move the skin over the underlying structures. Avoid sliding on the client's skin or clothes. The term *deep* does not denote hard pressure but rather the effect of moving the skin and superficial fascia over deeper structures.

Superficial Friction

A warming, stimulating stroke, superficial friction is applied with the palms of one or both hands in a rapid back-and-forth movement over the clothed client. A variation is to use the ulnar sides of the hands in a sawing motion. This variation is effective for reducing muscular tension around the shoulder joint on either side of the spine and across the top of the upper trapezius.

Pétrissage

Pétrissage involves grasping, lifting, and kneading the tissues or rolling the tissues between the thumb and fingers. This massage movement is used primarily in the neck and upper trapezius.

Effleurage

Effleurage is applied over the client's clothing for relaxation and sedation. Nerve strokes, a variation of effleurage, can also be used.

Tapotement

Toward the end of the seated massage, tapotement can be used on the back, head, arms, and hips. Hacking (using the ulnar [little finger] edge of the hands) and loose fist beating (using the ulnar side of loosely clenched fists) are best for the torso, hips, and arms, whereas tapping with the fingertips is best on the scalp.

ADAPTIVE PROFESSIONAL COMMUNICATION

Because eye contact is impossible when the client is in the face cradle, a method of communication must be established in the initial interview before beginning the treatment. The following guidelines are recommended for establishing communication:

When it hurts. Explain that you will be examining the tissues of the back, neck, and arms, looking for areas that are tight and contracted. When these areas are located, they will be tender. You should suggest, "Be sure to tell me whenever I find a tender area. Will you do that for me?" Not only does this give the client permission to tell you that something is tender, but he or she also agrees to do so.

When it gets better. Continue by saying, "When I find these tender places, I will stop and maintain the pressure. This will cause the nervous system to respond by relaxing the tender area. It may feel to you like I am letting up on the pressure, or it is beginning to feel better. Will you let me know when it gets better?"

If it refers. You should then add, "When I am examining or maintaining pressure on an area of tissue, you may experience sensation somewhere else. It could be a pain, tingling, numbness, aching, or other sensation somewhere besides right where I am massaging. These are trigger points. Will you tell me if you feel any sensation radiating anywhere other than where I am working?"

If it is too hard. Say, "If at any time I am working too hard, be sure and tell me right away. Will you do that?" This request is important because it gives the client permission to tell you that you are working too hard. In many instances, the client will not tell you because he or she thinks you are the professional and you must be doing it right. The client may think it is supposed to hurt. Some clients will endure anything if they believe it may make them better. You can also say, "Let me know if what I am doing feels good or if it hurts, especially if it hurts, because this work should not be painful."

During onsite massage, the massage area may be noisy, which makes hearing the client difficult. In this case, ask the client to communicate by raising his or her hand if pain is felt. If more specific information is needed regarding pain, then establish a pain-measuring system on a scale from 1 (no pain) through 5 (excruciating pain). You will know, by the number of fingers raised, how the client is responding to the pressure (Figure 15-3). This system also may be used in quiet places.

Some people will not tell you that something hurts. They may be accustomed to denying pain. However, the body never lies. You can tell that you are working too hard when the client begins to pull away from you or unconsciously contracts muscles to limit your access into the tissues. If he or she is tensing up, squirming, or pulling away, then *you are using too much pressure.*

RECORD KEEPING

Have your clients fill out an intake form and obtain consent. The initial interview with your client may be brief, but the form should ask questions regarding eye conditions that might be affected by the face cradle (e.g., contacts), and any medical conditions for which the person is being treated. Establish your client's primary and secondary treatment goals and screen for possible contraindications using the PPALM assessment and treatment planning method outlined in Chapter 10.

Clinical application of seated massage requires more detailed records. Treatment notes document progress and remind the therapist of what procedures were performed and which treatments were helpful. In legal situations, proper documentation is helpful for you and your clients. Additionally, unless you give each client a receipt, it may not be considered a legal transaction by taxation authorities. To save time, receipts may be preprinted and prepared in advance, with a place to fill in the client's name, date, and amount.

SAMPLE SEATED MASSAGE ROUTINE

The following basic routine is a suggested protocol that you can accomplish in 15 minutes. Use it as a guide, but remain creative and intuitive. Accomplish as much as you can for each client within the time allowed. Concentrate the major part of the session on the client's primary area of complaint, which is usually the neck, shoulders, and lower back. Start with some general strokes to acquaint clients with your touch and to establish their individual sensitivity in receiving; gradually become more specific as you go on. You cannot resolve everything from which a client has been suffering for years in one treatment. Even recent injuries usually require multiple treatments (see Chapter 14 for information about clinical massage). One 15-minute session can reduce the main complaint and accomplish some general relaxation; therefore you will have performed a great service for the client in that amount of time.

Upper Back and Neck

Begin the treatment with compression strokes to the paraspinal muscles. Use the heels of the hands or loosely clenched fists. Having the client breathe in rhythm with the compression is important. Ask your client to take a deep

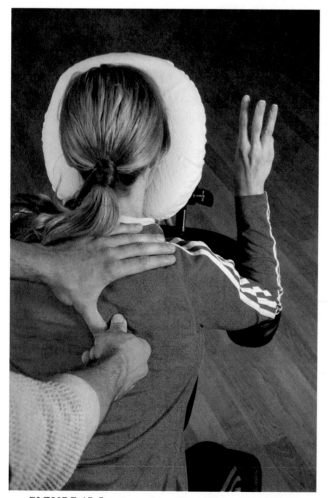

FIGURE 15-3 Client raising three fingers of one hand.

breath and exhale. As he or she exhales, apply firm pressure to the tissues on either side of the spine (ideally, the therapist breathes in the same pattern as the client). Begin between the scapulas and move inferiorly a handwidth at a time until the ilium bones are reached. Then move back superiorly a handwidth at a time until the starting point is reached. This technique establishes contact with the client, introduces relaxation, and gets him or her into a regular deep-breathing pattern.

You should be standing directly behind the center of the client's back. Keep your arms outstretched with just a slight bend in the elbows, back straight, head erect, moving from the pelvis in a lunge position. If you are using the heels of the hands, the wrists will be significantly extended. If pressure applied with the heels of the hands creates discomfort in your wrists, then switch to a loosely clenched fist. Using a loose fist to apply compression keeps the wrist straight as you apply pressure with the proximal phalanges.

Repeat this pattern using loosely clenched fists but with a circular deep frictioning stroke. Make four to eight circles with each hand, working simultaneously down and up the sides of the spine. If massaging in circles with both hands at the same time is too difficult or tiresome, then you may choose to switch to cross-fiber or chucking friction. Apply four friction strokes medially to laterally over the paraspinal muscles, then four friction strokes superiorly to inferiorly, and then move a hand width and repeat.

Every few minutes, ask the client how he or she perceives the pressure, using the guidelines discussed in the "Adaptive Professional Communication" section.

Grasp the upper trapezius muscle with one or both hands, using a pincerlike grip. Begin just lateral to the base of the neck, at approximately the center of the upper trapezius (see Figure 7-15, *B*), and perform pétrissage between the thumb and fingers. Work laterally to the acromion process, then work medially to the base of the neck, and continue as far superior on the neck as you can while still isolating the trapezius fibers. The trapezius fibers will typically become too small to grasp at the third cervical (C3) level. When tender areas or trigger points are encountered, stop and maintain the pressure for 8 to 10 seconds. If your pressure is appropriate for the person, then the client will feel it relax within 10 seconds; if he or she does not, then you are applying too much pressure. Slowly release the pressure and move to another area, returning to the tender area in approximately 1 minute. Trigger points in the upper fibers of the trapezius commonly refer to the back of the head and up to the temple area.

You may now move to the side of the client; grasp and perform pétrissage to the back of his or her neck in the lamina groove (Figure 15-4). Work all the way up to the occipital bone and back down to the shoulder. Because the thumb is more sensitive and powerful, you may choose to go to the other side and repeat this step. This decision is based on the sensitivity found in the tissues the first time you pass over them and the client's main complaint. If the

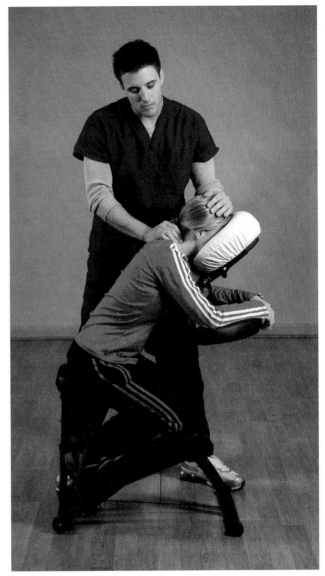

FIGURE 15-4 Therapist massaging back of client's neck.

main complaint is the neck and shoulders, then you will want to be thorough in this area. If the main complaint is in the lower back, then less time will be spent in the posterior cervical region.

Tilt the face cradle forward to place the head and neck in 45 degrees of flexion. While standing at the side of the client, use the thumb and second finger of one hand to apply deep frictioning to the tissues between the occiput and C2. Work from lateral to medial and back. These tissues can be tender; be sure to check with the client about appropriate pressures when working this area.

Using the heel of the hand or fingertips, examine the rhomboid muscles and the posterior surface of the scapula with deep circular friction. When massaging the posterior region of the scapula, support the anterior aspect of the shoulder with the other hand. If this area is the client's primary complaint, more specific treatment of these tissues

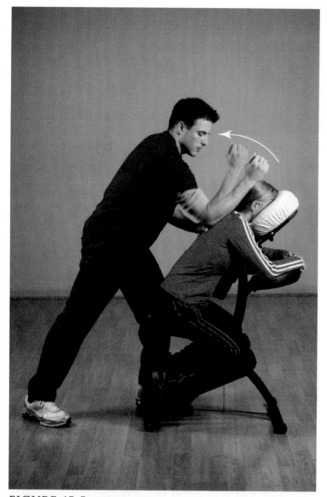

FIGURE 15-5 Guided elbow technique, becoming deeper and more specific by bending the elbow.

can then be done with the thumbs or a guided elbow. For a broader, less specific pressure, use the blade of the ulna. To apply more precise pressure, the elbow is slightly bent (Figure 15-5). For the most precise and deepest pressure, flex the elbow so only the olecranon process is contacting the tissue. Always guide the elbow with the other hand for control, precision, and better sensitivity. When this area is complete, move lateral to the shoulder joint and treat the rotator cuff tendons with circular friction.

Apply circular friction to the area below the scapulas using the heels of the hands, working both sides of the spine at once. This action addresses the latissimus dorsi muscle and paraspinal muscles in the midback.

Lower Back

Moving your hand inferiorly, use circular friction to address the lower back. The quadratus lumborum muscle can be examined and treated effectively in the seated position. This muscle is responsible for many complaints of lower back pain. Trigger points in the quadratus lumborum often mimic hip and sciatic nerve pain. Palpate the client's waistline,

being careful not to elicit a tickle response. After locating the lateral end of the twelfth rib, apply deep friction with your thumbs or the heel of your hand in a lateral to medial direction along its inferior surface. As you move medially, you will encounter a hard structure; this is the spine, specifically the lateral aspect (the "tip") of the transverse process of L1. This is often more lateral than expected. Change directions of pressure to 45 degrees medial anterior. Using circular friction, examine the edge of the lumbar spine in the area of the transverse processes. Using deep circular friction, massage this area in thumbwidth increments from L1 to the ilium bone. Change the direction of pressure to inferior anterior, and treat the superior surface of the ilium laterally to the midline of the body.

The lower portion of the paraspinal muscles can now be examined more thoroughly using fingertips, thumbs, or a guided elbow. Treat one side at a time with deep circular or cross-fiber friction, using sustained pressure on tender areas and trigger points. Apply friction on this area from medial to lateral, allowing the client to rock slightly in the chair. This technique is effective and relaxing. With clients in acute lower back pain, side-to-side rocking may aggravate the condition and cause pain. Be sure to ask the client if the rocking feels good. If it does not, stop and use a different technique.

Arm and Forearm

Because no surface is available against which to compress the biceps and triceps during seated massage, the therapist is limited to pétrissage, rolling, jostling, nerve strokes, or squeezing the tissues of the upper arm with one or two hands.

Facing the front of the chair, slightly to one side, place the client's forearm with the palm down on the armrest to treat the forearm muscles. Apply compression to the extensor muscle group using the heel of your hand, working from wrist to elbow. Repeat this sequence three times, then rotate the forearm, palm up, and apply three sets of compression to the flexor muscles.

Roll the forearm over, with the hand palm down, and instead of compression, repeat this pattern using circular friction applied with the heel of your hand, with your fingers pointed toward the elbow of the client. Work from wrist to elbow in 1- or 2-inch intervals, making 5 to 10 circles on each spot. Repeat this sequence three times. Rotate the forearm, palm up, and repeat the circular friction moves on the flexor muscles of the forearm.

Using the thumbs, apply circular friction to all sides of the wrist. Grasp the client's hand, shake out the arm, and return it to the armrest. Repeat this sequence on the other arm.

Face and Scalp

Facial and scalp massage feels great while in a chair; however, many people do not want their hair or makeup disturbed, so obtain permission first. Using the pads of the fingers, apply circular friction to the temples, jaw, face, and forehead. During scalp massage, the tissue can be shifted back and forth across the cranium using deep friction in any direction. Gentle tapping or pincement tapotement also works well on the scalp, especially as part of the general finishing strokes. Avoid this step if your client has a headache.

> ⊝volve *Log on to the Evolve website to view a demonstration of scalp massage.* ∎

Stretches

Stretches are useful in seated massage. Because most individuals spend much of their time in a flexed position, the anterior cervical region and pectoral regions of the body are typically contracted. Most clients also have chronically internally rotated shoulders. Passive and active-assisted stretches can relax and lengthen these habitually contracted tissues. Massage therapists should use only the specific systems of stretching in which they are trained and must always be careful not to overstretch the client's soft tissue and to avoid bouncy (ballistic) or prolonged stretching. Stretches for the forearm, wrist, and hand can be done with the client in the usual position on the massage chair. Stretches for the cervical and shoulder regions are best done with the client sitting up straight in the chair. This actually allows for a more complete stretching routine than can be done on a massage table—another advantage (and opportunity) of chair massage.

Final Procedure

As the seated massage session draws to a close, return to general strokes. If the goal is to leave the client relaxed and sedated, then finish with some effleurage and slow downward nerve strokes on the back and shoulders. If the client is returning to work and needs to be more alert, finish with tapotement, superficial (palmar) friction, and brisk nerve strokes. Tapping tapotement on the head and hacking or loose fist beating on the shoulders and back, as well as over the hips and lateral thighs, is a stimulating way to finish the massage.

When the treatment is complete, tell the client, and ask him or her to get off the chair slowly and carefully. Remain with the client a few moments because many people, especially older adults, may feel unsteady. Some people actually doze off during the massage and may need time to become fully oriented. Be ready to assist your client as needed.

Be sure your client is in possession of any personal items such as eyeglasses, keys, or cell phones.

Always have your appointment calendar handy to schedule appointments and your business cards ready to distribute. As you collect your fee from the client or just thank the person and say good-bye, suggest that the client schedule another appointment. Also appropriate is to mention that, if the client liked your work, he or she should recommend you to others.

On completion of all transactions with the client, sanitize your hands, disinfect the chair, write your case notes (if appropriate), take a few deep breaths, and get ready for the next client.

E-RESOURCES

⊝volve

http://evolve.elsevier.com/Salvo/MassageTherapy
- Chapter challenge
- Flash cards
- Photo gallery
- Weblinks

▶ **DVD**

- 15-1: Seated massage

BIBLIOGRAPHY

Benjamin P, Tappan F: *Tappan's handbook of healing massage technique*, ed 4, Upper Saddle River, NJ, 2004, Prentice Hall.

Benjamin PJ: Seated massage in history, *Massage Ther J* 42(1):144, 2003.

Field T: Massage therapy reduces anxiety and enhances EEG pattern of alertness and math computations, *Int J Neurosci* 86:197-205, 1996.

Fritz S: *Fundamentals of therapeutic massage*, ed 3, St Louis, 2003, Mosby.

Holland PM, Anderson SK: *Chair massage*, St Louis, 2011, Mosby.

Ironson G et al: Massage therapy is associated with enhancement of the immune system's cytotoxic capacity, *Int J Neurosci* 84:205-218, 1996.

Mattes A: *Active isolated stretching*, Sarasota, Fla, 1995, self-published.

Palmer D: *How to market on site massage*, Santa Rosa, Calif, 1986, Living Earth Crafts.

Palmer D: *The bodywork entrepreneur*, San Francisco, 1990, Thumb Press.

Parfitt A: *Seated acupressure bodywork: a practical handbook for therapists*, Berkeley, Calif, 2006, North Atlantic Books.

Stephens R: *Seated therapeutic massage*, vol I-III video seminars, Cedar Rapids, Iowa, 1996, Ralph Stephens Seminars.

Stephens R: *Therapeutic chair massage*, Baltimore, 2005, Lippincott Williams & Wilkins.

Travell JG, Simons D: *Myofascial pain and dysfunction, the trigger point manual*, Baltimore, 1992, Williams & Wilkins.

MATCHING I

Place the letter of the answer next to the term or phrase that best describes it.

A. Amma
B. Antimicrobial disposable towelettes
C. Benefits of chair massage
D. Convenient and affordable
E. David Palmer
F. Desktop face support
G. Dr. Tiffany Field
H. Factors in buying a massage chair
I. Hand sanitizer
J. Lubricant
K. Protection of the face cushion
L. Sit in the chair

_____ 1. Type of seated massage equipment that can be clamped to or balanced on the edge of a counter, desk or table

_____ 2. Examples are massage chairs that are lightweight, easy to set up and take down, and adjust to fit a variety of body styles

_____ 3. Massage product NOT used in seated massage

_____ 4. What the therapist should do first when explaining to a first-time client the proper way to sit in a massage chair

_____ 5. Should be used to clean the chair fabric between client sessions

_____ 6. Individual who helped conduct research indicating that seated massage increases cognitive ability and performance on math tests

_____ 7. Examples of reasons why seated techniques have made massage more accessible to the mainstream public

_____ 8. Replaces traditional hand washing at on-site massage locations

_____ 9. Traditional Japanese system of massage from which chair massage techniques were derived

_____ 10. What a nurse bouffant cap, paper covers, paper towels can provide

_____ 11. Individual who introduced seated massage in the workplace in the early 1980s

_____ 12. Examples are uses as a promotional tool; takes up less space than a massage table; easier to take on-site than a massage table

MATCHING II

Place the letter of the answer next to the term or phrase that best describes it.

A. 5 to 15 minutes
B. Are you comfortable?
C. Bouncy or ballistic
D. Client pulls away
E. Deep friction
F. Lunge
G. Pelvis
H. Raising fingers
I. Shoulders
J. Stacking the bones
K. Sustained pressure compression
L. Tapotement

_____ 1. Technique used in seated massage that is usually applied with a finger, thumb, elbow, or hand-held tool

_____ 2. Part of the client's body that should not be raised if the armrest is positioned properly

_____ 3. Where therapist movements and pressure are generated

_____ 4. Stance most commonly used by therapists performing seated massage

_____ 5. One possible therapist observation if applied pressure is too deep

_____ 6. Method to help the therapist maintain proper thumb alignment

_____ 7. Question asked by the therapist once initial chair adjustments are completed

_____ 8. Length of a typical seated massage session

_____ 9. Techniques usually applied toward the end of the seated massage session; can be performed on the back, head, arms, and hips

_____ 10. Technique that engages and moves the skin over the underlying structures and can be applied using the thumb, finger, elbow, loosely clenched fist, palm, or heel of the hand

_____ 11. Pain-measuring system using a scale of 1 to 5 that a client can use to communicate with the therapist in a noisy area

_____ 12. Type of stretch the therapist avoids using

CASE STUDY

Chair Massage During Pregnancy

Cyndi saw her obstetrician a few days ago because she has been feeling fatigued. She's 40 years old and going to give birth to her first child in 3 months. Admittedly, she feels a little nervous. Well, maybe more than just a little. "Will the baby's room be ready? Are the crib, stroller and car seat safe? Disposable diapers are easier, but what about the environment? Will my husband really be able to take a week off from work after the delivery? Am I too old to have a baby? Will my mother and mother-in-law be helpful or stressful? When will I ever find time to take a shower?"

During her visit, while Cyndi expressed her list of concerns, Dr. Grayson noticed her patient fidgeting, clenching her fists, with a stressed look on her face. She took her blood pressure for a second time in that visit and, as she suspected, Cyndi's blood pressure was slightly higher than at the beginning of the visit. Cyndi's concern about the birth were beginning to have physiologic effects that could develop into complications.

Cyndi's obstetrician referred her to a massage therapist with training in pregnancy massage. She suggested that a weekly massage could help relax her nerves, keep her blood pressure in a healthy range, and may even help empower her to believe that she can handle the pregnancy, delivery, and raising her child one day at a time.

Cyndi agrees that massage therapy may be a great health care option. Unfortunately, the massage therapist Dr Grayson recommended doesn't hold office hours during the times that Cyndi is able to schedule. On the bright side, her employer recently began a wellness program that allows each employee to have two 10-minute chair massages each month at the employer's expense, with the option of paying out of pocket for additional minutes, or for additional sessions, at a rate of $1/minute. Dr. Grayson agrees that this is a good option so long as the therapist available to her is qualified to provide prenatal massage for women with risk factors.

Cyndi learned that Clara, one of the three massage therapists hired by her employer, is certified in prenatal massage and has advanced training for treating women at risk.

Should Cyndi opt for the chair massage? If so, how often and of what duration?

What should the treatment goals for Cyndi's sessions be?

If she chooses weekly chair massage, what considerations need to be made for positioning Cyndi on the chair?

Based on Cyndi's position on the massage chair, what adjustments, if any, should Clara make to ensure proper body mechanics?

Should Clara provide a simple consent form for Cyndi, or is a more detailed intake form necessary?

Does the therapist need clearance from Dr. Grayson? Should Clara and Dr. Grayson communicate with each other directly?

CRITICAL THINKING

When would seated massage be more advantageous over table massage?

CHAPTER 16

Energy-Based Bodywork Therapy: Shiatsu and Ayurveda

Kenneth G. Zysk, PhD, DPhil

LEARNING OBJECTIVES

After completing this chapter, the student should be able to:

- Describe the unifying concepts in shiatsu and Ayurveda.
- Contrast and compare Asian and Western medicine.
- Define Asian bodywork therapy.
- Describe the theory of yin and yang and their major correspondences.
- Name the 12 regular channels, and delineate their paths in the human body.
- Define tsubos and their role in shiatsu.
- Contrast and compare zang organs to fu organs.
- State and describe the five element theory and its major correspondences.
- Contrast and compare creation cycles with control cycles.
- Discuss the concepts of kyo and jitsu and how they are used in treatment.
- Apply appropriate techniques when addressing ki (qi) deficiency/yin and/or excess/yang in the channels while using proper body mechanics.
- State the definition of shiatsu.
- Incorporate the Zen Shiatsu principles of touch during a session.
- Demonstrate the techniques of thumbing and palming.
- Explain hara evaluation, and define its purpose.
- Describe the three doshas.
- State the Hindu meaning of prakriti.
- Outline the seven chakras and their characteristics.

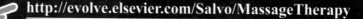

INTRODUCTION

This chapter provides the student an overview of Asian Bodywork Therapy, with a focus on shiatsu, a Japanese bodywork therapy. The chapter also examines Ayurveda, an Indian science of health. Both systems are rooted in the philosophy of traditional Asian medicine.

The Asian bodywork therapy principles are simple to understand and practice at a basic level. This chapter provides this basis. However, the professional practice of Asian bodywork therapy requires training and guidance from an instructor who is experienced in Asian principles and methods. Should the material presented stimulate your curiosity, seek further training to expand the information provided in these pages. Asian bodywork therapy is a profession in itself, with nationally recognized standards of education.

TRADITIONAL ASIAN MEDICINE MODEL OF HEALTH

The central idea that runs through traditional Asian medicine is the concept of *energy*. Imagine a tree: The concept of energy is the trunk of the tree, and different ways to organize and to assess energy are its branches (Figure 16-1). Traditional Asian medicine provides a basic model illustrating

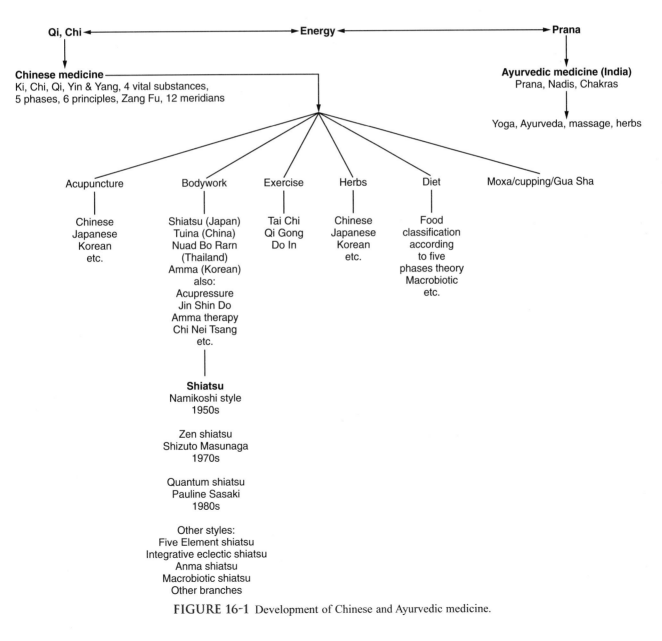

FIGURE 16-1 Development of Chinese and Ayurvedic medicine.

this concept. The concept further branches out, following different styles that have originated in various Asian regions (e.g., China, Japan, India) and have developed under the influence of many great teachers.

WHAT IS ASIAN BODYWORK THERAPY?

The American Organization for Bodywork Therapies of Asia (AOBTA) defines **Asian bodywork therapy** (ABT) as the use of traditional Asian techniques and strategies to treat the human body, mind, and spirit (this includes the electromagnetic or energetic field that surrounds, infuses, and brings that body to life). Asian bodywork is based on traditional Chinese medicine (TCM) for assessing and evaluating the energetic system. Pressure and/or manipulation may also be used to maintain or restore health and to balance the human body, emotions, mind, energy field, and spirit.

Many different bodywork therapies share the Asian origins and the definition mentioned previously—for example, shiatsu from Japan, Nuad Bo Rarn (Thai massage) from Thailand, amma from Korea, Tui na from China, and other styles such as acupressure, Chi Nei Tsang, Jin Shin Do, Jin Shin Jyutsu, and so forth. Many of these styles developed further in countries such as the United States but maintain the same principles and philosophy originated in Asia more than 2500 years ago.

ABT is one of the three branches of traditional Asian medicine, as recognized by the National Certification Commission on Acupuncture and Oriental Medicine (NCCAOM). The other two branches are acupuncture and oriental herbology. We might say that bodywork, acupuncture, and herbs are tools that can be used to apply the principles of traditional Asian medicine to restore and maintain health. The same principles of traditional Asian medicine can be applied through other means such as exercise (e.g., tai chi, qi gong), traditional Asian medicine dietary principles, *moxibustion* (stimulation of *acupoints* [see discussion in next section] with heat from burning an herb called mugwort or moxa applied above or on the acupoints), and other techniques such as *Gua Sha* (a skin-scraping technique to help expel excess heat or remove energy stagnation) and *cupping* (a method in which a warmed cup is placed upside down directly on the skin, creating a vacuum that suctions the skin to relieve energy stagnation). Additionally, liniments, compresses, herbal baths, and essential oils are applied on acupoints.

Herbs, foods, and essential oils have their own particular energetic qualities that have affinity for particular organs and functions of the body. They can be used to strengthen certain physiological functions and help resolve symptoms of disease. Only a qualified and experienced practitioner should use herbs. Consult your state laws to be sure you are within your scope of practice before using any method on your clients.

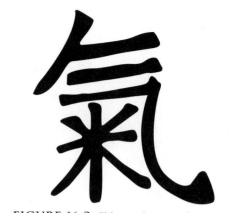

FIGURE 16-2 Chinese character for energy.

ENERGY

Energy, or **ki** (in Japanese), **qi** (sometimes spelled *ch'i*, or **chi**—all variations pronounced "chee"—in Chinese), or *ojas* (in Sanskrit), also known as life force, is the element that creates and binds together all things and phenomena existing in the universe (Figure 16-2). This includes everything that manifests physically in nature and in the human body, as well as the emotions, thoughts, and spirit.

Energy demonstrates itself as *movement* and *vibration*. Solid material and seemingly inanimate objects also have vibration that can be scientifically observed at a microscopic level in the vibration and movement of the atoms that form all things. Electrons spin around protons, and they constantly collide against each other and other atoms, releasing energy. The force of attraction and rejection between the protons and electrons and the space between them are also manifestations of energy in the form of a magnetic field that binds them. The human body also generates a magnetic field that can be measured.

Scientific studies done on particles of light determined that any given particle can be observed as a particle of matter or a wave of energy at the same time. This interchangeability between matter and wave (nonmatter) introduces the *concept of relativity,* which is further expanded on in the field of quantum physics. This concept provides a scientific model for the theories of Asian medicine.

Pauline Sasaki, a disciple of the renowned teacher Shizuto Masunaga and the creator of quantum shiatsu, describes the observable energetic phenomena as variations in the speed of vibration in which the material aspects have the slowest speed of vibration (therefore easier to see with the naked eye), and the spiritual aspects have the fastest. The faster the vibration is, the harder it is to observe its manifestations, although by increasing the development of our sensory system, we are able to sense them. In any case, we can observe the effects of these faster vibrations the same as in the case of electricity, in which we cannot see electricity itself, but we can see how a light turns on as we flip the switch.

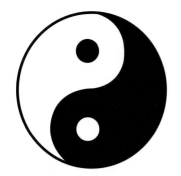

FIGURE 16-3 Tai Ji: Symbol of yin and yang.

YIN AND YANG

The *Yellow Emperor's Inner Classic* (*Huang Di Nei Jing* in Chinese) is the highly regarded text of Chinese medicine that dates from 300 to 100 BCE. It is here that the theories of yin and yang are first mentioned and the model for the creation of ki is provided. The symbol of the Tai Ji, which represents yin and yang, is formed by a complete circle or the one, meaning completeness. The circle is divided in two sides symbolizing duality, or the dynamic struggle between opposites. One is black and one is white, each containing a smaller circle of the opposite color, symbolizing the nonabsolute quality of all things within itself (Figure 16-3). Hence yin contains a speck of yang, and vice versa.

The two sides are moving toward each other in a *circular* motion. In the same way, during the day (yang), the light of the sun decreases to make way to the darkness of the night (yin), and dawn comes to end the night by bringing light (yang) into the darkness (yin). The constant movement of one thing into its opposite is what generates ki. In this example, keep in mind that a moment of the day exists, after sunset or before sunrise, called twilight, when it is difficult to tell whether it is day or night. Day and night are relative to each other and also relative to the point where the observer is placed.

Yin and *yang* literally mean in Chinese "the dark (shadow) side of the hill" and "the light (sunny) side of the hill." The Tai Ji poetically and graphically represents a dynamic that can be observed not only in the duality of the day-night or lightness-darkness cycle, but also in all aspects of nature. Male and female, up and down, inside and outside, slow and fast, matter and energy, passive and active, and contraction and expansion are just some of the possible yin and yang pairs. An illustration of the sunny and dark sides of a hill can be seen on the Evolve website accompanying this text.

On the sunny side of the hill, more light, warmth, activity, and movement exist. Plants grow easily and have foliage and seeds that attract insects and birds. On the shadowy side of the hill, it is darker, the temperature is cooler, plants grow more slowly, more dampness can be found, and less activity overall exists compared to the sunny side.

When comparing yin and yang qualities, remember that one is not *better* than the other and that one is not necessarily

TABLE 16-1 Relative Correspondences of Yin and Yang

YIN	YANG
Feminine	Masculine
Dark	Light
Cold (numb)	Hot (inflamed)
Moist	Dry
Interior	Exterior
Chronic	Acute
Anterior	Posterior
Medial	Lateral
Inferior	Superior
Community	Competition
Earth	Heaven
Water	Fire
Moon	Sun
Slow (still, lethargic)	Fast (restless, energetic)
Static, storing, conserving	Transforming, changing
Substantial	Nonsubstantial
Matter	Energy
Soft, mushy tissue	Hard, congested tissue
Concave	Convex
Passive (inhibited)	Active (excited)
Pale tongue	Red tongue
Thin pulse	Full pulse
Contraction	Expansion
Deficiency	Excess
Pain is dull, achy, stiff	Pain is sharp or moving
Deep	Shallow (on the surface)
Client says "Mm-mm-mm."	Client says "Ouch!"

right and the other *wrong*. They are simply different aspects of the same oneness: ki (Table 16-1). They mutually create and balance each other; thus the one is necessary for the other to exist. They have equal value relative to one another. In this way, health is a dynamic equilibrium between yin and yang.

Given that energy is movement, to get in contact with the movement of yin energy, we can focus on the contractive phase such as movement from the periphery to the center and from the top to bottom. To get in contact with yang energy, we can focus on the expansive phase of energy such as movement from the center to the periphery and from below to above. These phases can also be illustrated by how air expands and rises when heated, and then contracts and moves downward when cooled. These phases are exhibited as *tendencies,* always in movement; they are not static.

The concept of direction of energy movement between yin and yang is often best understood with a picture, since as we know "a picture is worth a thousand words." Log on to the Evolve website using your student account to see this image and more.

In ABT, a symptom such as pain, for example, can be assessed energetically as being either predominantly yin or predominantly yang in nature and treated accordingly. Pain, as a manifestation of a yang imbalance, is a feeling of heat, agitation, and restlessness; the area appears red, is warm to touch, feels hard and inflamed. If symptoms are in the upper part of the body, the pain is sharp and moves around. The person may feel additional pain if the affected area is touched.

Pain as a manifestation of a yin imbalance is a feeling of cold, weakness, weight, and lethargy; the pain is dull rather than sharp, and it feels deep. The skin is discolored or dark, and it feels good if the area is touched directly. Yang type of pain can be observed in acute phases of injury; yin type of pain can be observed in chronic and prolonged phases of disease.

Therapeutically, a yang condition would be addressed with soothing (yin) techniques that would help *disperse the excess energy.* In the case of a yin imbalance, it is desirable to bring in a bit more movement (yang) to break up the stagnation of energy or *tone up* or *strengthen the deficiency or weaknesses.* Using a bit of the opposite quality, the practitioner helps to restore the movement between yin and yang. This method will help the client regain balance at all levels. If a person is living with persistent physical pain, over time he or she will become impatient, angry, or depressed, which are emotional aspects. Also affected are the client's self-perception, ability to succeed in life's pursuits, and outlook on life, which are examples of mental aspects. Even the person's relationships with others and to the universe, which are spiritual aspects, will be affected. ABT offers a coherent theory to affect all aspects of the client's life.

"All of me, why not take all of me."
—Billie Holiday

CHANNELS

Energy circulates in the body through **channels** or *meridians,* which are pathways of energy and vessels. It helps move the *vital substances*—ki, essence, blood, body fluids, and Spirit—to the *zang* and *fu,* which are organ systems (discussed in a later section). The channels are the connections of the material body to the nonmaterial body (e.g., energy field surrounding the body). Channels distribute, balance, and connect the ki of the interior organs with the surface and exterior of the body.

Channels help "move the ki and blood, regulate the yin and the yang, moisten the tendons and the bones, and benefit the joints…" *(Yellow Emperor's Inner Classic).* Ki circulates through the channels in a fixed direction, one channel ending where the following one starts, making one continuous interconnected channel.

Channels meet at the distal ends of the extremities. The order of the flow follows the *Chinese Clock,* a system based in the circadian or biologic cycle in which each organ has a time of the day when its energy is at its peak of activity, starting with the lung and ending with the liver (Figure 16-4).

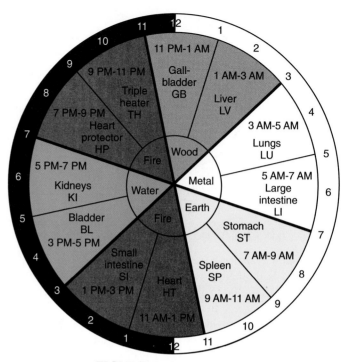

FIGURE 16-4 Chinese clock.

Names of organ systems and channels are depicted in capital letters (e.g., *Heart*) to differentiate them from the anatomic organs (i.e., the heart). If you find that a client has a Heart channel imbalance, this does not mean that there is an illness or disease of the heart, so avoid making statements such as "You have a problem with your heart." This statement may cause unnecessary anxiety in the client about a possible medical condition affecting the heart; and it clearly falls outside your scope of practice.

The most important channels are the 12 regular channels, which are bilateral and symmetric, and the 8 extraordinary vessels. The 12 regular channels are named after the organ systems associated with them and occur in yin and yang pairs.

1. Yin organ *lung* (LU): 3 to 5 AM (Figure 16-5)
   Yang organ *large intestine* (LI): 5 to 7 AM (Figure 16-6)
2. Yang organ *stomach* (ST): 7 to 9 AM (Figure 16-7)
   Yin organ *spleen* (SP): 9 to 11 AM (Figure 16-8)
3. Yin organ *heart* (HT): 11 AM to 1 PM (Figure 16-9)
   Yang organ *small intestine* (SI): 1 to 3 PM (Figure 16-10)
4. Yang organ *bladder* (BL): 3 to 5 PM (Figure 16-11)
   Yin organ *kidney* (KID): 5 to 7 PM (Figure 16-12)
5. Yin organ *heart protector* (HP) or *pericardium* (P): 7 to 9 PM (Figure 16-13)
   Yang organ *triple heater** (TH): 9 to 11 PM (Figure 16-14)

---

*Triple heater, or triple warmer, refers to three "heaters" or "burners" in the body. According to traditional Chinese medicine, the upper heater is in the chest, where blood is made; the middle heater is in the central abdominal area, where food is processed; the lower burner involves the intestines, where the pure is separated from the impure products and where waste is eliminated.

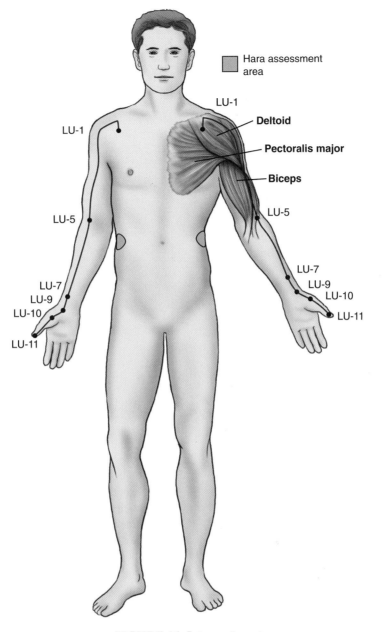

FIGURE 16-5 Lung channel.

6. Yang organ *gallbladder* (GB): 11 PM to 1 AM (Figure 16-15)
   Yin organ *liver* (LIV): 1 to 3 AM (Figure 16-16)

When an imbalance occurs in an organ, symptoms may flare up at the time of either the most or the least activity of the day for that organ system. For example, if someone wakes up every night between 1 and 3 AM, then it may point to a liver imbalance.

The eight extraordinary vessels work as reservoirs for the regular channels, supplementing their function and pooling and storing ki as needed to preserve balance in the whole system. The conception (Ren), governing (Du),

penetrating (Chong), and belt (Dai) vessels are particularly important in the formation and support of the embryo.

TSUBOS

Along the channels are specific points at which the energy concentrates and surfaces as vortices of ki. These points are called **tsubos** (Japanese for "container" or "vase"). Channel charts map the location of the tsubos related to each channel. The tsubos have specific actions when stimulated with pressure (shiatsu, acupressure), the insertion of needles

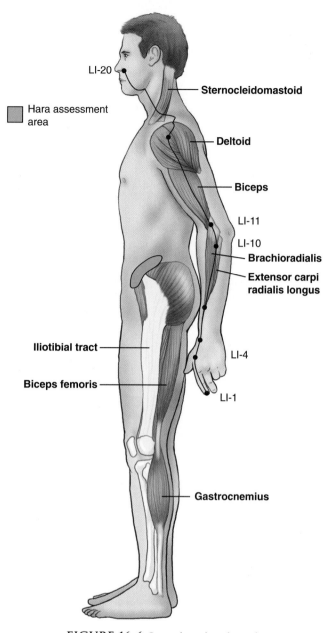

LI-20

Hara assessment area

Sternocleidomastoid

Deltoid

Biceps

LI-11

LI-10

Brachioradialis

Extensor carpi radialis longus

Iliotibial tract

LI-4

Biceps femoris

LI-1

Gastrocnemius

FIGURE 16-6 Large intestine channel.

CHAT ROOM

To find the location of the tsubos, distance is measured in cun (pronounced *soon*), which is the body inch unit (see illustration). This is a system of proportional measurement that is determined by the client's body, not the practitioner's body. For example, ST36 *(leg three miles)* is located *3 cun below the lower edge of the patella, 1 cun lateral to the crest of the tibia.* Each cun is measured by the width of the client's own thumb knuckle.

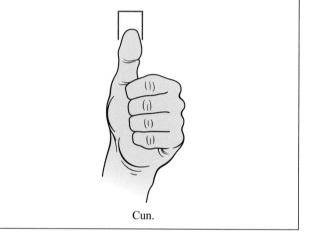

Cun.

Kyo and Jitsu

When you palpate or lean on a tsubo, it will feel neutral, full, or empty. Kyo and jitsu are terms used to describe the quantity of energy or the activity in a tsubo. **Kyo** means empty, yin, depleted or not enough ki. **Jitsu** means full, yang, excess, or too much ki. Jitsu also means the quality of the ki such as responsive or sluggish, soft or hard, expansive or contractive.

In most instances, when you lean on a kyo tsubo or area of the body, it feels as though you can go deep. It can feel soft, cooler, nonresponsive, or sluggish; energy in the tsubo is lacking. Thus the ki that is projected in the form of pressure through your hand is welcome. While focusing on it, you are calling ki to that particular tsubo, helping to draw energy towards it. This technique is called *tonification*. The ki that pours into the tsubo comes from other places in the system of the client where it is not needed or has an excess amount, and from the universe. When you feel something start to stir or move, move on to another point.

By bringing the attention to the tsubo, your own ki initiates a process of transformation. This does not mean that you are pouring your own ki into the tsubo, as in a gasoline filling pump. By respecting the Zen Shiatsu principles of touch (see later discussion), your own energy field will be expanded. Because of this expansion, you should not feel drained at the end of a session.

A jitsu tsubo feels full of energy. The point may feel hard, warm, and superficial. Your pressure feels pushed out or resisted to the extent that it feels as if you cannot stay there long. The intention in this case should be to disperse the excess ki in the tsubo. This technique is called *sedation*.

(acupuncture), heat (moxibustion), essential oils, and even the vibration of tuning forks placed on them.

Tsubos are identified with the name of the channel plus numbers that increase sequentially in order from the origin to the end of the channel pathway (SP1, SP2, SP3, and so forth). They also have Chinese names that sometimes evoke geologic features, such as for KI1 *(bubbling spring),* LI4 *(union valley),* and HP7 *(great mound).*

Knowing the indications for these points, you can include them in your treatment plan, according to the symptoms presented by the client. You can obtain reference guides with the names, locations, indications, and actions of the 361 tsubos of the body.

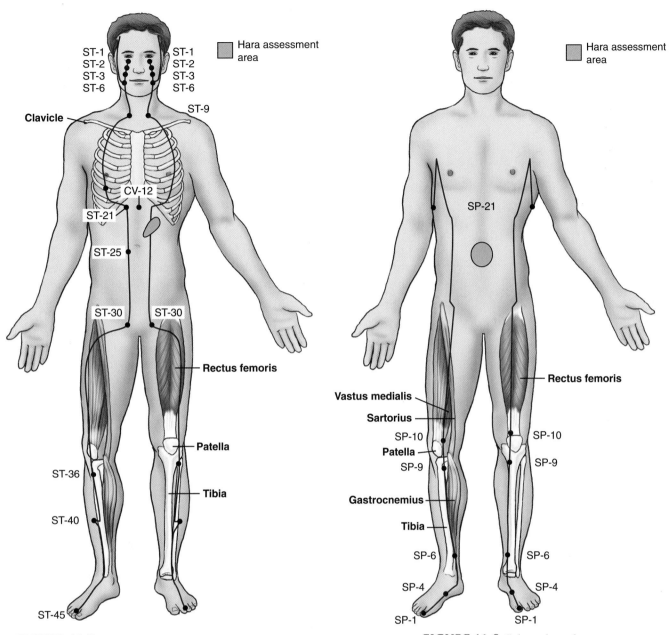

FIGURE 16-7 Stomach channel. CV = Conception vessel.

FIGURE 16-8 Spleen channel.

This entire system is designed to be self-regulating. As with yin and yang, kyo and jitsu are relative to each other. Every jitsu has a corresponding kyo somewhere down the line, the depletion of which is bankrolling the excess; and every kyo has a jitsu that needs to overwork to balance the deficiency. You will sometimes find kyo and jitsu points next to each other on the same channel.

In fact, you will often find channels that are predominantly kyo or predominantly jitsu. In a hara assessment, the most kyo and the most jitsu channels are determined. While other channels may be addressed during treatment, the focus will be on balancing out the most kyo and the most jitsu channel.

Through tonification and sedation, the goal is to even out or harmonize the ki in the whole channel. This process will balance the ki throughout the system. The difference between tonification and sedation techniques is the practitioner's intention. Pressure is applied to areas of kyo and jitsu perpendicular into the channel. However, with kyo areas, the pressure will most likely be applied longer as the ki gathers; in jitsu areas, the pressure will most likely be applied just long enough to disperse the excess ki.

The practitioner should first address the need (kyo) wherever it is found because this action will initiate balance in the whole system. If you push the ki away from a jitsu area or tsubo, without first identifying and tonifying the kyo,

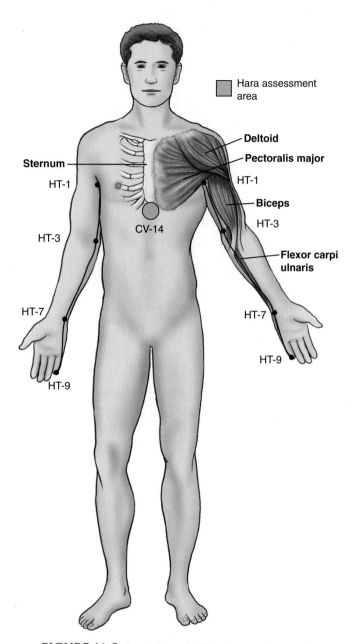

Hara assessment area

Deltoid

Pectoralis major

Sternum

HT-1

HT-1

Biceps

HT-3

HT-3

CV-14

Flexor carpi ulnaris

HT-7

HT-7

HT-9

HT-9

FIGURE 16-9 Heart channel. CV = Conception vessel.

it may feel temporarily better, but the results will not be long-lasting. In fact, probably by the time you go back to the first identified jitsu area or tsubo, it will have already started to change before it is touched again.

Therefore, the treatment strategy is to

1. Identify kyo and jitsu.
2. Tonify the kyo.
3. If necessary, disperse or sedate the jitsu.
4. Check for changes until ki evens out throughout the whole channel or system.

---

evolve *Technique tips for ABT practitioners, as well as hara assessment tips, are located on the Evolve web site for this chapter.* ∎

ZANG AND FU

The *zang* and *fu* are the organ systems, divided into yin and yang organs. They include their internal organs and associated channels. The functions of the organ systems are physical (e.g., digestion, or transformation of foods for nourishment in the case of the stomach and the spleen) and also include the emotional, mental, and spiritual aspects of human existence. Emotional nourishment is as important for the full development of a child as food is. Mental stimulation and nourishment, such as learning, is vital for the development of intellectual capabilities. It is the same as nourishing your relationships with yourself, others, and the universe to help you have a spiritually rich life. This applies to all the other functions of the body (e.g., respiration, elimination, detoxification, assimilation).

Zang are the yin organ systems: heart, liver, lungs, kidney, pericardium, and spleen. They tend to be *solid* organs. *Fu* are the yang organ systems: small intestine, gallbladder, large intestine, bladder, triple heater, and stomach. The anatomic organs of this group tend to be *hollow*. The zang and fu also have correspondences with and associations to other organs; elemental forces in nature (discussed under the theory of the five phases); climatic conditions such as dampness, heat, cold, dryness, colors, sounds, flavors, smells, times of the day, seasons; and other characteristics.

A good flow of energy through the channels and vessels to the whole system keeps the zang and fu and the body nourished, which is the foundation for health. An imbalance anywhere in the system—or an interruption, blockage, or depletion of the flow of energy—will affect not only the area, but also the system as a whole. ABT can be used as a preventive measure by identifying the imbalances and helping to restore the energy flow before symptoms become manifest. When an ABT practitioner works with this system, he or she must remember that the aim is not just to fix the particular problem or symptom that might need immediate attention but rather to restore a smooth flow of energy overall. This action, in itself, will help ensure that the functions of the zang and fu are performed properly, and in turn any imbalances or symptoms will tend to be resolved.

"Fish will be the last one to discover water."
—Einstein

THE FIVE PHASES OR FIVE ELEMENTS

Another way to classify the information observed from natural phenomena is by using the theory of five phases (also translated from Chinese as "five elements"), which results from centuries of careful observation of life cycles and nature. The term *phases* is used here because it best describes a dynamic rather than a static state of the energy. Health is an expression of the state in which all five phases are in harmony with each other.

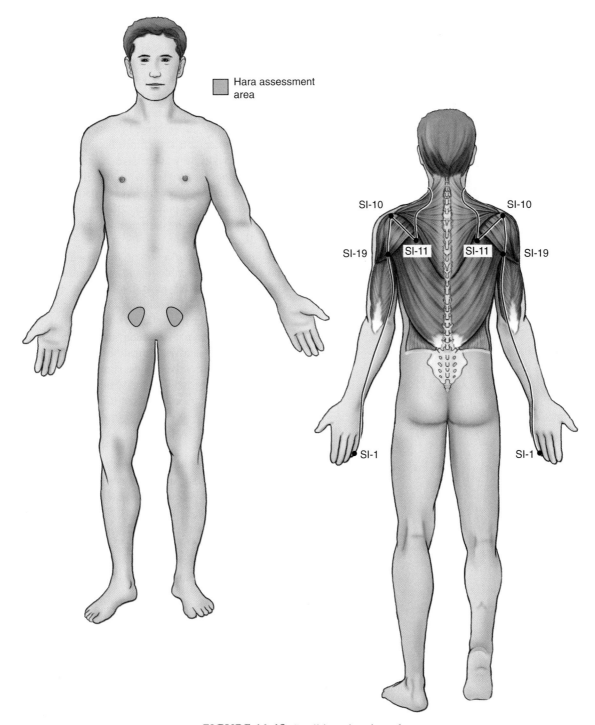

Hara assessment area

SI-10   SI-10
SI-19   SI-11   SI-11   SI-19
SI-1   SI-1

FIGURE 16-10 Small intestine channel.

The phases appeared later in history than the theory of yin and yang. Knowledge of the phases helps the practitioner understand what is going on with the client. Each phase has particular characteristics and interacts with the other phases in certain ways.

The five phases, or elements, are *earth, wood, fire, metal,* and *water*. They can be correlated, for example, with the different stages in the biologic cycle of birth, growth, climax, decay, and death. Another example is the seasons of the year. A fifth season is identified as late summer, or the transition between seasons. Each of these seasons has particular qualities. The phases refer mainly to the process of how energy behaves at these different stages.

Each phase has influence over, and is influenced by, its associated bodily organs; sense organs; bodily secretions, colors, flavors, smells, sounds; seasons of the year; times of

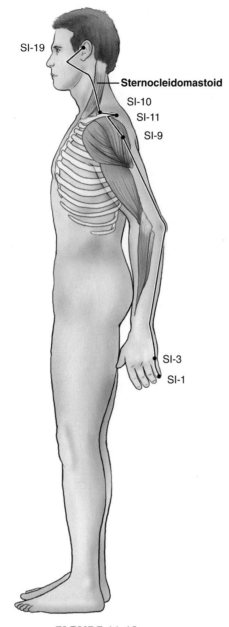

FIGURE 16-10, **cont'd**

the day; emotions; and by its general body-mind-spirit function.

Wood

The wood phase is associated with the exuberance and fast growth observed in spring as seeds sprout, new and flexible shoots appear on the branches of the trees, and the activity that had decreased during the winter suddenly picks up. Green, the color of foliage at its peak, is the color associated with the wood phase. People also react to the influence of the spring; and the wood phase is observed in the renewed hope and bursts of energy often experienced with the first sunny days after a long winter. Strong winds are common

in spring. Wind is associated with the wood phase and is recognized as an element of its influence. In a person, this dynamism can be observed as the emotional irritation that develops when exposed to a draft of air for a long time. In addition, a burst of anger has a similar behavior to a burst of wind. It pushes and breaks things for a few moments and then suddenly disappears—the same as when anger calms down once it has been vented (from Latin *ventus*, meaning "wind"). Frustration, which can be repressed anger, is also associated with the wood phase. Anger and frustration are also emotions associated with the liver and gallbladder organ systems. By working liver or gallbladder channels or their corresponding points on the surface of the skin, you can help someone with chronic anger to change or moderate his or her behavior.

People who have a lot of the wood element in their makeup tend to be athletic and in charge. For example, an Olympic triathlete is most likely has a lot of the wood element, as do chief executives of Fortune 500 companies. Accordingly, liver stockpiles or stores ki for decisive action, distributes ki where it is needed, and is involved in the functions of planning and detoxification. The gallbladder together with the liver is involved in decision making and affects the sides of the body and the eyes. Sour flavor and the craving for oils and fats are also related to wood.

Fire

The fire phase rules the heart, small intestine, heart protector (pericardium), and triple heater (triple warmer) organ systems. Fire provides light, warmth, and spark, a lively and colorful dynamic.

The fire phase is associated with the color red, summer, heat, bitter flavor, the tongue, the circulatory system and blood vessels, the emotion of joy, speech, sweat, meditation, insight, and inspiration. When this phase is imbalanced, a craving for alcohol may exist.

The main functions of fire's organ systems are (1) heart, emotional stability, (2) small intestine—assimilation, (3) heart protector—circulation, and (4) triple heater—protection. Together they are the *interpreters of experience*.

People who have a lot of fire tend to be the life of the party. They are engaging and charismatic and like to connect with people. Most entertainers have a lot of fire in their bodily makeup.

Earth

Being "down to earth" is an expression that sums up the centering, stable quality of the earth phase. Between all the other phases, a moment of transition exists that is ruled by the earth.

All foods come from the soil and therefore are associated with earth. The act of eating has a calming, satisfying, and comforting effect. People eat "comfort foods" when sick or depressed. These foods are those that remind us of home,

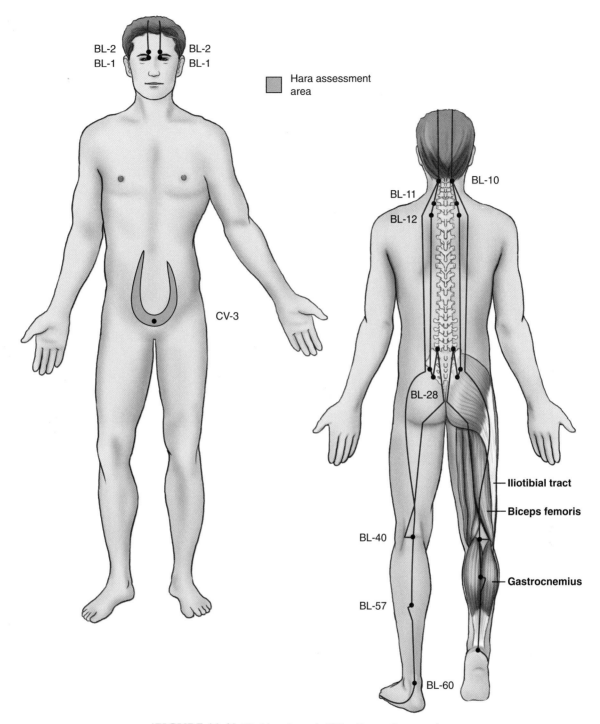

FIGURE 16-11 Bladder channel. CV = Conception vessels.

with its warmth, safety, sweet smells, and the figure of the mother. Mother Earth in her bountiful generosity, fertility, receptivity, and patience provides everything we need.

The yellow color associated with earth comes from the color of the soil in the region of northern China, where the theory of five phases supposedly originated (cf. Huang He, Yellow River). Carefully observing a person's face can sometimes reveal a yellow hue or coloring that can point to

an earth phase imbalance, probably affecting the spleen or stomach, the organ systems associated with earth.

People who have a lot of earth in their makeup love home and family. They tend to be the ones who like to have everyone home for the holidays, and will make the big holiday dinner. They are concerned that everyone's needs are being met. Accordingly, the main functions of the stomach and the spleen are digestion and transformation for nourishment.

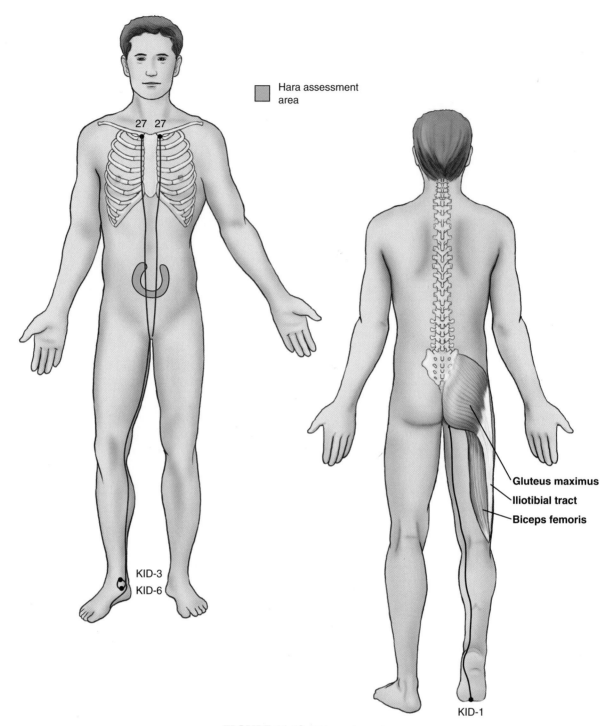

FIGURE 16-12 Kidney channel.

This phase is associated with fertility, reproductive organs, moisture, singing, sweet flavor, the flesh and lips, and saliva. Craving sugar is a sign of imbalance pointing to these organ systems.

Metal

From the soil deep in the earth, minerals are extracted to make strong and valuable metals. During our history as human beings, the metal blade of swords and of other weapons has shaped much of our civilization. The borders of countries have been determined by wars fought with metal weapons or by the influence of commerce based on precious metals. Gold is the agreed-upon measure of material worth in many societies. Value, worth, structure, shape, and border are some of the words associated with the metal phase. The border of our body, the skin, and keeping healthy psychological boundaries are necessary to protect ourselves

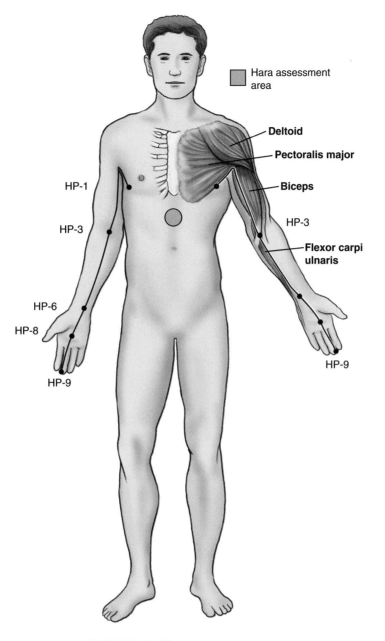

FIGURE 16-13 Heart protector channel.

from unwanted, outside influences. A sense of self-worth (metal), for example, is gained and supported from the grounded (earth) knowledge of ourselves.

The lungs and large intestine organ systems are also associated with metal. In TCM, lung gathers ki from the air and creates wei (protective) ki, which circulates along the surface of the body as a barrier of defense. Our first breath and last breath mark the beginning and end boundaries of our life in physical form. The large intestines' function of elimination or letting go is what helps rid the body of waste. It also applies to unwanted emotional or mental structures we no longer need.

Those who have a lot of metal in their makeup like to sort, organize, and eliminate what is not necessary. They crave an orderly existence. As children, they most likely insisted on coloring inside the lines, and tend to gravitate toward occupations such as accounting or professional organizing. The nose, pungent and spicy flavors, the color white, autumn, grief, mucus, dry climate, and imbalanced craving for protein are also associations with the metal phase. The figure of the father is traditionally associated with this element. The main functions of these organ systems are (1) lungs—intake of ki and (2) large intestine—elimination.

Water

Water takes the shape of whichever vessel contains it, be it a river or a glass, but at the same time keeps its very unique

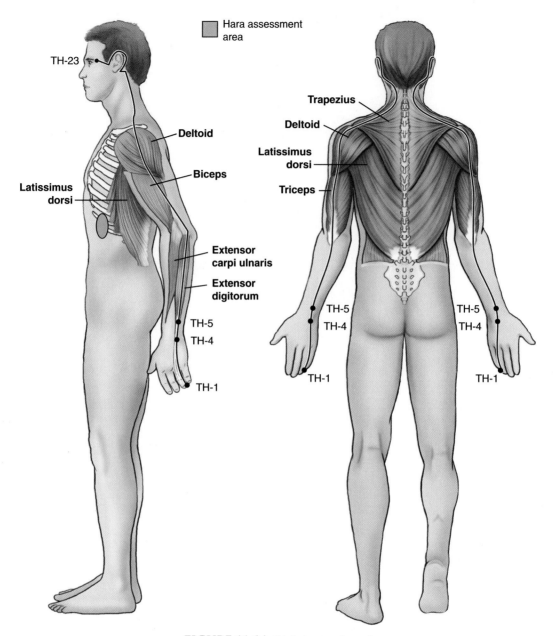

FIGURE 16-14 Triple heater channel.

characteristics. It always moves toward the lowest point. Fluidity and adaptability are some of its defining characteristics.

This characteristic is what gives water its power and energy, as with a stream coming down the mountain. If the mountain slopes are gentle, then water will move smoothly and easily in a continuous flow. If rocks and branches interrupt the stream, then water will go around, jump over, or carve into the obstacles until it finds its way through. Willpower is a trait associated with the water phase.

Water rules the functioning of the kidney and bladder, whose task is to provide the impetus (the "get up and go" energy for life). Water is a precious and essential element for survival because our bodies are mostly water. The water

element is sensitive to the pressures of stress in modern life. The adrenal glands that provide adrenaline for the *fight-or-flight* response when we are frightened are also part of this organ system.

People who have a lot of water in their makeup like to spend time alone, preferably doing something creative such as writing poetry or doing art; most artists have a great deal of water in their makeup. Kidney and bladder are in charge of the purification process and the balance of water in the body. The bones, bone marrow, teeth, central nervous system, ears, hearing, the emotion of fear, winter, black or dark blue color, urine, groaning sound, and craving for stimulants are all correspondences to the water phase.

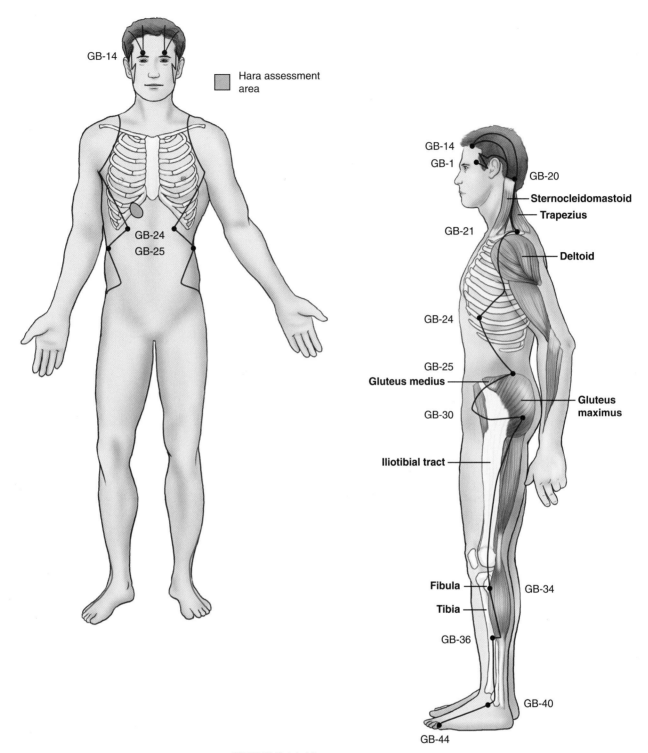

FIGURE 16-15 Gallbladder channel.

It is important to note that everyone has all five phases within them. While one phase tends to be more dominant, paying attention to the other phases is equally important to maintain balance in life.

Please see Table 16-2 for a list of associations and correspondences of the five phases.

THE CYCLES

While contemplating the five phases, it is important to consider underlying cycles that contribute to its balance or imbalance.

The *creative* or *generative cycle* feeds, nourishes, or generates the next cycle in line. It describes the previous phase

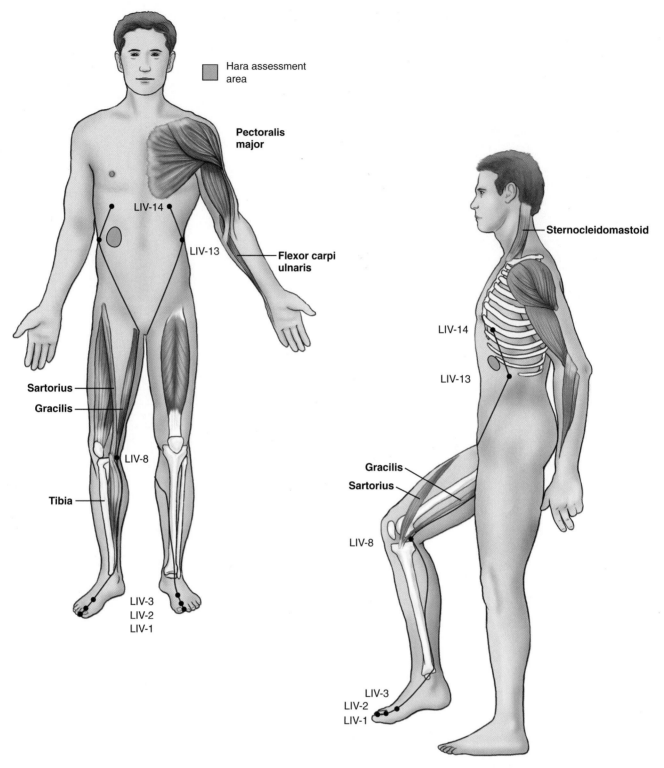

FIGURE 16-16 Liver channel.

TABLE 16-2 Five Phases (Elements) Correspondences

ELEMENT	ORGAN SYSTEMS	SEASON	COLOR	SENSE ORGAN	FUNCTION	EMOTION
Fire	SI/TH HT/HP	Summer	Red	Tongue	Emotional stability Assimilation Circulation Protection	Joy
Earth	SP/ST	Late summer	Yellow	Mouth	Digestion Nourishment Support	Pensiveness
Metal	LU/LI	Autumn	White	Nose	Respiration Intake of ki Letting go (LI)	Grief
Water	KID/BL	Winter	Black/dark blue	Ears	Purification Impetus	Fear
Wood	LIV/GB	Spring	Green	Eyes	Gather ki for decisive action	Anger Frustration

HT/SI, Heart, small intestine; *P/TH*, pericardium, triple heater; *SP/ST*, spleen-pancreas, stomach; *LU/LI*, lung, large intestine; *KID/BL*, kidney, bladder; *LIV/GB*, liver, gallbladder.

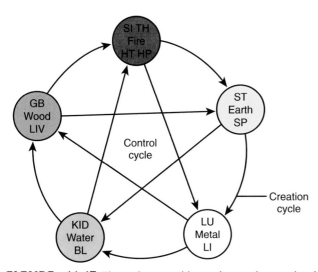

FIGURE 16-17 Five phases with cycles and associated channels.

in the same way in which a mother generates or creates the child phase (Figure 16-17).

The *control cycle* is a system of checks and balances, which keeps any one phase from overacting.

The *overacting cycle* is a stronger version of the creative cycle; excessive control weakens or suppresses the phase being controlled.

The *counteracting* or *insulting cycle* inverts or goes in the opposite order of the creative cycle. The following examples are presented to illustrate use of the cycles in evaluation of the client.

Wood Creates Fire

In a client who has a lot of fire-associated symptoms, such as redness in the face, agitation, and inappropriate emotional responses, the practitioner checks not only the fire channels but also the wood channels.

In this case, wood is the mother that creates or generates fire, which is described as the child. Too much wood can generate too much fire. In this case, for example, the fire phase might be tamed by controlling the amount of fuel (wood) that stokes the flame.

The reverse situation might also happen. A client without "sparkle" and who has a pale face and is constantly feeling cold and showing other signs of lack of fire, might be treated by strengthening the mother phase, in this case wood.

Earth Controls Water

Since the beginning of time, farmers along riverbanks know that when the river rises and floods its banks, it may have dire consequences for their crops and livelihood. A strong earth element will keep water under control, just as a dam or riverbank does. If the water phase (ruling the bladder, kidney, and the water balance in the body) overacts, then it can *swamp* the earth-ruled function of the stomach and spleen, dampening stomach's function. This action can slow down digestion and increase bloating, tiredness, and edema, under which conditions fluids become backed up in the interstitial space between the cells. A strong earth phase helps keep everything in its place (one of the spleen functions). A person with this kind of imbalance would do well to exercise; eat cooked foods such as stews, grains, and soups; and receive treatments that strengthen the stomach and spleen organ systems.

WAYS TO EVALUATE ENERGETIC IMBALANCES

Shiatsu practitioners have different tools that, used together, can help them guide their intuition to form an idea of what might be happening with their clients. Clients might be experiencing physical or emotional aspects of one of the five phases, or have an affinity or aversion that can point to a particular phase. They might have either a more yin or a more yang type of condition. They may have weakness or excess in a certain channel. All these ideas put together, plus the valuable addition of the practitioner's hunches or gut feelings about what is going on, can help the practitioner tailor the session to the specific needs of the client.

An illustration titled "What Is Balance?" is found on the Evolve website under course materials for this edition and shows one way of depicting balance.

There are four main assessments a practitioner can use to determine the best approach for the client: Looking, listening and smelling, palpating, and asking.

Looking

By observing how the client looks and behaves, his or her physical constitution, body proportions, posture, gait, mannerisms, level of activity, and strength in movement, the practitioner can tell a lot about the person's state of health and personality.

You can check the face color (hue), circles under eyes, condition of hair and nails, redness or discoloring of the skin, and "sparkle" in the eyes. Looking at the tongue, or tongue diagnosis, is an art regularly used by TCM practitioners to determine internal conditions of the body. Redness on the tip of the tongue, for example, points to heat in the heart. A thick white coating or fur at the back of the tongue might point to coldness in the kidney or bladder. Deep cracks at the center might point to deficiency in the stomach or spleen.

When looking at a person, you should be discreet as you observe details. Keeping your gaze relaxed is important; this increases your peripheral vision. Thus you can have a one-shot look and impression of the whole person, instead of parts or specific details. The details will later fit into the big picture. Another way is to look at the space larger than just the physical body of the client. This space contains the physical body and the energy field around the client.

Listening and Smelling

Listening refers not only to what the person is saying but also to how it is being said, what is not being said, and the tone of the voice. Is a complaining, angry, sad tone heard? Is the client talking in a hushed voice, growling, or shouting? Does it sound as though the person is holding the breath? Does he or she have a dry mouth?

You can sometimes distinguish a particular smell associated with the person such as sweet (relating to earth), burnt (relating to fire), damp (relating to earth and water), rancid (relating to wood), metallic (relating to metal), or urinelike (relating to water).

Palpating

You can check specific reflex areas in the abdomen, or hara, and compare energetic states of different organ systems (see hara evaluation section). Many TCM practitioners rely on feeling the pulses at three different places on each of the client's wrists. This skill gives information on the ki, zang and fu, and channels. As the practitioner works, he or she checks skin texture and firmness, temperature changes, and areas of pain in the client's body. Areas of pain are called *Ah shi* points. Ah shi, which means "that's it," elicits a reaction from a client when touched. Other points that are palpated for assessment are Shu and Yu (transporting) points on the back and Bo or Mu (alarm) points on the front of the body.

Asking

The practitioner can specifically inquire about the client's symptoms, sleep patterns, elimination, digestion, appetite, diet, exercise, menstruation patterns, and health history, as well as climatic likes or dislikes. For example, a person might strongly dislike cold, heat, or drafts of air, or a symptom might worsen on damp or rainy days.

> *"In the beginner's mind there are many possibilities, but in the expert's mind there are only a few."*
> —Shunryu Suzuki

SHIATSU

Shiatsu, a Japanese Asian bodywork therapy, uses pressure on the surface of the skin along energy pathways called *channels* or *meridians* to restore, maintain, or balance the harmonic flow of energy throughout the body-mind-spirit. The term *shiatsu* literally means "finger (*shi*) pressure (*atsu*)," but hands, elbows, knees, and feet are also used and, when appropriate, joint mobilizations and stretches. Along the channels are points called *tsubos,* also known as *acupoints* (although *acupoint* is more of an acupuncture term), which are energetic vortices on the surface of the skin where the energy of the channel can be accessed.

From this perspective, health is a state of harmonious flow of the body-mind-spirit's energy (ki) along the channels. Symptoms of poor health can be interpreted as an imbalance of ki flow. According to a person's state of health and any symptoms, and depending on constitution and general energy levels, the shiatsu practitioner uses a variety of techniques to improve the energy flow. As the quality of ki changes with the application of shiatsu, the symptoms associated with lack of ki flow will gradually resolve, facilitating pain relief, as well as improved digestion, breathing, elimination, and sleep patterns; increased mobility; and reduced anxiety and depression. Following a treatment, increased vitality is often experienced; and the person may feel invigorated yet relaxed.

SHIZUKO YAMAMOTO

Born: June 1, 1924

"Carefully observe your activities of thinking, breathing, movement, diet, sex, and sleep, for these are the six fundamentals of health. Within this realm lies success or failure in your physical health and emotional happiness."

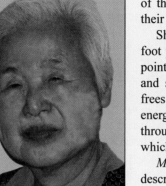

Shizuko Yamamoto is a bodyworker, author, and founder of the International Macrobiotic Shiatsu Society. What she believes, teaches, and practices is at once simple and sublime. In a nutshell, she advises us to return to nature as a means to promote health and well-being. Of course this isn't a new idea. Around 400 BC Hippocrates taught that violating nature's laws brought disharmony in the form of physical or emotional sickness. The cure was to recreate balance, so that the patient could cure the self.

Centuries after Hippocrates, Chinese medicine made its way to Japan and with it came the art of massage. But unlike the full spectrum of treatment practiced in Chinese medicine, massage soon became viewed as a pleasurable indulgence for the wealthy—much like the way Westerners have viewed massage for generations. But there were those practitioners who stuck to the old, more holistic ways of healing. A segment of this group branched out and named their form of massage *shiatsu.*

Shiatsu is finger, forearm, elbow, or foot pressure and stimulation to certain points on the body, and includes rotation and stretching of joints. This pressure frees any blockage in the normal route of energy as it moves from organ to organ throughout the body and balances the *ki,* which means life force in Japanese.

Macrobiotic is an ancient term that describes healthy people who live a long life. Macrobiotic shiatsu is a blend of hand and barefoot shiatsu, diet, exercise, breathing, stretching, postural rebalancing, and use of medicinal plant foods to create balance, and thus health, in individuals. Basic macrobiotic principles are as follows:

1. Health is the natural condition of human beings. It is our birthright.
2. Illness and unhappiness are unnatural conditions.

(Continued)

Although traditional shiatsu is done on a floor mat, it can also be done on a massage table or with the person seated. Given that the client is fully clothed and no oils or ointments are used, shiatsu is adaptable to almost any environment and situation. It is popular not just for relaxation and well-being but also in pregnancy, during labor, in critical care of patients in hospitals, for emergency relief support, and in corporate, military, and other settings.

Based in TCM, shiatsu had been used in Japan for centuries until it was banned, alongside other folk medicine methods, during the U.S. occupation of Japan after World War II. In the 1950s, Tokujiro Namikoshi created a style of shiatsu that used Western anatomic references instead of traditional Chinese-Japanese nomenclature. Thanks to his effort, the Ministry of Health in Japan approved his style of shiatsu as medical treatment. The Namikoshi Shiatsu school, which he created, is still open today; and this style of shiatsu is very popular in Japan.

Shizuto Masunaga, creator of Zen Shiatsu, studied with Namikoshi but took a different approach. He trained at the university as a psychologist but also studied the ancient Chinese medicine texts in which mind-spirit references to clinical practice were commonplace. After meticulous research, Masunaga came up with an expanded model of health in which emotional and mental aspects of the person were taken into consideration and blended into the physical touch technique of shiatsu. He called his form of shiatsu *Zen Shiatsu.* He created a new chart of channels that extended the classical pathways, and contributed hara (abdominal) assessments of the channels. Widely used in shiatsu schools throughout the world today, hara assessment of the channels provide a focus for treatment. Hara diagnostic areas are also featured for each of the 12 sets of channels in Figures 16-5 through 16-16.

ZEN SHIATSU PRINCIPLES OF TOUCH

As discussed previously, Zen Shiatsu is a type of shiatsu developed by Masunaga. The *Zen* part of Zen Shiatsu means

SHIZUKO YAMAMOTO (*continued*)

3. Health or sickness is not an accident or something inexplicable.
4. Sickness arises from how we live as a result of our own actions and thoughts.
5. Food is one of the very important factors in determining sickness.
6. We should eat seasonal foods that grow in our own environment.

One of the most enlightening gems you can receive from learning more about macrobiotic shiatsu makes you feel like the scene in the *Wizard of Oz* when Toto revealed that the great wizard was nothing but a mere man. Illness is not so much shrouded in mystery as it is a function of how you think, breathe, move and sleep, your diet, and your relationship with others. To a certain degree, you can influence your own health, even though it may not be as easy as clicking your heels together three times.

Shizuko Yamamoto was born in Tokyo, the youngest of three brothers and one sister. Her father had his own company; her mother was a homemaker. After World War II, a generous cousin made it possible for her to be trained in yoga, shiatsu, aikido, and Chinese acupuncture. But it was a bout with ill health that changed her life. She had leukemia, lost her eyesight, and had absolutely no energy. She was advised to eat only fresh, organic foods and whole grains—no animal products and no sugar. She began walking for exercise and doing corrective breathing exercises. One month later she felt much better, something that 12 operations hadn't done.

Now she shares her experience and expertise with others the world over.

"We are nature's creation. Our bodies should be organic. We need clean water and a good environment. We are not just existing as ourselves; we are part of the planet, otherwise we cannot survive."

Survive she has. With gusto. She travels all over the world, teaches and counsels at a pace that might be grueling for someone half her age. She is sturdy and exudes energy and warmth. But at a mere 5 feet 3 inches, she worked on many people who were much larger than she when she started her practice in the states. Her clients weren't just bigger, they were also less flexible, which she attributes to a higher consumption of animal fats and protein. She worked on so many people for so many years, her hands would get to the point that they couldn't move. To compensate for her size difference and to continue a strong practice for years to come, she developed barefoot shiatsu, a simple yet effective routine wherein the client lies on the floor and the practitioner stands and uses primarily the feet to deliver the treatment.

Yamamoto outlines her advice to beginning massage therapists: "I don't think about money. I concentrate on how I can help." She also recommends being sensitive to clients' needs, maintaining good health, and using good judgment. Increase your knowledge of your craft, then practice, practice, practice. And naturally her last bit of advice is, "Maintain a healthy balance in your life."

---

meditation or contemplation, and is the state of mind in which the Zen Shiatsu practitioner must be in order to perceive and be in contact with the ki of both the client and the self. The *Zen* part of Zen Shiatsu does not have a religious connotation, as in Zen Buddhism.

The emphasis of Zen Shiatsu techniques is to have an in-the-moment understanding of the quality and movement of ki. Although the functions and actions of the individual tsubos are essential to learn and use in practice, the more inclusive concept is of the entire channel, for it is what guides the practitioner during the session.

The Zen Shiatsu principles of touch are designed to provide a way for the practitioner to be relaxed and aware throughout the session while maintaining a clear mind. One of the ways to help the practitioner and the client stay centered is to be present and pay attention to the process as it unfolds moment to moment. One of the practitioner's hands

receives feedback and reactions from the client as he or she works. The practitioner should be able to interpret this information so he or she can adapt a technique to what is going on with, and what is appropriate for, the client at that precise moment in time. Although the practitioner will follow a certain routine, especially at the beginning of his or her training, no two sessions will be the same because the practitioner will tailor shiatsu treatments to the unique circumstances of each client.

The principles of Zen Shiatsu are:
- Relaxation
- Use of body weight, not force
- Moving from the hara
- Using two-handed connection
- Stationary, perpendicular penetration
- Projection of ki
- Continuity

Relaxation

Some bodywork styles emphasize the practitioner's muscular strength as a way to perform techniques and therefore are rather vigorous and quite physical. To have muscular strength, the practitioner's muscles have to be contracted. Of course, once muscle contraction reaches a threshold, it cannot be sustained for prolonged periods. The practitioner can push the threshold to sustain more and more contraction with practice, just like weight lifters, but there is a point at which the muscles need to relax before they can contract again. It is difficult for a practitioner to keep high levels of contraction throughout the hour or more of a typical session, never mind doing many sessions in a day. In addition, if the practitioner's effectiveness is tied to his or her muscular strength, then much stress is continually placed on muscles to remain in a contracted state.

Zen Shiatsu is based on the opposite principle—namely, that the practitioner must be relaxed to be effective. Being relaxed does not mean that the practitioner's touch will be too light or ineffective. He or she can perform any task that demands physical power while keeping a sense of openness and relaxation. Think of the grace of a top class dancer or skater, whose muscular effort is guided by a prevailing sense of calmness and fixed attention even in the midst of a challenging performance.

Being aware of the body, consciously releasing areas of tension, breathing fully, having a comfortable posture, and adjusting it to keep relaxed and open during the session are some of the ways to ensure that the practitioner does not use muscular force in a purely contractive way. Besides, helping clients to relax is impossible if the therapist is not relaxed.

As the practitioner relaxes, his or her own energy field expands, and so does the awareness of the surrounding space. The perception of the client increases as does what is needed during the session. The expansion of his field happens in all directions at the same time. As the practitioner's energy field expands downward, the connection to the earth increases. As the practitioner's field expands forward, connection with the client increases. As the practitioner expands upward, a connection is made with the cosmic ki that might help inspire and guide the session.

When the practitioner relaxes and expands his or her energy field, coming in contact with the client's ki in the channels is relatively easy and more effective.

Use Body Weight, Not Force

Using the weight of the practitioner's body to apply pressure is not only the most effective way to ensure a supportive and effective touch but will also help him or her better perceive the client's reaction.

Effective body mechanics include having an aligned spine; a good connection of the legs, and knees; feet to the floor; and arms extended with elbows slightly flexed or unlocked. Good alignment also protects the practitioner from injury.

Move from Your Hara

The hara, a Japanese word to describe the lower abdomen, is the center of balance of the body. More precisely, a point in the hara called the *Dan Tien*—located three fingerwidths distance below the navel, also called the *sea of ki*—is traditionally described as the center of focused power and action. It is where all bodily movement originates. In Japan, a person is said to "have a good hara" when he or she enjoys good health, stability, and strength. Several qi gong and tai chi exercises and meditations can be used to develop the dan tien because it is the center of power for the practice of martial arts. It is the point at which the person physically embodies the ki of the earth as his or her own state of being, allowing it to permeate every action he does.

Moving from the hara means the practitioner's body is connected to the earth and that he works from a grounded sense of self. Simple exercises such as bringing your breathing down to the hara can help you center yourself and feel grounded very quickly.

Zen Shiatsu practitioners relax their hara and face it toward the area on the client's body on which they are working.

Use Two-Handed Connection

Having both hands in contact with the client as you work is a good way to give stability, support, and continuous connection. Throughout the session, the practitioner's hands become more yin (receptive, feeling, slower, supportive) or more yang (active, faster, directive). The practitioner's more yin *mother hand* is the one that stays in one place, supporting and feeling the reaction of the work. The *child hand* is the more yang and active hand that moves along the channel. Ideally, both of the practitioner's hands are on the same channel or pathway. As the practitioner moves, one hand remains on the client as long as possible.

Feeling the reaction underneath the mother hand is relatively easy if the practitioner's hand and wrist are relaxed. The practitioner's hands connect through the client's channel, forming a closed circuit that includes hara, mother hand, and child hand, and the client's channel or area worked. The practitioner's awareness of the client's subtle reactions is increased by visualizing a sphere of ki within this closed circuit.

Stationary, Perpendicular Penetration

Probably the most defining principle in the Zen Shiatsu technique, approaching the area of work *perpendicularly* allows the practitioner to connect energetically with ki in the channels. Touch that approaches the surface of the skin nonperpendicularly creates tissue resistance, bringing up dense, slow vibrations of ki. This approach restricts the practitioner's work to only the physical range of ki. It can be effective, but it is "hit or miss," and the effect will be localized. When leaning with the body weight perpendicularly into the channel, the practitioner reaches the full range of vibrations of the channel—emotional, mental, spiritual, and the physical, thus stimulating the whole channel at once.

The practitioner adjusts the angle of pressure, adapting to the different curvatures of the body. He or she leans perpendicularly into the channel until the ki is contacted; then pressure is released before proceeding to the next area. Circling, rubbing, or moving the thumb or palm on the area restricts the practitioner's work to the physical and local aspects of the area.

Project Ki

By relaxing the body weight perpendicularly into a channel, the practitioner allows his or her ki to project itself beyond the point of contact with the surface of the client's skin, allowing a better contact with the client's ki. The practitioner can visualize the area as a sphere and project ki toward the center of the sphere.

Continuity

As a rule of thumb, the practitioner follows along the same channel instead of jumping back and forth from different channels or areas of the body. The practitioner continues along the entire channel, moving around the client in a logical, fluid manner.

TECHNIQUES: PALMING AND THUMBING

There are two main techniques used in Zen Shlatsu: palming and thumbing.

Palming

Palming is a yin technique and is done with relaxed hands placed on the body of the client. The practitioner extends the arms and brings the body weight forward so he or she feels the pressure under the hands. Without moving the hands, and as he moves the body weight backward, the pressure is relieved from underneath the hands. Palming is a good way to feel and evaluate the quality of the ki in the channel, comparing the different sensations on each area as he works. The *mother* hand and the *child* hand switch positions as needed.

Thumbing

This technique should be done with extended arms and thumbs, and relaxed fingers. The elbows are slightly flexed or unlocked and the shoulders relaxed or dropped. The thumb should be aligned with the wrist, elbow, and shoulders. The practitioner should be mindful of not flexing the distal phalanx of the thumb, but instead, keep the distal interphalangeal joint extended. The point of contact of the thumb with the channel should be midway between the pad and the nail of the thumb, taking care not to be too close to the nail. Thumbing can be done effectively only if the practitioner's nails are clipped short.

When thumbing, the practitioner uses the *child* hand, and keeps the *mother* hand in the palming position, for self-stabilization and support of the client as well.

Direction of Techniques. Palming and thumbing should be done rhythmically while following the direction of the flow of ki in the client's channels:
   Client Supine:
- From the hara down the legs to the feet along the yang channels on the lateral aspect of the legs
- From the chest out to the arms along the yin channels
- From the chest up the throat, neck, and face, to the head
   Client Prone:
- From the base of the neck, laterally to shoulders and arms
- From the base of the neck down along the back toward the sacrum
- From the sacrum down each leg to the feet

HARA EVALUATION

By palpating the different reflex areas of the channels on the hara, the practitioner can compare the overall energetic state of the client and gain a clearer picture of where the imbalance may be. The aim is to find the kyo-jitsu pair of channels that will be the focus of the client's treatment. Working the kyo and jitsu pair of channels is the fastest and most direct way to balance the client's whole system.

The following is how a Zen Shiatsu practitioner performs a hara assessment:
- Sits in a comfortable position by the client's hara so all the channel assessment areas are easily reached.
- Aligns his or her the spine and centers him or herself by bringing attention to the connection of the legs to the earth, and breathing from to the lower abdomen.
- Places the *mother* hand on the side of the client's trunk.
- With the other hand, he or she gently and perpendicularly palpates each of the client's hara assessment areas with relaxed fingertips (Figure 16-18). The pressure should be light and comfortable for the client but still deep enough to be present and make contact with the ki.
- Feels for the client's most kyo assessment area, comparing all the areas with even pressure and for an equal amount of time.
- Feels for the client's most jitsu assessment area, comparing all the areas with even pressure and for an equal amount of time.

To find the kyo and jitsu reaction, the practitioner:
- Places the *mother* hand's fingertips on the client's most kyo area, making contact with the ki.

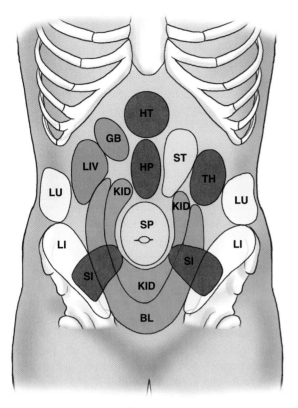

FIGURE 16-18 Hara assessment map.

- Places the *child* hand on the client's most jitsu area and feels for a reaction in the most kyo area, underneath his or her *mother* hand. There may be a feeling of subtle movement or change under the fingertips.

If the practitioner does not get a reaction of any kind with the most jitsu area, the *mother* hand is left on the client's most kyo area, and with the *child* hand, the practitioner makes another round of the remaining assessment areas, this time going in gently but a bit deeper than before until the area that reacts is found. This will be the jitsu channel used during the client's treatment.

Some guidelines for hara assessment:
- Channels such as kidney, bladder, large intestine, small intestine, and lung have either broad or bilateral diagnostic areas in the hara. They need to be palpated evenly. If one side feels jitsu and the other side of the same channel assessment area feels kyo, then the practitioner should discard them and look for an alternative one that has a consistent kyo or jitsu feeling throughout the whole area to be assessed.
- One channel of a yin and yang pair (LV/GB, LU/LI, HT/SI, and so forth) cannot be the most kyo and the other the most jitsu.

> *"Kindness can become its own motive.*
> *We are made kind by being kind."*
> —Eric Hoffer

INTRODUCTION TO TRADITIONAL AYURVEDA

India's traditional healing modality of Ayurveda is one of the world's oldest healing systems currently practiced. It has absorbed the fundamental principles of Hinduism along with some ideas that probably derive from the ancient Middle East. More specifically, modern **Ayurveda** is a science of health and medicine designed to maintain or improve health through measures such as dietary modification, massage, yoga, and use of herbal preparations. Health care practitioners who find themselves drawn to Ayurveda deserve the most reliable and up-to-date information about it. Therefore this section discusses the fundamental principles and practices of traditional Ayurveda as understood from their original Sanskrit sources and traditional practitioners.

Indian medical history is necessary to understand the development of this traditional system of medicine. Based on available literary sources, the history of Indian medicine occurred in four main phases. The first, or *Vedic,* phase dates to approximately 800 BCE. Information about medicine during this period is obtained from numerous incantations and references to healing found in the *Atharvaveda* and the *Rigveda,* two religious scriptures that reveal a *magico-religious* approach to healing.

The second, or *classical,* phase is marked by the advent of the first Sanskrit medical treatises, the *Caraka* and *Sushruta Samhitas,* which probably date from a few centuries before to several centuries after the start of the Christian era. This period includes all subsequent medical treatises dating from before the Muslim invasions of India at the beginning of the eleventh century, given that these works tend to follow the earlier classical compilations closely and provide the basis of traditional Ayurveda.

The third, or *syncretic,* phase is marked by clear influences on the classical paradigm from Islamic or Unani, and other nonclassical medical systems. Sarngadhara's fourteenth century *Sarngadhara Samhita* is one text that reveals the results of these influences, which includes diagnosis by examination of pulse and urine. This phase extends from the time of the Muslim incursions to the present era.

The final or current phase is called *New Age Ayurveda,* wherein the classical paradigm is being adapted to the world of modern science and technology, including quantum physics, mind-body science, and advanced biomedical science. This recent manifestation of Ayurveda is most visible in the Western world, although much of New Age Ayurveda is filtering back to India.

From its beginnings during the Vedic era, Indian medicine has always adhered closely to the principle of a fundamental connection between microcosm and macrocosm. Humans are the microcosm, or tiny representations of the universe, which is the macrocosm. Contained within each person is everything that makes up the surrounding world. The interconnectedness of humans and their world makes it impossible to understand one completely without the other.

THE DOSHAS

According to Ayurveda, the cosmos consists of five basic elements: earth, air, fire, water, and space or ether. Certain forces caused these elements to interact, giving rise to all that exists. In humans, these five elements combine in such a way as to produce the three *doshas*, psychophysic elements and forces that, along with the seven *dhatus* (tissues) and three *malas* (waste products), make up the human body.

The Sanskrit word *dosha*, means a "fault" or "defect." Recalling that the five elements combine and give rise to the doshas, the three doshas are, therefore, the combination of the five elements in the human body; and when they are not balanced, they cause bodily malfunctions because they disrupt the normal functioning of the organism. The three active doshas, or *tri-doshas,* are called vata (wind), pitta (bile), and kapha (phlegm).

The three doshas occur in varying amounts in every human body, and the proportion that is in an individual's body is due to the relative quantities he is born with. This is called the person's innate, natural state, or *prakriti,* which is unique for each person. When they are in their natural proportions in the body, the three doshas are balanced and maintain health, but when an imbalance occurs among them, they disrupt the normal functioning of the body, leading to the manifestation of disease. An imbalance indicates an increase or decrease in one, two, or all three of the doshas.

The qualities of each dosha help determine the individual's basic bodily and mental makeup and provide the basis for ascertaining which dosha or combination of doshas is responsible for a disease.

Vata

Vata, or *vayu,* meaning "wind," is composed of the elements air and space. It is the principle of kinetic energy and is responsible for all bodily movement, evacuation, and nervous functions. Vata is located below the navel and in the bladder, large intestines, nervous system, pelvic region, thighs, bone marrow, and legs; its principal seat is the colon. When disrupted, its primary manifestation is gas and muscular or nervous energy, leading to pain.

The qualities of vata are dryness, cold, light, irregularity, mobility, roughness, and abundance. Dryness occurs when vata is disturbed and is a side effect of motion. Too much dryness produces irregularity in the body and mind.

Pitta

Pitta, or "bile," is made up of the elements fire and water or, according to some references, just fire. It governs enzymes and hormones and is responsible for digestion, pigmentation, body temperature, hunger, thirst, sight, courage, and mental activity. Pitta is located between the navel and the chest, and in the stomach, small intestines, liver, spleen, skin, and blood; its principal seat is the stomach. When disrupted, its primary manifestation is acid and bile, leading to inflammation.

Pitta is hot, light, intense, fluid, liquid, putrid, pungent, and sour. Heat appears when pitta is disturbed, resulting from a change caused by pitta. The intensity of excessive heat produces irritability in the body and mind.

Kapha

Kapha, or *shleshman,* meaning "phlegm," is made up of the elements of earth and water. It connotes the principle of cohesion and stability. Kapha regulates vata and pitta and is responsible for keeping the body lubricated and maintaining its solid nature, tissues, sexual power, and strength. It also controls patience. The normal locations of kapha are the upper part of the body, the thorax, head, neck, upper portion of the stomach, pleural cavity, fat tissues, and areas between joints; its principal seat are the lungs. When it is disrupted, its primary manifestation is fluids and mucus, leading to swelling, with or without discharge.

Kapha is heavy, cold, stable, dense, soft, and smooth. Heaviness occurs when kapha is disturbed and results from firmness caused by kapha. The viscosity of excessive kapha produces slowness in body and mind.

THE DHATUS

The seven *dhatus*, or tissues, are responsible for sustaining the body. Each dhatu is responsible for the one that comes next in the following order:

1. *Rasa*, meaning "sap" or "juice," includes the tissue fluids, chyle (in Western science, chyle is lymph and fats formed in the small intestine), lymph, and plasma. It functions as nourishment and comes from digested food.
2. Blood includes the red blood cells and functions to invigorate the body.
3. Flesh includes muscle tissue and functions as stabilization.
4. Fat includes adipose tissue and functions as lubrication.
5. Bone includes bone and cartilage and functions as support.
6. Marrow includes red and yellow bone marrow and functions as filling in the bones.
7. *Shukra* includes male and female sexual fluids and functions in reproduction and immunity.

THE MALAS

The *malas* are the waste products of digested and processed food and drink. Ayurveda delineates three principal malas: urine, feces, and sweat. A fourth category of other waste products includes fatty excretions from the skin and intestines, ear wax, mucus of the nose, saliva, tears, hair, and nails. According to Ayurveda, an individual should evacuate the bowels once a day and eliminate urine six times a day.

Ayurveda considers digestion to be the most important function that takes place in the human body. It provides all that is required to sustain the organism and is the principal cause for all maladies from which an individual may suffer. The process of digestion and assimilation of nutrients is discussed under the topics of the agnis (enzymes), ama (improperly digested food and drink), and the srotas (channels of circulation).

The Agnis

The *agnis,* literally means "fires," are enzymes that assist in the digestion and assimilation of food. They are divided into three types, as follows:

Jatharagni. Jatharagni are the enzymes that are active in the mouth, stomach, and gastrointestinal tract and help break down food. The waste product of feces results from this activity.

Bhutagnis. The five enzymes located in the liver are the bhutagnis. They adapt the broken-down food into a homologous chyle according to the five elements and assist the chyle to assimilate with the corresponding five elements in the body. The homologous chyle circulates in the blood channels as rasa, nourishing the body and supplying the seven dhatus.

Dhatvagnis. The seven enzymes, or dhatvagnis, synthesize the seven dhatus from the assimilated chyle homologized with the five elements. The remaining waste products result from this activity.

AMA

Ama, one of the major causes of disease, is formed when a decrease in the activity of the three agnis occurs. A product of improperly or incompletely digested food and drink, it takes the form of a sticky sludge that travels through the same channels as the chyle.

Because of its density, however, it lodges in different parts of the body, blocking the channels. Ama often mixes with the doshas that circulate through the same pathways and usually gravitates to a weak or stressed organ or to a site of a disease manifestation. Because all diseases invariably come from ama, the word *amaya*, meaning "coming from ama," is a synonym for disease. Internal diseases begin with ama, and external diseases produce ama.

In general, ama can be detected by a coating on the tongue, turbid urine with foul odor, and feces that are passed with undigested food, an offensive odor, or abundant gas. The principal course of treatment in Ayurveda involves the elimination of ama, by means of the fivefold purification therapy called *panchakarma*, and the restoration of the balance of the doshas through diet, regimen, and herbal-based medicines.

SROTAS

The *srotas* are the vessels or channels of the body through which all substances circulate. They are either large, such as the large and small intestines, uterus, arteries, and veins, or small, such as the capillaries. A healthy body has open and free flowing channels. Blockage of the channels, usually by ama, results in disease. The 13 srotas are as follows:

1. Pranavahisrotas convey vitality and vital wind or breath (*prana*) and originate in the heart and alimentary tract.
2. Udakavahisrotas convey water and fluids and originate in the palate and pancreas.
3. Annavahisrotas convey food from the outside and originate in the stomach.
4. Rasavahisrotas convey chyle, lymph, and plasma and originate in the heart and in the ten vessels connected with the heart. Ama primarily accumulates within them.
5. Raktavahisrotas convey red blood cells and originate in the liver and spleen.
6. Mamsavahisrotas convey ingredients for muscle tissue and originate in the tendons, ligaments, and skin.
7. Medovahisrotas convey ingredients for fat tissue and originate in the kidneys and fat tissues of the abdomen.
8. Asthavahisrotas convey ingredients for bone tissue and originate in the hipbone.
9. Majjavahisrotas convey ingredients for marrow and originate in the bones and joints.
10. Shukravahisrotas convey ingredients for the male and female reproductive tissues and originate in the testicles and ovaries, respectively.
11. Mutravahisrotas convey urine and originate in the kidney and bladder.
12. Purishavahisrotas convey feces and originate in the colon and rectum.
13. Svedavahisrotas convey sweat and originate in the fat tissues and hair follicles.

This broad outline indicates that Ayurveda understands that the human body's anatomic parts are composed of the five basic elements that have undergone a process of metabolism and assimilation in the body.

Humans differ from one another in their natural bodily constitution, or *prakriti*, which is determined at the moment of conception and remains until death. The four factors that influence constitutional type are (1) the father, (2) the mother (particularly her food intake), (3) the womb, and (4) the season of the year. A large imbalance of the doshas in the mother will affect the growth of the embryo and fetus, and a moderate excess of one or two of the doshas will affect the constitution of the child.

PRAKRITI

A person's constitution is called the *prakriti*. Seven normal body constitutions exist and are based on the three doshas: vata, pitta, kapha, vata-pitta, pitta-kapha, vata-kapha, and sama. The last is a state in which all three occur in equal proportions. It is the best condition but is extremely rare.

Most people are a combination of doshas, in which one dosha predominates. In general, vata type of people tend to be anxious and fearful, exhibit light and "airy" characteristics, and are prone to vata diseases. Pitta type of people are aggressive and impatient, exhibit fiery and hotheaded characteristics, and are prone to pitta diseases. Kapha type of people are stable and entrenched, if not sluggish at times; they exhibit heavy, wet, and earthy characteristics and are prone to kapha diseases.

These concepts are the principal factors that help the ayurvedic physician determine the correct course of treatment to be administered to a client for a particular ailment.

NADIS

Similar to the traditional Chinese channels, the *nadis*, which are known from traditions of yoga, are channels in which prana energy flows (Box 16-1). Although the concept of the bodily winds or pranas occurs in Ayurveda, the development of the notion of the nadis is restricted to the system of yoga in India. Nadis are sometimes viewed as extending only to the skin of the body but are often thought to extend to the boundary of the aura.

The three main nadis include *sushumna, ida,* and *pingala,* but a total of 72,000 nadis are said to exist in the body. Nadis start from the central channel along which they are located and radiate from the chakras to the periphery, then where the nadis gradually become thinner.

The nadis are stimulated through the practice of pranayama, or breath control, which involves alternate breathing through left and right nostrils, which stimulate, respectively, the left and right sides of the body.

BOX 16-1

The Pranas

Atmospheric wind (*vata*) becomes *prana* when it enters the human body. There are five pranas.

Prana. The wind that passes upward and is located in the eyes, the ears, the mouth, and the nose.

Apana. The wind that passes downward and is located in the organs of excretion and generation.

Smana. The wind that is located in the middle of the body and equalizes in distribution throughout the body what is consumed as food.

Vyana. The wind that moves in the channels of the body and supports the prana and apana.

Udana. This rises up from the central channel (*sushumna*) and is the wind between the vyana and samana. It belches forth and swallows down what is eaten and drunk.

"The job of the physician is merely to amuse the patient while the body heals itself."
—Voltaire

CHAT ROOM

Eastern Anatomic Position

In the Eastern anatomic position, the arms are raised above the head, with palms facing forward. The yang channels descend from the ceiling downward along the backside of the body, and the yin channels ascend from the feet upwards to the hands along the front and trunk of the body.

CHAKRAS

The word **chakra** comes from a Sanskrit word meaning wheel or circle, referring to the seven energy centers in the body, located along the central channel (*sushumna*). The functions of the chakras are to receive, process, and distribute energy and to keep the spiritual, mental, emotional, and physical health of the body in balance.

The earliest mention of chakra, found in *Rigveda*, dating from about 1500 BC, refers to the wheel of a carriage or of the Sun's chariot. An early reference to it as an energy center in the body is found in *Yoga Upanishads* (circa 600 AD). The chakra system came to be an integral part of the Tantric yoga philosophy and practice.

The main text about chakras came to the West in a translation by the Englishman Sir John Woodroffe, alias Arthur Avalon, in a book entitled *The Serpent Power,* published in 1919. The book lists seven basic chakras, and they all exist within the subtle body, present along with the physical body.

Chakras are described as being located in ascending order from the base of the spine to above the head (Figure 16-19), even though they may express themselves externally at points along the front of the body (navel, heart, throat, and so forth). All chakras are associated with a color, an element, a sound, a symbol (a different number of lotus petals in each chakra), and many other distinguishing characteristics.

Although some discrepancies exist, here are the more traditional chakra characteristics. Information on how to use essential oils associated with the chakras are located in Chapter 12.

The Root Chakra (First Chakra)

Location: in the perineum at base of spine
Sanskrit name: Muladhara
Gland: adrenal medulla
Symbol: four-petaled lotus
Color: blood-red
Element: earth

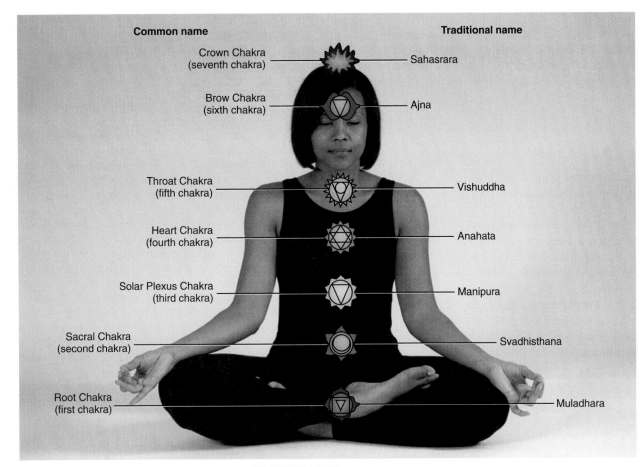

Common name

Crown Chakra (seventh chakra)
Brow Chakra (sixth chakra)
Throat Chakra (fifth chakra)
Heart Chakra (fourth chakra)
Solar Plexus Chakra (third chakra)
Sacral Chakra (second chakra)
Root Chakra (first chakra)

Traditional name

Sahasrara
Ajna
Vishuddha
Anahata
Manipura
Svadhisthana
Muladhara

FIGURE 16-19 The chakras.

Qualities: grounding, patience, structure, stability, security, survival
Essential oils: cinnamon, garlic, sandalwood
Gem: ruby
Herb: mugwort
Musical note: C

The Sacral Chakra (Second Chakra)

Location: sacrum, 2 inches below the navel and 2 inches into the pelvis
Sanskrit name: Svadhisthana
Gland: gonads
Symbol: six-petaled lotus
Color: orange
Element: water
Qualities: well-being, sexuality, sensuality, pleasure, abundance, seat of the emotions
Essential oils: jasmine, neroli, orange blossom
Gem: moonstone
Herb: cedar
Musical note: D

The Solar Plexus Chakra (Third Chakra)

Location: directly below the sternum and just above the navel
Sanskrit name: Manipura
Gland: pancreas
Symbol: 10-petaled lotus
Color: yellow
Element: fire
Qualities: self-worth, self-esteem, confidence, personal power, mentality
Essential oils: lemon, grapefruit, juniper
Gem: yellow sapphire, topaz, citrine
Herb: rosemary
Musical note: E

The Heart Chakra (Fourth Chakra)

Location: middle of chest
Sanskrit name: Anahata
Gland: thymus
Symbol: 12-petaled lotus
Color: green

Element: air
Qualities: unity, love, peace, purity, and innocence
Essential oils: rose, carnation, lily of the valley
Gem: emerald, rose quartz
Herb: lavender
Musical note: F

The Throat Chakra (Fifth Chakra)

Location: throat
Sanskrit name: Vishuddha
Gland: thyroid
Symbol: 16-petaled lotus, circle
Color: blue or turquoise
Element: ether (contains all elements)
Qualities: communication, will, creativity, truthfulness, integrity
Essential oils: blue chamomile, gardenia, ylang-ylang
Gem: blue sapphire, blue pearl
Herb: wintergreen
Musical note: G

The Brow Chakra (Sixth Chakra)

Location: between the eyebrows (third eye or eye of psychic vision)
Sanskrit name: Ajna
Gland: pineal
Symbol: two-petaled lotus
Color: indigo
Element: the cosmos
Qualities: intuition, discernment, wisdom, imagination, knowledge
Essential oils: camphor, sweet pea
Gem: amethyst
Herb: sage
Musical note: A

The Crown Chakra (Seventh Chakra)

Location: top of skull (some say just above the skull)
Sanskrit name: Sahasrara
Gland: pituitary
Symbol: 1000-petaled lotus
Color: white (sometimes purple) or white streaked with purple
Element: the cosmos
Qualities: enlightenment, grace, beauty, serenity, oneness with all that is
Essential oils: violet, lavender, lotus
Gem: alexandrite
Herbs: frankincense and myrrh
Musical note: B

CHAT ROOM

Differences and Similarities Between Traditional Chinese Medicine and Yoga and Ayurveda

Although the concept of energy is the same in India and China, the yogic, the ayurvedic, and TCM models of reference differ in how this energy can be observed and organized for therapeutic uses.

In India, the Hindu tradition of the deities—the male Shiva (contracting, manifesting, downward stream of prana) and the female Shakti (expansive, liberating, upward stream of prana)—embodies a similar dynamic as in the Chinese theory of yin and yang (see later discussion). Likewise, the nadis, subtle energy pathways in yoga, have a resemblance to the channel system in TCM.

The chakras, as centers of energy, are of pivotal importance in yoga. They receive, process, and distribute energy in the body. They have their own system of correspondences that are the points of reference for some types of bodywork and energy healing systems, even beyond yoga. Seven major chakras of yoga exist along the centerline of the body (Sushumna). Three doshas of Ayurveda and their various combinations help detect tendencies toward disease or weaknesses. Each chakra has its own correspondence with sounds, colors, elements, body organs, foods, and psychologic and physiologic functions, among other things. Ayurvedic massage, yoga, meditation, diet, and herbology are used to prevent and treat imbalances and to support optimal functioning of the body.

Within both Chinese medicine and Ayurveda are *five elements* and *vital substances* theories, but they differ considerably.

E-RESOURCES

⊖volve

http://evolve.elsevier.com/Salvo/MassageTherapy

- Chapter challenge
- Flash cards
- Photo gallery
- Additional information
- Weblinks

Special thanks goes to Diego Sanchez and Georgia Tetlow for their past contributions to this chapter.

BIBLIOGRAPHY

American Organization for Bodywork Therapies of Asia (AOBTA) (website): http://www.aobta.org/. Accessed May 2, 2010.

Anderson SK: *The practice of shiatsu,* St Louis, 2008, Mosby.

Beinfeld H, Korngold E: *Between heaven and earth: a guide to Chinese medicine,* New York, 1992, Random House.

Beresford-Cooke C: *Shiatsu theory and practice: a comprehensive text for the student and professional,* St Louis, 2002, Churchill Livingstone.

Brennan BA: *Light emerging: the journey of personal healing,* New York, 1993, Bantam Books.

Connelly D: *Traditional acupuncture: the law of the five elements,* Laurel, Md, 1994, Tai Sophia Institute.

Dash B, Lalitesh K: *Basic principles of Ayurveda,* New Delhi, 1980, Asia Book Corp of America, Concept Publishing.

Dash VB: *Fundamentals of Ayurvedic medicine,* Twin Lakes, Wis, 1990, Lotus Press.

Dubitsky C: *Bodywork shiatsu; bringing the art of finger pressure to the massage table*, Rochester, Vt, 1997, Inner Traditions International.

Ellis A: *Fundamentals of Chinese acupuncture*, Brookline, Mass, 1994, Paradigm Publications.

Ferguson P: *Take five: the five elements guide to health and harmony*, Dublin, 2000, Gill & MacMillan.

Holland A: *Voices of Qi: an introductory guide to traditional Chinese medicine*, ed 2, Berkeley, Calif, 1999, North Atlantic Books.

Jolly J: *Indian medicine*, New Delhi, 1977, Munshiram Manoharial Publishers Private.

Judith A, Ravenwolf S: *Wheels of life: a journey through the chakras*, Woodbury, Minn, 1999, Llewellyn Worldwide.

Kaptchuk TJ: *The web that has no weaver: understanding Chinese medicine*, Lincolnwood, Ill, 2000, NTC Publishing Group.

Lad V: *Ayurveda: the science of self-healing*, Twin Lakes, Wis, 1990, Lotus Press.

Leggett D: *Recipes for self-healing*, London, 1999, Meridian Press.

Leslie CM, Young AH: *Paths to Asian medical knowledge*, Berkeley, Calif, 1992, University of California Press.

Lundberg P: *The book of shiatsu: a complete guide to using hand pressure and gentle manipulation to improve your health, vitality, and stamina*, New York, 2003, Simon & Schuster.

Maciocia G: *Tongue diagnosis in Chinese medicine*, Vista, Calif, 1995, Eastland Press.

Maciocia G: *Foundations of Chinese medicine: a comprehensive text*, St Louis, 2005, Churchill Livingstone.

Masunaga S, Ohashi W: *Zen shiatsu: how to harmonize yin and yang for better health*, Tokyo, 1997, Japan Publications.

Matsumoto K: *Extraordinary vessels*, Brookline, Mass, 1983, Paradigm.

Meulenbeld G, Wujastyk JM, Wujastyk D: *Studies on Indian medical history*, Amsterdam, 2001, Egbert Forsten.

Nadkarni AK: *Indian materia medica*, New Delhi, 1989, Popular Prakashan.

Namikoshi T: *Complete book of shiatsu therapy: health and vitality at your fingertips*, Tokyo, 1981, Japan Publications.

Pitman V: *On the nature of the whole, Indian medical tradition series*, vol 7, New Delhi, 2004, Motilal Banarsidass.

Sasaki P: Personal communication, 1989.

Sharma HM, Clark C: *Contemporary Ayurveda: medicine and research in Maharishi Ayur-Veda*, St Louis, 2002, Churchill Livingstone.

Sharma PV: *Essentials of Ayurveda*, New Delhi, 1999, Motilal Banarsidass.

Svoboda R: *Prakriti: your Ayurvedic constitution*, Twin Lakes, Wis, 1998, Lotus Press.

Svoboda RE, Lade A: *Tao and dharma: Chinese medicine and Ayurveda*, Twin Lakes, Wis, 1995, Lotus Press.

Tsu L: *Tao Te Ching*, New York, 1989, Knopf (Translated by G Fu Feng and J English).

Upadhyay SD: *Nadivijana (ancient pulse science)*, Delhi, India, 1986, Chaukhamba Sanskrit Pratisthan.

Xinnong C: *Chinese acupuncture and moxibustion*, Beijing, 2002, Beijing Foreign Languages Press.

Zimmermann F: *Jungle and the aroma of meats: an ecological theme in Hindu medicine*, New Delhi, 1999, Motilal Banarsidass.

Zysk KG: *Asceticism and healing in ancient India. Medicine in the Buddhist monastery*, Revised edition: New Delhi, 1997, 2000, Motilal Banarsidass. Vol 2 of Indian Medical Tradition.

Zysk KG: *Conjugal love in India. Ratisastra and Ratiramana*, Text, translation, and notes. Leiden, 2002, E.J. Brill. Sir Henry Wellcome Asian Series, vol 1.

Zysk KG: *Medicine in the Veda*, New Delhi, 1996, 2009, Motital Banarsidass. Vol 1 of Indian Medical Tradition.

Zysk KG: New age Ayurveda or what happens to Indian medicine when it comes to America, *Tradit South Asian Med* 6:10-26, 2001.

Zysk KG: The bodily winds in ancient India revisited, *J R Anthropol Inst* 13:105-115, 2007.

Zysk KG: The science of respiration and the doctrine of the vital winds in ancient India, *J Am Orient Soc* 113(2):198-213, 1993.

Zysk KG: *Siddha medicine in Tamil Nadu.* Copenhagen, 2008, National museet.

Zysk KG: Traditional medicine in India: Ayurveda and Siddha. In: Micozzi M, ed: *Fundamentals of complementary and alternative medicine*, ed 4, St. Louis, 2010, Saunders.

MATCHING I

Place the letter of the answer next to the term or phrase that best describes it.

A. Asian Bodywork Therapy
B. Channels
C. Dan tien
D. Five Phases
E. Hara
F. Jitsu
G. Ki
H. Kyo
I. Movement and vibration
J. Qi or chi
K. Shiatsu
L. Tsubos

_____ 1. Examples are earth, wood, fire, metal, and water

_____ 2. Examples of how energy demonstrates itself

_____ 3. Japanese bodywork therapy that uses pressure on the surface of the skin along energy channels to regain and maintain a harmonic flow of energy throughout the body-mind-spirit

_____ 4. Japanese term to meaning full, yang, excess, or too much ki

_____ 5. Japanese term to meaning empty, yin, depleted, or not enough ki

_____ 6. Traditional Asian techniques and strategies to treat the human body, mind, and spirit

_____ 7. Chinese term for energy or life force

_____ 8. Japanese term for energy or life force

_____ 9. Pathways of energy and vessels that distribute, balance, and connect ki of the interior organs with the surface and exterior of the body

_____ 10. Japanese term used to describe energetic vortices on the surface of the skin where energy of a channel can be accessed

_____ 11. Japanese term for the geographic center of balance of the body located in the lower abdomen

_____ 12. Area located three fingerwidths distance below the navel; traditionally described as the center of focused power and action

MATCHING II

Place the letter of the answer next to the term or phrase that best describes it.

A. Ayurveda
B. Chakras
C. Dosha
D. Kapha

E. Moxibustion
F. Nadis
G. Pitta
H. Prakriti

I. Prana
J. Tri-doshas
K. Vata
L. Zang/fu

_____ 1. Technique that uses heat from burning mugwort to stimulate acupoints

_____ 2. Examples are vata, pitta, and kapha

_____ 3. In Ayurveda, a person's unique constitution or the innate, natural state

_____ 4. In Chinese medicine, term used to describe the organ systems, both yin and yang

_____ 5. In Ayurveda, the dosha composed of the elements air and space

_____ 6. In Ayurveda, the combination of five elements and forces in the body

_____ 7. In Ayurveda, the energy of the body-mind-spirit; becomes atmospheric wind when it enters the human body

_____ 8. Term used to reference the body's seven energy centers located along the central channel

_____ 9. In Ayurveda, the dosha made up of the elements of earth and water

_____ 10. In yoga, channels in which prana energy flows

_____ 11. In Ayurveda, the dosha made up of the elements fire and water (or just fire)

_____ 12. India's traditional healing modality defined as the science of health and medicine designed to maintain or improve health through the use of measures such as dietary modification, massage, yoga, and herbal preparations

CASE STUDY

Synergy

Marcia is a cashier at her local grocery store. She stands for 8 hours per day, 5 days per week. She has been having pain in her foot, primarily around the medial malleolus and medial heel, which sometimes extends up the leg or into the arch, and is sometimes accompanied by tingling. Increasingly over the past few months, her lower back and shoulders become so achy that she just wants to lie down. She has sprained her ankle twice – once as a child and once about 2 years ago. She rested and iced the ankle both times, but had no treatment. Marcia's doctor recommended manual therapy, and gave her contact information for Gerry, a massage therapist, and Sarah, a shiatsu practitioner. After researching both, Marcia was unable to determine which would be better so she scheduled appointments with both.

Gerry focused his treatment on reducing scar tissue that developed following the sprains, and lengthening and deactivating trigger points in the tibialis posterior, flexor digitorum longus, and flexor hallucis longus, to reduce supination of the ankle, and reduce compression of

CASE STUDY—cont'd

the tibial nerve in the tarsal tunnel. For two full days following treatment, Marcia experienced a reduction in episodes of tingling around the ankle, and felt stronger when standing and walking. She felt minor relief in her back, but the pain continued to fatigue her.

Sarah focused her treatment on the Kidney and Bladder channels, where she found stagnation that may be the result of Marcia's standing for long hours, and that may explain the back pain. For the next two days her back pain was reduced and she felt a surge in energy and focus that she hadn't experienced in years.

Marcia wishes to continue seeing both therapists, but wants to be certain that their treatment goals are synergistic, and that one's approach does not contradict the goals of the other. She noticed that both of them

spent considerable time treating the medial leg. While she felt no negative effects after the first round of treatment, she is slightly concerned about overtreatment. She understands that as treatment progresses, treatment goals may change.

What can Marcia do to ensure that the treatment goals are synergistic?

Explore the anatomic structures and channels described above to understand better why practitioners with different treatment goals are focusing in the same areas.

Discuss the possible relationship between tsubos and trigger points.

If the tsubos and trigger points are in the same or similar places, will the combined treatments result in overtreatment?

Discuss options for avoiding overtreatment to the medial leg.

CRITICAL THINKING

Western medicine and Chinese medicine have both been evolving for centuries, but within different cultures. How might one objectively contrast and compare each approach to health and disease?

Business, Marketing, Accounting, and Finance

LEARNING OBJECTIVES

After completing this chapter, the student should be able to:

- Identify your primary values.
- Write a vision and a mission statement.
- Define professionalism, and list qualities of a professional massage therapist.
- List several employment opportunities for massage therapists.
- Explain differences between an employee and an independent contractor.
- Contrast and compare types of business entities.
- Outline pertinent licenses, permits, and registrations required to operate a professional practice.
- List types of insurance and describe their purpose.
- Identify several marketing and advertising strategies.
- Prepare a résumé.
- List business resources, and explain their importance.
- Describe a typical day for a massage therapist.
- Describe and demonstrate proper telephone etiquette for business-related calls.
- Create a plan to avoid professional burnout.
- Delineate financial aspects of the business, such as how to determine fees, bartering, tips and gifts, start-up costs, and how to manage NSF transactions.
- List ways to diversify income.
- Discuss insurance reimbursement for professional services.
- Describe aspects of accounting practices, such as the use of checking accounts, petty cash accounts, and payroll.
- List financial reports and describe their purpose.
- Identify taxes the professional massage therapist is responsible for paying and appropriate tax deductions.
- Devise a plan for building a cash reserve and investing toward retirement using securities and retirement accounts.
- Develop a business plan.

http://evolve.elsevier.com/Salvo/MassageTherapy

INTRODUCTION

Having a gratifying career in massage therapy happens in several ways: from monetary compensation to personal satisfaction. Many students enter this profession because they felt "drawn" or "called" to become a massage therapist. For some, the attraction is simply a matter of the personal success achieved as a massage client. What does a career in massage mean to you?

- Personal fulfillment from helping others
- Financial reward of a part-time or full-time job
- More free time without loss of income
- Personal recognition
- Travel opportunities
- Being your own boss
- Flexible hours
- Retirement career

According to the American Massage Therapy Association, while therapists work in a variety of work environments, 96% are sole practitioners or independent contractors. This chapter presents an overview of the business knowledge needed to build a prosperous practice, such as how to write a business plan, employment, types of business entities, business licenses and permits, insurance, marketing, how to deal with professional burnout, finances, and accounting. There is even a section on investing. This chapter is both a tool kit and a survival kit.

BUSINESS FOUNDATIONS

Massage therapists have two main choices of employment: (1) they can work for someone else or (2) they can become self-employed. A majority of therapists, even those who start out working for someone else, eventually become self-employed. Starting your own business can be a daunting process, but broken down into steps and taken one step at a time, it can be accomplished by anyone.

Why does a massage business fail? The same reason other businesses fail. Dun and Bradstreet, the world's largest business database manager, claims that 90% of all businesses fail because of lack of planning (not lack of professional skills). The American Massage Therapy Association agrees with Dun and Bradstreet, stating that when massage therapists leave the profession, the number one reason is lack of ability to "grow" a business.

This section will help you with both business planning and development. First, you will conduct a survey of personal values by listing your dreams and desires and stating the purpose of your business. Building a practice requires a vision, a mission, and a working plan. This will help bring into focus your course of action after licensure and help you set the course for your business.

> *"Careers, like rockets, don't always take off on schedule. The key is to keep working the engines."*
> —Gary Sinise

What Do You Value?

Your massage practice will reflect who you are. Who you are (your character) and how you behave (your personality) come naturally from your needs, desires, attitudes, and beliefs about life and death. A big part of your success is, and will be, embedded in your personal, business, and spiritual philosophies. If your work is not an extension of your self—that is, if your inner life and outer life are not congruent—then you will experience a mental and emotional tug of war.

Identifying what you value is often difficult because values themselves are abstract concepts. However, as experience teaches us and scientific research tells us, we spend time and energy on things we value or on acquiring things we value. Using a backdoor approach, the following activity may help you identify important elements about yourself.

Activity. List 15 to 20 things you like or want to do. These activities can range from cooking to hiking to reading to small children, to watching television, baby-sitting, or to getting *or* receiving massages. After reading over your list, assign a *value* to the right of each activity. For example, cooking may be linked to spending time with family, creative expression, or nurturing. This evaluation may take some time, but the underlying motivation of each activity should emerge. During this exercise, you will be shifting the focus from things you like or want to do to things you value.

Next, create a new list from the values you have identified in the previous section. From the most important to the least important, number each value. Although it may feel as though you are soul-searching, this exercise is often liberating because it helps you identify your most important values, making it easier to make decisions involving *your time* and *your money*—two of your most valuable assets. This list will change to reflect your changing needs. (I do this activity annually, usually on New Years Day.)

Copy the new list on several sheets of paper, and tape the list where you can see it, such as on the bathroom mirror, on the refrigerator door, or on the dashboard of your car. This exercise is also a beneficial activity to teach clients about stress reduction. If your clients feel stressed out and overwhelmed, ask them to go through this process and help them identify what is important to them and make decisions regarding their time and money accordingly.

> *"Things which matter most must never be at the mercy of the things which matter least."*
> —Goethe

Vision Statement

Every business follows a path. It is important to recognize that this path is largely designed by you, either consciously or unconsciously. Yes, it is the "self-fulfilling prophecy" and beliefs often predict behavior; behaviors determine future events. When envisioning your career path, think about what you want, not what you don't want. It is okay to experience worries, anxieties, or fears; just do not dwell on them.

The harsh truth is that if you do not consciously design your business vision, circumstances will. Unless you give thought to it and create your vision, you will be trying to navigate your business without an idea about where you are and where you are headed.

A vision statement embraces what you want—the desires for your business. Influenced by your value list, your business vision should create excitement as well as energize you. This vision is not necessarily a preview of the future but is rather a glimpse of how things might be if certain obstacles were removed, such as time, money, training, experience, and so on.

Activity. Embark on a *vision quest* of your ideal practice setting, and describe it on paper. What do you see? How do you look? What type of office and work setting are you in? How busy are you? What methods are you trained in?

Be as descriptive and specific as you want (color, smell, sound). As you create your vision, notice how it makes you feel. If it does not feel right, then alter the vision until it does. Note whether you must make any changes within yourself to fulfill your business vision. Also, when talking to others about your business, speak of it affectionately and not with impatience.

Once your vision is clear, move on to writing your mission statement and then on to the business plan. The business plan will help you turn your dreams into a reality.

> *"Argue for your limitations and they're yours."*
> —Richard Bach

Mission Statement

A *mission statement*, or statement of purpose, briefly and succinctly defines your type of business and its objective. Mission statements give businesses direction. The U.S. Constitution can be viewed as a mission statement. When writing your mission statement, you might say that you are in the massage industry, and your mission is to help people relax or be healthier. This textbook has a mission, too; its mission is to assist in the educational process of individuals who wish to become knowledgeable, well-informed, and competent massage therapists.

There are a few guidelines for writing a mission statement. First, it must be short. If it is not, you are probably not going to remember it or read it often; being able to recite it by memory is a good idea. Next, it must focus on meeting the needs of other people while not conflicting with your own. Every successful massage therapist will tell you the same thing—when your focus is serving humanity, opportunities are never in short supply. Last, your mission statement must be totally compatible with your most important

values. It will evolve as you evolve, so it must be flexible and revised as needed.

> *"To accomplish great things, we must not only act, but also dream; not only plan, but also believe."*
> —Anatole France

PROFESSIONALISM

Professionalism is the adherence to a set of values and obligations, formally agreed-upon codes of conduct, and reasonable expectations of clients, colleagues, and co-workers. Key values of professionalism include fiduciary responsibility (acting in the client's best interest), maintaining standards expected of other members of the profession, and staying current with changes and discoveries in the field. These standards include ethical aspects such as integrity, decency, accountability, responsibility, and honor. Health care professionals should possess psychosocial and humanistic qualities such as caring, empathy, humility and compassion, social responsibility, and sensitivity to the culture and beliefs of others.

Knowing and abiding by the laws and standards that govern the profession are part of our responsibilities as massage therapists. Aspects of professionalism incorporate confidentiality, scope of practice, codes of ethics, and standards of a professional massage practice (Box 17-1). Professionalism needs to be understood, practiced, and refined as much as one's technique.

Professional Image

Although creating a reputable image clearly serves the therapist, it also serves the profession and promotes trust. The massage therapist aspires to develop and maintain a professional image that is credible (Figure 17-1). Projecting a favorable image includes acting within professional boundaries. Additionally, business cards, brochures, and how clients report your work to others all reflect professional image.

Professional image also involves how the therapist is dressed. Wearing a uniform or clothing that separates the therapist from the client not only makes a statement regarding how we feel about our profession and ourselves, but it also helps create a professional atmosphere. In fact, no second chance to make a first impression exists. Avoid wearing clothing that is too revealing or distracting to clients and co-workers. One rule of thumb: If you have to question whether what you are wearing is appropriate, it probably isn't.

For more information, see "Appearance" in the section on boundaries in Chapter 2.

> *"In the end, we will conserve only what we love, we will love only what we understand, we will understand only what we are taught."*
> —Baba Dioum (Senegalese conservationist)

BOX 17-1

Qualities of a Professional Massage Therapist

Massage therapists should have knowledge of techniques and principles that include an understanding of legal and ethical issues. They must also acquire a working knowledge of, and tolerance for, human nature and individual characteristics, given that daily contact with a wide variety of people with a host of problems and concerns is a significant part of our work. Courtesy, compassion, and common sense are often cited as the *three Cs* most vital to the success of a massage therapist.

In fact, the first responsibility of a massage therapist is always to provide competent, courteous, and compassionate health care to clients. Other characteristics of a professional massage therapist include:

- Has an aptitude for working with his or her hands
- Is computer literate
- Has good communication skills that include writing, speaking, and listening
- Maintains professional boundaries and integrity
- Avoids dual relationships
- Is trustworthy and exhibits a sense of responsibility

- Prepares and maintains client records
- Keeps client information confidential
- Leaves private concerns at home
- Has patience in dealing with others and the ability to work as a member of a team
- Practices with competence and within the scope of practice determined by state law
- Projects a favorable image
- Possesses expertise that comes through three main sources: technical competence, social validation (through a formal recognition of training and status), and reputation
- Exhibits a relaxed attitude when meeting new people
- Starts and ends each session on time and lets nothing interrupt a session
- Has an understanding of and empathy for others
- Uses appropriate guidelines when releasing information
- Uses tact when resolving conflicts
- Has a willingness to learn new skills and techniques

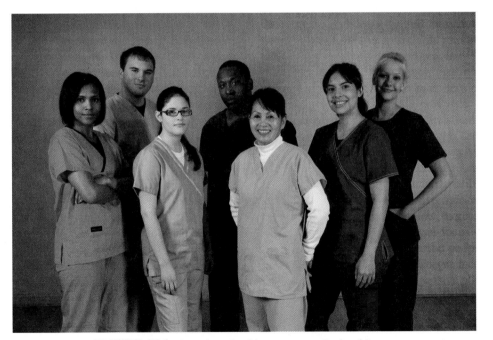

FIGURE 17-1 Therapists should portray a professional image.

EMPLOYMENT OPPORTUNITIES

A career in massage therapy offers many employment opportunities for working with people in the health and fitness industry, beauty and spa industry, travel and recreation industry, and health care industry. Massage can be incorporated in almost any setting, such as:

- Acupuncture clinics
- Airports
- Athletic teams and dance companies
- Casinos
- Chiropractic clinics
- Corporate wellness programs

BENNY VAUGHN

Born: October 11, 1951

"Success is to be measured not so much by the position that one has reached in life as by the obstacles which he has overcome while trying to succeed."
—Booker T. Washington

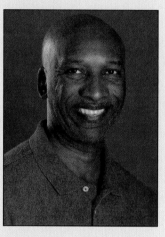

Benny Vaughn grew up in Georgia. His father was an Army cook, earning his GED while in service to his country. His mother was a food service worker with a seventh grade education. In the early years of his life, Benny and his family had to ride at the back of public buses, drink from segregated water fountains, sit in segregated seating at public venues, and attend segregated movie theaters. Being black in the Deep South at that time was a constant challenge, one that could result in arrest, beatings, and sometimes death.

"As a black man in America, my personal and professional challenges have always been accented by the color of my skin. That is to say, I always had to work harder, perform better, and do more than my white American counterparts just to be afforded an equal opportunity."

Benny's view of the world and the possibilities ahead of him changed in 1960 when his father was transferred to Crailsheim, Germany, with the 4th Armored Division. In a 24-hour period, Benny and his siblings were plucked from a segregated society and placed into an integrated society. His mother had to explain to her children that they would be living in an apartment building with white families, attending school with white children and white teachers, and most importantly that this was okay. They would not be arrested, shot, or beaten for being black. His mother did a masterful job of helping her children adjust to a culture with equal opportunity in a time when black citizens in America were dying for that right.

Vaughn attended the University of Florida in 1969 on a full athletic scholarship. It was while competing in track that he first read about the use of massage therapy in Europe to help athletes recover from training and competition. This intrigued him and he discovered a few massage schools and books written on the subject. Benny

- Cruise lines
- Day spas
- Dentist offices
- Facial, nail, and beauty salons
- Golf, tennis, and country clubs
- Gyms and health clubs
- Hospitals
- Hotels
- Nursing homes
- Onsite massage in offices
- Pain management clinics
- Physical therapy, rehab, and sports medicine clinics
- Private practice (in office or out-call)
- Psychiatric treatment centers
- Resorts
- Rodeos
- Shopping malls
- Upscale grocery stores
- Veterinarians and race tracks (animal massage)

Employees and Independent Contractors

The two main areas of employment are to work for someone else and to work for yourself. When working in an office different from your own, you may be classified as an employee or independent contractor. These classifications have legal and tax consequences.

If you are classified as an employee, an employer sets your hours and provides the place for massage services. Employers generally provide the tools and materials required to perform the service and exercise at least a measure of control and supervision over how the employee goes about his or her tasks. The employer fixes the rates for the services. The employee agrees, by virtue of that relationship, to act as the agent for the employer, upholding all instructions by the employer unless illegal or out of scope of practice. In addition the employer is responsible for the collection of all taxes and must provide compensation coverage for the employee. The employment relationship continues for an indefinite period (i.e., term of employment).

BENNY VAUGHN (*continued*)

was amazed that using his hands could have such a great impact on the health and welfare of another human being. He graduated from the College of Health and Human Performance, with a degree in Health Education and a certification in Health Promotion and Wellness.

After attending the American Institute of Massage Therapy in Florida, he took a job as a "masseur" at the Gainesville Executive Health Club under the mentorship of his teacher Bruce Simer. In addition to teaching techniques, Simer emphasized the importance of customer satisfaction and encouraged him to educate his clients on the benefits of massage therapy.

At that time, making a living as a massage therapist was challenging enough. But in addition, Vaughn was a black male working in the South. He had to be impeccably professional, and patient in overcoming apprehensions that many customers had about people of color. Inspired by such strong figures as Muhammad Ali, Willie Mays, Nelson Mandela, Martin Luther King, Jr., and Malcom X, Vaughn was committed to his personal success despite the societal challenges.

As a result, Benny Vaughn became recognized internationally as an expert in massage therapy and sports massage. He is a Certified Athletic Trainer and a Certified Strength and Conditioning Specialist. Vaughn was a member of the sports medicine staff for the USA Track and Field team at the 2003 World Championships in France, the 2004 Summer Olympics in Greece, and the 2007 World Championships in Japan.

Vaughn has always considered himself a clinician first. Teaching became a way for him to improve his clinical skills, develop better strategies of care for clients, and inspire students who want to become professional massage therapists. "Education is nourishing for the soul. Our profession is measured by how well we educate ourselves. Teachers play a most important role in the development and continuation of a society, and of a profession."

After 35 years as a massage therapist, Vaughn still goes to his office each day to treat a full schedule of clients. He continues to review cases and create treatment plans that will make a difference for the client, and to develop new ideas and information to share with others. He believes that good massage therapy is not about technique; it is about the plan of care.

"In the end, the names that we use for massage techniques really indicate belief systems and philosophies. Simply calling it something other than touch or massage does not make the outcome better for that individual client. It is the combination of skill, experience, and compassion of the massage therapist that carries powerful results for the client."

Independent contractors, in most cases, receive a fee based on completion of the task. That fee is fixed by you as the independent contractor, not the person to whom you are providing the service, or the person who contracted with you to provide the service. Independent contractors have special skills, training, or licensure that allows operation without detailed supervision by others. Independent contractors often provide their own tools and equipment. They generally determine the precise time for performing services and work in more than one place of business.

Contracting businesses occasionally attempt to mischaracterize employees as independent contractors. This temptation may arise from wanting to avoid employers' responsibilities such as withholding income taxes on wages, contributing to social security, paying unemployment compensation insurance, and obtaining worker's compensation coverage.

However, a mischaracterization can expose an employer to interest and penalties for missing tax payments. An employee treated as an independent contractor may take legal action for gaps in Social Security and unemployment compensation coverage. Even worse, if the employee has failed to pay income taxes due, the employer may have to pay the employee's taxes to the extent of the tax-withholding shortfall. A massage therapist who is considering an independent contractor relationship should obtain tax advice from a lawyer or accountant to confirm that a proper characterization of the relationship exists.

MINI-LAB

In your own words, define *success* and *security.*

BUSINESS ENTITY

Business enterprises may take many forms. Common choices in for-profit businesses include *proprietorships, partnerships,* and *corporations.* The choice of entity has compliance, tax, and liability consequences. Be sure to consult with your lawyer, accountant, and other experts to help you make a decision on which to use.

Sole Proprietorship

Sole proprietorship, or *proprietorship,* involves a single owner. Legally, no distinction exists between the business and the owner. It is the simplest and least expensive type of business to open. The owner provides all the capital and receives all the profits. Creditors look to both the owner's personal assets and the business assets to satisfy their claims. The sole proprietor is responsible for the filing and payment of all taxes, licenses, fees, and insurance needed to operate. Additionally, people injured by an employee of the proprietorship, or by products used by that employee, or injuries received on the property used by that employee during the course of employment, may pursue a claim against the owner of the proprietorship and attach all of the proprietor's personal assets to the claim.

In the case of a sole proprietorship that uses a different name from that of the owner, the proprietor often must make a filing under local statutes to protect the use of the assumed name, which is referred to as *doing business as* (DBA).

Advantages
- It is easy to start, and easy to terminate.
- You own it, and you control it.
- Profit and loss are reported on Schedule C with your individual Form 1040 tax return.

Disadvantages
- You are personally liable; any court judgment may affect your personal assets.
- If you decide to expand, locating financial resources (loan or credit) depends on your personal credit history and net worth.
- Self-employment taxes are paid by you, and all necessary insurance and fees are paid by you.

What You Will Need to Do
- Obtain an occupational license, which is issued by the city, county, or parish in which you operate.
- In some states, establishment licenses are required in addition to a local occupational license, and in addition to a massage license.
- Acquire professional liability insurance (malpractice). Check the policy; if you are using additional treatment products, such as hot stones, you may need additional coverage.
- Acquire business liability insurance (for slips and falls).

Partnerships

Partnerships are owned by two or more people working toward a common goal. Investment expense is usually shared among the partners. Business partnerships are similar to domestic partnerships in that both parties agree to share both the responsibilities and the rewards of the business. Also, it helps if business partners have good chemistry; similar to domestic partnerships, business partnerships have approximately a 50% "divorce" rate. Additionally, as with domestic partners who choose not to formally marry, two people can enter the business relationship without a formal written agreement. However, having a written agreement drawn up and reviewed by an attorney is advisable.

There are three types of partnerships: general, limited, and limited liability. In *general partnerships*, which are the most common type, members share equally in decision making, profit sharing, and personal liability. In *limited partnerships*, members may be silent (also called a silent partner) in which he or she does not actively participate in business management, but still receives profit and is liable only up to the amount of personal investment. In *limited liability partnerships,* a member(s) can limit their liability to their equity in the company and are not held liable for another partner's misconduct or negligence. State laws control the particulars of the legal protections offered by limited liability partnerships. And, in some jurisdictions, limited liability partnerships may require that one partner's personal liability is *not* limited.

Advantages
- It is easy to start.
- Start-up costs are divided between two or more people.
- It provides a broader base of skills and interest (two heads are better than one).

Disadvantages
- Decision making must be shared with one or more partners.
- As with a sole proprietorship, the partners are liable for business-related mistakes.
- Unlike a sole proprietorship, one partner can be personally liable for suits against another partner (the exception to this would be a limited liability partnership).
- Although a partnership is only a tax-reporting rather than a tax-paying entity, it must still file a tax return.
- Think carefully about entering into a partnership with your best friend; many business partnerships end in dispute.

What You Will Need to Do
- Obtain an occupational license, which is issued by the city, county, or parish in which you operate.
- In some states, establishment licenses are required in addition to local occupational license, and in addition to a massage license.
- Acquire professional liability insurance (malpractice). Check the policy; if you are using additional treatment products, such as hot stones, you may need additional coverage.
- Acquire business liability insurance (for slips and falls).
- File forms for the type of partnership required.
- Consider drawing up an operating agreement.
- Acquire federal and state identification employee numbers.

Corporations

A corporation is a business entity that is granted a charter recognizing it as a separate legal entity having its own privileges and liabilities distinct from those of its members. A properly organized and operated corporation limits the owner's liability. Limiting liability is the principal reason most small-business owners organize in the corporate format. After the corporation is organized by the articles of incorporation with the secretary of state or other appropriate state (and, if applicable, local) officers, shares of stock are issued to the stockholders.

Shareholders elect (or reelect) a board of directors annually, which oversees business operations. Corporate officers who run the daily affairs of the business can be elected or appointed by the board.

For Internal Revenue Service (IRS) purposes, a small business may be either a C corporation or an S corporation. A *C corporation* pays federal taxes on its taxable income. Subject to exceptions, the income or loss of an *S corporation* flows to its shareholders in proportion to share ownership.

Advantages
- You are not liable to third parties and your personal assets cannot be attached in a lawsuit against the business.
- The practice can continue in the event an owner leaves or dies.
- Because of its limited liability and accounting requirements, the corporate structure is attractive to a broader range of financial resources; over time, a profitable corporation is an attractive risk to banks and investors.
- Your financial risk is generally limited to the amount you pay for your stock.

Disadvantages
- A corporation is the most legally complicated business structure, and creating a corporate entity requires the assistance of an attorney.
- C corporations pay taxes separately from its shareholders (Form 1120); if the corporation pays dividends to its shareholders, then such payments are not tax deductible to the corporation, but the shareholders are required to pay tax on the dividend distribution.
- Most states charge a corporate franchise tax each year.

What You Will Need to Do
- Employ an attorney to help draw up articles of incorporation.
- File the articles of incorporation with the state where you wish to be incorporated (usually the secretary of state); you may ask the attorney you hire to take care of this task.
- Obtain an occupational license, which is issued by the city, county, or parish in which you operate.
- In some states, establishment licenses are required in addition to local occupational license, and in addition to the massage license.
- Acquire professional liability insurance (malpractice). Check the policy; if you are using additional treatment products, such as hot stones, you may need additional coverage.
- Acquire business liability insurance (for slips and falls).
- Acquire federal and state employee tax identification numbers.

LICENSES, PERMITS, AND REGISTRATIONS

Various licenses, permits, and registrations may be required before starting your business. Each state, county (or parish), and municipality differ in how and when these are issued. Contact your local city hall for the proper procedure. The local Small Business Administration (*www.sba.gov*) also may be of assistance.

If you do not know whether your state has a massage licensing board, then contact your state attorney's office or the secretary of state. If no massage board or a state licensing program is available for massage, then contact the Federation of State Massage Therapy Boards (*www.fsmbt.org*) or the National Certification Board for Therapeutic Massage and Bodywork (*www.ncbtmb.org*) for more information about peri- or post-graduation examinations that may help you obtain additional credentials.

If your state does have a licensing board, contact them and request information. Most often, this is listed on the board's website. Carefully read state requirements, and ensure that your educational program meets or exceeds these requirements. Preparation for licensure may include successfully completing an approved course of study and an internship program. Most states require not only a minimum number of hours but also a number of hours in specific subject areas.

Obtain a copy and read your state's massage therapy laws, as well as the rules and regulations (usually a separate document). These documents are often found at your local library or can be downloaded from the board's website.

Provisional License

In most states, a massage therapist must obtain a state license before he or she is allowed to practice. However, because of time between graduation and licensure, many states offer a provisional license to graduates who have completed prelicensing requirements. Although not mandatory, a provisional license allows the therapist to practice legally for a specified period. This time frame may be for a fixed period such as 1 month, or it may be flexible, being valid until the next scheduled state testing date. An additional application and fee usually are required.

The provisional license assumes that the graduate is fully trained and will be able to pass the state examination. In some states, the required provision is that a licensed therapist must sponsor the graduate and be willing to supervise all professional activities. In this way, if a problem situation arises, the provisional therapist can ask the licensed therapist for guidance. Check with your own state or regional statutes for specifics.

State License

Once you have graduated from a massage therapy program, obtain an application for professional licensure from your

---

BOX 17-2

Certification, Licensure, and Registration

The terms *licensed, certified,* and *registered* are used to describe massage therapists. Credentials and identifying titles are important parts of professionalism and allow therapists to promote himself or herself as qualified and competent to the general public. These terms are often confusing because different agencies that issue the right to use these descriptions often have different requirements.

Certification is the voluntary process by which a nongovernmental organization grants certification to an individual that possesses certain skills or abilities relevant to a field of practice. Certification requirement may include graduation from an educational institution that sets criteria for attendance and successful passing of examinations. The validity of any type of certification depends upon the integrity and authority of the certifying organization.

Licensure is a mandatory process in which a license is granted, and permission given, to perform an activity. Licenses are usually issued to regulate activities that require a certain level of skill or that may be a threat to the person (i.e., client) or the public. In most cases, licenses are issued by the state government. *Professional licensure* grants the licensee permission to perform certain professional activities within a scope of practice. This scope varies from profession to profession.

Some states that grant the right to participate in a particular profession require members to be *registered* rather than licensed. However, the meaning is basically the same. The state granting the privilege maintains an official registry or record, listing the names of persons in an occupation who have satisfied specific requirements.

---

state board and fill it out completely. An incomplete application may delay or void your testing date and may cost you a resubmission fee (Box 17-2). If your application is approved, you may then be able to apply for a provisional license while you are waiting to pass your licensing examination. If not, then do not practice massage for compensation until you have received your state license. There are serious penalties for practicing without a license. The licensing procedure varies from state to state; therefore obtain specific instructions from your state board.

If your state accepts the Massage and Bodywork Licensing Examination (MBLEx) offered by the Federation of State Massage Boards (*www.fsmtb.org*), or the National Examination for State Licensure (NESL) offered by the National Certification Board for Therapeutic Massage and Bodywork (*www.ncbtmb.org*), you may take your examination while you are still enrolled in massage school. The advantage of this is expediting the licensing process after graduation (if you pass the examination, of course).

If you take and pass the NESL to meet licensing requirements, you can convert it to a national certificate after graduation. Contact the National Certification Board for Therapeutic Massage and Bodywork for more information.

Your state board of massage therapy exists to protect the public. Informing you of proposed or current changes in the law is not its responsibility. Each massage therapist must keep abreast of changes in the state law by attending open board meetings or local massage therapy association meetings or by reading notices posted on the state board's website.

Occupational License

In most cities, you must acquire a business or occupational license to operate any kind of business. Contact the clerk of court, city planning department, or appropriate public office in your area. Typically, part of the procedure of obtaining your business license is to have your business location approved through the city zoning department and the fire marshal. This process is required for a home or cottage business. Your occupational license is displayed in a public place.

Sales Tax Permit

If you plan to sell products, you may then be required to obtain a sales tax permit through a state or county (parish) taxing authority. You will receive a taxpayer identification number and instructions on how to pay your sales tax, which usually involves monthly or quarterly payments. Some municipalities tax services such as massage, whereas others do not.

Registration of a Business Name

Some therapists trade on their own name. Many therapists chose a new name under which their business is conducted. This is called a business or trade name, or a "doing business as" (*DBA*) name. Be sure to register your business name with the city or county (parish) clerk's office. This process protects you from other businesses that may use your business name and also ensures that you are not using a name currently registered by someone else in your area.

"A true definition of an entrepreneur comes closer to: a poet, visionary, or packager of social change."
—Robert Schwartz

INSURANCE

Find out which type of insurance is required by law for your business to operate. Additionally, an insurance agent should be contacted to discuss your individual insurance needs. Some types of insurance can be obtained through professional massage organizations.

Professional Liability Insurance

Also referred to as *malpractice insurance* and *errors and omission insurance,* professional liability covers liability costs arising from your professional activities. Liability claims may be filed when a massage therapist causes injury to a client in the course of providing a massage. This includes burns from hot stones and other physical injuries resulting from professional activities.

Professional liability insurance is required in most states and is available through professional associations. Professional liability insurance can be purchased while you are a student. If you operate a home-based practice, most homeowner's policies do not cover professional activities.

General Liability Insurance

Also referred to as *premise liability,* general liability covers liability costs that are a result of bodily injury, property damage, and personal injury incurred when the client is on your premises. An example would be if your client slips and falls on your property or if a tree limb falls and damages a client's parked car.

Business Personal Property Insurance

Business insurance covers the cost of business property such as a desk, massage table, chairs, and stereo equipment in your business location. Again, your homeowner's policy probably does not cover the costs of your business property if you operate a home-based business. An inexpensive rider can usually be purchased under your homeowner's policy to cover these costs in the event of flood, fire, or theft.

Automobile Insurance

Some states require that you have an automobile policy that is rated for business use if you travel to and from a client's home or office.

Health Insurance

Medical expenses such as physician visits and hospitalization are covered with health insurance. If you are self-employed, then this type of insurance can be purchased through the National Association for the Self-Employed (*www.nase.org*).

Life Insurance

If you have dependents, then life insurance provides your loved ones with financial support in the event of your death. *Term life* is the least expensive choice and is the insurance policy most frequently purchased.

Disability Insurance

Disability insurance provides you with income in the event that you cannot work as a result of a disability resulting from illness or injury. Considering that most massage therapist are self-employed, even a short period of time without regular income could be a great inconvenience. For this reason it is advisable to look into purchasing disability insurance. The premiums are based on the rate that is payable to you when injured, and the rate is determined by your income level. So this insurance grows with your practice, but protects you from day one.

"Luck is talent meeting opportunity."
—Monica Reno

MARKETING

Marketing comprises ideas, strategies, and activities to aid in attracting and retaining clients. Marketing strategies include:

- Paid television or radio advertising
- Passing out business cards at a local country club
- Using a website to promote your services
- Giving gift certificates to potential referral sources
- Sending a proposal to a hospital for massage services
- Setting up a booth at a local heath fair
- Sending a résumé to a prospective employer

Essentially, marketing is everything you do to get clients in your door and on your table (or chair). Effective marketing is an important tool to help you achieve both your business goal and your client's therapeutic goals.

Advertising is a form of communication used to make your business noticeable to the public. Most often, it includes developing the message, and then using forms of media to deliver the message, usually at a cost to you. Massage therapists often use media in the form of Internet advertising (appearing in search engine results), phone book advertising, newspaper and newsletter advertising (display or classified), radio or television commercials, or direct mailing.

Advertising also creates your image, the picture created mentally when people read or see your business name. You have a lot of control over this, so really think about how your advertising looks, sounds, and feels. Soliciting the help of advertising agencies or specialists would be helpful.

Advertising lets people know who you are and what services you provide. *General advertising* announces or reminds current or potential clients about your business. *Specific advertising* targets an objective such as gift certificate sales or increasing the sale of a new or pre-existing service, such as body wraps or reflexology. By determining your target group, you can decide what advertising and promotional strategies are most effective because the most effective advertisements target a specific population. Keep in mind that a lag time always exists between action and results, and you cannot always predict the results.

Most forms of media (methods of mass communication) sell advertising and offer prospective customers a media kit. Media kits include the coverage area and market information. It may also include population statistics by groups (women, men, teens, and children); information about households with computers, cable, and cell phones; and demographics about household income, education level, and occupation. Also included are a price sheet; history of the company; its mission statement, owners, and stock listing; and any advantages regarding buying this particular medium over other media.

All forms of advertising should include your contact information including your website address or URL (acronym for *uniform resource locator*).

It is also helpful to ask clients where and how they heard about your business so you can better understand which advertising is most effective. You can better allocate limited financial resources to the methods that work best.

evolve Therapists often use print advertising to promote their business. Log on to the Evolve website to view several sample ads. Use your imagination to create future ads. ∎

Business Cards

Business cards let people know who you are and how to contact you. Having a business card also indicates that you are serious about your work. Be generous and hand your business cards out often. They serve no purpose in a box on the shelf. As you give them to people, introduce yourself and clearly state what business you practice. People will often remember what you do rather than your name, which is another reason why business cards are important.

When you hand someone a business card, make a good impression (Figure 17-2). You want them to remember you days later when he or she comes across your card in a pocket or billfold.

Business cards may also be used for appointment cards. You may even use your business card as part of an incentive program by writing something on the back, such as "$10 off next massage." Be creative and have fun, but remember, this is your *business face*.

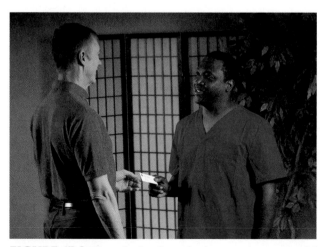

FIGURE 17-2 Therapist handing a business card to a potential client.

Your card should be well spaced and not overcrowded with words or graphics; beauty lies in simplicity. Be sure the font is easy to read. Note these examples. Be sure to compare both the letters and the numbers.

SUSAN G. SALVO
123.455.6868

SUSAN G. SALVO
123.455.6868

SUSAN G. SALVO
123.455.6868

SUSAN G. SALVO
123.455.6868

Be sure to proofread all information before it goes to print. If you have a logo, then use it on your business card and on every other piece of advertising.

▌ MINI-LAB

Design your own business card, letting it reflect your area of specialty.

Brochures

The purpose of a brochure is to explain to prospective clients, in some detail, about you and your services. Brochures are obviously more expensive than business cards, but because of added space, they can describe your business more adequately. If you have a computer, printer, and proper computer program, you can design and print your own brochures. The most popular format is a trifold, which is printed double-sided on an 8.5-inch × 11-inch sheet of paper. This size can also be used as a mailer.

Begin your brochure with an attention grabber that conveys some benefit of massage, such as "Feel comfortable in your body again." Then describe the benefits people often experience (in your clients' words). Next, describe what you actually do and give a short autobiography. In your autobiography, state a brief description of your qualifications and, if appropriate, include years of experience: "Since 1990" is preferred over "20 years of experience" as the latter limits your use of the brochure to the year of publication. Your telephone number or primary means of contact such as email should be large and readable. If you use social media such as Facebook to promote your business, be sure to state this on your brochure as well.

Use vivid language, appealing to vision, hearing, and emotion—for example, "One part therapy, one part luxury" or "Visit the tranquil place." Note that you do not have to say things directly, as with "Must be experienced to be fully understood," or "Relax under pressure." What are the mental images that come to mind when you read those words? A brochure is easier to read if you use bullet points and attractive graphics instead of paragraphs of text. This principle also applies to text on a computer screen.

If you include your fees and menu of services, then print them on a separate sheet of paper that slips into your brochure as an insert. Use facsimile machines and electronic mail to send out your brochure when someone calls you with an inquiry.

Once you have a rough draft, give it to three trusted friends and ask for feedback. Revise it as often as needed. Ensure that after reading your brochure, a potential client will know what needs you can fulfill and how you are different from others providing a similar service.

Résumé

A **résumé**, or *curriculum vitae* (CV), is an autobiographical sketch that documents your achievements, including occupational, avocational, academic, and any relevant personal information. This information is made available to a prospective employer or business contact. Even if you are self-employed, a résumé can help you in business meetings, with developing business relationships, and in acquiring a referral base. A well-written résumé lets your business contacts know who you are and what you can offer their employers, members, clients, or patients.

Before you sit down to write your résumé, take time to reflect on your life. What are the accomplishments of which you are proud? What are the things that have brought you the most joy? Your list of accomplishments may include acting in a community play, assisting with a political campaign, or being a successful blogger. Now, study the list. You might notice a pattern of personal strengths or interests emerging. You may find that you are a natural leader or that you work best with groups of people. This information can help you write your personal data section.

The most widely used format is the *reverse chronologic format,* which emphasizes your education and work experience from most recent to earliest. Begin by posting your name, address, telephone number, and e-mail address at the top center of the page in a larger font than the rest of the text.

> ⓔvolve   *I keep my résumé as a Word document and update it annually. A sample résumé is on the Evolve website under course materials for Chapter 17. Research other formats and choose the one that works best for you.* ∎

Education. List all of your academic achievements in reverse chronologic order. If you did not attend college, then list your high school; if you did attend college, omit your high school in this section. Also include the name of the educational institution, any college degrees, postgraduate degrees, certificates, and any awards or honors. Also include schools you attended and any major and minor courses that have helped you as a massage therapist (e.g., psychology,

anatomy and physiology, kinesiology). If you have attended any postgraduate workshops, then list them after your formal educational achievements.

Work Experience. Starting with the most recent, list all of the jobs held within the last 10 years. Include the names of your employers, titles or positions held, job descriptions, and starting and termination dates. Focus on your field experience while you were at school. Did you provide sports massage for athletes? Did you massage residents in a skilled care facility? Select the activities that enhance your qualifications, such as hobbies, sports, and professional affiliations.

Personal Data. Although not necessary, this section is your opportunity for the reader to know about you. List your marital status, number and ages of your children, your general health status, and whether you are a nonsmoker. Use only the personal information that will help you project the positive image that you began to formulate in the preceding sections. You might even mention that you like to coach baseball or that you enjoy playing chess. These activities may create a pleasant image of you to the reader.

Cover Letter. Finally, prepare your cover letter. At the top, list all contact information such as your mailing address, e-mail address, and phone numbers. The letter should contain a maximum of four paragraphs. Use the first paragraph to state the position you are applying for and how you heard about it. The second paragraph elaborates on your skills, experience, and suitability for the position. Do not simply repeat what is in your résumé. Make it more personal while still remaining professional. Creating a portrait of yourself; mention qualities that make the best impression. Relate these qualities to any advertised requirements. Paragraph three is about why you are interested in the position and what your contributions are. The final paragraph contains information on your availability for an interview. Be sure it suggests the action you want the prospective employer to take.

Keep your writing style simple. After you have proofread it once, let three other people proofread it for you. This approach is a good system for reducing grammar and spelling errors.

If you have a specific employer in mind, send it by e-mail or regular mail. If invited to an interview or a business meeting, then call the day before to confirm. On the day of the interview or meeting, arrive 15 minutes early. Within a week, send a thank you note mentioning how much you enjoyed the opportunity to share ideas.

Another very popular method of introducing yourself to prospective employers and business contacts is a brief video. Video résumés, while offering an opportunity to show your creativity, still must serve to inform future employers of your employment skills and history. When making a video résumé, be sure to keep the video short—1 to 2 minutes is standard. The video should be focused, just like responses in an interview. Be confident and clear, but be yourself. Recognize that this is not a commercial and you are not acting. Always keep the video professional—talk mostly about your work experience. Once the video is made and handed over, it could end up anywhere. For this reason, it is usually suggested to not include any contact information on a video, especially a personal phone number. There are many examples, both good and bad, of video résumés available online by simply searching. Watch a few and decide which ones you like and why.

Websites

Although radio and television advertising are occasionally cost-prohibitive for people with small practices, an Internet website can be an inexpensive way to reach large numbers of clients. It allows you to communicate with them at their convenience. The exposure can range from a free listing on established massage sites to creating and publishing your own website.

To have a website, you must first obtain a domain name. This name is registered with one of several companies (we use *www.domainname.com*). Next, you design your website (or have it designed by someone else).

Once your website is ready to launch, you must hire a company or someone to host your website. Cost depends on the size of your website and additional services such as accepting payments for sales. Basic hosting services will run between $25 and $40 per month. Larger massage associations offer design and hosting services as part of their membership benefits.

Six guidelines for designing your website are as follows:

1. ***Color scheme.*** If you have a logo or preferred colors on business cards and stationery, that is a good start. If you do not, then choose two or three complementary colors and stay with them—do not change colors on every page. If you are unsure, then surf the Web and find a website that you like. The current most popular color schemes are:
   - Red, yellow, and white
   - Blue and white
   - Red, gray, and white
   - Blue, orange, and white
   - Yellow, gray, and white
2. ***Use a template.*** Most website design software (such as SharePoint and Dreamweaver) includes some templates, or you can check out some websites that specialize in designing templates. Visit:
   - http://www.templatesbox.com
   - http://www.templatemonster.com
   - http://freesitetemplates.com
   - http://www.freelayouts.com
3. ***Easy navigation system.*** An easy-to-navigate site is one of the most important considerations. Be sure visitors can find information easily. Most websites display a navigation bar on the left or at the top. Include a navigation bar at the bottom of each page to save your visitors from having to scroll back to the top.
4. ***Limit special effects.*** Although including one or two special effects to spice up a website is nice, avoid rotating graphics, because they serve to distract from the site's content and slow download time. Less patient visitors may move off your site even before your spinning logo finishes loading.
5. ***Backgrounds.*** Use a background color that contrasts well with your text and links. The default for links in most programs is blue (before being visited) and burgundy (after being visited).

Be sure that your website is up to date, especially if you include prices or special sales. An outdated site not only is unprofessional but can cost you clientele if what you promoted is no longer available. If you close your business, or merge with another one, always take down your site.

E-mail

E-mail can be a great way for you to communicate with clients. It is free and accessible at your convenience, which is ideal for a massage therapist. If your website lists an e-mail address, be sure to make it professional sounding (no "babyluv_thang@" addresses) and check it often. E-mail can also be a great way to send out notices to your clientele about any specials you may be offering. Plus, they may forward the information to friends (prospective clients).

"You've achieved success in your field when you don't know whether what you're doing is work or play."
—Warren Beatty

Social Networking Sites

One of the most powerful tools available in modern times is social networking. Social networking sites are a broad expanse of generally free websites that connect a community of people together. Some sites are designed for a specific interest, organization, or profession, but many are free of such parameters. Such sites may allow for personal profiles of individual members, forum boards for discussions, site-specific e-mail accounts, or photo, audio, and video sharing. Popular social networking sites include Facebook, MySpace, and YouTube.

The benefit of such sites is they offer a free means of connecting with countless new potential clients and staying connected with established clientele. Industry-specific sites, such as www.MassageProfessionals.com, can offer a network of support and potential collaboration between colleagues. Most of these sites have a relatively simple registration process and are highly accessible. If you have a professional website, simply listing your website address with a link on your social network profile can increase your website traffic immensely at minimal effort or cost.

The primary drawback of social networking sites is that they lack the element of control offered by a professional website. Your profile page may display ads not congruent to your message, or links to other sites you may not want associated with your business. It is a tricky balance. Most social networking sites operate under a very casual regimen, and may contain inappropriate imagery, text, or humor-dependent upon the site.

Video sites, such as YouTube, can be an especially useful tool. A majority of people today prefer imagery to printed information—wouldn't you rather be watching a video right now? Video sites can allow you to upload essentially commercials for your business, not only free of charge, but depending on the popularity of your video, you can even make a profit on people viewing it.

Here are a few tips for creating and uploading videos:

- Think of an accurate title for the video, but also one containing words likely to be searched often. For example, the term "Swedish" will not be searched nearly as often as "relaxation" or "relaxing."
- Make sure your video conveys the image you want to portray. A darkly lit, poorly shot video can do more to hurt your business than help it. Keep in mind that this video may be the first impression a potential client has of your business.
- If you have a personal profile, be careful to keep it separate from your business profile. A link to your personal profile on your business page or video can take a client from viewing your professional image to a picture of your Friday night out on the town. Exercise caution with anything you post online—remember, you are your business image.

It is important to use discretion in creating any social networking page, profile, or video. There is a fine line between being fun and being unprofessional; however, when maintained properly, electronic advertising can expand your business in unprecedented ways.

CHAT ROOM

Security in Electronic Media

There are many ways your information can be misused on the Internet. This could negatively impact your business. Keep in touch with what is written about you and attributed to you. One easy way to do this is to Google yourself often. Make sure you flip 6 to 10 pages back to be sure you have seen even the most obscure entries or postings.

Other Ideas

Depending on your business location and demographic, there are other marketing techniques that may work for your business. Knowing your surrounding culture is key; if you work in a predominantly Spanish-speaking community, bilingual advertisements may be a good idea. Other ideas include press releases and publicity, discussed next.

Press Releases. These are short pieces used to inform the public on local ongoings. A press release should contain newsworthy information such as a class or lecture being held or an award or honor that has been bestowed upon you. This tactic provides a subtle reminder of who you are and gives the message that you are active in your community and your profession. A press release is not an advertisement. If yours has the sound of an advertisement, then the editor of the newspaper will not publish it. Contact your local paper or website about the specifications and guidelines for press releases.

Publicity. Simply put, publicity is free media exposure. One good option is becoming the expert. This can be in the form of writing an article about massage for a local paper, answering questions about massage on a television program, or giving public lectures related to massage or stress. Volunteering is another great way to attract attention and participate in community services. Sports events, health fairs, or donating gift certificates to charities are all great ways to advertise your business, while promoting a positive image. Donating your time to public servants, such as police officers and fire fighters, can be beneficial to your business. Volunteerism is also a way to give back to the community that supports your practice. Through donations of time and talent, massage can touch lives.

BUSINESS RESOURCES

Resources and support are vital for the health of any business. One person cannot know everything about managing a business. It is important to reach out to others and ask for advice. The saying "two heads are better than one" definitely applies here. Learning from the experience and mistakes of others can save you a lot of trouble, as well as time and money. Several methods are available for accomplishing this task.

Preceptor

While you are in school, your massage instructors teach you the knowledge and skills of your trade. They are also there to answer your questions. After graduation, you will still have lots of questions. To help you, locate a preceptor. A *preceptor* is someone who guides you during your post-graduate practice; this person is a kind of mentor. Participating in a preceptorship can be rewarding for both parties. Your preceptor may be physically on the premises while you engage in your professional activities, or he or she may be available to be contacted as you have questions such as how to handle certain situations. This person may be one of your instructors but most often is a veteran massage therapist—someone who was once a massage student and new graduate who understand your concerns.

Business Coach

A business coach can be another important resource. This person is not always in the massage business, but acts more as a consultant and a teacher, someone who helps you bridge the gap between where you are and where you want to be. A business coach may offer honest, direct feedback and professional advice. Your business coach may be a chiropractor, physical or occupational therapist, banker, or self-employed person. Do not be afraid to approach people from whom you would like to learn. These individuals can act as a sounding board if you need help in making decisions. The following is a list of keys to finding and keeping a business coach relationship:

1. Find someone you admire.
2. Find someone who is successful.
3. Find someone who is willing to be a coach.
4. Be willing to learn from the person's mistakes.
5. Give something back to the person. Money is probably not appropriate in this circumstance, but find a service that he or she needs, such as cooking or baby-sitting, or give a gift such as flowers, a book, or even a massage. Show the person how much he or she is appreciated.
6. Remember that, regardless of what advice is offered, the decision and responsibility are ultimately your own.

Other Business Resources

Additional business resources may include:
- Business organizations, such as the Small Business Administration (SBA)
- Civic organizations, such as the Service Corps of Retired Executives (SCORE)
- Local university business or marketing departments. Volunteer your business as a project for graduate students who must analyze and prepare business proposals.
- Professional massage organizations. Belonging to a massage association helps you keep up with current trends, exchange ideas with the only people who truly understand your problems, and actively support the industry as a whole. Attend massage conferences and conventions often. Nothing is quite as inspiring as hundreds of people gathered together who share a common experience.

Contracts and Proposals

When embarking on a new business venture, you may be asked to write a business contract or a proposal. Both contracts and proposals outline your ideas, help to avoid communication problems, state specifically how problems will be handled and who will handle them when they do arise, and help keep both parties focused.

Contract. A *contract* is a written voluntary agreement between two or more parties that communicates expectations, duties, and responsibilities. A signed and dated contract is enforceable by law. Ideally, all parties should draw up a rough draft outlining what they perceive as a reasonable agreement. Be sure your draft (1) clarifies the business relationship of each party (e.g., lessor or lessee, employer or employee, partner or independent contractor); (2) states the duration of the contract (e.g., 6 months, 1 year); and (3) predetermines on what grounds the contract can be terminated, if before the previously agreed-on time. Use these rough drafts to develop the official contract. It is best to have your attorney look it over before signatures are collected. Everything is negotiable, but negotiate before signing.

Proposal. A *proposal* is a written idea put forward for consideration, discussion, or adoption. Many massage therapists entering the field have the opportunity to approach businesses that do not offer massage therapy and create a position for themselves or for other therapists. The following elements should be included when writing a proposal to a sports group, skilled care facility, or any other business endeavor where you wish to be hired or volunteer your services.

- *Cover Letter.* See the section on cover letter writing under Résumé.
- *Objective.* The objective is a broad statement that encompasses the aim and expected results of the project, or both—for example, "Providing stress-reduction services for employees of 'said' corporation to improve employee productivity and reduce absenteeism." Then discuss the significance and need for this project; compare your project with other projects in the same field and other geographic locations (when applicable). Last, state any anticipated outcomes and methods of evaluating and reporting these outcomes.
- *Logistics.* Logistics consists of the managing details of the operation—that is, the what, when, and where section of the proposal. If you are familiar with the facility, recommend a specific location at which services will be provided. Briefly discuss physical arrangements such as room dimensions, bathroom location, lighting, equipment, and supplies. Mention which of these items as well as which services you are providing. Are you proposing full-time or part-time work? Will services be available during the day, evenings, or weekends? One idea is to propose a part-time availability and to increase your hours as demand increases. What hours of the day will services be offered, and who will pay for them? State which person in the company will be responsible for managing the project, and identify your organization's contact person, if different from the person negotiating the proposal. Specify how you can be reached. Also include who should be contacted as ideas are developed and problems arise, and a mutually agreed-on mediator (third party) to help settle disputes in cases of irreconcilable differences.

- *Qualifications*. Include a brief outline of your training and experience. If you do not have postgraduate experience, then focus on the field experience you acquired while you were in school. Introduce other people (e.g., staff, volunteers) who are key to the project, and provide their backgrounds. Mention any professional affiliations such as with the American Massage Therapy Association (AMTA), National Certification Board for Therapeutic Massage and Bodywork (NCBTMB), and Associated Bodywork and Massage Professionals (ABMP) and whether participating massage therapists are insured.
- *Funding*. This important section outlines the proposed budget for the project and includes the amount you are contributing, if any; the names and amounts of funds received from other participants; and the amount you are requesting from the agency or corporation. If needed, suggest plans for additional fund-raising. The budget should include both expenses and revenues for the entire proposed project. If revenue is generated by this project, then outline who will benefit financially. This section should also include payment schedules and payment method.
- *Summary*. The summary, or closing remarks, should summarize your proposal and convey a sense of warmth, camaraderie, confidence, and willingness to be part of this project. Also helpful is to include a brief synopsis on a separate sheet of paper listing or bulleting all of the elements in your proposal, outlining their contents, which can be used during the meeting in which your proposal is presented before the board members. Do not use complete sentences but rather provide a brief descriptions of what each element entails, which is similar to using note cards for a speech; it will keep you on track and allow others to follow your presentation easily. PowerPoint presentations are also effective ways of delivering your proposal at meetings.

MINI-LAB

Using the guidelines outlined in this chapter, write a proposal and a contract.

"A ship in harbor is safe—but that is not what ships are for."
—John A. Shedd

AN AVERAGE DAY

There is no such thing as an average day, but it's a good idea to examine events in which you are likely to be involved. It is also important to consider responsibilities that coincide with these events. Just remember that experience is your best teacher. By palpating, listening, questioning, and massaging, you will further develop your skill and knowledge, which promotes competence and confidence. You will learn that mastery comes not only in the doing but also in the deciding. Many small decisions are made in the course of a workday. Let this section serve as a guide.

Before the Client Arrives

This section is concerned with the time frame beginning when you report to work until the client arrives. If possible, arrive at least 60 minutes before your first appointment. Check your incoming messages and take care of any calls or business-related e-mails (Box 17-3). You may want to contact each person the day before the scheduled massage to verify the appointment; this reduces confusion about appointment times and minimizes "no-shows." Look over your schedule; pull and review client intake forms and past notes for any clients scheduled that day. If you are expecting a first-time client, then have a new intake form and pertinent literature ready.

Next, check your massage table. Are the knobs that connect the table legs to the tabletop loose? If so, then tighten them. Dress your massage table and ready the room—view your room as a client would. If you have prepared your massage room the day before, then inspect the room for any unexpected items (e.g., dead insects). When your client enters the massage room, have the music playing, the lighting dim and indirect, and the room warm. Having the massage area visually appealing and ready to go (i.e., bolsters, linens, lubricant) is a mark of professionalism.

Using a mirror, critique your own appearance. Is your hair in place? Are your lips and nose clean? Next, are your nails trimmed, neat, and clean? Is your breath fresh? Are your pockets empty of keys and change? Have you removed your jewelry? Is your cell phone turned off or set to "vibrate"?

MINI-LAB

Visit a massage therapist's office. What is the initial impression you have on approaching the door? List the words that describe how you feel. Is the mood serene, business-like, busy, chaotic, impersonal, or cluttered? What do you hear or smell?

When the Client Arrives

Greet your client with a smile, making eye contact and calling him or her by name. Introduce yourself (if this is your first time as his or her therapist), and escort the person to the area where the intake will take place (Figure 17-3). Be calm, confident, friendly, and courteous while in the presence of your client. The therapeutic relationship will evolve over time spent with the client and is built on a foundation of trust and good communication skills, which build rapport (see Chapter 2). To show respect for the client and the relationship, avoid using tobacco in any form while in the company of a client. The smell of tobacco is often offensive to nonsmoking clients. Although many smoking

BOX 17-3

Telephone Etiquette

Telephone etiquette is the behavior used when on the telephone communicating for social or professional activities. Here are some tips:

General Telephone Standards

- Answer between the second and third ring.
- Speak slowly and use a pleasant, expressive tone of voice; smile as you talk.
- Give the caller or person you are calling your undivided attention; do not carry on two conversations at once.
- Say "please," "thank you," and "you're welcome."
- Do not chew while on the telephone.
- End each call with a sincere closing remark.
- Keep your promises, and follow up on the call.
- Return calls within 24 hours; this is known as the *sundown rule.*

Placing a Call

- Identify yourself by name and business or title (if applicable).
- Be cordial, and explain the purpose of the call.
- Have all necessary information handy before placing the call.

Answering a Call

- Begin with "Good morning," "Good afternoon," or "Good evening," followed by your name, the name of your establishment, and an inquiry. For example, "Good afternoon. This is Jane at the Downtown Spa. How may I help you?"
- Find out the caller's name, and use it as you speak to him or her.
- Be a good listener; find out what the caller wants first.
- Let the caller end the conversation, allowing him or her to hang up first.

Putting a Caller on Hold

- If you must place the caller on hold, ask permission and wait for a reply. For example, "May I put you on hold?"

- If the caller concurs, then do not leave him or her on hold for more than 30 seconds. If the caller must be on hold longer than that, offer to return the call. The caller may choose to continue holding.
- Always thank the caller for holding.
- If the caller says no, get his or her name and number and say that you will return the call shortly. Keep this promise.

Taking Messages

- Clearly write down the date, time the call was received, who called, why the person called, and a return telephone number and extension (if applicable).
- Be sure you understand the message.
- Repeat all the information to the caller, and check for accuracy before hanging up.
- Give the message to the proper person as soon as possible.

Massage Inquiries by Telephone

- Inform the caller of available services and fees.
- State appointment times that are available. Avoid telling the caller times that are not available.
- If the caller schedules an appointment, recommend that he or she avoid eating 1 hour before the scheduled appointment.
- If your client comes directly from his or her work, suggest that he or she bring alternate clothing to wear after the session.
- If you require that the client bring special items such as shorts, a swimsuit, or a towel, inform him or her at this time.
- Suggest that the client schedule *downtime,* or time to relax, after the session.
- If you have a cancellation or late policy, then let him or her know about it at this time.
- Verify the appointment day and time.
- Give the client directions to your establishment and any other information that you deem necessary.
- Finally, ask if he or she has any questions.

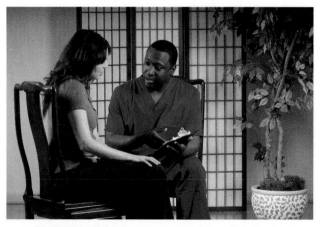

FIGURE 17-3 Therapist performing a client intake.

therapists are unaware of their tobacco odor, it can be detected on their clothes, hands, hair, and linens.

Ask the new client to fill out an intake form (see Chapter 10). Obtain consent for treatment. If the person is a previous client, then review the health history information and record any changes. Perform any assessments related to treatment, and prioritize the client's needs based on the interview. Explain to the client what will be done during the session and why. Ask if the client has any questions, and answer them to the best of your ability.

If any special considerations need to be addressed, then discuss how the massage will be adapted to suit the client's special needs (see Chapter 11). The client may be overwhelmed by all the information that is needed to prepare for a safe and well-tailored massage session. Asking the client to show up 15 minutes early for the first appointment may be helpful, or you may want to mail out in advance the intake form.

You may wish to direct your client to the music selection, telling him or her what is currently playing and asking the client to make a selection if he or she prefers a different kind of music. Next, direct the client to your massage lubricant selection, and ask him or her to make a choice (see Chapter 3). Point out the most popular lubricant so as to make the selection process easier. Take into consideration any skin sensitivities and allergies. You may need to obtain an ingredient list in large type so the client can read the ingredients. The use of aromatherapy can also help the client to unwind (see Chapter 12).

Even though draping is discussed in the premassage consultation, many emotions are often associated with disrobing and touch that distort the new client's perspective, making directions and instructions difficult to hear. Simple and concise instructions assist the client in the transition from the mental focus of the consultation to the physical and emotional focus of a massage session. Be sure to allow the client time to settle into the space provided for him or her before giving directions on the use of linens, positioning himself or herself on the table, indicating when you will return to begin the massage (see Chapter 7). Every precaution should be taken to ensure the client's comfort, physical and emotional safety, and privacy.

Before you exit the room, address any comfort needs your client may have. Offer the client a glass of water, and suggest a trip to the toilet. Show the client where to place clothes and personal items, and explain to the client any special procedures you use to handle these items. Explain to the client how to lie on the table (i.e., underneath the top drape). Tell the person that you are going to leave the room so he or she may disrobe in privacy and that, when you reenter the room, you will knock before you open the door. This precaution alleviates any apprehension he or she may have about your unannounced return.

CHAT ROOM

Client empathy is one of the reasons that you, as the therapist, should receive massages from other therapists. By staying in touch with how it feels to be a client, you will be a more attentive and sensitive therapist.

Clients often wear jewelry and may bring a purse, wallet, cell phone, or other items to the massage office. Because most jewelry is removed before the massage begins, care must be taken to safeguard these items. Large articles, such as purses, should not leave the client's sight. For smaller items such as rings, use a large envelope, small basket, or small bowl to accommodate the client's belongings. A portable container allows these items to remain with the client if he or she must move from one room to another. A locker may also be used to store these items safely during the massage.

MINI-LAB

Once you have learned a basic massage routine, perform a massage blindfolded. The recipient on the table may have to assist with the draping and turning aspects of the massage because these tasks may be too difficult for you without your sense of sight. This activity will help you get out of your head and intellect, and into your hands and feeling skills.

Before the Session

Wash and dry your hands and forearms or use a sanitizing agent (see Chapter 9). Warm your hands by rubbing them together if they have become cooled by this procedure.

Spend a little time preparing yourself mentally and physically. Grounding and centering yourself before the massage should be an integral part of your therapy session. If you feel distracted and not present with your client, then you will not be able to give the best massage possible. Learning how to clear your thoughts, how to prepare your body, and how to ground and center yourself will help you be a more sensitive and responsive therapist (see Chapter 4).

Breathing and performing body movements are some techniques you can use to prepare yourself (see Figure 4-4). Before you enter the massage room, move and stretch your body while taking deep breaths. If all you have is a few seconds, then simply squat down to stretch your lower back (only if your knees can do this comfortably) and stand up to shake out your entire body. Relaxation allows achievement of a calm state. A therapist who is calm will more easily project professionalism, confidence, and peace to the client with both presence and touch.

Some therapists choose to incorporate elements of their own spirituality into the massage. This may involve turning the direction of the massage over to the care of God (or a higher power). A simple prayer, verbal or silent, of gratitude for the opportunity to work with this client helps to create a healing atmosphere (most massage therapists who pray prefer to pray in silence).

Some clients will ask you how many massages you have done today and if you are tired, or after noting the physical nature of your work, they will ask if your hands become tired. What they may really be asking is "Do you have enough energy for me?" Assure them that you have stamina and endurance built up from frequently doing massage and that when your hands do feel tired, you massage them back to happiness. At this point, they seem to be greatly relieved.

MINI-LAB

When feasible, get a massage from a therapist you do not know. During the massage intake, do not reveal to the therapist that you are a massage therapist or student of massage therapy. In this way, you will more fully experience of how it feels to be a client. Along with helping you learn what to do and what not to do, this activity will also reinforce the things you are doing that work well for the client. Role reversal can be an eye-opening experience.

The Massage Session

Before you begin the massage, address the client's care and comfort needs once more. Ask if the room temperature is comfortable. Adjust if needed as relaxing is difficult if you feel chilled. Encourage your client's proper body alignment with the placement of bolsters or pillows underneath the areas of the body that require support (e.g., neck, knees, ankles; see Chapter 7). Remind the client about the importance of being relaxed and offering feedback during the massage.

Initial Contact. Begin by making physical contact with the client, perhaps with quiet, motionless touch. Help your client relax by asking him or her to take a few deep breaths. Once you and the client are ready, proceed with the massage routine. The dozens of methods for massaging the body, each effective in its own way, are best learned in the classroom under a skilled and caring instructor.

Structured Time. The length of treatment is determined by the client. The client schedules the session, often in 30- to 90-minute increments. If the client is undecided about the length of the session, tell him or her that you will schedule a half-hour session but will block out a full hour. When 30 minutes is up, let the client know, and he or she can then decide if the massage will continue.

Focus on the client's areas of complaint as well as areas of tension and tenderness you find through palpation. Address the client's concerns first (e.g., back, neck, shoulder) so as to avoid running out of time accidentally. Although the session is confined to a specific duration, try not to let the massage feel hurried.

Communication. Communicating during the massage may be challenging because eye contact is infrequent. When the client is lying prone, the head is to one side or in a face cradle; when the client is supine, either the eyes are closed or a client must strain the neck muscles to lift the head to obtain eye contact. Consider establishing a method of communication during the interview. Massage therapist Ralph Stephens developed the following system of communication.

When It Hurts or If the Pressure Is Too Deep – Tell the client, "Be sure to tell me whenever I find a tender area. Will you do that for me?" or "If at any time I am working too deep, be sure to tell me right away. Will you do that?" Quantitative measuring scales you can use are as follows:

- Ask the client to simply raise a hand if pain is felt.
- Use the 1-to-10 scale, with 1 being barely felt and 10 being the most pain imaginable. The goal is to apply pressure that registers as a 5, 6, or 7.
- Establish a thumbs up, thumbs down, "OK" gesture system. Thumbs up means that the pressure is too great. Thumbs down means that more pressure is requested. An "OK" symbol (index finger touching thumb with other fingers extended) means the pressure is perfect.

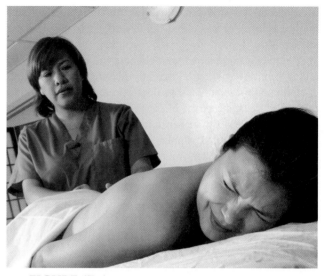

FIGURE 17-4 Therapist noticing signs of discomfort.

When It Gets Better – Tell the client, "When I find these tender places, I will stop and maintain pressure. After a while, the tenderness usually subsides and it may feel to you like I am letting up on the pressure or that it is beginning to feel better. Will you let me know when it gets better?"

If It Refers – Tell the client, "When I am examining or maintaining pressure on an area, you may experience some sensation somewhere else. It might be a pain, tingling, numbness, aching, or some other sensation, somewhere besides right where I am massaging. These may be trigger points that also need to be massaged. Will you tell me if you feel anything other than pressure where I am working?"

Nonverbal Feedback – Regardless of which system of feedback you use for assessing pain and pressure, use your peripheral vision and look for physical signs of discomfort (Figure 17-4). Some clients do not volunteer verbal feedback about pain. However, the body rarely lies. Body gestures that may indicate you are working too deep include

1. The client pulling away from you or contracting muscles to limit your access into the tissues,
2. General squirming,
3. Raising eyebrows or frowning,
4. Holding the breath,
5. White knuckles, and
6. Raising the head or foot up off the table.

When you suspect you are working too deep from the client's gestures, respond initially by changing your pressure or rhythm. If the client does not relax, then ask for verbal feedback. Reiterate how important communication is during the massage. You may discover that the client is ticklish or is in pain and is therefore splinting, or contracting, his or her muscles. The client may also have to use the restroom. Address his or her needs, and then continue with the massage. Be patient and caring.

Regarding conversation during the massage, less is better. Ask questions related to the massage, or answer questions your client asks. Being too talkative may prevent your client from relaxing. Also, limit the exchange of personal information unrelated to the therapeutic relationship.

Giving Directions – Use tactile cues and gestures when giving a client direction during the massage. For example, when you ask your client to scoot over to the edge of the table, gently touch his or her shoulder or tap the tabletop on the side toward which you want him or her to move. This method can be used when you need the client to move up or down the table and also when to turn the head to one side or another. If you need the client to raise the head, feet, or knees to accommodate a bolster, then use a gentle lifting motion with your hand. Your client may be so relaxed that verbal directions are processed slowly. Tactile cues help the client understand what you need him or her to do.

When asking your client to turn over, if eye contact is possible, supinate or pronate your hand to indicate the direction he or she should roll. When giving directions in which a client should place the arms or other body part a certain way, demonstrate this positioning, too.

Conclusion

When you are finished with the massage, remove the bolsters and wipe off any excess lubricant from the soles of your client's feet. Avoid hurrying your client off the massage table. In fact, invite the client to rest a few minutes. Because the client has been in one position for an extended period, asking the person to roll over on their side and bend the knees to the chest is often helpful. Place a soft pillow under your client's head, and ask him or her to lie in this position for a few minutes before getting up to dress. If the client is afraid of falling asleep and losing track of time, then state that you will be back in 5 minutes to remind him or her to get up. This short rest period allows the client some quiet time devoid of stimuli to integrate the physical and emotional aspects of the massage. It also allows transition time to move from internal focus to external focus before rescheduling an appointment, leaving your facility, and driving away.

You may need to instruct the client on how to get up off the table. Once the person is lying on his or her side, suggest allowing the legs to slide off the edge of the table. The client can then use the arm that is not lying against the massage table to push the upper body up into a seated position. Avoid letting the client sit straight up from a supine position because he or she may strain the lower back and neck. Remind the client that the best way to get off the massage table is also the best way to get out of bed in the morning. Your client may require assistance getting off the table (see Chapter 7).

A portion of the population (approximately 10%) finds difficulty in standing up after lying down for an extended period. This circumstance is the result of a brief decrease in blood pressure when moving from a lying-down position to an upright position, causing dizziness (the medical term for this is orthostatic or postural hypotension). In severe cases, fainting may occur. With this in mind, either (1) remind him or her to move slowly and carefully and to sit up for a few moments before standing, or (2) assist him or her into a standing position, pausing for a few moments to be sure he or she is oriented in the upright position.

If you remove your client's eyeglasses while he or she is on the massage table, or if a client gives you his or her eyeglasses before the massage, hand them back to the client before he or she gets off the massage table and before you leave the massage room to allow the person time to redress. If you neglect this important procedure, you may then be liable if your client trips or falls in your massage room and incurs injuries because he or she was unable to see clearly.

If your client removed jewelry or wristwatches, be sure they leave with these items. You may need to tell the client where these items have been placed before leaving the room for him or her to dress. In the case of a client who is physically unable to put the jewelry back on him or herself, offer assistance.

As you leave the massage room, let the client know if he or she is to wait in the room for you to return or if he or she needs to exit the room to find you in another area.

After the Session

While your client is dressing, wash or sanitize your hands and write any case notes. Be sure the lighting in the postmassage area is not too bright or too noisy because this type of environment is not relaxing. Provide a transitional space. Take a few deep breaths, and prepare to greet your client with a smile.

Avoid challenging or ego-driven statements such as "Do you feel better?" or "Was that good?" Instead, ask the client for information that is usable in documentation such as "Do you feel any change?", "Could you express it in a percent?", "Has your pain decreased?", "Is your hip moving more freely?", or "Can you pick an adjective that describes the change?"

Clients may be disoriented after a massage and may accidentally forget some of their belongings. If you do discover personal articles in a room after a massage, then you should place them inside an envelope and seal it. Write the date, the item, and the owner of the item, contact the client, and let him or her know. If you do not know who owns the item, then call the clients who were there that day and ask them if they left anything in your studio. Letting them tell you what they are missing and give you a complete description before returning the item is generally best.

Client Information. Have ready any parting information that you wish to give your client. Information sheets can be anything ranging from tips on how to use ice, self-massage, relaxation techniques, and theories about muscle soreness to how to preserve and prolong the effects of the massage (Box 17-4). Without the educational element of massage therapy,

> ## BOX 17-4
>
> ### Ten Daily Steps for Preserving and Prolonging the Effects of Your Massage
>
> - Drink at least 0.5 oz of fresh water per 1 lb of body weight.
> - Maintain a neutral sleeping posture by using pillows to bolster the extremities to keep the spine straight.
> - Stretch.
> - Apply ice packs on painful areas (for 20 minutes).
> - Be aware of your posture during the day.
> - Decrease the intake of caffeine and sugar as much as possible (these neurostimulants can increase pain perception and dehydrate the body).
> - Breathe slowly, extending the exhale.
> - Develop a positive attitude.
> - Simplify and prioritize, and take stress breaks.
> - Love yourself.

the massage session may be no more than an expensive aspirin or bandage. Avoid just putting out fires; show clients how to prevent them. Clients really appreciate this added service of valuable information on topics such as how to alter sleeping positions or how to sit in a chair comfortably to reduce muscle strain.

Some clients report becoming sore after a massage because it may produce a mild inflammatory response. However, this usually resolves within 48 hours. Some reasons for this reaction are the amount of pressure used during the massage, the length of time spent massaging an area, the health of the client's tissues, lack of client hydration, client inactivity, exposure to environmental toxins, and lack of postmassage care. If you worked an area deeply or for an extended period, or if you suspect a client may be sore, then recommend that the client drink lots of fresh water (at least 0.5 oz of water per 1 lb of body weight) and ice the area for 20 minutes.

Rescheduling. Collect fees if you have not already done so, and ask the client if he or she would like to reschedule. How often a client schedules a massage can be influenced by the therapist but is determined by the client. Massage rarely resolves issues in one session that have been bothering the client for years. Typically, clients schedule (1) once a week, (2) once a month, or (3) only when they are in pain, such as a headache or stiff shoulder. The latter client may become a regular client if he or she begins to see massage as keeping pain from occurring. If a client asks you to decide when you think he or she should come back, politely tell him or her that only when everything you have shown him or her (e.g., stretching, self-massage, cold and hot packs) fails to work. This approach builds trust and confidence between client and therapist by empowering the client.

Offer the client another glass of water before he or she departs. After the client has gone, ready your room for your next client, then breath deeply and stretch.

Some clients may want to stay and talk after the massage. If the conversation is related to the massage and the client's health and progress, then make some time to address his or her concerns. If, on the other hand, the conversation is just a friendly chat, you may have other priorities. There are often calls or e-mails to return, linens to be washed, a massage room that needs your attention, or you may need to eat. Usually, walking your client to the door, perhaps even stepping outside with him or her, saying thank you and good-bye, and walking back in the office will be enough. You may have to say something such as "I really enjoy talking with you, but I have a few things to take care of." Setting a boundary is necessary to take care of yourself and to serve other clients you have scheduled for the rest of your day (see Chapter 2).

PROFESSIONAL BURNOUT

Burnout is the condition of being tired of, or unhappy with, one's work. Burnout affects everyone from teachers to neurosurgeons. Symptoms of burnout can include simple disinterest in the job, dreading your next client, boredom, restlessness, inability to remain focused, fatigue, and outright hatred of a job or associates. Burnout can include depression, lack of productivity, increased tardiness, increased absenteeism, decline of social skills, workaholism, and a decline in professional boundaries. The added stress can also affect your health.

Burnout affects people for different reasons. Many massage therapists are "natural" entrepreneurs and are highly motivated, hardworking people. Many self-employed people have difficulty setting limits on their time. Because delineating a 40-hour week can be difficult, self-employed people may overwork, which may lead to burnout.

If burnout is the result of overwork, it is necessary to schedule time for yourself to receive nurturing because you have given so much of it away. Set aside a small amount (e.g., 1%) of your daily net income towards that time off. Burnout can be managed or prevented by working toward balance in our own lives first, and then assisting others who are struggling to do the same. A few suggestions for managing burnout follow.

Nurture Yourself

Eat right, get enough rest, and exercise. Spend time with people you like, read a book, or take a class in something you enjoy such as photography or painting. Rediscover things you like to do, or try new things that you might enjoy. Write down 10 things you currently like to do and how long it has been since you have done them. This activity may be quite revealing. List each activity on a separate strip of paper and place the strips in a jar. When you feel excessively stressed or on the verge of burnout, pick one of the activities from the jar and do it. This exercise is also a great stress-reduction activity to recommend for your clients. Refer to Chapter 4 for other ideas on self-care.

Stimulate Yourself

Some therapists experience burnout from the boredom of repetitive routines and lack of challenge. If this is the case, take a continuing education workshop. Workshops also bring you together with your colleagues. Online forums and social networks are another way to stay connected and energized. Whether it is a local group or an international one, social networks offer a means to meet new people and be introduced to new ideas. Or, take a class in something interesting and outrageous, not just massage technique and anatomy.

Sojourn

Scheduling a certain amount of time off is extremely important for massage therapists. If your massage days are Monday through Friday, then take off Saturday and Sunday; or if everyone wants Saturday massages, then take off Sunday and Monday. Remember that you cannot give away what you do not have and that recharging your own batteries is necessary. Do not forget to vacation at least once a year. Get away from the office, especially if you work out of your home. If you feel the need, then take a break from massage altogether. Shift gears and take a sabbatical. Use this time not only to recharge your batteries but also to reevaluate important decisions or situations.

Relax with Massage

Get massages yourself (Figure 17-5). Regular massages are a necessity because of the tremendous physical requirements of this job. The recommended minimum is one massage per month. No maximum number exists.

"I am indeed rich, since my income is superior to my expense, and my expense is equal to my wishes."
—Edward Gibson

FINANCES

Now that your business planning has begun and you have learned some ways to nurture and promote it, you need to know strategies for staying in business. The economics of private practice usually move in a spiral, not a linear, pattern. This and the next several sections explore ideas for diversifying your income, adding insurance billing and reimbursement to your practice, and monitoring the pulse of your business through basic accounting and financial reports. Also included are discussions of taxes and tax deductions, handling insufficient funds, and investing in your future. But first, you must decide what to charge for your services.

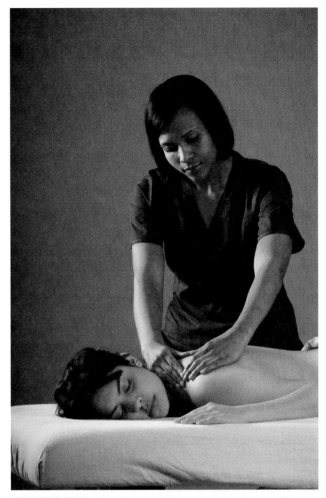

FIGURE 17-5 Therapist receiving a massage from a colleague.

Determining Fees

If you work for yourself, you need to determine your fees and establish a fee schedule. Most therapists charge for time, often in 30-, 60-, or 90-minute increments. The price per minute (increment) is usually lowered as the session time increases. For example, a therapist may charge $40 for 30 minutes, then $60 for 60 minutes, and $80 for 90 minutes.

Some therapists charge a fee for a relaxing massage and then a higher fee for deeper pressure or for specialized methods, such as manual lymphatic or neuromuscular techniques.

Several things are factored into determining fees. For example, massage usually cost more in metropolitan areas and less in rural areas where the cost of living is lower. A therapist with experience or specialized training may charge more than a newly graduated therapist. House calls cost more because they require additional expense and time.

Be sure your clients know, in advance, how much their session will cost and the methods of payment you accept such as cash, checks, or credit/debit cards. Charging more in certain circumstances, such as when an insurance company is involved or using credit/debit cards, is unethical and illegal.

Prepayment plans are frequently offered by massage therapists such as pay for X and get X free. One therapist sells what she calls a 6-pack and a 12-pack. When you purchase a 6-pack, you are prepaying for 5 sessions at full price and in advance, and receive the sixth session free. Or when you purchase a 12-pack, you are prepaying for 10 sessions at full price and receive the eleventh and twelfth sessions free. Have a time of year in mind when promoting these packages to match your desire to increase or stabilize cash flow. Offering a 6-pack for "summer," Memorial Day to Labor Day, gets clients in during a slow season. A "New Year of Wellness" 12-pack sold at Christmas with a coupon good for each month of the year secures this year's steady client who will come once a month. Avoid offering packages that will do nothing more than allow steady clients to get a reduced price massage.

Consider offering something besides a massage (e.g., salt glow, lotion) as the bonus item for prepurchases. If the service or item is something your client has not tried, it may be purchased in the future. The service or item can be from another business (e.g., facial, eyebrow waxing). This is a great way to build relationships with other professionals.

You must clearly indicate the time frame in which prepaid services can be redeemed. This includes expiration dates on gift certificates. As of November 1, 2008, the federal government requires all businesses that sell gift cards or certificates to have an expiration date of no sooner than 5 years from the date the card is issued.

Bartering

Bartering is the practice of exchanging goods or services for other goods or services without the use of money. Therapists often barter massage sessions for things they need or want. This ranges from haircuts to appliances.

It is important to realize that the fair market value of the bartered goods or services must be included as part of your income. For example, if you have bartered $1000 worth of services in exchange for a boat valued at $1000, you are required to include 100% bartered services (in this case $1000) as income on your tax return (1099-B form).

The reciprocating party is required to do the same. Your client who bartered the boat valued at $1000 is required to report its fair market value (in this case $1000) as barter exchange income on his or her tax return via a 1099-B form.

Tips and Gifts

In massage therapy, tips (gratuities) are small gifts, usually of money, given to the therapist who provided the service. The amount, which is determined by the client, is an addition to the cost of the session ($70 [massage] + $14 [20% tip] = $84). Tips are a common occurrence in personal service occupations. By contrast, tips are not commonly given to therapists who work in a medical or rehabilitative setting such as physical therapy or chiropractic care.

In settings where tipping is customary, the person who owns the business or who is self-employed and receive the full price of the massage is not usually tipped. Tipping is meant to be a way to compensate people who receive only a portion of the service fee and to thank them for good service. Therefore employees or independent contractors who receive a portion of the price of the massage may accept tips.

Tips should not be solicited by the therapist. Be sure that tippers and nontippers receive the same level of care. Good tippers should not receive preferential treatment.

Gifts, nonmonetary tokens of appreciation, may be given to therapists during special occasions, such as holidays or birthdays. The general rule when accepting tips or gifts is that they do not exceed the price of the massage. Also, do not accept gifts from a client who you suspect has a romantic or sexual intention (i.e., gifts of lingerie).

The IRS considers tips taxable income. Keep a record of your tips and report them as income when filing your income tax return.

Start-up Costs

Start-up costs vary from person to person and from one geographic region to the next. Take a realistic look at how much money you will need to open your doors. The following discussion assumes that you will be working for yourself.

Once you have made your initial calculations, you can make adjustments before purchases are made if you find that the figures are high. For example, you may decide that asking another therapist to share certain expenses with you will be advantageous financially. High overhead and maintaining an office are risky when you are just starting out and do not have many steady clients. Some costs, such as advertising and printing, must eventually be repeated. Box 17-5 is a worksheet that helps clarify start-up costs.

Insufficient Fund Transactions

When you receive an insufficient ("not sufficient") funds (NSF) transactions, call your client as soon as possible and politely explain the situation. Tell the client that you are mailing him or her a certified letter to serve as official notification, and ask him or her for a specific time and date when he or she can make payment. Write this information down. Send a copy of the letter by regular mail too (i.e., send two identical letters—one by certified mail with return receipt requested and one by regular mail). Receive payment for the NSF transactions in cash or money order. Most businesses also collect an additional NSF check fee (e.g., an extra $20 to $30) to cover costs associated with collection and bank charges. Yes, you are now spending your time and money collecting a debt.

BOX 17-5

Determining Start-Up Costs

Opening a business checking account _____

Equipment and machinery (massage tables, stereo, telephone) _____

Room furnishings and fixtures (shelves, lamp, chair) _____

Office rent (first and one month's rent plus security deposit) _____

Telephone deposit and installation costs _____

Utility deposits and installation costs _____

Legal and professional services (accountant, attorney) _____

Personnel _____

Insurance (auto, general liability, malpractice, property) _____

Professional society membership (may be an insurance payment) _____

Initial licenses and permits _____

Remodeling _____

Initial office supplies (appointment book, stapler, pens) _____

Initial massage supplies (linens, massage lubricants) _____

Advertising and promotion _____

Printing cost (business cards, gift certificates, stationery, forms) _____

Petty cash _____

Miscellaneous _____

TOTAL _____

If you have not received payment within 10 days after receiving verification that the certified letter was claimed, or if your certified letter was returned unclaimed or refused, then contact your local district attorney's office. Do not open the certified letter if it is returned to you. The district attorney's office may require the returned item, a copy of the certified letter, your returned receipt card, or the unopened returned certified letter.

If you accepted a postdated check and it was returned, then you have accepted a check knowing the person did not have money in his or her bank account. In this case, the district attorney's office may not be able to help you.

In any case, be pleasant, patient, understanding, and persistent. See Evolve for a sample letter to be used in these circumstances.

Diversifying Your Income

The business world is a jungle, and the law of the jungle is survival of the fittest. One way to survive in the ever-changing business environment is by diversifying your income. Diversification helps minimize the effects of fluctuation in the market (whether its the consumer market or the stock market); diversification helps reduce financial stress while you are building a clientele. The idea of diversity follows the same idea as in financial investments: Do not put all your eggs in one basket. Finding 10 places to scrape up $1000 each year is easier than finding one place that provides $10,000. Diversify your income by using different strategies for producing revenue. Here are a few ideas to protect you from extinction.

Retail Sales. Selling products at retail cost helps to increase your revenue. Clients may choose to buy individual containers of massage cream; massage tools; relaxation music; essential oils, candles, or bath salts; and eye, neck, and back pillows. If you are going to sell retail goods, then be sure that you have the proper license requirements. You may also need to collect and pay sales tax regularly. The following should be considered:

- Be sure that many, if not most, items are easily affordable. Clients may buy a $7 item; few will buy a $50 item.
- Sell items at a significant markup. Common markups are between 50% and 100% above wholesale price.
- The items should be related to massage or relaxation. Do not sell candy and cigarettes.
- Sell what you use yourself or what you would recommend.

Be sure to record when these items were purchased, how much you paid for them (wholesale), and how much they sold (retail). Your **inventory** is the unsold items you have on hand.

Selling products to clients creates a dual relationship and possible conflicts of interest. See Chapter 2 for a complete discussion.

Expand Your Services. Offer clients a variety of treatment options. Some therapists offer whirlpool baths, steam rooms, saunas, salt scrubs, hot stone massage, and other services. Or perhaps, take a new technique or method you learned at a worshop and teach an introductory version at the local massage school. Offer a low-cost class in massage therapy or relaxation techniques at your local college or university or community center for people who want to learn massage to work on a family member or friend.

Specialized Training. This is a good way to attract new business and expand your client base. Most states require massage therapists to obtain continuing education each year. Training in a new area of expertise may be worthwhile. Learn an approach or technique that is unique to your community—something that will fill a gap in the existing market. For example, if you practice relaxation massage, then you might want to attend a workshop in hydrotherapy, get some experience in the field, and open a day spa facility.

Work in More than One Location. Locate part-time work a couple of afternoons a week for a chiropractor or physical or occupational therapist. Offer chair massage at the local health food store or busy office building. Offer foot massage at shoeshine booths, and share the proceeds with the owner.

Insurance Reimbursement

Insurance billing is another aspect of expanding your practice and increasing your income. Massage has been proved to be effective in treating musculoskeletal and myofascial pain, and physicians are referring clients to massage therapists. Physical and occupational therapists are hiring massage therapists to work in their offices. When the time-consuming work of massage is handled by massage therapists, the physical and occupational therapist becomes free to perform the more technically demanding tasks of evaluations, assigning exercise protocols, and so on. Chiropractors also are taking advantage of the success of massage therapy by employing therapists within their practices and billing insurance for massage services.

Many rewards and frustrations exist related to insurance reimbursement. The therapist must be willing and able to prepare and submit all required documents related to client care and wait for reimbursement, which may take months or even years, at which time the therapist's bill may be reduced or even denied.

"If I had really wanted to do all this damned secretarial work, I'd have gone to secretarial school."
—S. Devillier

Health maintenance organizations (HMOs) and preferred provider organizations (PPOs) will cover services provided by therapists who are on an approved list. As of 2011, federal insurance programs such as Medicare and Medicaid do not cover massage. Most major medical policies issued by insurance companies do not include massage therapy. The types of cases most likely to cover the cost of massage therapy are personal injury (PI) cases, automobile medical insurance and automobile liability, and worker's compensation.

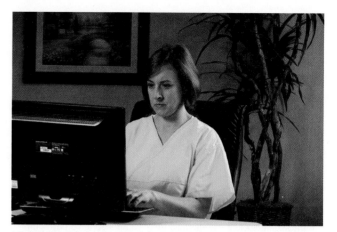

FIGURE 17-6 Therapist downloading needed forms from the Internet.

Additional signed documents are needed in these cases—not only a completed client intake form but a medical release form (see Box 10-9) as well. These forms allow the therapist to communicate legally with the client's health care providers, as well as agents of the insurance company, about the client's injuries. Also obtain a physician's prescription.

When submitting a claim, include the client's name, date of services, fees for services, payments and adjustments, previous and current balance due, Current Procedural Terminology (CPT) codes, the therapist's contact information and provider number (if applicable), and the therapist's tax identification number. Avoid using a social security number as a tax identification number because of identification theft issues. This claim form, an HCFA 1500 form, can be purchased in most stationery supply stores or downloaded from the Internet (Figure 17-6).

Accurate documentation is essential when expecting insurance reimbursement. Progress notes for each session document the course and progress of treatments and are required to establish the validity of massage and to help determine whether to approve current and future treatments, because insurance companies pay only for services that are deemed medically necessary. The first priority here is that these clients are now patients; a prescription for their care has been ordered by a physician, who is now the primary caregiver. You must communicate with this individual and the insurance representative. You must possess the necessary skills to handle the condition that this patient presents with, and be able to accurately describe your evaluation procedure, treatment plan, and verify your progress objectively. If you feel confident to do this, then proceed. If not, refer the client to a different therapist.

From a business perspective, the first rule of insurance filing is to never compromise your cash flow. In other words, do not take insurance cases over cash-paying clients. Realize that insurance clients may be seen as often as three times a week; therefore you must be sure you have the time in your current schedule to accommodate the needs of a patient. And if you want to work a personal injury claim, you should be good with paperwork.

The second rule is to be aware that attorneys are often involved in these cases; the legal considerations involved typically represents additional work for you and some possible risks. These claims are the most challenging regarding payment. Personal injury cases that involve an attorney will include having you sign a lien. This will stipulate that if the patient is not successful in winning their case you may not get paid, or you may be paid a portion of your claim, and you will not be able to bill the patient for the outstanding amount. With an attorney involved, you will not get payment until the case is settled, which can sometimes take years.

The upside is if your service fees include work performed under prescription with a responsible price to cover all additional work considerations, and you perform these services for the 2 or sometimes 3 years it may take to conclude, and the patient recovers considerable damages, you will (finally) get a check that will cover your next vacation and the paint job the office needed.

It is all a matter of what kinds of services you wish to provide.

Paperwork for insurance claims is time-consuming and runs up costs because it takes away from time with your regular clientele. You can also hire a medical billing company to take care of treatment authorization and filing for you. These companies get paid per sheet of claims they file, and bill monthly. So you need to be prepared to pay them before you receive your insurance reimbursement.

HCFA 1500 Form. The Health Care Financing Administration created the HCFA 1500 form as a method of standardizing claims, eliminating the confusion of different forms for different insurance companies. Medicare and Medicaid use the Centers for Medicare & Medicaid Services (CMS) form, which is identical to the HCFA 1500 form and therefore interchangeable. Both forms are designed to be read by an optical character-recognition program to assist in the processing of insurance claims.

When filing a claim, insurance companies require a diagnosis code, or ICD-9 code, identifying the attending physician's diagnosis. ICD-9 is an acronym for Internal Classification of Disease, ninth edition. The U.S. Health Services and U.S. Health Care Financing Administration publish these codes. Only a physician can provide a medical diagnosis and its corresponding ICD-9 code.

Also required for filing are procedural codes, or current procedural terminology (CPT) codes, identifying services provided to the client. CPT codes are published annually by the American Medical Association. These codes are arranged according to their specialty; massage is classified as physical medicine. Because CPT codes do change, consult the most recently published list or consult with the client's physician's office or an insurance agent. A few current codes are:
97010—Hot and cold packs
97124—Massage (soft tissue mobilization)

97140—Myofascial release
97139—Therapeutic procedure
97112—Neuromuscular reeducation

Most procedures are applied in 15-minute increments.

Once the claim is submitted, the insurance company has 30 days to respond. If 6 weeks have lapsed and the insurance company has not contacted you, then you should contact the insurance company. Document the inquiry by stating the time and date of the telephone call, as well as the names of the person(s) to whom you spoke and what was said.

If no reasonable action has been taken after the second inquiry, then contact the client's attorney (if one is available) or file a compliant with your state insurance commissioner. If the claim was denied, then contact the client and inform him or her of the insurance company's decision and that he or she is now responsible for the balance due. A signed agreement stating this before treatment begins is standard protocol.

ACCOUNTING

Accounting is the art of interpreting, measuring, and describing economic activity. Whether you are preparing a household budget, balancing a checkbook, preparing an income tax return, or running your massage practice or a major corporation, you are working with accounting concepts (Box 17-6). Accounting has often been called the language of business.

BOX 17-6

Accounting Terminology

Accounting. The art of interpreting, measuring, and describing economic activity.

Accounts payable. Money you owe to suppliers.

Accounts receivable. Money owed to you or your business.

Assets. Economic resources that offer value to your business.

Balance sheet. A summary of all of your business assets and liabilities and the owner's equity at an exact point in time, usually at the end of a quarter or a fiscal year.

Cash flow. Movement of money into and out of a business.

Depreciation. The process of spreading out the deduction for the cost of an asset over time.

Equity. The difference between your total assets and your liabilities; also called net worth.

Gross income. All the money a person or business makes before subtracting expenses or taxes.

Liabilities. Debts that your business owes.

Net income. The amount of money a person or business has left after subtracting expenses and taxes.

Petty cash. Cash used to pay for incidental expenses. Usually set up and treated like a separate account.

Profit and loss statement. Summary of your income and expenses over a fixed period, indicating whether your business made a profit or sustained a loss.

Business Checking Account

Begin by opening up a business checking account. If the account will be in a business name rather than your personal name, a DBA (doing business as) designation issued from the courthouse is usually required.

Use this account when depositing all money earned as a result of your business and paying business expenses. Avoid combining personal transactions (deposits or withdrawals) with business transactions.

If you are sharing expenses with another therapist, then avoid commingling funds to maintain your separate business entity.

Petty Cash

Petty cash is cash that is used to pay for incidental expenses. Petty cash is usually set up and treated like a separate account. Establish your petty cash account by writing yourself a check and cashing it. Most businesses keep $100 to $200 in this fund. Keep this money in a separate envelope or small lock box. Do not put cash received from clients in this account.

Use this account when purchasing small incidental business-related expenses you pay in cash (e.g., paper, mailing certified letters). Be sure to write petty cash on any cash receipts and file them in a secure location. When the fund dwindles, total the receipts from petty cash transactions and write yourself another check equal to the amount of the receipts. This exchange will replenish the fund to its original balance.

At any given time, you should be able to count the money and receipts and balance back to the originally established total.

Accountant Versus Accounting Software

Acquiring an accountant or a bookkeeper can help you with record keeping, financial statements, and preparation of tax forms. A good accountant can help you save money and evaluate tax consequences of tax deductions and major purchases.

Accounting software packages such as Peachtree or Quickbooks Pro (the latter is what I use) can be used to help with your accounting needs.

If you have an accountant or plan to get one, ask which software program he or she recommends, because you will be giving him or her electronic copies of files throughout the year.

Payroll

If you have employees, then you need to keep track of their payroll. Payroll is the total of all salaries, taxes (state, federal, and Social Security), deductions, and bonuses paid to employees as well as local, state, and federal governments.

When filing reports related to payroll, you must acquire an employer identification number (EIN). Also called a federal tax identification number, your EIN is a nine-digit number that begins with the prefix 72.

FINANCIAL REPORTS

Financial information is used to prepare three key financial reports: cash flow statement, profit and loss statement, and balance sheet. The accuracy of these reports reflects the accuracy of the financial information you collect and record throughout the year. These reports will help you track business and financial trends and spot potential problem areas that may need attention. If you are trying to get a business loan or have another financial need, then you will probably need to produce these reports.

Cash Flow Statements

Cash flow is the movement of money into and out of a business. Cash flow statements measure this activity over a finite period of time, such as a month, quarterly (every 3 months), or annually (every 12 months). If more money comes into the business than is distributed, the cash balance increases and the business is said to have a positive cash flow. Conversely, if the cash balance decreases, the business has a negative cash flow.

Because cash flow is regarded as the life-giving blood of a business, keeping track of these amounts and having the opportunity to regulate these amounts may make the difference between whether your business thrives or not.

Profit and Loss Statements

Profit and loss (P&L) statements, also called income statements, summarize your income and expenses over a fixed period, indicating whether your business made a profit or sustained a loss. Most businesses prepare these statements monthly, quarterly, or annually.

Balance Sheets

Balance sheets, also called statements of financial condition, summarize all of your businesses assets and liabilities and the owner's equity at an exact point in time, usually at the end of a quarter or a fiscal year.

Terms Used in Financial Reports

Understanding the following terms will assist you when reviewing your financial reports.

Assets. In business, **assets** are economic resources that offer value to your business. Assets are divided into current and fixed assets. *Current assets* are cash on hand, including petty cash; money in checking and savings accounts;

accounts receivable (money owed to you or your business); prepaid expenses such as deposits on rent, utilities, and insurance; and the value of your inventory. *Fixed assets* are purchases that are needed to continually operate your business, including machinery, equipment, and furniture such as a massage table, computer, and computer desk. Vehicles, property, and buildings that are owned by the business are also fixed assets.

Liabilities. **Liabilities** are debts that your business owes. Liabilities can be classified as current liabilities and long-term liabilities. Examples of *current liabilities* are accounts payable (what you owe to suppliers); payments you owe on business loans that will be paid off within 1 year; accrued expenses such as salaries, wages, and commissions that you owe but have not paid; and taxes that you owe but have not paid. Examples of these taxes are payroll, sales, income, property, and self-employment taxes. *Long-term liabilities* are expenses that extend beyond 1 calendar year and include mortgage payments on your business location and promissory notes taken out on behalf of the business for major purchases.

Equity. Also called net worth, **equity** is the difference between your total assets and your liabilities. If your assets outweigh your liabilities, you are said to have positive equity. Conversely, if your liabilities outweigh your assets, you have negative equity.

Gross Income. **Gross income** is all the money a person or business makes before subtracting expenses or taxes.

Net Income. **Net income** is the amount of money a person or business has left after subtracting expenses and taxes. Net income is often called the *bottom line* because it is the last line of a person's or business's P&L statement.

> *"Though I am grateful for the blessings of wealth, it hasn't changed who I am. My feet are still on the ground. I'm just wearing better shoes."*
> —Oprah Winfrey

CHAT ROOM

Debt-to-income ratio (DTI) is the relationship, stated as a percentage, between your monthly gross income and your monthly payments on loans, including payments made on your home, car, and credit cards. DTI is often used by financial institutions when determining loan eligibility. One bank I called said that for home loans, loan officers accept a DTI of 28%. For consumer loans, you need DTI of 40%. Each financial institution will use a different percentage when calculating loan eligibility. There are calculators available on the Internet if you would like to know your DTI.

TAXES

All businesses and individuals pay tax. Taxes are paid on income, sales, inventory, property, capital gains, just to name a few. Tax laws change periodically; consult your accountant about current tax information.

Income Tax

Taxes must be paid on the net income (or profits) you or your business earns. The percentage you pay depends on your tax bracket. If your net income is low (let us say $7000), your tax bracket is often low (e.g., 10%). If your net income is high (let's say $200,000), your tax bracket is often higher (e.g., 33%). The amount paid to state and local governments varies from region to region. Contact your state and local departments of revenue for more information.

Track how much profit (or loss) you are generating throughout the year. If you notice a large profit during the year, then begin preparing for a sizable income tax payment by saving money or by making quarterly estimated tax payments.

Self-Employment Tax

When you are an employee, your employer deducts a percentage of your wages (usually 7.65%) for Social Security and Medicare tax. The employee then matches the amount deducted (usually 7.65%) and pays this (now 15.3%) to the IRS. At the end of the year, your employer issues you a W-2 form, which includes your total wages, tips, and compensation, as well as withholdings. When you prepare your income tax return, you will determine if you owe additional tax or if you are entitled to a tax refund.

When you are self-employed, you are required to pay both the employer's and the employee's portion of Social Security and Medicare taxes, which is currently 15.3%. Most self-employed individuals pay self-employment tax quarterly, but check with a tax consultant to be sure.

Sales Tax

If you sell products, you may be required to collect sales tax. These collected taxes are paid to state and local governments on a regular basis, usually once a month. Some municipalities tax services such as massage, whereas others do not.

Be sure to obtain a sales tax number. Use this number on all payment vouchers. Contact your local department of revenue and taxation for more information.

Tax Deductions

Anyone who is self-employed (files a Schedule C with Form 1040) or operates as a corporate business can deduct the amount of any business-related expenses from their gross income. Tax deductions, or tax-deductible expenses, lower your overall taxable income and thus lower the amount of tax paid. As stated previously, the exact amount of tax savings is dependent on your tax bracket.

Let us say rent on your building is $600 per month ($7200 annually). If you are in the 10% tax bracket, you will pay $720 less income tax annually. If you are in the 33% tax bracket, you will pay $2376 less income tax annually.

Tax Bracket	10%	33%
Annual Income	$15,000	$100,000
Taxes Due	$1500	$33,000
Subtract Rent	−$7200	−$7200
Adjusted Income	$7800	$92,800
Adjusted Taxes Due	$780	$30,624
Taxes saved	$720	$2376

The IRS says that you may deduct any ordinary and necessary items from your business; therefore you may deduct needed items that may not be common in other businesses but that make your business function efficiently.

For tax purposes, keep all your business receipts, past income tax returns, and documents related to your tax returns for 7 years. Be sure to consult with your accountant to help you make timely decisions when purchasing assets (from a tax liability perspective). Examples of tax deductions are as follows:

- Accounting and bookkeeping fees
- Accounting or computer courses (may be deductible as continuing education)
- Advertising and promotion
- Bank service charges and card merchant fees
- Books and periodicals
- Business-related insurance
- Continuing education and professional development
- Conventions and conferences of business and trade organizations
- Depreciation on major purchases
- Gifts to and entertaining current or prospective clients (IRS limits apply)
- Health insurance
- Interest on business and investment loans; business bank card interest and annual fees incurred
- Laundry and cleaning services
- Legal, consulting, and professional services
- License fees
- Mileage (IRS mileage cost per mile can be used or deduct actual cost, but not both), excluding travel to and from work; keep a mileage log if you deduct cost per mile
- Office supplies (including lubricants)
- Postage and shipping charges
- Printing and duplication
- Rent (home office; use a ratio of office space to total square footage)
- Repairs to office or equipment

- Uniforms and protective clothing
- Utilities and telephone service (home office; unless you have a business-dedicated meter, use a percentage of utilities; should be the same percentage used to determine rent amount; cannot deduct personal telephone line but can deduct business-related long distance calls or get a separate business line)

Keep a record of your fixed assets such as equipment, machines, furniture, computer and computer peripherals, vehicles, and other business-related property. The value of these items may need to be depreciated. **Depreciation** is the process of spreading out the deduction for the cost of an asset over time. Some fixed assets can be deducted in one fiscal year. Check with your tax consultant to see whether it is tax advantageous for you to take the deduction in one or multiple years.

INVESTING IN YOUR FUTURE

A business plan will help you chart your business course (see Business Plan section). Also important is putting away money for a rainy day because cash flow fluctuates from day to day and from year to year. You need to build a cash reserve to get you through tough times when more money is going out than coming in, when you are unemployed, or when any other financial disasters occur.

Do not wait until you have a goal (college for children, retirement) to start investing in your future.

10% Rule

Once a week to once a month, pay yourself 10% of your gross income. Yes, you have bills, so consider yourself a creditor you must pay. You will always have bills, so do not wait until you have extra money to begin saving. Do it. 10%. No excuses.

Cash Reserve

Put this money in a liquid account (e.g., savings account, interest-bearing checking account) so you can access it quickly and easily. When you have enough money saved to pay for 6 months of living expenses, you have reached your goal of an adequate cash reserve to be used in emergencies and when you are ready to begin your next financial goal, investing.

Invest for the Long Term

After you have your cash reserve in place, continue with the 10% rule (pay yourself 10% of your gross income). This time, instead of putting money into a liquid account, put it in an investment vehicle in your financial portfolio such as stock, bonds, funds, certificates of deposits, or a retirement account. If done properly, this money will grow over time. A **financial portfolio** is all of the various investments held by an individual investor. What you choose to buy will depend on your need for income, your personality (whether you can handle it when the stock, bond, or fund price fluctuates), and your risk tolerance. The following investment guidelines can help you with market investing.

Invest Systemically. When you invest in stocks or funds, buying when they are at their lowest price is almost impossible (unless you have a crystal ball). But if you invest the same amount systematically and periodically over a specific time period (such as $50 monthly) in a particular investment, more shares are purchased when prices are low and fewer shares when prices are high. This lowers the total average cost per share. This strategy is called *dollar-cost averaging.*

Diversify. Do not put all your eggs in one basket. If you allocate your money among several different sectors of the market (energy, consumer goods, pharmaceuticals), or different types of securities (stocks, bonds, mutual funds), your portfolio performs better. Many investors use the *diversity by five* strategy, which means carefully selecting five companies (names you know such as Coca Cola, Wal-Mart, or Exxon Mobil) and purchase stock from these companies methodically. Odds are that three of these will perform well, one will offer a stellar performance, and one will be disappointing.

Consider Using Professional Advice. Finding a good financial advisor is tricky. Brokers make their living whether you make money or not; they get a commission if you buy or sell. Many horror stories have been told about unscrupulous financial advisors who recommend purchasing something for an exorbitant fee that only later you discover never performed even though you were charged. If you wish to consult with a financial advisor, ask around for someone who gives you the pros and cons of an investment and lets you make the decision. It is important that you like and trust this person. Ask for references, too.

SECURITIES

Securities are the instruments that represent financial value. Types of securities are stocks and bonds. A *mutual fund* contains many types of securities (but mostly stocks). Unless money is invested in a retirement account or other tax shelter, you will owe tax on income gained from your investments (i.e., capital gains tax).

Stocks

Stock is a type of security issued in the form of shares. Shares represent ownership in a company. As a stockholder (or shareholder), you reap rewards of the company's profits but also suffer the company's losses. Most companies pay their stockholders dividends. A *dividend* is a portion of a company's profits distributed at regular intervals to its shareholders. Money derived from dividends can be reinvested to buy more shares or can be paid to you in cash.

A *stock market* is a public market used for trading company stock. A *stock exchange* is a facility where stocks listed on the stock market are bought and sold (e.g., the New York Stock Exchange on Wall Street). Most stock trading is done by stock brokers.

The stock market does not move in one direction all year, but historically the stock market moves up over time, even with relatively sharp downturns.

Recommendations for how much of your portfolio is in the stock market varies with age (i.e., people close to retirement will usually have less of their portfolio in the stock market than persons in their 30s). Regardless of your age, if you cannot sleep at night worrying about your investments, then you probably should not be investing in the stock market or you are in the wrong sector of the market (e.g., consumer goods, utilities, health care, technology).

Bonds

A bond is loan in which you (the investor) are the lender. The borrowers range from the government (government bonds), municipalities (municipal bonds or "munis"), and corporations (corporate bonds). In exchange for your money, the borrower agrees to pay you interest at a predetermined rate. Interest earned on municipal and government bonds is often tax free.

The proceeds of the bond issue are used for many purposes such as to fund infrastructure (bridges, roads), expand operations, or develop an area of a city.

When the bond matures (after a period ranging from 1 to 40 years), the borrower returns your initial investment. Most people who buy bonds need to receive a regular income, such as individuals who are already retired.

Funds

A mutual fund contains a variety of securities. An investment firm pools money from many investors. Then a manager, often someone within the firm, manages the fund. The fund manager trades the pooled money on a regular basis. The net proceeds or losses are distributed to the investors either quarterly or annually.

Equity funds, which consist mainly of stocks, are the most common type of mutual fund. Other types of mutual funds are bond funds and money market funds.

Some mutual funds charge a fee to join and to withdraw; other funds are no-load funds, which mean no fee is charged when shares are bought or sold.

Index funds are unmanaged mutual funds that seek to replicate the performance of established market indices. Some well-known indexes include the Dow Jones Industrial Average, Standard & Poor's 500 Index and the NASDAQ Composite Index.

RETIREMENT ACCOUNTS

The federal government wants you to save for your own retirement, too. In fact, they help you by allowing you to treat all or part of your contributions to an individual retirement account (IRA) as a tax deduction (the exception is the Roth IRA). The income you earn from a traditional IRA is tax-deferred; therefore taxes are not due until you begin withdrawing the money during retirement. At this future time, you will probably be in a lower tax bracket.

Money in an IRA can be invested in a wide variety of securities (certificates of deposit [CDs], stocks, bonds, or funds). You have until April 15 to make contributions for the previous year. In 2010, the maximum deductible contribution is $5000. For individuals 50 years of age or older, an additional $1000 can be contributed for a total of $6000; this is known as a catch-up contribution. Please consult your accountant or your financial advisor for current information.

If you withdraw funds from a retirement account before you qualify (usually age-dependant), then you have 90 days to replace it or you may pay income tax on the amount withdrawn plus a penalty.

However, the federal government does allow you to withdraw the money under certain conditions (e.g., education, down payment on primary residence). Under these conditions, you are taxed on the distribution but not penalized. You can sometimes borrow against retirement accounts; thus it can be regarded as an asset and therefore loan collateral.

A Roth IRA, which was created through the Taxpayer Relief Act of 1997, does not allow you to write off contributions, but income derived as a result of distributions during retirement is tax-free.

BUSINESS PLAN

No chapter on business is complete without discussing business plans. These are essentially tools in which you gather data to answer questions related to aspects of a current to prospective business. This will assist you in (1) identifying your business parameters and (2) developing a better understanding of what areas need attention. The components of a basic business plan are personal information; general description of your business; services, fees, and pricing; competition; your location and operations; and your management and personnel.

Personal Information
1. What is my experience in this business, if any?
2. What do I love about my work?
3. What are my weaknesses and shortcomings?
4. What are my strengths and talents?
5. What is special and distinct about me as a massage therapist? Why will these attributes appeal to clients?
6. What are my values?

7. What have I learned about this business from fellow therapists, teachers, trade journals, and trade suppliers?

General Description of Business
1. What is my vision statement?
2. What is my mission statement?
3. What services do I or will I offer? Describe these services and the benefits of these services.
4. For what purpose will people buy my services?
5. Am I willing to change what I offer, to some extent, to meet my clients' changing needs?

Operating Procedures
1. What types of licenses are required to operate my business?
2. What will be the opening date of my business? What hours of the day and days of the week will I be in operation?
3. What will my office policies be for late clients, cancellations, out-of-date gift certificate redemption, insufficient funds checks, and credit/debit card sales?

Management and Personnel
1. What is my management experience?
2. What do I predict my legal structure will be?
3. Who will be the other key figures in my business? Include an organizational chart, list of duties and backgrounds of key individuals, outside consultants or advisers, and board of directors.
4. How will services be provided? Will I do all the work, or will I use employees or independent contractors?
5. What are the types of support that my business may require? Include child care, janitorial service, lawn and garden care, and bookkeeping and accounting.
6. What are the wages and benefits I can offer each employee and support person?

Insurance Needs
1. What are my insurance needs? These may include professional and general liability, business personal property, automotive, life and health insurance, and disability insurance.
2. Have I contacted an agent to discuss what types of policies they offer, and the cost and benefit of each?

Marketing and Competition
1. What do I want my business identity to be? Describe the image you want to project. You never get a second chance to make a first impression.
2. What do I want people to say to others about my services?
3. Who is my target market? Who will want to buy my services? Identify important characteristics such as age, gender, occupation, income, and so on.
4. Who else provides a similar service? In order of their strength in the market, list your five closest competitors

by name and address. Next, describe each competitor's strengths and weaknesses.

5. What have I learned from my competitors' operations and from their advertising?
6. What will my fee schedule look like? How have I determined these fees? Will this price cover my material costs, labor costs, and overhead?
7. What are my competitors charging?
8. How am I different from my competitors in ways that matter to potential clients?

Advertising, Promotion, and Location

1. How can I get the attention of the people I want to reach? Which advertising media are appropriate for my business and targeted clients?
2. What other channels such as social networking, referrals, and publicity will I use to reach clients?
3. How can I discover whether a promotion is working?
4. What is my advertising budget for 6 months? Include specific media you will use and the cost of each.
5. What type of location does my business require? Describe the type of building your business needs, including office and studio space, parking, exterior lighting, security needs, and proximity to other businesses for added exposure.
6. Where do I plan to locate my business? Is this location right for my business and me?
7. What geographic area will my business serve? Are sufficient numbers of potential clients located there?
8. What type of physical layout is needed for my business? Include layout for reception area, restroom, hydrotherapy and spa room (if applicable), retail and inventory areas, and gift certificate sales.

Financial Projections

1. How much money do I have to begin this business?
2. What is the cost of my capital equipment, supply list, and other start-up items?
3. If money is to be borrowed, do I have a bank and loan officer in mind?
4. How will my business be profitable? Produce an income projection [profit and loss statements], balance sheet, cash flow statement, and break-even analysis. The projection should cover 3 years—that is, the first year projects monthly and the next 2 years project quarterly.
5. Based on these documents, how much money will I need to make to stay in business?
6. What are the growth opportunities?

E-RESOURCES

Ⓔvolve

http://evolve.elsevier.com/Salvo/MassageTherapy

- Chapter challenge
- Flash cards
- Photo gallery
- Additional information
- Weblinks

BIBLIOGRAPHY

Allen L: *One year to a successful massage therapy practice*, Philadelphia, 2009, Lippincott Williams & Wilkins.

AMTA (website): http://www.amtamassage.org/articles/2/PressRelease/detail/2146.

Ashley M: *Massage: a career at your fingertips*, ed 2, Mahopac Falls, NY, 2005, Enterprise.

Associated Bodywork and Massage Professionals: *Successful business handbook*, Evergreen, Colo, 2001, ABMP.

Barnhart T: *The five rituals of wealth: proven strategies for turning the little you have into more than enough*, New York, 1996, HarperCollins.

Beck MF: *Theory and practice of therapeutic massage*, ed 4, Clifton Park, NY, 2006, Thomson Delmar Learning.

Benjamin PJ: *Pearson's massage therapy: blending art with science*, Pearson Education (in press).

Boldt LG: *Zen and the art of making a living: a practical guide to creative career design*, New York, 1999, Penguin Books.

Individual Retirement Accounts (website): http://www.schwab.com/. Accessed May 11, 2010.

Consumer Reports (website): http://www.consumerreports.org/health/free-highlights/manage-your-health/alternative_therapies.htm Accessed November 4, 2010.

Dechow M: *New requirements for gift cards and gift certificates*, AFPD (website): http://www.afpdonline.org/index2.php?option=com_content&do_pdf=1&id=225. Accessed March 9, 2010.

Denning E: Massage therapy medical codes for 2002, *Massage Bodyw* Feb/Mar: 144-145, 2002.

Downes J, Goodman JE: *Barron's dictionary of finance and investment terms*, ed 5, Hauppauge, NY, 1995, Barron's Educational Services.

Edward Jones: Retirement Planning (website): http://www.edwardjones.com/. Accessed May 11, 2010.

Fritz S: *Business and professional skills for massage therapists*, ed 4, St Louis, 2010, Mosby.

Fritz S: *Mosby's fundamentals of therapeutic massage*, ed 4, St Louis, 2009, Mosby.

Gaedeke R, Tootelian D: *Small business management*, ed 3, Needham Heights, Mass, 1991, Simon & Schuster.

Grodzki L: *Building your ideal private practice: how to love what you do and be highly profitable too!* New York, 2000, WW Norton.

Harrison BJ: *Business practices: a guide to starting your massage therapy practice in New Mexico*, 1994, Albuquerque, NM.

IRS: *Retirement plans: FAQs regarding hardship distribution* (website): http://www.irs.gov/retirement/article/0,,id=162416,00.html. Accessed March 12, 2010.

Meigs WB, Roberts F: *Accounting: the basis for business decisions*, ed 13, New York, 2004, McGraw-Hill.

Olympic Massage: *About Benny Vaughn* (website): http://massagemag.com/massage-blog/olympic-massage/about/. Accessed March 20, 2010.

Palmer DA: *The bodywork entrepreneur*, San Francisco, 1990, Thumb Press.

Sohnen-Moe C: *Business mastery: a guide for creating a fulfilling, thriving business and keeping it successful*, ed 3, Tucson, 1997, Sohnen-Moe Associates.

MATCHING I

Place the letter of the answer next to the term or phrase that best describes it.

A. Accounts receivable
B. Advertising
C. Balance sheet
D. Contract

E. Curriculum vitae
F. Gross income
G. Marketing
H. Media

I. Net income
J. Professional liability
K. Publicity
L. Sole proprietorship

_____ 1. Methods of mass communication

_____ 2. All money a person or business makes before subtracting expenses or taxes

_____ 3. Term used to describe a business of a single owner

_____ 4. Financial statement that summarizes all of a company's assets, liabilities, and owner's equity at an exact point in time, usually at the end of a quarter or a fiscal year

_____ 5. Free media exposure

_____ 6. Term synonymous with *malpractice insurance*

_____ 7. Amount of money a person or business has left after subtracting expenses and taxes

_____ 8. Autobiographical sketch that documents your achievements: occupational, avocational, and academic, as well as any personal information; also called a résumé

_____ 9. Written agreement between two or more parties that is enforceable by law

_____ 10. Money owed to you or your business

_____ 11. Ideas, strategies, and activities used to attract and retain clients

_____ 12. Form of communication that includes developing a message and then using forms media to deliver the message, usually at a cost

MATCHING II

Place the letter of the answer next to the term or phrase that best describes it.

A. Cash flow
B. Depreciation
C. Dividend
D. Equity

E. Financial portfolio
F. General advertising
G. Inventory
H. IRA

I. Liabilities
J. Profit and loss statement
K. Securities
L. Specific advertising

_____ 1. Type of advertising that announces or reminds current or potential clients about your business

_____ 2. Financial report that summarizes income and expenses over a fixed period

_____ 3. Acronym for a tax-deferred retirement account

_____ 4. Term used to describe the movement of money into and out of a business

_____ 5. Outlines various investments held by an individual investor

_____ 6. Also called net worth, the difference between total assets and liabilities

_____ 7. Unsold retail items you have on hand

_____ 8. Debts in which your business owes

_____ 9. Portion of a company's profits distributed at regular intervals to its shareholders

_____ 10. Instruments that represent financial value such as stocks, bonds, and funds

_____ 11. Type of advertising that targets an objective such as gift certificate sales or increasing the purchase of a new or existent service, such as body wraps or reflexology

_____ 12. Process of spreading the deduction for the cost of an asset over time

CASE STUDY

Scope of Practice

Mike has been working at a chiropractic clinic for 10 years as a massage therapist. Elmer is a patient at the clinic, who has been seeing one of the doctors for chiropractic adjustments and Mike for massages for the last 3 years. Elmer comes in with pain in the wrist and proceeds to receive a massage from Mike. The doctors are away from the clinic to attend a chiropractic association meeting; there is no one at the clinic but Mike and the office staff.

During the massage, Elmer asks Mike if he has ever had one of the doctors adjust his wrist. Mike replies "Sure! In this business, you tend to weight bear with your hands and sometimes the carpal bones become misaligned." Elmer replies, "Well see if *you* can adjust my wrist. I know you can do it. I trust you. I won't tell anyone." Mike is hesitant, but enjoys the compliment. Mike has always wanted to be a doctor and have the admiration and respect that go with the title. "Come on," says Elmer, "you know that you know as much about the body as they do…" Mike smiles, and grasping Elmer by the right wrist, he pulls down and out and sharply whips the wrist as he has seen his employers do for years. There is an audible pop! And Elmer's face whitens, "My hand is numb!" he says. "Will this go away? What did you do?"

How might Mike respond to Elmer's inquiry?

Is Mike liable for any damage to Elmer's wrist as a result of his desire to help Elmer?

Should Mike get the office staff involved and document the incident?

How might Mike tell the doctors about the incident when they return?

Is this an ethics issue? Why or why not?

Is this a legal issue? Why or why not?

CRITICAL THINKING

Why is it important for massage therapists to understand business practices as they begin their career in massage therapy?

UNIT TWO

ANATOMY AND PHYSIOLOGY

CHAPTER 18

Introduction to the Human Body: Cells, Tissues, and the Body Compass

"Not all who wander are lost."

—J.R.R. Tolkien

LEARNING OBJECTIVES

After completing this chapter, the student should be able to:

- Define anatomy and physiology.
- Discuss the importance of learning the terminology of science and medicine.
- Place the levels of organization in a hierarchy from least to most complex.
- Identify and discuss cellular anatomy, physiology, and metabolism.
- Discuss embryonic tissue development, tissue types, and give examples of each tissue type.
- Outline the phases of tissue repair.
- Describe types of membranes, and state their secretions.
- Define homeostasis.
- Name the body systems, outlining the anatomy and physiology of each.
- Describe or stand in the Western anatomical position.
- Indicate the planes of reference.
- Differentiate among the main body cavities, their subdivisions, and the organs contained within them.
- Identify the abdominal quadrants and regions.
- State the terms used to describe anatomical directions; use them to express the location of body structures.
- Name and locate body regions using terminology provided in this chapter.
- Identify terms used to describe the position of a reclining person.

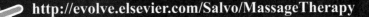
http://evolve.elsevier.com/Salvo/MassageTherapy

INTRODUCTION

You are about to embark on an unforgettable journey—a new path of self-discovery—into your own interior. To begin, you have to learn a few terms used in science and medicine, many of which are in Latin and Greek. Basic terminology is crucial to your understanding of the anatomy and physiology that follows; to be an effective and skillful massage therapist, you must have a comprehensive knowledge of this material. And these terms and concepts will be reinforced many times during your studies. The key to learning is repetition.

A clear visual picture of the many arrangements of cells and tissues will help you feel what is beneath your hands. As massage therapists, you will be manipulating and comparing numerous types of tissues. You will be gliding across the epidermis (epithelial and nervous tissues), compressing and stretching fascia (connective tissue), kneading the deltoids (muscle tissue), and chucking metacarpals (connective tissue).

Our bodies are all physiologic masterpieces. As you read this text, your heart is pumping blood, your lungs are moving air, your pupils are adjusting to reading conditions, and your nerves are monitoring both internal and external environments. These processes occur within us at every moment. During your study of anatomy and physiology, many wonders will be revealed. The philosopher Plato once noted that the "acquiring of knowledge is just a form of recollection." Learning anatomy and physiology is simply becoming aware of who you are already.

Anatomy and physiology are inseparable. Structure is determined by its function, and function is carried out through its structure. Another way of looking at this concept is that *form follows function*. For example, consider the form (or structure) of the lungs, a pair of thin-tissue organs. Lung tissue is suited for gas exchange. What organ (structure), with its thick, muscular walls, is suited for pumping fluids (function)? The heart, of course.

This chapter is also designed to serve as a reference as you continue your studies in anatomy, physiology, and massage. Here, you will learn about cells, tissues, and their membranes. You will also be introduced to organ systems. Additionally, terms used to navigate your way around the body are presented. These terms of reference, which are called the *body compass*, are used in learning planes (e.g., midsagittal), cavities (e.g., abdominopelvic), quadrants (e.g., upper right), direction (e.g., proximal), and regions (e.g., antebrachial).

ANATOMY AND PHYSIOLOGY

Anatomy is the study of the structures of the human body and their positional relationship to one another (the head bone is connected to the neck bone, and so on). The study of anatomy can be approached in several ways. *Gross anatomy* is the study of larger body structures such as bones, muscle, and organs. *Microscopic anatomy* is the study of smaller structures that can best be seen through a microscope. These structures include cells and tissues, which make up the larger structures of gross anatomy. *Applied anatomy* studies body structures and the changes they undergo during the diagnosis and treatment of disease. *Comparative anatomy* studies the structures of all life forms to indicate a progression from the simplest to the most highly specialized. *Surface anatomy* studies structural relationships of the body's surface and how they relate to internal structures.

Physiology is the study of how the body and its individual parts function in normal body processes. As with anatomy, different ways are used to approach the study of physiology. *Comparative physiology* is the study of similarities and differences in vital processes. *Developmental physiology* is the study of embryonic development. *Pathophysiology*, or pathology, is the study of the processes of disease (see Chapter 9 for more information on pathology).

Biology is defined as the scientific study of life. Both anatomy and physiology are subdivisions of this very broad area of science. To understand the relationship between anatomy and physiology better, a theater metaphor may be helpful: The stage, props, and cast of characters are the structures of the play (anatomy). How the characters relate to one another and the plot of the play is its function (physiology).

Nearly everyone has some understanding of basic anatomy and physiology, if not from prior education classes, then from practical experience of one's own body. As we begin our study, getting a good definition of anatomic terms based on the medical model is important so that everyone speaks a common language.

TERMINOLOGY

Science and medicine have their own language. These were born in 18th century universities in which Greek and Latin were the languages used during lectures and in textbooks. Hence most scientific and medical words are based on Greek or Latin.

Medical terms possess one or more parts: a prefix, a root, and a suffix. Once you have become familiar with medical terminology, looking at a new term and determining its meaning will be easier.

A **root** is the main part of a word, or its foundation. Some words combine two roots, such as *cardi-*, Greek for "heart," and "vascular," Latin for "vessel." In most cases, a vowel is used to combine two roots to aid in pronunciation. The most common combining vowel is the letter *o*. After combining the two example roots, the new term is *cardiovascular*.

A **prefix** is a syllable or syllables placed before a root to alter its meaning. For example, *pre-* is a prefix that means "before" or "front." Add *pre-* before the root *cancerous* and it becomes *precancerous,* denoting a stage of tumor growth that is likely to develop, but has not yet developed, into cancer. (See Vocabulary Builder: Prefixes.)

A **suffix** is a syllable or syllables placed after a root to alter its meaning. For example, *-ectomy* is a suffix that means "to cut out," usually in surgery. Add *-ectomy* behind the word *appendix,* and the new term is *appendectomy,* or surgical removal of the appendix. See the following Vocabulary Builder: Suffixes and Vocabulary Builder: Commonly Used Plural Endings.

As you study anatomy and physiology, you will become familiar with prefixes, suffixes, and roots. To assist in learning pronunciations, echo back (either mentally or subvocally) terms as your instructor says them aloud. Along with correct pronunciation, correct spelling is crucial because many medical and scientific terms look or sound similar. For example, *ileum* is a section of the small intestine and *ilium* is a section of the pelvis. When in doubt, use a medical dictionary or electronic medical spell-checker.

Learning medical terms can be daunting initially, but with time and practice, you will reap many rewards, including better marks on examinations. You will soon discover that medical terminology makes sense and is easy to understand, once you are familiar with basics.

Vocabulary Builder: Prefixes

PREFIX	MEANING	EXAMPLE
a-, an-	Lacking, without, not	Asymptomatic, anaerobic
ab-	Away from, absent, decrease	Abduction, abnormal
ad-	Toward, near to, increase	Adduction, adjust
adeno-	Gland	Adenoma, adenitis
angio-	Vessel	Angiogram, angioma
ante-	Front, before, toward	Anterior, ante mortem
anti-	Against, opposed	Antifungal, antibody
auto-	Self	Autoimmune, autonomic
bi-, di-	Twice, double, two	Biceps, diencephalon
bio-	Life	Biology, biohazard
cephal-	Head	Cephalitis, cephalalgia
circum-	Around	Circumduction, circumcision
contra-	Opposite, against	Contraindication, contralateral
cryo-	Extreme cold	Cryotherapy, cryoablation
cyto-	Cell	Cytoplasm, cytomegaly
de-	Separate, away from, down	Decapitate, decompose
dia-	Through	Diaphragm, diarrhea
dis-	Apart, away	Dislocation, dissection
dors-	Back	Dorsal, dorsiflexion
dys-	Difficult, bad, labored	Dysfunction, dysplasia
ecto-, exo-, ex-	On the outer side	Ectoderm, exocrine, excise
endo-	Within, inside	Endometrium, endocardium
epi-	Upon, over, in addition to	Epicondyle, epicardium
extend-	Straighten	Extension, extensor
flex-	Bend	Flexion, flexibility
glu-, gly-	Sugar, sweet	Glucose, glycosuria
histo-	Tissue	Histology, histamine
hetero-	Dissimilar	Heterocellular, heterogeneous
homeo-, homo-	Like, same	Homeopathy, homosexuality
hydro-	Water or hydrogen	Hydromassage, hydrophobia
hyper-	Over, above, excessive	Hyperextension, hypertension
hypo-	Under, below, deficient	Hypodermic, hypovolemia
hyster-	Uterus, womb	Hysterectomy, hysteroscopy
infra-	Under, below, beneath	Infraspinatus, infrahyoid
inter-	Between, together, midst	Intercostal, interarticular
intra-	Within	Intravenous, intravascular
lipo-	Lipid, fat	Lipoma, liposuction
meso-	Middle	Mesentery, mesoderm
meta-	Beyond, after, change	Metabolism, metacarpals
micro-	Small	Microvilli, microscope
mono-	One, single	Mononuclear, monoaxial
multi-	Many	Multifidus, multipennate
narco-	Sleep, numbness, stupor	Narcolepsy, narcotic
necro-	Death	Necrosis, necropsy
ophthalmo-	Eye	Opthalmic, ophthalmologist
ot-	Ear	Otitis, otologist
para-	Alongside, beside	Parasympathetic, paranormal
patho-	Disease	Pathology, pathogen
peri-	Around, about	Periosteum, periodontal
post-	Rear, after, behind	Posterior, postmortem
pre-, pro-	Before, front	Prenatal, protuberance
quad-	Four	Quadriceps, quadratus
re-	Again, back	Realign, retract
recto-	Straight	Rectum, rectus
retro-	Backward	Retroperitoneal, retroverted
sub-	Under, beneath, below	Subscapular, subcutaneous
super-, supra-	Above, over	Superficial, supraspinatus
syn-, sym-	Together, with, joined	Synarthrotic, symbiotic
therm-	Heat	Thermal, thermotherapy
trans-	Across, over, beyond, through	Transverse, transfusion
tri-	Three	Triceps, triaxial
uni-	One	Unilateral, uniaxial

Vocabulary Builder: Suffixes

SUFFIX	MEANING	EXAMPLE
-algia	Pain	Fibromyalgia, neuralgia
-blast	Bud or sprout	Osteoblast, collagenoblast
-cele	Tumor, herniation	Meningocele, rectocele
-clast	Destroy or break down	Angioclast, osteoclast
-cyte	Cell	Hemocyte, osteocyte
-ectomy	Excision or to cut out	Tonsillectomy, mastectomy
-emia	Blood condition	Hyperemia, lipidemia
-gen	Produce	Carcinogen, fibrinogen
-gram	To record	Electrocardiogram, angiogram
-ia, -osis, -ism	State or condition	Anemia, cyanosis, embolism
-iatry	Healing	Psychiatry, podiatry
-itis	Inflammation	Arthritis, tonsillitis
-megaly	Great, large	Cardiomegaly, splenomegaly
-oid	Shaped	Rhomboid, osteoid
-ologist	Specialist in a particular study	Biologist, histologist
-ology	Study of	Urology, oncology
-oma	Tumor	Neuroma, lipoma
-osis	Condition	Lordosis, sclerosis
-otomy	Incision or to cut into	Colostomy, lumpectomy
-penia	Poverty	Osteopenia, thrombocytopenia
-plasia	To form	Hyperplasia, dysplasia
-rrhage, -rrhea	Abnormal or excessive flow	Hemorrhage, diarrhea
-scopy	To view or examine	Orthoscopy, cystoscopy
-stasis	Control, stopping	Homeostasis, hemostasis
-trophy	Nourish, grow, develop	Hypertrophy, dystrophy
-tropy	Turning	Thixotropy

Vocabulary Builder: Commonly Used Plural Endings

SINGULAR	PLURAL
-a; scapula	-ae; scapulae
-en; foramen	-ina; foramina
-is; testis	-es; testes
-is; iris	-ides; irides
-nx; larynx	-ges; larynges
-on; mitochondrion	-a; mitochondria
-um; bacterium	-a; bacteria
-us; nucleus	-i; nuclei
-x; thorax	-ces; thoraces
-y; cavity	-ies; cavities

LEVELS OF ORGANIZATION

The human body can be regarded as a universe made up of small components organized to function as a unit. This organization follows a hierarchy based on level of complexity. The levels are *chemical, cellular, tissue, organ, organ system*, and *organism* (Figure 18-1).

Chemical level. The chemical level encompasses the chemical elements that make up the body (e.g., water, oxygen, iron, deoxyribonucleic acid [DNA]).

Cellular level. The cellular level includes cells, which are composed of organelles. Cells perform functions vital to life (e.g., skin cells, blood cells).

Tissue level. The tissue level is composed of groups of cells that perform specific functions. Different tissue types possess their own unique properties (e.g., connective, nervous).

Organ level. The organ level involves structures composed of two or more specialized groups of tissue that carry on specific functions (e.g., stomach, brain).

Organ system level. Related organs with complementary functions arrange themselves into organ systems that can perform certain necessary tasks (e.g., respiration, digestion).

Organism level. The organism level is the highest level of organization, representing living entities composed of several organ systems. All organ systems provide functions that promote life. The total of all structures and functions is a living individual (Table 18-1).

ⓔvolve *Log on to the Evolve website to play the game "Name That Word Part."* ■

Think of these levels as the building materials of a house. The cells are similar to the individual parts such as nails, studs, bricks, and mortar. These materials are put together to make walls, floors, and ceilings, which correspond to the tissues of the body. Then put these "tissues" together, and you get a room, which is similar in nature to an organ. Several rooms may function as an organ system; the bedrooms might constitute one organ system; the bathrooms and kitchen constitute another. These systems are all linked together into one house, which is akin to the organism level. To understand the body, the smallest components are examined first, and then we proceed up to the organism level. Let us take a look at our cellular level.

MINI-LAB

In small groups or as a class, discuss the concept of being *alive*. Use a board or overhead projector to list all the ideas that accumulate. As you will discover, the concept of being alive is a very complex set of ideas.

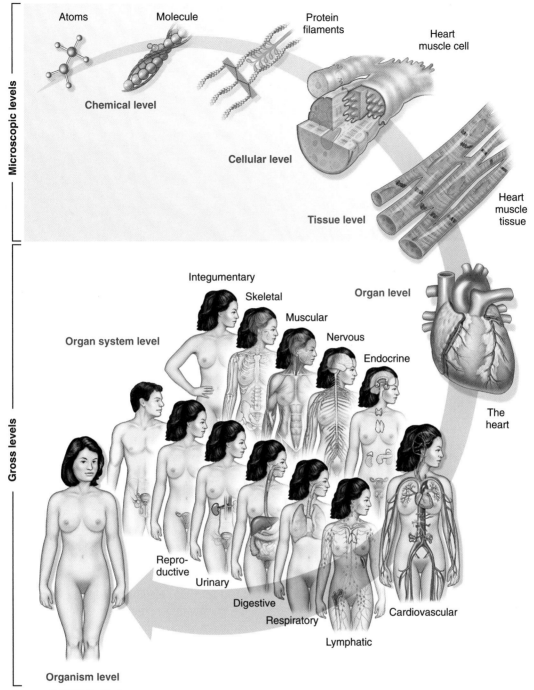

FIGURE 18-1 Levels of organization of the body, from the chemical level to the organism level.

TABLE 18-1 Levels of Organization

LEVEL	DESCRIPTION	EXAMPLES
Chemical	Biochemistry of the body	Atoms, molecules, compounds, water, hormones, DNA, oxygen, iron
Cellular	Basic unit of life	Bone cell, muscle cell, nerve cell
Tissue	Groups of cells that share a similar structure and function	Epithelial, connective, muscular, nervous
Organ	Complex structures of two or more tissue types performing a specific function	Heart, kidney, brain, lung
Organ system	Related organs with complementary functions that perform certain tasks	Circulatory, urinary, nervous, respiratory
Organism	Living entities composed of several organ systems; most complex level	*Homo sapiens*, fish, frog, butterfly

DNA, Deoxyribonucleic acid.

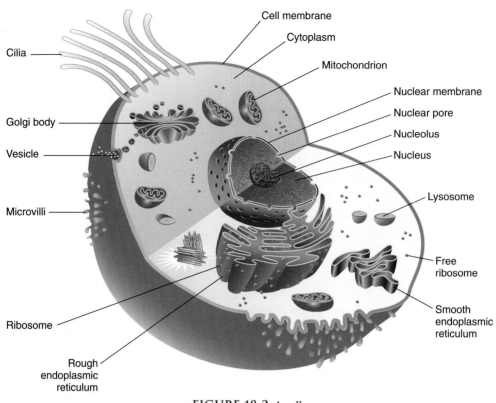

FIGURE 18-2 A cell.

"Dance like nobody's watching; love like you've never been hurt. Sing like nobody's listening; live like it's heaven on earth."
—Mark Twain

CELLS

The **cell** is the fundamental unit of all living organisms and is the simplest form of life that can exist as a self-sustaining unit. Cells are the building blocks of the human body (Figure 18-2). Scientists estimate that between 75 and 100 trillion active, living cells are present in the body at any given moment.

All forms of matter, whether it is living or nonliving, are made up of chemical building blocks called *elements*. Cells consist of four main elements: (1) carbon, (2) oxygen, (3) hydrogen, and (4) nitrogen. *Trace elements* are elements that are present in tiny amounts. Trace elements include iron, sodium, and potassium, among others. These trace elements are extremely important for cellular functions: Calcium is needed for blood clotting; iron is necessary to make hemoglobin, which carries oxygen in the blood; and iodine is needed to make thyroid hormones, which control metabolism. Besides these elements and trace elements, water makes up approximately 60% to 80% of all cells.

Cell Anatomy

A cell contains a membrane, cytoplasm, and organelles. Organelles include the nucleus, mitochondria, ribosomes, endoplasmic reticulum, Golgi body, and lysosomes (Table 18-2). The specialized nature of body tissues reflects the specialized function of their cellular makeup.

Cell Membrane

The cell (*plasma*) membrane separates the cytoplasm from the surrounding external environment. The membrane creates a semipermeable boundary, meaning that some materials can freely pass, and others cannot. This function governs the exchange of nutrients and waste materials. This movement takes place by active and passive processes, which are discussed later. The cell membrane can respond to changes outside the cell or stimuli.

Cell membranes may contain projections such as *microvilli, cilia,* or *flagella,* which help protect the cell and aid in its mobility.

Cytoplasm

Consisting primarily of water, cytoplasm (*cytosol*) is the gel-like intracellular fluid within the cell membrane. Floating in cytoplasm are cellular structures called organelles, which provide special functions. Functions of cytoplasm are to provide cellular nutrition and to support the organelles.

TABLE 18-2 Cell Structures and Functions

PART OF CELL	ACTION
Cell membrane	Governs exchange of nutrients and waste materials
Cytoplasm	Provides cellular nutrition and supports organelles
Organelles	
Nucleus	Control center of the cell; directs nearly all metabolic activities; contains DNA and RNA
Ribosome	Synthesizes proteins
Endoplasmic reticulum	Synthesizes proteins and lipids; assists in the transportation of these materials
Golgi body	Packing and shipping plant of the cell; alters proteins and lipids, packs and stores them till needed
Mitochondrion	Power plant of the cell, responsible for cellular respiration; provides most of the cell's ATP
Lysosome	Engulfs and digests bacteria, cellular debris, and other organelles

ATP, Adenosine triphosphate; *DNA,* deoxyribonucleic acid; *RNA,* ribonucleic acid.

The total water of the body can be subdivided into two major compartments: extracellular fluids and intracellular fluids. *Extracellular fluids* include fluid portion of blood called plasma, the fluid between tissues, or interstitial fluid, and fluid of the lymphatic system called lymph. These fluids provide a constant environment for cells and help in the transportation of substances to and from them. *Intracellular fluids* lie within cells and is called cytoplasm. Most body fluid is intracellular (see Figure 30-6).

Organelles. Within the cell are organelles ("little organs"). Each organelle possesses distinct structures and functions. Some organelles function in reproduction, some store materials, and some metabolize nutrients.

Nucleus. The nucleus, the largest organelle, is the control center of the cell, directing most metabolic activities. All cells have at least one nucleus at some time in their existence. Red blood cells lose their nuclei (they are *anucleate*) as they mature, and skeletal muscle cells possess many nuclei (they are *multinucleate*). The shape of the nucleus is usually spherical. Each nucleus contains clusters of proteins, ribonucleic acid (RNA), and DNA, which make up chromosomes (our genetic code). Humans possess 23 pairs of chromosomes, although abnormalities can exist. A discussion of chromosomes is found in Chapter 25.

Nucleoli within the nucleus produce ribosomes (discussed later).

Endoplasmic reticulum. A complex network of membranous channels is endoplasmic reticulum. These structures often extend from the cell membrane to the nuclear membrane and may extend to other organelles. Endoplasmic reticulum functions in the synthesis of protein and lipids and assists in the transportation of these materials from one part of the cell to another. Endoplasmic reticula are classified as *rough* or *granular* (ribosomes are attached to the surface) or as *smooth* or *agranular* (ribosomes are absent).

Ribosomes. Ribosomes are small granules of RNA and protein. Their function is to synthesize protein for use within the cell and to produce other proteins that are exported outside the cell. Ribosomes may bind to rough endoplasmic reticulum or may float in the cytoplasm and are called *free ribosomes.*

Golgi body. The Golgi body, or *Golgi apparatus*, is a series of four to six horizontal membranous sacs. Referred to as the "packing and shipping plants" of the cell, Golgi bodies can alter proteins and lipids and then pack and store them until needed. Once this process is complete, they are wrapped in a piece of the Golgi body's membrane, or vesicle, and jettisoned to the desired area, often out of the cell.

Mitochondria. An oval organelle, the mitochondrion is considered the cell's "power plant" because it is a site for cellular respiration and provides most of a cell's adenosine triphosphate (ATP), which is the body's energy molecule. Mitochondria consist of an inner and outer membrane; the outer shell is smooth, and the inner, convoluted membrane contains many projections called *cristae*. These inner chambers increase the surface area to enhance mitochondrion's metabolic properties.

Lysosomes. Lysosomes engulf pathogens, cellular debris, and other organelles. Because they contain enzymes, they can digest these materials. The lysosome can also cause self-digestion when a decrease in number of cells in an organ is needed, such as reduction in the size of the uterus after childbirth. Lysosomes also release their digestive enzymes at injury sites to help dispose of cellular debris.

CHAT ROOM

One way to view a cell is as a city. The organelles represent the city's infrastructure and many essential services. For example, the *nucleus* is the city hall that contains records of the city's history (or genetic information). The *endoplasmic reticulum* is the factory that manufactures proteins. The *ribosomes* are the factories that synthesize proteins. The post office, or *Golgi body*, represents the place where molecules are packed and shipped. The *mitochondria* are the power plants of the cell that generates "electricity" for the city. And the vital sanitation department is operated by the *lysosomes*.

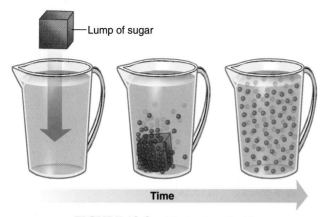

FIGURE 18-3 Diffusion in a liquid.

CHAT ROOM

In the late 1600s, Robert Hooke was examining plant tissue samples through a primitive microscope. He identified structures that reminded him of the long rows of cell rooms in a monastery. He named these cubelike structures *cells*.

Cell Physiology

To survive, a cell must be able to carry on a variety of functions. These include the ability of substances to move across the cell membrane. These processes can be classified as passive or active processes.

Passive processes include diffusion, filtration, and osmosis. These processes occur without the expenditure of energy of the cell, usually by means of gradients of temperature, pressure, or concentration. The gradient or difference in levels of temperature, pressure, or concentration is the driving force behind the exchange of particles or fluid across the cell's membrane.

Active processes require energy and use either pump mechanisms or vesicles to carry out cellular functions and include endocytosis and exocytosis.

Passive Processes

Diffusion – Diffusion is the movement of molecules from an area of high concentration to an area of low concentration. This passive process continues until the distribution of particulates is equal in all areas (Figure 18-3).

Diffusion can be easily demonstrated by filling a long baking pan with cool water and setting it somewhere where no vibration or movement can disturb the pan. Open a packet of colored soft drink mix (e.g., Kool-Aid), and gently sprinkle the powder in one corner of the pan. Even though no true currents are in the pan, the colored powder diffuses across the pan. When kinetic energy, or speed, of the particles is increased (e.g., by raising the temperature), the rate of diffusion also increases. The greater the energy is, and the higher the gradient is, the faster the rate of diffusion will

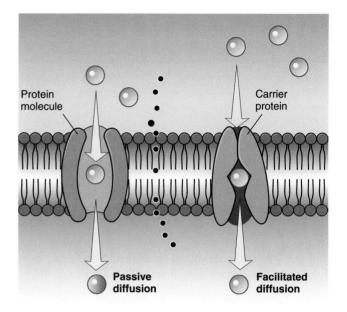

FIGURE 18-4 Passive and facilitated diffusion.

be. Try the Kool-Aid experiment with a pan of hot water or by gently shaking the pan, and see how the rate of the diffusion process increases.

Facilitated diffusion is a special type of diffusion that uses a carrier protein or channels to facilitate the diffusion process (Figure 18-4). Carrier proteins and channels are within the cell membrane. Sometimes molecules in a solution are too large to cross the cell membrane. When the fluid outside the cell membrane has a high concentration of large molecules, the carrier proteins in the cell membrane assist the large molecules in crossing the membrane. The number of available carrier proteins limits facilitated diffusion. Channels are specific as to what can pass through them, such as certain types of ions. For example, sodium channels open to allow only sodium ions through, which is a crucial aspect of nerve impulse conduction. Many of the nutrients inside our digestive tract enter our bloodstream through diffusion or facilitated diffusion through the cells of the digestive tract.

Filtration – Filtration is the movement of particles across the cellular membrane because of pressure. A pressure gradient across a cell membrane is the force that drives the filtration process. The air filter on your furnace or central air conditioning unit is a good example. The vacuum created by the suction of the fan lowers the pressure behind the filter. The atmospheric pressure in the room is then greater than that behind the filter. The air flows through the pores of the filter, which is selective and traps the larger particles of dust, pet dander, and smoke. An example of filtration occurs in the kidneys. Waste from the blood moves across a special membrane, ultimately resulting in urine.

Osmosis – Similar to diffusion, osmosis is the movement of a pure solvent such as water through a selectively permeable membrane from an area of low concentration (most

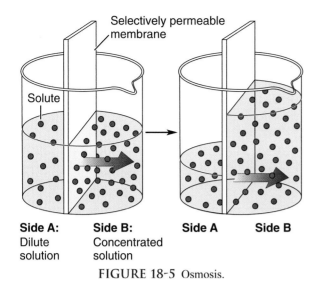

Side A:
Dilute
solution

Side B:
Concentrated
solution

Side A   Side B

FIGURE 18-5 Osmosis.

dilute) to an area of high concentration (least dilute). This action continues until the two concentrations equalize (Figure 18-5). In osmosis, water moves instead of particles to create equilibrium.

Unlike filtration, osmotic movement does not depend on pressure but rather on the concentration of dissolved elements that lie in the solutions on each side of a cell membrane or vessel wall. When the solutions contain particles that are too large to cross the membrane, diffusion cannot occur. Even though a cell membrane does not permit the particles to pass through its walls, the solvent fluid is still able to move across the membrane. When your fingers are wrinkled from being in water too long, it is because water has been moved by osmosis from your body toward the particles in the water in which your hands have been.

Active Processes

Active Transport – Active transport moves important atoms and molecules, such as ions, amino acids, and sugars, against the concentration gradient from low levels to high levels. The mechanisms of active transport are both chemical and physical. The chemical part of the mechanism involves the breakdown of ATP to produce the energy needed for the transport. Scientists estimate that at least 40% of the ATP in the human body is used solely for active transport. The two major types of active transport involve transport by pumps and transport by vesicles.

Transport by pumps. Pumps are carrier proteins that are part of a cell's membrane. Certain ions are attracted to the protein molecule. The outside of the carrier protein opens, in the same manner as a clamshell, and the ion is drawn inside and binds to it. The binding causes the chemical breakdown of ATP, which again transforms the shape of the carrier protein. The clamshell closes, and then the opposite side of the carrier protein opens again to release the ion to the inside of the cell. This process is similar to an air lock in that only one door can be opened at a time and represents the physical component of the pump.

For example, sometimes ions move through the cell membrane by facilitated diffusion via channels and other times they move through the membrane by active transport via pumps. During nerve impulse conduction, sodium ions move into nerve cells through channels. Once the impulse is over, the sodium ions need to be actively transported back out and potassium ions need to be actively transported back into the cell (Figure 18-6, *A*, p. 390). The mechanism that performs this process is called the sodium-potassium pump.

Transport by vesicles. Vesicles are small, spherical sacs that transport various substances within cells, as well as import and export materials into and out of the cell.

Endocytosis – Endocytosis is a process that moves large particles across the cell membrane into the cell. The two main types of endocytosis are phagocytosis and pinocytosis, both of which are vital to the immune defense systems of the body.

In endocytosis the plasma membrane forms around extracellular material, trapping it in a vesicle within the cell. The basic mechanism of endocytosis is summarized in Figure 18-6, *B*, p. 390.

Phagocytosis. Phagocytosis, or *cell eating,* is a specialized type of endocytosis in which certain cells ingest harmful microorganisms and cellular debris, break them down, and expel the harmless remains back into the body. Phagocytosis is chiefly characteristic of leukocytes found in the blood and throughout body tissues. In fact, one type of leukocyte is called a *macrophage* because it is a huge cell that is exceptional at devouring pathogens and wastes. The process includes five steps. Once the leukocyte locates the microbe through chemical attraction and targeted for destruction, it forms extensions to surround it. Next, it engulfs the microbe. Third, a vesicle is formed around the microbe as it becomes internalized. Fourth, lysosomal enzymes destroy the material. Finally, the digested microbial products are released.

Pinocytosis. Pinocytosis, or *cell drinking,* is almost identical to phagocytosis except that the target is liquid. In this process, the cell membrane surrounds the fluid and draws it inside, trapped in a vesicle. Pinocytic cells are more common than phagocytic cells.

Exocytosis – Exocytosis releases materials from a cell. Membrane enclosed vesicles form inside the cell, fuse with the plasma membrane, then release their contents outside the cell (see Figure 18-6, *C*). All cells carry out exocytosis, but it is especially important in cells that secrete digestive enzymes, hormones, and mucus, as well as nerve cells that release chemicals called *neurotransmitters.* Neurotransmitters are discussed in more detail in Chapter 23.

Transcytosis – Transcytosis is the process in which substances are moved into, through, and out of a cell by transport vesicles. The vesicles undergo endocytosis on one side of the cell, move across the cell, then undergo exocytosis on the other side, releasing their contents into fluid surrounding the cell. Antibodies from a pregnant mother's blood cross the placenta and enter the baby's blood via transcytosis.

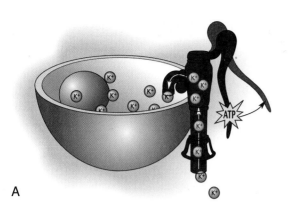

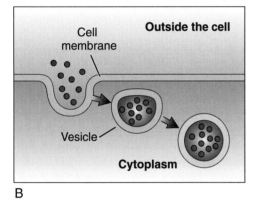

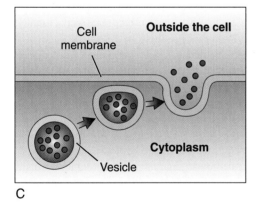

FIGURE 18-6 Active transport: Moving potassium or K+ into a cell **(A)**, endocytosis **(B)**, and exocytosis **(C)**. *ATP*, Adenosine triphosphate.

Cellular Metabolism

Metabolism is the total of all physical and chemical processes that occur in an organism (i.e., those that are considered to be signs of life). Metabolic reactions harvest the chemical energy stored in food (with the use of oxygen) and use the energy for the body's growth, repair, and other energy needs such as nerve impulse conduction, muscle contraction, elimination of wastes, and so forth. Excess energy released during metabolism that is not needed by the body is released as heat.

Metabolism occurs in two phases: anabolism and catabolism.

Anabolism. The constructive phase in which smaller, simpler molecules (e.g., amino acids) are built up into larger molecules (e.g., proteins).

Catabolism. The destructive phase in which larger, more complex molecules (e.g., carbohydrates) are converted to smaller, simpler molecules (e.g., glucose).

Metabolic Rate. This is the overall rate at which metabolic reactions use energy. Exercise, elevated body temperature, hormonal activity, digestion and pregnancy can all increase the metabolic rate. Everyone has a particular baseline metabolic rate, referred to as basal metabolic rate. Basal metabolic rate (BMR) is discussed in Chapter 29.

> ⊖volve   *Log on to your student account on the Evolve website to view animations of carbohydrate metabolism and a really cool organ system 3-D turntable.* ∎

TISSUES

Tissues are defined as groups of similar cells that act together to perform a specific function. Only four major types of tissues are present in the human body: (1) epithelial, (2) connective, (3) muscle, and (4) nervous (Figure 18-7).

Tissues organize themselves into organs. *Organs* are defined as groups of two or more tissue types that act together to perform a specific common function and have a consistently recognizable shape.

Embryonic Tissue Development

Tissue development begins early in the embryo. By day 16, the inner cell mass of the blastocyst begin to differentiate into three primary germ layers. From superficial to deep, these layers are *ectoderm, mesoderm,* and *endoderm.* These layers will develop into all tissues and organs of the body.

Ectoderm. The outermost layer, the ectoderm, gives rise to structures of the nervous system, including the special senses (e.g., retina, taste buds, olfactory bulb, inner ear), mucosa of the mouth and anus, the epidermis of the skin, and epidermal tissues such as fingernails, hair, skin glands, and the pituitary (Figure 18-8).

Mesoderm. The middle layer, the mesoderm, develops into the muscles and connective tissues of the body. Examples of connective tissue structures are fascia, tendons, retinaculum, ligaments, cartilage, bone, mesenteries, dermis,

DEANE JUHAN, MA

Born: April 18, 1945

"The principle is elegantly simple. We learn to love by being loved, we learn gentleness by being gentle, we learn to be graceful by experiencing the feeling of grace."

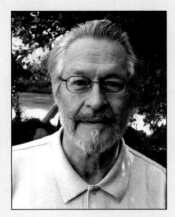

Deane Juhan is a bodyworker, one of the first Trager-trained instructors, an anatomy teacher and lecturer for the Trager Institute, and author of *Job's Body: A Handbook for Bodyworkers*. As the title suggests, the book offers an answer to the age-old question of *why* regarding the Old Testament book of Job . . . but that is just for starters. The book explores "the various ways through which intuitive and informed touch can positively affect a wide variety of symptoms and help to change people's lives for the better." The book was 9 years in the making, which is surprising, considering the manner in which Juhan's words easily flow during casual conversation.

Born to a woman who had "poor taste in men" and a soldier who did not hang around to become a father, Juhan was later adopted, growing up as an only child in Glenwood Springs, Colo. His father worked for the state and never drew a large salary, but his parents were wise about using resources and were determined that their only child's education would receive top priority in their lives.

Juhan describes himself as an underachiever in high school. The University of Colorado introduced him to a whole new way of living, and he admits to being caught up in the novelty of its hip, liberal atmosphere until his junior year, when "his rudder finally bit the water," he says. At this point in his life, he became interested in the aspects of art, science, and civilization.

Juhan learned about Esalen, a workshop and meeting place for developing human potential in Big Sur, Calif., while working on his dissertation in literature. He actually managed to sneak in and start doing massage. He was so good at it. Juhan's first experience in anatomy was developing slides and lectures for *Structural Integration for Rolfing* lectures, but when he witnessed Milton Trager at work, he was hooked and abandoned all other methods to learn the Trager approach.

"It was love at first sight," says Juhan. "I was attracted to his quality of being. It was his rich avuncular benevolence without all the preliminary folderol that made me want to learn to do what he did, so I threw myself into it and gave it my all."

Learning the approach did not come easy though for this hard-pushing 6-footer. His strength had always been, well, his strength. Nonetheless, Juhan broke down and cried when he saw his first Trager demonstration. Then, as he clumsily applied himself to unlearning everything he ever thought he knew about bodywork, Trager reduced his ego to ashes, yelling at him during training, slapping his hand away and taking over, always admonishing him to work lighter and softer and to quit trying so hard to get the job done.

Juhan points out that Trager's use of inducing a meditative state during a session, which has been called *hook-up*, is one of the things that sets Trager apart and makes the work so effective. During this hook-up, messages are communicated that have nothing to do with verbal and nonverbal interaction as we know it, and this exchange is the key to long-term change.

For the bodywork session, the goal is to connect with the client's sensory information, and then help the client *wake up* to the possibility for long-term change through movement. The therapist lays down new patterns by repeating a movement message again and again. The feeling finally becomes etched on the client's awareness, creating an experience of longitudinal, relaxation, and pain-free movement.

Juhan writes in *Job's Body: A Handbook for Bodyworkers:* "For Job this was revelation—the perception that God was in his very flesh, in the throbbing of his heart, in the singing of his nerves, in the coiling of his muscles, to be touched and felt more intimately than an embrace."

As a beginning massage therapist, you are probably not seeking a revelation so much as you are a direction. You can probably guess that Juhan's advice is to look within. Choose the method or modality that will, according to Juhan, "flower in your psyche or experience. Look for what turns you on, look for what you love, not what the market says is hot."

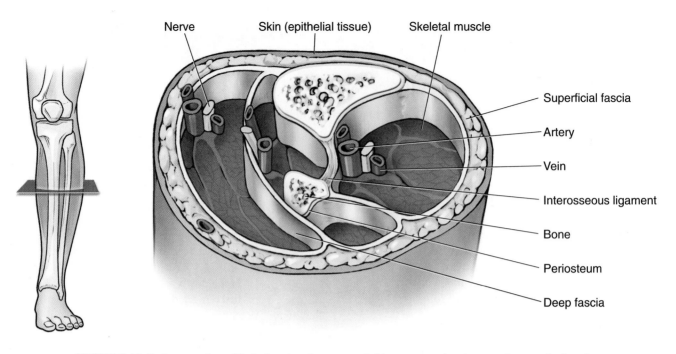

FIGURE 18-7 Cross section of limb denoting tissue types (white = connective tissue; red = muscle tissue).

and hypodermis. Blood, lymph and related vessels, as well as the pleurae of the lungs, the pericardium, peritoneum, and the urogenital tract are all derived from mesoderm.

Endoderm. This is the innermost cell layer, from which the lining of the gastrointestinal tract, lining of the respiratory passages, and most tissues of organs and glands arise. Thus the endoderm makes up the lining of the body's passages and the covering for most of the internal organs.

CHAT ROOM

It is important to recognize that the skin's epidermis and the entire nervous system (i.e., brain, spinal cord, sense organs of smell, taste, hearing, and vision) arise from ectoderm. These structures keep the organism informed about what is going on in its environment. Because of the ectoderm connection, the skin is considered exposed neural tissue, and, in contrast, the brain is immersed skin. We can therefore regard the skin as a superficial nervous system. Hence massage techniques can relax or stimulate the nervous system, depending on how they are used.

Epithelial Tissue

Epithelial tissue, or epithelium, lines or covers the body's external surface such as the skin; internal organs/glands such as the liver and thyroid; lines blood vessels and body cavities; and lines the digestive, respiratory, urinary, and reproductive tracts (Figure 18-9). Functions of this tissue include protection, absorption, secretion, excretion, and sensation.

Generalized protection is the most important function of epithelium. The digestive and respiratory epithelium allows for the absorption of nutrients and exchange of gases. Some epithelium secretes substances such as hormones, mucus, digestive juices, and sweat. Epithelial lining of the urinary system provides excretion of urine. Some epithelial structures found in skin, the nose, eyes, and ears, are adapted for sensory functions. Epithelium has a high rate of cell division and regenerates quickly.

Epithelial tissues are classified according to their arrangement (*simple* [one-layer], *stratified* [multiple layers]) or the shape of the cells (*squamous* [flat], *cuboidal* [cube-shaped], *columnar* [column-shaped]). In many cases, these two classifications are combined to describe epithelium (*simple squamous* [as in lung epithelium], *stratified cuboidal* [as in oral epithelium]).

Pseudostratified epithelium appears to have multiple layers, but it is actually a single layer of cells of various heights, giving the appearance of more than one layer. *Transitional epithelium* is a unique arrangement that combines all cell shapes in a stratified sheet of tissue. This tissue type permits stretching and is found in the ureters and bladder.

Connective Tissue

Connective tissue is the most abundant and diverse tissue type, and it surrounds almost every organ. This tissue serves a wide variety of functions. Connective tissue connects, supports, transports, and defends. It connects tissues to each other (e.g., muscles to muscles, muscles to bones, bones to bones). It forms a supporting framework for the whole body, as well as for organs and glands. Blood, one connective

CHAT ROOM

More on Fascia

One type of connective tissue, fascia, deserves further discussion because it relates directly to a massage therapist's work. The two types of fascia are (1) *superficial fascia,* which is immediately under the skin, and (2) *deep fascia,* which surrounds muscles, holding them together and separating them into functioning groups. The main difference between superficial and deep fascia is location. Some therapists view fascia as a single, but complex, body covering or membrane.

Ground substance is the material in which the fibers and cells of connective tissues are embedded. The ground substance in fascia possesses two physical states: (1) a relatively thin fluid or *sol state* and (2) a thicker, more gelatinous fluid or *gel state.* Fascia in its sol state has a fluid quality, is more pliant and elastic, and offers less-restricted movements. Fascia in the gel state is tougher, more inflexible, and can restrict the body's movements.

The physical state of fascia, to some degree, can be altered because it possesses a property called thixotropism. The word *thixotropy* comes from the Greek root words meaning "to touch" and "turning." This term refers to fascia's ability to change the ground substance in the matrix from one state to the other. Through touch and/or friction, fascia can *change* or *turn* the state of its ground substance in the matrix from a gel state to a sol state.

When the body is not in efficient posture, as in forward head posture, the spine no longer adequately supports the head in space. The muscles and fascia become the supportive tissue, adapting to the situation by becoming firmer. The fascia in the neck can turn from liquid to gel to help hold the head in this physically stressful position. The stiffness that the client feels is partly due to fascia's gel state. This restricted fascia must be addressed during the massage in order for the client to benefit from the treatment.

As we apply pressure and heat, either by friction or local and general application, thixotropy occurs, converting the gel state to the sol state. The fascia loosens, melts, and becomes more flexible and elastic. This softening of the fascia that surrounds the muscles allows the muscles to be manipulated to their fullest resting length, increases joint range of motion, and frees the body from restrictions of movement. Thixotropism also occurs when the body is warmed by physical work, exercise, and stretching.

---

tissue type, transports nutrients and wastes. Several kinds of connective tissue cells provide defense mechanisms, such as blood clotting and inflammatory responses (Figure 18-10, p. 396).

Connective tissue is highly vascularized, providing nutrition and oxygen to itself and nearby tissues such as skin and muscle. One exception is cartilage. This is why it takes cartilage a long time to heal from injury—little blood supply.

All connective tissue is composed of connective tissue cells scattered in an extracellular matrix. The matrix itself is a gelatinous liquid that is primarily composed of a ground substance and fibers (collagenous, reticular, or elastic). Collagenous fibers are made up of long protein strands called *collagen.* Collagen is the main component of connective tissue. Reticular fibers are made up of a special type of collagen called *reticulin.* Reticulin are crosslinked to form a mesh used to support tissues in organs, glands, and bone marrow. Elastic fibers are made of a protein called *elastin.* Elastin returns to its original length after being stretched. The arrangement of these fibers and the ratio of collagen to ground substance is the primary factor for determining the different types of connective tissues. Blood and lymph are dilute and have high amounts of a fluid ground substance. Bone has a very high ratio of collagen arranged to trap the mineral salts, resulting in a solid ground substance that gives it density and firmness. The ligaments and fascia have a ratio of collagen to ground substance that is somewhere in the middle, giving it both durability and elasticity.

The ground substance is mostly water with some suspended solids, giving some connective tissue viscosity. Within the ground substance are stem cells called *fibroblasts,* which are precursors for cells specializing in tissue healing and metabolism. Examples of cells arising from fibroblasts are chondroblasts (immature chondrocytes or cartilage cells) and osteoblasts (immature osteocytes or bone cells).

The main types of connective tissue are *fibrous, bone, cartilage,* and *liquid.* Each category contains several different subtypes that possess similar structural characteristics (Table 18-3).

Fibrous. Fibrous connective tissue is regarded as the packing material of the body. It attaches the skin to underlying structures in a basement membrane, serves to wrap and support the body cells, fills in the spaces between structures such as organs and muscles, and helps keep them in their proper places. The following are types of fibrous connective tissue.

Loose (Areolar) – Loose connective tissue is one of the most widely distributed connective tissues and has little tensile strength. Along with adipose tissue, loose connective tissue forms the subcutaneous layer of the skin (superficial fascia), which attaches the skin to its underlying tissues and structures.

Adipose – Adipose tissue, or fatty tissue, is specialized for fat storage. This connective tissue, which includes yellow bone marrow, also insulates the body against heat loss, provides fuel reserves for energy, and provides a cushion around certain structures such as the heart, kidneys, and some joints.

Reticular – Reticular connective tissue forms the supportive framework of bones and of certain organs, such as the liver and spleen.

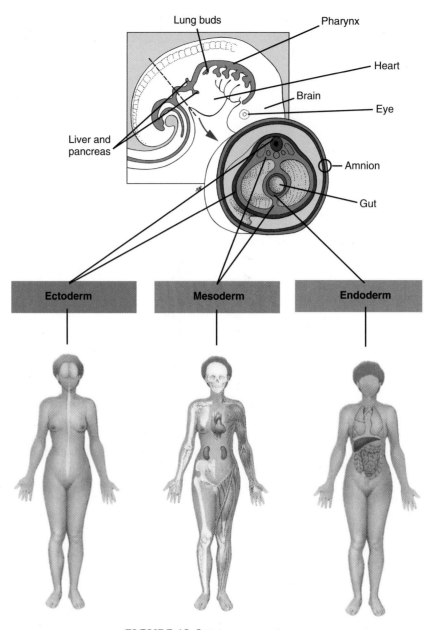

FIGURE 18-8 Primary germ layers.

Dense – Dense fibrous connective tissue consists of compact, strong, inelastic bundles of parallel collagenous fibers that have a glistening white color. The two types of dense connective tissue are irregular and regular.

Dense irregular fibrous tissue resists pulling forces in several different directions; examples of dense irregular connective tissue are deep fascia, dermis of the skin, periosteum, and the capsules of organs.

Dense regular fibrous tissue offers great strength and can resist pulling forces, generally in two directions; examples are ligaments, tendons, retinacula, and aponeuroses.

Bone. The hardest, most dense connective tissue is *bone,* or *osseous tissue.* Bones are permeated by many blood vessels and nerves and are enclosed in membranous periosteum. Long bones contain yellow marrow in longitudinal cavities and red marrow in their articular ends. Blood cells are produced in active red marrow. Types of bone are compact and spongy. Bones are also discussed in Chapter 19.

Compact – This type tissue forms the hard outer shell of bone. It contains few spaces and is the strongest form of bone tissue.

Spongy (Cancellous) – Within many bones is a lattice of thin beams called trabeculae. The spaces between the trabeculae give this type of tissue its spongy appearance. They also lighten the bone and, in some bones, are filled with red bone marrow (see Figure 19-2).

Epithelial Tissue

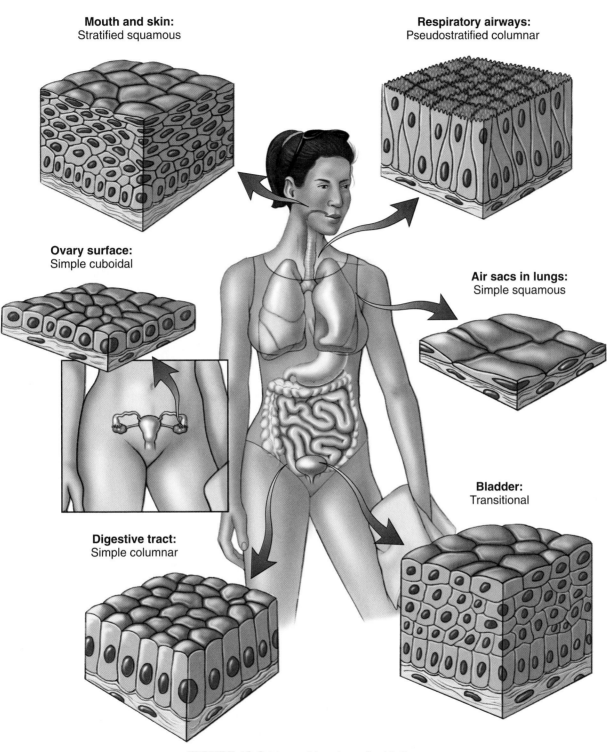

Mouth and skin:
Stratified squamous

Respiratory airways:
Pseudostratified columnar

Ovary surface:
Simple cuboidal

Air sacs in lungs:
Simple squamous

Bladder:
Transitional

Digestive tract:
Simple columnar

FIGURE 18-9 Types of locations of epithelium.

Cartilage. Cartilage is an avascular, tough, protective tissue capable of withstanding repeated stress and is found chiefly in the thorax, joints, and certain rigid structures of the body (trachea, larynx, nose, ears). Temporary cartilage, such as most of the fetal skeleton at an early stage, is later replaced

by bone. Permanent cartilage remains unossified, except in certain diseases and, sometimes, in advanced age.

Hyaline – Hyaline cartilage (gristle) is an elastic, rubbery, smooth type of cartilage composed of cells in a translucent, pearly-blue matrix. The most common type of cartilage,

Connective Tissue

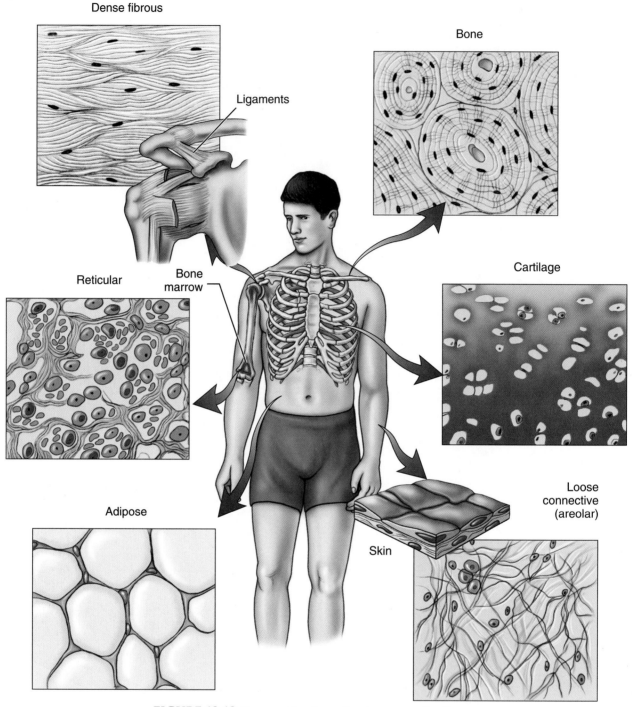

Dense fibrous

Bone

Ligaments

Reticular

Bone marrow

Cartilage

Adipose

Skin

Loose connective (areolar)

FIGURE 18-10 Types and locations of various connective tissues.

hyaline thinly covers the articulating surfaces of bones, connects the ribs to the sternum, and supports the nose, the trachea, and part of the larynx. The early fetal skeleton is mostly of this cartilage type.

Fibrocartilage – Fibrocartilage has the greatest tensile strength of all cartilage types; it consists of a dense matrix of white collagenous fibers. Fibrocartilaginous disks are found between the vertebrae, in the knee joint, and between the pubic bones.

Elastic – Elastic cartilage (yellow) is the softest and most pliable of all three kinds of cartilage, consisting of elastic fibers in a flexible fibrous matrix. It gives shape to the external nose and ears and internal structures such as the epiglottis, part of the larynx, and the auditory tubes.

TABLE 18-3 Connective Tissue Types

TYPE	CHARACTERISTICS
Fibrous	
Loose (areolar)	Most widely distributed; forms the superficial fascia
Adipose	Specialized for fat storage; insulates the body against heat loss; provides fuel reserves for energy; provides cushion around structures
Reticular	Forms the framework for bones and organs
Dense	Types are dense irregular and dense regular
Bone	
Compact	Forms the hard outer shell of bone
Cancellous (spongy)	Lattice of thin beams within bone
Cartilage	
Hyaline	Most common type; elastic, rubbery, and smooth; covers articular surfaces of bones and part of the larynx and nose; forms the C-shaped rings of the trachea
Elastic	Soft and pliable, giving shape to the external nose and ears and the epiglottis and auditory tubes
Fibrocartilage	Greatest tensile strength of all cartilage types; found in the intervertebral disks, meniscus of the knee, and between the pubic bones
Liquid	
Blood	Fluid medium (plasma) containing blood cells
Lymph	Fluid medium containing lymphocytes

Liquid. Liquid, or fluid, connective tissues exist in a liquid stage and include blood and lymph. They contain a distinctive collection of cells floating in their liquid matrix.

Blood – Blood is composed of red blood cells, white blood cells, and platelets suspended in a liquid called plasma. Plasma makes up about 55% of whole blood, and blood cells compose about 45%. Blood is also discussed in Chapter 26.

Lymph – Lymph is the liquid portion of the lymphatic system; this liquid contains white blood cells called lymphocytes. These cells are largely responsible for the body's immune responses. Lymph is also discussed in Chapter 27.

Muscle Tissue

Muscle tissue is regarded as the movement specialist of the body. This highly elastic tissue is unique in that it has both *contractility* (ability to shorten) and *extensibility* (ability to stretch and lengthen). Muscle tissue also possesses properties of *excitability* (ability to respond to a stimulus) and *elasticity* (ability of muscle fibers to return to their original shape after movement). Types of muscle tissue are smooth, skeletal, and cardiac (Table 18-4).

Smooth. Smooth muscle (involuntary) forms the walls of hollow organs such as the stomach, bladder, and uterus as well as tubes such as blood vessels. Consuming little energy, these cells are adapted for long, sustained contractions (Figure 18-11). Smooth muscle cells are spindle-shaped (pointed at both ends), and each contains one oval-shaped nucleus. Smooth muscle receives additional coverage in Chapter 29.

Skeletal. Skeletal muscle (voluntary) fibers are cigar-shaped and are multinucleate; many nuclei are located on the periphery of the cell. Each skeletal muscle fiber contains bands of red and white material, which causes it to appear

TABLE 18-4 Muscle Histology

| | HISTOLOGICAL CHARACTERISTICS | | |
	SMOOTH	SKELETAL	CARDIAC
Synonyms	Visceral	Heart	Voluntary
Striations	No	Yes	Yes
Number of nuclei	Mononucleate	Mononucleate (can be multinucleate)	Multinucleate
Location of nuclei	Centrally located	Centrally located	Peripherally located
Shape of nuclei	Oval-shaped	Oval shaped	Small, elongated
Shape of fibers	Spindle-shaped	Y- or H-shaped	Cylindrical
Voluntary or involuntary	Involuntary	Involuntary	Voluntary
Distinguishing characteristics	Shape of fibers	Intercalated disks	Striations
Fatigue rate	Slow	None	Rapid
Discussion	Forms the walls of hollow organs and tubes (e.g., stomach, bladder, blood vessel); controls the transport of materials, moving them along or restricting their flow	Located in the myocardium; possesses intercalated disks, which operate like an electrical synapse	Attaches to bones or related structures; is the *flesh* of the body; stimulated by a nerve impulse to contract

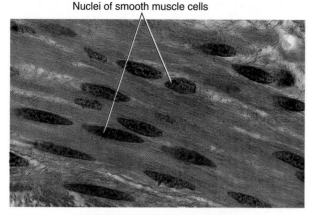

Nuclei of smooth muscle cells

FIGURE 18-11 Smooth muscle.

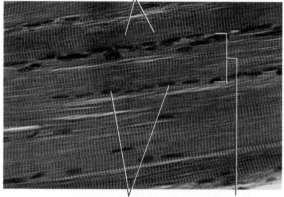

Cross striations of muscle cell

Nuclei of muscle cell   Muscle fiber

FIGURE 18-12 Skeletal muscle.

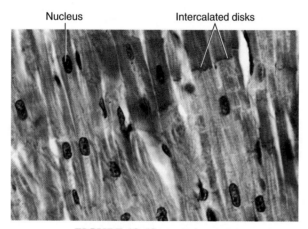

Nucleus   Intercalated disks

FIGURE 18-13 Cardiac muscle.

striped or striated under a microscope (Figure 18-12). Muscle contraction is stimulated by a neural impulse. Skeletal muscles are studied in detail in Chapter 20.

Cardiac. Cardiac muscle (involuntary-striated) is located in the heart wall, and its fibers are **Y**- or **H**-shaped (Figure 18-13). These shapes allow the cells to fit together like

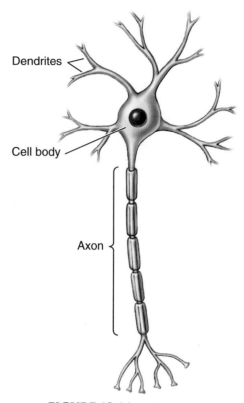

Dendrites

Cell body

Axon

FIGURE 18-14 Basic neuron.

clasped fingers and help create the spherical shape of the heart. Between each cardiac muscle cell is a structure known as the *intercalated disk.* These disks assist in the transmission of a nervous stimulus so that the cardiac muscle fibers contract in a synchronized fashion. More information on cardiac muscle can be found in Chapter 26.

Nervous Tissue

Nervous tissue consists of oddly shaped cells called *neurons,* which can detect and transmit electrical signals by converting stimuli into nerve impulses. Located in the brain, spinal cord, and peripheral nerves, nervous tissue possesses characteristics of *excitability* (the ability to generate a nerve impulse) and *conductibility* (the ability to transmit nerve impulses).

The three principal parts of a neuron are (1) the cell body, which contains the nucleus and other standard cell machinery; (2) the dendrites, which transmit impulses to the cell body; and (3) the axon, which transmits impulses away from the cell body (Figure 18-14). Neurons are also discussed in Chapter 23.

Neurons detect changes both inside and outside the body, interpret the perceived information and provide a response such as muscular contractions or glandular secretions, and are involved in higher mental processing and emotional responses.

HOMEOSTASIS

Within the study of anatomy and physiology is an important concept called homeostasis. **Homeostasis** is constancy of the body's internal environment. It represents a relatively stable condition of the body's internal environment within a limited range. Even when the outside conditions change, the body's internal environment needs to stay relatively consistent. Every body structure, from microscopic cells to complex organ systems, helps keep the internal environment within normal limits.

Homeostasis is maintained primarily by neural and hormonal control systems, which are featured in Chapters 23 and 24.

TISSUE REPAIR

As stated previously, homeostasis is the body's constant migration toward physiological balance. It is a controlled condition, one of relative constancy and equilibrium. When a person sustains an injury, homeostasis is disturbed. Tissue damage stimulates healing processes and begins with the same initial response—inflammation.

Inflammation

The purpose of inflammation is to contain the damage and prepare tissues for repair. Blood flow to the area increases and local capillaries become more permeable; these changes cause the cardinal signs and symptoms of inflammation, which can be remembered by the acronym SHARP. SHARP stands for *S*welling, *H*eat, *A* loss of function, *R*edness, and *P*ain (Figure 18-15). The increased blood flow and capillary permeability bring oxygen and nutrients necessary for rebuilding tissue to the area, as well as leukocytes cells that phagocytize foreign particles and debris from damaged tissues. If blood vessel damage has occurred, platelets form a clot to stop the loss of blood through the damaged area (Figure 18-16). How long inflammation lasts varies

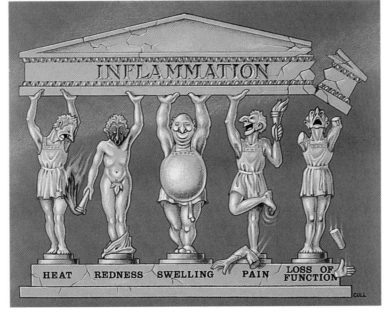

FIGURE 18-15 Cardinal signs of inflammation.

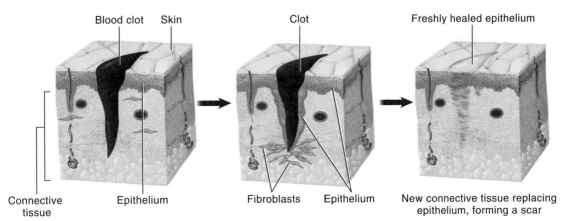

FIGURE 18-16 Stages of tissue repair and healing.

depending on the severity of the initial trauma and the strength of the person's immune system.

Regeneration

Damaged capillaries regrow; tissue structure is restored as collagen fibers are laid down and granulation tissue forms to provide a framework for the new tissue to grow into. Granulation tissue is fragile and can easily be reinjured. The swelling reduces as excess interstitial fluid enters the lymphatic system. If the injury only affects the more superficial layers, no scarring will result. If the injury is deep enough into connective tissues, scarring may result. Scar tissues can form adhesions. **Adhesions** are abnormal tissue connections that can restrict the normal movement of tissues, limiting the strength and motion of the body.

Remodeling

Inflammation has subsided and damaged blood vessels have regrown. The tissues are almost completely healed and, depending on the extent of the original damage, tissue function returns as much as is possible. The collagen fibers become more organized and scars diminish somewhat.

CHAT ROOM

One effect of deep friction is to manually assist the collagen fibers in becoming more aligned and to loosen adhesions.

Factors That Affect Tissue Repair

Several factors affect tissue repair. Nutrition is important because the healing process requires increased amounts of nutrients. For example, dietary protein is important because most of the structural components of tissues are proteins. Vitamin C is directly necessary for the normal production and maintenance of tissue components, especially collagen. It also strengthens and promotes new blood cell formation.

The condition of the wound is another factor. A clean, sutured wound heals faster. Suturing of a wound not only places the edges of the wound in contact with each other for improved healing but also supports tissue healing by reducing the stress placed on it by the pulling tissues (e.g., skin, muscle) in different directions.

Infection can slow or halt the rate of recovery.

Proper blood circulation is essential so that oxygen, nutrients, white blood cells, and platelets are transported to the injured site. Blood and lymph flow also remove excess tissue fluid, bacteria, foreign bodies, and debris which promote the healing process.

Different types of tissue have different rates of healing. Epithelial tissue has cells that divide rapidly and regenerate the tissue quickly and easily. On the other end of the spectrum, cartilage repairs slowly owing to its lack of blood supply. Muscle has an extensive blood supply and can heal

relatively quickly, whereas bone tissue takes longer to heal, and tendons and ligaments take even longer because they have a sparse blood supply.

Tissues heal faster and leave less obvious scars in people who are younger. The younger body is generally in a better nutritional state, there is a better blood supply to the tissues, and the body cells have a higher metabolic rate. This means the cells in a younger person's body can synthesize needed materials and divide more quickly to repair tissues.

"I don't believe in failure. It is not failure if you enjoyed the process."
—Oprah Winfrey

MEMBRANES

Membranes are thin, soft, pliable sheets of tissue that cover the body, line tubes or body cavities, cover organs, and separate one part of a cavity from another. Types of membranes are epithelial and connective. *Epithelial membranes* are composed of epithelium and an underlying layer of connective tissue. Types of epithelial membranes are cutaneous, mucous, and serous. *Connective tissue membranes* are composed exclusively of various types of connective tissue, such as synovial membranes (Figure 18-17). Another type of connective tissue membrane is meninges, which surrounds the brain and spinal cord. Meninges are discussed in Chapter 23.

Cutaneous. Both tough and supple, cutaneous membranes, or skin, cover the entire surface of the body. Skin, the largest organ of the body by weight, is discussed in Chapter 22.

Mucous. Membranes that line open body cavities are called mucous membranes or *mucosae*. Essentially, skin continues into various parts of the body as epithelium, such as in the lining of nose and mouth leading to the digestive respiratory tracts, the urethra leading to the urinary tract, and the vagina leading to the uterus. Mucous membranes secrete *mucus*, a fluid that lubricates and protects associated structures.

Serous. Serous membranes line closed body cavities that do not open to the outside of the body. Examples of serous membranes are the pericardium, the pleura, peritoneum, and mesenteries. These membranes consist of two layers, a *parietal layer*, which lines the wall of body cavities, often adhering to it, and a *visceral layer*, which provides a covering to organs in closed body cavities. Serous membranes secrete a lubricating *serous fluid* between the parietal and visceral layers. This fluid lubricates organs and reduces friction between the organs.

Synovial. Lining the joint cavities of freely moving joints (shoulder, hip, knee) are the synovial membranes or *synovium*. These membranes secrete *synovial fluid*, a viscous liquid that provides nutrition and lubrication to joints so that they can move freely without undue friction.

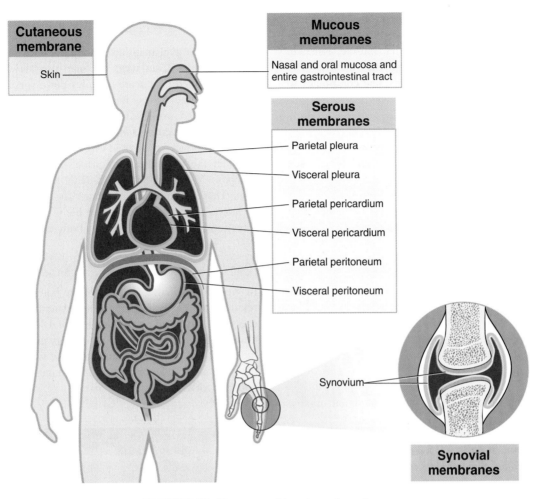

FIGURE 18-17 Types and locations of membranes.

BODY SYSTEMS

To review, the human body is made up of small components organized to function as a unit. The levels are chemical, cellular, tissue, organ, organ system, and organism (see Figure 18-1). Body systems make up the entire organism. Basic anatomy and physiology of each body system are featured next.

Skeletal System

Anatomy. Bones, cartilage, joints, and ligaments.

Physiology. Supports the body, protects vital organs, provides movement through muscle attachments, produces blood cells, stores fats and vital minerals.

Muscular System

Anatomy. Skeletal muscles, related fascial structures (e.g., tendons, aponeurosis).

Physiology. Provides movement and helps move substances, produces heat, and maintains posture.

Integumentary System

Anatomy. Skin, hair, nails, and skin glands.

Physiology. Provides protection, absorption, sensation, body temperature regulation, waste elimination, vitamin D synthesis, and immunity.

Nervous System

Anatomy. Brain, spinal cord, meninges, cranial and spinal nerves, special senses, cerebrospinal fluid, and neurotransmitters.

Physiology. Provides sensory input, interpretive functions, motor output, and higher mental processing and emotional responses.

Endocrine System

Anatomy. Hypothalamus, pituitary, pineal, thyroid, parathyroids, thymus, adrenals, pancreatic islets, ovaries, testes, and hormones.

Physiology. Produces and secretes hormones, regulates metabolic activities, regulates the activity of other organs and glands as well as smooth and cardiac muscle, assists in adaptation during times of stress, regulates the chemical composition and volume of body fluids, and contributes to the reproductive process.

Reproductive System

Anatomy. Gonads, gametes, ducts, male and female sex organs and accessory glands.

Physiology. Produces offspring, releases hormones that regulate reproduction and other body processes.

Cardiovascular System

Anatomy. Heart, blood vessels, and blood.

Physiology. Transportation of substances, protection by fighting disease, and combats hemorrhage.

Lymphatic System

Anatomy. Lymph, lymph vessels, lymph glands and organs, lymph nodes, and lymphocytes.

Physiology. Transports lipids from the digestive tract to the blood, provides the immune response, and maintains homeostasis.

Respiratory System

Anatomy. Nose and nasal cavity, pharynx, larynx, trachea, bronchi and bronchioles, alveoli, lungs, and diaphragm.

Physiology. Exchange of gases, olfaction (smell), produces sounds, and maintains homeostasis.

Digestive System

Anatomy. Oral cavity, pharynx, esophagus, stomach, small and large intestines, salivary glands, pancreas, liver, and gallbladder.

Physiology. Ingestion, digestion, absorption, and defecation.

Urinary System

Anatomy. Kidneys, ureters, urethra, and urinary bladder.

Physiology. Eliminates wastes and foreign substances, regulates blood pressure, and maintains homeostasis by regulating pH balance, blood volume, and fluid balance.

BODY COMPASS

Every good travel map has a compass drawing to indicate north, south, east, and west. The map also has some distance reference, such as a scale of miles per a specific measure. Any map without these items is of little or no use. Imagine trying to read a map if you cannot understand terms or phrases such as *south, 5 miles, 1 block,* or *by the lake.* Think of the anatomic drawings in this textbook as your map, and consider the following sections of this chapter as a body compass. You will learn terms denoting position and direction. These terms include names for planes of the body, locations that are relative to the body planes, regional and directional designations, and the body cavities.

ANATOMIC POSITION

In Western medicine, all parts of the body are described in relation to other body parts using a standard body position called the **anatomic position** (Figure 18-18). In this position, the body is upright and facing forward, the arms are at the sides, the palms are facing forward with the thumbs to the side, and feet are about hip distance apart with toes pointing forward.

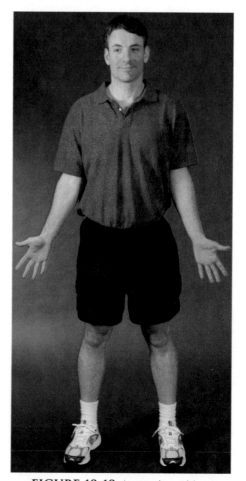

FIGURE 18-18 Anatomic position.

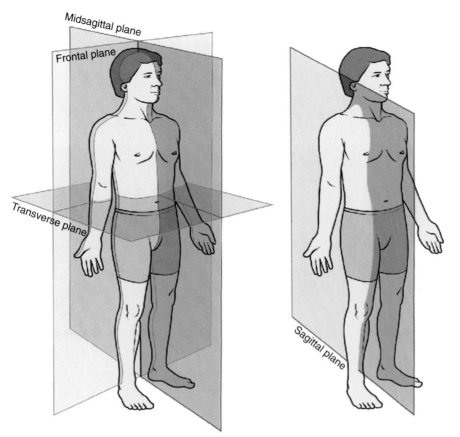

FIGURE 18-19 Planes of the body.

PLANES OF REFERENCE

A **plane** is a flat surface determined by three points in space such as height, depth, and width. These planes lie at right angles to one another (Figure 18-19). These terms are used to describe the location of a specific body part.

Midsagittal/Median. The midsagittal plane runs longitudinally or vertically down the body, anterior to posterior, dividing the body into equal right and left sections.

   Sagittal – A plane that passes through the body parallel to the midsagittal plane is called the sagittal plane.

Frontal/Coronal. The frontal plane passes through the body side to side to create anterior and posterior sections.

Transverse/Horizontal. The transverse plane passes through the body to create superior and inferior sections.

BODY CAVITIES

A **cavity** is a hollow space within a larger structure. The two main body cavities are the dorsal and the ventral cavities (Figure 18-20).

Dorsal. The dorsal cavity is located on the backside or posterior aspect of the body. The dorsal cavity is divided into the *cranial cavity* (contains the brain) and the *spinal* or *vertebral cavity* (contains the spinal cord).

Ventral. The larger ventral cavity is located on the front side or anterior aspect of the body. The ventral cavity is divided by the diaphragm into the *thoracic* and *abdominopelvic cavities.*

   Thoracic – The thoracic cavity contains the *pleural cavities,* which surround the lungs, and the *mediastinum,* which is the area between the lungs and includes the pericardium, heart, great vessels, esophagus, and trachea.

   Abdominopelvic – The abdominopelvic is actually two cavities in one. The *abdominal cavity* contains the digestive organs and the *pelvic cavity* contains the reproductive and urinary organs.

ABDOMINAL QUADRANTS AND REGIONS

To assist in locating abdominal organs or describing symptoms in these areas, there are two ways of dividing the abdomen. One method uses a grid made up of four quadrants and the other uses a grid of nine regions (Figure 18-21).

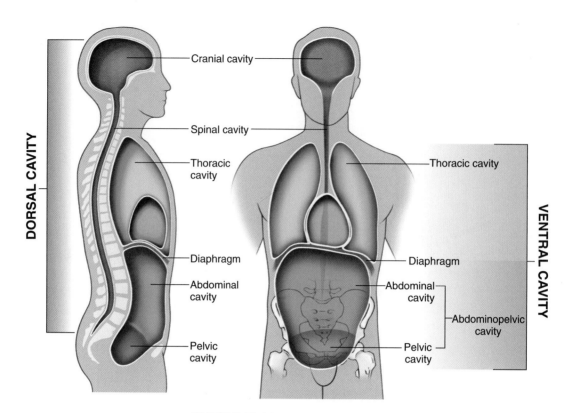

FIGURE 18-20 Major body cavities.

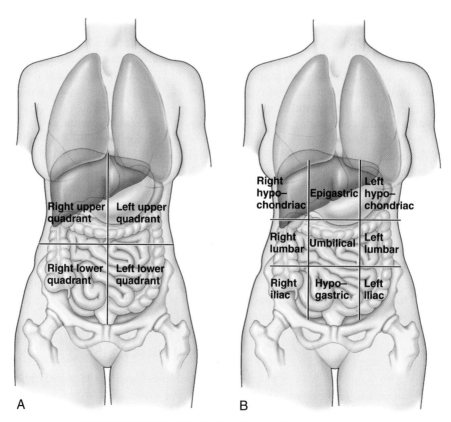

FIGURE 18-21 Abdominal quadrants (**A**) and regions (**B**).

Abdominopelvic Quadrants

One horizontal line and one vertical line divide the abdomen into four quadrants. From right to left, and from top to bottom, they are:

1. Right upper quadrant
2. Left upper quadrant
3. Right lower quadrant
4. Left lower quadrant

Abdominal Regions

Two horizontal and two vertical lines divide the body into a tic-tac-toe–like grid of nine abdominal regions. From right to left, and from top to bottom, they are:

1. Right hypochondriac region
2. Epigastric region
3. Left hypochondriac region
4. Right lumbar region
5. Umbilical region
6. Left lumbar region
7. Right iliac (inguinal) region
8. Hypogastric region
9. Left iliac (inguinal) region

DIRECTIONAL TERMS

The following terms describe location and direction on one body part with respect to another (Figure 18-22).

Left. To the left of the body or structure (not your left, the subject's left). *The heart is located primarily on the left side of the body.*

Right. To the right of the body or structure. *The liver is located primarily on the right side of the body.*

Superior (Cranial, Cephalic). Situated above or toward the head end. *The jaw is superior to the neck.*

Inferior (Caudal). Situated below or toward the tail end. *The sacrum is inferior to the skull.*

Anterior (Ventral). Pertaining to the front side of a structure. *The heart is anterior to the vertebral column.*

Posterior (Dorsal). Pertaining to the back of a structure. *The vertebral column is posterior to the sternum.*

Medial. Oriented toward or near the midline of the body. *The nose is medial to the ears.*

Lateral. Oriented farther away from the midline of the body. *The ribs are lateral to the vertebral column.*
   Note – Medial and lateral may be used to refer to structures that are on a larger structure such as the trunk.

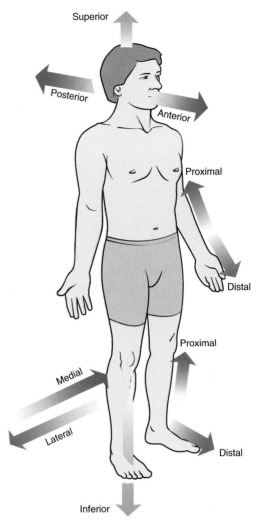

FIGURE 18-22 Directional terminology.

Ipsilateral (Homolateral). Related to the same side of the body. *The right hand is homolateral to the right elbow.*

Contralateral. Related to opposite sides of the body. *The right foot is contralateral to the left foot.*

Proximal. Nearer to the point of reference, usually toward the trunk of the body. *The hip is proximal to the knee.*

Distal. Farther from the point of reference, usually away from the midline. *The foot is distal to the knee.*
   Note – Proximal and distal refer to structures located on the extremities.

Terms Related to Organs and Structures

These terms are often used to describe anatomical relationships among organs or regions within the organ.

Deep (Central). Pertaining to or situated at a center of the body. *The heart is centrally located.*

Superficial (Peripheral). Pertaining to the outside surface, periphery, or surrounding external area of a structure. *The skin is superficial to the muscles.*

Internal. Nearest the inside (within) of a body cavity. *The stomach is an internally located organ.*

External. Nearest the outside of a body cavity. *The skin is located on the external surface of the body.*

Medullary (Medulla). Inner region of an organ or structure. *The medullary cavity is the inner region of long bones.*

Cortical (Cortex). Outer region of an organ or structure. *The cerebral cortex is the outer region of the brain.*

Lumen. In anatomy, the inside space of a tubular structure, such as an artery or intestine. *During vasodilation, the arterial lumen enlarges.*

REGIONAL TERMS

This section identifies regions associated with body areas such as the head and neck, upper and lower extremities, and anterior and posterior torso (Figure 18-23).

Head and Neck

Buccal. Lower cheek.

Cervical. Neck.

Cephalic. Head.

Cranial. Upper skull.

Facial. Face.

Frontal. Forehead.

Mandibular. Lower jaw.

Mental. Chin.

Nasal. Nose.

Nuchal. Posterior neck.

Occipital. Back lower part of skull.

Oral. Mouth.

Orbital (Ophthalmic). Eye.

Otic (Auricular). Ear.

Temporal. Side of skull.

Zygomatic. Upper cheek.

Upper Extremity

Acromial. Top of shoulder.

Antebrachial. Forearm; between wrist and elbow.

Antecubital. Front of elbow/bend of elbow.

Axillary. Armpit.

Brachial. Arm; between the shoulder and elbow.

Carpal. Wrist.

Clavicular. Collar bone.

Cubital. Elbow.

Deltoid. Curve of the shoulder and upper arm formed by the deltoid muscle.

Digital (Phalangeal). Fingers and/or toes.

Olecranal. Back of elbow.

Palmar (Volar). Anterior surface of hand.

Pollex. Thumb.

Anterior Torso

Abdominal. Abdomen; superior region of the abdomino-pelvic cavity.

Costal. Ribs.

Inguinal (Groin). Area between thigh and abdomen.

Mammary (Pectoral). Breast/upper anterior thorax.

Mediastinal. Between the lungs.

Pelvic. Pelvis; inferior region of the abdominopelvic cavity.

Perineal. Region between the anus and the genitals.

Pubic. Region of the pubic symphysis or genital area.

Thoracic. Chest, between neck and diaphragm.

Umbilical. Navel (scar left from the umbilical cord).

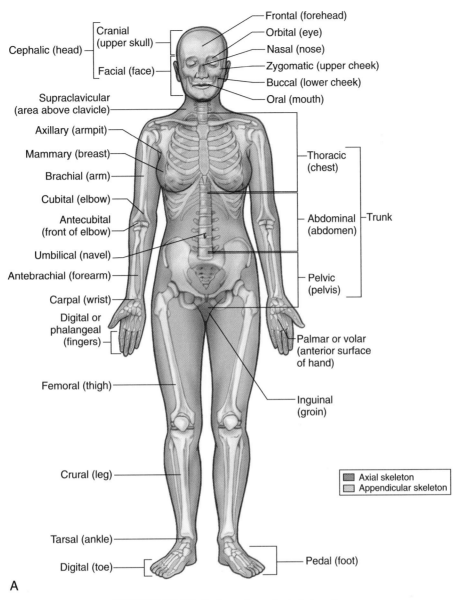

FIGURE 18-23 Body regions. **A**, Anterior view.

Posterior Torso

Coccygeal. Bottom of the spinal column or coccyx; upper region of the gluteal cleft.

Dorsal. Back.

Flank. Lateral trunk.

Gluteal (Buttock). Curve of the buttocks formed by the gluteal muscles.

Lumbar. Loin or lower back; between ribs and hips.

Sacral. Sacrum of the spinal column.

Sacroiliac. Between the sacrum and pelvic bone.

Scapular. Shoulder blade.

Vertebral. Vertebrae of the spinal column.

Lower Extremity

Calcaneal. Heel.

Calf (Sural). Posterior leg.

Coxal. Hip.

Crural. Leg; between knee and ankle.

Digital (Phalangeal). Fingers and/or toes.

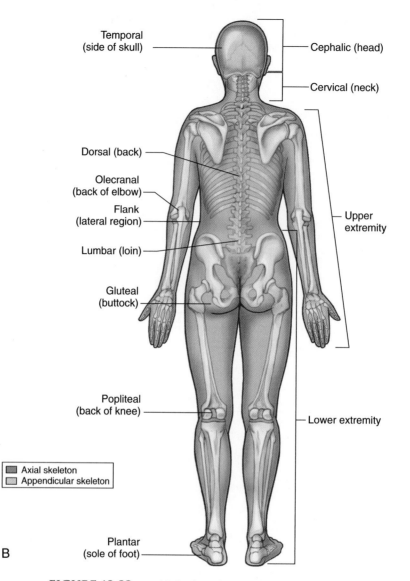

Temporal (side of skull)

Cephalic (head)

Cervical (neck)

Dorsal (back)

Olecranal (back of elbow)

Flank (lateral region)

Lumbar (loin)

Gluteal (buttock)

Upper extremity

Popliteal (back of knee)

Lower extremity

Axial skeleton
Appendicular skeleton

Plantar (sole of foot)

B

FIGURE 18-23, cont'd Body regions. **B,** Posterior view.

Dorsum. Top of foot.

Femoral. Thigh; between hip and knee.

Hallux. Great toe.

Patellar. Kneecap.

Pedal. Foot or feet.

Plantar (Volar). Bottom or sole of foot.

Popliteal. Posterior knee.

Tarsal. Ankle.

BODY POSITIONS

The following terms are used in describing a person lying down or reclining (Figure 18-24, p. 409). The knees may be bent while the subject is in any of these body positions.

Prone. Lying face down.

Supine. Lying face up.

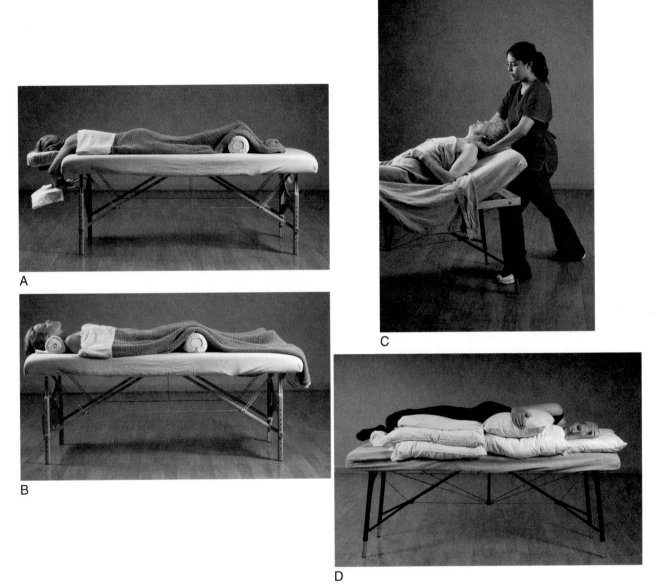

FIGURE 18-24 Body positions. **A,** Prone; **B,** Supine; **C,** Semireclining; **D,** Side lying.

Semi-reclining. A semi-upright sitting position. This is also called the *Fowler position* (upper body elevated 80 to 90 degrees) or semi-Fowler position (upper body elevated 30 to 45 degrees).

Side Lying. Lying on the left or right side. This is also called the *lateral recumbent position* (left lateral or right lateral recumbent). The term recumbent means lying back.

E-RESOURCES

ⓔvolve

http://evolve.elsevier.com/Salvo/MassageTherapy

- Chapter challenge
- Flash cards
- Photo gallery
- Educational animations
- Weblinks

BIBLIOGRAPHY

Abrahams P, Marks S, Hutchings R: *McMinn's color atlas of human anatomy*, St Louis, 2003, Mosby.

Applegate EJ: *The anatomy and physiology learning system*, ed 3, Philadelphia, 2006, Saunders.

Beers MH, Berkow R: *The Merck manual of diagnosis and therapy*, Whitehouse Station, NJ, 2006, Merck Research Laboratories.

Crawley J, Van De Graaff KM: *A photographic atlas for anatomy and physiology*, Englewood, Colo, 2002, Morton.

Ferri FF: *2003 Ferri's clinical advisor, instant diagnosis and treatment*, St Louis, 2003, Mosby.

Gould BE: *Pathophysiology for the health-related professionals*, ed 3, Philadelphia, 2006, Saunders.

Goldberg S: *Clinical anatomy made ridiculously simple*, Miami, 2004, Medmaster.

Grafelman T: *Graf's anatomy and physiology guide for the massage therapist*, Aurora, Colo, 1998, DG Publishing.

Gray HT, Pickering P, Howden R: *Gray's anatomy*, ed 29, Philadelphia, 1974, Running Press.

Guyton A: *Human physiology and mechanisms of disease*, ed 6, Philadelphia, 1996, WB Saunders.

Haubrich WS: *Medical meanings: a glossary of word origins*, New York, 1984, Harcourt Brace Jovanovich.

Herlihy B: *The human body in health and illness*, ed 3, Philadelphia, 2007, Saunders.

Jacob S, Francone C: *Elements of anatomy and physiology*, Philadelphia, 1989, WB Saunders.

Juhan D: *Job's body: a handbook for bodyworkers*, ed 3, Barrington, NY, 2003, Station Hill Press.

Kalat JW: *Biological psychology*, ed 8, Belmont, Calif, 2003, Wadsworth.

Kapit W, Elson LM: *The anatomy coloring book*, ed 3, New York, 2002, Benjamin Cummings.

Kapit W, Macey R, Meisami E: *The physiology coloring book*, ed 2, New York, 1999, HarperCollins.

Lauderstein D: *Putting the soul back in the body: a manual of imaginative anatomy for massage therapists*, Chicago, 1985, self-published manual.

Marieb EN: *Essentials of human anatomy and physiology*, ed 8, New York, 2005, Benjamin Cummings.

Martini FH, Bartholomew EF: *Essentials of anatomy and physiology*, ed 3, New York, 2003, Benjamin Cummings.

Merck manual, ed 17, Whitehouse Station, NJ, 1998, Merck and Co.

Moore KL: *Clinically oriented anatomy*, ed 5, Baltimore, 2005, Lippincott Williams & Wilkins.

Mosby's dictionary of medicine, nursing & health professions, ed 8, St Louis, 2009, Mosby.

Mosby's medical, nursing, and allied health dictionary, ed 6, St Louis, 2002, Mosby.

Myers TW: *Anatomy trains: myofascial meridians for manual and movement therapists*, New York, 2001, Churchill Livingstone.

Netter FH: *Atlas of human anatomy*, ed 3, Teterboro, NJ, 2003, Icon Learning Systems.

Premkumar K: *The massage connection: anatomy and physiology*, ed 2, Philadelphia, 2004, Lippincott Williams & Wilkins.

Salvo SG: *Mosby's pathology for massage therapists*, ed 2, St Louis, 2009, Mosby.

Thibodeau G, Patton K: *Anatomy and physiology*, ed 7, St Louis, 2010, Mosby.

Thibodeau G, Patton K: *Structure and function of the body*, ed 12, St Louis, 2004, Mosby.

Tortora GJ: *Introduction to the human body: the essentials of anatomy and physiology*, ed 5, Hoboken, NJ, 2000, John Wiley & Sons.

Tortora GJ, Grabowksi SR: *Principles of anatomy and physiology*, ed 12, New York, 2009, John Wiley & Sons.

Venes D, Thomas CL, Taber CW: *Taber's cyclopedic medical dictionary*, ed 20, Philadelphia, 2005, FA Davis.

MATCHING I

Place the letter of the answer next to the term or phrase that best describes it.

A. Anatomy
B. Cell
C. Cytoplasm
D. Diffusion
E. Filtration
F. Metabolism
G. Mitochondrion
H. Nucleus
I. Phagocytosis
J. Physiology
K. Ribosome
L. Semipermeable

_____ 1. Organelle that is the cell's control center, directing most metabolic activities

_____ 2. Total of all physical and chemical processes that occur in an organism

_____ 3. Organelle that is the cell's power plant and site for cellular respiration

_____ 4. Study of how the body and its individual parts function in normal body processes

_____ 5. Cellular membrane property in which some materials can freely pass and others cannot

_____ 6. Gel-like intracellular fluid

_____ 7. Fundamental unit of all living organisms and the simplest form of life that can exist as a self-sustaining unit

_____ 8. Study of human body structures and their positional relationships

_____ 9. Organelle that synthesizes and produces proteins, some of which are exported outside the cell

_____ 10. Cellular process that includes movement of particles across cellular membranes through pressure differences

_____ 11. Cellular process of ingesting, breaking down, and expelling harmful microorganisms and cellular debris

_____ 12. Cellular process that includes movement of molecules from an area of high to low concentration

MATCHING II

Place the letter of the answer next to the term or phrase that best describes it.

A. Adipose
B. Blood
C. Connective
D. Epithelium

E. Fibrocartilage
F. Homeostasis
G. Hyaline
H. Inflammation

I. Mucous
J. Muscle
K. Nervous
L. Remodeling

_____ 1. Tissue repair stage in which tissue is almost completely healed and function returns as much as possible

_____ 2. Body's constant migration toward physiologic balance; controlled condition of relative constancy and equilibrium

_____ 3. Tissue type that produces movement

_____ 4. Tissue type that lines or covers internal and external organs, blood vessels, body cavities, and digestive, respiratory, urinary, and reproductive tracts

_____ 5. Cartilage that covers articulating surfaces of bones, connects ribs to the sternum, and supports the nose, trachea, and part of the larynx

_____ 6. Initial stage of tissue repair that seeks to contain the damage and prepare the area for further healing

_____ 7. Cartilage found between the vertebrae, in the knee, and between the pubic bones

_____ 8. Connective tissue type specialized for fat storage

_____ 9. Tissue type that detects and transmits electrical signals by converting stimuli into impulses

_____ 10. Liquid connective tissue

_____ 11. Most abundant and diverse tissue type; serves in nutrient transport, defense, blood clotting, and organ protection

_____ 12. Membrane that lines open body cavities

MATCHING III

Place the letter of the answer next to the term or phrase that best describes it.

A. Anatomic position
B. Anterior
C. Contralateral
D. Deep

E. Distal
F. Frontal
G. Inferior
H. Ipsilateral

I. Midsagittal
J. Posterior
K. Proximal
L. Superior

_____ 1. Pertains to or situated at a center of the body

_____ 2. Means same side of the body

_____ 3. Situated above or toward the head end

_____ 4. Plane passing side to side through the body, creating anterior and posterior sections

_____ 5. Pertains to the front side of a structure

_____ 6. Means opposite side of the body

_____ 7. Situated below or toward the tail end

_____ 8. Plane dividing the body into equal right and left sections

_____ 9. Nearer to the point of reference, usually toward the trunk; used only in referencing the extremities

_____ 10. Pertains to the back of a structure

_____ 11. Body position in which the individual is standing upright, facing forward, arms at the side, palms facing forward with thumbs to the side, and feet about hip distance apart with toes pointing forward

_____ 12. Farther from the point of reference, usually away from the midline; used only in referencing the extremities

MATCHING IV

Place the letter of the answer next to the anatomic term or phrase that best describes it.

A. Antebrachial
B. Antecubital
C. Axillary
D. Brachial

E. Carpal
F. Cervical
G. Clavicular
H. Mental

I. Oral
J. Orbital
K. Otic
L. Pollex

_____ 1.   Ear

_____ 2.   Mouth

_____ 3.   Collar bone

_____ 4.   Posterior neck

_____ 5.   Eye

_____ 6.   Armpit

_____ 7.   Forearm

_____ 8.   Arm

_____ 9.   Thumb

_____ 10. Wrist

_____ 11. Front of elbow

_____ 12. Chin

MATCHING V

Place the letter of the answer next to the regional term or phrase that best describes it.

A. Calcaneal
B. Costal
C. Coxal
D. Crural

E. Dorsum
F. Hallux
G. Lumbar
H. Mediastinal

I. Plantar
J. Popliteal
K. Sacroiliac
L. Sural

_____ 1.   Lower back; between ribs and hips

_____ 2.   Ribs

_____ 3.   Between the lungs

_____ 4.   Between the sacrum and pelvic bone

_____ 5.   Calf

_____ 6.   Leg

_____ 7.   Great toe

_____ 8.   Bottom or sole of foot

_____ 9.   Top of foot

_____ 10. Hip

_____ 11. Posterior knee

_____ 12. Heel

CASE STUDY

A Friend in Need Is a Friend Indeed!

Janet was just starting her massage therapy career. She was excited about helping people in pain and providing healthy service. Occasionally, Janet offered her services free of charge at community events.

Janet was happy to give free massages to a health fair at her local church. It was a rainy day; not many people attended the health fair, but she felt the response was very good. She remembers a man named Richard in particular. Richard looked like he was down on his luck. His clothes seemed old and a little dirty; his hair was unkempt, and Janet noticed Richard watching her give the other participants' massages. She felt a little uncomfortable as he approached her asking if he, too, could get a massage. Janet agreed, and when she was finished, he noticed her business cards on the table and asked if he could have one. With an uneasy feeling she could not explain, Janet handed him one of her business cards.

CASE STUDY—cont'd

A couple of weeks went by and Janet forgot all about Richard until one day her phone rang. The man on the other end of the phone asked if she remembered him and Janet recognized his voice instantly. Richard explained that he did not have many friends, and he did not make a habit of reaching out to strangers, but he had a drug addiction and needed a friend.

What positive outcomes might come from Janet's reaching out to Richard?

What negative outcomes might occur from giving Richard a hand?

If you were Janet, how would you feel about Richard's request? How might Janet respond to Richard's request?

Is there anyway to create a win-win situation?

CRITICAL THINKING

Why is it important for the massage therapist to know all the components of a body—from the cellular level to the whole body—and how they work? How does this knowledge benefit the client?

CHAPTER 19

Skeletal System

"Opportunity is missed by most people because it is dressed in overalls and looks like work."
—Thomas Edison

LEARNING OBJECTIVES

After completing this chapter, the student should be able to:

- List the anatomy and physiology of the skeletal system.
- Classify bones according to their shape.
- Discuss the types of bone tissue and bone marrow.
- Name the parts of a long bone.
- Describe the process of bone development and bone remodeling.
- Discuss the effects of aging and exercise on bone health.
- Group the bones of the body into either the axial skeleton or the appendicular skeleton.
- Describe the structural and functional classifications of joints.
- List the structures of a synovial joint.
- Name the types of synovial joints.
- Name and describe various skeletal pathologic conditions and massage considerations of each.

INTRODUCTION

The skeletal system is composed of individual and fused bones and their associated ligaments and cartilage. Bones are living tissue. The skeletons in anatomy classes, laboratories, and museums are the mineral salts that remain after death. Second to tooth enamel, bones possess the hardest tissue in the body, yet they are relatively light, somewhat flexible, and able to resist tension and other external forces of stress.

The human body has 206 bones. Bones are the steel girders of the body, forming its internal framework. Mammals ranging from humans to bats to elephants have remarkably similar skeletal systems. For example, seven vertebrae are in the human cervical spine and are also in the long-necked giraffe and the no-necked whale.

The study of the skeletal system is multifaceted. Besides the basic structure and function of bone, this chapter also reviews bone classifications, types of bone tissue, long bone anatomy, bone development, skeletal system divisions, types of joints, and skeletal pathological conditions.

ANATOMY

Basic structures of the skeletal system are:

- Bones
- Joints
- Cartilage
- Ligaments

IT'S ALL GREEK TO ME

Amphi	*Gr.* on both sides
Arthr, arthro	*Gr.* joint
Blast	*Gr.* germ cell or bud
Bursa	*Gr.* a leather sac
Chondr	*Gr.* cartilage
Clast	*Gr.* to break
Crepitus	*L.* crackling or rattling (sound)
Diarthrotic	*Gr.* two; joint
Epiphysis	*Gr.* upon, over; to grow
Haversian	Havers, British physician and anatomist (1650-1702)
Ligament	*L.* to bind or a band
Ossicle	*L.* little bone
Os, ossi	*Gr.* bone
Osteo, osseo	*L.* bone
Periosteum	*Gr.* around, about; *L.* bone
Sesamoid	*Gr.* sesame seedlike; shaped
Sharpey	Scottish anatomist (1802-1880)
Skeleton	*Gr.* dried up
Symphysis	*Gr.* together with, joined; to grow
Synarthrotic	*Gr.* together; joint
Volkmann	German physician (1800-1877)

Fr., French; *Gr.,* Greek; *L.,* Latin.

PHYSIOLOGY

The functions of the skeletal system are:

- **Support.** The skeletal system provides support for the rest of the body through a bony framework.
- **Protection.** Bones help protect vital organs of the body.
- **Movement.** On the surface of bones are attachment sites for tendons of skeletal muscles. As muscles contract, they pull on bones, causing movement at joints. Hence, bones and their associated joints along with muscle contractions constitute levers needed for movement to occur (see Chapter 20 for information regarding levers).
- **Blood cell production (hemopoiesis).** Blood cells are produced in the red marrow of certain bones, especially long bones.
- **Fat storage.** Fats are stored in yellow bone marrow and are released when needed.
- **Mineral storage.** Vital minerals (e.g., phosphorus, magnesium, sodium) and mineral compounds (e.g., calcium phosphate, calcium carbonate) are stored in bone and released when needed.

CLASSIFICATION OF BONES

Bones are classified according to their size and shape (Figure 19-1).

Long. These bones are longer than they are wide. Examples are the humerus (arm), femur (thigh), and tibia (leg).

Short. Short bones are generally small and cube-shaped and contain multiple articulating surfaces. Examples are most of the carpal (wrist) bones and tarsal (ankle) bones.

Irregular. Consider this a catch-all category for bones that do not fit in other categories. Examples of irregular bones are facial bones and vertebrae (individual bones of the spinal column).

Flat. These bones possess a broad flat surface for muscle attachment or protection of underlying organs. The sternum (breast bone), scapula (shoulder blade), ribs, and most cranial bones are flat bones.

Sesamoid. Sesamoid bones are small, round bones that are embedded in certain tendons. They are often found in the hands and feet. The largest sesamoid bone is the patella (kneecap).

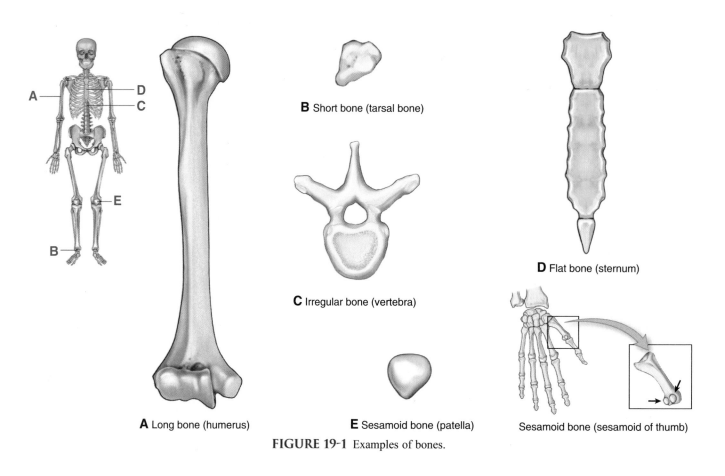

A Long bone (humerus) B Short bone (tarsal bone) C Irregular bone (vertebra) D Flat bone (sternum) E Sesamoid bone (patella) Sesamoid bone (sesamoid of thumb)

FIGURE 19-1 Examples of bones.

BONE TISSUE

Bone can be classified according to its tissue type (Figure 19-2, *B*). The two types are compact and spongy bone.

Compact. Compact bone forms the hard outer shell of all bones and a portion of the shaft bulk of long bones. Compact bone consists of mature bone cells (called *osteocytes*) almost completely surrounded by dense material made of calcium and phosphate. Compact bone provides protection and support and resists the stresses of weight and movement.

Spongy (cancellous) bone. Within many bones is a lattice of thin beams, giving it a spongy appearance. Such lattices lighten the bone and are filled with red marrow.

Bone Marrow

There are two types of bone marrow: red and yellow. At birth, all bone marrow is red. With age, some red marrow is converted to yellow marrow. This process continues until about half of all adult bone marrow is yellow and half is red.

In some cases, such as with severe blood loss, the body can convert yellow marrow back to red marrow to increase blood cell production.

Red Bone Marrow. Contains blood forming cells and found mainly in flat bones and in spongy bone located at the ends of long bones (e.g., humerus, femur).

Yellow Bone Marrow. Contains mainly fat cells and is found in the medullary cavity (discussed next).

ANATOMY OF A LONG BONE

Parts of a long bone and their associated structures are listed next (Figure 19-2, *A*).

Diaphysis. The diaphysis is the long cylindrical shaft of the bone.

Epiphyses. The two ends of a long bone, which are usually wider than the diaphysis, are the epiphyses (*sing.,* epiphysis). The epiphyses are also where the bone grows in length.

Articular cartilage. Articular surfaces of the epiphyses are covered with hyaline cartilage, a type of connective tissue.

Periosteum. The fibrous, dense, vascular tissue sheath that surrounds the diaphysis and is noticeably absent on the epiphyses. It is the bone's life support system, containing

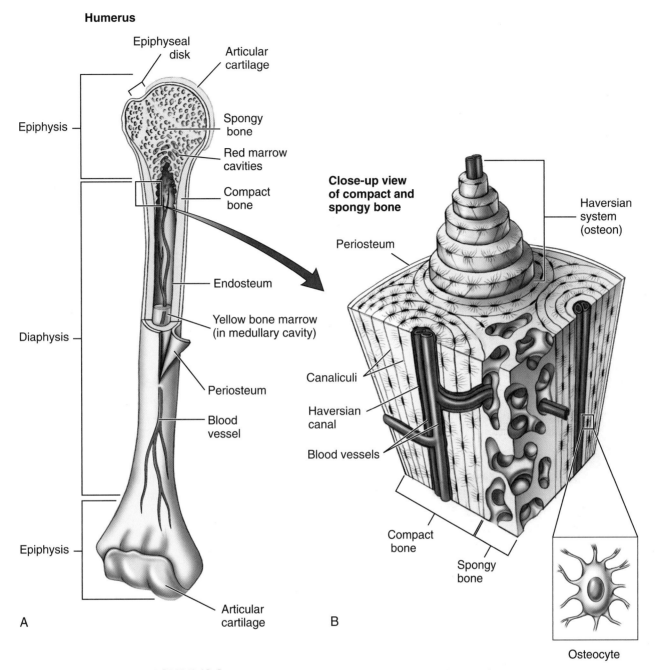

FIGURE 19-2 Bone. **A,** Long bone anatomy **B,** Compact and spongy bone.

blood and lymphatic vessels, nerves, and bone-forming cells (osteoblasts) for growth and healing of fractures. Periosteum is attached to the underlying bone via perforating fibers called *Sharpey fibers*.

Medullary cavity. The medullary cavity is the hollow space within the center of the bone shaft filled with yellow bone marrow.

Haversian canals. These tiny vascular canals run longitudinally through the bone.

Volkmann canals. These canals connect to the Haversian canals and run horizontally through the bone.

Metaphysis. Metaphyses contain the growth portion of the bone and is located where the diaphysis joins the epiphysis. Depending on the bone's age, it can contain the epiphyseal disk or the epiphyseal line.

Epiphyseal disk. In growing bone, the epiphyseal disk is a thin layer of cartilage where new bone is formed. This is also known as the *growth plate* or *epiphyseal plate*.

Epiphyseal line. Replaced by bone, the epiphyseal disk becomes the epiphyseal line when bone growth is complete.

Many long bones, such as ones located in the forearm and leg, are connected by a tough membrane. This *interosseous membrane* (also called *interosseous ligament*) connects select bones by attaching to their periosteum (see Figure 21-8). This structure also provides muscle attachment.

⊖volve *Be sure to log onto your student account to access activities and additional resources.* ■

BONE DEVELOPMENT, REMODELING, AND BONE HEALTH

Bone Development

The processes contributing to bone development, or **ossification**, begin between the sixth and seventh week of embryonic life and continue throughout adulthood. The two mechanisms of ossification replace preexisting connective tissue with osseous or bone tissue. The two types of ossification are:

Intramembranous ossification. This process involves bone formation from membranes and is found in flat bone development. A summary of events follows: development of an ossification center, calcification, formation of trabeculae, and finally the development of the periosteum.

Endochondral (cartilaginous) ossification. This type of bone formation begins from cartilage and occurs in most bones of the body. A summary of events follows: development of a cartilage model, growth of the cartilage model, development of a primary ossification center, development of the medullary (marrow) cavity, development of secondary ossification center, and then the formation of articular cartilage and epiphyseal disks.

Bone Remodeling

After bone growth has ceased, bones undergo a process of remodeling throughout life. This process can alter a bone's thickness and width.

The process of remodeling involves two phases: bone resorption and bone deposition. Bone remodeling is accomplished by the combined actions of osteoblasts and osteoclasts.

Osteoblasts. These bone-forming cells, found just beneath periosteum, continuously deposit bone on its external surface (i.e., moving calcium found in blood to the bone). This is the *bone deposition* or *formation phase* of bone remodeling.

Osteoclasts. These bone-destroying cells, found in the lining of the medullary cavity, break down bone tissue to maintain blood calcium levels (i.e., moving calcium found in bone to the blood). This is the *bone resorption* phase of bone remodeling.

Bone Health

Exercise promotes bone health. During exercise, bones become stressed from mechanical forces (e.g., gravity, pulling force of tendons, ligaments). The body responds to the demands of physical activity by secreting a hormone (calcitonin [see Chapter 24]), which moves blood calcium into the bones. Osteoblasts are stimulated to create more bone tissue and thus stronger bones. The fact that bones must be physically stressed to remain strong and healthy cannot be overemphasized. When we remain physically active, when muscles and gravity exert force on skeletal bones, they respond by becoming stronger.

To maintain mineral homeostasis, the osteoclasts break down the bone's minerals and move them into the blood, while osteoblasts replace the bone lost to metabolism. Both processes occur at approximately the same rate; thus density in healthy bones is relatively constant.

Both estrogens in women and testosterone in men stimulate osteoblast activity. However, the production of estrogens in women declines greatly at menopause. The decreased hormone level causes osteoblasts to become less active. As a result, osteoclasts break down bone faster than osteoblasts can rebuild it; therefore a decrease in bone mass may occur. Bone mass can become so depleted that the skeleton can no longer withstand mechanical stress.

This lack of bone replacement makes the bones porous, resulting in the condition known as osteoporosis. Testosterone decreases gradually and only slightly in older men. This coupled with the fact that men tend to have more massive bones than women means that relatively few men develop osteoporosis.

DIVISIONS OF THE SKELETAL SYSTEM

To make the study of the skeletal system easier, it can be divided into the following two distinct regions (Figure 19-3): (1) *axial skeleton,* consisting of the bones associated with the central axis of the body (skull, vertebrae, sternum, ribs); and (2) *appendicular skeleton,* composed of the extremities (upper and lower extremities) and shoulder and pelvic girdles. See Chapter 21 for specific locations.

Axial Skeleton (80 Bones)

Skull. 29 bones.
- 8 bones in the cranium (frontal [1], parietal [2], temporal [2], occipital [1], sphenoid [1], ethmoid [1])
- 14 bones in the face (maxilla [2], zygomatic [2], palatine [2], mandible [1], lacrimal [2], nasal [2], inferior concha [2], vomer [1])
- 6 ear ossicles (malleus [2], incus [2], stapes [2])
- 1 hyoid bone (some texts do not consider the hyoid a skull bone)

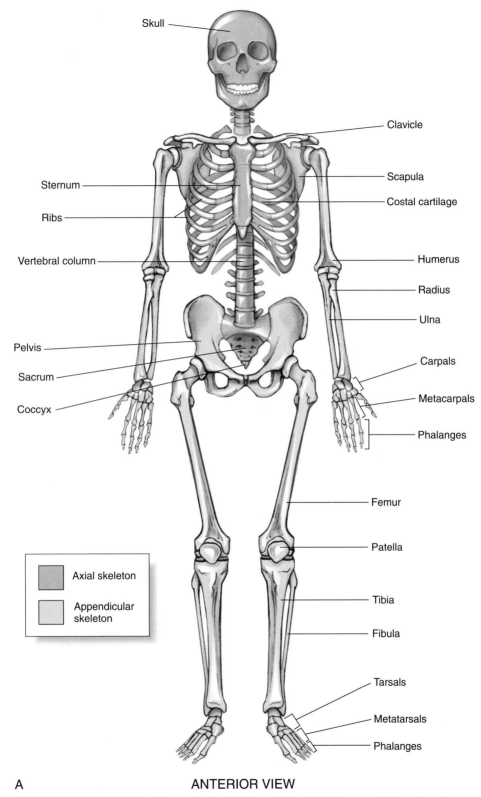

Skull

Clavicle

Sternum

Scapula

Costal cartilage

Ribs

Vertebral column

Humerus

Radius

Ulna

Pelvis

Carpals

Sacrum

Metacarpals

Coccyx

Phalanges

Axial skeleton

Appendicular skeleton

Femur

Patella

Tibia

Fibula

Tarsals

Metatarsals

Phalanges

A   ANTERIOR VIEW

FIGURE 19-3 Axial and appendicular divisions of the skeletal system. **A,** Anterior view.

Continued

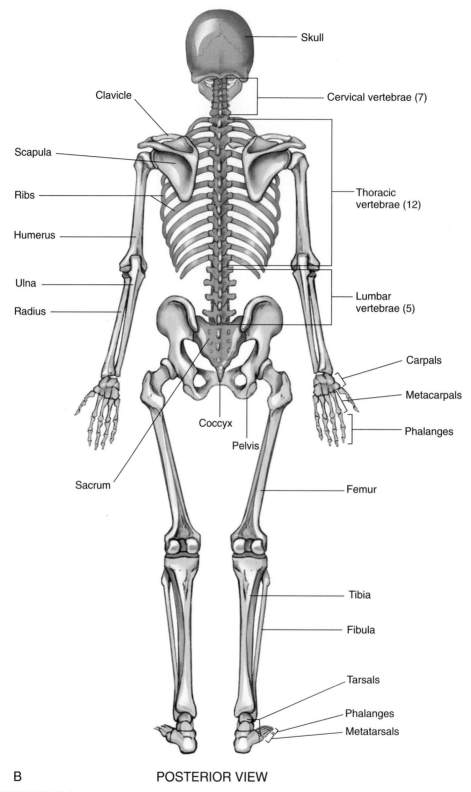

B POSTERIOR VIEW

FIGURE 19-3, cont'd Axial and appendicular divisions of the skeletal system. **B,** Posterior view.

Vertebral Column. 26 bones.
- 7 cervical vertebrae
- 12 thoracic vertebrae
- 5 lumbar vertebrae
- 1 sacrum (5 fused vertebrae)
- 1 coccyx (3 to 5 fused vertebrae)

Sternum. 1 bone.

Ribs. 24 bones (12 pairs).
- 14 true ribs (7 pairs)
- 6 false ribs (3 pairs)
- 4 floating (2 pairs, some texts regard floating ribs as false ribs)

Appendicular Skeleton (126 Bones)

Shoulder Girdle. 4 bones; the shoulder girdle or *pectoral girdle.*
- 2 scapulae
- 2 clavicles

Upper Extremities. 60 bones (30 on each side).
- 2 humeri
- 2 ulni
- 2 radii
- 16 carpals
- 10 metacarpals
- 28 phalanges

Pelvic Girdle. 2 bones; the pelvic girdle or pelvis (6 fused bones [2 each of ilium, ischium, pubic bones]).

Lower Extremities. 60 bones (30 on each side).
- 2 femurs
- 2 patellae
- 2 tibias
- 2 fibulas
- 14 tarsals
- 10 metatarsals
- 28 phalanges

> *"Why would you waste energy to do badly*
> *what is so easy to do well."*
> —Anonymous

Bony Markings

Located on the bones are bony markings where muscles, tendons, and ligaments attach and where nerve and blood vessels pass. These marks are called bony landmarks or surface markings (see Box 21-1). Examples of bony markings are:

Condyle. Rounded projection that forms a joint; knuckle shaped. *Lateral condyle of the femur*

Fossa. Shallow depression in a bone. *Glenoid fossa of the scapula*

Head. Rounded end of a bone. *Fibular head*

Process. General term for any prominence or prolongation from a bone. *Styloid process of the radius*

Tuberosity. Large, rounded rough projection. *Deltoid tuberosity*

JOINTS

Joints, or **articulations**, are where bones come together or join. Another term for a joint is an arthrosis (*pl.*, arthroses). Joints serve one main purpose, to enable the body to move. Other functions of joints are to bear the weight of the body and to provide stability.

Every bone in the human skeleton articulates with at least one other bone, except the hyoid bone. Where a joint exists, so does joint movement. This movement may be limited, as sutures in the cranium, or the joint may be highly mobile, as the ball-and-socket joint of the shoulder.

Joints can be classified according to their structure or by their function (i.e., amount of movement allowed).

Structural Classification

The following classifies joints based on structural characteristics. Its corresponding functional classification is included in italics.

Fibrous. Fibrous joints are connected by dense fibrous connective tissue, consisting mainly of collagen. See *synarthroses* in next section for examples of fibrous joints.

Cartilaginous. Cartilaginous joints are connected by cartilage. See *amphiarthroses* in next section for examples of cartilaginous joints.

Synovial. Synovial joints are the most common and most movable type of joint in the body. These joints contain a capsule surrounding articulating surfaces. The cavity with the capsule contains a lubricating (synovial) fluid. See *diarthroses* in next section for examples of synovial joints.

Functional Classification

The following classifies joints based on the range or degree of movement that is allowed. Its corresponding structural classification is included in italics (Figure 19-4).

Synarthroses. Movement in synarthrotic joints, also known as *fibrous joints,* is extremely limited. Examples of synarthroses are the joints between bones in the cranium and face (sutures), the joints that hold the teeth into their sockets (gomphoses), and the joints located at the proximal ends of the leg (tibiofibular joints [syndesmoses]).

Amphiarthroses. Also known as *cartilaginous joints,* these joints are slightly movable. Examples are the joints of the ribs (costochondral joints), joint between the pubic bones (pubic symphysis), and the joints between the vertebral bodies (intervertebral disk joints), all of which move apart only a few millimeters.

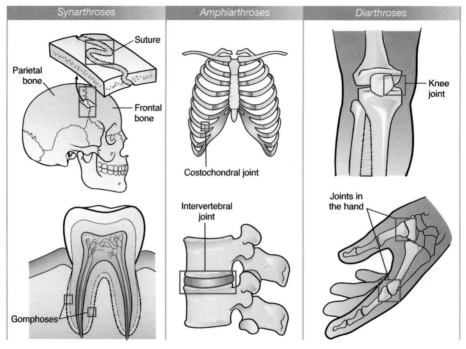

FIGURE 19-4 Functional classification of joints.

Diarthroses. Also known as *synovial joints,* these joints are freely movable joints. Synovial joints differ from fibrous synarthrotic joints and cartilaginous amphiarthrotic joints in that they have a space between the articulating bones called the *joint cavity.* Diarthrotic joints allow movement in one, two, or three planes. Many synovial joints also feature associated structures such as bursa sacs (bursae) filled with synovial fluid. Examples of synovial joints include knees (tibiofemoral joints), elbows (humeroulnar/humeroradial joints), hips (iliofemoral joints), and shoulders (glenohumeral joints).

SYNOVIAL JOINTS

The following structures are associated with synovial joints (Figure 19-5).

Articular cartilage. In synovial joints, articulating surfaces are covered with hyaline cartilage. It is smooth and slippery, decreases friction, and helps absorb shock.

Joint capsule. The capsule of synovial joints is a double-layer structure. The outer layer is fibrous and forms ligaments, which connect the bones in the joint together.

Joint cavity. The inner region of the capsule is called the joint cavity. It is lined with a **synovial membrane** and filled with synovial fluid. Synovial membranes also line synovial sheaths and bursae. **Synovial fluid,** or *synovia,* is a viscous fluid and provides nutrition and lubrication so the joint can move freely without undue friction. The amount produced depends on the physical activity of the joints.

The following structures are associated features that are not present in all synovial joints:

Bursae. A bursa is a saclike flattened structure with an interior lining of synovial membrane containing synovial fluid. When present, they are usually found between ligaments and joint capsules, providing a cushion that protects a muscle's tendon from rubbing against bone during muscular contraction. Examples of joints in which bursae are found are the knees (tibiofemoral joints) and shoulders (glenohumeral joints). Many bursae also have villi (additional folds to increase the surface area).

Synovial sheaths. Synovial sheaths are similar to bursae in that they are lined with synovial membranes. However, instead of being flat, they are tubular. These structures surround long tendons and increase their gliding capacity. They are found mainly in the tendons located in the wrists, hands, ankles, and feet.

Menisci. These are fibrocartilage pads found in select joints such as the knee (tibiofemoral) and jaw (temporomandibular). Menisci help the joint to move smoothly and serve as a shock absorber.

TYPES OF SYNOVIAL JOINTS

Synovial joints can be classified by their movement potential around axes (Figure 19-6). An *axis* is an imaginary line around which the joint moves.

IDA PAULINE ROLF, PhD

Born: May 18, 1896; died: March 19, 1979

*"God didn't come down and tell me; I had to find it out through many years of experience.
The work came first; the inspiration came later."*

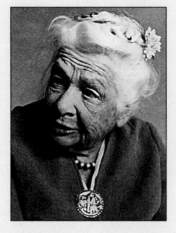

It was the middle of World War II, and most of America's men were far from home. Women began to fill roles they had never dreamed they would. One such young woman, Ida Pauline Rolf, accepted a position with the Rockefeller Institute, even though her father was dead set against it. War or peace, a proper lady stayed home where she belonged. After all, her family had money; she did not need to earn her way.

Rolf had a mind of her own. She earned a doctorate in biochemistry. She was just as passionate about philosophy and general semantics as she was about studying the science of the body; thus she explored homeopathy, was heavily influenced by osteopathy, and practiced yoga under the direction of a tantric yogi. Perhaps even more integral to her success than any other factor was that she was not afraid to pursue new directions.

Rolf's studies led her to Amy Cochran, an osteopath who claimed to have received her special abilities through a psychic encounter with Dr. Benjamin Rush, the physician who signed the Declaration of Independence. When Rolf returned to New York, she began work on a 45-year-old woman who had endured physical disabilities since the age of 8 years. Within a few years, the woman was up and walking.

Rolf believed that bodies are created balanced and comfortably supported by gravity, but injuries, overwork of one muscle group, or other postural dysfunctions result in fasciae that are too tight or loose. Thus our bodies expend energy inefficiently and fight gravity, rather than allowing it to support us. She also believed that anything that made individuals feel fear or guilt could exhibit itself in bad physiologic characteristics. For her, both mental and physical health make up two sides of the same coin.

Rolfing methodically restructures connective tissue through work on one body section at a time, gradually working deeper and deeper. The technique that we know today as *Rolfing* was first called structural integration. When the container is aligned properly, the *stuff* inside functions as it should. Structural integration helps achieve homeostasis. Rolf's vision went beyond physical change because she believed that this tissue reorganization of the body was necessary to achieve spiritual growth.

One of the most lasting impressions of rolfing seems to be that sessions must be painful to be effective. This was never Rolf's goal, and because of the body's reactive mechanism to pain, too much force may have a negative effect on results. In fact, Rosemary Feitis, Rolf's longtime assistant, quotes her as saying, "Don't just go in there as though you were a locomotive charging in at a 100 miles an hour. In general, if there is trouble going on inside the body, fascia on the outside will be so tight it will tend to protect the area that's in trouble. So don't barge through fascia. If you are doing the right thing, and there isn't some deep pathology, the fascia will let go—let you in."

Rolf tried to teach others what she had discovered and, at the same time, attempted to preserve the integrity of her work, but her commitment was singular. Not everyone shared her enthusiasm, work ethic, or understanding of the body. She taught whomever she could and cautioned them to wait until they were experienced before considering themselves *Rolfers*.

Eventually, an invitation to present her work at Esalen, a California resort proving ground for new movements, landed Rolf in the midst of a new type of student. She began to teach her work to those with no preconceived notions and a variety of backgrounds. The world began to take notice of her work. Research established its effectiveness. Articles were published. The Rolf Institute, formerly the Guild for Structural Integration, was created in the early 1970s.

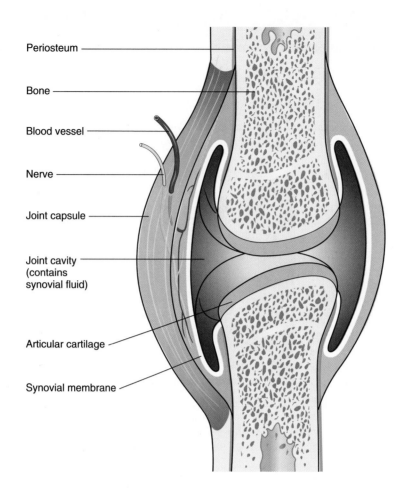

Periosteum

Bone

Blood vessel

Nerve

Joint capsule

Joint cavity
(contains
synovial fluid)

Articular cartilage

Synovial membrane

FIGURE 19-5 Synovial joint structures.

See Chapter 21 for a more detailed discussion and illustrations of the actions listed next.

Hinge (monaxial/uniaxial). Movements of hinge joints are limited to flexion and extension, as in the elbow, ankle, and joints within fingers and toes (interphalangeal joints). These joints possess one convex articular surface fitting into one concave articular surface.

Pivot (monaxial/uniaxial). Pivot joints allow rotation only. Examples of these joints are the joint between the first and second cervical vertebrae (atlantoaxial joint) and the joints located within the elbow and wrist (proximal and distal radioulnar joints). Pivot joints usually possess one rounded or pointed surface that fits into a ring formed in part by bone and in part by a ligament.

Ellipsoidal/condyloid (biaxial). Ellipsoidal joints are essentially slightly altered ball-and-socket joints. These joints contain one oval convex surface and one concave surface, allowing flexion, extension, abduction, adduction, and circumduction, but not rotation. Examples of ellipsoidal joints are radiocarpal joints (wrists), and the metatarsophalangeal and metacarpophalangeal joints (knuckles).

Saddle (biaxial). These joints resemble a rider in a saddle and allow movements of flexion, extension, abduction, adduction, opposition, reposition, and circumduction, but not rotation. The articulating surfaces are concave in one direction and convex in the other. An example of a saddle joint is the thumb joint between the carpal bone and the metacarpal bone (carpometacarpal joint of the thumb).

Ball and socket (multiaxial/triaxial). Ball and socket joints, such as the hips (iliofemoral joints) and shoulders (glenohumeral joints), permit all movements except gliding and offer the greatest range of motion. In these joints, one articular surface is rounded, fitting into a cuplike cavity provided by the second bone.

Gliding/planar (nonaxial). Movement in these joints is limited to a gliding movement and is permitted in all planes. Examples of gliding joints are the wrists (intercarpal joints), feet (intertarsal joints) and the joints between the articular facets of adjacent vertebrae (facet or zygapophyseal joints). Both articular surfaces are flat or slightly curved.

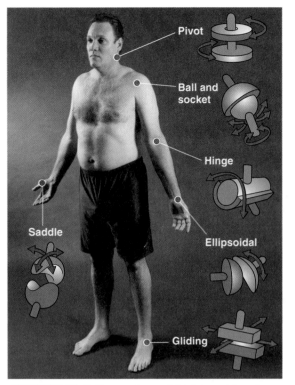

FIGURE 19-6 Types of synovial joints and locations.

PATHOLOGIES INVOLVING THE SKELETAL SYSTEM

Skeletal Disorders

Osteoporosis. Osteoporosis occurs with loss of normal bone density causing an increased susceptibility to fractures. The most frequent cause of bone loss is decreased estrogen levels commonly seen in women after menopause (both normal and surgically induced). Spinal deformities are common, especially kyphosis.

Joint mobilizations and compression should be avoided or administered carefully and without any twisting or torquing movements. Use lighter-than-normal pressure, especially over areas of known bone loss (asking about recent bone scan and the results will help make this determination). Be sure to position the client for comfort, especially in cases of kyphosis.

Paget Disease. Paget disease occurs with excessive bone remodeling resulting in weak enlarged and deformed bones. Bone deformity may result in kyphosis, bowlegs, and a larger, misshapen skull. The latter may compress cranial nerves and cause headaches and hearing loss. Paget disease is seldom seen before the age of 40 and becomes more common with advancing age. This disease is more common in men than in women.

Joint mobilizations and compression should be avoided or administered carefully and without any twisting or torquing movements. Use lighter-than-normal pressure, especially over affected areas.

Spinal/Postural Deviations

Kyphosis. Kyphosis is an exaggeration of the normal posterior curvature of the thoracic spine. Persons are often asymptomatic until a hump becomes obvious. By then, there may be mild back pain and decreased mobility of the spine. In more severe cases, the chest appears caved in, the arms tend to hang in the front of the body, and the head hangs forward.

Take care not to overstretch the spine. If the cause is osteoporosis, a lighter massage is indicated. Some relief can be gained by massage of pectoralis major/minor, serratus anterior, rhomboids major/minor using techniques such as deep gliding and deep friction.

Lordosis. Lordosis, or swayback, is an exaggeration of the normal anterior curvature of the lumbar spine. The most common cause of this condition is postural compensation for added abdominal mass and girth, such as seen in advanced pregnancy or obesity.

Position the client for comfort, which may include use of a knee bolster to reduce the anterior curve while the client is lying supine. The lumbar spine should not be overstretched. Be sure to address the quadratus lumborum, iliopsoas, hamstrings, and paraspinals. Techniques such as deep gliding strokes, deep friction, and myofascial release techniques can be helpful.

Scoliosis. Scoliosis is the lateral curvature in the normally straight vertical line of the spine, usually in the thoracic region, but the lumbar region may be involved. More serious cases require bracing to stabilize the spine and, as a last resort, spinal fusion.

Position your client for comfort. The spine should not be overstretched. Address the iliopsoas, quadratus lumborum, and the paraspinal muscles; expect to find tightness on both sides of the spine. Deep gliding strokes, deep friction, myofascial release techniques, and gentle stretches are indicated.

Joint Disorders

Patellofemoral Syndrome. Patellofemoral syndrome is the degeneration of the articular cartilage between the patella and the femur. It is most commonly seen in athletes involved in sports and in adults older than 65 years of age. In athletes, patellofemoral syndrome is often due to overuse, injury, or misalignment associated with improper patellar tracking. In older adults, patellofemoral syndrome is usually related to arthritic changes in the knee joint. Patellofemoral syndrome is also called chondromalacia patellae (CMP) or runner's knee.

If the knee is swollen, inflamed, or painful, local massage is contraindicated. Otherwise, massage is indicated, especially on the hamstring and quadricep groups. Before working on these muscles, flex the knees (use a bolster under the knees for a supine client and under the ankles for a prone client). Rework these muscles with the knees extended (i.e., remove the bolster).

Ganglion Cyst. Ganglion cyst is a common benign mass that appears as a smooth raised round lump just under the skin. In 90% of cases, ganglion cysts are located over or near the wrist and can range in size from a pea to an inch in diameter.

Local massage is contraindicated because pressure can cause pain or burst the cyst.

Baker Cyst. A Baker cyst is an accumulation of fluid behind the knee. Persons with a Baker cyst will have a palpable mass behind the knee (popliteal space); it may feel soft like a balloon or hard like a baseball. Baker cysts usually disappear spontaneously.

Local massage is contraindicated because pressure over the area may be painful. Use an extrasoft bolster behind the knees while the client is supine.

Bursitis. Inflammation of the bursae is called bursitis. There are two types: acute and chronic (most common). Acute bursitis has a sudden onset. Chronic bursitis results from longstanding bursitis and may be caused from overuse, prolonged repetitive motion, and excessive pressure. Musculoskeletal conditions such as scoliosis or rotator cuff injury can cause or contribute to bursitis.

In the acute stage, local massage is contraindicated until inflammation has subsided. In such cases, the therapist can use ice packs over the affected areas while massaging unaffected areas. In chronic bursitis, massage is indicated. Position the client for comfort and avoid the side-lying position in cases of trochanteric bursitis.

Temporomandibular Joint Dysfunction. Temporomandibular joint dysfunction (TMJD) is a generalized term to describe disorders affecting the jaw joint, its musculature, or both. Chief symptoms are facial pain (jaw pain, headaches, earaches, toothaches), which become worse when opening the mouth. Clicking, popping, or grating sounds may be heard while opening the mouth or while chewing.

Advanced techniques that require donning of disposable gloves to address some of the intraoral jaw musculature can be helpful. Be sure to massage the masseter, temporalis, medial and lateral pterygoids, and neck and shoulder muscles. Because most TMJD cases are associated with bruxism, which is often stress-related, relaxation massage can also be helpful.

Arthritis

Osteoarthritis. The most common form of arthritis, osteoarthritis (or *degenerative joint disease*) is characterized by progressive damage and eventual loss of articular cartilage especially on weight-bearing joints. This disease is common in the elderly and almost universal in those older than 75. It affects both peripheral and central joints of the body. Pain, along with joint stiffness and decreased range of motion, becomes more severe as disease progresses.

Ascertain from the client the joints affected by osteoarthritis. Avoid joints that are red or hot to the touch. On other affected joints, use only moderate pressure and gentle stretching. Joint mobilizations of the cervical area are best omitted or carried out with extreme caution.

Spondylosis. Spondylosis is a term used to describe any degenerative changes in the spine. Also called *arthritis of the spine* or *spinal osteoarthritis*, spondylosis most commonly affects the neck and lower back. By the age of 60 years, 70% of women and 85% of men will have signs of spondylosis in the cervical or lumbar spine. The disease may also result in abnormal growths, called *bone spurs*, which can put pressure on spinal nerves or the spinal cord.

Ask your client about the severity of the condition. Modify your massage accordingly. Gentle to moderate massage of the back using gliding strokes can be helpful. Joint mobilizations of the spine (including the cervical area) are best omitted or carried out with extreme caution.

Rheumatoid Arthritis. Rheumatoid arthritis is a chronic, inflammatory, and systemic form of arthritis. It often affects the small joints of fingers first, and then progresses to other joints. The course of disease is marked by exacerbations and remissions. Joints eventually become red, warm, swollen, and painful, and tender to touch. Over time, joints become deformed, especially in hands, and joint motion is lost.

Massage is contraindicated during periods of exacerbation as massage will only worsen the inflammation. When the client's rheumatoid arthritis is in remission, massage can be administered safely while avoiding areas and nodules that are painful and tender to touch. Mobilizations of affected joints are best omitted or carried out with caution.

Ankylosing Spondylitis. Ankylosing spondylitis is a chronic, systemic, inflammatory arthritis leading to calcification and fusion (ankylosis) of the joints, usually the spine and sacroiliac joints. As the spine becomes fibrosed and calcified, intervertebral discs are replaced with bony material, causing the spine to lose mobility. Rib cage expansion during inspiration is reduced if costovertebral joints are affected. When joints have completed ankylosing, they are permanently fused.

Avoid elevating the client's upper body while they are supine because this may cause back pain. Ankylosed joints should not be forced into movement, and compression over the rib cage should be avoided.

Gouty Arthritis. Gouty arthritis, or *gout*, is a type of inflammatory arthritis resulting from the accumulation of uric acid crystals in joints. When these crystals settle in joints, it causes inflammation. The first symptom is usually pain in the joint of the great toe (metatarsophalangeal joint). During flare-ups (or attacks), affected joints are warm, red, and painful. Slight fever, chills, headache, or nausea can accompany an attack. Between attacks, the person is usually symptom-free. As the disease progresses, affected joints become deformed.

During attacks, massage is postponed if the client is feverish or nauseated. If these symptoms are not present, massage can be performed while avoiding affected joints. Between attacks, massage is indicated, but joint mobilizations are contraindicated over deformed joints in persons with chronic gout. Avoid using a drape over the affected foot while your client is supine.

Lyme Disease. Lyme disease (or *Lyme arthritis*) is a recurrent form of arthritis that affects not only joints, but the skin, heart, and nervous system. Large joints, such as the knee and hip, are most commonly involved. Lyme disease is caused by the *Borrelia burgdorferi* bacterium, which is introduced into the body by a tick bite. This tick is carried by deer or by mice. A rash develops several weeks to a month after a tick bite that is red and circular with a clear center, resembling a bull's eye on a target (called *bull's eye rash* or *target lesion*).

Massage is postponed if the client is experiencing widespread inflammation indicated by fever. Otherwise, tailor the massage to the client's individual symptoms. For example, avoid any skin lesions and red, swollen joints. Passive stretching and joint mobilizations are cautiously applied, within the client's tolerance. Because a person with Lyme disease tends to have recurrent episodes, inquire about symptoms before each massage and adjust the treatment plan accordingly.

Skeletal Injuries

Dislocation. A dislocation is temporary displacement of two or more bones at a joint. The most common cause of dislocations is trauma, usually by a fall, motor vehicle accident, or sports injury. If the contact between the two articulating surfaces is only partially lost, the injury is called a *subluxation* or *separation*.

Local massage and joint movements are contraindicated for recent dislocations. Once inflammation has subsided and healing is complete, deep cross-fiber friction movements can help reduce the ill effects of scarring. Because dislocations often leaves the affected joint with permanent ligament laxity, avoid traction and mobilizations of the joint indefinitely.

Fracture. Any disruption or break in the continuity of bone is called a fracture. Fractures are broadly classified as complete or incomplete and as open or closed. *Complete fractures* occur when the bone breaks all the way through; *incomplete fractures* occur when the bone is damaged, but is still in one piece. *Open fractures* are fractures in which the skin is broken. In *closed fractures*, the skin over the broken bone is intact.

While the bone is immobilized, treat the area as a local contraindication. Massage proximal and distal to the fracture area can help maintain circulation and reduce edema. If located on a limb, elevate the affected area to help fluid drainage. Once healing is complete and bone union has occurred (physician determined) massage can begin slowly and gently for about a week. Gradually increase pressure to the client's tolerance.

If the client is wearing a soft cast or splint, do not reduce or remove it. To prevent fluid accumulation beneath the cast or splint, avoid heat application or techniques that drain tissues distal to the cast.

Sprain. Joint trauma that stretches or tears ligaments is called a sprain. Sprains can be classified into three grades or degrees of severity: first, second, and third degree. In a *first degree sprain*, the affected tissues are over-stretched and damaged microscopically, but not actually torn. In a *second degree sprain*, affected tissues are partially torn. In a *third degree sprain*, there is a complete rupture of the involved structures with significant damage and joint instability.

Ask how recent the injury is. If the injury is less than 72 hours old, avoid the affected area. During this time, use ICE (ice, compression, elevation) while massaging noninjured areas.

After 72 hours has passed, use light gliding and friction strokes over the area, gradually increasing pressure while staying within the client's tolerance. Initially, treatments of shorter duration are indicated and can become longer as the area becomes more accustomed to pressure. Avoid overstretching the injured area.

Adhesive Capsulitis. Adhesive capsulitis, or *frozen shoulder*, occurs when the shoulder is initially inflamed and eventually becomes stiff or frozen. Continued disuse of the shoulder often leads to a vicious cycle of more stiffness and disuse, which perpetuates the problem. Typically, only one shoulder is affected, but not always. Most often, the cause is idiopathic.

Local massage is contraindicated until inflammation has resolved. Afterward, appropriate goals are to gradually increase range of motion by relaxing and stretching surrounding muscles. This can be done by stretching/tractioning the capsule with the client's arm hanging over the side of the massage table. Shoulder girdle and rotator cuff muscles should all be addressed during the massage, especially the subscapularis (also known as the frozen shoulder muscle). Gentle stretching and joint movements are helpful, all within the client's tolerance.

SPOTLIGHT ON RESEARCH

Research suggests that massage therapy may:
- Increase range of motion (ROM)
- Improve bone grown in preterm infants
- Reduce pain, depression, and promote a higher quality of life in persons with osteoarthritis
- Reduce symptoms of juvenile rheumatoid arthritis

E-RESOURCES

⊜volve

http://evolve.elsevier.com/Salvo/MassageTherapy
- Chapter challenge
- Flash cards
- Photo gallery
- Weblinks

BIBLIOGRAPHY

Abrahams P, Marks S, Hutchings R: *McMinn's color atlas of human anatomy*, St Louis, 2003, Mosby.

Applegate EJ: *The anatomy and physiology learning system*, ed 3, Philadelphia, 2006, Saunders.

Beers MH, Berkow R: *The Merck manual of diagnosis and therapy*, Whitehouse Station, NJ, 2006, Merck Research Laboratories.

Como D, editor: *Mosby's medical, nursing, and allied health dictionary*, ed 6, St Louis, 2002, Mosby.

Crawley J, Van De Graaff KM: *A photographic atlas for anatomy and physiology*, Englewood, Colo, 2000, Morton.

Damjanov I: *Pathophysiology for the health-related professions*, ed 3, Philadelphia, 2006, Saunders.

Dominguez R, Gajda R: *Total body training*, New York, 1984, Warner Books.

Ferri FF: *2003 Ferri's clinical advisor, instant diagnosis and treatment*, St Louis, 2003, Mosby.

Frazier MS, Drzymkowski JW: *Essentials of human diseases and conditions*, ed 3, Philadelphia, 2004, Saunders.

Goldberg S: *Clinical anatomy made ridiculously simple*, Miami, 2004, Medmaster.

Gould BE: *Pathophysiology for the health professions*, ed 3, Philadelphia, 2006, Saunders.

Grafelman T: *Graf's anatomy and physiology guide for the massage therapist*, Aurora, Colo, 1998, DG Publishing.

Guyton A: *Human physiology and mechanisms of disease*, ed 6, Philadelphia, 1996, Saunders.

Haubrich WS: *Medical meanings, a glossary of word origins*, New York, 1984, Harcourt Brace Jovanovich.

Herlihy B: *The human body in health and illness*, ed 3, St Louis, 2007, Saunders.

Huether SE, McCance KL: *Understanding pathophysiology*, ed 3, St Louis, 2004, Mosby.

Jacob S, Francone C: *Elements of anatomy and physiology*, Philadelphia, 1989, Saunders.

Kapandji IA: *The physiology of the joints*, ed 5, New York, 1988, Churchill Livingstone.

Kapit W, Elson LM: *The anatomy coloring book*, ed 3, New York, 2002, Benjamin Cummings.

Kapit W, Macey R, Meisami E: *The physiology coloring book*, ed 2, New York, 1999, HarperCollins.

Kordish M, Dickson S: *Introduction to basic human anatomy*, Lake Charles, La, 1985, McNeese State University Press.

Kumar V, Abbas A, Fausto N: *Robbins and Cotran physiologic basis of disease*, ed 7, St Louis, 2005, Mosby.

Luttgens K, Wells K: *Kinesiology: scientific basis of human motion*, ed 7, Philadelphia, 1990, Saunders College Publishing.

Marieb EN: *Essentials of human anatomy and physiology*, ed 8, New York, 2005, Benjamin Cummings.

Martini FH, Bartholomew EF: *Essentials of anatomy and physiology*, ed 3, New York, 2003, Benjamin Cummings.

McAleer N: *The body almanac*, Garden City, NY, 1985, Doubleday.

McAtee R: *Facilitated stretching*, ed 2, Colorado Springs, Colo, 1999, Human Kinetics.

McCance K, Huether S: *Pathophysiology: the biological basis for disease in adults and children*, St Louis, 2006, Mosby.

Merck manual, ed 17, Whitehouse Station, NJ, 1998, Merck and Co.

Moore KL: *Clinically oriented anatomy*, ed 5, Baltimore, 2005, Lippincott Williams & Wilkins.

Muscolino JE: *The muscular system manual: the skeletal muscles of the human body*, ed 3, St Louis, 2010, Mosby.

Muscolino JE: *Kinesiology: the skeletal system and muscle function*, St Louis, 2006, Mosby.

Netter FH: *Atlas of human anatomy*, ed 3, Teterboro, NJ, 2003, Icon Learning Systems.

Newton D: *Pathology for massage therapists*, ed 2, Portland, Ore, 1995, Simran.

Patton KT, Thibodeau GA: *Anatomy and physiology*, ed 7, St Louis, 2006, Mosby.

Platzer W: *Color atlas and textbook of human anatomy: locomotor system*, vol 1, ed 3, New York, 1984, Thieme.

Premkumar K: *Pathology A to Z, a handbook for massage therapists*, Baltimore, 1999, Lippincott Williams & Wilkins.

Salvo SG, Anderson SK: *Mosby's pathology for massage therapists*, ed 2, St Louis, 2009, Mosby.

Solomon EP, Phillips GA: *Understanding human anatomy and physiology*, Philadelphia, 1987, WB Saunders.

Souza TA: *Differential diagnosis and management for the chiropractor*, ed 2, Gaithersburg, Md, 2001, Aspen Publications.

Thibodeau G, Patton K: *Structure and function of the body*, ed 12, St Louis, 2004, Mosby.

Tortora GJ: *Introduction to the human body: the essentials of anatomy and physiology*, ed 5, Hoboken, NJ, 2000, John Wiley & Sons.

Tortora GJ, Grabowksi SR: *Principles of anatomy and physiology*, ed 11, New York, 2005, John Wiley & Sons.

Venes D, Thomas CL, Taber CW: *Taber's cyclopedic medical dictionary*, ed 20, Philadelphia, 2005, FA Davis.

MATCHING I

Place the letter of the answer next to the term or phrase that best describes it.

A. Arthrosis
B. Articular cartilage
C. Bony markings
D. Diaphysis

E. Epiphysis
F. Metaphysis
G. Osteoblast
H. Osteoclast

I. Periosteum
J. Red marrow
K. Sesamoid
L. Synovial joint

_____ 1. Cylindrical shaft of a long bone

_____ 2. Where blood cell production occurs in a bone

_____ 3. Small, round bone embedded in certain tendons

_____ 4. Term synonymous with *joint*

_____ 5. Most movable type of joint and characterized by having a joint cavity

_____ 6. Bone-destroying cells

_____ 7. Covers the articular surface of the epiphyses

_____ 8. Dense, fibrous sheath surrounding the diaphysis

_____ 9. End of a long bone

_____ 10. Growth portion of a long bone

_____ 11. Places on bones where muscles, tendons, and ligaments attach and where nerve and blood vessels pass

_____ 12. Bone-forming cell

MATCHING II

Place the letter of the answer next to the term or phrase that best describes it.

A. Amphiarthroses
B. Appendicular skeleton
C. Axial skeleton
D. Ball and socket joint

E. Bursa
F. Diarthroses
G. Fossa
H. Head

I. Hinge joint
J. Menisci
K. Pivot joint
L. Process

_____ 1. Saclike flattened structure lined with synovial membrane containing synovial fluid that provides protection from a muscle's tendon rubbing against bone during muscular contraction

_____ 2. General term for any prominence or prolongation from a bone

_____ 3. Fibrocartilage pads found in joints that help it to move smoothly; also serves as a shock absorber

_____ 4. Skeletal region that includes the skull, vertebrae, sternum, and ribs

_____ 5. Synovial joint type that offers the greatest range of motion

_____ 6. Slightly movable joints or cartilaginous joints

_____ 7. Shallow depression in a bone

_____ 8. Synovial joint type limited to flexion and extension movements

_____ 9. Skeletal region that includes the upper and lower extremities, and the shoulder and pelvic girdles

_____ 10. Synovial joint type that allows rotation only; examples are the proximal and distal radioulnar joints

_____ 11. Term synonymous with synovial joints

_____ 12. Rounded end of a bone; a bony marking

CASE STUDY

Rheumatoid Arthritis

Betty is a 52-year-old woman who was diagnosed with rheumatoid arthritis 10 years ago. Her hands have become deformed, and she experiences periods during which joints in her hands are warm, swollen, and tender to touch. During this time, hand movements are painful. Because of inactivity during times when her symptoms are more severe, she has lost overall muscle strength; her leg muscles show evidence of atrophy.

To help slow disease progression, Betty began taking corticosteroids and immunosuppressants to control flare-ups.

Betty has scheduled a massage appointment with you on Tuesday. How should you proceed?

What are appropriate modifications you might implement for her? What home self-care would you suggest, if any?

CRITICAL THINKING

The pain associated with many of the skeletal and joint conditions discussed in this chapter is often managed with antiinflammatory and analgesic medication. What are some massage considerations for clients taking these kinds of drugs? See Chapter 10 for "Medication Guidelines."

Muscular System

LEARNING OBJECTIVES

After completing this chapter, the student should be able to:

- List the anatomy and describe the physiology of the muscular system.
- Describe how muscle cells are organized into muscle organs.
- Categorize connective tissue components of the muscular system.
- Identify characteristics and properties of muscle cells.
- Explain the mechanisms involved in muscle contraction.
- Describe thresholds and strength of muscle contraction.
- State how a muscle relaxes.
- List and discuss muscles' energy sources.
- Contrast and compare types of skeletal muscle fibers.
- Identify possible arrangements of muscle fibers.
- State parts of a skeletal muscle.
- Discuss lever systems.
- State how skeletal muscles act together to coordinate movement.
- Demonstrate and explain types of muscle contraction.
- Discuss the receptors involved in stretching.
- Discuss the importance of good posture and muscle tone.
- Name types of pathologic conditions of the muscular system, giving characteristics and massage considerations for each.

INTRODUCTION

Knowledge of the muscular system is essential to massage therapists because skeletal muscles and their related fascia are a primary focus in the application of effective massage therapy treatments. Chapter 19 examined the body's framework and joints that allow movement. However, bones cannot move themselves; they must be moved by something—namely, skeletal muscles. This chapter examines the muscular system, explores the types of muscle cells, and describes the mechanism of skeletal muscle contraction. Origins and insertions (muscle attachments), as well as actions and innervations of skeletal muscle, are discussed in Chapter 21. Definitions of the terms origin and insertion are presented in this chapter.

The thought of being alive brings to the forefront the idea of movement—the heartbeat, facial expression, and the rise and fall of the chest with each breath. These visible signs of life are all created by muscle contractions.

Years ago, physiologists believed that skeletal muscles contracted by folding, similar to an accordion, or by changes in the diameter of each cell. Some researchers hypothesized that muscles just grew or perhaps moved the way springs move. In 1969, Hugh Huxley, a British biologist, discovered that contraction does not occur by folding or springing. Shortening or lengthening of a muscle results from a change in the relative positions of one muscle fiber to another. To understand contraction, we will examine muscle fibers themselves.

ANATOMY

Basic anatomy related to skeletal muscles includes:
- Skeletal muscles
- Related fascial structures including tendons and aponeurosis

PHYSIOLOGY

Functions of skeletal muscle are:
- **Movement.** Skeletal muscle contractions produce movement of the body as a whole (locomotion) or movement of its parts.
- **Posture maintenance.** Skeletal muscles must contract to maintain static postures, such as in sitting and standing. Muscles also contribute to joint stability.
- **Moving substances.** Contraction of skeletal muscles promotes lymphatic flow and blood flow from the extremities to the heart.
- **Heat production.** Muscle contractions produce and release heat. Skeletal muscles are the most metabolically active structures in the body and produce a significant amount of heat. This mechanism is called *thermogenesis* and is important for maintaining body temperature. Additionally, when the body becomes chilled, skeletal muscles contract rapidly (seen as shivering) to produce additional heat.

IT'S ALL GREEK TO ME

antagonist	*Gr.* to struggle against
aponeurosis	*Gr.* away from; nerve; condition
atrophy	*Gr.* lacking, without, not; to grow
concentric	*L.* toward the middle
eccentric	*Gr.* away from the middle
fatigue	*L.* to tire
fascia	*L.* strong central structural unit or band
fasciculus	*L.* little bundle
flaccid	*L.* flabby
Golgi tendon organs	Golgi, Italian histologist (1844-1926)
hypertrophy	*Gr.* over, above, excessive; to grow
isometric	*Gr.* same or equal measure
isotonic	*Gr.* same or equal tension
myo	*Gr.* muscle
pennate	*L.* feather
retinaculum	*L.* a halter
sarco	*Gr.* flesh
spasm	*Gr.* a convulsion
synergist	*Gr.* together, work
tendon	*L.* to stretch

Gr., Greek; *L.,* Latin.

ORGANIZATION: MUSCLE CELLS INTO MUSCLE ORGANS

Muscle cells are referred to as **muscle fibers** because of their threadlike, slender shape. These fibers usually run the length of the muscle. Each muscle fiber contains thin strands called **myofibrils**. Within each myofibril are numerous **sarcomeres**. Sarcomeres are lined, end to end, in repeating compartments and run the length of a myofibril. Each sarcomere consisting of thinner protein strands called **myofilaments** (actin and myosin; discussed later).

Muscle fibers are arranged in bundles called **fasciculi** (*sing.* fascicle) and often lie in parallel rows. Groups of fasciculi form muscle organs or skeletal muscles (Figure 20-1). The progression from microscopic to macroscopic is as follows:

myofilaments → sarcomere → myofibril → muscle fiber (cell) → fascicle → skeletal muscle (organ)

Connective Tissues

Muscles are strong, but muscle fibers themselves are quite fragile. Therefore they are arranged and protected by a series

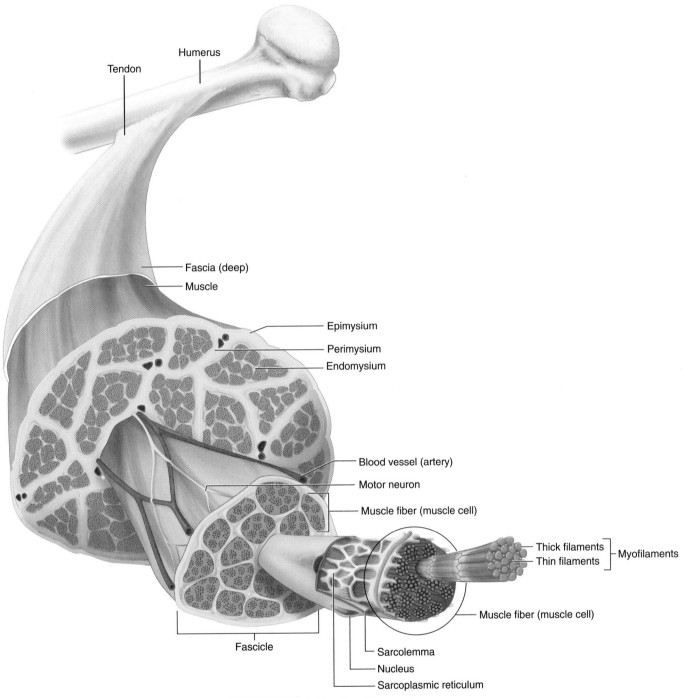

FIGURE 20-1 Structure of a muscle organ.

of connective tissue wrappings. The connective tissue layer that surrounds individual muscle fibers is called *endomysium*. This important fascial covering allows for muscular vascularization and innervation. The connective tissue layer that surrounds fasciculi is called *perimysium*. Finally, the connective tissue layer surrounding an entire muscle is called *epimysium* (see Figure 20-1).

Fibrous bands of connective tissue that surround muscle groups are often called *deep fascia*. In contrast with deep

fascia, *superficial fascia* is the fascial layer beneath the skin (see Figure 18-7). *Myofascial* refers to the skeletal muscles and related fascia in the muscular system. It is important to understand that all fascial structures are continuous with one another; that is, their fibers blend together.

Let us also review the connective tissue coverings of muscle cells and actual muscles:

Endomysium (surrounds muscle fibers or myofibrils) → perimysium (surrounds muscle bundles or fasciculi) →

epimysium (surrounds entire muscle) → deep fascia (surrounds muscle groups).

When deep fascia forms a cord, anchoring the ends of muscle to bone, it is called a **tendon.** A broad, flat tendon is called an **aponeurosis** and attaches skeletal muscle to bone, another muscle, or to the skin. Tendons and aponeuroses are both tough, collagenous structures and differ only in shape. When tendons cross multiple joints, as in the hands and feet, they are wrapped in *tendon sheaths*. These tubular structures resemble little sleeves lined with a synovial membrane. Synovial fluid secreted by this membrane reduces friction as the tendons glide back and forth within the sheath.

Retinacula, bandagelike retaining bands of connective tissue, help keep tendons and tendon sheaths in place. Retinacula are found primarily around the elbows, knees, ankles, and wrists. The retinaculum may also act as a pulley for tendons.

MUSCLE CELLS

Skeletal muscle cells are long, cylindrical, striated, and possess unique characteristics such as numerous nuclei and mitochondria (see Table 18-4). Most structures are the same as other cells, but include sarco- as part of many terms to indicate that they are related to muscle. *Sarco-* is Greek for "flesh."

Sarcoplasm. The cytoplasm within muscle cells is called *sarcoplasm.*

Sarcolemma. This is the cell membrane and encases the sarcoplasm and the organelles (Figure 20-2).

Sarcoplasmic Reticulum. The sarcoplasmic reticulum, a fluid-filled system of sacs, is similar to, but not identical with, the endoplasmic reticulum of typical cells.

Sarcoplasmic reticula play a crucial role in muscular contractions by storing and releasing calcium ions.

T-tubules. Transverse tubules, or T-tubules, are so named because they run transversely across the sarcoplasmic reticulum, forming inward channels. T-tubules transport stored calcium ions from the sarcoplasmic reticulum into the interior of the muscle cell. This action causes the depolarization phase of a nerve impulse (see Chapter 23).

Sarcomere. Positioned within each myofibril are small contractile units called sarcomeres. Each sarcomere contains myofilaments, mainly actin and myosin. Myofilaments and sarcomeres are discussed next.

CHAT ROOM

Other types of muscle, such as smooth and cardiac, are featured in Chapter 18.

Myofilaments

Sarcomeres are located within each muscle cell. Sarcomeres, a muscle's contractile unit, contain numerous rows of thick and thin myofilaments.

Thin Myofilaments. Thin myofilaments, or filaments, are made of a combination of three proteins; actin, tropomyosin, and troponin. *Actin* molecules are strung together, resembling a twisted double strand of beads (Figure 20-3, *A*). Actin contains binding sites that are used during muscle contraction. *Tropomyosin* molecules lie across actin strands and block access to actin's binding sites. *Troponin* is spaced at regular intervals along thin myofilaments and keep tropomyosin molecules in place over binding sites while the muscle is at rest.

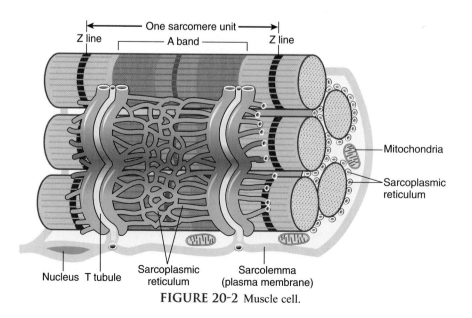

Z line — One sarcomere unit — Z line
A band
Mitochondria
Sarcoplasmic reticulum
Nucleus   T tubule   Sarcoplasmic reticulum   Sarcolemma (plasma membrane)

FIGURE 20-2 Muscle cell.

Thick Myofilaments. The thick myofilaments are made almost entirely of myosin protein. Myosin molecules are shaped like golf clubs with the golf shafts bundled together, making up the bulk of the thick myofilament. Sticking out of the shaft is a structure called a *myosin head* (Figure 20-3, *B*). While a muscle is at rest, these myosin heads angle toward the tropomyosin—covered binding sites located on thin myofilaments.

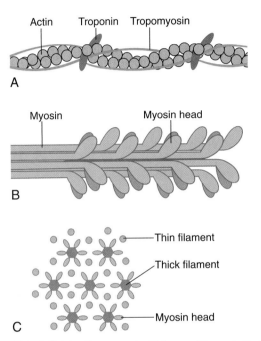

FIGURE 20-3 Myofilaments. **A,** Thin myofilament. **B,** Thick myofilament. **C,** Cross section of several myofilaments to show relative positions and myosin head extensions.

Sarcomeres

Defining the ends of a sarcomere are *Z lines* or Z disks, appearing as thin longitudinal columns. Z lines are so called because of their jagged Z-like appearance. Thin myofilaments attach to Z lines located at both ends of a sarcomere and extend only part way toward the sarcomere's center. In other words, the center of a sarcomere, known as the *H zone*, is devoid of thin myofilaments (Figure 20-4).

The *A band* runs the entire length of the thick myofilaments and includes the H zone. The absence of the myosin at either end of the sarcomere is known as the I band. So the *I band* includes the Z line and the thin myofilaments where they do not overlap thick myofilaments or myosin. When muscle length shortens, Z lines move toward the H zone.

Sarcomeres lie in parallel rows in a honeycomb arrangement (see Figure 20-3, *C*). Note that myosin does not run the entire length of the sarcomere. Because the myofilament arrangement is slightly staggered, myofilaments overlap in some areas (dark stripe) and not in others (light stripe), which gives it a striated appearance. Hence, skeletal muscle is also called striated muscle.

To review:
- **Z line.** Ends of the sarcomere
- **H zone.** Center of sarcomere, myosin only
- **A band.** Length of the myosin
- **I band.** Thin myofilament only

ⓔvolve *To see a muscle cell progressing from microscopic up to a macroscopic image, log on to the Evolve website and access this animation in Chapter 20 using your student account.* ▪

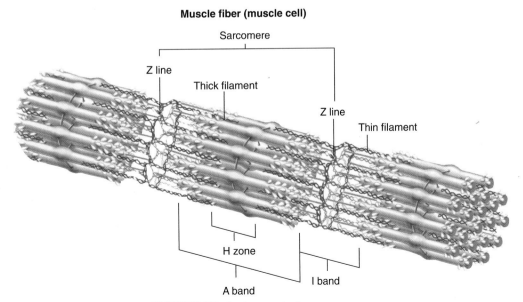

FIGURE 20-4 Close-up look at a sarcomere.

Muscle Cell Properties

Muscle cells possess the following characteristics that give them the ability to change their length:

Excitability. Meaning muscle fibers can respond to a stimulus

Contractility. Meaning muscle fibers can shorten

Extensibility. Meaning muscle fibers can lengthen

Elasticity. Meaning muscle fibers can return to their original shape after movement

MECHANISM OF CONTRACTION

Excitation of the Sarcolemma

The contraction of skeletal muscle begins with a nerve impulse. A special type of neuron, a **motor neuron**, is responsible for sending the impulse to muscle cells (see Chapter 23). Motor neurons are responsible for carrying messages of contraction (or inhibition of contraction) to a muscle.

One motor neuron may branch off and connect to other individual muscle fibers (2 or up to 2000). A single motor neuron plus all the muscle fibers to which it attaches is called a **motor unit** (Figure 20-5, *A, B*). Each skeletal muscle is composed of many motor units.

Motor neurons terminate at folded sections of the sarcolemma called a *motor end plate*. The junction between the motor neuron and the motor end plate is called the **neuromuscular junction** (see Figure 20-5, *B*). This space occupying the neuromuscular junction is called a **synaptic cleft** characterized by a narrow gap or cleft.

When a nerve impulse reaches the end of a motor neuron axon, neurotransmitters stored in synaptic vesicles are released and enters the synaptic cleft. The principal neurotransmitter involved in muscle contraction is **acetylcholine (ACh)**. When ACh crosses the synaptic cleft, it binds with receptor sites on the motor end plate located on the sarcolemma. This binding is similar to a key in a lock.

When this connection is made, the impulse created in the muscle cell travels from the sarcolemma into the T-tubules, and then to sarcomeres (see Figure 20-2). This triggers the release of calcium ions from the sarcoplasmic reticulum.

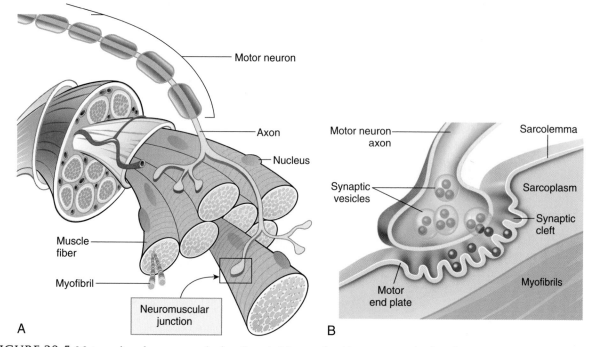

FIGURE 20-5 Motor unit and neuromuscular junction. **A,** Motor unit with neuromuscular junction. **B,** Neuromuscular junction.

Calcium ions assist in the binding of myosin to actin so muscle contraction can occur.

Contraction

To review, positioned on thin myofilaments are two protein molecules: troponin and tropomyosin. Recall that troponin normally holds tropomyosin strands in place, the latter covering myosin binding sites. Without these regulatory proteins, muscles would be in a constant state of contraction.

When calcium binds to troponin, it alters them in a way that tropomyosin slides off and exposes the site for a myosin head to attach. The connection between the myosin heads on thick myofilaments and thin myofilaments creates a *cross-bridge* effect. Myosin heads, which are hinged at their base, then toggle in a mechanism similar to that of a light switch. This is called a *power stroke*. This action causes thin myofilaments to slide toward the H zone located in the center of the sarcomere (recall that thin myofilaments are attached to the Z lines). The sarcomere shortens, causing the muscle fiber to shorten.

If adenosine triphosphate (ATP) is present, myosin heads then detach themselves, bind to the next exposed site, and pull again (Figure 20-6). This model of muscle contraction is appropriately named the **sliding filament mechanism**. Now muscle contraction has occurred, taking just a few thousandths of second.

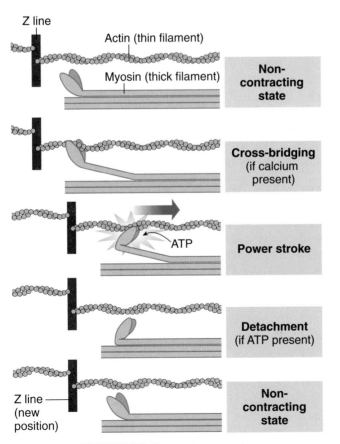

FIGURE 20-6 Muscle contraction.

Thresholds and Strength of Contraction

When a motor neuron delivers a stimulus of contraction, all the muscle fibers of the motor unit receive the same signal at the same time. If the stimulus is sufficient, all muscle fibers associated with the motor unit will contract to its fullest extent; there is no partial contraction. Conversely, if the stimulus is not sufficient (subthreshold stimulus), muscle contraction will not occur and muscle fibers will remain at its full resting length. This principle is known as the **all-or-none response**.

This all-or-none response is true only for motor units, not the entire muscle. Numerous motor units are linked to a single skeletal muscle. The nervous system regulates the amount of muscular contraction by activating only the motor units needed to perform a given action. If more strength is required, additional motor units are recruited, and the muscle contraction is stronger. For example, more motor units are required to pick up a hammer than to pick up a nail. This process of motor unit activation based on need is known as **recruitment**.

Relaxation

Almost immediately after the sarcoplasmic reticulum releases calcium ions into the sarcoplasm, it begins to actively pump them back into its sacs. Within a few milliseconds, much of calcium is recovered. Freed from its chemical bond with the calcium ions, the tropomyosin slides back to cover the myosin binding sites on thin myofilaments. This action releases the myosin heads and returns them to their precontraction state. The muscle is now at rest.

CHAT ROOM

A goal for massage therapy can be to release muscular spasm. One of the components of a spasm is a leakage of calcium from the sarcoplasmic reticulum without nerve stimulation, which can occur as a result of a tear from an injury or exercise. Calcium ions trigger contraction, and this action can create spasms, unless something flushes calcium out of the cells. Massage can assist in this flushing and may remove not only calcium but also metabolic wastes. As an added bonus, massage also brings oxygen and other essential nutrients to the tissues.

MINI-LAB

Hold your hands 18 inches from your face, palms facing you. Extend your thumbs up and interlace your extended fingers. Let your thumbs represent the Z-lines, and your fingers represent thick and thin myofilaments. Slide your fingers toward the middle. Notice how the spaces between your thumbs, or Z-lines, move closer together. As the spaces between the thumbs shorten, do your fingers shorten? This exercise illustrates how the sarcomere within a muscle creates movement by shortening.

*"All of us invent ourselves. Some of us
have more imagination than others."*
—Cher

ENERGY SOURCES FOR CONTRACTION

Adenosine Triphosphate

The energy needed for muscle contraction comes from ATP, which is produced by the body's cells. When ATP's energy bonds are broken, the released energy allows myosin heads to return to their original position.

Between contractions, myosin is in a "cocked" position, ready for action. When calcium ions move tropomyosin from the binding sites, the sites become exposed. Myosin then binds to thin myofilaments, releases ATP's stored energy, and causes the myosin head to spring back to its original or cocked position. Once the myosin head is released, it moves into its resting position again—ready for the next pull. The cycle repeats as long as ATP is available and binding sites are exposed on thin myofilaments.

This action pulls thin myofilaments toward the center of the sarcomere, which shortens the sarcomere and ultimately the muscle itself.

Oxygen and Glucose

Besides ATP, skeletal muscle contraction requires two other essential ingredients, glucose and oxygen.

During rest, oxygen is stored in muscle cells. It is stored on large protein molecules called myoglobin. *Myoglobin is* a red respiratory pigment similar to hemoglobin in red blood cells. Like hemoglobin, myoglobin contains iron that attracts oxygen and holds it temporarily.

When oxygen within muscles cells decreases rapidly, as it does in exercise, it is quickly replenished as a result of myoglobin. Muscle fibers that contain large amounts of myoglobin take on a deep red appearance and are often called *red muscle*. Muscle fibers with little myoglobin are lighter in color and are often called *white muscle*. Most muscles contain a mixture of red and white fibers. Additional information can be found next under "Types of Skeletal Muscle Fibers."

Normal ATP concentration in muscle cells is very low because ATP is used as rapidly as it is made. In fact, ATP can sustain approximately 10 to 15 additional seconds of muscle activity. To continually produce ATP, the body breaks down sugars—namely, glucose. If there is plenty of glucose in the blood, muscle cells are able to take in a steady supply. Excess glucose is stored as glycogen predominantly in liver and muscle cells. When blood levels of glucose are low, muscle cells transform glycogen back into glucose so that they can continue to generate ATP.

The breakdown of glucose, or glycolysis, occurs in two stages. The first stage is called *anaerobic* because oxygen is not used. The second stage, when physical activity becomes even more vigorous, is called *aerobic respiration* because oxygen is used to produce even more energy. Let us consider each step individually.

Almost as soon as muscle contraction starts, the anaerobic process also begins. Anaerobic glycolysis does not contribute a large amount of energy (energy equivalent of 2 ATP molecules), and its contribution is likely to last 30 to 60 seconds. Lactic acid is formed as the end product of anaerobic glycolysis. Lactic acid may accumulate in muscle tissue during exercise, causing local fatigue and a burning sensation. Some lactic acid eventually diffuses into the blood and is delivered to the liver, where an oxygen-consuming process converts it back into glucose.

This process is one of the reasons that, after heavy exercise, a person may still continue to breathe heavily. The body is repaying the so-called *oxygen debt* by using the extra oxygen gained by heavy breathing to process the lactic acid that was produced during exercise.

The second stage is aerobic glycolysis, creating the equivalent of 36 ATP molecules. Oxygen is brought in and carbon dioxide is expelled from the muscle cell through mitochondrial cellular respiration (see Chapter 18). This process of energy production can continue as long as enough oxygen is available through cellular respiration.

TYPES OF SKELETAL MUSCLE FIBERS

As discussed in Chapter 18, there are three types of muscle tissue: smooth, cardiac, and skeletal. Both smooth and cardiac muscle tissue are the same throughout the body. However, skeletal muscle can be classified into three types: slow twitch (red), fast twitch (white), and intermediate twitch (pink). Although each muscle organ contains a mix of all three, the ratio of slow twitch to fast twitch is unique to each individual, but some commonalities exist, as is described in the following:

Slow Twitch. Also known as *red muscle,* slow-twitch fibers are fatigue resistant. They react at a slow rate, and because they contract slowly, slow-twitch fibers are usually able to produce ATP quickly enough to keep up with the muscle's energy needs and thus avoid fatigue. This effect is enhanced by a good blood supply, a large number of mitochondria, and the rich oxygen supply provided by myoglobin. Most postural or core muscles are slow-twitch muscles. A high ratio of slow-twitch muscles is present in the legs of world-class long-distance runners.

Fast Twitch. Also known as *white muscle,* fast-twitch fibers contain very little myoglobin, few mitochondria, and few capillaries; thus they appear light in color. White muscles contract more rapidly than slowly because they possess a type of myosin that moves faster and because their system of T-tubules and sarcoplasmic reticulum is more efficient at delivering stored calcium. The price of a more rapid contraction is a quick depletion of ATP and fibers that fatigue quickly. Muscles of the arm contain many fast-twitch fibers.

Intermediate. Intermediate fibers are classified in between slow-twitch and fast-twitch fibers and are referred to as *pink muscle*. They contain large amounts of myoglobin, many mitochondria, and numerous capillaries. These fibers also generate copious amounts of ATP aerobically. However, they break down ATP quickly. They are more fatigue resistant than fast-twitch fibers and can generate more force more quickly than slow-twitch fibers. This muscle type predominates in muscles that both provide postural support and are occasionally required to generate rapid powerful contractions. Many world-class sprinters have a high ratio of intermediate fibers in their leg muscles, and world-class boxers have a high ratio in their arms.

CHAT ROOM

The presence of myoglobin in skeletal muscles makes them appear darker. Notice that the dark meat of chickens is the legs and the thighs. Ducks, by contrast, have dark breast meat. This difference is because, in general, chickens run around a chicken yard, and ducks fly powered by their breast muscles.

MUSCLE FIBER ARRANGEMENT

Muscle fibers are arranged in several ways. Some muscles have their fibers running parallel to a bone's long axis. Some muscles converge to a narrow attachment. Their fibers can be obliquely arranged or curved. Other muscle fibers appear in featherlike arrangements coming off one or both sides of a tendon. Differences between muscle fiber arrangements affect their shape and size (Figure 20-7). Some muscles can

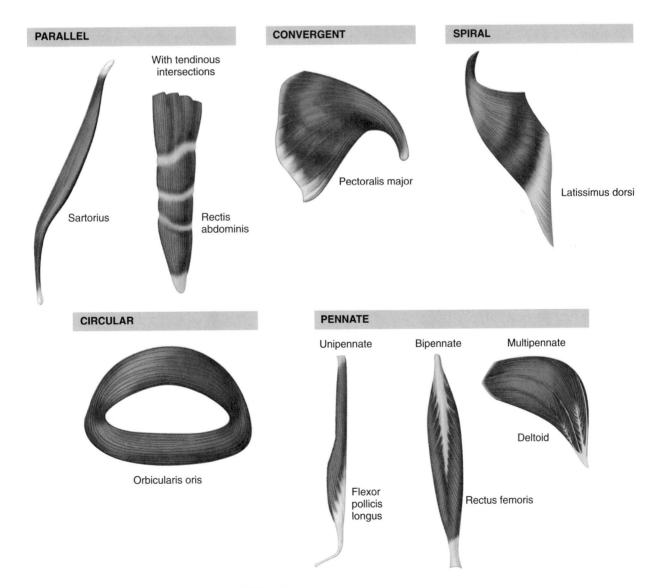

FIGURE 20-7 Muscle fiber arrangement.

fall into several categories. For example, the pectoralis major muscle of the chest wall can be classified as convergent and spiral. The following five muscle shapes are often used to describe skeletal muscles.

Parallel. The fibers in this arrangement run parallel to the long axis of the muscle and are usually spindle-shaped. Spindle-shaped muscles are also called fusiform. Most skeletal muscles have parallel architecture. They vary in length (from the smallest muscle in the body, stapedius in the middle ear, to the longest muscle in the body, sartorius on the anterior thigh). The rectus abdominis muscle, which runs the length of the anterior abdominal wall, is a parallel muscle that contains tendinous intersections to help maintain its length and to add strength.

Convergent. A convergent muscle has fibers converging at one end with fibers spreading out like blades of a fan at the other end. The muscles can pull in several directions rather than in one direction. An example of a convergent muscle is the pectoralis major in the chest wall.

Spiral. These muscles have fibers that twist between their points of attachment. Examples of spiral muscles are the latissimus dorsi of the lower back, the levator scapulae of the lateral neck, and the pectoralis major of the chest wall.

Circular. These muscles have a circular arrangement. Examples are the orbicularis oris muscle that surrounds the mouth and the orbicularis oculi muscles that surround the

eyes. Sphincters, discussed in Chapter 29, are circular-shaped muscles.

Pennate. These muscles are arranged with a central tendon and muscle fibers extending from the tendon diagonally, giving the muscle a featherlike appearance. Types are *unipennate* (fibers come off one side of the tendon), *bipennate* (fibers are arranged on both sides of the tendon), and *multipennate* (having several tendons within the belly with fibers run diagonally between them). Examples of unipennate muscles are the flexor hallucis longus muscle located in the leg, which flexes the great toe, and the extensor digitorum longus in the leg, which extends the toes. An example of a bipennate muscle is rectus femoris in the thigh, which extends the knee joint. Examples of multipennate muscles are the deltoid and subscapularis, which act on the shoulder joint.

PARTS OF A SKELETAL MUSCLE

Most skeletal muscles cross at least one joint and attach to articulating bones. At the simplest level, when contraction occurs and a muscle shortens, one bone moves while the other stays fixed. There are three main parts of a muscle (Figure 20-8, *A*).

Belly. The muscle belly is the wide central portion. The muscle belly contains sarcomeres, the functional contractile units of the muscle discussed previously. The muscle produces movement by shortening during contraction. This action pulls on tendons and moves a muscle's attachment sites closer together.

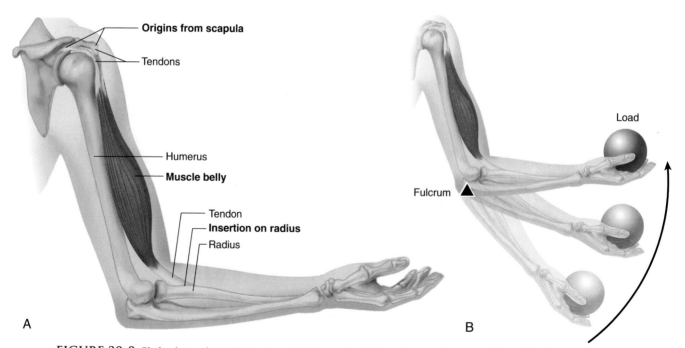

A

B

FIGURE 20-8 Skeletal muscle. **A,** Parts of a skeletal muscle. **B,** Insertion moving toward the origin (biceps brachii).

Origin. The origin is the tendinous attachment on the less movable bone (or other structure) during contraction. It is usually located as the medial attachment on the trunk or as the proximal attachment on the extremities. The origin also tends to be the more extensive or largest point of attachment.

Insertion. The insertion is the tendinous attachment on the more movable bone (or other structure) during contraction. It is usually located as the lateral attachment on the trunk or as the distal attachment on the extremities. The insertion tends to be the more confined or smaller point of attachment.

Muscle contraction usually moves bones, which serve as levers, and acts on joints, which serve as fulcrums for those levers. When a muscular contraction occurs, the insertion commonly moves toward the origin (see Figure 20-8, *B*).

The terms *origin* and *insertion* provide useful points of reference. Generally, the insertion moves toward the origin; however, the roles can be reversed. Some muscles possess the property of *functional reversibility*. For example, you can lean over, bringing your torso toward your thigh, or you can lift your thigh, bringing it toward your torso. Both cause flexion of the hip. Thus the terms *origin* and *insertion* do not always provide the necessary information needed to ascertain a muscle's action. Skeletal muscles and their actions are discussed in Chapter 21.

When a muscle crosses a joint, it acts on that joint. Muscles may cross one or more joints and are referred to as *uniarticular*, *biarticular*, and *multiarticular*.

Uniarticular. Muscles that cross one joint.

Biarticular. Muscles that cross two joints, acting on both joints.

Multiarticular. Muscles that cross more than two joints acting on all joints crossed.

LEVER SYSTEMS

For the muscular system to produce movement at joints, it uses the skeletal system for leverage. A lever (bone) is a rod that is moved by at a fulcrum (joint) (Figure 20-8, *B*). Lever systems have three parts: (1) *load* or resistance, or weight of the body and/or an object, and (2) *pull*, force, or effort (muscular contraction) which then moves around a (3) *fulcrum* or fixed point.

Levers are categorized into three classes according to how the fulcrum, pull, and load are arranged (Figure 20-9).

Class 1. Class 1 levers resemble a seesaw or pair of scissors. The fulcrum is positioned between the pull and the load. The cranium sitting on top of the vertebral column is an example of a class 1 lever. In this example, the *pull*

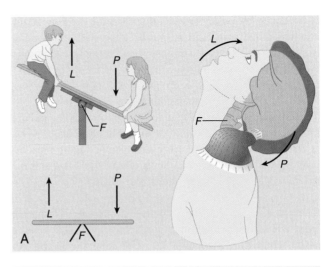

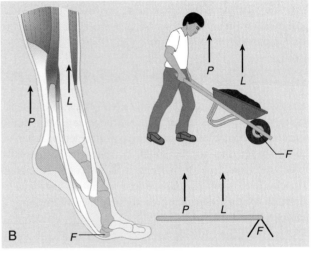

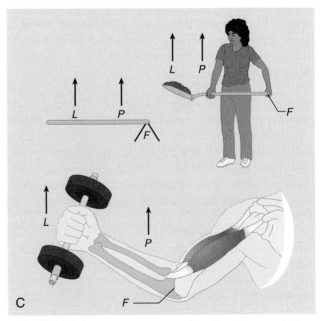

FIGURE 20-9 Lever systems. **A,** First class. **B,** second class. **C,** third class. *L,* load or resistance, *P,* pull or force, and *F,* fulcrum or fixed point.

is produced by posterior neck muscles, the *fulcrum* is the atlantooccipital joint, and the *load* is the weight of the anterior portion of the head. This lever class is the least common type of lever in the body.

Class 2. Class 2 levers function as would a wheelbarrow. The fulcrum is at one end, the load is in the middle, and the pull is at the opposite end. One example of a class 2 lever is rising up on the toes. Here the plantar flexor muscles provide the *pull,* the *load* is the weight of the body, and the *fulcrum* is at the metatarsophalangeal joints.

Class 3. Class-3 levers are the most common and resemble using a shovel. The fulcrum is at one end, the pull is located in the central portion, and the load is at the opposite end. An example of a class 3 lever is flexing the elbow during a bicep curl. The *fulcrum* is the elbow joint, the *pull* is provided by arm muscles (mainly biceps brachii and brachialis), and the *load* is the weight of the barbell.

MUSCLE ACTIONS

Almost all skeletal muscles work in groups instead of separately. Most muscles are arranged in opposing pairs; some muscles are contracting to perform a specific action, whereas others are lengthening (Figure 20-10). Muscles assume different responsibilities to perform a variety of movements. Muscles may function as prime movers, antagonists, synergists, or fixators, depending on their role in performing a particular task.

Prime Mover. The muscle that is responsible for causing a specific or desired action is the prime mover, also called the *agonist.* By concentric contraction, the movement produced by the prime mover describes the action or function of the muscle. For example, the brachialis is a prime mover in elbow flexion.

Antagonist. The opposing muscle, or antagonist, must relax and lengthen or eccentrically contract and lengthen to allow the actions of the prime mover to occur. The antagonist usually lies on the opposite side of the joint and can cause the opposite joint action when it contracts and shortens (see Figure 20-10, *A*). An example of a prime mover-antagonist relationship is that of the brachialis-triceps brachii (see Chapter 21).

Synergist. To help things run smoothly by stabilizing movements, other muscles, called synergists, contract at the same time as prime movers. For example, pronator teres is a synergist for biceps brachii (see Figure 20-10, *B*).

Fixators. Fixators are specialized synergists and are also referred to as *stabilizers.* They generally stabilize joints in a given position so that a prime mover can exert its action. For example, deltoid stabilizes the shoulder joint so that

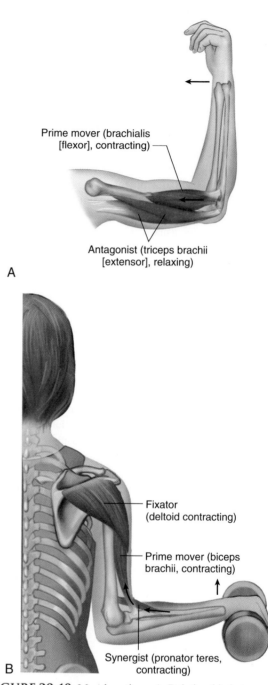

Prime mover (brachialis [flexor], contracting)

Antagonist (triceps brachii [extensor], relaxing)

A

Fixator (deltoid contracting)

Prime mover (biceps brachii, contracting)

Synergist (pronator teres, contracting)

B

FIGURE 20-10 Muscle actions: **A,** Relationship between prime movers and their antagonists. **B,** Relationship between prime movers and their synergists.

biceps brachii can flex the shoulder joint and the elbow (see Figure 20-10, *B*).

To review:
- **Prime mover:** muscle causing the specific action
- **Antagonist:** muscle opposing the prime mover
- **Synergist:** muscle that aids the prime mover by causing same movement
- **Fixator:** muscle that stabilizes a joint so the prime mover can exert its action

TYPES OF MUSCLE CONTRACTIONS

Muscles contractions are classified as either isotonic or isometric. Most movements include both types of contractions.

Isotonic Contractions

During isotonic, or *dynamic,* contractions, muscle tone or tension remains almost constant as the length of the muscle changes. Isotonic contractions are the most common type of muscle contraction. When a muscle is involved in isotonic contractions, it can shorten or lengthen (Figure 20-11).

Concentric. The muscle contracts and shortens. An example of a concentric contraction is shortening of biceps brachii to flex the elbow during the lifting phase of a biceps curl. Muscles involved in providing forward movement that concentrically contract are also known as accelerators or spurt muscles.

Eccentric. The muscle contracts and lengthens. An example of an eccentric contraction is the lengthening of biceps brachii during the lowering phase of a biceps curl. Repeated eccentric contraction causes more muscle damage and muscle soreness than concentric contraction; your quads are more tender and sore from running downhill than your hamstrings. Muscles engaged in eccentric contractions are also known as decelerators or shunt muscles because they slow down the powerful concentric contractors.

Isometric Contractions

Muscles do not always shorten or lengthen when they contract. If you attempt to pick up a weight that is too heavy, do the muscles still shorten? No. In isometric contractions, the muscle length remains the same while the muscle tension increases (Figure 20-12). Isometric contractions do work by *tightening* to resist a force, but they do not produce movement. The tension produced by the *power stroke* of the myosin heads pulling thin myofilaments toward a sarcomere center cannot overcome the load placed on the muscle (see Lever Systems section). Isometric contractions often occur in fixators or stabilizers because they stabilize joints so that prime movers and synergists can perform their actions (see "Muscle Actions").

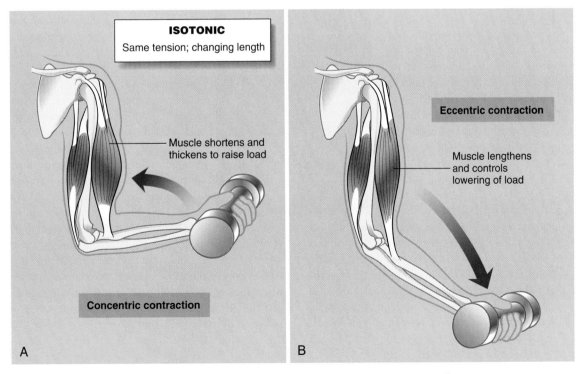

ISOTONIC
Same tension; changing length

Muscle shortens and thickens to raise load

Concentric contraction

Eccentric contraction

Muscle lengthens and controls lowering of load

A

B

FIGURE 20-11 Isotonic contractions. **A,** Concentric. **B,** Eccentric.

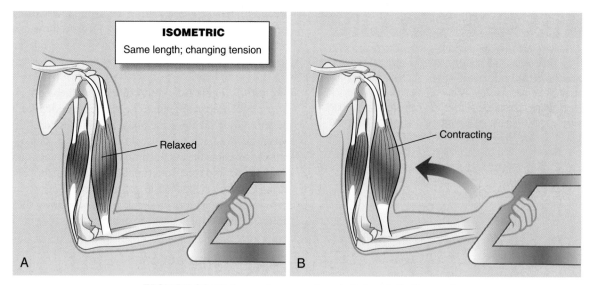

FIGURE 20-12 Isometric contraction. **A,** Relaxed. **B,** Contracting.

JUDITH DeLANY

Born: April 5, 1956

"What am I doing, watching, reading, saying, and thinking? What does all that have me becoming? Is that okay with me?"

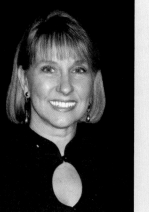

Judith DeLany, the youngest of six children, grew up in a rural Florida farming community. Her parents had little formal education, but passed on their love of learning and passion for knowledge to their children. Her father's resourcefulness taught the children that they could accomplish anything. Something broken can be made to work again, often using only what could be found around the home. Although he only had a fifth-grade education, Judith's father could roll out the plans for a new house and set to work building it. Judith remembers her mother sitting in a rocker, reading the encyclopedia as most people read novels. One of her favorites was a multivolume set about the human body, from which she would recite the description of a body system, disease, or glandular process to her children. Her mother used these moments to teach her children, asking questions like "Do you know how your finger works?" and then suggesting that they use the books to figure it out and then let her know.

Judith was athletic and loved music, playing in the school band and singing in the church choir. She considers herself fortunate to have had teachers and band leaders who set a high standard of excellence and instilled a strong work ethic in their students. She was profoundly impacted by her high school anatomy teacher, who assigned experiments such as revealing the skeleton of a dead animal and then reconstructing it into a posed form. She graduated as salutatorian of her high school class in 1974.

In 1981, Judith fell off a ladder, injuring her neck and low back. Although not severe at the time, the symptoms progressively worsened over the next year. Walking became difficult, and it grew nearly impossible to run, dance, or continue participating in the activities she loved. One day a massage therapist noticed her limping from the pain that was now radiating down her leg and into her foot, and suggested that neuromuscular therapy could help. In just a few treatments, Judith was out of pain and moving well. She

Isometrics is the therapy of choice when a client fears pain during movement and refuses to move an injured part. However, it only strengthens muscles when done in the position of the actual contraction. Isometric contractions are the key component of muscle energy techniques. Isometrics is great for building muscle bulk or increasing strength in certain positions, but these exercises do not increase the efficiency or endurance of skeletal muscles.

Isometric contraction can also be used clinically to reset tone on muscles that are weak from nonuse. Isometrics is often the first method of rehabilitation after surgery or injury because isometric contractions are relatively painless and increase local blood circulation without stretching tissues.

Many texts have stopped using the term *isotonic* and list three types of contractions only: concentric, eccentric, and isometric. I may do this next edition.

"Pain is inevitable. Suffering is optional."
—Kathleen Casey Theisen

STRETCHING AND STRETCH RECEPTORS

Although stretching is discussed in Chapter 8, it is important enough to warrant a brief mention here. Stretching can extend a muscle to its full length and, to some degree, elongates surrounding connective tissues. How far you can stretch a muscle depends on several factors. Most factors are out of our control (e.g., genetics, movement capability of a joint). What can be changed is the amount of tension in a muscle during a voluntary stretch.

Extensibility, the ability of muscles and other soft tissues to lengthen, can be improved by regular stretching. Stretching can also improve joint range of movement because it influences the physiologic characteristics of the muscle, tendons, ligaments, and other structures surrounding the joint. Hyperflexibility (hypermobility) is flexibility beyond

JUDITH DeLANY (continued)

was so profoundly changed by his work that she followed his advice to enroll in massage school.

At the time she was still working for the international company and had no intention of becoming a full-time massage therapist. She planned instead to use massage to help family and friends. Destiny, however, had a different plan. In 1982, just as Judith got her massage therapy license, the real estate company closed and she found herself unemployed. This thrust her, full time, into massage therapy as a career.

After her first neuromuscular therapy course, Judith knew that she had found her profession. She spent a day at the Institute for Natural Health in the clinical practice of Paul St. John, and by the end of that day, St. John offered Judith a position. Clinical reasoning came easily, the clinical results were successful, and her enthusiasm for learning turned into a passion to teach. At first, DeLany cotaught with St. John, and later became the first additional instructor approved to teach his method. In 1989, St. John and DeLany separated their work, he teaching the St. John Method of neuromuscular therapy (NMT) and DeLany simply referring to her method as NMT.

In 1994, Dr. Leon Chaitow invited Judith to contribute to a book project intended to introduce the U.S. method of NMT, and compare it with European

techniques. They later decided to distinguish their work and chose a distinct name for her method—NMT American version™. The publisher then invited Chaitow and DeLany to combine their work into two comprehensive volumes, *Clinical Application of Neuromuscular Techniques,* which propelled them into 15 years of coauthorship. DeLany later assisted Chaitow in his creation of the *Journal of Bodywork and Movement Therapies* (JBMT), the first peer-reviewed journal for massage therapists.

Life has tested DeLany's core principles constantly since 1996, when, as she turned 40, her daughter, Kaila, was born. As a mother, she began to see the world through the eyes of a child. Looking more simply at virtually everything gave her a new perspective on the world, politics, and yes, even the human body. In 1999 Judith was named "Massage Therapist of the Year" by the Florida Chiropractic Association.

"The most distinct change in my own approach through the years was to move from knowing into not knowing," states DeLany. "I now understand that it is human nature to want a definitive answer, to understand a precise cause, and to be rooted in a particular, often deeply etched track. However, where pain and dysfunction are concerned, there usually is more than one factor causing the problem."

a joint's normal range of motion and contributes to joint instability.

Proprioceptors are sensory receptors located in muscles, tendons, and joints (see Chapter 23). They detect information about the body's static position in space and the dynamic movement through space. Two proprioceptors that can be stimulated during a stretch are muscle spindles and Golgi tendon organs.

Muscle Spindles

These stretch receptors are located within the muscle belly (see Figure 23-22). If the muscle is stretched too rapidly, in a maneuver called a ballistic stretch, muscle spindles detect the sudden motion, and the nervous system responds by reflexively contracting the muscle. This reflex is a protective mechanism that is intended to safeguard the muscle from overstretching. This reflex is also important for maintaining posture.

Golgi Tendon Organs

These are located in the musculotendinous junctions (see Figure 23-23) and detect tension applied to the tendon during slow, static stretching. The nervous system responds by inhibiting contraction, which reduces damage to the tendon. This action allows the muscle to relax and stretch. It works the exact opposite of a muscle spindle and represses contraction and prevents muscle tearing or avulsion of the tendon from its attachment.

CHAT ROOM

Massage therapists can use information about stretch receptors when applying or instructing clients in stretching. To enhance flexibility, apply only slow, static stretches. Movements that are perceived by the nervous system as dangerous will be met with resistance.

MINI-LAB

Hold a shoestring by the two coated ends with both of your hands. Slowly begin to pull the ends apart. Watch what happens to the individual strands in the string. Do the fibers spread apart or draw closer together? Imagine that this string is a muscle and the two ends are tendinous attachments. Within this muscle is a spasm. Pull the ends again. As the muscle is being stretched, is the spasm released? Note that separation in the muscle fibers does not occur when the muscle is stretched, which helps explain why stretching does not release local muscle spasms.

POSTURE AND MUSCLE TONE

The term *posture* refers to body position. Good posture implies many concepts. Good posture reduces strain on muscles, ligaments, and bones. Good posture helps keep the body's center of gravity over its base. Poor posture places stress on most body structures and may lead to soreness and fatigue. As a massage therapist, you should demonstrate body mechanics that reflect good posture.

Muscles help maintain posture and help keep joints stabilized because muscles must exert a pull on bones to counteract the force of gravity. The continued partial contraction of skeletal muscles is called *muscle tone*, or *tonus*. This baseline tone enables us to stand, sit, and maintain relatively stable body postures while performing gait actions such as walking, running, hopping, and skipping. Muscles with less tone than normal are described as *flaccid* and are often in the first stage of muscular atrophy. Muscles with more than normal tone are called *spastic*.

Tonus is a characteristic of the muscles that normal individuals have when they are awake. However, muscle tone is lessened during sleep; we cannot sleep standing up. Hence good posture while asleep is also important. A neutral sleeping posture is best maintained by using pillows to support the neck and extremities to keep the spine straight.

SPOTLIGHT ON RESEARCH

Research suggests that massage therapy may:

- Decrease tension within the muscle-tendon unit
- Assist in the treatment of tendinitis
- Increase scar tissue strength to aid in tendon healing
- Increase range of motion (ROM)
- Decrease delayed-onset muscle soreness (DOMS)
- Decrease electromyography (EMG) activity, suggesting increased muscle relaxation and decreased muscle fatigue
- Decrease pain and activate the parasympathetic nervous system, causing relaxation and reduction of trigger point activity
- Reduce chronic tension headaches
- Reduce lower back pain
- Reduce pain and other symptoms of fibromyalgia

MUSCULAR PATHOLOGIES

Headaches and Muscular Pathologies

Tension Headaches. The most common headache type is the tension headache. Many things cause or contribute to tension headaches such as stress; anxiety; depression; contraction of jaw, neck, and shoulder muscles; holding your head in one position for a long time (like at a computer or microscope); eyestrain; or sleeping in an uncomfortable position. Using alcohol or recreational drugs can also make you more susceptible to them. Headaches can be a side effect of medication use.

The goals of massage are to relax the involved head, neck, shoulder, and back muscles. A cranial base release is indicated for headaches in the occipital or suboccipital region (see Chapter 14).

Fibromyalgia Syndrome. Fibromyalgia is a chronic generalized syndrome characterized by the presence of multiple tender points. There are no signs of inflammation or degeneration in the tissues and the disease is characterized by periods of exacerbation and remission. It is one of the most common conditions affecting muscles. The most prominent symptom is pain often described as aching, burning, or gnawing; a "migraine headache of the muscles."

Massage should be tailored to how your client is feeling at the time of treatment because symptoms vary daily. Evidence suggests that although many clients request deep pressure, this often provokes strong reactions for several days following treatment. A very slow increment in depth of massage strokes, from session to session, with careful deactivation of tender areas, is recommended.

Myofascial Pain Syndrome. Myofascial pain syndrome is associated with the presence of localized trigger points. The points are best described as a taut band that is exquisitely tender when pressed. Touching these points can produce referred pain. The person often experiences reduced range of motion and muscle weakness in involved muscles.

Ascertain from the client the areas of pain. Once they are identified, massage these areas and their adjacent areas. Deep, slow, gliding pressure over trigger points can help deactivate them. Avoid oscillating movement such as percussion and vibration as these movements can cause stimulation of muscle spindles, leading to localized contractions. Moist heat can be used to soften fascia around the trigger point before massage.

Muscular Injuries

Strain. A strain occurs when muscle or its tendons become overstretched or torn. Strains can be classified into three grades or degrees of severity: first, second, and third degree. In a *first-degree strain*, the affected tissues are overstretched and damaged microscopically, but not actually torn. In *second-degree strain*, affected tissues are partially torn. In *third-degree strain*, there is a complete rupture of the involved structures with significant damage.

Ask how recent the injury is. If the injury is less than 72 hours old, avoid the affected area. During this time, use ICE (ice, compression, elevation) while massaging noninjured areas.

After 72 hours has passed, use light gliding and friction strokes over the area, gradually increasing pressure while staying within the client's tolerance. Then, cross-fiber frictions are used to create a more appropriate scar. Initially, treatments of shorter duration are indicated; treatments can become longer as the area becomes

more accustomed to pressure. Avoid overstretching the injured area.

Tendinitis. Inflammation of a tendon is referred to as tendinitis. Tendinitis can occur in any tendon, but the most commonly involved areas are the wrists, elbows, shoulders, knees, and heels (Achilles). The most common cause of tendinitis is chronic overuse. The second most common cause is injury.

If tendinitis is the result of injury, local massage is contraindicated for 72 hours because of inflammation. During this time, ICE (ice, compression, elevation) of the injured area is appropriate while massaging noninjured areas. Otherwise, use deep gliding and cross-fiber friction strokes on the involved tendons. Follow this up with 20 minutes of icing. Initially, treatments of shorter duration are indicated and can become longer as the area becomes more accustomed to pressure.

De Quervain Tenosynovitis. De Quervain's tenosynovitis results in inflammation of a tendinous sheath located on the radial side of the wrist. This tendon sheath surrounds two muscles of the thumb, abductor pollicis longus and extensor pollicis brevis. De Quervain's tenosynovitis is often related to a repetitive motion injury. The affected person may experience difficulty with certain thumb movements, such as gripping.

If the area is inflamed, local massage is contraindicated. Otherwise, massage can loosen the affected muscles located in the hand's thenar eminence (thumb pad).

Osgood-Schlatter Disease. Osgood-Schlatter disease is patellar tendinitis in immature bone of adolescents at the tibial tuberosity. The tibial tuberosity is where the quadriceps insert (see Figure 21-109). In mild cases, the tibial tuberosity is inflamed; in severe cases, there is a complete separation of the tibial tuberosity from the bone.

Avoid massage and movement of the affected area during the acute phase because of pain and inflammation. Once inflammation has abated, friction around the knee can reduce adhesions. Massage of the quads can reduce muscle tension. Be sure the knees are flexed during part of the massage to the thigh (use a bolster under the knee). This will assure that the thigh muscles will be massaged in at least two positions (shortened and lengthened).

Torticollis. Torticollis, or wryneck, is a disorder involving spasms of the sternocleidomastoid (SCM) muscle. Because this condition is often unilateral, the head is tilted or may be pulled forward or backward, and the chin is elevated.

If torticollis is the result of injury, ask the client how recent the injury was; if less than 72 hours old, avoid the affected areas till 72 hours has passed. Otherwise, local massage can be helpful after positioning the client for comfort (this may mean avoiding the prone position). Along with SCM, massage of the trapezius, scalenes, and the splenius muscles may also help torticollis. Muscles can be stretched, but not forced.

Whiplash. Whiplash is a sprain or strain of the cervical spine and surrounding musculature. The most frequent cause of whiplash is injury from being pushed or struck from behind such as being rear-ended in a motor vehicle accident. This causes the head and neck to snap backward and then forward. The upper four vertebrae act as the lash and the lower three act as the handle of a whip—hence the term *whiplash*. The head motion may also be lateral (side to side), depending on the direction of impact.

Ascertain from the client how the whiplash occurred. If due to injury, local massage is contraindicated for first 72 hours. Then proceed with massage, within the client's tolerance. If it is an anterior-posterior whiplash, the muscles involved could include longus colli, scalenes, splenius muscles, sternocleidomastoid, levator scapulae, trapezius, and suboccipitals. If it is a lateral whiplash, scalenes, trapezius, and sternocleidomastoid could be the primary muscles involved. All of these muscles can be stretched, but not forced.

Shin Splints. Shin splints is a term used to describe pain along the tibia. This condition is often bilateral and is common among people who participate in sports and exercises that involve running and jumping. It may occur during the first few weeks of a new exercise program or after a sudden increase in the amount of exercise in an ongoing fitness program.

If the client indicates that the pain is severe, treat as a local contraindication and use ice on the affected area while massaging nonaffected areas. If the symptoms are not severe, elevation and massaging muscles of the leg are helpful, using ice applications afterward. Dorsiflex and plantarflex the ankle to stretch leg muscles; be careful not to overstretch them.

Plantar Fasciitis. Plantar fasciitis is a chronic inflammation of the plantar fascia. The most frequent cause of plantar fasciitis is prolonged repetitive motion, and is a recurrent problem for people who participate in sports that involve running. Symptoms are pain and tenderness in the heel and/or pain on dorsiflexion.

If foot pain is exquisitely tender, treat as a local contraindication. Otherwise, cross-fiber friction on the plantar surface of the foot, within the client's tolerance, may help reduce adhesions. Muscles of the leg should be massaged thoroughly first, using deep gliding and kneading strokes. Ensure that the client's ankle is not excessively dorsiflexed by using a bolster while the client is prone.

ⓔvolve *Use your student account to access online resources for Chapter 20, such as flash cards.* ∎

E-RESOURCES

ⓔvolve

http://evolve.elsevier.com/Salvo/MassageTherapy

- Chapter challenge
- Flash cards
- Photo gallery
- Educational animations
- Weblinks

BIBLIOGRAPHY

Abrahams P, Marks S, Hutchings R: *McMinn's color atlas of human anatomy*, St Louis, 2003, Mosby.

Applegate EJ: *The anatomy and physiology learning system*, ed 3, Philadelphia, 2006, Saunders.

Ardion C: Certified manual lymphatic drainage practitioner, personal communication, 2010.

Beers MH, Berkow R: *The Merck manual of diagnosis and therapy*, Whitehouse Station, NJ, 2006, Merck Research Laboratories.

Como D, editor: *Mosby's medical, nursing, and allied health dictionary*, ed 6, St Louis, 2002, Mosby.

Crawley J, Van De Graaff KM: *A photographic atlas for anatomy and physiology*, Englewood, Colo, 2002, Morton.

Damjanov I: *Pathophysiology for the health-related professions*, ed 3, Philadelphia, 2006, Saunders.

Ferri FF: *2003 Ferri's clinical advisor, instant diagnosis and treatment*, St Louis, 2003, Mosby.

Frazier MS, Drzymkowski JW: *Essentials of human diseases and conditions*, ed 3, Philadelphia, 2004, Saunders.

Goldberg S: *Clinical anatomy made ridiculously simple*, Miami, 2004, Medmaster.

Gould BE: *Pathophysiology for the health-related professionals*, ed 3, Philadelphia, 2006, Saunders.

Grafelman T: *Graf's anatomy and physiology guide for the massage therapist*, Aurora, Colo, 1988, DG Publishing.

Guyton A: *Human physiology and mechanisms of disease*, ed 6, Philadelphia, 1996, Saunders.

Haubrich WS: *Medical meanings: a glossary of word origins*, New York, 1984, Harcourt Brace Jovanovich.

Huether SE, McCance KL: *Understanding pathophysiology*, ed 3, St Louis, 2004, Mosby.

Jacob S, Francone C: *Elements of anatomy and physiology*, Philadelphia, 1989, Saunders.

Juhan D: *Job's body: a handbook for bodyworkers*, ed 3, Barrington, NY, 2003, Station Hill Press.

Kapit W, Elson LM: *The anatomy coloring book*, ed 3, New York, 2002, Benjamin Cummings.

Kapit W, Macey R, Meisami E: *The physiology coloring book*, ed 2, New York, 1999, HarperCollins.

Kordish M, Dickson S: *Introduction to basic human anatomy*, Lake Charles, La, 1985, McNeese State University.

Kumar V, Abbas A, Fausto N: *Robbins and Cotran physiologic basis of disease*, ed 7, St Louis, 2005, Mosby.

Marieb EN: *Essentials of human anatomy and physiology*, ed 8, New York, 2005, Benjamin Cummings.

Martini FH, Bartholomew EF: *Essentials of anatomy and physiology*, ed 3, New York, 2003, Benjamin Cummings.

Mattes A: *Active isolated stretching*, Sarasota, Fla, 1995, self-published.

McAleer N: *The body almanac*, Garden City, NY, 1985, Doubleday.

McCance K, Huether S: *Pathophysiology: the biological basis for disease in adults and children*, St Louis, 2006, Mosby.

Merck manual, ed 17, Whitehouse Station, NJ, 1998, Merck Co.

Moore KL: *Clinically oriented anatomy*, ed 5, Baltimore, 2005, Lippincott Williams & Wilkins.

Muscolino JE: *Kinesiology: the skeletal system and muscle function*, ed 2, St Louis, 2011, Mosby.

Muscolino JE: *The muscular system manual: the skeletal muscles of the human body*, ed 3, St Louis, 2010, Mosby.

Netter FH: *Atlas of human anatomy*, ed 3, Teterboro, NJ, 2003, Icon Learning Systems.

Newton D: *Pathology for massage therapists*, ed 2, Portland, Ore, 1995, Simran.

Patton KT, Thibodeau GA: *Anatomy and physiology*, ed 7, St Louis, 2010, Mosby.

Platzer W: *Color atlas and textbook of human anatomy: locomotor system*, vol I, ed 5, New York, 2003, Thieme.

Premkumar K: *Pathology A to Z, a handbook for massage therapists*, Baltimore, 1999, Lippincott Williams & Wilkins.

Salvo SG: *Mosby's pathology for massage therapists*, ed 2, St Louis, 2009, Elsevier Mosby.

Solomon EP, Phillips GA: *Understanding human anatomy and physiology*, Philadelphia, 1987, Saunders.

Souza TA: *Differential diagnosis and management for the chiropractor*, ed 2, Gaithersburg, Md, 2001, Aspen.

Thibodeau G, Patton K: *Structure and function of the body*, ed 12, St Louis, 2004, Mosby.

Tortora GJ: *Introduction to the human body: the essentials of anatomy and physiology*, ed 5, Hoboken, NJ, 2000, John Wiley & Sons.

Tortora GJ, Grabowksi SR: *Principles of anatomy and physiology*, ed 11, New York, 2005, John Wiley & Sons.

Travell JG, Simons D: *Myofascial pain and dysfunction, the trigger point manual*, Baltimore, 1992, Lippincott Williams & Wilkins.

Venes D, Thomas CL, Taber CW: *Taber's cyclopedic medical dictionary*, ed 20, Philadelphia, 2005, FA Davis.

MATCHING I

Place the letter of the answer next to the term or phrase that best describes it.

A. Acetylcholine
B. Actin
C. Aponeurosis
D. Contractility

E. Extensibility
F. Muscle fibers
G. Myosin
H. Retinacula

I. Sarcolemma
J. Sarcomere
K. Sliding filament
L. Tendon

_____ 1. Used to describe the mechanism of muscle contraction at the microscopic level

_____ 2. Thick myofilament

_____ 3. Muscle's contractile unit; located within myofibrils

_____ 4. Property that describes the muscle fibers ability to lengthen

_____ 5. Cordlike connective tissue structure attaching muscle to bone

_____ 6. Term synonymous with muscle cells

_____ 7. Broad, flat tendon

_____ 8. Property that describes the muscle fiber's ability to shorten

_____ 9. Retaining bands of connective tissue found around elbows, knees, ankles, and wrists

_____ 10. Thin myofilament

_____ 11. Cell membrane of a muscle fiber

_____ 12. Principal neurotransmitter involved in muscle contraction

MATCHING II

Place the letter of the answer next to the term or phrase that best describes it.

A. All-or-none response
B. Antagonist
C. Concentric
D. Eccentric

E. Fast-twitch
F. Insertion
G. Muscle spindle
H. Origin

I. Oxygen debt
J. Prime mover
K. Recruitment
L. Slow-twitch

_____ 1. Type of isotonic contraction in which the muscle shortens

_____ 2. Fibers that fatigue quickly; also known as white muscle

_____ 3. May occur during heavy exercise when anaerobic glycolysis is required

_____ 4. Only the motor units needed to perform a given action are activated; if more strength is required, more motor units are activated

_____ 5. Muscle causing desired action; also known as the agonist

_____ 6. Muscle attachment that is relatively fixed and immovable during contraction

_____ 7. Fatigue-resistant fibers; also known as red muscle

_____ 8. Muscle opposing an action of the prime mover

_____ 9. Type of isotonic contraction in which the muscle lengthens

_____ 10. Stretch receptor that detects sudden motion, causing reflexive muscle contraction

_____ 11. Refers to the fact that muscle fibers contract to their fullest extent or not at all

_____ 12. Muscle attachment undergoing the greatest movement during contraction

CASE STUDY

Christine is a 58-year-old woman who was diagnosed with fibromyalgia five years ago. She takes yoga classes three times a week. Christine also takes medication daily which helps manage her pain. A few days ago, she had decided to stop drinking coffee to reduce caffeine intake. This was recommended by her physician. Today, she is experiencing a headache that she attributes to caffeine withdrawal.

Christine has an appointment with you today. She has never had a massage before. During the intake, she states that her neighbor receives deep tissue massage and he finds it beneficial. She would like a deep tissue massage today.

Should Christine receive this type of massage? Why or why not? What techniques are appropriate for her? Cite research studies to support your choice of techniques.

CRITICAL THINKING

During a massage, you realize that your client's muscles seem weak and underused. How will you assess the client's condition to determine the best therapeutic approach?

CHAPTER 21

Kinesiology

"The map is not the territory."
—Alfred Korzbyski

LEARNING OBJECTIVES

After completing this chapter, the student should be able to:

- Define kinesiology.
- Name, locate, and palpate bones and bony markings listed in Lessons One and Two.
- Name, locate, and palpate bones, bony markings, and related structures listed in Lessons Three, Four, and Five.
- Name, locate, palpate, and produce movements of muscles listed in Lessons Six and Seven.
- Name, locate, palpate, and produce movements of muscles listed in Lessons Eight and Nine.
- Name, locate, palpate, and produce movements of muscles listed in Lessons Ten and Eleven.
- Name, locate, palpate, and produce movements of muscles listed in Lessons Twelve, Thirteen, and Fourteen.

http://evolve.elsevier.com/Salvo/MassageTherapy

INTRODUCTION

Massage therapists come to know the bones, muscles, and body movements well. This chapter addresses skeletal nomenclature, articulations, body movements, and muscular nomenclature. This collection of information is needed to understand the study of human motion, or **kinesiology**.

Bones contain landmarks for locating muscles and other soft tissue structures (Box 21-1). Many of the terms in earlier chapters are repeated here. For example, the thigh bone is called the *femur* because it is located in the *femoral* region of the body (see Figure 18-23).

Not all bones, bony markings, joints, or muscles are featured—just those that are important in the practice of massage therapy.

Illustrations are included to locate these important structures (Figure 21-1). Use anatomic models, diagrams, and a willing classmate to locate these structures in class.

Your own body and all the bodies with which you will be working are the best teachers. Instead of thinking, "I am massaging the arm," say to yourself silently or aloud structures of the arm, such as *humerus, triceps brachii, biceps brachii,* and *brachialis.* This exercise continually reinforces your new vocabulary. Use *scapula* instead of "shoulder blade" or *olecranon process* instead of "tip of the elbow."

The lesson layout for this chapter is:

Lesson One: Bones of the Upper Extremity
Lesson Two: Bones of the Lower Extremity
Lesson Three: Bones of the Skull
Lesson Four: Bones of the Thorax and Vertebral Column
Lesson Five: Actions and Articulations
Lesson Six: Muscles of Scapular Movement
Lesson Seven: Muscles of Shoulder Joint Movement
Lesson Eight: Muscles of the Elbow and Proximal Radioulnar Joint
Lesson Nine: Muscles of the Forearm, Wrist, and Hand
Lesson Ten: Muscles of Hip and Knee Joint Movement
Lesson Eleven: Muscles of the Ankle and Foot
Lesson Twelve: Muscles of the Head and Neck
Lesson Thirteen: Muscles of the Trunk and Vertebral Column
Lesson Fourteen: Muscles of Respiration

BOX 21-1

Bony Markings

Bones are not smooth but are marked with projections, holes, and depressions. These markings are located where muscles, tendons, and ligaments attach and where nerve and blood vessels pass. These marks are called bony markings, bony landmarks, or surface markings. Here is a list of common markings, their descriptions, and examples:

Angle. Projecting corner of a bone. *Mandibular angle*

Border. Linear ridge, often the edge of a bone. *Medial border of the scapula*

Condyle. Knuckle-shaped rounded projection that often forms a joint. *Lateral condyle of the femur*

Crest. Prominent linear elevation. *Iliac crest*

Epicondyle. Projection over a condyle. *Medial epicondyle of the humerus*

Facet. Small, shallow depression articulating with another bone. *Vertebral articular facet*

Foramen. Hole for blood vessels and nerves to pass. *Foramen magnum of the occipital bone*

Fossa. Large shallow depression in a bone. *Glenoid fossa of the scapula*

Groove. Depression that accommodates a structure. *Intertubercular groove*

Head. Rounded end of a bone. *Fibular head*

Line. Narrow ridge that is less prominent than a crest. *Superior nuchal line*

Meatus. Tubelike opening that forms a tunnel or canal. *External auditory meatus of the temporal bone*

Notch. Deep indention or a narrow gap. *Trochlear notch*

Process. General term for any prominence or prolongation from a bone. *Styloid process of the radius*

Protuberance. Knoblike protrusion of a bone. *External occipital protuberance*

Ramus. Long branchlike prolongation of a bone. *Superior pubic ramus*

Ridge. Elongated projection on a bone. *Supracondylar ridge*

Spine. Sharp, slender projection of a bone. *Spine of the scapula*

Trochanter. Large rough process found only on the femur. *Greater trochanter*

Tubercle. Rounded projection usually blunt and irregular. *Lesser tubercle of the humerus*

Tuberosity. Large, rounded rough projection. *Deltoid tuberosity*

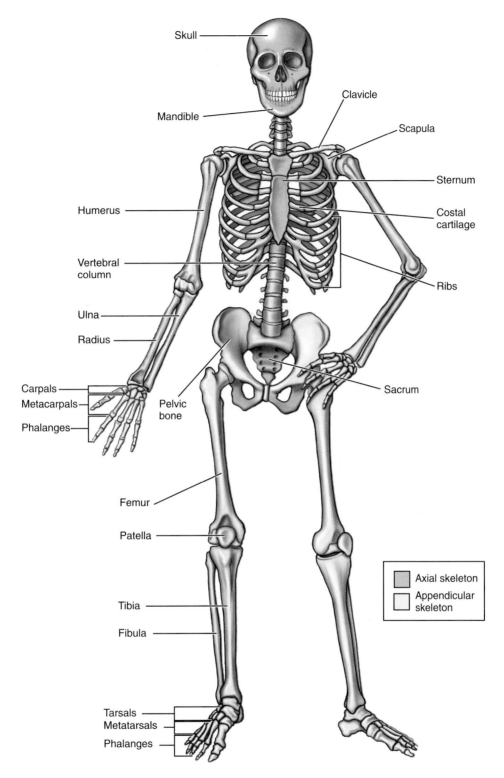

Skull

Mandible

Clavicle

Scapula

Sternum

Humerus

Costal
cartilage

Vertebral
column

Ribs

Ulna

Radius

Carpals

Metacarpals

Phalanges

Pelvic
bone

Sacrum

Femur

Patella

Axial skeleton

Appendicular
skeleton

Tibia

Fibula

Tarsals

Metatarsals

Phalanges

FIGURE 21-1 Bones of the skeletal system or skeletal nomenclature. Anterior view.

IT'S ALL GREEK TO ME

Term	Meaning
acetabulum	*L.* vinegar, saucer, or bowl; small
acromion	Gr. extremity; topmost; the shoulder
atlas	*Gr.* to bear (as the giant of Greek mythology holding up the world)
axis	*Gr.* an axis; an axle
bifid	*L.* cleaved or split in two; twice
carpus	*Gr.* wrist
calcaneus	*L.* heel
clavicle	*L.* little key
coracoid	*Gr.* like a crow's beak
coronal	*L.* shaped as a corona or crown around the head
costal	*L.* rib
crural	*L.* leg
cuneiform	*L.* wedge-shaped
digit	*L.* resembling a finger or toe
dens, dent	*L.* toothlike
ethmoid	*Gr.* sievelike; shaped
femur	*L.* thigh
glenoid	*Gr.* shaped as a socket
hamate	*L.* possessing a small hook
humerus	*L.* shoulder
hyoid	*Gr.* U-shaped
ilium	*L.* flank
ischium	*L.* hip
lambdoidal	*Gr.* shaped as the Greek letter Λ
lamina	*L.* a plate
linea	*L.* line
malleolus	*L.* hammer or mallet; small
mandible	*L.* to chew
manubrium	*L.* a handle
mastoid	Gr. breastlike; shaped
meniscus	*Gr.* crescent; small
metacarpal	Gr. after or beyond; wrist
metatarsal	*Gr.* after or beyond; foot
navicular	A ship; small
obturator	*L.* to obstruct, close, block up, or plug
odont	*Gr.* toothlike
olecranon	*Gr.* skull or tip of the elbow
ossicle	*L.* small bone
parietal	*L.* a wall or partition
patella	*L.* a little dish
pectoral	*L.* breast or chest
pedicle	*L.* small foot
pelvis	*L.* a basin
phalanx	*Gr.* a line of soldiers
pisiform	*L.* pea-shaped
poples	*L.* ham
prominens	*L.* prominent or projecting
pterygoid	*Gr.* shaped as a wing
pubic	*L.* grownup
sacrum	*L.* sacred
sagittal	*L.* an arrow
scaphoid	*Gr.* shaped as a boat
sphenoid	*Gr.* shaped as a wedge
spine	*L.* spiny or thorny plant
stapes	*L.* a stirrup
suture	*L.* to sew; a seam
styloid	*Gr.* shaped as a pillar
talus	*L.* ankle
tarsal	*L.* broad, flat surface; foot
temporal	*L.* time
ulna	*L.* elbow
vertebrae	*L.* turning joint
Wormian	Olaus Worm, Danish Anatomist, 1588-1655
xiphoid	*Gr.* shaped as a sword
zygomatic	*Gr.* a yoke or bar

L., Latin; *Gr.,* Greek.

LESSON ONE—BONES OF THE UPPER EXTREMITY

Clavicle, Scapula, Humerus, Ulna, Radius, Carpals, Metacarpals, Phalanges

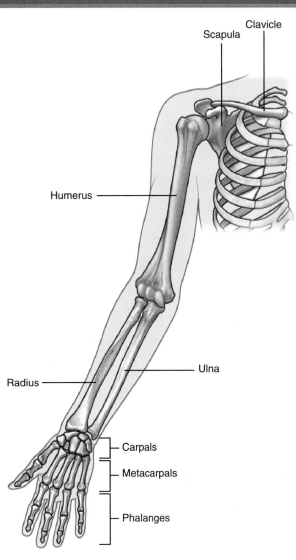

Anterior View

FIGURE 21-2 Bones of the right upper extremity.

Notes: Part of the upper extremity is the *shoulder* (*pectoral*) *girdle*. It consists of the clavicle and the scapula. The shoulder girdle lacks a posterior attachment to the axial skeleton; this permits a wide range of motion of the shoulder. Its only attachment to the axial skeleton is at the sternum, where it joins to the medial end of the clavicle (i.e., sternoclavicular joint).

CLAVICLE

Latin: Little key

BONY MARKING	SIGNIFICANCE
Medial (sternal) end	Joint formation
Lateral (acromial) end	Joint formation

Notes: The clavicle is the collarbone. A helpful mnemonic to learn the name of this bone is *C and C*; **C**ollarbone is the **C**lavicle. The clavicle's medial end articulates with the sternum (sternoclavicular joint) and the cartilage of the first rib, and its lateral end articulates with the acromion of the scapula (acromioclavicular joint). The clavicle acts as a brace to hold the arm away from the top of the thorax. The clavicle is the most commonly fractured bone. When the clavicle is broken, the entire shoulder region caves in medially. This consequence demonstrates its function as a brace.

Lateral end   *Medial end*

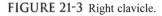

Superior View

FIGURE 21-3 Right clavicle.

SCAPULA

Latin: Shoulder

BONY MARKING	SIGNIFICANCE	BONY MARKING	SIGNIFICANCE
Superior border	Landmark	Acromion (process)	Muscle attachment and joint formation
Medial (vertebral) border	Muscle attachment	Coracoid process	Muscle attachment
Lateral (axillary) border	Muscle attachment	Glenoid cavity (fossa)	Joint formation
Superior angle	Muscle attachment	Supraspinous fossa	Muscle attachment
Inferior angle	Muscle attachment	Infraspinous fossa	Muscle attachment
Spine of the scapula	Muscle attachment	Subscapular fossa	Muscle attachment
Root of spine	Muscle attachment	Supraglenoid tubercle	Muscle attachment
		Infraglenoid tubercle	Muscle attachment

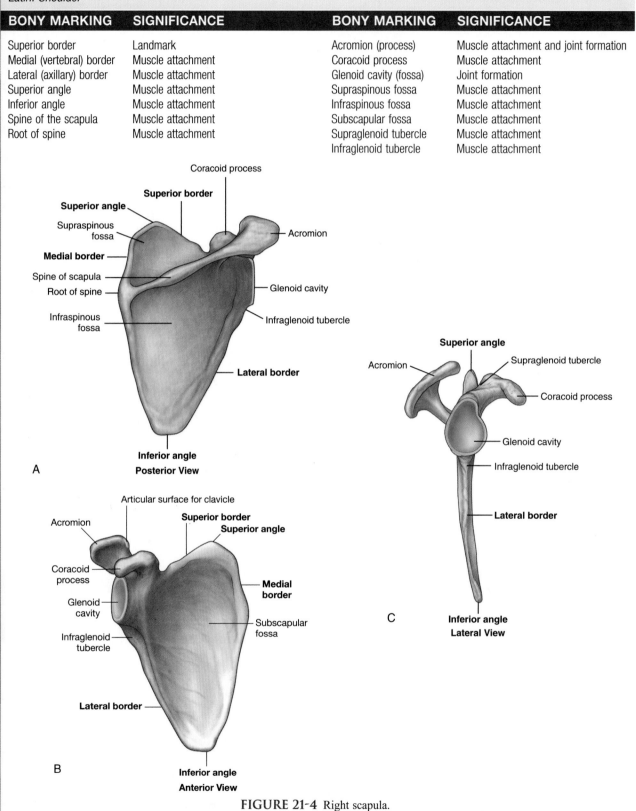

FIGURE 21-4 Right scapula.

Notes: The scapula is the shoulder blade. A helpful mnemonic to learn the name of this bone is *S and S; S*houlder blade is the *S*capula. The scapula articulates with the clavicle forming the acromioclavicular (AC) joint and with the humerus forming the glenohumeral (shoulder) joint. This triangular-shaped bone is located between the second and the seventh ribs. When the scapula is set in motion, it slides against the posterior rib cage.

HUMERUS

Latin: Shoulder

BONY MARKING	SIGNIFICANCE
Humeral head	Joint formation
Anatomical neck	Landmark
Surgical neck	Landmark (where most humeral fractures occur)
Greater tubercle	Muscle attachment
Lesser tubercle	Muscle attachment
Intertubercular (bicipital) groove	Muscle attachment (medial and lateral lips)
Deltoid tuberosity	Muscle attachment
Radial fossa	Joint formation
Olecranon fossa	Joint formation
Coronoid fossa	Joint formation
Capitulum	Joint formation
Trochlea	Joint formation
Medial epicondyle	Muscle attachment
Lateral epicondyle	Muscle attachment
Supracondylar ridge	Muscle attachment (medial and lateral sections)

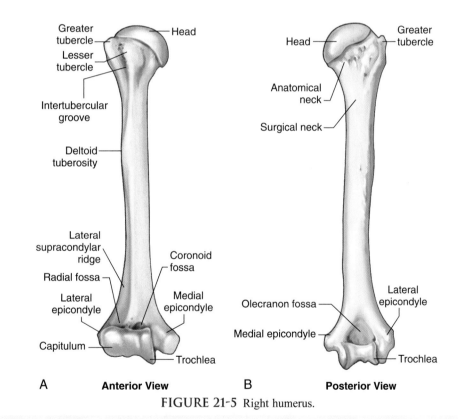

FIGURE 21-5 Right humerus.

Notes: The humerus is the arm bone. Its proximal end articulates with the scapula forming the glenohumeral (shoulder) joint, and its distal end articulates with the radius and the ulna forming a portion of the humeroulnar/humeroradial (elbow) joint. The humerus is also called the *funny bone* or *crazy bone* because hitting the elbow in a certain way makes it feel funny, or *humorous*. These sensations are caused by stimulation of the ulnar nerve where it passes posterior to the medial epicondyle of the humerus.

ULNA

Latin: Elbow

BONY MARKING	SIGNIFICANCE
Olecranon (process)	Muscle attachment
Trochlear (semilunar) notch	Joint formation
Radial notch	Joint formation
Ulnar tuberosity	Muscle attachment
Coronoid process	Muscle attachment
Styloid process	Landmark

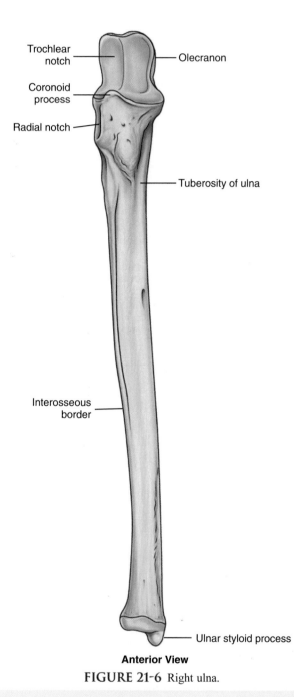

Anterior View

FIGURE 21-6 Right ulna.

Notes: The ulna is one of two forearm bones. In the anatomic position, the ulna is located on the medial, or little finger, side of the forearm. The ulna's proximal end articulates with the humerus, forming the humeroulnar joint (part of the elbow joint), and at its distal end with the triquetrum (carpal bone), forming the ulnomenisco-triquetral portion of the wrist joint.

RADIUS

Latin: Staff or spoke of a wheel

BONY MARKING	SIGNIFICANCE
Radial head	Joint formation
Radial neck	Landmark
Oblique line	Muscle attachment
Radial (bicipital) tuberosity	Muscle attachment
Ulnar notch	Joint formation
Styloid process	Muscle attachment

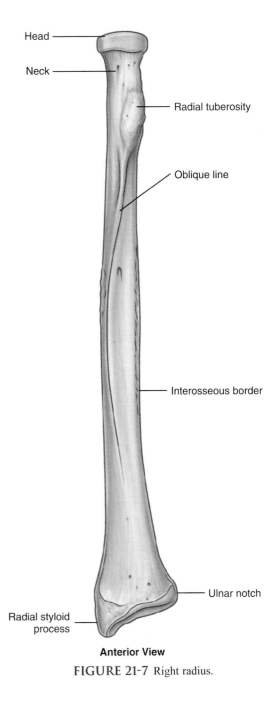

Anterior View

FIGURE 21-7 Right radius.

Notes: The radius is the lateral forearm bone, located on the thumb side of the forearm. The proximal end of the radius articulates with the humerus, forming the humeroradial joint (part of the elbow joint). Its wide distal end articulates with the ulna and with the lunate and scaphoid (carpal bones), forming the radiocarpal (wrist) joint.

To help differentiate the location of radius from the ulna, palpate your radial pulse. You palpate the radial pulse by gently pressing the radial artery against the distal end of radius. Another way to remember the name of this bone is to remember that the Radius always Rotates on the ulna (during supination and pronation [these movements are featured later]).

ADDITIONAL INFORMATION: INTEROSSEOUS MEMBRANE

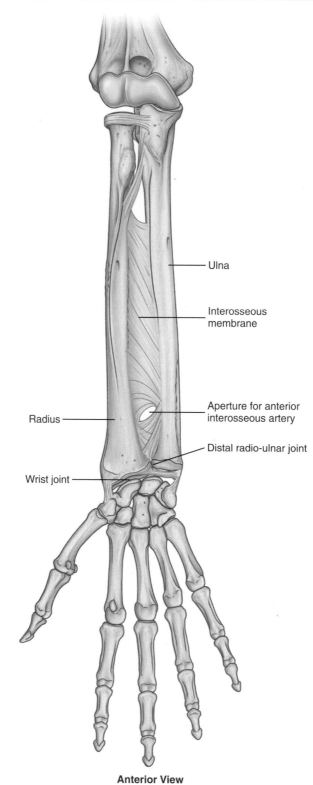

Anterior View

FIGURE 21-8 Right radius and ulna with interosseous membrane.

Notes: An interosseous membrane connects the ulna and the radius with bands of tough connective tissue (Figure 21-8). This anatomic arrangement gives the forearm lightness and mobility and provides attachment sites for the many muscles of the forearm and hand. An interosseous membrane is also located between the tibia and fibula (Lesson Two).

CARPALS

Greek: Wrist

BONE	SIGNIFICANCE
Scaphoid	Largest bone in the proximal row; most commonly fractured carpal bone
Lunate	Crescent moon-shaped bone; most commonly dislocated carpal and the second most commonly fractured carpal
Triquetrum	Triangular or pyramid-shaped bone
Pisiform	Pea-shaped bone; smallest carpal bone; a sesamoid bone
Trapezium	Triangular bone
Trapezoid	Four-sided bone with two parallel sides
Capitate	Largest carpal bone; has a round head
Hamate	Bone has an anterior hook (hook of hamate)

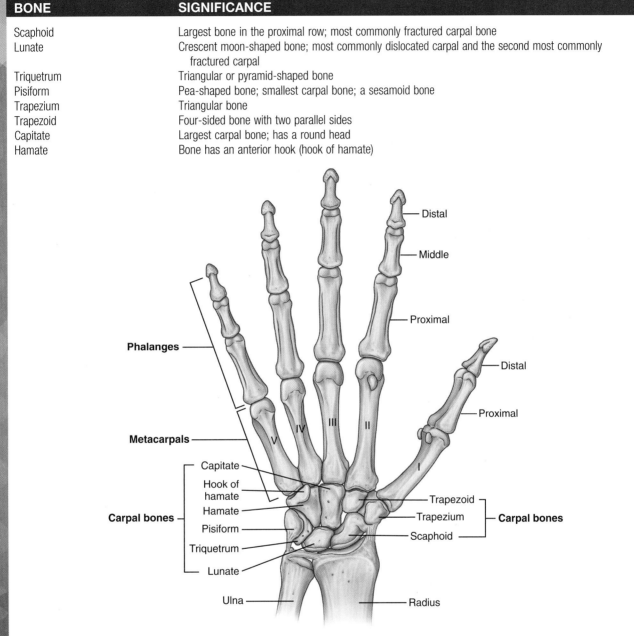

Posterior View

FIGURE 21-9 Right hand.

Notes: The eight carpal bones of the wrist are arranged in two rows of four bones (proximal row and distal row) that are linked together by ligaments and bound in a joint capsule. The carpal bones in the proximal row from lateral to medial are the scaphoid (largest carpal), lunate, triquetrum, and pisiform. The carpal bones in the distal row from lateral to medial are trapezium, trapezoid, capitate, and hamate. The carpal bones function as ball bearings.

To help you learn the names of the capal bones, learn the following sentence: Steve Left The Party To Take Cathy Home. The first letter of each word is also the first letter of each of the carpal bones: Scaphoid-Lunate-Triquetrum-Pisiform-Trapezium-Trapezoid-Capitate-Hamate.

METACARPALS

Greek: After or beyond; wrist

Notes: The metacarpals are located in each hand and are numbered I through V, starting from the thumb (I) to the little finger (V). Each metacarpal has a base (proximal end), shaft, and head (distal end).

When the hand is clenched to make a fist, heads of metacarpals II-V become obvious as the knuckles (see Figure 21-9).

PHALANGES

Greek: A line of soldiers

Notes: In each hand, the fingers and thumb, or digits, contain the 14 phalanges (see Figure 21-9). Each finger has three, and the thumb has two. Depending on their location, the phalanges are referred to as *proximal, middle,* and *distal.* The thumb, or pollicis,

has only a proximal and distal phalanx (singular of phalanges). As with the metacarpals, each phalanx has a base (proximal end), shaft, and head (distal end).

ADDITIONAL INFORMATION: CARPAL TUNNEL

The eight carpal bones of the wrist are arranged in two rows of four bones (proximal row and distal row) that are linked together by ligaments and bound in a joint capsule. The carpal bones in the proximal row from lateral to medial are the *scaphoid, lunate, triquetrum,* and *pisiform.* The carpal bones in the distal row from lateral to medial are *trapezium, trapezoid, capitate,* and *hamate.* The carpal bones function as ball bearings.

To help you learn the names of the carpal bones, learn the following sentence: **S**teve **L**eft **T**he **P**arty **T**o **T**ake **C**athy **H**ome. The first letter of each word is also the first letter of each of the carpal bones: **S**caphoid-**L**unate-**T**riquetrum-**P**isiform-**T**rapezium-**T**rapezoid-**C**apitate-**H**amate.

Notes: A tunnel, or carpal tunnel, is produced by the carpal bones and bound by the *transverse carpal ligament* or the *flexor retinaculum.* This ligament creates a pulley system important for hand functions. Many muscles of the thumb and little finger originate on the transverse carpal ligament.

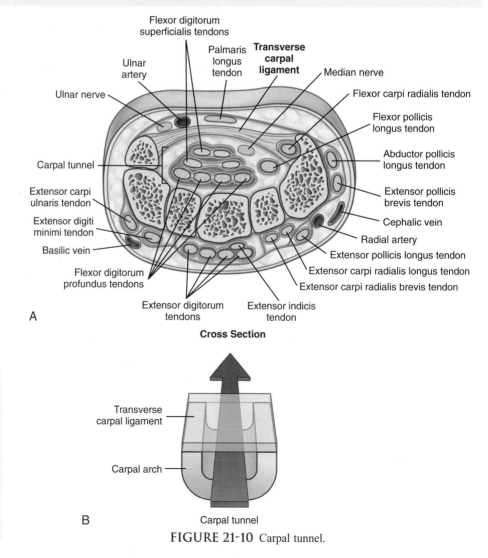

FIGURE 21-10 Carpal tunnel.

LESSON TWO—BONES OF THE LOWER EXTREMITY

Pelvic Bone, Femur, Patella, Tibia, Fibula, Tarsals, Metatarsals, Phalanges

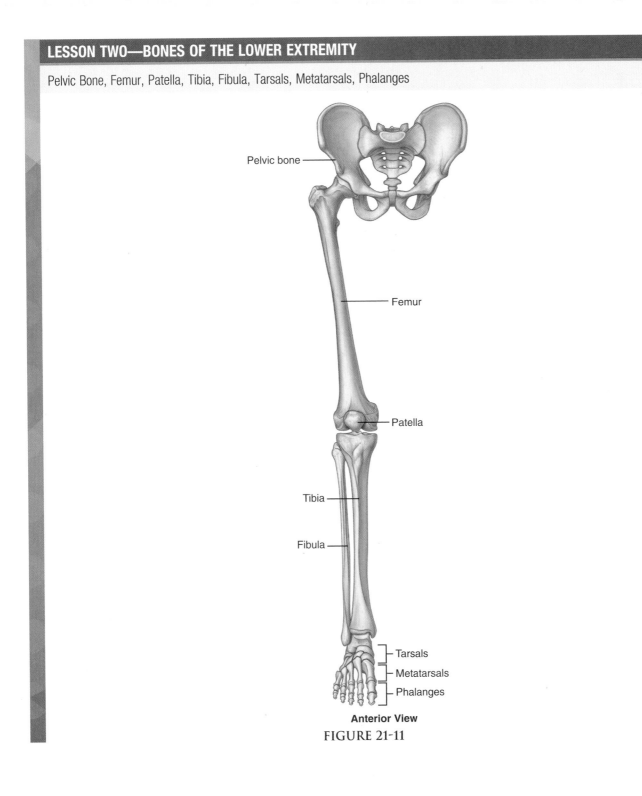

Pelvic bone

Femur

Patella

Tibia

Fibula

Tarsals

Metatarsals

Phalanges

Anterior View

FIGURE 21-11

PELVIC BONE

Latin: A basin

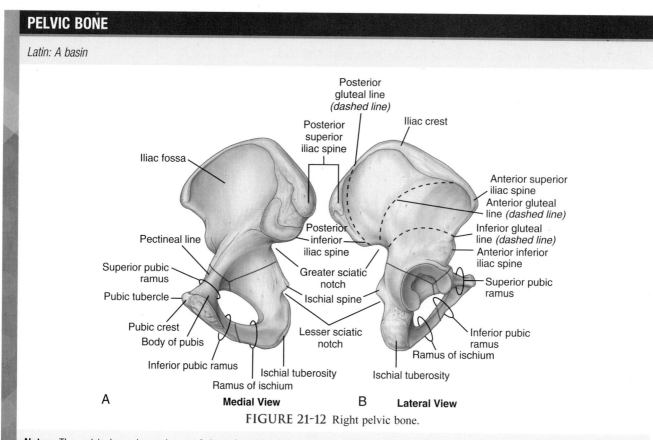

FIGURE 21-12 Right pelvic bone.

Notes: The pelvic bone is made up of three fused bones: ilium, ischium, and pubis. The two pelvic bones together make up the *pelvic girdle*. The pelvic girdle is also known as the *os coxa, coxal bones, hip bones,* or *innominate bones*. The pelvic girdle articulates anteriorly at the pubic symphysis and posteriorly with the sacrum at the sacroiliac (SI) joints. The SI joints are where the lower extremities join the axial skeleton.

The *pelvis* is formed by the two pelvic bones and the sacrum.

ADDITIONAL INFORMATION: PELVIC STRUCTURES

Notes: The *acetabulum*—acetabular cavity, or hip socket—provides a deep socket for the femoral head and forms the iliofemoral joint or hip joint. Each acetabulum is made up of equal portions of the three fused pelvic bones.

The *obturator foramen* is located inferior to the acetabulum. In a living skeleton, the obturator membrane *obstructs* most of the foramen and provides attachment sites for the muscles of the hip and thigh.

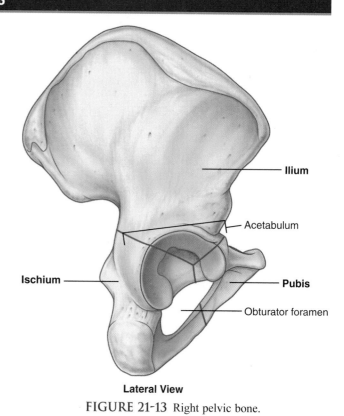

Lateral View

FIGURE 21-13 Right pelvic bone.

ILIUM

Latin:
Flank

BONY MARKING	SIGNIFICANCE
Iliac crest	Muscle attachment
Iliac fossa	Muscle attachment
Anterior superior iliac spine (ASIS)	Muscle attachment
Anterior inferior iliac spine (AIIS)	Muscle attachment
Posterior superior iliac spine (PSIS)	Muscle attachment
Posterior inferior iliac spine (PIIS)	Muscle attachment
Posterior gluteal line	Muscle attachment
Anterior gluteal line	Muscle attachment
Inferior gluteal line	Muscle attachment
Greater sciatic notch	Passage of sciatic nerve

Note: The ilium is the most superior pelvic bone and resembles a broad, expanding blade.

ISCHIUM

Latin:
Hip

BONY MARKING	SIGNIFICANCE
Ischial tuberosity	Muscle attachment
Ischial spine	Muscle attachment
Ischial ramus (ramus of the ischium)	Muscle attachment
Greater sciatic notch	Passage of sciatic nerve
Lesser sciatic notch	Passage of obturator internus

Note: The ischium is the most inferior and most posterior pelvic bone. Correcting sitting posture involves sitting on the ischial tuberosity rather than the sacrum.

PUBIS

Latin:
Grownup

BONY MARKING	SIGNIFICANCE
Superior pubic ramus	Muscle attachment
Inferior pubic ramus	Muscle attachment
Pubic tubercle	Muscle attachment
Pubic crest	Muscle attachment
Pectineal line	Muscle attachment
Pubic body (body of pubis)	Landmark

Note: This is the most anterior pelvic bone.

FEMUR

Latin: Thigh

BONY MARKING	SIGNIFICANCE
Femoral head	Joint formation
Femoral neck	Landmark (where most femoral fractures occur)
Greater trochanter	Muscle attachment
Lesser trochanter	Muscle attachment
Intertrochanteric line	Muscle attachment
Intertrochanteric crest	Muscle attachment
Linea aspera	Muscle attachment (medial and lateral lips)
Gluteal tuberosity	Muscle attachment
Adductor tubercle	Muscle attachment
Medial condyle	Joint formation
Lateral condyle	Joint formation
Medial epicondyle	Muscle attachment
Lateral epicondyle	Muscle attachment

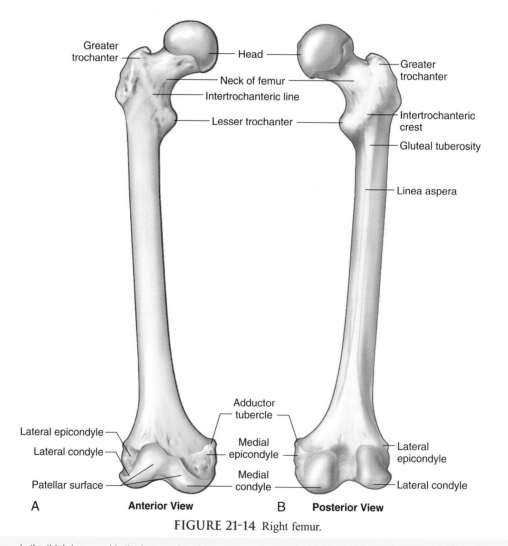

FIGURE 21-14 Right femur.

Notes: The femur is the thigh bone and is the longest, heaviest, and strongest bone in the body. It has a ball-like head at the proximal end and two ball-like condyles at its distal end. The femur articulates proximally with the hip joint at the acetabulum, forming the iliofemoral or acetabulofemoral (hip) joint, and distally with the patella and the tibia, forming the patellofemoral joint and the tibiofemoral (knee) joint.

PATELLA

Latin: A little dish

Notes: The patella, or kneecap, is the largest sesamoid bone in the body and articulates with the distal end of the femur (see Figure 21-11). The patella is embedded in the tendon of the quadriceps femoris muscle group. Its main function is to assist knee extension by increased leverage of the quadriceps tendon. However, the patella is not always considered part of the knee joint.

TIBIA

Latin: Shinbone

BONY MARKING	SIGNIFICANCE
Medial condyle	Joint formation
Lateral condyle	Joint formation
Tibial tuberosity	Muscle attachment
Crest	Landmark
Soleal line	Muscle attachment
Medial malleolus	Landmark

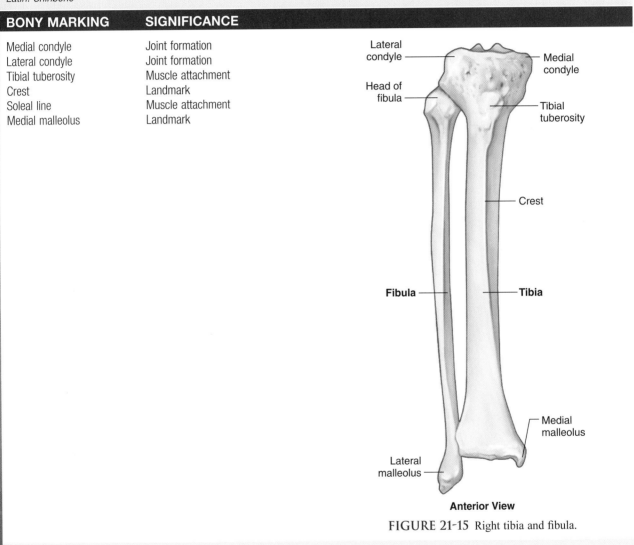

Anterior View

FIGURE 21-15 Right tibia and fibula.

Notes: The tibia is the medial leg bone. Also called the shin bone, the tibia is the stoutest and straightest long bone in the body. The tibial shaft is triangular-shaped. Its proximal aspect articulates with the femur at the tibiofemoral (knee) joint and the fibula. Its distal end articulates with the talus, forming the talocrural (ankle) joint and the fibula. The tibial crest is also called the anterior border.

FIBULA

Latin: Clasp or pin of a brooch

BONY MARKING	SIGNIFICANCE
Fibular head	Muscle attachment
Lateral malleolus	Landmark

Notes: The fibula is the lateral leg bone (see Figure 21-15). The fibula is much smaller in diameter than the tibia and supports only approximately 10% of the body's weight. The proximal end of the fibula articulates with the tibia and is not involved with the knee joint (proximal tibiofibular joint). The distal end of the fibula articulates with the talus and the tibia (talocrural joint and distal tibiofibular joint).

As with the ulna and radius of the forearm, an interosseous membrane connects the tibia and the fibula and provides muscle attachments.

TARSALS

Latin: Broad, flat surface; foot

BONES

Talus (astragalus)
Cuneiforms: I (medial), II (intermediate), III (lateral)
Navicular
Cuboid
Calcaneus

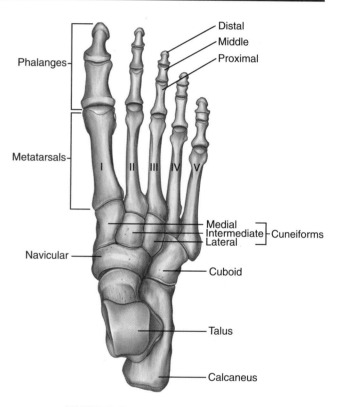

FIGURE 21-16 Right foot, dorsal view.

Notes: The seven tarsal bones are the *talus, calcaneus, cuboid, navicular,* and the three *cuneiforms.*

To help you learn the names of the tarsal bones, learn the following sentence: **T**he **C**rayon **N**ow **M**arks **I**nside **L**ines **C**learly. The first letter of each word is also the first letter of each of the tarsal bones: **T**alus-**C**alcaneus-**N**avicular-**M**edial cuneiform-**I**ntermediate cuneiform-**L**ateral cuneiform-**C**uboid. Each tarsal bone slides minutely over the next tarsal bone to collectively provide motion. This characteristic is similar to the way the spine creates movement.

METATARSALS

Greek: After or beyond; foot

Notes: Five metatarsals, numbered I through V, are in each foot starting from the great toe (I) to the little toe (V). The metatarsals articulate proximally with cuboid and cuneiform and distally with the phalanges (see Figure 21-16). The length of the metatarsals determines shoe size. Each metatarsal has a base (proximal end), a shaft, and a head (distal end). When you flex your toes dorsally and look at your knuckles, you are actually looking at the heads of the metatarsals. The distal ends articulate with the phalanges, forming the metatarsophalangeal joints.

PHALANGES

Greek: A line of soldiers

Notes: The phalanges are also known as the *digits,* or *toes* (see Figure 21-16). The great toe, or hallux, has two phalanges (proximal and distal phalanx) while each of the other toes has three (i.e., middle phalanx). As with the metatarsals, each phalanx has a base (proximal end), a shaft and a head (proximal end). At the distal end of each distal phalanx is a tubercle.

ADDITIONAL INFORMATION: FOOT ARCHES

MEDIAL LONGITUDINAL ARCH

The calcaneus, talus, navicular, cuneiform I-III, and the heads of metatarsals I-III constitute contribute to this arch. This is the arch usually referred to when people mention an arch of the foot.

LATERAL LONGITUDINAL ARCH

The calcaneus, cuboid, and the heads of metatarsals IV and V make up this arch.

TRANSVERSE ARCH

This arch runs from side-to-side and is formed by the cuboid, cuneiforms I-III and the metatarsal heads.

Notes: For walking, running, and jumping to be springy, our feet must absorb shock. To help accomplish this task, the foot uses a system of arches. Together, these arches resemble a geodesic structure. This shape helps to distribute weight.

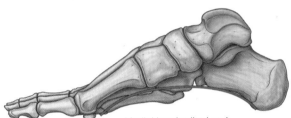

Medial longitudinal arch

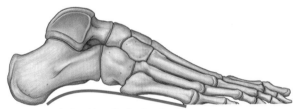

Lateral longitudinal arch

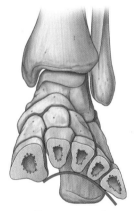

Transverse arch

FIGURE 21-17 Arches of the foot.

LESSON THREE—BONES OF THE SKULL

This lesson examines the bones of the skull, which include the cranial and facial bones. The hyoid bone is usually included with bones of the skull but is not actually part of the skull (see later discussion). The eye sockets, or *eye orbits*, are made up of several skull bones. Except for the movable joints between the jawbone and the rest of the skull (temporomandibular joint), all skull bones are joined by sutures.

SKULL

Greek: Skull

CRANIAL BONES	BONY MARKING AND/OR SIGNIFICANCE
Frontal bone	Non-applicable
Parietal bones	Non-applicable
Temporal bones	Styloid process (ligament attachment)
	External auditory meatus or ear canal (contains the malleus [hammer], incus [anvil], and stapes [stirrup]).
	Mastoid process (muscle attachment)
Ethmoid bone	Non-applicable
Sphenoid bone (articulates with all other cranial bones)	Sella turcica (pituitary location)
	Pterygoid plate (muscle attachment)
	Greater wings (muscle attachment)
Occipital bone	Foramen magnum (passage for spinal cord)
	Superior nuchal line (muscle attachment)
	Inferior nuchal line (muscle attachment)
	External occipital protuberance or *inion* (landmark and muscle attachment)
	Occipital condyles (joint formation)

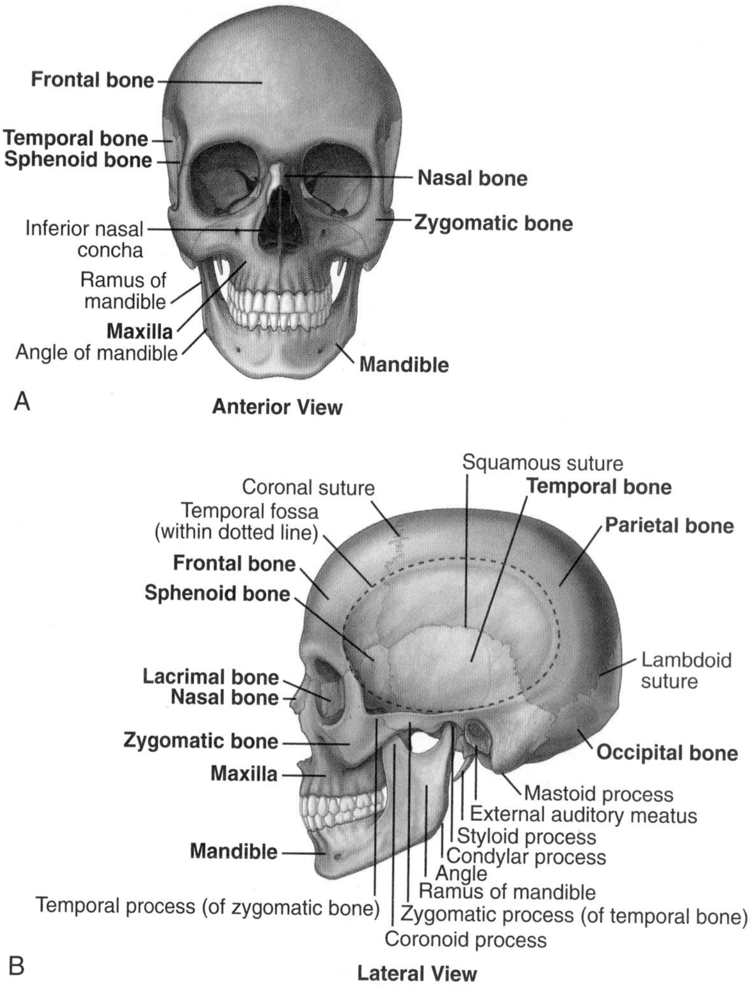

FIGURE 21-18 The skull.

SKULL, CONT'D

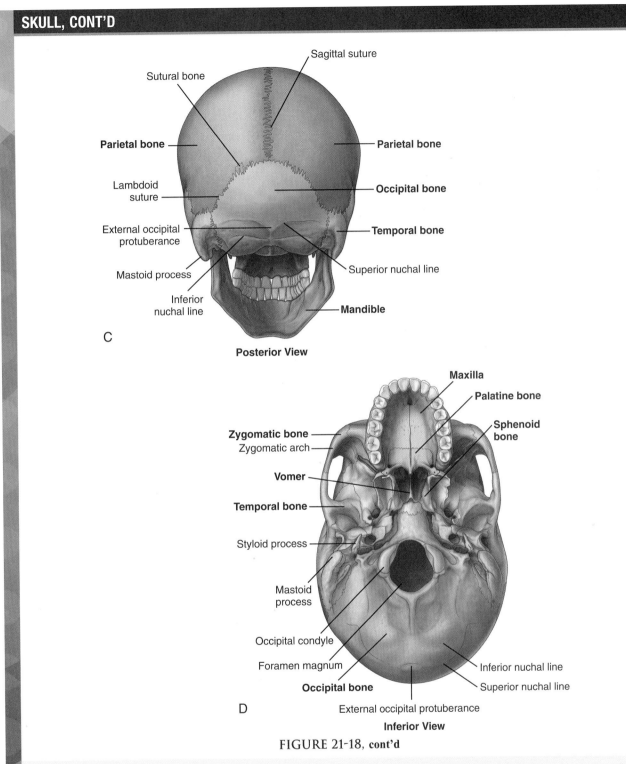

Posterior View

Labels (posterior view):
- Sagittal suture
- Sutural bone
- **Parietal bone**
- **Parietal bone**
- Lambdoid suture
- **Occipital bone**
- External occipital protuberance
- **Temporal bone**
- Mastoid process
- Superior nuchal line
- Inferior nuchal line
- **Mandible**

C

Inferior View

Labels (inferior view):
- **Maxilla**
- **Palatine bone**
- **Zygomatic bone**
- **Sphenoid bone**
- Zygomatic arch
- **Vomer**
- **Temporal bone**
- Styloid process
- Mastoid process
- Occipital condyle
- Foramen magnum
- **Occipital bone**
- External occipital protuberance
- Inferior nuchal line
- Superior nuchal line

D

FIGURE 21-18, cont'd

Notes: The cranium contains eight bones: frontal bone (forehead), two parietal bones, two temporal bones, ethmoid bone, sphenoid bone, and occipital bone. This bony region protects the brain and provides a bony passageway for the spinal cords, various nerves, blood vessels, and organs of sight, taste, hearing, and smell. The occipital bone articulates with the first cervical vertebra (C1) and forms the atlantooccipital joint. External auditory meatus or ear canal (contains the malleus [hammer], incus [anvil], and stapes [stirrup]).

FACIAL BONES

Old English: Of the face

BONES	BONY MARKING
Nasal bones	Non-applicable
Vomer bone	Non-applicable
Zygomatic bones	Non-applicable
Lacrimal bones	Non-applicable
Inferior nasal concha bones	Non-applicable
Palatine bones	Non-applicable
Maxillae	Non-applicable
Mandible	Mandibular ramus (muscle attachment)
	Mandibular angle (muscle attachment)
	Coronoid process (muscle attachment)
	Condylar process (muscle attachment and joint formation)

Notes: The face has 14 bones: the vomer bone, two nasal bones, two zygomatic bones (cheekbones), two lacrimal bones, two inferior nasal concha bones, two palatine bones, two fused maxillae, one mandible (jawbone). Facial features are largely a result of facial bone and cartilaginous structures. Facial and cranial bones articulate with one another by means of sutures, discussed in the next section.

ADDITIONAL INFORMATION: SUTURES

Latin: To sew; a seam

SAGITTAL SUTURE
Joins the two parietal bones.

CORONAL SUTURE
Joins the frontal bone to the parietal bones. Shaped like a corona, or crown, around the head.

LAMBDOIDAL SUTURE
Joins the parietal bones to the occipital bone.

SQUAMOSAL SUTURE
Joins the parietal bones to the temporal bones.

Notes: Sutures are located anywhere skull bones articulate (see Figure 21-18). The only exception is the temporomandibular (TMJ) joint. Very little movement exists in these sutural regions. Sutures may be named by the bones between which they sit (e.g., frontonasal suture lies between the frontal and nasal bones), but some have specialized names. *Sutural bones*, also known as *Wormian bones*, are irregular bones found in the sutures between bones of the skull. The number of sutural bones varies considerably from person to person.

HYOID

Greek: U-shaped

Notes: Inferior to the skull at the level of C3 is the hyoid bone. It is shaped similar to a miniature mandible (body and greater horns) with two canine teeth (lesser horns). This bone does not articulate directly with any other bone and, and therefore is really not a skull bone. However, it relates to the skull because it is suspended from the styloid process of the temporal bone by ligaments. These ligaments serve as support for the tongue and provide muscle attachments for the tongue, neck, and pharynx. This bone is important in forensic medicine. When it is found broken, it may mean the victim has been strangled or hanged.

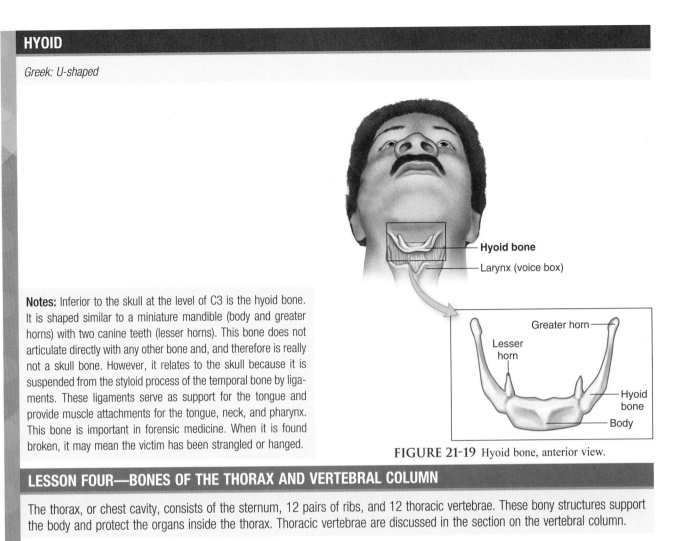

FIGURE 21-19 Hyoid bone, anterior view.

LESSON FOUR—BONES OF THE THORAX AND VERTEBRAL COLUMN

The thorax, or chest cavity, consists of the sternum, 12 pairs of ribs, and 12 thoracic vertebrae. These bony structures support the body and protect the organs inside the thorax. Thoracic vertebrae are discussed in the section on the vertebral column.

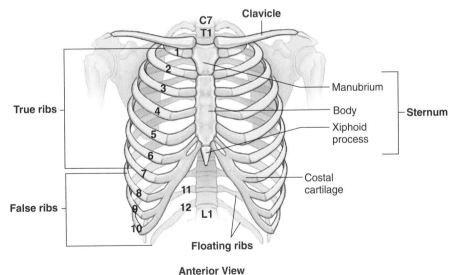

Anterior View

FIGURE 21-20 The thorax.

STERNUM

Greek: Chest, breast, breastbone

BONY MARKING	SIGNIFICANCE
Manubrium	Muscle attachment and joint formation
Sternal body	Muscle attachment and joint formation
Xiphoid process	Muscle attachment and joint formation

Notes: The sternum, or breastbone, forms the central portion of the anterior chest wall. In the adult, the sternum is a single bone made up of three bones: the manubrium, body, and xiphoid process (see Figure 21-20). The manubrium articulates with the medial end of the clavicle at the sternoclavicular (SC) joint and with the first rib at one of several sternocostal joints.

RIBS

Old English: To roof, cover

BONES	SIGNIFICANCE
True ribs (7 pairs)	Articulate directly with the sternum via their costal cartilages
False ribs (3 pairs)	Articulate indirectly with the sternum via costal cartilages of rib seven
Floating ribs (2 pairs)	Does not articulate with the sternum

Notes: The ribs are 24 individual (12 pairs) long, flat, curved bones that articulate posteriorly with the thoracic vertebrae (see Figure 21-20). Anteriorly, the first seven pairs of ribs have their costal cartilages articulate directly with the sternum and are known as the *true ribs*. The first rib is short and thick, and the great vessels and main nerves run over it.

The next five pairs are called the *false ribs*. Ribs 8, 9, and 10 attach indirectly to the sternum by borrowing the costal cartilage of rib seven. The last two pairs of false ribs are designated *floating ribs* as they do not attach to the sternum at all.

VERTEBRAL COLUMN

Latin: Turning joint

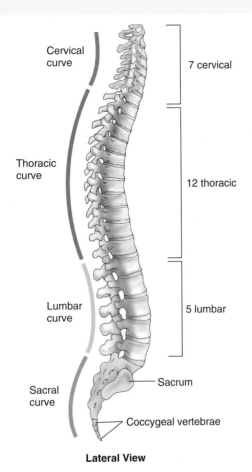

Lateral View

FIGURE 21-21 Vertebral column and regions.

REGIONS	TRAITS
Cervical (C1-C7)	Most possess bifid spinous processes and transverse foramina
Thoracic (T1-T12)	Possess demifacets for articulating ribs
Lumbar (L1-L5)	Possess large vertebral bodies
Sacrum (S1-S5—fused)	Triangular-shaped
Coccyx (Co1-Co3 to Co5—fused)	Tail shaped

NORMAL CURVATURES	
Cervical	Curves anteriorly
Thoracic	Curves posteriorly
Lumbar	Curves anteriorly
Sacrococcygeal	Curves posteriorly

Notes: The vertebral (spinal) column consists of 26 individual bones. It provides support for the spinal cord and the head, articulates with the ribs, and provides attachment sites for muscles.

The spinal column of an infant is C-shaped, arching posteriorly. A cervical curvature occurs when the baby learns to hold its head up, and lumbar curvature occurs as the child learns to walk. In an adult, the vertebral column bends anteriorly to posteriorly and back to anteriorly a total of four times (in normal spines). These curvatures are required for a functional upright posture, to help support the weight of the body, and to help provide balance.

One way to remember the number of vertebrae in each region is breakfast at seven (7 cervical vertebrae) lunch at twelve (12 thoracic vertebrae), and dinner at five (5 lumbar vertebrae).

VERTEBRA

Latin: Turning joint

VERTEBRAL ELEMENT	SIGNIFICANCE
Vertebral body	Joint formation
Pedicle	Attaches arch to body
Transverse processes	Muscle attachment
Lamina	Lamina groove
Spinous process	Muscle attachment

Notes: Bones of the vertebral column are called the vertebrae. They differ slightly in their shape and size from region to region. Each weight-bearing portion of the vertebra (i.e., vertebral body) gradually increases in size so that the lumbar vertebrae are much larger than the cervical or upper thoracic vertebrae.

Most vertebrae have two main regions: a body and an arch. The vertebral arch is the circle of bone that extends out from the body and is formed by the pedicles and the laminae on either side. The transverse process projects laterally from the arch and the spinous process projects posteriorly. Each vertebra varies only in location, shape, and size.

Just posterior to the intervertebral disk is a large central hole, or *vetebral canal*, for the spinal cord to pass. Each vertebra articulates with another vertebra by *articular facets*. As vertebrae are stacked as a column, an opening, or *intervertebral foramen*, is created at the pedicles for spinal roots to pass.

These stacked vertebrae also create a trench in the lamina region of the spine, or the *lamina groove*.

Between each unfused vertebral body is a fibrocartilage disk called the *intervertebral disk*. Its function is to maintain joint spaces, assist with spinal movements, and absorb vertical shock. The disk has two parts: *annulus fibrosus*, or the outer ring for shock absorption, and *nucleus pulposus*, or the soft, gel-like center that adjusts to weight distribution throughout the column. The disk loses some of its elasticity with age; it can also become compressed and herniate.

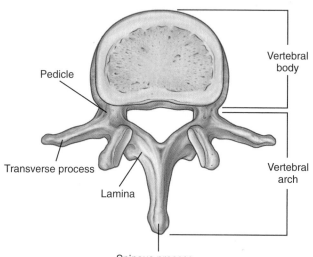

Superior View

FIGURE 21-22 Typical vertebra.

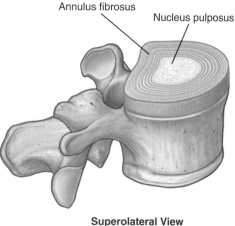

Superolateral View

FIGURE 21-23 Intervertebral disk.

ADDITIONAL INFORMATION: MAJOR SPINAL LIGAMENTS

NUCHAL LIGAMENT

Located in the posterior region of the neck, the nuchal ligament extends from the occipital bone at the external occipital protuberance to all the spinous processes of the cervical vertebrae and offers the neck both stability and muscle attachment sites.

SUPRASPINOUS LIGAMENT

The supraspinous ligament connects the spinous process of C7 to L5 and offers strength and stability. In reference, the supraspinous ligament lies superficial to the nuchal ligament.

SACROTUBEROUS LIGAMENT

The sacrotuberous ligament runs from the sacrum to the ischial tuberosity and provides stability to the vertebrae and pelvis (see Figure 21-87, B).

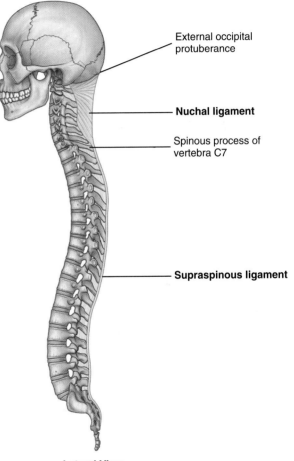

External occipital protuberance

Nuchal ligament

Spinous process of vertebra C7

Supraspinous ligament

Lateral View

FIGURE 21-24 Supraspinous and nuchal ligaments.

ADDITIONAL INFORMATION: ATYPICAL VERTEBRA AND CHARACTERISTICS OF THORACIC AND LUMBAR VERTEBRAE

C1

The first cervical vertebra, also known as the *atlas*, or C1, is shaped as a bony ring. The atlas possesses no body, pedicles, or laminae (Figure 21-25, *A*). The spinous process has been reduced to a posterior tubercle. Facets on the superior surface articulate with the occipital bone and permit head nodding. On the inferior surface, facets articulate with the second cervical vertebrae. This and most other cervical vertebrae possess a *transverse foramen* (hole in the transverse processes for the passage of the vertebral artery).

C2

The second cervical vertebra is often referred to as the *axis,* or *C2.* The axis has a spinous process that is thick and strongly bifurcated (forked). The *odontoid process*, or *dens*, is a bony extension that projects superiorly through the ring of the atlas and permits rotation of the head (Figure 21-25, *B*). Theories suggest that the dens evolved from the old body of the atlas.

C7

The *vertebra prominens*, typically C7, has a spinous process that is long and projects posteriorly approximately 70% of the time (Figure 21-24). The vertebral prominens can be easily palpated at the base of the neck. This vertebra is the only cervical vertebra that does not possess a transverse foramen; the vertebral artery passes directly over the transverse process.

The vertebral prominens is occasionally C6 approximately 20% of the time and T1 approximately 10% of the time.

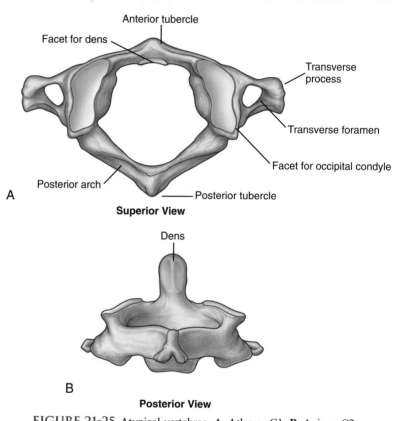

Superior View

Posterior View

FIGURE 21-25 Atypical vertebrae. **A,** Atlas or C1. **B,** Axis or C2.

ADDITIONAL INFORMATION: ATYPICAL VERTEBRA AND CHARACTERISTICS OF THORACIC AND LUMBAR VERTEBRAE, CONT'D

T1-T12

Located on the body and transverse processes of the thoracic vertebrae is an extra pair of facets called demifacets for articulating ribs (Figure 21-26, A).

L1-L5

Lumbar vertebrae contain a large vertebral body. The spinous process and transverse processes that are short and thick (Figure 21-26, B).

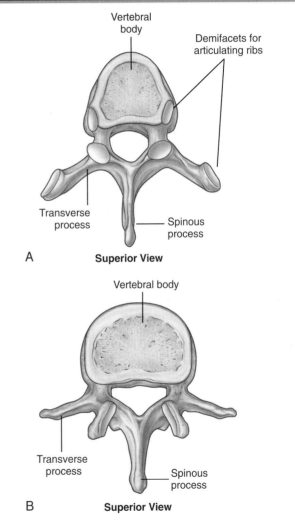

A   **Superior View**

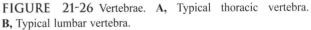

B   **Superior View**

FIGURE 21-26 Vertebrae. **A,** Typical thoracic vertebra. **B,** Typical lumbar vertebra.

LESSON FIVE—ACTIONS AND ARTICULATIONS

This lesson examines action terminology and the articulations, or joints that produce them.

Action Terminology

The following movements are provided by joints of the body with the anatomic position used as the reference point or beginning point of movement (see Figure 18-18).

Flexion. Bends or decreases the angle of a joint. It is usually performed in the midsagittal plane (see Figure 18-19). Exceptions are flexion of the thumb and side bending or *lateral flexion* of the axial skeleton, which are carried out in the coronal plane.

The movements at the ankle joint are referred to as *plantar flexion* (moving the sole of the foot inferiorly) and *dorsiflexion* (moving the dorsal surface of the foot superiorly). These movements are featured later in this section.

Extension. Straightens or increases the angle of a joint. As with flexion, extension is usually performed in the sagittal plane and has exceptions. *Hyperextension* is a continuation of extension beyond anatomic position, as in bending the head backward (Figure 21-27, *A–K*).
- Digital
- Elbow
- Hip
- Knee
- Neck
- Shoulder
- Spinal
- Wrist
- Neck
- Spinal

Abduction. Movement away from the median plane. This movement usually occurs in the coronal plane, with the exception of thumb adduction, which is moving the thumb away from the palm. Abduction of the fingers is movement away from an imaginary line through the third digit, and in the toes, through the second digit. *Horizontal abduction* refers to abduction performed when the arm is flexed approximately 90 degrees rather than from the anatomic position.

Adduction. Movement toward the median plane. *Horizontal adduction* is the opposite movement of horizontal abduction (Figure 21-28, *A–F*).
- Digital. The median plane for finger abduction and adduction is the middle digit.
- Hip
- Shoulder
- Wrist. Wrist abduction is also referred to as *radial deviation* or *radial flexion*. Wrist adduction is referred to as *ulnar deviation* or *ulnar flexion*.

   Notes: Both ulnar and radial deviations occur around an axis that passes through the capitate. To help remember the difference between radial and ulnar deviation, note that the letter *L* is in both *ulnar* and *little finger*. Hence, during u*L*nar deviation, the *L*ittle finger moves toward the ulna.

Supination. Lateral (outward) rotation of the forearm so that the palm is turned up. A good way to remember this movement is that s*UP*ination has an *UP* in it, or think of it as holding a cup of soup (Figure 21-29).

Pronation. Medial (inward) rotation of the forearm so that the palm is turned down and therefore prone to spill the soup (see Figure 21-29).

Plantar Flexion. Extension of the ankle so that the toes are pointing downward, increasing the ankle angle anteriorly (Figure 21-30).

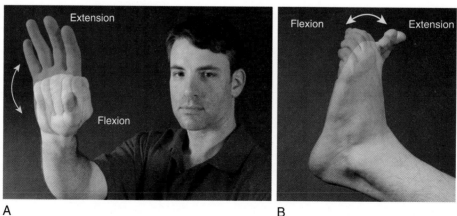

A   B

FIGURE 21-27 **A,** Finger flexion and extension. **B,** Toe flexion and extension.

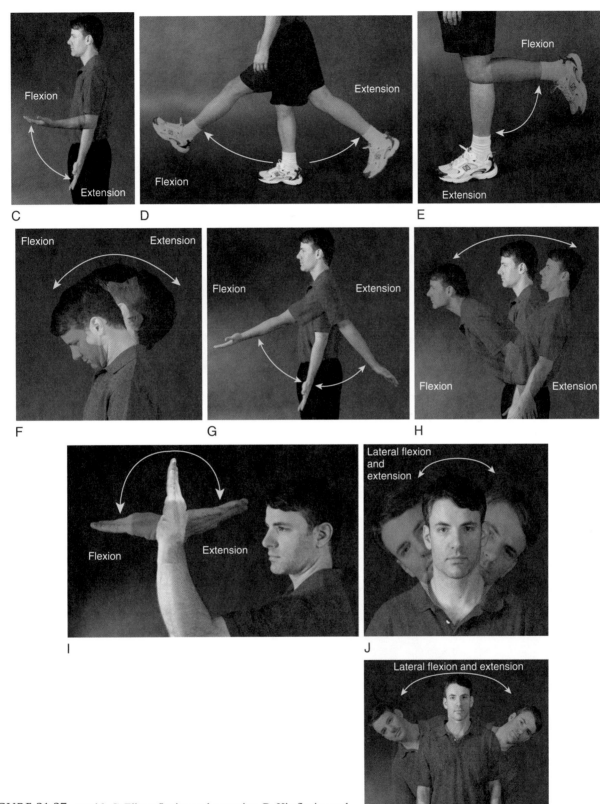

FIGURE 21-27, **cont'd C,** Elbow flexion and extension. **D,** Hip flexion and extension. **E,** Knee flexion and extension. **F,** Neck flexion and extension. **G,** Shoulder flexion and extension. **H,** Spinal flexion and extension. **I,** Wrist flexion and extension. **J,** Neck lateral flexion and extension. **K,** Spinal lateral flexion and extension.

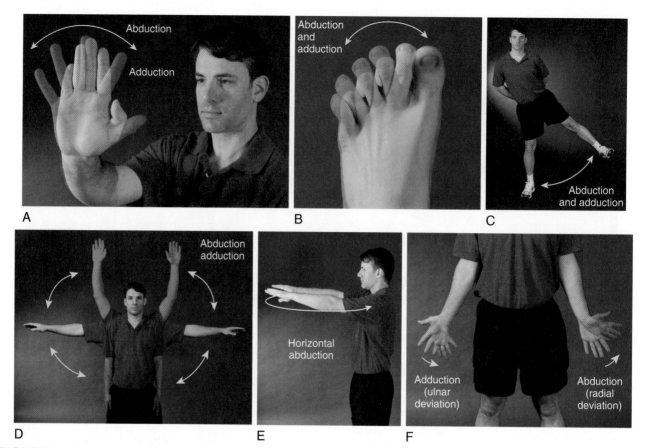

FIGURE 21-28 **A,** Finger abduction and adduction. **B,** Toe abduction. **C,** Hip abduction and adduction. **D,** Shoulder abduction and adduction. **E,** Shoulder horizontal abduction. **F,** Wrist abduction and adduction.

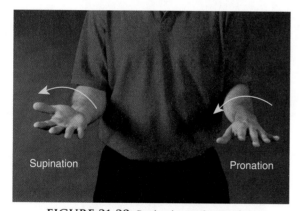

FIGURE 21-29 Supination and pronation.

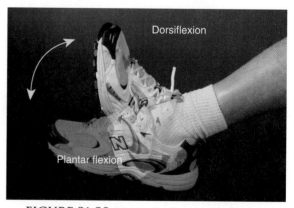

FIGURE 21-30 Plantar flexion and dorsiflexion.

Dorsiflexion. Flexing the ankle dorsally so that the toes are moving toward the shin, as in walking on the heels (see Figure 21-30).

Inversion. Elevation of the medial edge of the foot so that the sole is turned inward (or medially). When both feet are inverted, the soles of the feet face each other (Figure 21-31).

Eversion. Elevation of the lateral edge of the foot so that the sole is turned outward (or laterally). When both feet are everted, the soles of the feet do not face each other (see Figure 21-31).

Circumduction. The distal end of a structure moves in a circle and the proximal end is relatively fixed; it can be described as cone-shaped range of motion but is actually a combination of several movements including flexion, extension, adduction, and abduction (Figure 21-32, *A–C*).

- Shoulder
- Hip
- Digital

Rotation. Circular movement when a bone moves around its own central axis. You may refer to this movement as axial rotation.

Left and *right* rotation refers to the direction of rotation and is reserved for joints that lie within the median axis, such as the head, neck, and spine.

Lateral and *medial rotation* refers to the direction of rotation and is used for joints that lie outside of the median axis, such as the shoulder, hip, and knee (the knee can be rotated slightly when flexed).

Upward (lateral) and *downward (medial)* rotation are terms reserved for the scapula. In scapular rotation, the point of reference is its glenoid cavity. During upward rotation, the glenoid cavity faces upward. During downward rotation, the glenoid cavity faces downward (Figure 21-33, *A–F*).

- Neck
- Spinal

- Shoulder
- Hip
- Knee
- Scapular

Elevation. Raising or lifting a body part, moving superiorly.

Depression. Lowering or dropping a body part, moving inferiorly (Figure 21-34, *A, B*).

- Mandibular
- Scapular

Protraction. Movement forward or anteriorly.

Retraction. Movement backward or posteriorly (Figure 21-35, *A, B*).

- Mandibular
- Scapular

Opposition. Movement in which the tip of the thumb comes into contact with the tip of any other digit on the same hand (Figure 21-36).

Lateral Deviation. Side-to-side movement, in the transverse plane is often used when discussing mandibular movements (Figure 21-37).

Pelvic Tilt

A pelvic tilt refers to an anterior or posterior tilting of the *entire* pelvis in the frontal plane around a mediolateral axis. In describing pelvic tilts, the reference point is the ilium (Figure 21-38, *A* and *B*). However, some kinesiologists choose to use specific bony markings on the ilium, such as the anterior and posterior iliac spines or the iliac crest. Caution is needed in applying these terms because they do not always delineate whether they are describing pelvic displacement or joint movement.

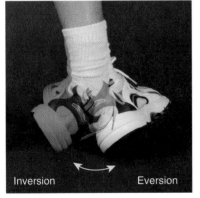

FIGURE 21-31 Inversion and eversion.

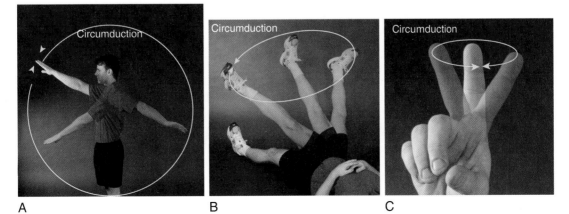

FIGURE 21-32 **A,** Shoulder circumduction. **B,** Hip circumduction. **C,** Finger circumduction.

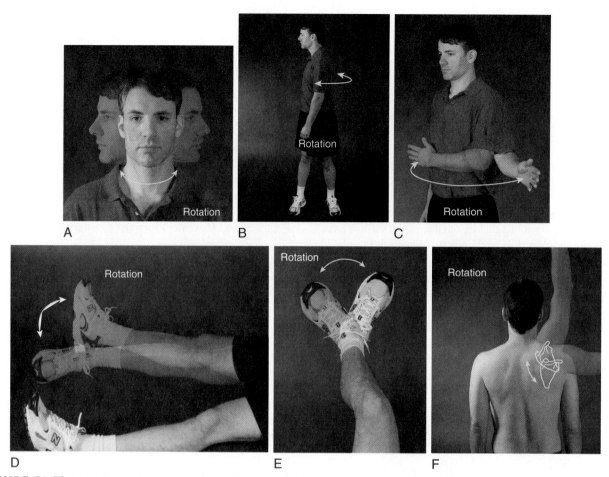

FIGURE 21-33 **A,** Neck rotation. **B,** Spinal rotation. **C,** Shoulder rotation with elbow flexed. **D,** Knee rotation. **E,** Ankle rotation. **F,** Scapular rotation.

Anterior Tilt. During an anterior tilt, the iliums are tilted forward. A common example is that of a person with lordosis, giving the lumbar spine an exaggerated anterior curve.

Posterior Tilt. During a posterior tilt, the iliums are tilted backward. A common example is that of a person who is seated slouched in a chair.

Synovial Joint Types

Joints were discussed briefly in Chapter 19, including synovial joints. This section expounds on this information and features types of synovial joints. These joint types can also be classified according to the number of axes or planes in which movement occurs, such as monoaxial, biaxial, or triaxial (Figure 21-39).

Hinge Joints (Monoaxial). Movements are limited to flexion and extension. These joints possess one concave and one convex surface. Examples of hinge joints are the knees, elbows, and interphalangeal joints.

Pivot Joints (Monoaxial). Movement that is limited to rotation. These joints possess one conical surface and one depressed surface. Examples of pivot joints are the atlanto-axial joint and the proximal radioulnar joints.

Saddle Joints (Biaxial). Movements of flexion, extension, abduction, adduction, opposition, reposition, and circumduction are permitted, but not rotation. The joints contain a concave surface in one direction and convex in the other, like a saddle. The only saddle joint is the carpometacarpal of the thumb.

Ellipsoidal Joints (Biaxial). Allows movements of flexion, extension, abduction, and adduction, but rotation is not permitted. These are essentially reduced ball and socket joints, with one convex surface and one concave surface. Examples of ellipsoidal joints, often called condyloid joints, are radiocarpal joints located in the wrist and joints between the metacarpals and metatarsals and the phalanges.

Gliding Joints (Triaxial). Permit all movements but are limited to gliding. Both articular surfaces are nearly flat.

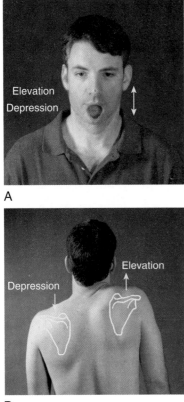

A

B

FIGURE 21-34 A, Mandibular elevation and depression. **B,** Scapular elevation and depression.

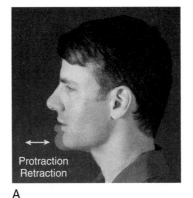

A

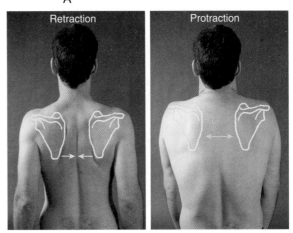

B

FIGURE 21-35 A, Mandibular protraction and retraction. **B,** Scapular protraction and retraction.

Examples of gliding joints are intercarpal and intertarsal joints.

Ball and Socket Joints (Triaxial). Permit all movements and offer the greatest range of motion of all joints. One surface is rounded, fitting into a cuplike cavity. Examples of ball and socket joints are shoulders and hips.

Naming Joints

Most joint names provide information about their articulating bones (Figure 21-40). For example, the sacroiliac joint is between the sacrum and the ilium. The temporomandibular joint is between the temporal bone and the mandible. The radiocarpal joint is between the radius and the carpal bones. The tibiofemoral joint is between the tibia and the femur. See Table 21-1 for names of select joints classified by type.

Some joint names refer to bony markings rather than specific bones. For instance, the glenohumeral joint is between the glenoid cavity of the scapula and the humerus. The acromioclavicular joint is between the acromion of the scapula and the clavicle.

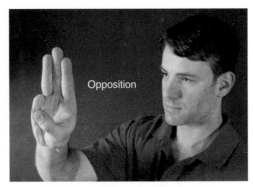

FIGURE 21-36 Thumb opposition.

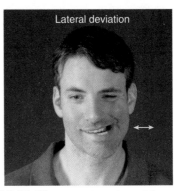

FIGURE 21-37 Lateral deviation of the mandible.

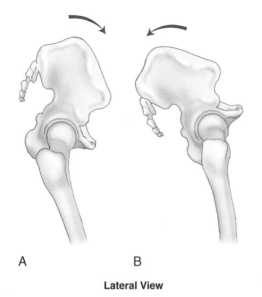

Lateral View

FIGURE 21-38 Anterior (**A**) and posterior (**B**) pelvic tilts.

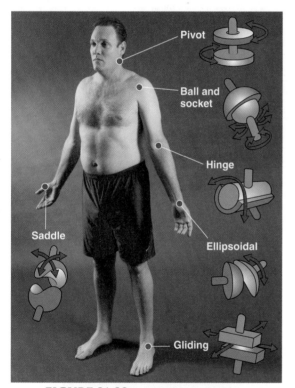

FIGURE 21-39 Types of synovial joints.

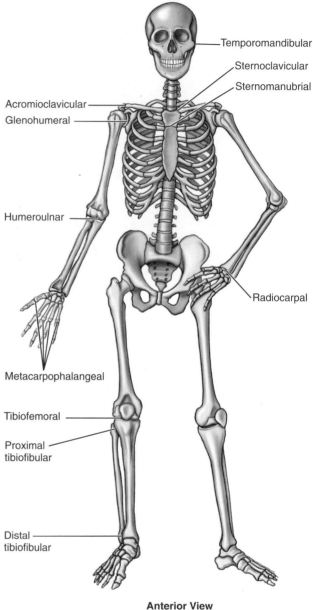

Anterior View

FIGURE 21-40 Select joints.

MUSCLES

Massage therapists must learn about muscles since so much of their work involves direct application to muscle tissue. One of the best approaches to learning muscles is to reduce the task into bite-size pieces. This section groups muscles into lessons six through fourteen. When learning the muscles in each lesson, consider using a five-phase approach.

Phase I: Decode muscle names in each lesson and learn pronunciations.
Phase II: Learn general locations of muscles.
Phase III: Learn specific muscle locations using attachment sites.
Phase IV: Learn muscle actions using a multisensory approach.
Phase V: Apply knowledge.

In *phase I*, look over all the muscles in each lesson and learn exactly how they were named. Use the information in the next section to familiarize yourself with ways muscles are named. Listen to how your instructor pronounces each muscle, and repeat it back to yourself, silently or aloud.

TABLE 21-1 Synovial Joints

SCIENTIFIC NAME	COMMON NAME
Ball and Socket	
Glenohumeral (scapulohumeral) joint	Shoulder joint
Iliofemoral (coxal) joint	Hip joint
Hinge	
Humeroulnar/humeroradial joint	Elbow joint
Tibiofemoral joint	Knee joint
Talocrural joint	Ankle joint
Interphalangeal joint	IP joint
Interphalangeal joint (proximal)	PIP joint
Interphalangeal joint (distal)	DIP joint
Temporomandibular joint	TMJ, jaw joint
Pivot	
Atlantoaxial joint	"No-no" joint
Radioulnar joint (proximal)	Non-applicable
Saddle	
Carpometacarpal joint of the thumb	Non-applicable
Ellipsoidal	
Radiocarpal joint	Wrist joint
Metacarpophalangeal joint	MCP joint
Metatarsophalangeal joint	MTP joint
Atlantooccipital joint	"Yes-yes" joint
Gliding	
Intervertebral facet joint	Facet joints
Atlantooccipital joint	Non-applicable
Acromioclavicular joint	AC joint
Sternoclavicular joint	SC joint
Intercarpal joint	Non-appliable
Carpometacarpal joint	CM joint
Lumbosacral facet joint	Non-applicable
Patellofemoral joint	Non-applicable
Tarsometatarsal joint	TM joint
Intertarsal joint	Non-applicable

Next, look at each muscle in each lesson, place your hand on the muscle, and say its name. As your teacher lectures, place your hand on the muscle and repeat its name silently or aloud. *Phase II* familiarizes you with their general locations on the body (Figure 21-41, *A* and *B*).

Phase III adds an important dimension to understanding muscle location by focusing on attachment sites. Using an articulated skeleton, find each bony attachment site. Using a piece of colorful yarn or cord, touch the origin and insertion at once. This exercise gives you a graphic idea of the muscles.

You can make up flash cards; on the front of each card, write the name of the each muscle; the back then states the attachment sites. Drawing muscles on a real body is helpful; this body may belong to one of your classmates, or you can recruit someone else such as a friend or family member. Use nontoxic, water-soluble markers.

Muscles commonly attach to the bony markings (see Box 21-1). However, muscles can also attach to ligaments (e.g., nuchal, inguinal, transverse carpal), fascia (e.g., palmar, superficial, abdominal, thoracolumbar, iliotibial band), membranes (e.g., obturator, interosseous), and specialized tendinous structures (e.g., galea aponeurotica, linea alba).

Phase IV is designed to teach muscle actions. To understand muscle actions, you need to know some things about the muscle. For example, to which bones do the muscles attach? Which joint does it cross? Begin to deduce a muscle's action by applying the general principle that the insertion, or *I,* moves toward the origin, or *O.* Also remember that the action refers to movement in anatomic position. You can learn actions by rote memory or by a multisensory approach. If you have chosen the latter, go back to the phase III learning strategy; place yarn on the *O* and *I* of an articulated skeleton, and shorten the string. This activity will produce the action of the muscle.

Another useful technique is to say aloud the name of the muscle while you are doing the action with your own body. You can even touch the muscle, say the muscle name aloud, and perform the action. The muscle producing the action will feel hard and become short and thick.

Again, make flash cards. On the front, write the name of the muscle; on the back, write the name of the action.

To assist you in learning the muscles, please review the following information. Ask your instructor for additional suggestions:

- Origins are generally located medial or proximal to their insertions.
- Muscles on the anterior side of the body generally flex (except thigh muscles).
- Muscles on the posterior side of the body generally extend (except thigh muscles).
- Muscles on the medial aspect of the body generally adduct.
- Muscles on the lateral aspect of the body generally abduct.
- Muscles with fibers running superior to inferior generally flex and extend.
- Muscles with oblique running fibers generally rotate.
- If a muscle crosses two joints, then it has an action on both joints.
- Most muscles have at least two actions, which include primary action and secondary actions.
- Prime movers and antagonists are generally situated opposite each other and often have the same insertion.

Phase V is to APPLY, APPLY, APPLY! With your instructor's help, learn how to palpate these muscles using

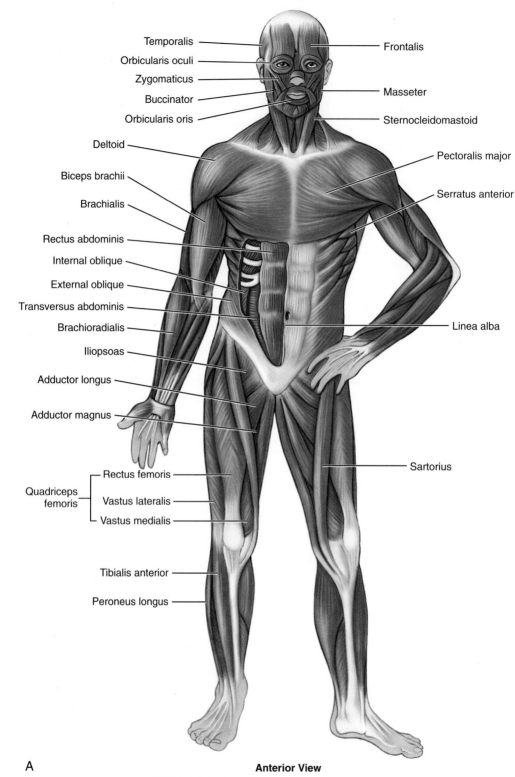

Temporalis
Orbicularis oculi
Zygomaticus
Buccinator
Orbicularis oris
Deltoid
Biceps brachii
Brachialis
Rectus abdominis
Internal oblique
External oblique
Transversus abdominis
Brachioradialis
Iliopsoas
Adductor longus
Adductor magnus
Quadriceps femoris
Rectus femoris
Vastus lateralis
Vastus medialis
Tibialis anterior
Peroneus longus

Frontalis
Masseter
Sternocleidomastoid
Pectoralis major
Serratus anterior
Linea alba
Sartorius

A

Anterior View

FIGURE 21-41 Superficial muscles of the body.

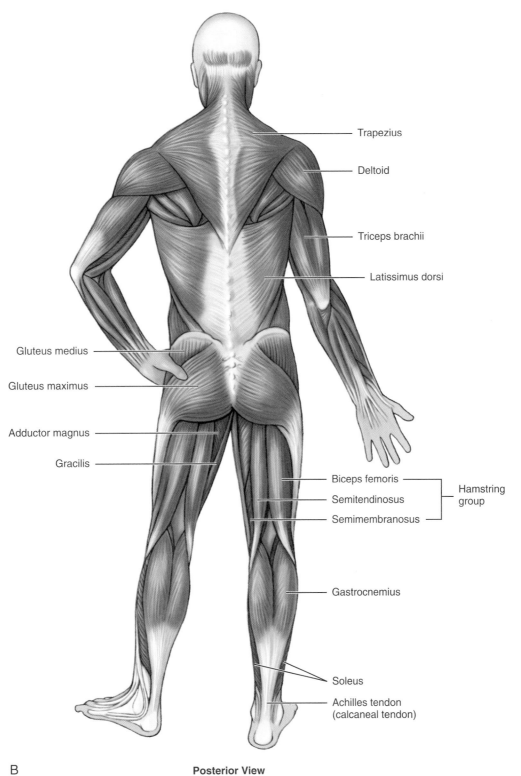

Trapezius

Deltoid

Triceps brachii

Latissimus dorsi

Gluteus medius

Gluteus maximus

Adductor magnus

Gracilis

Biceps femoris
Semitendinosus
Semimembranosus

Hamstring group

Gastrocnemius

Soleus

Achilles tendon
(calcaneal tendon)

 B

Posterior View

FIGURE 21-41, cont'd

BOX 21-2

How to Palpate Muscles

- **Locate attachment sites.** Using yourself or a subject, find the attachment sites of the muscle you wish to palpate. You may need to reposition the body to allow neighboring muscles to relax. Note that the muscle may not have accessible attachment sites.
- **Sink in slowly.** Make contact with the skin and allow your hand to sink into the tissues over the muscle. Now you can go for depth slowly and with purpose.
- **Move back and forth.** Allow your fingers to move back and forth. This strumming motion allows for better identification as the structure moves under your fingertips.
- **Action.** Perform or ask your subject to perform the muscle's action(s). This will contract the muscle and make it easier to locate. Ask your subject to relax, and repeat the contraction.

---

the information in Box 21-2, How to Palpate Muscles. Use all of this anatomic information in massage class, and use the names of these muscles with your clients. Use the anatomic terminology as much as you can so it becomes part of *you*. As the names, locations, and actions of the muscles become more fixed in your brain, your confidence will grow.

Remember, repetition is the key to learning; repetition is the key to learning; repetition is the key to learning.

Many muscles are part of a larger group. In some instances, the term used to denote the muscle group is more commonly used than individual muscle names. Examples are hamstrings, quadriceps, adductors, and glutes. Because of this regularity, muscle groups have been featured before individual muscles.

In researching muscle origin, insertion, action, and nerve supply information, the authors discovered numerous variations, inconsistencies, and disagreements on the subject of muscle nomenclature. This issue should be noted as you read and work with the information found in this chapter. Collect the books mentioned in the reference section and many other books concerning this fascinating subject to aid in the process of learning.

Important Note: In the figures that follow, bones where a muscle's origin and insertion are located are shaded blue. The white arrows denote the featured muscle's action. Furthermore, generally muscles are drawn on only the right side of the body.

Naming Muscles

Muscle names are essentially Latin and Greek words. But muscle names are more logical and therefore easier to learn when the reasons behind the names are understood. Muscles can be named by the following features:

Attachment Sites or Origin and Insertion. An example is sternocleidomastoid, which is attached to the sternum, clavicle, and mastoid process.

Action or Function. The action is usually named first, followed by the body part on which the action takes place. Examples are flexor pollicis longus (flexes the thumb), levator scapulae (elevates the scapula), and erector spinae (keeps the spine erect).

Number of Origins. Here, the number of origins, or heads, is given first and the body part is given next. Examples are biceps brachii (two-headed muscle of the arm), triceps brachii (three-headed muscle of the arm), and quadriceps femoris (four-headed muscle of the thigh).

Relative Shape and Size. Examples are gluteus maximus (large), gluteus minimus (small), adductor longus (long), and deltoid (triangular).

Location and/or Direction of Fibers. Examples are temporalis (temporal bone [location]), frontalis (frontal bone [location]), rectus femoris (straight [location and direction of fibers]), internal obliques (slanted [location and direction of fibers]), latissimus dorsi (dorsum or posterior [location]), and transverse abdominis (across [location and direction of fibers]).

Combinations. Many muscles are named using a combination of the aforementioned, such as extensor digitorum longus (long muscle that extends the digits or fingers) and flexor digitorum profundus (deep muscle that flexes the fingers).

LESSON SIX—MUSCLES OF SCAPULAR MOVEMENT

Trapezius, Levator Scapulae, Rhomboids Major and Minor, Serratus Anterior, Pectoralis Minor

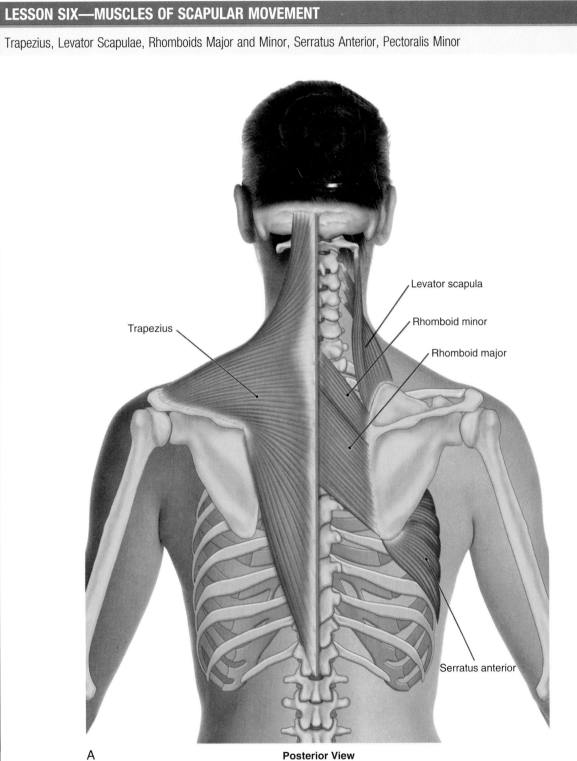

Levator scapula

Rhomboid minor

Rhomboid major

Trapezius

Serratus anterior

A

Posterior View

FIGURE 21-42

LESSON SIX—MUSCLES OF SCAPULAR MOVEMENT, CONT'D

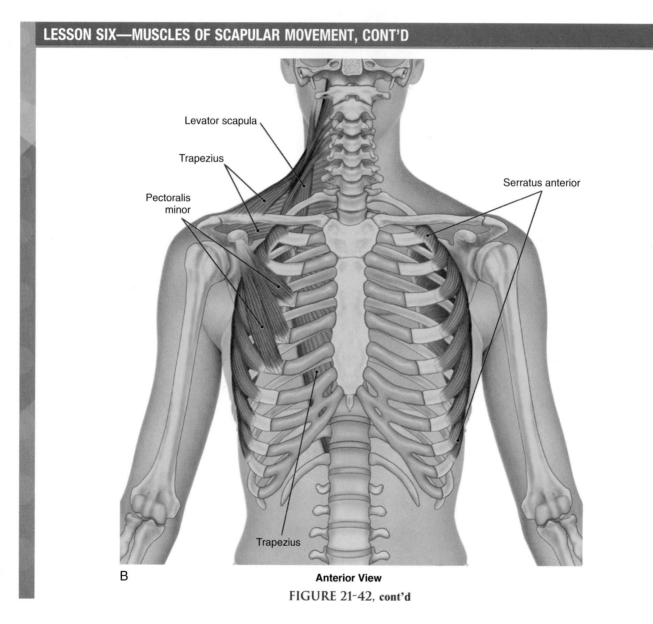

Levator scapula

Trapezius

Pectoralis
minor

Serratus anterior

Trapezius

B

Anterior View

FIGURE 21-42, cont'd

TRAPEZIUS

Greek: trapezoeides—tablelike

ORIGINS
External occipital protuberance
Superior nuchal line
Nuchal ligament
Spinous processes of C7-T12
Supraspinous ligament of C7-T12

INSERTIONS
Lateral third of the clavicle
Acromion process
Scapular spine

ACTIONS
Extends the neck and head (upper fibers)
Elevates the scapula (upper fibers)
Upwardly rotates the scapula (upper fibers)
Retracts the scapula (middle fibers)
Depresses the scapula (lower fibers)
Laterally flexes the neck (unilateral contraction)
Rotates the head (unilateral contraction)
Stabilizes the scapula

NERVES
Spinal accessory nerve (cranial nerve XI)
Midcervical nerves

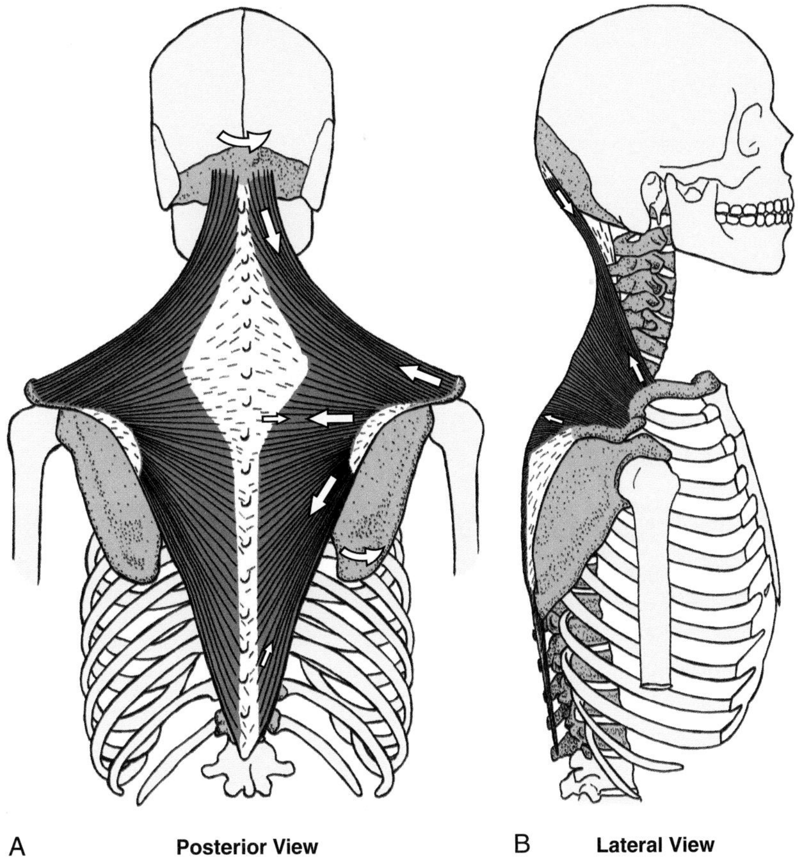

A **Posterior View**   B **Lateral View**

FIGURE 21-43

Notes: Trapezius is also known as the "coat hanger muscle" because clothes hang from it, similar to a coat hanger. This muscle functions like three muscles in one with the upper, middle, and lower fibers capable of performing three separate actions. Note that this muscle can be an antagonist to itself. Trapezius muscles, or *traps,* are to the neck and head what erector spinae muscles are to the back (see later discussion).

LEVATOR SCAPULAE

Latin: levator—a lifter
scapulae—shoulder blade

ORIGINS
Transverse processes of C1-C4

INSERTION
Medial border of the scapula (superior angle to root of spine)

ACTIONS
Elevates the scapula
Downwardly rotates the scapula
Laterally flexes the neck
Stabilizes the scapula

NERVES
Dorsal scapular nerve
Midcervical nerves

Notes: Levator scapulae lies between two muscles discussed later—splenius capitis and scalenus posterior. The body may shift its fascial structure from sol state to gel state so as to reinforce this muscle's actions, one of which is stabilizing the scapula, acting as a fixator. In its gel state, upon palpation, "crunches" can be felt as it flips over the insertion. The levator scapulae muscles are the only neck muscles that move the scapulae.

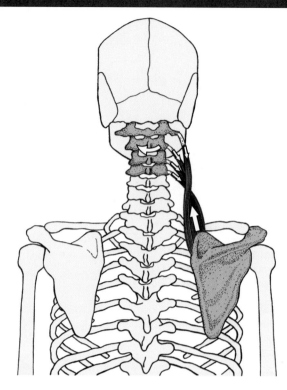

Posterior View
FIGURE 21-44

RHOMBOIDS MAJOR AND MINOR

Latin: rhombus—all sides even
major—larger
minor—smaller

ORIGINS
Spinous processes of C7-T1 (minor)
Spinous processes of T2-T5 (major)

INSERTIONS
Medial border of the scapula from the superior angle to the root
  of the scapular spine (minor)
Medial border of the scapula from root of scapular spine to the
  inferior angle (major)

ACTIONS
Retracts the scapula
Downwardly rotates the scapula
Stabilizes the scapula

NERVE
Dorsal scapular nerve

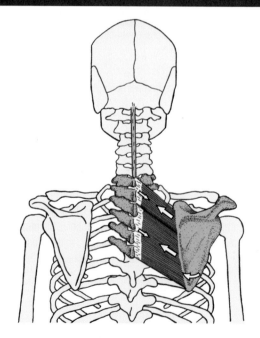

Posterior View
FIGURE 21-45

Notes: *Rhomboids* is the name given for rhomboid major and rhomboid minor, but they occasionally fuse to form one muscle. Both rhomboids lie deep to trapezius; rhomboid minor is superior to rhomboid major. They are also known as the *Christmas tree muscles* because the fiber direction is obliquely arranged, similar to Christmas tree branches.

SERRATUS ANTERIOR

Latin: serratus—notched or jagged, similar to a saw
ante—before

ORIGINS
Ribs 1 through 8 or 9 (lateral to costal cartilage—exterior
surface of the rib)

INSERTION
Anterior medial border of the scapula

ACTIONS
Protracts the scapula
Upwardly rotates the scapula
Depresses the scapula

NERVE
Long thoracic nerve

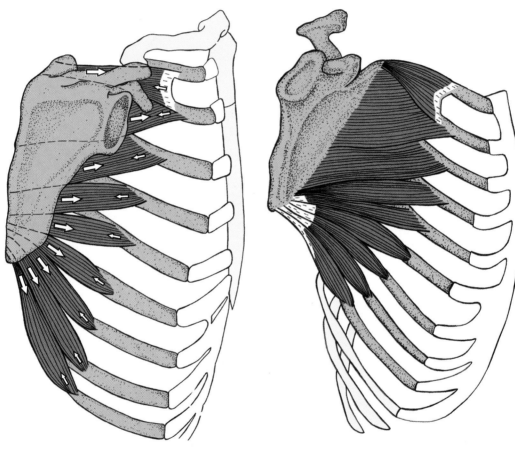

Lateral View

FIGURE 21-46 In the right image, the scapula has been lifted medially.

Notes: Serratus anterior, along with triceps brachii, is called the *boxer's muscle* because the protraction of the scapula enables a boxer to deliver a punch. Note that this muscle is antagonist to the rhomboids. Serratus anterior often interlaces with external obliques on the lateral aspect of the trunk. Full or partial paralysis of serratus anterior produces a *winged scapula,* leading to difficulty in lifting the arm above the shoulder.

PECTORALIS MINOR

Latin: pectoralis—pertaining to the chest
minor—smaller

ORIGINS
Ribs 3 through 5 (lateral to costal cartilage)

INSERTION
Coracoid process of the scapula

ACTIONS
Depresses the scapula
Protracts the scapula
Downwardly rotates the scapula
Assists in forced inspiration (elevates ribs)

NERVES
Medial pectoral nerves (C8 and T1)

Note: Pectoralis minor, along with scalenes, is known as the *neurovascular entrapper* because this muscle, which forms a bridge over the axillary artery and brachial plexus, can entrap them and cause arm and hand pain, numbness, and/or weakness.

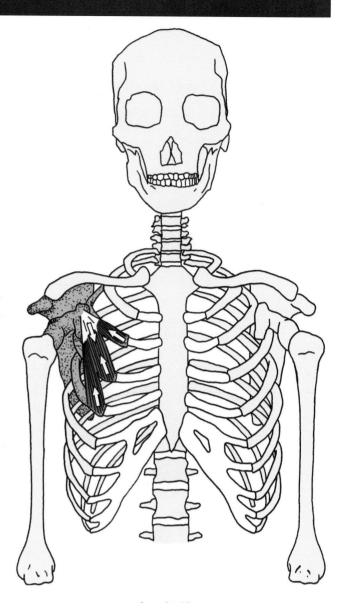

Anterior View

FIGURE 21-47

LESSON SIX REVIEW—MUSCLES OF SCAPULAR MOVEMENT

ELEVATION	DEPRESSION	UPWARD ROTATION	DOWNWARD ROTATION	PROTRACTION	RETRACTION
Trapezius (upper fibers)	Trapezius (lower fibers)	Trapezius (upper fibers)	Levator scapulae	Serratus anterior	Trapezius (middle fibers)
Levator scapulae	Serratus anterior	Serratus anterior	Rhomboids	Pectoralis minor	Rhomboids
	Pectoralis minor		Pectoralis minor		

LESSON SEVEN—MUSCLES OF SHOULDER JOINT MOVEMENT

Latissimus Dorsi, Teres Major, Supraspinatus, Infraspinatus, Teres Minor, Subscapularis, Deltoid, Pectoralis Major, Coracobrachialis, Biceps Brachii (Lesson Three), Triceps Brachii (Lesson Three)

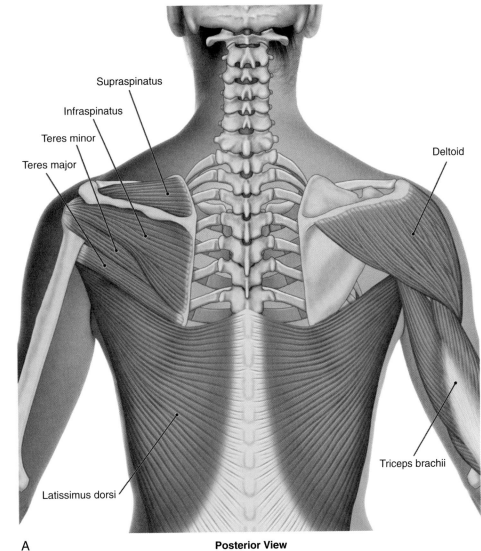

A

Posterior View

FIGURE 21-48

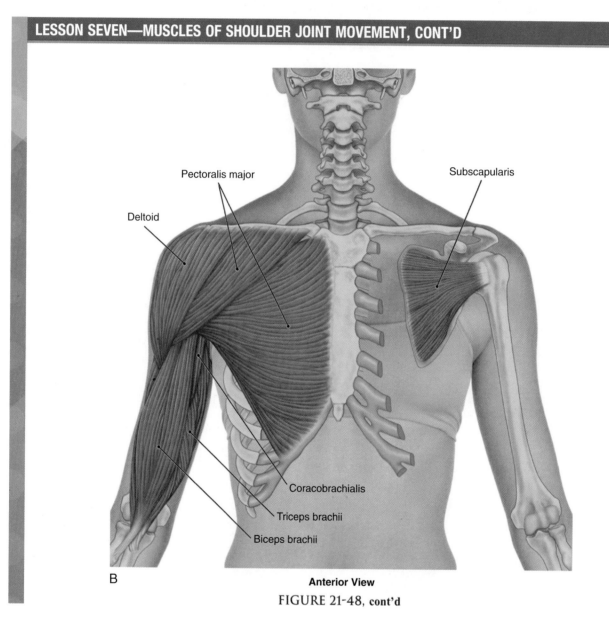

B

Anterior View

FIGURE 21-48, cont'd

LATISSIMUS DORSI

Latin: *latus—broad*
dorsum—back

ORIGINS
Spinous processes of T7-L5
Ribs 9 through 12 (posterior surface)
Posterior iliac crest
Posterior sacrum

INSERTION
Intertubercular groove of the humerus (medial lip)

ACTIONS
Extends the humerus
Medially rotates the humerus
Adducts the humerus

NERVE
Thoracodorsal nerve

Notes: Latissimus dorsi muscles, or *lats*, are also known as the *swimmer's muscle* because it allows us to extend our arm and propel us in water. It is widest muscle of the body. Elevation and anterior tilting of the hip are assisted with this muscle. In some cases, latissimus dorsi interlaces with external obliques on the lateral aspect of the trunk.

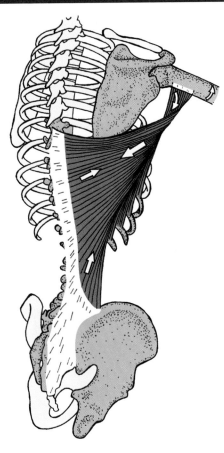

Posterolateral View

FIGURE 21-49

TERES MAJOR

Latin: *teres—round*
major—larger

ORIGIN
Inferior third of the lateral border of the scapula

INSERTION
Intertubercular groove of the humerus (medial lip)

ACTIONS
Extends the humerus
Medially rotates the humerus
Adducts the humerus

NERVE
Lower subscapular nerve

Notes: Teres major is a synergist to latissimus dorsi and it is often called *lat's little helper*. This muscle may merge with the lats and, in some cases, is completely absent. Teres major may assist in upward rotation of the scapula.

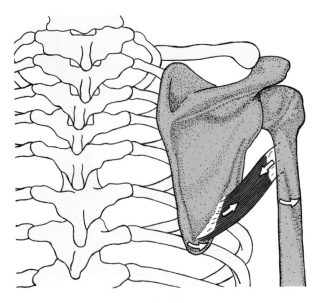

Posterior View

FIGURE 21-50

ROTATOR CUFF

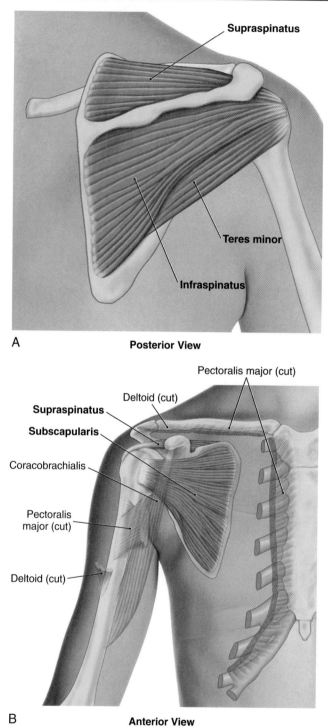

A   **Posterior View**

B   **Anterior View**

FIGURE 21-51

Notes: Also known as musculotendinous cuff, the *rotator cuff is a* group of muscles deep to the deltoid. They are also called the *SItS muscles: S*upraspinatus, *I*nfraspinatus, *t*eres minor, and *S*ubscapularis. The lower case *t* helps you remember that teres *minor*, not teres *major*, is part of this group. Three of the four muscles arise from scapular fossae (supraspinatus, infraspinatus, subscapularis). Three of the four muscles attach to the greater tubercle (supraspinatus, infraspinatus, teres minor). These muscles do a great deal for the stability of the shoulder joint and may function as ligaments.

SUPRASPINATUS

Latin: supra—above
spinatus—spine

ORIGIN
Supraspinous fossa of the scapula

INSERTION
Greater tubercle of the humerus

ACTION
Abducts the humerus

NERVE
Suprascapular nerve

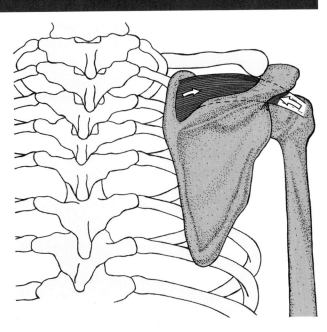

Posterior View
FIGURE 21-52

Notes: Supraspinatus muscle is the only muscle of the musculotendinous cuff that does not rotate the humerus. This muscle initiates shoulder abduction and continues to act throughout the entire abduction, assisting the deltoid. The supraspinatus also prevents downward dislocation of the humerus in tasks such as carrying, for example, a heavy portable massage table.

INFRASPINATUS

Latin: infra—beneath
spinatus—spine

ORIGIN
Infraspinous fossa of the scapula

INSERTION
Greater tubercle of the humerus

ACTION
Laterally rotates the humerus

NERVE
Suprascapular nerve

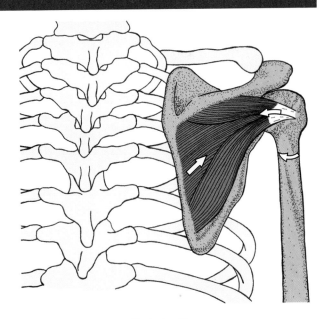

Posterior View
FIGURE 21-53

TERES MINOR

Latin: teres—round
minor—smaller

ORIGIN
Superior two thirds of the lateral border of the scapula

INSERTION
Greater tubercle of the humerus

ACTIONS
Laterally rotates the humerus
Adducts the humerus

NERVE
Axillary nerve

Note: Teres minor is the synergist to infraspinatus and may be fused with it.

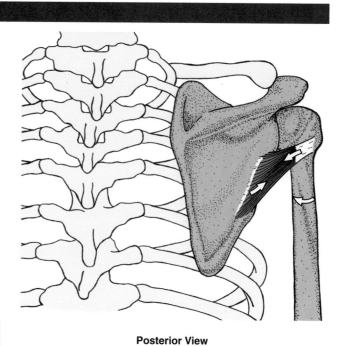

Posterior View
FIGURE 21-54

SUBSCAPULARIS

Latin: sub—below
scapulae—shoulder blade

ORIGIN
Subscapular fossa of the scapula

INSERTION
Lesser tubercle of the humerus

ACTION
Medially rotates the humerus

NERVE
Subscapular nerve

Note: Dr. Janet Travell, one of the authors of *Myofascial Pain and Dysfunction,* refers to subscapularis as the "frozen shoulder" muscle.

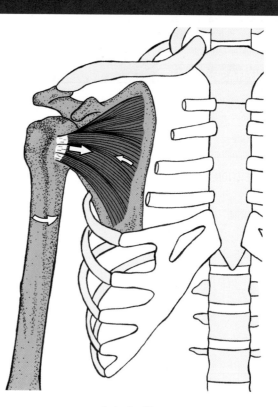

Anterior View
FIGURE 21-55

DELTOID

Greek: delta—triangular

ORIGINS
Lateral third of the clavicle
Acromion process
Scapular spine

INSERTION
Deltoid tuberosity

ACTIONS
Flexes the humerus (anterior fibers)
Medially rotates the humerus (anterior fibers)
Abducts the humerus (middle fibers)
Extends the humerus (posterior fibers)
Laterally rotates the humerus (posterior fibers)

NERVE
Axillary nerve

Notes: Dr. Mary Kordish, biology professor at McNeese State University, said that if the deltoid were discovered today, it would be considered three independent muscles. The anterior, middle, and posterior fibers of deltoid function as three separate muscles. Because of this fact, the deltoid regions are commonly referred to as the anterior deltoid, the middle deltoid, and the posterior deltoid. Structurally, they resemble gluteals. Deltoid is the most important abductor of the shoulder joint. This muscle can be an antagonist to itself.

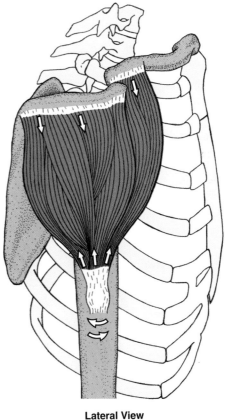

Lateral View

FIGURE 21-56

PECTORALIS MAJOR

Latin: pectoralis—pertaining to the chest
major—larger

ORIGINS
Medial half of the clavicle
Edge of the sternal body
Ribs 1 through 7 (costal cartilages)

INSERTION
Intertubercular groove of the humerus (lateral lip)

ACTIONS
Adducts the humerus
Medially rotates the humerus
Flexes the humerus
Extends the humerus

NERVE
Medial and lateral pectoral nerves

Notes: Pectoralis major muscles, or *pecs,* forms the upper anterior chest wall and anterior axillary fold. This muscle possesses clavicular, sternal, and costal regions. Tightness in these muscle may cause constriction of chest and angina-like pain or postural distortions such as rounded shoulders.

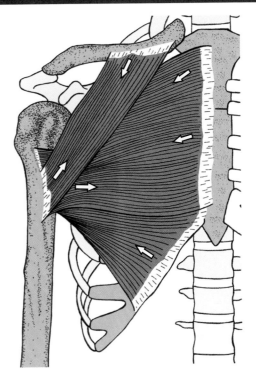

Anterior View

FIGURE 21-57

CORACOBRACHIALIS

Greek: korax—crow's beak
Latin: bracchium—arm

ORIGIN
Coracoid process of the scapula

INSERTION
Medial humeral shaft (middle region)

ACTIONS
Flexes the humerus
Adducts the humerus

NERVE
Musculocutaneous nerve

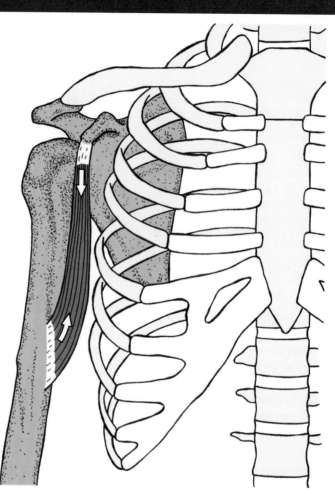

Anterior View

FIGURE 21-58

LESSON SEVEN REVIEW—MUSCLES OF SHOULDER JOINT MOVEMENT

FLEXION	EXTENSION	MEDIAL ROTATION	LATERAL ROTATION	ABDUCTION	ADDUCTION
Anterior deltoid	Latissimus dorsi	Latissimus dorsi	Infraspinatus	Supraspinatus	Latissimus dorsi
Pectoralis major	Teres major	Teres major	Teres minor	Middle deltoid	Teres major
Coracobrachialis	Posterior deltoid	Subscapularis	Posterior deltoid		Teres minor
Biceps brachii	Pectoralis major	Anterior deltoid			Pectoralis major
	Triceps brachii	Pectoralis major			Coracobrachialis
					Triceps brachii

LESSON EIGHT—MUSCLES OF THE ELBOW AND PROXIMAL RADIOULNAR JOINT

Biceps Brachii, Brachialis, Brachioradialis, Triceps Brachii, Anconeus, Pronator Teres, Pronator Quadratus, Supinator, Flexor Carpi Radialis (Lesson Four)

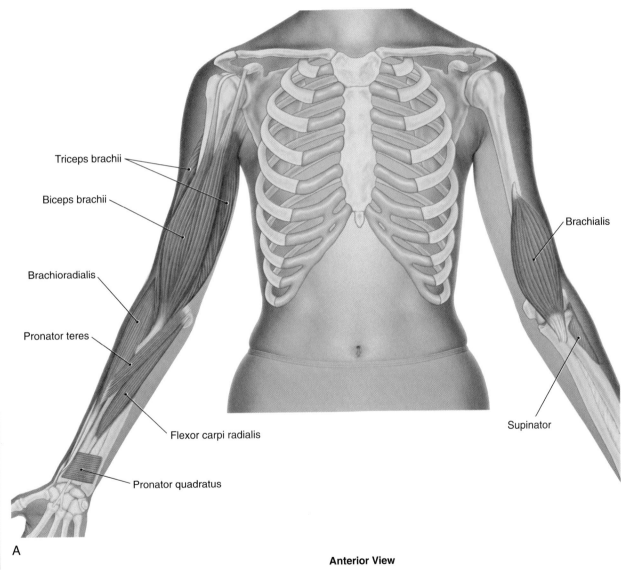

Anterior View

FIGURE 21-59

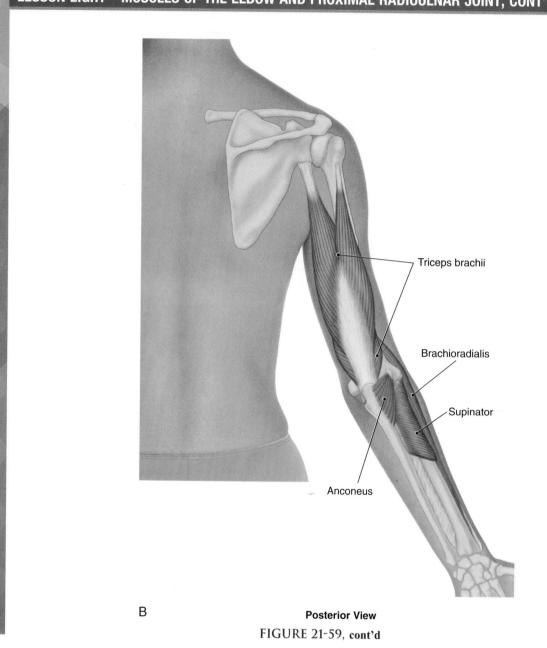

Triceps brachii

Brachioradialis

Supinator

Anconeus

B

Posterior View

FIGURE 21-59, cont'd

BICEPS BRACHII

*Latin: bis—twice + caput—head
bracchium—arm*

ORIGINS
Supraglenoid tubercle of the scapula (long head)
Coracoid process of scapula (short head)

INSERTIONS
Radial tuberosity
Bicipital aponeurosis

ACTIONS
Flexes the elbow
Supinates the forearm
Flexes the humerus

NERVE
Musculocutaneous nerve

Notes: Biceps brachii is called the *corkscrew muscle* because two of its actions mimic uncorking a wine bottle. The tendon of the long head passes within the intertubercular groove of the humerus and also passes through the capsule of the shoulder joint itself. This muscle may have an additional head attaching to the midshaft of the humerus (approximately 10% of cadavers).

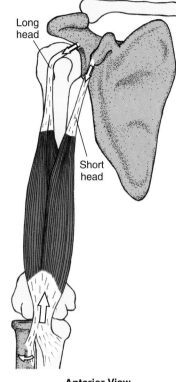

Anterior View

FIGURE 21-60

BRACHIALIS

Latin: bracchium—arm

ORIGIN
Distal half of anterior humeral shaft

INSERTIONS
Ulnar tuberosity
Coronoid process of the ulna

ACTION
Flexes the elbow

NERVE
Musculocutaneous nerve

Notes: Brachialis is the most effective arm flexor because of its mechanical advantage, lying deep to biceps brachii. Additionally, when you flex your forearm to *show off* your biceps brachii, a great deal of this display is actually the brachialis *pushing up* on the biceps brachii.

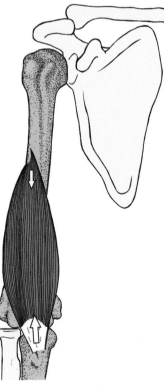

Anterior View

FIGURE 21-61

BRACHIORADIALIS

Latin: bracchium—arm
radialis—spoke of a wheel

ORIGIN
Lateral supracondylar ridge of the humerus

INSERTION
Styloid process of the radius

ACTION
Flexes the elbow

NERVE
Radial nerve

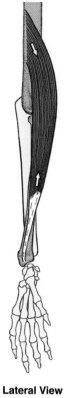

Notes: The bulge you can palpate on the radial side of your forearm is the brachioradialis. The radial pulse is located between the tendons of the brachioradialis and the flexor carpi radialis.

Lateral View
FIGURE 21-62

TRICEPS BRACHII

Greek: treis—three
Latin: bracchium—arm

ORIGINS
Infraglenoid tubercle of the scapula (long head)
Posterior proximal humeral shaft (lateral head)
Posterior distal humeral shaft (medial head)

INSERTION
Olecranon process

ACTIONS
Extends the elbow
Extends the humerus
Adducts the humerus

NERVE
Radial nerve

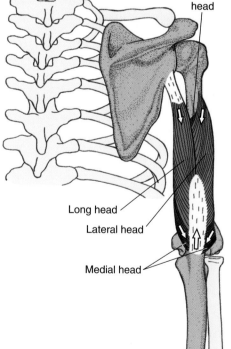

Medial head

Long head
Lateral head

Medial head

Note: This muscle, along with the serratus anterior, is called the *boxer's muscle* because it delivers a straight-arm knockout punch.

Posterior View
FIGURE 21-63

ANCONEUS

Greek: angkon—elbow

ORIGIN
Lateral epicondyle of the humerus

INSERTIONS
Olecranon process
Superior eighth of posterior ulnar shaft

ACTION
Extends the elbow

NERVE
Radial nerve

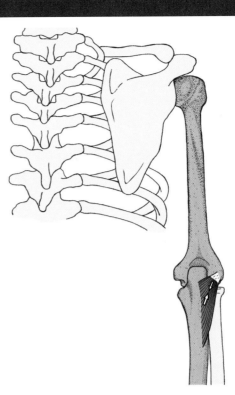

Posterior View
FIGURE 21-64

PRONATOR TERES

Latin: pronus—downward
teres—round

ORIGINS
Medial epicondyle of the humerus via the common flexor tendon
Coronoid process of the ulna

INSERTION
Midlateral radial shaft

ACTIONS
Pronates the forearm
Flexes the elbow

NERVE
Median nerve

Notes: The *common flexor tendon* is a common proximal attachment for five muscles—pronator teres, flexor carpi radialis, palmaris longus, flexor carpi ulnaris, and flexor digitorum superficialis. These last four muscles are featured later in the chapter.

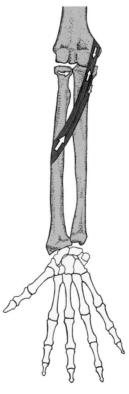

Anterior View
FIGURE 21-65

PRONATOR QUADRATUS

Latin: pronus—downward
quadratus—four sided

ORIGIN
Anterior distal quarter of the ulnar shaft

INSERTION
Anterior distal quarter of the radial shaft

ACTION
Pronates the forearm

NERVE
Median nerve

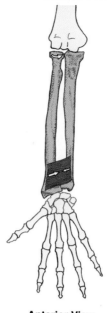

Anterior View

FIGURE 21-66

SUPINATOR

Latin: supinatus—bent backward

ORIGINS
Lateral epicondyle of the humerus
Proximal eighth of ulnar shaft
Radial collateral ligament
Annular ligament

INSERTION
Proximal lateral radial shaft

ACTION
Supinates the forearm

NERVE
Radial nerve

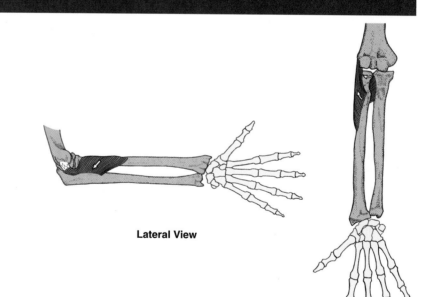

Lateral View

Anterior View

FIGURE 21-67

LESSON EIGHT—MOVEMENTS OF THE ELBOW AND PROXIMAL RADIOULNAR JOINT

FLEXION	EXTENSION	PRONATION	SUPINATION
Biceps brachii	Triceps brachii	Pronator teres	Biceps brachii
Brachialis	Anconeus	Pronator quadratus	Supinator
Brachioradialis			
Pronator teres			
Flexor carpi radialis			

Flexor Carpi Radialis, Flexor Carpi Ulnaris, Palmaris Longus, Flexor Digitorum Superficialis, Flexor Digitorum Profundus, Extensor Carpi Radialis Longus and Brevis, Extensor Carpi Ulnaris, Extensor Digitorum, Extensor Digiti Minimi, Extensor Indicis, Extensor Pollicis Longus and Brevis, Flexor Pollicis Longus and Brevis, Opponens Pollicis, Abductor Pollicis Longus and Brevis, Flexor Digiti Minimi, Abductor Digiti Minimi, Opponens Digiti Minimi

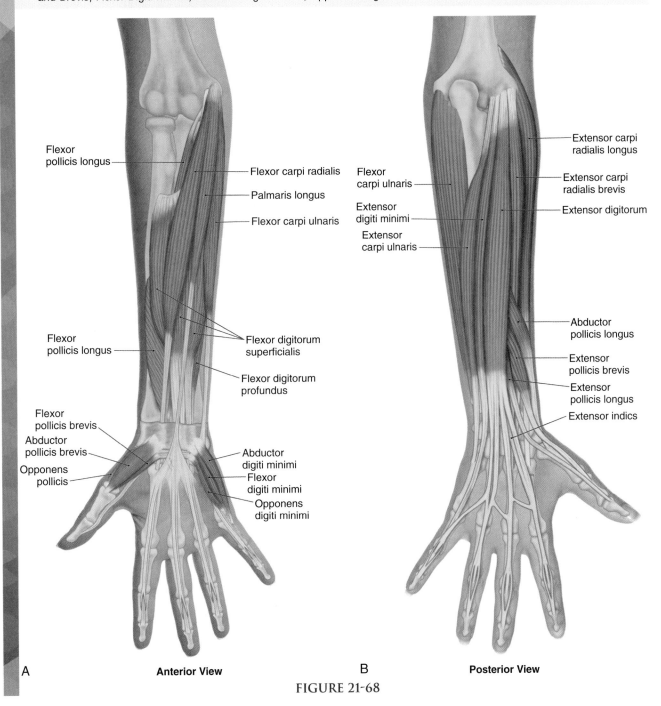

A   **Anterior View**   B   **Posterior View**

FIGURE 21-68

FLEXOR CARPI RADIALIS

Latin: flexus—bent
karpos—wrist
radialis—spoke of a wheel

ORIGIN
Medial epicondyle of the humerus via the common flexor tendon

INSERTIONS
Bases of metacarpals II and III

ACTIONS
Flexes the wrist
Abducts the wrist
Flexes the elbow

NERVE
Median nerve

Notes: Notice how this muscle and the next three (flexor carpi ulnaris, palmaris longus, and flexor digitorum superficialis) all flex the wrist and all originate on the medial epicondyle of the humerus. Wrist flexors lie on the anterior side of the forearm. These muscles can become inflamed at their origin of the common flexor tendon resulting in *golfers elbow*; the medical term for this condition is *medial epicondylitis*. The radial pulse is located between the tendons of flexor carpi radialis and brachioradialis.

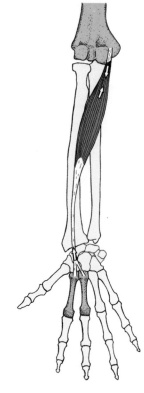

Anterior View

FIGURE 21-69

FLEXOR CARPI ULNARIS

Latin: flexus—bent
karpos—wrist
ulna—elbow

ORIGINS
Medial epicondyle of the humerus via the common flexor tendon
Medial olecranon
Posterior proximal two thirds of the ulna

INSERTIONS
Base of metacarpal V
Pisiform
Hook of hamate

ACTIONS
Flexes the wrist
Adducts the wrist

NERVE
Ulnar nerve

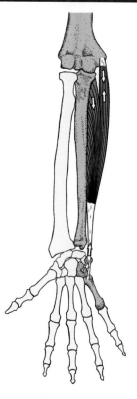

Anterior View

FIGURE 21-70

PALMARIS LONGUS

Latin: palma—hand
longus—long

ORIGIN
Medial epicondyle of the humerus via the common flexor tendon

INSERTION
Palmar aponeurosis

ACTIONS
Flexes the wrist
Cups (tenses) the palm

NERVE
Median nerve

Note: This muscle is absent in approximately 10% of cadavers.

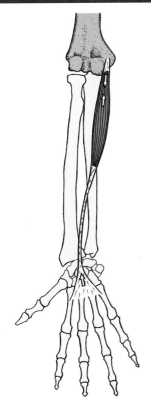

Anterior View
FIGURE 21-71

FLEXOR DIGITORUM SUPERFICIALIS

Latin: flexus—bent
digitus—finger
superficialis—toward the surface

ORIGINS
Medial epicondyle of the humerus via the common flexor tendon
Anterior proximal radial shaft (upper region)
Coronoid process of the ulna

INSERTIONS
Middle phalanges of digits II through V

ACTIONS
Flexes the wrist
Flexes the fingers at the proximal interphalangeal (PIP) and
    metacarpophalangeal (MP) joints

NERVE
Median nerve

Note: Flexor digitorum superficialis is also called flexor digitorum
sublimis.

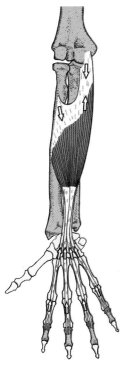

Anterior View
FIGURE 21-72

FLEXOR DIGITORUM PROFUNDUS

Latin: flexus—bent
digitus—finger
profundus—deep

ORIGINS
Anterior proximal three fourths of the anterior ulnar shaft
Interosseus membrane

INSERTIONS
Distal phalanges of digits II through V

ACTIONS
Flexes the wrist
Flexes the fingers at the distal interphalangeal (DIP), PIP, and
MP joints

NERVES
Ulnar nerve
Median nerve

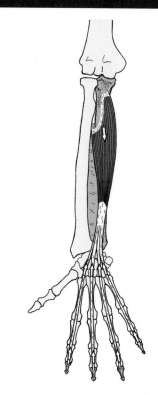

Anterior View

FIGURE 21-73

EXTENSOR CARPI RADIALIS LONGUS

Latin: extensio—to extend
karpos—wrist
radialis—spoke of a wheel
longus—long

ORIGIN
Lateral supracondylar ridge of the humerus

INSERTION
Posterior base of metacarpal II

ACTIONS
Extends the wrist
Abducts the wrist

NERVE
Radial nerve

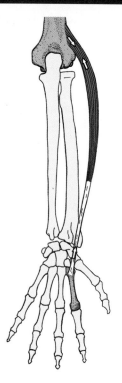

Posterior View

FIGURE 21-74

EXTENSOR CARPI RADIALIS BREVIS

Latin: extensio—to extend
karpos—wrist
radialis—spoke of a wheel
brevis—brief

ORIGIN
Lateral epicondyle of the humerus via the common extensor
   tendon

INSERTION
Posterior base of metacarpal III

ACTIONS
Extends the wrist
Abducts the wrist

NERVE
Radial nerve

Notes: The common extensor tendon is a common proximal attachment for four muscles—extensor carpi radialis brevis, extensor carpi ulnaris, extensor digitorum, and extensor digiti minimi. These last three muscles are featured next. Notice how these muscles and the next two (extensor carpi ulnaris and extensor digitorum) extend the wrist and originate on the lateral epicondyle of the humerus. Wrist extensors lie on the posterior side of the forearm and may become inflamed at the origin of the common extensor tendon in *tennis elbow*; the medical term for this condition is *lateral epicondylitis*.

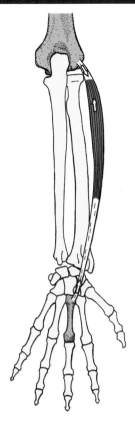

Posterior View

FIGURE 21-75

EXTENSOR CARPI ULNARIS

Latin: extensio—to extend
karpos—wrist
ulna—elbow

ORIGIN
Lateral epicondyle of the humerus via the common extensor tendon

INSERTION
Metacarpal V

ACTIONS
Extends the wrist
Adducts the wrist

NERVE
Radial nerve

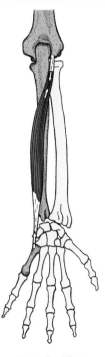

Posterior View

FIGURE 21-76

EXTENSOR DIGITORUM

Latin: extensio—to extend
digitus—finger

ORIGIN
Lateral epicondyle of the humerus via the common extensor tendon

INSERTIONS
Middle and distal digits II through V

ACTIONS
Extends the wrist
Extends the fingers at the DIP, PIP, and MP joints

NERVE
Radial nerve

Note: Extensor digitorum is sometimes called *extensor digitorum communis.*

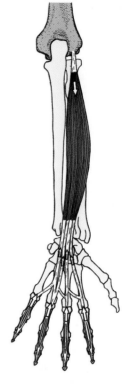

Posterior View
FIGURE 21-77

EXTENSOR DIGITI MINIMI

Latin: extensio—to extend
digitus—finger
minimum—least

ORIGIN
Lateral epicondyle of the humerus via the common extensor tendon

INSERTIONS
Posterior middle and distal digit V via tendon of extensor digitorum

ACTION
Extends the little finger (digit V)

NERVE
Radial nerve

Notes: Extensor digiti minimi is also known as the *tea drinker's muscle* because it extends the little finger while you raise the teacup to your lips. This muscle may also assist in extending the wrist.

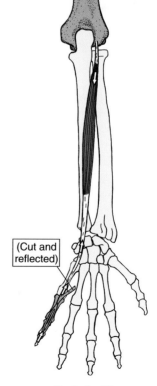

(Cut and reflected)

Posterior View
FIGURE 21-78

EXTENSOR INDICIS

Latin: extensio—to extend
indices—forefinger

ORIGINS
Posterior distal ulnar shaft
Interosseus membrane

INSERTIONS
Middle and distal digits of index finger (digit II)

ACTION
Extends the index finger (digit II)

NERVE
Radial nerve

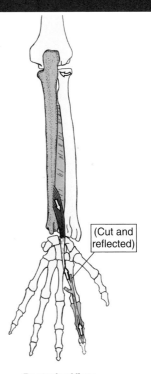

Posterior View

FIGURE 21-79

(Cut and reflected)

Note: This muscle may also assist in extending the wrist.

EXTENSOR POLLICIS LONGUS AND BREVIS

Latin: extensio—to extend
pollex—thumb
longus—long
brevis—brief

ORIGINS
Posterior ulnar shaft—middle region (longus)
Posterior radial shaft—distal region (brevis)
Interosseous membrane (brevis and longus)

INSERTIONS
Posterior distal phalanx of the thumb (longus)
Posterolateral proximal phalanx of the thumb (brevis)

ACTION
Extends the thumb (digit I)

NERVE
Radial nerve

Notes: These muscles may also assist in wrist extension (longus) and abduction (brevis). The tendons of extensor pollicis longus and brevis and abductor pollicis longus (featured next) form a space at the lateral wrist called the *anatomic snuffbox*. The reason that it is called the anatomic snuffbox is that snuff (powdered tobacco) could be put there and then inhaled (when this was popular, of course).

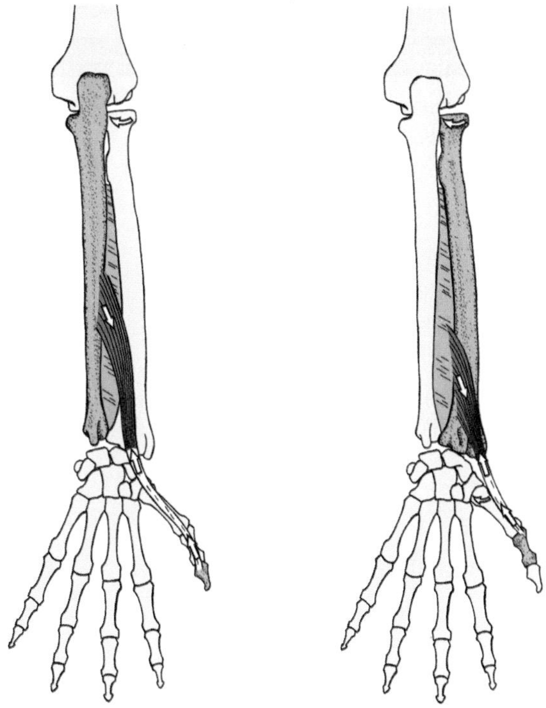

Extensor Pollicis Longus
Posterior View

Extensor Pollicis Brevis
Posterior View

FIGURE 21-80

FLEXOR POLLICIS LONGUS AND BREVIS

Latin: flexus—bent
pollex—thumb
longus—long
brevis—brief

ORIGINS
Anterior radial shaft—middle region (longus)
Interosseous membrane (longus)
Trapezium (brevis)
Transverse carpal ligament (brevis)

INSERTIONS
Anterior distal phalanx of the thumb (longus)
Proximal phalanx of the thumb (brevis)

ACTION
Flexes the thumb

NERVES
Median nerve (longus)
Median and ulnar nerves (brevis)

Notes: The flexor pollicis brevis, opponens pollicis, and abductor pollicis brevis (see latter two below) form the *thenar eminence*, or thumb pad located on the radial side of the palm.

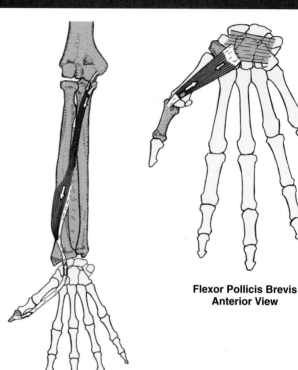

Flexor Pollicis Brevis
Anterior View

Flexor Pollicis Longus
Anterior View

FIGURE 21-81

OPPONENS POLLICIS

Latin: opponens—opposing
pollex—thumb

ORIGINS
Trapezium
Transverse carpal ligament

INSERTION
Anterior metacarpal I

ACTIONS
Opposes the thumb (adduction)
Flexes the thumb

NERVE
Median nerve

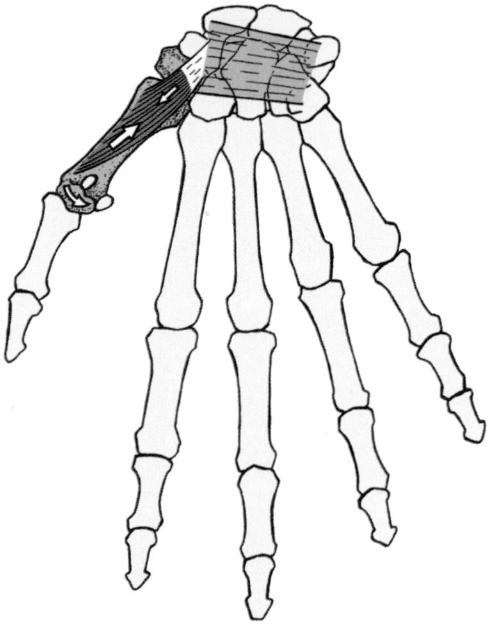

Anterior View

FIGURE 21-82

ABDUCTOR POLLICIS LONGUS AND BREVIS

Latin: abductus—led away
pollex—thumb
longus—long
brevis—brief

ORIGINS
Posterior ulnar shaft—middle region (longus)
Posterior radial shaft—middle region (longus)
Interosseus membrane (longus)
Trapezium (brevis)
Scaphoid (brevis)
Transverse carpal ligament (brevis)

INSERTIONS
Lateral metacarpal I (longus)
Lateral proximal phalanx of the thumb (brevis)

ACTION
Abducts the thumb (longus and brevis)

NERVES
Ulnar nerve (longus)
Median nerve (brevis)

Note: Abductor pollicis longus also assists in opposition.

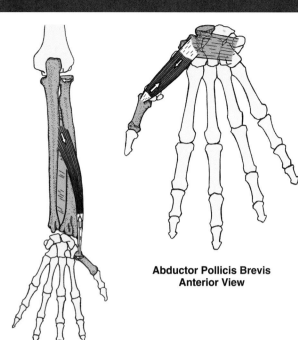

Abductor Pollicis Brevis
Anterior View

Abductor Pollicis Longus
Posterior View

FIGURE 21-83

FLEXOR DIGITI MINIMI

Latin: flexus—bent
digitus—finger
minimum—least

ORIGINS
Hook of hamate
Transverse carpal ligament

INSERTION
Proximal phalanx of the fifth finger (digit V)

ACTION
Flexes the little finger (digit V)

NERVE
Ulnar nerve

Notes: The flexor digiti minimi, abductor digiti minimi, and opponens digiti minimi (latter two muscles featured later) form the *hypothenar eminence,* a pad of tissue located on the ulnar side of the palm. Some texts distinguish flexor digiti minimi from flexor digiti minimi brevis in that the former is in the hand and the latter in the foot. Flexor digiti minimi is often absent.

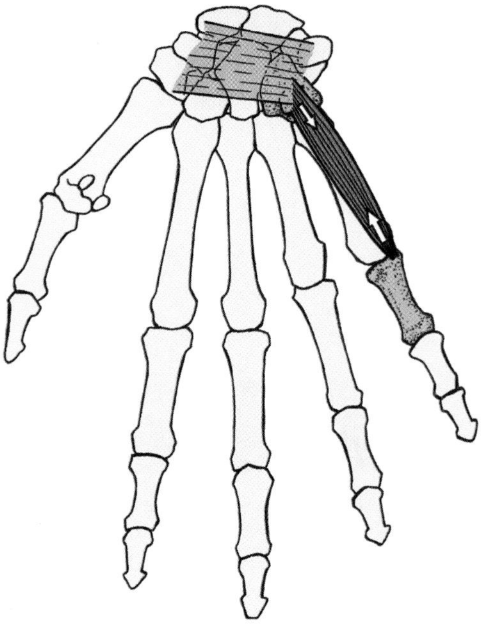

Anterior View
FIGURE 21-84

ABDUCTOR DIGITI MINIMI

Latin: abductus—led away
digitus—finger
minimum—least

ORIGINS
Pisiform
Tendon of flexor carpi ulnaris

INSERTION
Proximal phalanx of the fifth finger

ACTION
Abducts the fifth (little) finger

NERVE
Ulnar nerve

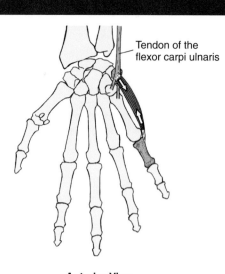

Tendon of the
flexor carpi ulnaris

Anterior View

FIGURE 21-85

OPPONENS DIGITI MINIMI

Latin: opponens—opposing
digitus—finger
minimum—least

ORIGINS
Hamate
Transverse carpal ligament

INSERTION
Metacarpal V

ACTION
Adducts the little finger (moves little finger into opposition)

NERVE
Ulnar nerve

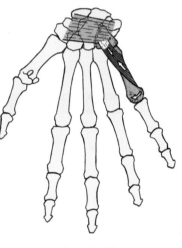

Anterior View

FIGURE 21-86

LESSON NINE REVIEW—MUSCLES OF WRIST MOVEMENT

FLEXION	EXTENSION	ABDUCTION	ADDUCTION
Flexor carpi radialis	Extensor carpi radialis longus	Flexor carpi radialis	Flexor carpi ulnaris
Flexor carpi ulnaris	Extensor carpi radialis brevis	Extensor carpi radialis longus	Extensor carpi ulnaris
Palmaris longus	Extensor carpi ulnaris	Extensor carpi radialis brevis	
Flexor digitorum superficialis	Extensor digitorum		
Flexor digitorum profundus			

LESSON TEN—MUSCLES OF HIP AND KNEE JOINT MOVEMENT

Psoas Major, Iliacus, Piriformis, Gemellus Superior, Gemellus Inferior, Obturator Internus, Obturator Externus, Quadratus Femoris, Gluteus Maximus, Gluteus Medius, Gluteus Minimus, Tensor Fascia Lata, Rectus Femoris, Vastus Intermedius, Vastus Medialis, Vastus Lateralis, Sartorius, Semimembranosus, Semitendinosus, Biceps Femoris, Gracilis, Adductor Magnus, Adductor Longus, Adductor Brevis, Pectineus, Gastrocnemius (Lesson Eleven), Plantaris (Lesson Eleven), Popliteus (Lesson Eleven)

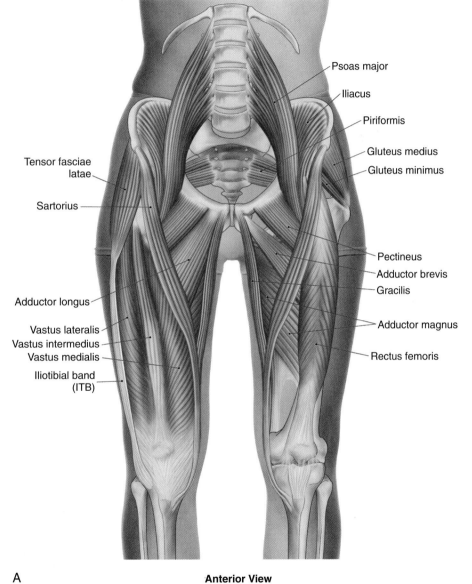

A

Anterior View

FIGURE 21-87

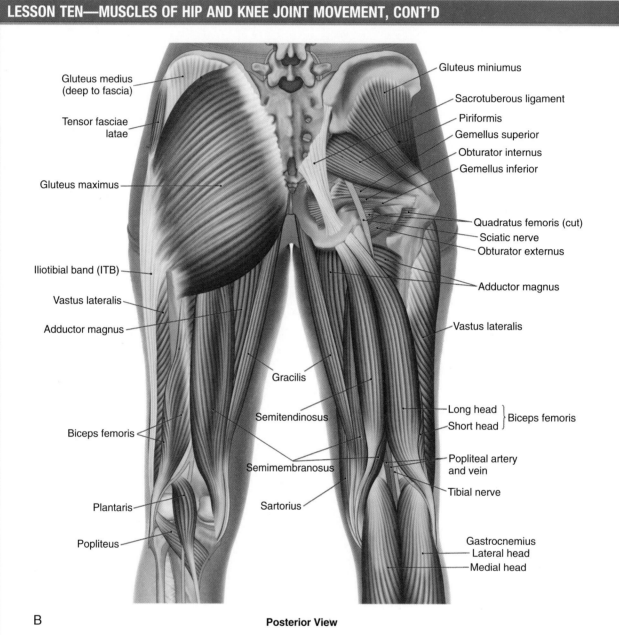

B

Posterior View

FIGURE 21-87, cont'd

ILIOPSOAS

Latin: ilium—flank
Greek: psoa—muscle of the loin

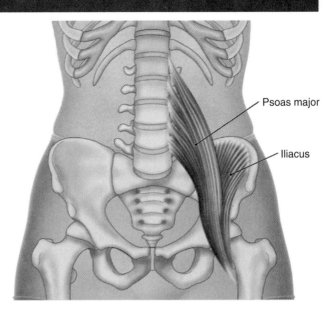

Anterior View
FIGURE 21-88

Notes: Psoas major and iliacus are usually referred to as *iliopsoas*. A third muscle, psoas minor, is absent in 50% of cadavers, and will not be included in this discussion. Iliopsoas is the main flexor of the hip. Tightness in this muscle can play a significant role in functional lordosis and scoliosis and may be a cause of lower back pain.

PSOAS MAJOR

Greek: psoa—muscle of the loin
major—larger

ORIGINS
Transverse processes of T12-L5
Vertebral bodies of T12-L5
Intervertebral disks of lumbar vertebrae

INSERTION
Lesser trochanter

ACTIONS
Laterally rotates the hip (unilateral contraction)
Flexes the hip (unilateral or bilateral contraction)
Flexes the vertebral column (bilateral contraction)
Anteriorly tilts the pelvis (bilateral contraction)

NERVES
Lumbar plexus

Note: Psoas major is the strongest hip flexor. Filet mignon is the psoas major muscle of a cow.

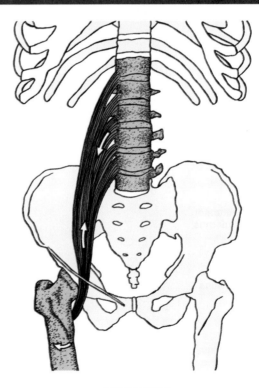

Anterior View
FIGURE 21-89

ILIACUS

Latin: iliacus—ilium

ORIGINS
Iliac fossa
Anterior inferior iliac spine

INSERTION
Lesser trochanter

ACTIONS
Flexes the hip (unilateral or bilateral contraction)
Laterally rotates the hip (unilateral contraction)
Anteriorly tilts the pelvis (bilateral contraction)

NERVE
Femoral nerve

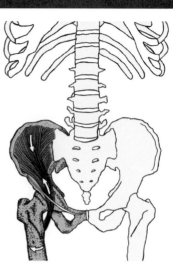

Anterior View
FIGURE 21-90

DEEP HIP OUTWARD ROTATORS

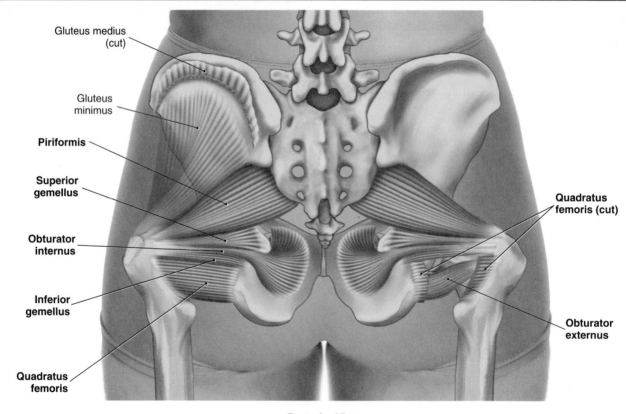

Gluteus medius (cut)
Gluteus minimus
Piriformis
Superior gemellus
Obturator internus
Inferior gemellus
Quadratus femoris
Quadratus femoris (cut)
Obturator externus

Posterior View
FIGURE 21-91

Notes: The six lateral hip rotators are located deep to the gluteal muscles (discussed later). These rotators correspond to some degree to the rotator cuff muscles of the humerus. To help you learn the names of the hip rotators, from superior to inferior, use the mnemonic phrase: **P**ieced **G**oods **O**ften **G**o **O**n **Q**uilts: **P**iriformis, **G**emellus superior, **O**bturator internus, **G**emellus inferior, **O**bturator externus, and **Q**uadratus femoris. Most of these muscles insert on the greater trochanter.

PIRIFORMIS

Latin: pirum—pear
forma—shape

ORIGIN
Anterior sacrum

INSERTION
Greater trochanter

ACTIONS
Laterally rotates the hip
Abducts the hip

NERVE
Sciatic nerve

Notes: Piriformis is the largest of all the lateral rotators and the most likely to become chronically shortened. Of the population, 15% has all or part of the sciatic nerve running *through* this muscle.

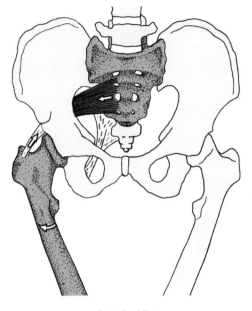

Anterior View

FIGURE 21-92

GEMELLUS SUPERIOR

Latin: gemellus—twin
superus—upper

ORIGIN
Ischial spine

INSERTION
Greater trochanter

ACTION
Laterally rotates the hip

NERVE
Sciatic nerve

Note: This muscle is occasionally absent.

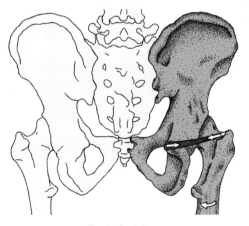

Posterior View

FIGURE 21-93

GEMELLUS INFERIOR

Latin: gemellus—twin
inferus—beneath

ORIGIN
Superior ischial tuberosity

INSERTION
Greater trochanter

ACTION
Laterally rotates the hip

NERVE
Sciatic nerve

Note: This muscle is occasionally absent.

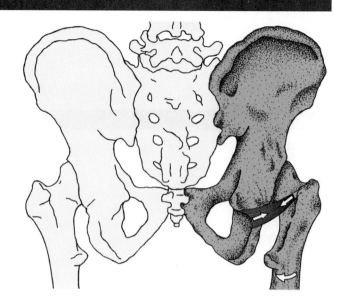

Posterior View

FIGURE 21-94

OBTURATOR INTERNUS

Latin: obturare—obstruct
internus—within

ORIGINS
Obturator membrane
Obturator margin

INSERTION
Greater trochanter

ACTION
Laterally rotates the hip

NERVE
Sciatic nerve

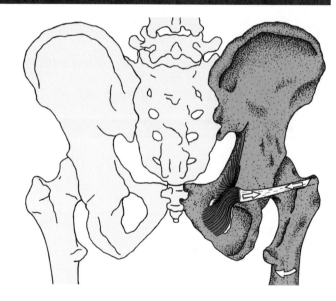

Posterior View

FIGURE 21-95

OBTURATOR EXTERNUS

Latin: obturare—obstruct
externus—outside

ORIGINS
Obturator membrane
Superior pubic ramus
Inferior pubic ramus
Ischial ramus

INSERTION
Greater trochanter

ACTION
Laterally rotates the hip

NERVE
Obturator nerve

Note: This muscle is occasionally absent.

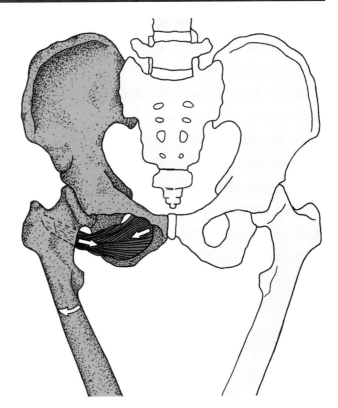

Anterior View
FIGURE 21-96

QUADRATUS FEMORIS

Latin: quadratus—four sided
femoralis—pertaining to the femur

ORIGIN
Lateral ischial tuberosity

INSERTION
Intertrochanteric crest

ACTIONS
Laterally rotates the hip
Adducts the hip

NERVE
Sciatic nerve

Note: This muscle is occasionally absent and may fuse with adductor magnus.

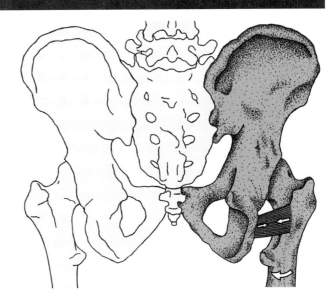

Posterior View
FIGURE 21-97

GLUTEALS

Greek: gloutous—buttock

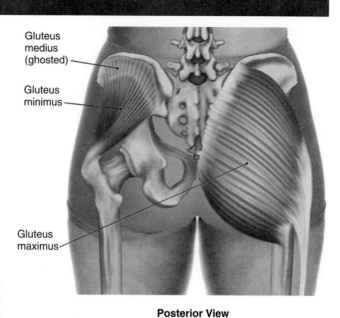

Gluteus medius (ghosted)

Gluteus minimus

Gluteus maximus

Posterior View

FIGURE 21-98

Notes: The gluteals, or *glutes,* refer to gluteus maximus, gluteus medius, and gluteus minimus. Note that these muscles can be antagonists to themselves.

GLUTEUS MAXIMUS

Greek: gloutos—buttock
Latin: maximus—greatest

ORIGINS
Posterior sacrum
Posterior coccyx
Posterior iliac crest
External ilium to the posterior gluteal line

INSERTIONS
Gluteal tuberosity (25%)
Iliotibial band (75%)

ACTIONS
Extends the hip
Laterally rotates the hip
Adducts the hip
Posteriorly tilts the pelvis

NERVE
Inferior gluteal nerve

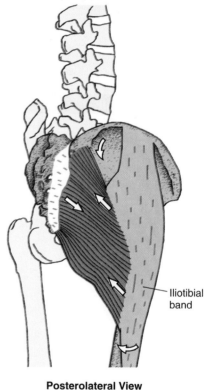

Iliotibial band

Posterolateral View

FIGURE 21-99

Notes: Gluteus maximus is the strongest hip extensor and one of the strongest muscles of the body; it is often more than 1 inch thick. This muscle is mainly used for power, as in climbing stairs, rising from a seated position, or running instead of walking.

Iliotibial band (ITB), or iliotibial tract, is a thickened lateral portion of the fascia lata. The *fascia lata* is a fascial tube that surrounds the thigh. The ITB stretches from the iliac crest to the tibia. The ITB, which assists in knee stabilization, serves as an insertion for gluteus maximus and tensor fasciae latae.

GLUTEUS MEDIUS

Greek: gloutos—buttock
Latin: medius—middle

ORIGIN
External ilium between the anterior and posterior gluteal lines

INSERTION
Greater trochanter

ACTIONS
Abducts the hip
Medially rotates the hip
Laterally rotates the hip
Anteriorly and posteriorly tilts the pelvis

NERVE
Superior gluteal nerve

Note: This muscle stabilizes the hip to give us the ability to stand on one leg.

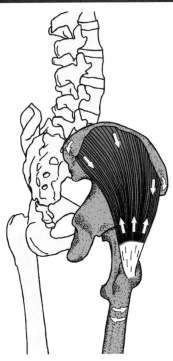

Posterolateral View
FIGURE 21-100

GLUTEUS MINIMUS

Greek: gloutos—buttock
Latin: minimum—least

ORIGIN
External ilium between the anterior and inferior gluteal lines

INSERTION
Greater trochanter

ACTIONS
Abducts the hip
Medially rotates the hip
Laterally rotates the hip
Anteriorly and posteriorly tilts the pelvis

NERVE
Superior gluteal nerve

Note: Gluteus minimus is the synergist to gluteus medius.

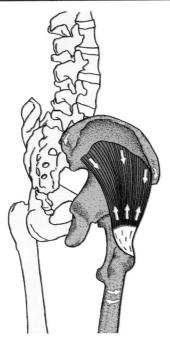

Posterolateral View
FIGURE 21-101

TENSOR FASCIAE LATAE

Latin: tensor—stretching
fascia—band
lata—broad

ORIGINS
Anterior iliac crest
Anterior superior iliac spine (ASIS)

INSERTION
Iliotibial band

ACTIONS
Abducts the hip
Flexes the hip
Medially rotates the hip

NERVE
Superior gluteal nerve

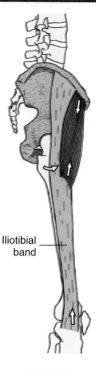

Iliotibial band

Lateral View

FIGURE 21-102

Note: As the name implies, tensor fasciae latae also helps tense the *fascia lata*, which is the fascial tube around the thigh.

ADDUCTORS

Latin: adductus—brought forward

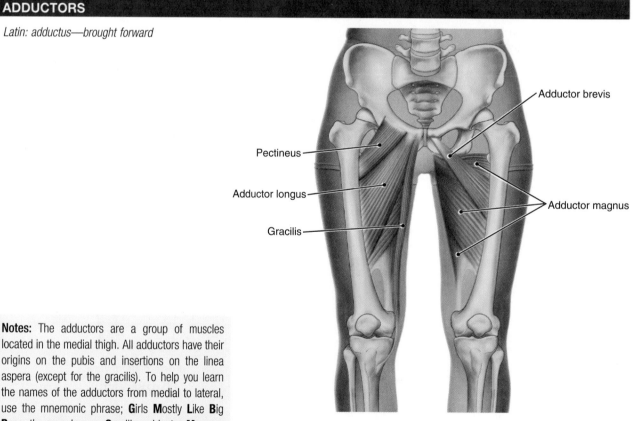

Pectineus

Adductor longus

Gracilis

Adductor brevis

Adductor magnus

Anterior View

FIGURE 21-103

Notes: The adductors are a group of muscles located in the medial thigh. All adductors have their origins on the pubis and insertions on the linea aspera (except for the gracilis). To help you learn the names of the adductors from medial to lateral, use the mnemonic phrase; **G**irls **M**ostly **L**ike **B**ig **P**ecs: the muscles are **G**racilis, adductor **M**agnus, adductor **L**ongus, adductor **B**revis, and **P**ectineus.

GRACILIS

Latin: gracilis—slender

ORIGIN
Inferior pubic ramus

INSERTION
Medial proximal tibial shaft (at the pes anserinus)

ACTIONS
Adducts the hip
Flexes the hip
Flexes the knee
Medially rotates the leg (when the knee is flexed)

NERVE
Obturator nerve

Notes: Gracilis is the most medial adductor and the only adductor that crosses both the hip and knee joints. Gracilis is one of the muscles of the pes anserine, which is discussed later in this section.

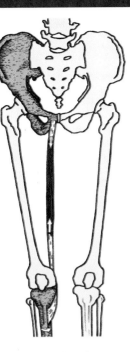

Anterior View

FIGURE 21-104

ADDUCTOR MAGNUS

Latin: adductus—brought toward
magnum—large

ORIGINS
Ischial tuberosity
Inferior pubic ramus
Ischial ramus

INSERTIONS
Linea aspera
Adductor tubercle of the femur

ACTIONS
Adducts the hip
Flexes the hip
Extends the hip

NERVES
Sciatic and obturator nerves

Notes: Adductor magnus lies deep to the hamstrings when viewed posteriorly. This muscle is divided into two sections: one on the linea aspera and one on the adductor tubercle. Between these two sections is an opening called the *adductor hiatus* for passage of the femoral artery and vein.

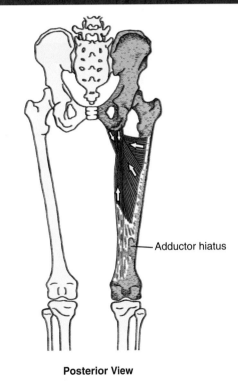

Adductor hiatus

Posterior View

FIGURE 21-105

ADDUCTOR LONGUS

Latin: adductus—brought toward
longus—long

ORIGIN
Anterior pubic body

INSERTION
Middle third of the linea aspera (medial lip)

ACTION
Adducts the hip

NERVE
Obturator nerve

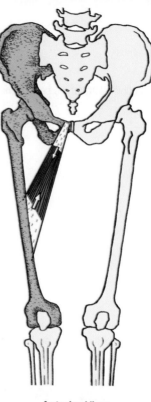

Anterior View
FIGURE 21-106

ADDUCTOR BREVIS

Latin: adductus—brought toward
brevis—brief

ORIGIN
Inferior pubic ramus

INSERTION
Proximal third of the linea aspera (medial lip)

ACTION
Adducts the hip

NERVE
Obturator nerve

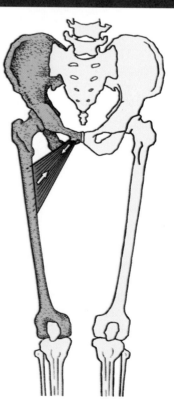

Anterior View
FIGURE 21-107

PECTINEUS

Latin: pecten—comb

ORIGINS
Superior pubic ramus
Pectineal line on pubis

INSERTION
Posterior proximal femoral shaft (inferior to lesser trochanter)

ACTIONS
Flexes the hip
Adducts the hip

NERVE
Femoral nerve

Notes: In relationship to pectineus, the femoral artery may lie medial to this muscle; in some cases, it may cross pectineus superficially. Additionally, this muscle is often regarded as an extension of the iliopsoas because of its insertion near the lesser trochanter and duplicate action of hip flexion.

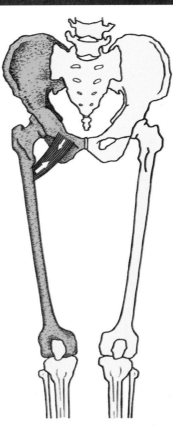

Anterior View

FIGURE 21-108

QUADRICEPS FEMORIS

Latin: quattuor—four
caput—head
femoralis—pertaining to the femur

Notes: Quadriceps femoris, or *quads*, is a group of four muscles sharing a common attachment site on the tibia. The four individual muscles are rectus femoris and three *V*asti—*V*astus intermedius, *V*astus medialis, and *V*astus lateralis. Lengthening and softening of quadriceps femoris may provide relief from knee problems because the quadriceps tendon crosses the knee joint. Conversely, overuse of quads may create knee problems.

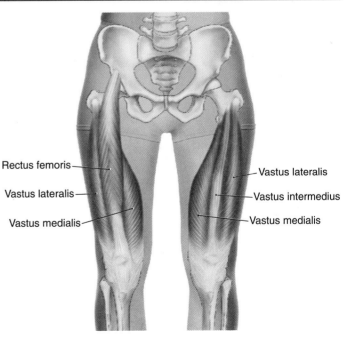

Rectus femoris
Vastus lateralis
Vastus medialis
Vastus lateralis
Vastus intermedius
Vastus medialis

Anterior View

FIGURE 21-109

RECTUS FEMORIS

Latin: rectus—straight
femoralis—pertaining to the femur

ORIGINS
Anterior inferior iliac spine (AIIS)
External ilium just superior to the acetabulum

INSERTION
Tibial tuberosity

ACTIONS
Flexes the hip
Extends the knee
Anteriorly tilts the pelvis

NERVE
Femoral nerve

Notes: Rectus femoris runs in a channel formed by the vastus muscles, and it overlies vastus intermedius. It is the only muscle of quadriceps femoris that crosses both the hip and knee joints.

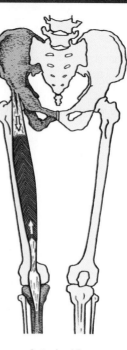

Anterior View
FIGURE 21-110

VASTUS INTERMEDIUS

Latin: vastus—immense
inter—internal
medius—middle

ORIGIN
Anterior lateral femoral shaft

INSERTION
Tibial tuberosity

ACTION
Extends the knee

NERVE
Femoral nerve

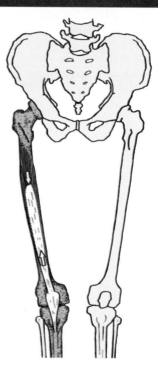

Anterior View
FIGURE 21-111

VASTUS MEDIALIS

Latin: vastus—immense
medius—middle

ORIGINS
Linea aspera (medial lip)
Intertrochanteric line

INSERTION
Tibial tuberosity

ACTION
Extends the knee

NERVE
Femoral nerve

Note: Vastus medialis is sometimes called the *teardrop* or *raindrop* muscle because of the way it appears when outlined by sartorius and rectus femoris.

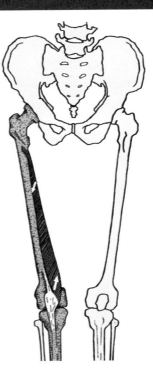

Anterior View

FIGURE 21-112

VASTUS LATERALIS

Latin: vastus—immense
lateralis—toward the side

ORIGINS
Linea aspera (lateral lip)
Gluteal tuberosity

INSERTION
Tibial tuberosity

ACTION
Extends the knee

NERVE
Femoral nerve

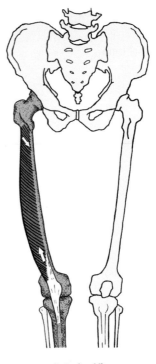

Anterior View

FIGURE 21-113

SARTORIUS

Latin: sartor—tailor

ORIGIN
Anterior superior iliac spine (ASIS)

INSERTION
Medial proximal tibial shaft (at pes anserine)

ACTIONS
Flexes the hip
Laterally rotates the hip
Abducts the hip
Flexes the knee
Medially rotates the leg (when the knee is flexed)

NERVE
Femoral nerve

Notes: Also known as the "tailor's muscle" because, in earlier times, tailors sat cross-legged with the hip flexed and laterally rotated, and the knee flexed while they sewed. Sartorius is the longest muscle in the body, crossing both the hip and knee, running superficially and obliquely across the quads. Sartorius is one of the muscles of the pes anserine, featured later in this section.

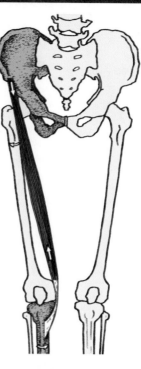

Anterior View
FIGURE 21-114

POPLITEUS

Latin: poples—hollow behind the knee

ORIGIN
Lateral condyle of femur

INSERTION
Posterior proximal tibial shaft

ACTIONS
Flexes the knee
Medially rotates the leg (when the knee is flexed)

NERVE
Tibial nerve

Notes: Popliteus is a weak flexor of the knee joint, but its function of unlocking the extended knee to initiate flexion is vital to the other stronger knee flexors. For this reason, it gets the nickname "the key that unlocks the knee."

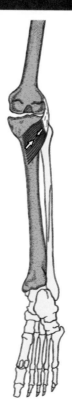

Posterior View
FIGURE 21-115

HAMSTRINGS

Anglo-Saxon: haun—haunch

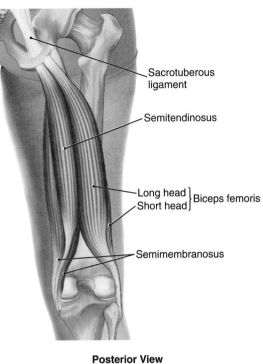

Sacrotuberous ligament

Semitendinosus

Long head ⎫ Biceps femoris
Short head ⎭

Semimembranosus

Posterior View

FIGURE 21-116

Notes: The term *hamstrings* comes from the fact that butchers in the eighteenth century used the tendons of the thighs and hips of pig carcasses to hang ham. Use the mnemonic **BMT** to remember their location on the posterior thigh (lateral to medial): **B**iceps femoris, semi**M**embranosus, semi**T**endinosus.

SEMIMEMBRANOSUS

Latin: semis—half
membrana—membrane

ORIGIN
Ischial tuberosity

INSERTION
Medial condyle of the tibia (posterior surface)

ACTIONS
Flexes the knee
Medially rotates the leg (when the knee is flexed)
Extends the hip
Medially rotates the hip
Posteriorly tilts the pelvis

NERVE
Tibial nerve

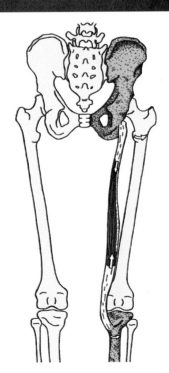

Posterior View

FIGURE 21-117

Notes: Use the mnemonic **M&M** to remember that the semi**M**embranosus is the most **M**edial hamstring muscle. On rare occasions, this muscle is absent or may fuse with semitendinosus.

SEMITENDINOSUS

*Latin: semis—half
tendinosus—tendinous*

ORIGIN
Ischial tuberosity

INSERTION
Medial proximal tibial shaft (at the pes anserinus)

ACTIONS
Flexes the knee
Medially rotates the leg (when the knee is flexed)
Extends the hip
Medially rotates the hip
Posteriorly tilts the pelvis

NERVE
Tibial nerve

Notes: SemiTendinosus is superficial to, or on Top of, semimembranosus. This muscle may contain obliquely arranged tendinous intersections within its belly. Semitendinous is one of the muscles of the pes anserinus, which is discussed later in this section.

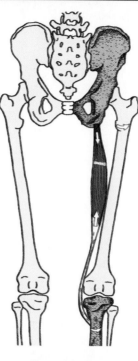

Posterior View
FIGURE 21-118

BICEPS FEMORIS

*Latin: bi—twice
caput—head
femoralis—pertaining to the femur*

ORIGINS
Ischial tuberosity (long head)
Linea aspera; lower lateral lip (short head)

INSERTION
Fibular head

ACTIONS
Flexes the knee
Laterally rotates the leg (when knee is flexed)
Extends the hip
Laterally rotates the hip
Posteriorly tilts the pelvis

NERVES
Tibial nerve (long head)
Common fibular/peroneal nerve (short head)

Notes: Biceps femoris occupies the lateral posterior thigh. The short head of biceps femoris does not cross the hip joint and, on rare occasions, is absent. There is occasionally an attachment to the lateral condyle, as shown in this figure.

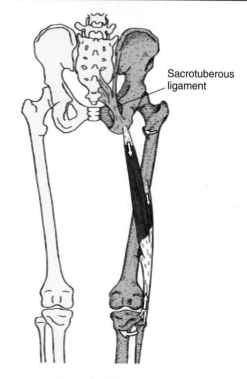

Sacrotuberous ligament

Posterior View
FIGURE 21-119

PES ANSERINUS

Latin: pes—foot
French: anser—a goose

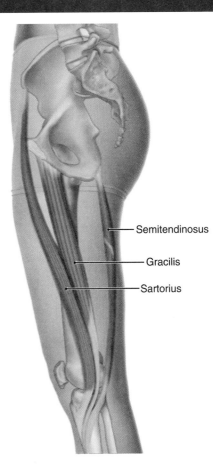

— Semitendinosus

— Gracilis

— Sartorius

Medial View

FIGURE 21-120

Notes: Pes anserinus is the tendinous expansion of **SA**rtorius, **GRAC**ilis, and semi**TE**ndinosus inserting at the medial proximal tibial shaft. Use the mnemonic phase **SA**y **GRAC**e before **TE**a, to assist you in remembering this trio of muscles contributing to the pes.

LESSON TEN REVIEW—MUSCLES OF HIP JOINT MOVEMENT

FLEXION	EXTENSION	ABDUCTION	ADDUCTION	MEDIAL ROTATION	LATERAL ROTATION
Psoas major	Gluteus maximus	Piriformis	Gluteus maximus	Gluteus medius	Psoas major
Iliacus	Semimembranosus	Gluteus medius	Gracilis	Gluteus minimus	Iliacus
Tensor fasciae latae	Semitendinosus	Gluteus minimus	Adductor magnus	Tensor fasciae latae	Gluteus medius
Rectus femoris	Biceps femoris	Tensor fasciae latae	Adductor longus	Semimembranosus	Gluteus minimus
Sartorius	Adductor magnus	Sartorius	Adductor brevis	Semitendinosus	Piriformis
Gracilis		Pectineus			Gemellus superior
Adductor magnus					Gemellus inferior
Pectineus					Obturator internus
					Obturator externus
					Quadratus femoris
					Gluteus maximus
					Sartorius
					Biceps femoris

LESSON TEN REVIEW—MUSCLES OF KNEE JOINT MOVEMENT

FLEXION		EXTENSION
Sartorius	Gracilis	Rectus femoris
Semimembranosus	Gastrocnemius	Vastus medialis
Semitendinosus	Plantaris	Vastus lateralis
Biceps femoris	Popliteus	Vastus intermedius

LESSON ELEVEN—MUSCLES OF THE ANKLE AND FOOT

Tibialis Anterior, Extensor Digitorum Longus and Brevis, Extensor Hallucis Longus, Fibularis Longus, Fibularis Brevis, Fibularis Tertius, Gastrocnemius, Plantaris, Soleus, Tibialis Posterior, Flexor Digitorum Longus, Flexor Hallucis Longus

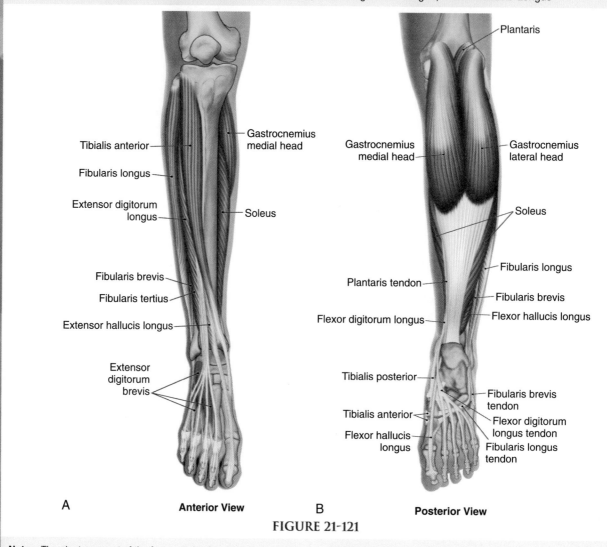

A   **Anterior View**   B   **Posterior View**

FIGURE 21-121

Notes: The plantar aspect of the foot contains four layers of muscles:
First (superficial) layer: Abductor hallucis, flexor digitorum brevis, abductor digiti minimi
Second layer: Quadratus plantae, lumbricals, (flexor hallucis longus tendon), (flexor digitorum longus tendon)

Third layer: Flexor hallucis brevis, adductor hallucis, flexor digiti minimi brevis
Fourth layer: Dorsal interossei, plantar interossei, (fibularis longus tendon), (tibialis posterior tendon)

TIBIALIS ANTERIOR

Latin: tibialis—shinbone
ante—before

ORIGINS
Proximal half of the lateral tibial shaft
Interosseous membrane

INSERTIONS
Metatarsal I
Cuneiform I (plantar surface)

ACTIONS
Dorsiflexes the ankle
Inverts the foot

NERVE
Deep fibular nerve

Notes: Tibialis anterior, along with fibularis longus (featured later), are referred to as *stirrup muscles* as their tendons cross the ankle on either side and attach to the bottom of the foot like stirrups.

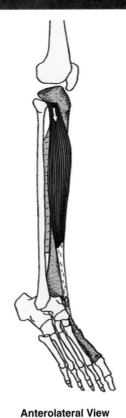

Anterolateral View

FIGURE 21-122

EXTENSOR DIGITORUM LONGUS AND BREVIS

Latin: extensio—to extend
digitus—finger or toe
longus—long
brevis—brief

ORIGINS
Fibular head (longus)
Proximal two thirds of the fibular shaft (longus)
Lateral condyle of the tibia (longus)
Interosseus membrane (longus)
Calcaneus (brevis)

INSERTIONS
Middle phalanges of toes 2-5 (longus)
Distal phalanges of toes 2-5 (longus)
Tendons of extensor digitorum longus to toes 2-4 (brevis)

ACTIONS
Extends toes 2-5 (longus)
Dorsiflexes ankle and everts the foot (longus)
Extends toes 2-4 (brevis)

NERVE
Deep fibular nerve (longus and brevis)

Note: Individual tendons may be absent.

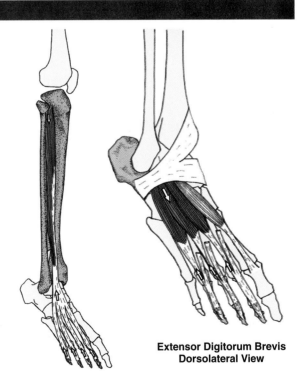

**Extensor Digitorum Brevis
Dorsolateral View**

**Extensor Digitorum Longus
Dorsolateral View**

FIGURE 21-123

EXTENSOR HALLUCIS LONGUS

Latin: extensio—to extend
hallux—large toe
longus—long

ORIGINS
Anterior fibular shaft (middle region)
Interosseous membrane

INSERTION
Distal phalanx of the great toe

ACTIONS
Extends the great toe
Dorsiflexes the ankle

NERVE
Deep fibular nerve

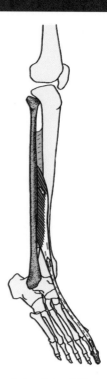

Anterolateral View
FIGURE 21-124

FIBULARIS LONGUS

Greek: fibula—pin
Latin: longus—long

ORIGINS
Fibular head
Lateral proximal half of the fibular shaft

INSERTIONS
Metatarsal I
Cuneiform I (plantar surface)

ACTIONS
Everts the foot
Plantar flexes the ankle

NERVE
Superficial fibular nerve

Notes: Fibularis longus and tibialis anterior are referred to as *stirrup muscles*, because their tendons cross the ankle on either side and attach to the bottom of the foot like stirrups. Fibularis longus is also known as *peroneus longus*.

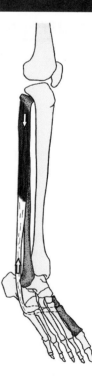

Anterolateral View
FIGURE 21-125

FIBULARIS BREVIS

Greek: fibula—pin
Latin: brevis—brief

ORIGIN
Lateral distal half of the fibular shaft

INSERTION
Metatarsal V

ACTIONS
Everts the foot
Plantar flexes the ankle

NERVE
Superficial fibular nerve

Note: Fibularis brevis is also known as *peroneus brevis.*

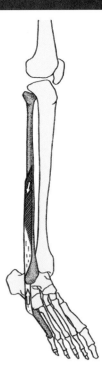

Anterolateral View
FIGURE 21-126

FIBULARIS TERTIUS

Greek: fibula—pin
Latin: tertiarius—third

ORIGINS
Lateral distal third of the fibular shaft
Interosseus membrane

INSERTION
Dorsal metatarsal V

ACTIONS
Everts the foot
Dorsiflexes the ankle

NERVE
Deep fibular nerve

Note: Fibularis tertius is also known as *peroneus tertius.*

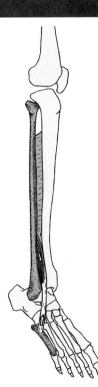

Anterolateral View
FIGURE 21-127

GASTROCNEMIUS

Greek: gaster—belly
kneme—leg

ORIGINS
Medial epicondyle of the femur
Lateral epicondyle of the femur

INSERTION
Calcaneus via the Achilles tendon

ACTIONS
Plantar flexes the ankle
Flexes the knee

NERVE
Tibial nerve

Notes: Gastrocnemius, or *gastroc*, is also known as the "toe dancer's muscle" because it helps ballerinas stand on their toes. The two actions of this muscle, ankle plantar flexion and knee flexion, are an *either-or* situation—gastrocnemius cannot perform both actions simultaneously. Occasionally, origins of this muscle are found on the joint capsule of the knee.

Gastrocnemius and soleus (discussed later) can be collectively called the *triceps surae*. These muscles share a common tendon of insertion and are viewed as the "triceps brachii" of the leg. Triceps surae lifts the weight of the body when moving forward, as in walking or running. Some references include plantaris as part of triceps surae.

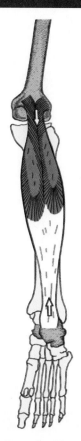

Posterior View

FIGURE 21-128

PLANTARIS

Latin: planta—sole

ORIGIN
Lateral epicondyle of the femur

INSERTION
Calcaneus via the Achilles tendon

ACTIONS
Plantar flexes the ankle
Flexes the knee

NERVE
Tibial nerve

Notes: Plantaris is regarded as a minigastrocnemius because of a common insertion and is occasionally missing in cadavers (approximately 10%). Plantaris tendon may be removed for grafting during reconstructive surgery of tendons of the hand.

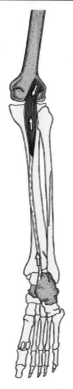

Posterior View

FIGURE 21-129

SOLEUS

Latin: solea—sole of the foot

ORIGINS
Superior posterior third of the fibular shaft
Soleal line of the tibia

INSERTION
Calcaneus via the Achilles tendon

ACTION
Plantar flexes the ankle

NERVE
Tibial nerve

Note: It has been rumored that soleus was so named because it resembled a sole fish from the Mediterranean Sea.

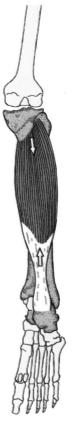

Posterior View

FIGURE 21-130

TIBIALIS POSTERIOR

Latin: tibialis—shinbone
posterus—behind

ORIGINS
Posterior tibial shaft
Posterior fibular shaft
Interosseous membrane

INSERTIONS
Tuberosity of navicular (plantar surface)
Cuneiforms I, II, and III
Cuboid
Calcaneus
Navicular
Bases of metatarsals II, III, and IV

ACTIONS
Inverts the foot
Plantar flexes the ankle

NERVE
Tibial nerve

Note: This muscle may be completely absent.

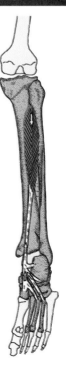

Posterior View

FIGURE 21-131

FLEXOR DIGITORUM LONGUS

Latin: flexus—bent
digitus—finger or toe
longus—long

ORIGIN
Posterior tibial shaft—middle region

INSERTIONS
Distal phalanges 2-5 (plantar surface)

ACTIONS
Flexes digits 2-5 at the DIP, PIP, and MP joints
Plantar flexes the ankle
Inverts the foot

NERVE
Tibial nerve

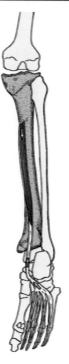

Posterior View

FIGURE 21-132

FLEXOR HALLUCIS LONGUS

Latin: flexus—bent
hallux—large toe
longus—long

ORIGINS
Posterior fibular shaft—middle region
Interosseus membrane

INSERTION
Distal phalanx of the great toe (plantar surface)

ACTIONS
Flexes the great toe
Plantar flexes the ankle
Inverts the foot
Supports the longitudinal arch

NERVE
Tibial nerve

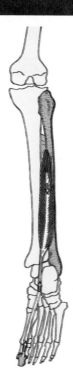

Posterior View

FIGURE 21-133

LESSON ELEVEN REVIEW—MUSCLES OF ANKLE AND FOOT MOVEMENT

PLANTAR FLEXION	DORSIFLEXION	INVERSION	EVERSION
Fibularis longus	Tibialis anterior	Tibialis anterior	Fibularis longus
Fibularis brevis	Extensor hallucis longus	Tibialis posterior	Fibularis brevis
Gastrocnemius	Fibularis tertius	Flexor digitorum longus	Fibularis tertius
Plantaris	Extensor digitorum longus	Flexor hallucis longus	Extensor digitorum longus
Soleus			
Tibialis posterior			
Flexor digitorum longus			
Flexor hallucis longus			

LESSON TWELVE—MUSCLES OF THE HEAD AND NECK

Occipitofrontalis, Orbicularis Oculi, Orbicularis Oris, Platysma, Temporalis, Masseter, Lateral Pterygoid, Medial Pterygoid, Longus Capitis, Longus Colli, Sternocleidomastoid, Scalenus Anterior, Scalenus Medius, Scalenus Posterior, Splenius Capitis, Splenius Cervicis, Rectus Capitis Posterior Major, Rectus Capitis Posterior Minor, Oblique Capitis Superior, Oblique Capitis Inferior, Levator Scapulae (Lesson Six), Trapezius (Lesson Six), Spinalis (Lesson Thirteen), Longissimus (Lesson Thirteen)

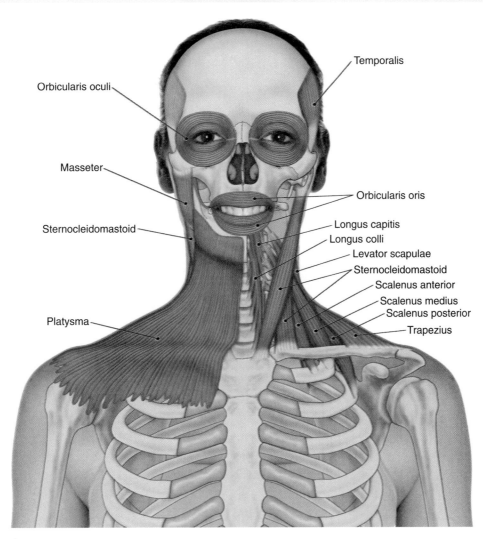

Anterior View

FIGURE 21-134

LESSON TWELVE—MUSCLES OF THE HEAD AND NECK, CONT'D

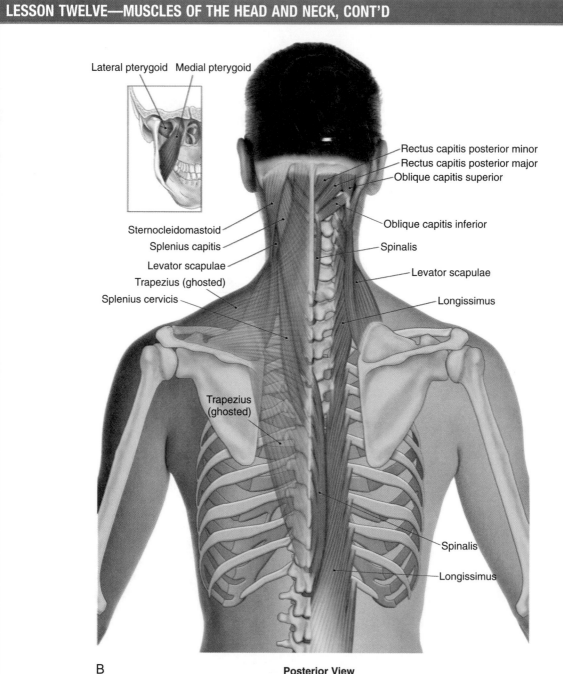

Lateral pterygoid   Medial pterygoid

Rectus capitis posterior minor
Rectus capitis posterior major
Oblique capitis superior

Sternocleidomastoid

Oblique capitis inferior

Splenius capitis

Spinalis

Levator scapulae

Levator scapulae

Trapezius (ghosted)

Longissimus

Splenius cervicis

Trapezius (ghosted)

Spinalis

Longissimus

B

Posterior View

FIGURE 21-134, cont'd

OCCIPITOFRONTALIS

*Latin: occipitalis—pertaining to the back of the head
frons—brow or referring to the frontal bone*

ORIGINS
Lateral two thirds of the superior nuchal line (occipitalis)
Galea aponeurotica (frontalis)

INSERTIONS
Galea aponeurotica (occipitalis)
Superficial fascia beneath the eyebrows (frontalis)

ACTIONS
Moves the scalp over the cranium (occipitalis)
Elevates the eyebrows (frontalis)
Horizontally wrinkles the skin over the forehead (frontalis)

NERVE
Facial nerve (cranial nerve VII)

Notes: The occipitofrontalis, or epicranius, contains *occipitalis* and *frontalis* and is connected by an extensive network of cranial fascia called the *galea aponeurotica*. The galea aponeurotica is firmly connected to the hypodermis and slides over the cranium. Frontalis muscle produces the expression of worry or concern. Occipitalis contributes to tension headaches.

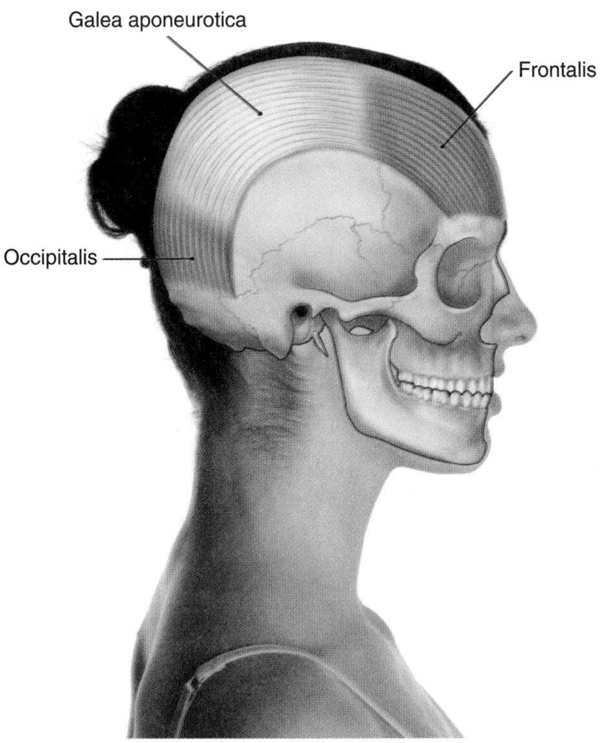

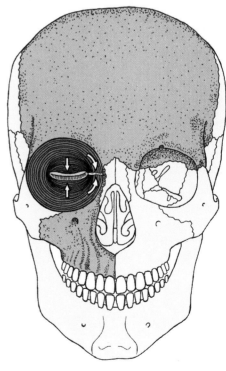

Lateral View
FIGURE 21-135

ORBICULARIS OCULI

*Latin: orbiculus—little circle
oculus—eye*

ORIGIN
Orbital margin

INSERTION
Superficial fascia beneath the upper eyelids

ACTIONS
Closes the eyelids
Folds the skin around the orbit (to protect eyeball and assist in
   tear transport)
Squints the eyelids

NERVE
Facial nerve (cranial nerve VII)

Notes: This is a very complex muscle with three main sections—orbital, palpebral, and lacrimal. Orbicularis oculi is also known as the *winking* or *blinking muscle,* as it closes the eyelid.

Anterior View
FIGURE 21-136

ORBICULARIS ORIS

Latin: orbiculus—little circle
oris—mouth

ORIGINS
Maxilla
Mandible

INSERTIONS
Mucous membranes of the lips
Muscles inserting into the lips

ACTIONS
Closes the lips
Protrudes and protracts the lips
Assists in dozens of activities such as eating, drinking, talking,
    and sucking

NERVE
Facial nerve (cranial nerve VII)

Notes: Also known as the *kissing muscle*, it protrudes the lips for a kiss.

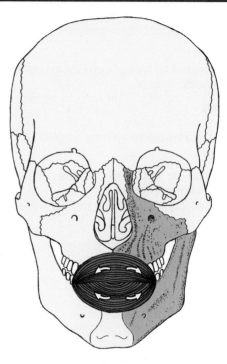

Anterior View
FIGURE 21-137

PLATYSMA

Greek: platysma—plate

ORIGINS
Superficial fascia of the deltoid
Superficial fascia of pectoralis major

INSERTIONS
Mandible
Muscles around angle of the mouth
Superficial fascia of the lower face

ACTIONS
Tenses the skin of the anterior neck (creating ridges)
Pulls the corner of the mouth downward and backward
Depresses the mandible

NERVE
Facial nerve (cranial nerve VII)

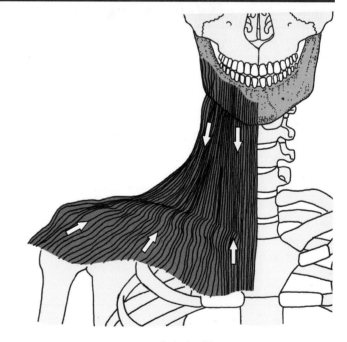

Anterior View
FIGURE 21-138

Notes: This muscle is the most superficial muscle of the anterior neck. Platysma is sometimes called the *pouting muscle* because it moves the corners of the mouth downward and back as in pouting. Additionally, this muscle is often referred to as the *lizard muscle* because when you contract platysma fully, you give the appearance of a lizard (this is enhanced if you dart your tongue in and out of your mouth quickly).

MUSCLES OF MASTICATION

Temporalis, Masseter, Medial and Lateral Pterygoids

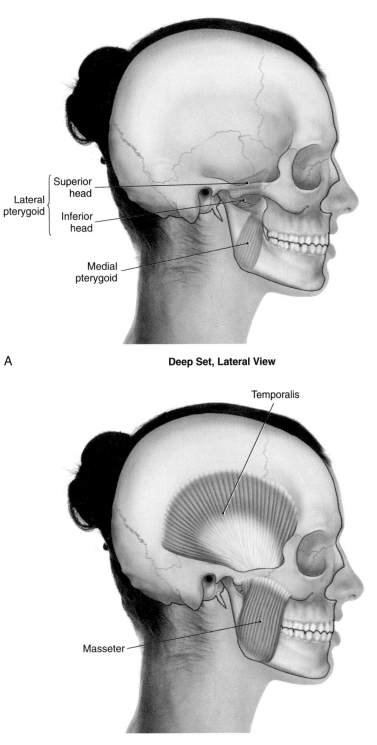

A   **Deep Set, Lateral View**

Lateral pterygoid
- Superior head
- Inferior head

Medial pterygoid

Temporalis

Masseter

B   **Superficial Set, Lateral View**

FIGURE 21-139 Muscles of mastication.

TEMPORALIS

Latin: temporalis—pertaining to the temporal bone

ORIGIN
Temporal fossa (frontal, parietal, and temporal bones)

INSERTION
Coronoid process and ramus of the mandible

ACTIONS
Elevates the mandible
Retracts the mandible

NERVE
Trigeminal nerve (cranial nerve V)

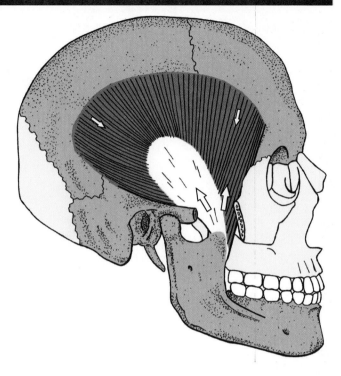

Lateral View

FIGURE 21-140

MASSETER

Greek: masseter—chewer

ORIGIN
Zygomatic arch*

INSERTIONS
Mandibular angle (superficial layer)
Mandibular ramus (deep layer)

ACTIONS
Elevates the mandible
Protracts the mandible

NERVE
Trigeminal nerve (cranial nerve V)

Note: Masseter possesses a superficial and a deep layer, and these may fuse. Masseter is essentially a mirror image of medial pterygoid.

*The zygomatic arch (see origin) is formed by two processes; one extending from the zygomatic bone and the other from the temporal bone.

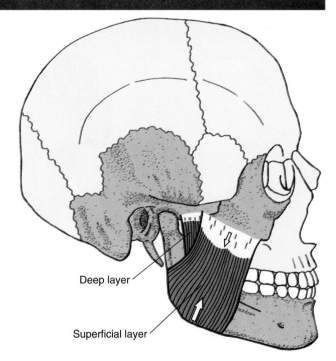

Deep layer

Superficial layer

Lateral View

FIGURE 21-141

LATERAL PTERYGOID

Latin: lateralis—toward the side
Greek: pterygodes—a wing

ORIGINS
Pterygoid plate of the sphenoid bone (lateral surface)
Greater wing of the sphenoid bone

INSERTIONS
Condylar process of the mandible
Temporomandibular joint capsule

ACTIONS
Produces lateral mandibular movements (unilateral contraction)
Depresses the mandible (bilateral contraction)
Protracts the mandible (bilateral contraction)

NERVE
Trigeminal nerve (cranial nerve V)

Notes: Lateral pterygoid has superior and inferior heads, which occasionally fuse. Some sources say that the superior head may also elevate the mandible.

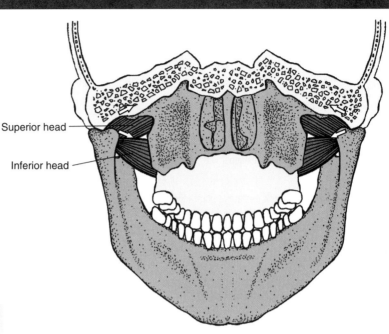

Superior head
Inferior head

Posterior View
FIGURE 21-142

MEDIAL PTERYGOID

Latin: medialis—toward the midline
Greek: pterygodes—a wing

ORIGIN
Pterygoid plate of the sphenoid bone (lateral surface)

INSERTIONS
Mandibular angle (interior surface)
Mandibular ramus (interior surface)

ACTIONS
Produces lateral mandibular movements (unilateral contraction)
Elevates the mandible (bilateral contraction)
Protracts the mandible (bilateral contraction)

NERVE
Trigeminal nerve (cranial nerve V)

Note: Medial pterygoid is essentially a mirror image of masseter.

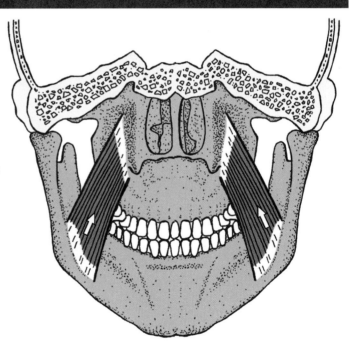

Posterior View
FIGURE 21-143

STERNOCLEIDOMASTOID

Greek: sternon—sternum
cleido—clavicle
mastos—breastlike

ORIGINS
Manubrium of the sternum (sternal head)
Medial third of the clavicle (clavicular head)

INSERTIONS
Mastoid process
Lateral half of the superior nuchal line

ACTIONS
Laterally flexes the neck (unilateral contraction)
Rotates the head to opposite side (unilateral contraction)
Flexes the neck (bilateral contraction)
Elevates the sternum to assist in forced inspiration (bilateral contraction)

NERVE
Spinal accessory nerve (cranial nerve XI)

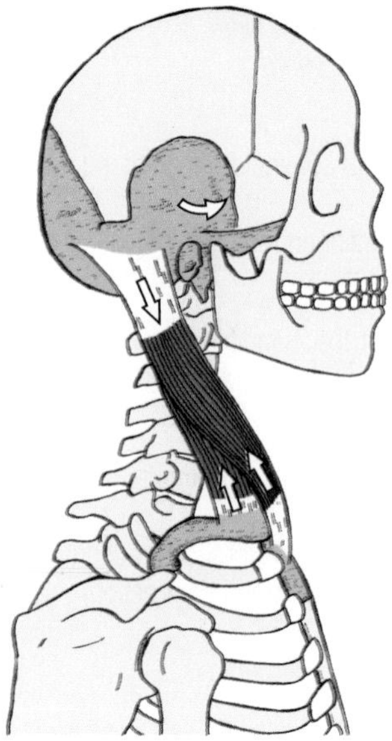

Lateral View

FIGURE 21-144

Notes: Sternocleidomastoid (SCM) feels similar to cables on both sides of the neck. SCM is the only muscle that moves the head but does not attach to any vertebrae. Bilateral contraction brings the head down in a bow, as in the position assumed while praying. Because of this action, SCM is also called the *praying muscle*.

The carotid artery lies deep and medial to SCM and the external jugular vein superficially. SCM is the mirror image of splenius capitis. A condition called *torticollis*, or *wryneck*, involves spasms of SCM. Spasms in this muscle may also cause vertigo because of the many sensory and positional receptors located here.

SCALENES

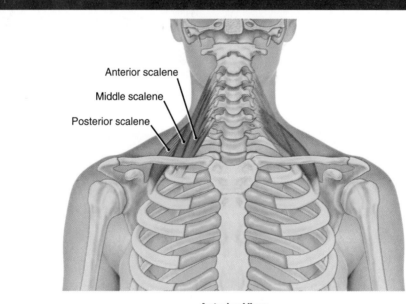

Anterior scalene

Middle scalene

Posterior scalene

Anterior View

FIGURE 21-145

Notes: Scalenes are a group of muscles consisting of scalenus anterior, scalenus medius, and scalenus posterior. These muscles, along with pectoralis minor, are known as the *neurovascular entrappers* because they can compress, or entrap, the subclavian artery and brachial plexus passing between scalenus anterior and scalenus medius. The scalenes are palpable in the posterior triangular of the neck between SCM and trapezius. Place your hands in this triangle, and inhale deeply. At the end of the inhalation, gasp quickly. This action forces the scalenes into noticeable contraction. Because of the relationship to breathing, scalenes represent the cranial continuation of the intercostals. Additionally, when the body is in motion, scalenes stabilize the neck by preventing side swaying. In approximately 30% of all cadavers, another scalene muscle, scalenus minimus, is found.

SCALENUS ANTERIOR

Greek: skalenos—uneven
Latin: ante—before

ORIGINS
Transverse processes of C3-C6

INSERTION
Rib 1 (superior surface)

ACTIONS
Flexes the neck (bilateral contraction)
Laterally flexes the neck (unilateral contraction)
Rotates the head (unilateral contraction)
Elevates the first rib during inspiration (bilateral contraction)

NERVES
Anterior rami of cervical nerves

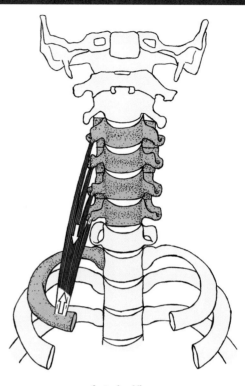

Anterior View

FIGURE 21-146

SCALENUS MEDIUS

Greek: skalenos—uneven
Latin: medialis—toward the midline

ORIGINS
Transverse processes of C2-C7

INSERTION
Rib 1 (superior surface)

ACTIONS
Flexes the neck (bilateral contraction)
Laterally flexes the neck (unilateral contraction)
Rotates the head (unilateral contraction)
Elevates the first rib during inspiration (bilateral contraction)

NERVES
Anterior rami of cervical nerves

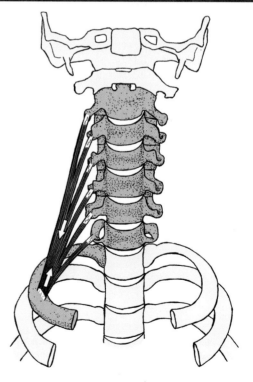

Anterior View

FIGURE 21-147

SCALENUS POSTERIOR

Greek: skalenos—uneven
Latin: posterus—behind

ORIGINS
Transverse processes of C5-C7

INSERTION
Rib 2 (superior lateral surface)

ACTIONS
Laterally flexes the neck (unilateral contraction)
Elevates the second rib during inspiration (bilateral contraction)

NERVES
Anterior rami of cervical nerves

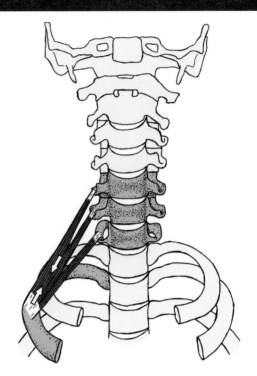

Anterior View

FIGURE 21-148

LONGUS CAPITIS

Latin: longus—long
caput—head

ORIGINS
Transverse processes of C3-C5

INSERTION
Occipital bone (just anterior to the foramen magnum)

ACTIONS
Laterally flexes the neck
Flexes the neck

NERVE
Anterior rami of cervical nerves

Note: Longus capitis and longus colli (featured next) are part of the prevertebral group and help maintain the anterior curve of the cervical spine.

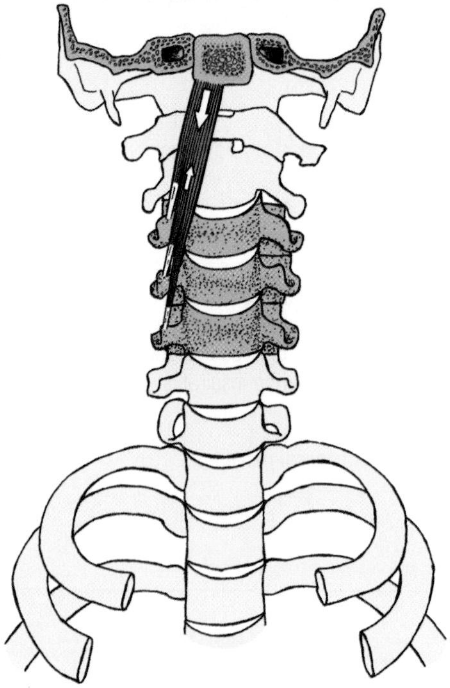

Anterior View

FIGURE 21-149

LONGUS COLLI

Latin: longus—long
colli—collar

ORIGINS
Anterior transverse processes of C3-C5 (superior oblique part)
Anterior vertebral bodies of T1-T3 (inferior oblique part)
Anterior vertebral bodies of C5-T3 (vertical part)

INSERTIONS
Anterior tubercle of C1 (superior oblique part)
Anterior transverse processes C5-C6 (inferior oblique part)
Anterior vertebral bodies C2-C4 (vertical part)

ACTIONS
Rotates the head
Flexes the neck
Laterally flexes the neck

NERVE
Anterior rami of cervical nerves

Note: Longus colli, similar to iliopsoas of the lower extremity, contains different portions: superior oblique, inferior oblique, and vertical.

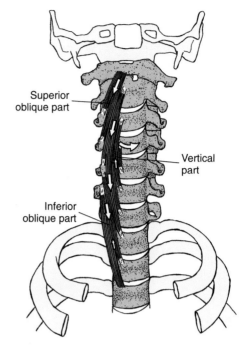

Anterior View
FIGURE 21-150

SPLENIUS CAPITIS

Greek: splenion—splint or bandage
caput—head

ORIGINS
Inferior nuchal ligament
Spinous processes of C7-T4

INSERTIONS
Mastoid process
Superior nuchal line—lateral region

ACTIONS
Rotates the head (unilateral contraction)
Laterally flexes the neck (unilateral contraction)
Extends the head (bilateral contraction)

NERVES
Posterior rami of the middle lower cervical nerves

Note: Splenius capitis is the mirror image of sternocleidomastoid.

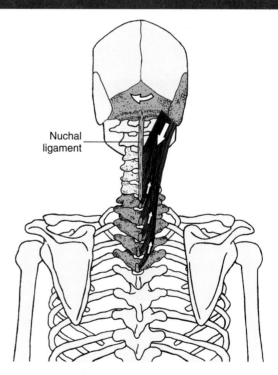

Posterior View
FIGURE 21-151

SPLENIUS CERVICIS

Greek: splenion—splint or bandage
cervicalis—neck

ORIGINS
Spinous processes of T3-T6

INSERTIONS
Transverse processes of C1-C3

ACTIONS
Rotates the head (unilateral contraction)
Laterally flexes the neck (unilateral contraction)
Extends the head (bilateral contraction)

NERVES
Posterior rami of middle lower cervical nerves

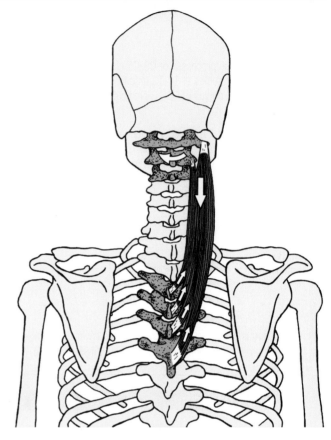

Posterior View

FIGURE 21-152

SUBOCCIPITALS

Latin: sub—below
occipitalis—pertaining to the back of the head

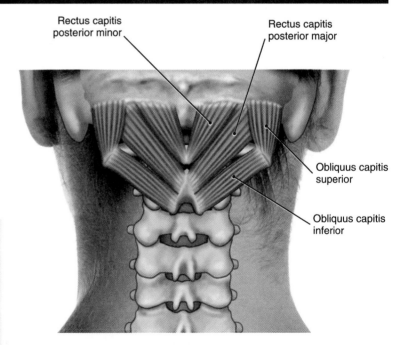

Rectus capitis posterior minor

Rectus capitis posterior major

Obliquus capitis superior

Obliquus capitis inferior

Posterior View

FIGURE 21-153

Notes: The suboccipitals include rectus capitis posterior major, rectus capitis posterior minor, oblique capitis inferior, and oblique capitis superior. Dr. Janet Travell (see her biography in Chapter 24) refers to the suboccipitals as the *ghost headache muscles* because the pain referred from these muscles seems to penetrate the skull and is difficult to locate. All suboccipitals attach on C1 and C2 and are responsible for initiating most head movements.

RECTUS CAPITIS POSTERIOR MAJOR

Latin: rectus—straight
caput—head
posterus—behind
major—larger

ORIGIN
Spinous process of C2

INSERTION
Lateral inferior nuchal line

ACTIONS
Extends the head
Rotates the head

NERVE
Suboccipital nerve

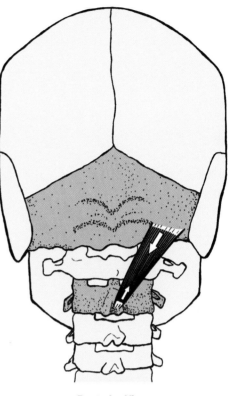

Posterior View

FIGURE 21-154

RECTUS CAPITIS POSTERIOR MINOR

Latin: rectus—straight
caput—head
posterus—behind
minor—smaller

ORIGIN
Posterior tubercle of C1

INSERTION
Medial inferior nuchal line

ACTION
Extends the head

NERVE
Suboccipital nerve

Notes: This muscle also attaches to the dura mater (connective tissue layer surrounding the brain and spinal cord). Tension in this muscle may cause headaches of a vascular and/or neurologic nature.

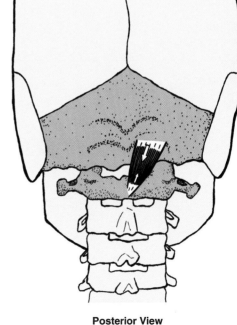

Posterior View

FIGURE 21-155

OBLIQUE CAPITIS SUPERIOR

Latin: obliquus—slant
caput—head
superus—upper

ORIGIN
Transverse process of C1

INSERTION
Inferior nuchal line

ACTIONS
Extends the head
Laterally flexes the head

NERVE
Suboccipital nerve

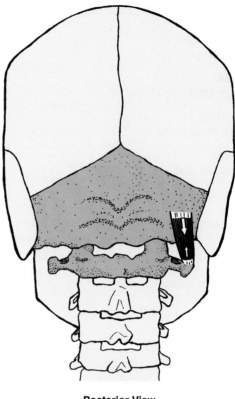

Posterior View

FIGURE 21-156

OBLIQUE CAPITIS INFERIOR

Latin: obliquus—slant
caput—head
infra—beneath

ORIGIN
Spinous process of C2

INSERTION
Transverse process of C1

ACTION
Rotates the head

NERVE
Suboccipital nerve

Note: Although the muscle includes the word *capitis,* it does not attach to the cranium.

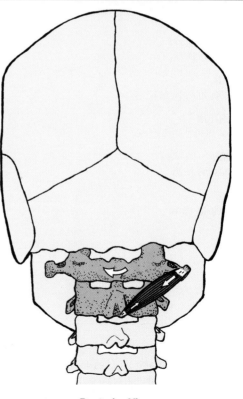

Posterior View

FIGURE 21-157

LESSON TWELVE REVIEW—MUSCLES OF MANDIBULAR MOVEMENT

ELEVATION	DEPRESSION	PROTRACTION	RETRACTION	LATERAL MOVEMENTS
Temporalis	Platysma	Masseter	Temporalis	Lateral pterygoid
Masseter	Lateral pterygoid	Lateral pterygoid		Medial pterygoid
Medial pterygoid		Medial pterygoid		

LESSON TWELVE REVIEW—MUSCLES OF NECK MOVEMENT

FLEXION	EXTENSION	LATERAL FLEXION	ROTATION
Longus capitis	Trapezius	Trapezius	Trapezius
Longus colli	Splenius capitis	Levator scapulae	Longus colli
Sternocleidomastoid	Splenius cervicis	Longus colli	Sternocleidomastoid
Scalenus anterior	Rectus capitis posterior major	Sternocleidomastoid	Scalenus anterior
Scalenus medius	Rectus capitis posterior minor	Scalenus anterior	Scalenus medius
	Oblique capitis superior	Scalenus medius	Scalenus posterior
	Spinalis	Scalenus posterior	Splenius capitis
	Longissimus	Splenius capitis	Splenius cervicis
		Splenius cervicis	Rectus capitis posterior major
		Oblique capitis superior	Oblique capitis inferior
		Oblique capitis inferior	
		Longus capitis	

LESSON THIRTEEN—MUSCLES OF THE TRUNK AND VERTEBRAL COLUMN

Rectus Abdominis, External Obliques, Internal Obliques, Transverse Abdominis, Quadratus Lumborum, Semispinalis, Rotatores, Multifidus, Spinalis, Longissimus, Iliocostalis (see Figure 21-159)

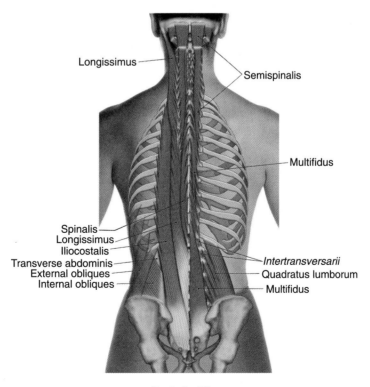

Posterior View

FIGURE 21-158

ABDOMINALS

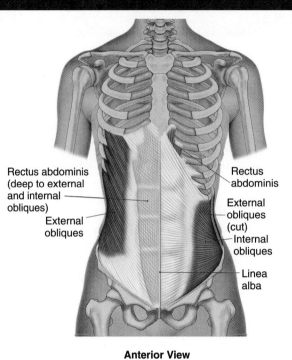

Anterior View

FIGURE 21-159

Notes: The abdominal muscles, or *abdominals*, are rectus abdominis, external and internal obliques, and transverse abdominis. Fiber arrangement of the abdominals run in four different directions. Think of this organization as the *plywood principle of anatomy*, used for added strength to hold in abdominal organs. Abdominals are also involved in forced expiration. The rectus sheath is formed by aponeurosis of the three lateral abdominal muscles. The *linea alba* is a tendinous structure located on the anterior abdominal wall between the two rectus muscles.

RECTUS ABDOMINIS

Latin: rectus—straight
abdomen—belly

ORIGINS
Pubic symphysis
Pubic tubercle

INSERTIONS
Ribs 5 through 7 (costal cartilage—anterior surface)
Xiphoid process

ACTIONS
Flexes the vertebral column
Laterally flexes the vertebral column
Compresses abdominal contents
Posteriorly tilts the pelvis

NERVES
Anterior rami of intercostal nerves (T7-T12)

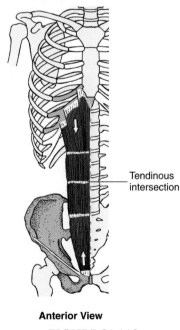

Tendinous intersection

Anterior View

FIGURE 21-160

Notes: Rectus abdominis goes a long distance without any skeletal attachment. To help keep its length relatively constant, this muscle contains horizontal layers of connective tissue called *tendinous intersections/inscriptions*. In well developed people, this muscle is often called the "six-pack (6-pack) muscle." There are, however, actually eight sections but it is usual that only six are well developed. Separation of this muscle, which may occur during advanced pregnancy, is called *rectus diastasis*.

EXTERNAL OBLIQUES

Latin: externus—outside
obliquus—slant

ORIGINS
Anterior iliac crest
Abdominal fascia or aponeurosis
Linea alba
Pubic crest

INSERTIONS
Ribs 5 through 12 (anterior lateral surface)

ACTIONS
Laterally flexes the vertebral column
Rotates the vertebral column
Flexes the vertebral column
Compresses abdomen contents
Posteriorly tilts the pelvis

NERVES
Anterior rami of intercostal nerves (T7-T12)

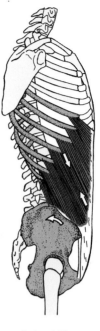

Lateral View
FIGURE 21-161

Notes: Fiber direction of this muscle is similar to the direction of your fingers when your hands are in the pockets of a jacket. The pockets of most jackets do not reach the midline. Similarly, external obliques do not reach the midline. They join the rectus sheath instead.

Tendinous intersections such as those in the rectus abdominis may be present. External obliques interlace with serratus anterior and latissimus dorsi on the lateral aspect of the trunk.

INTERNAL OBLIQUES

Latin: internus—within
obliquus—slant

ORIGINS
Iliac crest (anterior portion)
Thoracolumbar fascia
Inguinal ligament (lateral half)

INSERTIONS
Lower ribs 3 and 4 (anterior lateral surface)
Linea alba

ACTIONS
Laterally flexes the vertebral column
Rotates the vertebral column
Flexes the vertebral column
Compresses abdominal contents
Posteriorly tilts the pelvis

NERVES
Anterior rami of intercostal nerves

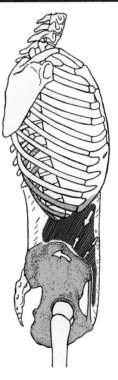

Lateral View
FIGURE 21-162

TRANSVERSE ABDOMINIS

Latin: transversus—lying across
abdomen—belly

ORIGINS
Ribs 7 through 12 (costal cartilage—inner surface)
Iliac crest
Thoracolumbar aponeurosis
Inguinal ligament

INSERTIONS
Abdominal aponeurosis
Linea alba

ACTION
Compresses abdominal contents

NERVES
Anterior rami of intercostal nerves

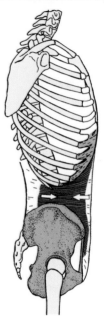

Lateral View
FIGURE 21-163

Notes: Transverse abdominis is the deepest abdominal muscle and wraps around the internal organs, similar to a cummerbund, and helps stabilize the lumbar spine. Lower fibers of rectus abdominis are enclosed by transverse abdominis, possibly for added strength. The inferior portion of this muscle may fuse completely with internal obliques. Because of its frequent variance, transverse abdominis is often called the *complex muscle.*

QUADRATUS LUMBORUM

Latin: quadratus—four-sided
lumbus—loins

ORIGIN
Posterior iliac crest

INSERTIONS
Rib 12 (inferior surface)
Transverse processes of L1-L4

ACTIONS
Laterally flexes the vertebral column (unilateral contraction)
Elevates the hip (unilateral contraction)
Extends the lumbar spine (bilateral contraction)
Anteriorly tilts the pelvis (bilateral contraction)

NERVES
Lumbar plexus

Notes: Also known as the "hip hiker muscle," quadratus lumborum (QL) *"hikes"* the hip.

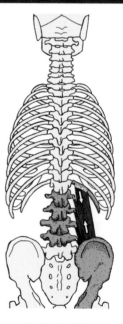

Posterior View
FIGURE 21-164

PARASPINALS

Greek: para—beside
Latin: spinatus—spine

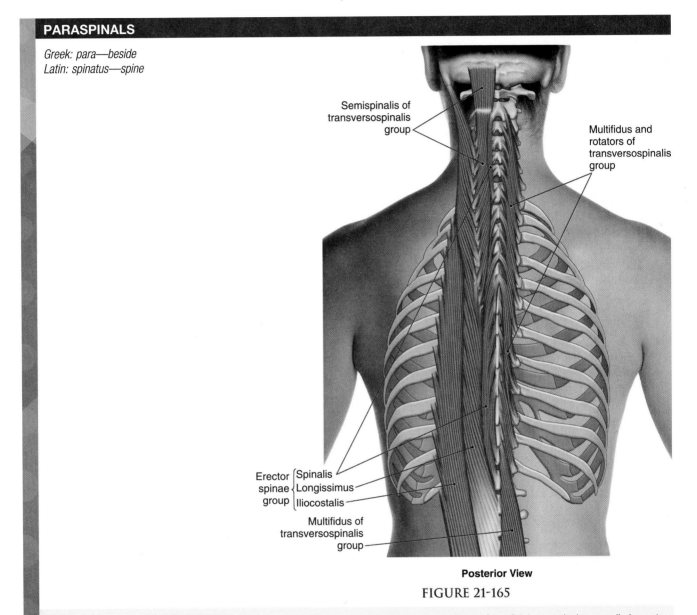

Semispinalis of
transversospinalis
group

Multifidus and
rotators of
transversospinalis
group

Erector
spinae
group
{ Spinalis
Longissimus
Iliocostalis

Multifidus of
transversospinalis
group

Posterior View

FIGURE 21-165

Notes: Paraspinals is the term given to a collection of back muscles. These can be divided into a deep and superficial set. Deep paraspinals are called *transversospinalis* and consist of semispinalis, rotatores, and multifidus. Superficial paraspinals are called *erector spinae* muscles, which consist of spinalis, longissimus, and iliocostalis

TRANSVERSOSPINALIS

Latin: transversus—lying across
spinatus—spine

Notes: *Transversospinalis,* or deep paraspinals, refers to the vertebral processes to which they attach—all attached to transverse or spinous processes. As stated previously, muscles of transversospinalis are *semispinalis, rotatores,* and *multifidus* (see Figure 21-165). Two of the muscle groups, semispinalis and rotatores, can be further subdivided. These subgroupings are semispinalis capitis, semispinalis cervicis, semispinalis thoracis, rotatores longus, and rotatores brevis. Multifidus has no subgroup. These muscles are stacked on top of one another and are composed of many short diagonal fibers.

Two other muscles, called segmental muscles, lie deep in the back. These muscles are *interspinales* and *intertransversarii.* They are called segmental muscles because they traverse a single vertebral segment. Interspinales attach to spinous processes, and intertransversarii attach to transverse processes.

SEMISPINALIS

Latin: semis—half
spinatus—spine

ORIGINS

Transverse process of one vertebral segment (cervical
   and thoracic regions)

INSERTIONS

Between superior and inferior nuchal lines
Spinous processes of the fifth, sixth, and seventh vertebral
   segments above (cervical and thoracic regions except C1)

ACTIONS

Rotates the vertebral column (unilateral contraction)
Extends the vertebral column (bilateral contraction)

NERVES

Posterior rami of cervical and thoracic spinal nerves

Notes: Semispinalis is the most **S**uperficial transversospinalis and runs in cervical and thoracic regions only. It contains subgroupings of capitus, cervicis, and thoracis. Semispinalis capitis often blends with the medial part of spinalis capitis of the erector spinae group.

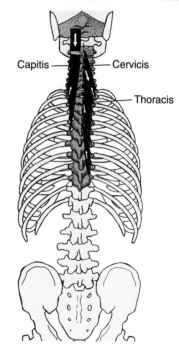

Posterior View

FIGURE 21-166

MULTIFIDUS

Latin: multus—many
fidus—to split

ORIGINS
Transverse process of one vertebral segment

INSERTIONS
Spinous processes of the second, third, and fourth vertebral
   segments above

ACTIONS
Rotates the vertebral column (unilateral contraction)
Laterally flexes the vertebral column (unilateral contraction)
Extends the vertebral column (bilateral contraction)

NERVES
Posterior rami of spinal nerves

Notes: **M**ultifidus is the **M**iddle transversospinalis and spans two to
four vertebrae. Multifidus lies over the rotatores and does not contain
subgroupings.

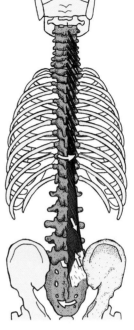

Posterior View

FIGURE 21-167

ROTATORES

Latin: rotare—to turn

ORIGINS
Transverse process of one vertebral segment

INSERTIONS
Spinous process of the first or second vertebral segment above

ACTIONS
Rotates the vertebral column (unilateral contraction)
Extends the vertebral column (bilateral contraction)

NERVES
Posterior rami of spinal nerves

Notes: Rotatores span one to two vertebrae. This is the deepest
transversospinalis and contains subgroupings of longus and brevis.

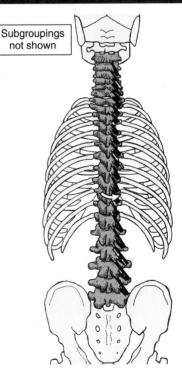

Subgroupings
not shown

Posterior View

FIGURE 21-168

ERECTOR SPINAE

Latin: erigere—to erect
spinatus—spine

Notes: The term erector spinae refers to the action of this muscle group—erection of the spine. From medial to lateral, the erector spinae muscles are *spinalis*, *longissimus*, and *iliocostalis* (see Figure 21-165). Each muscle can be further subdivided.

Also known as sacrospinalis, the erector spinae runs parallel to the spine, similar to a silo. The word **SILO** can be used as a mnemonic to recall the names of the erector spinae muscles: **S**pinalis, **IL**iocostalis, and **LO**ngissimus. These muscles lie next to one another, compared with the transversospinalis, which lie on top of one another.

SPINALIS

Latin: spinatus—spine

ORIGINS
Spinous processes of C4-T12
C7 and the nuchal ligament

INSERTIONS
Spinous processes of C2 and upper thoracic
Occipital bone (between the superior and inferior nuchal lines)

ACTIONS
Laterally flexes the vertebral column (unilateral contraction)
Extends the vertebral column (bilateral contraction)

NERVES
Posterior rami of thoracic and lower cervical spinal nerves

Notes: Spinalis is the most medial tract of the erector spinae group. The **spinalis hugs the spine** and lies in the lamina groove. The muscle's subgroupings are capitis, cervicis, and thoracis.

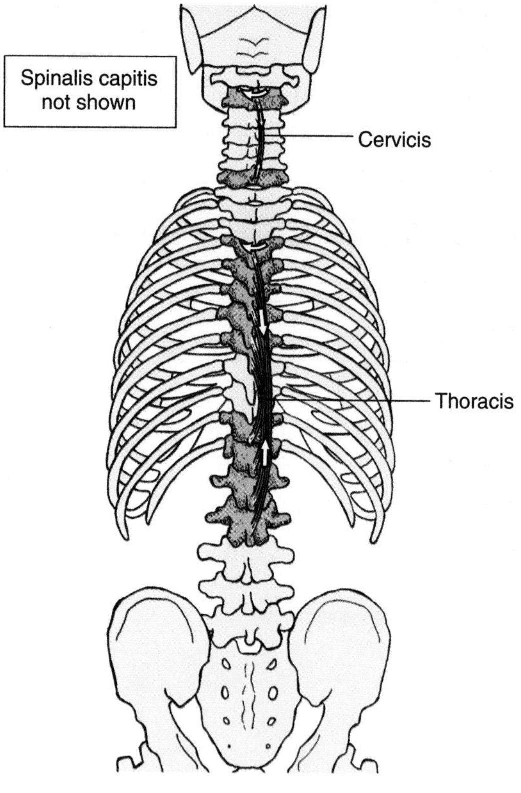

Spinalis capitis
not shown

Cervicis

Thoracis

Posterior View

FIGURE 21-169

LONGISSIMUS

Latin: longus—long

ORIGINS
Posterior sacrum
Transverse processes of T1-T5 and L1-L5
Transverse processes of C5-C7

INSERTIONS
Mastoid process
Transverse processes of C2-T12
Ribs 4 through 12 (posterior surface)

ACTIONS
Laterally flexes the vertebral column (unilateral contraction)
Rotates the vertebral column (unilateral contraction)
Extends the vertebral column (bilateral contraction)
Extends the head (bilateral contraction)

NERVE
Posterior rami of lumbar, thoracic, and lower cervical spinal
   nerves

Notes: *Longissimus* is the intermediate tract of erector spinae and covers a *long* territory stretching from sacrum to skull. This muscle's subgroupings are capitus, cervicis, and thoracis.

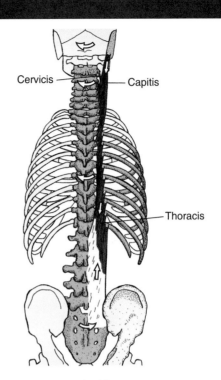

Posterior View

FIGURE 21-170

ILIOCOSTALIS

Latin: ilium—flank
costae—rib

ORIGINS
Posterior iliac crest
Posterior sacrum
Ribs 3 through 12 (posterior surface)

INSERTIONS
Ribs 1 through 12 (posterior surface)
Transverse processes of C4-C7

ACTIONS
Laterally flexes the vertebral column (unilateral contraction)
Extends the vertebral column (bilateral contraction)

NERVES
Posterior rami of upper lumbar, thoracic, and lower cervical
   spinal nerves

Notes: The iliocostalis is the lateral tract of the erector spinae group. The ilio*costal* hugs the *costals* (ribs). This muscle's subgroupings are the cervicis, thoracis, and lumborum.

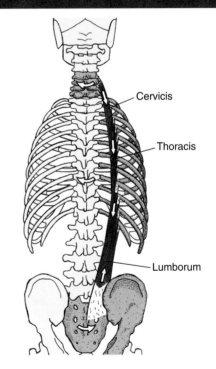

Posterior View

FIGURE 21-171

LESSON THIRTEEN REVIEW—MUSCLES OF VERTEBRAL COLUMN MOVEMENT

FLEXION	EXTENSION	LATERAL FLEXION	ROTATION
Psoas major	Quadratus lumborum	Rectus abdominis	External obliques
Rectus abdominis	Semispinalis	External obliques	Internal obliques
External obliques	Rotatores	Internal obliques	Semispinalis
Internal obliques	Multifidus	Quadratus lumborum	Rotatores
	Spinalis	Multifidus	Multifidus
	Longissimus	Spinalis	
	Iliocostalis	Longissimus	

LESSON FOURTEEN—MUSCLES OF RESPIRATION

Diaphragm, External Intercostals, Internal Intercostals, Serratus Posterior Superior, Serratus Posterior Inferior, Pectoralis Minor (Lesson Six), Scalenes (Lesson Twelve), Sternocleidomastoid (Lesson Twelve), Abdominals (Lesson Thirteen)

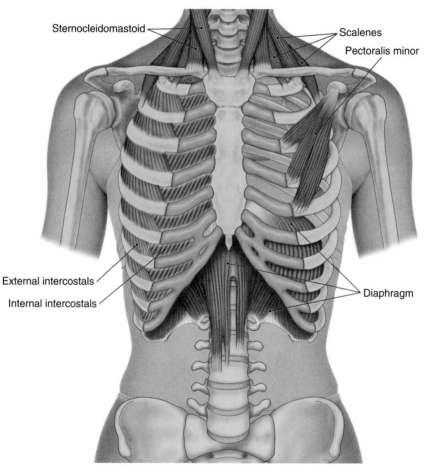

Anterior View

FIGURE 21-172 Select muscles of respiration.

DIAPHRAGM

Greek: diaphragma—a partition

ORIGINS
L1-L3
Lower six costal cartilages
Xiphoid process

INSERTION
Central tendon (cloverleaf-shaped aponeurosis)

ACTION
Expands the thoracic cavity during inhalation

NERVE
Phrenic nerve

Notes: The diaphragm divides the thoracic from the abdominal cavity and is the prime mover of inhalation. Because of its origins, the diaphragm possesses lumbar, costal, and sternal portions.

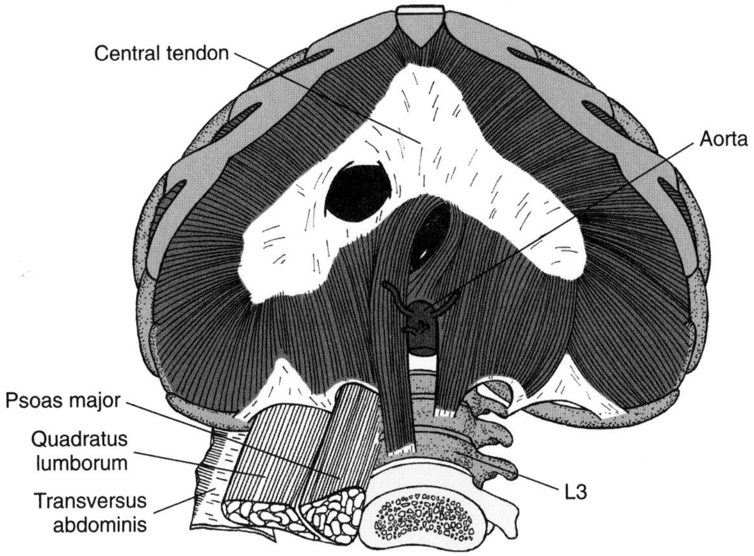

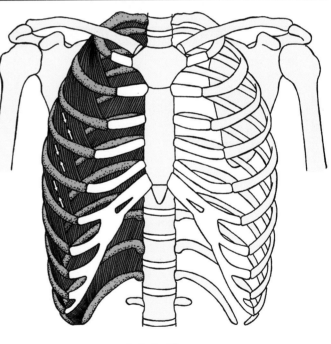

Inferior View

FIGURE 21-173

EXTERNAL INTERCOSTALS

Latin: externus—outside
internus—within
costae—rib

ORIGINS
Inferior border of rib (above)

INSERTIONS
Superior border of rib (below)

ACTIONS
Elevates the ribcage during inhalation
Maintains the intercostal spaces

NERVES
Intercostal nerves

Note: Fiber direction of external intercostals is the same as for external obliques.

Anterior View

FIGURE 21-174

INTERNAL INTERCOSTALS

Latin: internus—within
costae—rib

ORIGINS
Superior border of rib (below)

INSERTIONS
Inferior border of rib (above)

ACTIONS
Depresses the ribcage during exhalation
Maintains the intercostal spaces

NERVES
Intercostal nerves

Notes: As the name implies, internal intercostals are internal, or deep to, external intercostals and in between the ribs. Fiber direction of internal intercostals is the same as for internal obliques.

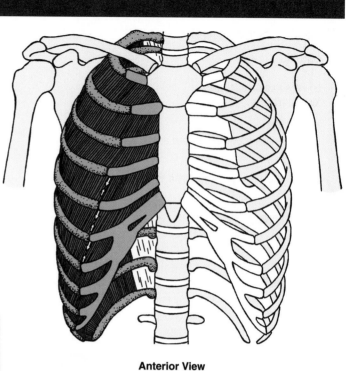

Anterior View

FIGURE 21-175

SERRATUS POSTERIOR SUPERIOR

Latin: serratus—notched or jagged, as a saw
posterus—behind
superus—upper

ORIGINS
Lower nuchal ligament
Spinous processes of C7-T3

INSERTIONS
Ribs 2 through 5 (posterior surface)

ACTION
Elevates the ribs during inhalation

NERVES
Intercostal nerves

Note: Deep to rhomboids, this and the following muscle aid in the process of labored breathing.

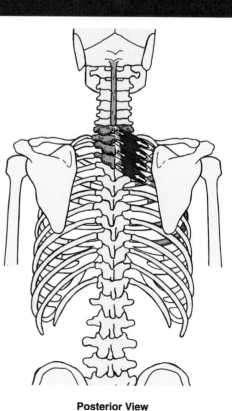

Posterior View

FIGURE 21-176

SERRATUS POSTERIOR INFERIOR

Latin: serratus—notched or jagged, as a saw
posterus—behind
infra—beneath

ORIGINS
Spinous processes of T11-L2

INSERTIONS
Ribs 9 through 12 (posterior surface)

ACTION
Depresses the ribs during exhalation

NERVES
Intercostal nerves (T9-T12)

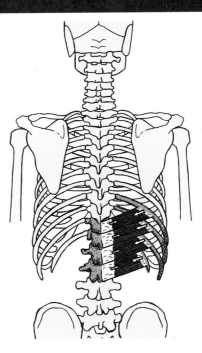

Posterior View
FIGURE 21-177

LESSON FOURTEEN: MUSCLES OF RESPIRATION

INHALATION	EXHALATION
Pectoralis minor	Internal intercostal
Scalenes	Serratus posterior inferior
Sternocleidomastoid	Abdominals (forced)
Diaphragm	
External intercostal	

E-RESOURCES

ⓔvolve

http://evolve.elsevier.com/Salvo/MassageTherapy

- Chapter challenge
- Flash cards
- Photo gallery
- Educational animations
- Weblinks

BIBLIOGRAPHY

Abrahams P, Marks S, Hutchings R: *McMinn's color atlas of human anatomy*, St Louis, 2003, Mosby.

Anderson SK: Personal communication, 2010.

Applegate EJ: *The anatomy and physiology learning system*, ed 3, Philadelphia, 2006, Saunders.

Ardoin W: *From a lecture on temporomandibular joint dysfunction given at the Louisiana Institute of Massage Therapy*, Lafayette, La, 1994, personal communication.

Biel A: *Trail guide to the body: how to locate muscles, bones, and more*, ed 3, Boulder, Colo, 2005, Books of Discovery.

Bowden B, Bowden J: *An illustrated atlas of the skeletal muscles*, Englewood, Colo, 2002, Morton.

Brossman AB: Some of the finer points about temporomandibular joint anatomy and physiology, CITYNET (website): http://www.ovnet.com/userpages/rebross/tmjoints.html. Accessed 8/12/10.

Como D, editor: *Mosby's medical, nursing, and allied health dictionary*, ed 6, St Louis, 2002, Mosby.

Crawley J, Van De Graaff KM: *A photographic atlas for anatomy and physiology*, Englewood, Colo, 2002, Morton.

Goldberg S: *Clinical anatomy made ridiculously simple*, Miami, 2004, Medmaster.

Grafelman T: *Graf's anatomy and physiology guide for the massage therapist*, Aurora, Colo, 1998, DG Publishing.

Gray H, Pick TP, Howden R: *Gray's anatomy*, ed 29, Philadelphia, 1974, Running Press.

Guyton A: *Human physiology and mechanisms of disease*, ed 6, Philadelphia, 1996, WB Saunders.

Haubrich WS: *Medical meanings: a glossary of word origins*, New York, 1984, Harcourt Brace Jovanovich.

Hoppenfeld S: *Physical examination of the spine and extremities*, Norwalk, Conn, 1976, Appleton-Century-Crofts.

Jacob S, Francone C: *Elements of anatomy and physiology*, Philadelphia, 1989, WB Saunders.

Juhan D: *Job's body: a handbook for bodyworkers*, ed 3, Barrington, NY, 2003, Station Hill Press.

Kapandji IA: *The physiology of the joints*, ed 5, New York, 1988, Churchill Livingstone.

Kapit W, Elson LM: *The anatomy coloring book*, ed 3, New York, 2002, Benjamin Cummings.

Kapit W, Macey R, Meisami E: *The physiology coloring book*, ed 2, New York, 1999, HarperCollins.

Kendall FP, McCreary EK: *Muscles: testing and function*, ed 3, Baltimore, 1983, Williams & Wilkins.

Kordish M, Dickson S: *Introduction to basic human anatomy*, Lake Charles, La, 1985, McNeese State University.

Lauderstein D: *Putting the soul back in the body: a manual of imaginative anatomy for massage therapists*, Chicago, 1985, self-published.

Lowe WW: *Functional assessment in massage therapy*, Corvallis, Ore, 1995, Pacific Orthopedic Massage.

Marieb EN: *Essentials of human anatomy and physiology*, ed 8, New York, 2005, Benjamin Cummings.

Martini FH, Bartholomew EF: *Essentials of anatomy and physiology*, ed 3, New York, 2003, Benjamin Cummings.

Mattes A: *Active isolated stretching*, Sarasota, Fla, 1995, self-published.

McAleer N: *The body almanac*, Garden City, NY, 1985, Doubleday.

McLaughlin C: *The bodyworker's muscle reference guide*, Bellevue, Colo, 1996, Bodyguide.

Merck manual, ed 17, Whitehouse Station, NJ, 1998, Merck Co.

Moore KL: *Clinically oriented anatomy*, ed 5, Baltimore, 2005, Lippincott Williams & Wilkins.

Muscolino JE: *Kinesiology: the skeletal system and muscle function*, ed 2, St Louis, 2011, Mosby.

Muscolino JE: *The muscular system manual: the skeletal muscles of the human body*, ed 3, St Louis, 2010, Elsevier Mosby.

Myers TW: *Anatomy trains: myofascial meridians for manual and movement therapists*, New York, 2001, Churchill Livingstone.

Netter FH: *Atlas of human anatomy*, ed 3, Teterboro, NJ, 2003, Icon Learning Systems.

Olsen A, McHose C: *Body stories: a guide to experiential anatomy*, Barrytown, NY, 2004, Station Hill Press.

Patton K, Thibodeau G: *Anatomy and physiology*, ed 7, St Louis, 2010, Mosby.

Platzer W: *Color atlas and textbook of human anatomy: locomotor system*, vol I, ed 5, New York, 2003, Thieme.

Rolf IP: *Rolfing: the integration of human structures*, New York, 1977, Harper & Row.

Sieg K, Adams S: *Illustrated essentials of musculoskeletal anatomy*, ed 3, Gainesville, Fla, 1996, Megabooks.

Solomon EP, Phillips GA: *Understanding human anatomy and physiology*, Philadelphia, 1987, WB Saunders.

Souza TA: *Differential diagnosis and management for the chiropractor*, ed 2, Gaithersburg, Md, 2001, Aspen.

St John P: *St John neuromuscular therapy seminars: manual I*, Largo, Fla, 1995, self-published.

Thibodeau G, Patton K: *Structure and function of the body*, ed 12, St Louis, 2004, Mosby.

Tortora GJ: *Introduction to the human body: the essentials of anatomy and physiology*, ed 5, Hoboken, NJ, 2000, John Wiley & Sons.

Tortora GJ, Grabowksi SR: *Principles of anatomy and physiology*, ed 11, New York, 2005, John Wiley & Sons.

Travell JG, Simons D: *Myofascial pain and dysfunction, the trigger point manual*, Baltimore, 1992, Lippincott Williams & Wilkins.

Venes D, Thomas CL, Taber CW: *Taber's cyclopedic medical dictionary*, ed 20, Philadelphia, 2005, FA Davis.

Warfel JH: *The extremities: muscles and motor points*, ed 6, Baltimore, 1992, Lippincott Williams & Wilkins.

Warfel JH: *The head, neck, and trunk*, ed 6, Baltimore, 1993, Lippincott Williams & Wilkins.

Wilson JM: *Doctoral dissertation: a natural philosophy of movement styles for theatre performers*, Madison, Wis, 1973, University of Wisconsin-Madison.

MATCHING I

Place the letter of the answer next to the term or phrase that best describes it.

A. Deltoid tuberosity
B. Glenoid cavity
C. Head
D. Humerus
E. Lunate
F. Olecranon process
G. Pectoral girdle
H. Radius
I. Scapula
J. Sternal
K. Thumb
L. Ulna

_____ 1. Composed of the clavicle and scapula

_____ 2. Medial forearm bone

_____ 3. Located on the lateral side of the scapula

_____ 4. Lateral forearm bone

_____ 5. Located on the lateral humerus

_____ 6. Term for the medial end of the clavicle

_____ 7. Term synonymous with *shoulder blade*

_____ 8. Located on the proximal end of the radius

_____ 9. Term synonymous with *arm bone*

_____ 10. Carpal bone

_____ 11. Possesses only a proximal and distal phalanx

_____ 12. Located on the proximal posterior ulna

MATCHING II

Place the letter of the answer next to the term or phrase that best describes it.

A. Acetabulum
B. Cuneiforms
C. Femur
D. Great toe

E. Iliac crest
F. Lateral malleolus
G. Linea aspera
H. Medial malleolus

I. Pelvic bone
J. Tibia
K. Tibial tuberosity
L. Transverse

_____ 1. Located on the superior portion of the pelvic bone

_____ 2. Located on the posterior femur

_____ 3. Located on the proximal tibia

_____ 4. Located on the distal tibia

_____ 5. Group of tarsals that include individual medial, intermediate, and lateral bones

_____ 6. Term synonymous with *hip socket*

_____ 7. Foot arch formed by the cuboid, cuneiformis I-III and metatarsal heads

_____ 8. Bone that includes the ilium, ischium and pubis

_____ 9. Located on the distal fibula

_____ 10. Medial leg bone

_____ 11. Possesses only a proximal and distal phalanx

_____ 12. Term synonymous with *thigh bone*

MATCHING III

Place the letter of the answer next to the term or phrase that best describes it.

A. 8
B. 14
C. Frontal bone
D. Hyoid bone

E. Mandible
F. Mastoid process
G. Occipital bone
H. Sagittal suture

I. Skull
J. Sphenoid bone
K. Temporal bone
L. Zygomatic bone

_____ 1. Does not articulate directly with any other bone

_____ 2. Includes the cranial and facial bones

_____ 3. Number of cranial bones

_____ 4. Bony marking on temporal bone

_____ 5. Cheekbone

_____ 6. Contains the foramen magnum

_____ 7. Joins the parietal bones

_____ 8. Contains the external auditory meatus

_____ 9. Number of facial bones

_____ 10. Forehead bone

_____ 11. Contains the sella turcica

_____ 12. Jawbone

MATCHING IV

Place the letter of the answer next to the term or phrase that best describes it.

A. 5
B. 12
C. Atlas
D. Axis

E. Coccyx
F. False
G. Intervertebral disc
H. Nuchal

I. Spinous process
J. Thorax
K. Vertebral canal
L. Xiphoid process

_____ 1. Part of the vertebra that projects posteriorly

_____ 2. Ligament that extends from the occipital bone to all spinous processes of the cervical vertebrae

_____ 3. Bone located at the inferior end of the vertebral column

_____ 4. Fibrocartilaginous tissue located between each unfused vertebral body

_____ 5. Number of lumbar vertebrae

_____ 6. Ribs that articulate indirectly with the sternum via costal cartilages

_____ 7. Term synonymous with *C1*

_____ 8. Located at the inferior portion of the sternum

_____ 9. Consists of the sternum, ribs, and thoracic vertebrae

_____ 10. Term synonymous with *C2*

_____ 11. Number of thoracic vertebrae

_____ 12. Vertebral structure for which the spinal cord passes

MATCHING V

Place the letter of the answer next to the term or phrase that best describes it.

A. Abduction
B. Anterior tilt
C. Biaxial joint
D. Elevation

E. Flexion
F. Knee
G. Plantar flexion
H. Retraction

I. Rotation
J. Shoulder
K. Supination
L. Triaxial joint

_____ 1. Movement backwards

_____ 2. Raising or lifting a body part

_____ 3. Lateral (outward) rotation of the forearm so that the palm is turned up

_____ 4. Term used to describe a forward tilt of the pelvis

_____ 5. Extension of the ankle so that the toes are pointing downward

_____ 6. Movement away from the median plane

_____ 7. Joint type that allows movement in two planes

_____ 8. Joint type that allows movement in three planes

_____ 9. Tibiofemoral joint

_____ 10. Movement around a central axis

_____ 11. Glenohumeral joint

_____ 12. Bending or decreasing the angle of a joint

MATCHING VI

Place the letter of the answer next to the term or phrase that best describes it.

A. Anterior medial border of scapula
B. Christmas tree muscles
C. Coracoid process of scapula
D. Depress the scapula

E. Downwardly rotate scapula
F. Insertions of trapezius
G. Levator scapulae
H. Pectoralis minor
I. Rhomboids, middle trapezius

J. Serratus anterior
K. Transverse processes of C1-C4
L. Trapezius

_____ 1. Lateral third of clavicle, acromion process, and scapular spine

_____ 2. Common action of levator scapulae, rhomboids, and pectoralis minor

_____ 3. Origin of levator scapula

_____ 4. Known as the neurovascular entrapper

_____ 5. Originates on ribs 1 through 8 or 9

_____ 6. Insertion of serratus anterior

_____ 7. Rhomboids major and minor

_____ 8. Retracts the scapula

_____ 9. Insertion of pectoralis minor

_____ 10. Muscle that is named for its action

_____ 11. Coat hanger muscle

_____ 12. Common action of lower fibers of trapezius, serratus anterior, and pectoralis minor

MATCHING VII

Place the letter of the answer next to the term or phrase that best describes it.

A. Adduct the shoulder joint
B. Coracobrachialis
C. Deltoid
D. Extend the shoulder joint
E. Infraspinous fossa

F. Latissimus dorsi
G. Medially rotate the shoulder joint
H. Pectoralis major
I. Rotator cuff muscles

J. Subscapularis
K. Supraspinatus, infraspinatus, teres minor
L. Teres major

_____ 1. Origin of infraspinatus

_____ 2. Common action of latissimus dorsi, teres major, subscapularis, anterior deltoid, and pectoralis major

_____ 3. Common action of latissimus dorsi, teres major, posterior deltoid, pectoralis major, and triceps brachii

_____ 4. Supraspinatus, infraspinatus, teres minor, and subscapularis

_____ 5. Attaches from the inferior third of the lateral border of the scapula to the intertubercular groove of the humerus

_____ 6. Inserts on the greater tubercle of the humerus

_____ 7. Attaches from the medial half of the clavicle, edge of the sternal body, and ribs 1 through 7 to the intertubercular groove of the humerus

_____ 8. Inserts on the coracoid process of the scapula

_____ 9. Common action of latissimus dorsi, teres major, teres minor, pectoralis major, coracobrachialis and triceps brachii

_____ 10. Swimmer's muscle; widest muscle of the body

_____ 11. Contains anterior, middle, and posterior fibers

_____ 12. Frozen shoulder muscle

MATCHING VIII

Place the letter of the answer next to the term or phrase that best describes it.

A. Biceps brachii
B. Brachialis
C. Brachioradialis
D. Common flexor tendon

E. Extend the elbow
F. Flex the elbow
G. Olecranon process
H. Pollicis

I. Pronator quadratus
J. Supinate the forearm
K. Supinator
L. Triceps brachii

_____ 1. Attaches from the lateral epicondyle of the humerus, proximal eighth of ulnar shaft, radial collateral ligament, and annular ligament to the proximal lateral radial shaft

_____ 2. Shared tendinous attachment for five muscles

_____ 3. Pronates the forearm

_____ 4. Term synonymous with *thumb*

_____ 5. Common action of triceps brachii and anconeus

_____ 6. Attaches from the lateral supracondylar ridge of the humerus to the styloid process of the radius

_____ 7. Boxer's muscle because it delivers a straight-arm knockout punch

_____ 8. Most effective arm flexor because of its mechanical advantage

_____ 9. Insertion of triceps brachii

_____ 10. Common action of biceps brachii and supinator

_____ 11. Common action of biceps brachii, brachialis, brachioradialis, pronator teres, and flexor carpi radialis

_____ 12. Corkscrew muscle

MATCHING IX

Place the letter of the answer next to the term or phrase that best describes it.

A. Extend the wrist
B. Extensor digiti minimi
C. Extensor indicis
D. Flex the fingers
E. Flex the wrist

F. Flexor digiti minimi
G. Lateral epicondyle of the humerus
H. Lateral epicondylitis

I. Medial epicondyle of the humerus
J. Medial epicondylitis
K. Opponens digiti minimi
L. Opponens pollicis

_____ 1. Term synonymous with *golfer's elbow*

_____ 2. Common action of flexor digitorum superficialis and flexor digitorum profundus

_____ 3. Extends the index finger

_____ 4. Where the common flexor tendon attaches

_____ 5. Common action of extensor carpi radialis longus and brevis, extensor carpi ulnaris, and extensor digitorum

_____ 6. Common action of flexor carpi radialis, flexor carpi ulnaris, palmaris longus, flexor digitorum superficialis and flexor digitorum profundus

_____ 7. Term synonymous with *tennis elbow*

_____ 8. Moves the little finger into opposition

_____ 9. Extends the little finger

_____ 10. Where the common extensor tendon attaches

_____ 11. Moves the thumb into opposition

_____ 12. Flexes the little finger

MATCHING X

Place the letter of the answer next to the term or phrase that best describes it.

A. Adduct the hip
B. Adductor magnus
C. Biceps femoris
D. Gluteus maximus

E. Iliopsoas
F. Medially rotate the hip
G. Pes anserine
H. Piriformis

I. Quadratus femoris
J. Rectus femoris
K. Sartorius
L. Tibial tuberosity

_____ 1. Common action of gluteus medius, gluteus minimus, tensor fasciae latae, semimembranosus, and semitendinosus

_____ 2. Insertion for the quadriceps femoris

_____ 3. Strongest hip extensor

_____ 4. Common action of gluteus maximus, gracilis, adductor magnus, adductor longus, and adductor brevis

_____ 5. Tailor's muscle

_____ 6. Lateral hamstring muscle

_____ 7. Only quadriceps femoris muscles that crosses both the hip and knee joints

_____ 8. Common tendinous insertion for sartorius, gracilis, and semitendinosus

_____ 9. Collective term used for the anterior thigh muscles

_____ 10. Main flexor of the hip

_____ 11. Attaches from the ischial tuberosity, inferior pubic ramus, ischial ramus to the linea aspera and adductor tubercle of the femur

_____ 12. Largest of all the hip lateral rotators

MATCHING XI

Place the letter of the answer next to the term or phrase that best describes it.

A. Calcaneus via the Achilles tendon
B. Evert the foot
C. Extensor digitorum longus and brevis
D. First layer of plantar aspect of foot
E. Flexor hallucis longus
F. Gastrocnemius
G. Metatarsal I and cuneiform I
H. Plantaris
I. Soleus
J. Third layer of plantar aspect of foot
K. Tibialis anterior
L. Triceps surae

_____ 1. Regarded as a mini-gastrocnemius because of its common insertion and missing about 10% of cadavers

_____ 2. Common action of fibularis longus, brevis and tertius, and extensor digitorum longus

_____ 3. Abductor hallucis, flexor digitorum brevis, and abductor digiti minimi

_____ 4. Insertions for both tibialis anterior and fibularis longus

_____ 5. Term used to describe gastrocnemius and soleus

_____ 6. Plantarflexes the ankle; known as the *toe dancer's muscle* because it helps ballerinas stand on their toes

_____ 7. Flexor hallucis brevis, adductor hallucis, and flexor digiti minimi brevis

_____ 8. Originates on the superior posterior third of the fibular shaft and soleal line of the tibia

_____ 9. Dorsiflexes the ankle and inverts the foot

_____ 10. Flexes the great toe

_____ 11. Extend toes 2-5

_____ 12. Common insertion for gastrocnemius, soleus, and plantaris

MATCHING XII

Place the letter of the answer next to the term or phrase that best describes it.

A. Facial nerve
B. Flex the neck
C. Muscles of mastication
D. Occipitofrontalis
E. Orbicularis oculi
F. Orbicularis oris
G. Platysma
H. Rotate the neck
I. Scalenes
J. Sternocleidomastoid
K. Suboccipitals
L. Trigeminal nerve

_____ 1. Common action of trapezius, longus colli, sternocleidomastoid, scalenes, splenius capitis and cervicis, rectus capitis posterior major, and oblique capitis inferior

_____ 2. Ghost headache muscles

_____ 3. Attaches from the manubrium of the sternum and medial third of the clavicle to the mastoid process and lateral half of the superior nuchal line

_____ 4. Assists in dozens of activities such as eating, drinking, talking, and sucking

_____ 5. What temporalis, masseter, and medial and lateral pterygoids are known as

_____ 6. Innervates occipitofrontalis, orbicularis oculi, orbicularis oris, and platysma

_____ 7. Known as the winking or blinking muscle

_____ 8. These, along with pectoralis minor, are known as the neurovascular entrappers; laterally flex the neck

_____ 9. Tenses the skin of the anterior neck, creating ridges

_____ 10. Common action of longus capitis, longus colli, sternocleidomastoid, scalenus anterior and scalenus medius

_____ 11. Innervates temporalis, masseter, and medial and lateral pterygoids

_____ 12. Term synonymous with *epicranius*

MATCHING XIII

Place the letter of the answer next to the term or phrase that best describes it.

A. Deep paraspinal muscles
B. Erector spinae muscles
C. Extend the vertebral column
D. Iliocostalis

E. Linea alba
F. Quadratus lumborum
G. Rectus abdominis
H. Ribs 5-12

I. Rotate the vertebral column
J. Segmental muscles
K. Semispinalis
L. Transverse abdominis

_____ 1. Most superficial transversospinalis and runs in cervical and thoracic regions only

_____ 2. Term used when referring to the interspinales and intertransversarii muscles

_____ 3. The most lateral erector spinae muscle

_____ 4. Term used to describe semispinalis, rotatores, and multifidus

_____ 5. Common action of external obliques, internal obliques, semispinalis, rotatores, and multifidus

_____ 6. Deepest abdominal muscle

_____ 7. Collective term for spinalis, longissimus and iliocostalis

_____ 8. A tendinous structure located on the anterior abdominal wall

_____ 9. Common action of quadratus lumborum, semispinalis, rotatores, multifidus, spinalis, longissimus, and iliocostalis

_____ 10. Attaches to the xiphoid process and the ribs; flexes the vertebral column

_____ 11. Hip hiker muscle

_____ 12. Insertion of external obliques

MATCHING XIV

Place the letter of the answer next to the term or phrase that best describes it.

A. Central tendon
B. Depress ribs during exhalation
C. Diaphragm
D. Elevate ribs during inhalation

E. External intercostals
F. Forced exhalation
G. Inferior border of rib above
H. Internal intercostals

I. Phrenic nerve
J. Serratus posterior inferior
K. Serratus posterior superior
L. Superior border of rib below

_____ 1. Originates on the spinous processes of T11-L2

_____ 2. Intercostal muscle that depresses the rib cage during exhalation

_____ 3. Innervates the diaphragm

_____ 4. Type of breathing that occurs when the abdominals contract

_____ 5. Intercostal muscle that elevates the rib cage during inhalation

_____ 6. Common action of scalenes, pectoralis minor, external intercostals, and serratus posterior superior

_____ 7. Insertion for internal intercostals

_____ 8. Originates on the lower nuchal ligament and the spinous processes of C7-T3

_____ 9. Prime mover of inhalation

_____ 10. Insertion of the diaphragm

_____ 11. Insertion for external intercostals

_____ 12. Common action of internal intercostals and serratus posterior inferior

CASE STUDY

Heal the Pain

About a month ago, Erik completed continuing education courses in orthopedic massage.

Jackie, one of Erik's regulars with chronic neck pain, is scheduled for a 1.5-hour treatment today. Erik is excited about applying his new knowledge and skills. When Jackie arrives, she is agitated. She tells Erik that her neck really hurts today. He immediately begins to notice imbalance in her feet and ankles. Jackie explains that it's been a difficult week, and that all she wants is to slip away for an hour and a half while Erik provides a full-body, general relaxation massage. Erik begins to explain what he's learned, and that he thinks treatment targeting more specific potential causes of her neck pain could be beneficial. Jackie shyly tells Erik that he's the expert and knows what's best, but Erik suspects that she's not as excited as he is about a clinical assessment and treatment. He feels so confident that he can make an informed assessment and develop a treatment plan that might just end her pain, but is today the day to start this treatment plan?

Reviewing the importance of intention, what do you think is the best way for Erik to proceed?

What consequences may result if Erik decides that the best thing to do is to treat her postural imbalance even though Jackie doesn't seem interested today?

If Erik decides not to push the specific treatment, will he fulfill any treatment goals with a general relaxation massage?

Review the concepts of speed, rhythm, and the therapeutic effects of Swedish massage strokes, and discuss which may be most appropriate to reduce Jackie's anxiety and to relieve her neck pain. Which should be avoided?

Can Erik incorporate other techniques discussed in this chapter that will allow him to provide some of the benefits of specific massage while allowing Jackie to remain completely relaxed during the session?

Should Erik continue to try to work with Jackie to plan specific treatment for her chronic pain? If so, when, and how?

CRITICAL THINKING

One of your clients tells you he has just had surgery to repair a torn rotator cuff. Where is this structure located, and why is it so susceptible to tearing? What type of motion or injury might have led to this tear?

CHAPTER 22

Integumentary System

> "The skin is no more separate from the brain than the surface of a lake is separate from its depths. They are two different locations in a continuous medium. To touch the surface is to stir the depths."
>
> —Deane Juhan

LEARNING OBJECTIVES

After completing this chapter, the student should be able to:

- List the anatomy and physiology of the skin.
- Define the regions of the skin and give characteristics of each.
- Identify and discuss several factors that contribute to skin color.
- Explain characteristics of hair.
- Contrast and compare sudoriferous and sebaceous glands.
- Name the main parts of a nail.
- Discuss the nervous system's role in touch and list touch receptors.
- Describe several pioneers in touch research.
- Name types of pathologic skin conditions, giving characteristics and the massage considerations for each.

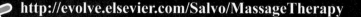

INTRODUCTION

The integumentary system includes the skin and its appendages such as the hair, nails, and glands that produce oil or sweat. The skin is the largest and heaviest organ of the body and it houses sensory receptors of pressure, pain, heat, cold, movement, and vibration. In fact, more than one-half million sensory receptors are found in the skin.

While the skin contains all types of tissue types, it is composed mostly of connective tissue underneath a layer of epithelial tissue. The skin is supported by a layer of fat, which is lost with aging. Absence of subcutaneous fat contributes to wrinkles and age spots.

The skin forms natural openings such as the mouth, external ear canal, nose, urethra, vagina, and anus. These passageways to the digestive, respiratory, urinary, and reproductive systems can be classified as extensions of the external environment. No other body system is more easily exposed to infections, disease, pollution, or injury than the skin, yet no other body system is as strong and resilient.

The appearance of the skin reflects our physiology. Information about a person's nutrition, hygiene habits, circulation, age, immunity, genetics, and environmental factors can be noted from the condition of the skin.

Not only does it reveal vital physiologic data (e.g., circulation, fever), but the skin also mirrors our emotional self. Through muscular expression and neurologic impulses, the skin, along with underlying muscles, has the power to reflect an ever-changing stream of emotions. How people feel about themselves and others is reflected on the surface of the skin.

CHAT ROOM

The skin covers an area of approximately 22 sq ft and weighs approximately 9 lb, making up 7% of body weight. A piece of skin the size of a quarter contains more than 3 million cells, 100 sweat glands, 50 nerve endings, and 3 feet of blood vessels. The skin is thinnest over the eyelids and thickest on the soles of the feet. The fingertips have approximately 700 touch receptors on 2 mm² of surface area.

ANATOMY

Basic anatomic structures of the integumentary system are:
* Skin
* Hair
* Nails
* Skin glands

PHYSIOLOGY

The functions of the integumentary system are:
* **Protection.** One of the functions of the skin is protection by acting as a physical, biologic, and chemical barrier.

The skin's physical barrier is essential for protecting underlying tissues from injury. The skin also provides limited protection from ultraviolet (UV) radiation through pigmentation. As a biologic barrier, intact skin is an effective barrier against many pathogens (e.g., bacteria). Secretions provided by the skin's glands inhibit growth of many pathogens by providing an acid mantle, which is a chemical barrier.

* **Absorption.** The skin has limited properties of absorption. Substances that can be absorbed by the skin are fat-soluble molecules (oxygen, carbon dioxide), fat-soluble vitamins (A, D, E, and K), steroids, resins of certain plants (poison ivy and poison oak), and salts of heavy metals (lead, mercury, and nickel). The use of topical medicated patches is based on the absorption properties of the skin.
* **Sensation.** The skin is considered an extension of the nervous system. It receives stimuli such as pressure, pain, and temperature.
* **Body temperature regulation.** An increase in blood circulation to the skin's surface is how skin plays a role in body temperature regulation. As blood moves to the skin's surface and blood vessels dilate, heat is discharged. Heat can also be dissipated through the evaporation of sweat produced by sweat glands. A limited amount of heat conservation is provided through shivering.
* **Waste elimination.** The skin functions as a mini-excretory system, eliminating wastes through sweating. Sweat, a waste product, is a mixture of 98% water and 2% solids (i.e., salt ions, lactic acid, and other metabolic wastes). By contrast, urine is 96% water and 4% solids.
* **Vitamin D synthesis.** Located in the skin are molecules that are converted to vitamin D by the UV rays in sunlight (with a little help from liver and kidney enzymes). Little UV light is required for this to occur. In fact, only 15 minutes of exposure to UV light daily is required for adequate amounts of vitamin D to be synthesized by the body; prolonged sunbathing is actually unnecessary.
* **Immunity.** Specialized cells, called *Langerhans cells*, trigger immunologic reactions.

REGIONS OF THE SKIN

The skin is composed of two major regions: the epidermis and the dermis. The epidermis consists of four or five layers (discussed later). Located beneath the epidermis is the dermis, which contains blood vessels, nerve receptors, hair follicles, and skin glands. A dermal-epidermal junction joins these two regions together. Underneath the skin is a layer of tissue known as the subcutaneous layer.

EPIDERMIS

The **epidermis** is the outer region of the skin and is composed of epithelial tissue. Cells within the epidermis are

IT'S ALL GREEK TO ME

acne vulgaris	*Gr.* point; common or ordinary common acne
bruise	*O. Fr.* to break
corium	*L.* leather, skin
cutaneous	*L.* skin
cuticle	*L.* little skin
decubitus	*L.* lying down
dermis	*Gr.* skin
eczema	*L.* to boil out
epidermis	*Gr.* upon or over skin
follicle	*L.* sac, small
boil	*AS.* sore
granulosum	*L.* grain, small
integument	*L.* a covering
Krause	German anatomist (1833-1910)
lacrimal	*L.* tear
lucidum	*L.* clear
Meissner	German histologist (1829-1905)
melano	*Gr.* black
Pacini	Italian anatomist (1812-1883)
palpate	*L.* stroke or touch
psoriasis	*Gr.* itching
Ruffini	Italian anatomist (1864-1929)
scleroderma	*Gr.* hard, skin
seborrhea	*L.* tallow, to flow
sebum	*L.* grease, tallow
stratum	*L.* a layer, cover, or spread
sudoriferous	*L.* sweat, to carry or bear
verruc	*L.* wart

Fr., French; *Gr.*, Greek; *L.*, Latin; *O.Fr.* Old French; *AS.* Anglo Saxon.

formed in the deeper layers. The epidermis itself is relatively avascular; therefore nutrients are provided by tissue fluids from the underlying dermis.

The epidermis is derived from ectoderm, the same embryonic cell layer that gives us the brain, spinal cord, and special senses. The epidermis also contains pores, which allow passage for hair and specialized glands.

Epidermal Cells

The epidermis contains several types of cells. These are keratinocytes, melanocytes, and Langerhans cells.

Keratinocytes. Keratinocytes are cells that produce *keratin*, a tough fibrous protein that gives the skin protection. Also, keratinocytes secrete a lipid substance that forms a waterproof barrier between cells. This liquid and the fibrous protein keratin help keep foreign entities out while keeping fluids in. Keratinocytes make up more than 90% of epidermal cells and form the principal structures of outer skin. Where the epidermis enters open body cavities (e.g., nasal or oral cavity), the mucous membrane simply lacks the skin's keratinization.

Melanocyte. These cells produce *melanin* or pigment, which contribute to skin color and serve to reduce the amount of UV light that can penetrate into the deeper layers of the skin. Melanocytes are also found in hair and the eye's iris. Both melanocyte-stimulating hormone from the pituitary and genetics determine the amount of melanin produced in an individual.

UV light stimulates the formation of melanin and causes darkening of the melanin granules. Melanin serves as a protective shield for the skin from the damaging effects of sunlight.

Langerhans Cells. These cells function, along with helper T cells, to trigger useful immunologic reactions. Langerhans cells originate in bone marrow but migrate to the deep layers of the epidermis in early life.

⊖volve *Use your student account from the Evolve website to view images of various skin pigmentations such as a freckled face, an albino child, vitiligo, and chloasma.* ∎

Epidermal Layers

Four epidermal layers, or *strata*, are typically found. However, in areas where friction is greatest (i.e., soles of the feet, palms of the hands) an extra layer of skin exists. From deepest to most superficial, these layers are the *stratum germinativum, stratum spinosum, stratum granulosum, stratum lucidum,* and *stratum corneum* (Figure 22-1).

- **Stratum germinativum:** This is the deepest epidermal layer. The stratum germinativum, or stratum basale, undergoes continuous cell division and generates all other layers. This layer also contains Merkel disks, which are pressure receptors.
- **Stratum spinosum:** The stratum spinosum, or *spiny layer,* is a bonding and transitional layer between the stratum granulosum and the stratum germinativum, possessing cells of both these layers.
- **Stratum granulosum:** This cell layer contains an accumulation of keratin granules, marking the beginning of skin drying and sloughing.
- **Stratum lucidum:** Found only in the thick skin of palms and soles, this translucent layer is found between the stratum corneum and stratum granulosum. In thin skin, the stratum lucidum is absent.

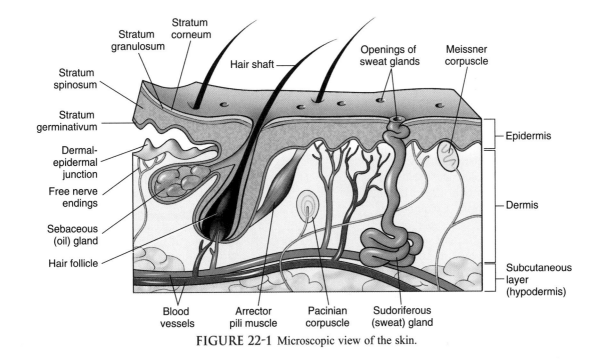

FIGURE 22-1 Microscopic view of the skin.

- **Stratum corneum:** This layer is the outermost layer of the skin. By the time the epidermal cells reach the surface, they have become completely keratinized, are no longer living, and are ready to be sloughed off.

Epidermal Growth

As surface cells of the stratum corneum are lost, replacement of epidermal cells by cell division is occurring in the stratum germinativum. New cells must be formed at approximately the same rate that old keratinized cells flake off to maintain a constant thickness of the epidermis. Cells push upward from the stratum germinativum into each consecutive layer, die, become keratinized, and eventually *desquamate* (fall away), as did their predecessors. Superficial epidermal cells are constantly being sloughed off in an endless renewal process. The entire life cycle of skin cells is 21 to 27 days.

Dermal-Epidermal Junction

Between the epidermis and the dermis is a specialized area where cells of the two regions meet. This basement membrane is called the dermal-epidermal junction and is easily identifiable with an electron microscope.

The dermal-epidermal junction not only cements the epidermis to the dermis but also provides support for the epidermis. Additionally, this junction serves as a partial barrier to the passage of some cells and large molecules.

DERMIS

Also known as the corium, or *hide,* the **dermis** is the inner region of skin. The dermis, or "true skin," contains blood vessels, sensory nerve receptors, hair follicles, muscles, sweat and oil glands, and connective tissue. Its rich vascular network plays a critical role in regulating body temperature (Figure 22-2). The dermis can contain as much as 5% of the blood in our bodies.

The dermis is generally thicker on the posterior aspect of the body and is thicker in men than it is in women; this difference may be the result of presence of certain hormones. More specifically, the dermis is thickest on the palms of the hands and soles of the feet and quite thin over the eyelids.

The connective tissue component of the dermis is mostly collagen and elastin fibers. Collagen constitutes approximately 70% of the dermis and offers support to the nerves, blood vessels, hair follicles, and glands. Within collagen fibers are the pliable *elastin fibers,* which give the skin its elasticity and resilience.

The loss of elasticity can be accelerated by excessive exposure to UV rays; perhaps one of the best ways to prevent premature wrinkling is to protect the skin from exposure to the sun. Avoiding the process of aging is impossible, but good nutrition, plenty of fluids, and daily skin care can retard the process.

Dermal Growth and Repair

The dermis does not continually shed and regenerate itself, in contrast with the cells of the epidermis. However, when

ASHLEY MONTAGU, PhD

Born: June 28, 1905; died: November 16, 1999

"To be kind, to be, to do, and to depart gracefully."

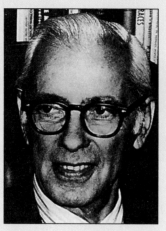

Born in London, Ashley Montagu studied at the University of London and the University of Florence before coming to the United States in 1927. He earned his doctorate from Columbia University in 1937. That same year, he published his first book, *Coming into Being Among the Aborigines*. Between 1937 and 1988, he authored more than 50 books.

Montagu's long and distinguished academic career included positions at some of the most respected schools in the country. He was a professor of anatomy at Hahnemann Medical College and Hospital, Philadelphia, from 1938 to 1949; chairman of the Department of Anthropology at Rutgers University from 1940 to 1955; and a lecturer at Princeton University from 1978 to 1983. During this period, Montagu held many other concurrent positions in education, professional associations, the United Nations, and the media.

Montagu realized that touch is an enormously important experience for every human being, not only from birth but also from the moment that life begins in the womb. As a professor of anatomy and anthropology, he was inspired to begin researching the effects of touch and nurturing after reading an article on the effects of thyroid surgery on two groups of rodents. The first group, with a 75% survival rate, was cared for by a female physician who caressed each rodent at feeding time. In the second group, the animals all died rapidly. They were cared for by a male laboratory attendant who threw food into the cages and roughly clanged the door. The article noted this difference in treatment but attached no significance to it; however, Montagu did. After he shared this study with a class that he was teaching, a student from a farming area told Montagu that everyone knows that newborn animals must be licked by their mother or they soon die. Notions such as these were the clues that led Montagu to begin his research on effective nurturing. As a scientist, Montagu scientifically solved the mysteries concerning the attributes that make up what we understand to be love. In his own words, "It [love] is the communication to another, by demonstrative acts, of your profound involvement in their welfare."

Montagu's works have emphasized that a healthy mental state results from effective nurturing. Of his own findings, he says, "the most surprising of all things was that doctors had rarely understood this."

Most of Montagu's written work deals in some way with the human condition. His book *Touching: The Human Significance of the Skin* is a must-read resource for all massage therapists. He is also well known for *The Elephant Man* and *Man's Most Dangerous Myth: The Fallacy of Race*.

Montagu's awards included the following:
- Distinguished Achievement Award from the American Anthropological Association (1987)
- Darwin Award from the American Association of Physical Anthropologists (1994)
- American Humanist of the Year Award (1995)

Montagu received more than a dozen major awards and two honorary doctoral degrees during his long and prolific career. When asked once what he would like future massage therapists to remember, he said, "To understand that what they are doing is very important indeed. That by caressing another human being's body, in which you are trained to do, I hope, by communicating this involvement in their welfare, what you are doing is what human beings should always be doing, all the days of their lives—caressing other people."

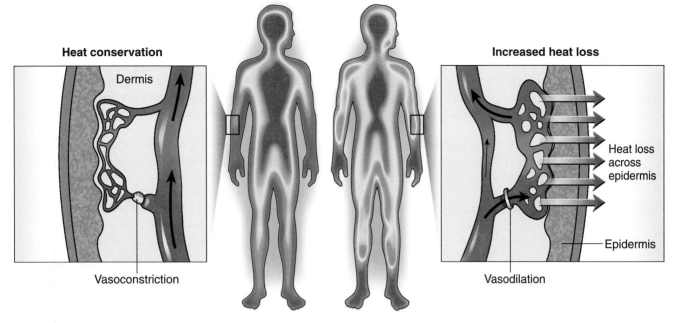

Heat conservation

Dermis

Vasoconstriction

Increased heat loss

Heat loss
across
epidermis

Epidermis

Vasodilation

FIGURE 22-2 Heat can be dissipated through the skin when superficial blood vessels dilate.

the dermis is injured, fibroblasts in the dermis quickly reproduce and begin forming a dense collection of new connective tissue called a *scar*.

If elastic fibers in the dermis are overstretched, such as may occur in the skin over the abdomen during later stages of pregnancy, these fibers may then weaken and tear. The result is an area of atrophy commonly referred to as a *stretch mark*. See Dermatologic Pathologies section for more information on scars and stretch marks.

SUBCUTANEOUS LAYER

Beneath the dermis is the *subcutaneous layer* or *hypodermis*. This is not a true layer of skin, but is often described along with the integumentary system. The subcutaneous layer consists of loose connective tissue and fat (or adipose; described next) and nerve receptors. This layer, known as the *superficial fascia*, sits above skeletal muscle and bone. When the superficial fascia surrounds deeper structures, it is referred to as deep fascia.

Located in the subcutaneous layer is a band of fatty tissue called the *panniculus adiposus*. Thickness of the panniculus adiposus varies with age, gender, and health. Infants and children have a uniform fat layer under the skin. Women have an extra thickness of adipose over the breasts, hips, and inner thighs. Men have an accumulation of fat on the nape of the neck, deltoid and triceps muscles, and abdominal region of the body.

SKIN COLOR

Skin color can range from almost black to nearly colorless. Skin color is determined primarily by pigment (melanin, carotene, abnormal levels of hemoglobin and bilirubin), blood flow, and hormones. Melanin production depends on factors such as genetics and UV light exposure (the latter causes melanin granules to darken). Freckles, moles, and age spots occur when melanin is concentrated in one area or from changes to melanocytes (Box 22-1). *Albinism* is a genetic condition in which the individual cannot produce melanin. *Vitiligo* is the partial or total loss of skin pigmentation, occurring in patches. Certain hormones such as those secreted during pregnancy can stimulate the synthesis of melanin, which can produce a dark line between the navel and pubic area or may give the childbearing woman *melasma*, or a mask of pregnancy, by darkening the skin of the face and throat.

Carotene gives a yellow-golden color to skin and is present in larger amounts in Asians. The amount of hemoglobin, blood's red respiratory pigment, can give light-colored skin a rosy cast.

Skin color is an indicator of the health of the individual and of the skin. Redness may indicate injury or a pathologic process and may be seen in people with inflammation, fever, or allergies. Increased blood flow, such as from exercise, blushing, or hot flashes can cause excessive redness called *hyperemia*. Lack of blood flow, called *ischemia*, or

BOX 22-1

Abnormal Moles

Abnormal moles should be avoided in massage and then reported to the client. Encourage your client to have abnormal moles medically evaluated as they may be malignant melanomas, a deadly skin cancer. **ABCDE** is a method of mole assessment to determine abnormal moles, which stands for:

Asymmetry. Asymmetry means that if a line were drawn down the middle, there would be not be two equal halves. Common moles are symmetrical and round. Malignant moles are asymmetrical.

Border. The edges or borders of early melanomas are uneven, often containing scalloped or notched edges.

Color. Different shades of brown or black are often the first sign of a problem. Common moles are evenly shaded brown.

Diameter. Common moles are usually less than one-quarter inch in diameter (6 mm), the size of a pencil eraser. Early melanomas tend to be larger.

Evolving. Common moles do not change much, if at all. Malignant moles evolve or change over a period of time, and may rapidly increase in size, indicating metastasis.

In addition, any lesion that does not heal properly may indicate malignancy.

---

excessive amounts of deoxygenated blood, called *hypoxemia*, can give skin the blue or purple cast of *cyanosis*. *Pallor*, or paleness of skin, is often seen in persons with anemia. Individuals with *jaundice* or liver disorders may have a yellow-gold color to their skin and eyes from increased levels of bilirubin.

CHAT ROOM

Because massage therapists use skin as the primary medium of contact, we can easily observe the client's skin, hair, and nails. This provides information about changes in the client's health. Undiagnosed skin conditions, especially sores, rashes, and changes in skin color and texture, often indicate disease. In these cases, bring such findings to your client's attention and suggest medical evaluation.

CHAT ROOM

Changes in Skin Caused by the Aging Process

Moisture: Skin becomes dryer and flakier.

Pigment: Skin color is paler in color.

Thickness: Wrinkling occurs, especially on face and arms. The skin takes on a parchmentlike appearance, especially over bony protuberances and on the back of the hands, feet, arms, and legs.

Texture: Not only does wrinkling occur, but the skin also feels rougher and may exhibit lines and creases.

Turgor: When pinched, the skin may tent (poor turgor).

HAIR

Hair is composed of keratinized filaments arising from pouchlike follicles located in the dermis. The hair shaft extends through a pore in the epidermis. The main function of hair is protecting the skin and body orifices. Hair protects the scalp from injury and UV radiation. Eyebrows and eyelashes guard the eyes from foreign particles; hair in the nostrils and external ear canals protects the nose and ears, respectively. Hairs also function in our sense of touch: a hair root plexus is a receptor that is stimulated each time hair is moved.

Hair comes in a variety of sizes and shapes. A round shaft of hair produces straight hair. When the hair shaft is oval, the person usually has wavy hair. If the hair shaft is flat and ribbonlike, then the hair is curly or kinky. In fine hair, no medulla (inner core) is present in the hair follicle. Genetics determine most of our hair characteristics, from hair color to texture.

Hair color originates from one or a combination of the three color pigments: brown, yellow, and black. Red hair is a combination of brown and yellow pigment. White hair often is the result of air in the hair follicle itself. Gray hair occurs when hair pigment decreases or is absent. Aging, emotional distress, certain chemical treatments (chemotherapy), radiation, excessive vitamin A, and certain fungal diseases can cause both graying and hair loss.

Hair covers most of the entire body. Only a few areas of skin are hairless, notably the palms of the hands and the soles of the feet. Hair is also absent from lips, nipples, and some areas of the genitalia. Heavier concentrations of hair are found in the axillae, on the scalp, on external genitalia, and above eyes and eyelids. Because of male hormones, men typically have extra hair growth on the face and chest.

CHAT ROOM

Hair follicles can sometimes become irritated during a massage, which may be caused by (1) an allergic reaction to the lubricant, (2) pulling of the hair, or (3) insufficient use of lubricant on the skin, causing undue friction.

Arrector Pili

Arrector pili are tiny muscles attached to hair follicles. These muscles contract to pull the hair upright. This may occur when you are cold or experiencing emotions such as fright or anxiety. During contraction, the skin may dimple, causing *goose bumps* or *goose flesh*. If an animal is cold, this action creates an insulating layer of air in the fur. Because humans do not have fur, this effect is relatively useless. If an animal is frightened, this added volume allows the animal to appear larger and possibly deter an enemy.

SKIN GLANDS

Sebaceous (Oil) Glands

Sebaceous glands, also known as *oil glands,* are connected to hair follicles by small ducts. These glands secrete *sebum,* rich in triglycerides, waxes, fatty acids, and cholesterol. Sebum is mildly antibacterial and antifungal, lubricating both the hair and the epidermis.

Overproduction of sebum, caused by hormones (mainly androgens) or disease, can make the skin appear oily; underproduction of sebum caused by nutritional factors and UV radiation makes the skin appear dry.

> ### CHAT ROOM
>
> Massage, especially friction, can stimulate the production of sebum, which adds additional natural oils to the skin.

Sudoriferous (Sweat) Glands

Sudoriferous glands, or *sweat glands*, secrete sweat, or perspiration. Their primary functions are to help regulate body temperature and to eliminate wastes. As perspiration evaporates, it carries large amounts of body heat away from the skin surface. In fact, the most rapid process of heat dissipation is evaporation of perspiration.

The skin's surface possesses approximately 2 million sweat glands. Approximately 1 pint of fluid and impurities is lost in each 8-hour period when a person is visibly sweating. When sweat production is high, replacement of lost minerals is essential. When the sweating is low, most of the sodium chloride present in the perspiration is reabsorbed in the skin. In this case, mineral depletion is minimal.

Sweat glands can be classified into two groups: (1) eccrine and (2) apocrine (Figure 22-3).

Eccrine Glands. These are the most numerous and help cool the body and provide minor elimination of waste products. They do not exist on the lips, in the ear canal, on the glans penis, and in nail beds.

Apocrine Glands. These are located in the axilla, the anogenital region, and the areola of the breast. These glands are larger than eccrine glands and open into hair follicles. Apocrine glands begin to function during puberty and may be similar to the sexual scent glands in other animals. In women, apocrine gland secretions show cyclic changes linked to the menstrual cycle. Odor produced by these glands is mainly the result of decomposition of the apocrine sweat by skin bacteria.

Within breasts are mammary glands, which are essentially modified sweat glands. These glands are most often studied in the reproductive system because of their function of lactation to feed the young.

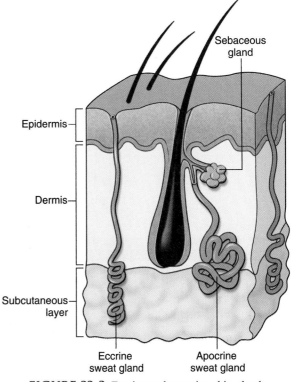

FIGURE 22-3 Eccrine and apocrine skin glands.

"It's not the age; it's the mileage."
—Harrison Ford as Indiana Jones in
Raiders of the Lost Ark

NAILS

Nails are compact keratinized cells that form the thin hard plates found on the distal surfaces of the fingers and toes. The two main functions of the nails are (1) protecting the ends of fingers and toes and (2) use as a tool for tasks such as digging, scratching, and manipulation of objects.

The *nail body* is the largest and most visible part of the nail. Nail production takes place in the *nail root.* The *nail bed* is the skin beneath the nail; it can be seen through the clear nail. The *lateral nail folds* are the edges of the nail where they meet the skin at the sides of the nail. This area is where hangnails occur. The *cuticle* is the tough ridge of skin that grows out over the nail from its base. Also located here is the *lunula,* which is the crescent-shaped white area at the nail base. The most distal portion of the nail is the *free edge,* which is trimmed as a result of nail growth (Figure 22-4).

Nails are typically transparent but appear pinkish because of blood vessels present in the dermis below. Nail changes, such as ridges and white spots, may occur as a result of poor nutrition or disease.

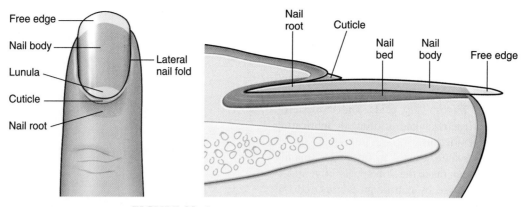

FIGURE 22-4 Nail from above and in cross section.

NERVOUS SYSTEM'S ROLE IN TOUCH

The sense of touch is actually a complex composition of specialized receptors found in the skin. These receptors detect sensations such as pressure, movement, heat, cold (or absence of heat), and pain. Touch is an amalgamation of many sensations.

Touch provides information about our surroundings. This sense also warns the body of danger or injury, such as the cooking pot is hot or your finger is in the way as you cut an orange with a sharp knife.

Information from the skin receptors makes their way to the central nervous system. The area of the brain that houses the sensation of touch is the postcentral gyrus in the parietal lobe of the cerebral cortex.

It is interesting to note the amount of tactile "brain space" dedicated to each area of the body, as shown in Figure 22-5. The more space devoted to an area in the postcentral gyrus, the more sensory receptors are found in the corresponding part of the body. The hands, face, lips, jaw, and tongue take up approximately 80% of this neural space. The more receptors that are located in that part of the body, the more sensitive is the body part. Note that the right postcentral gyrus represents the left side of the body and vice versa.

The following is a list of all currently known receptors and their functions. *Discriminative touch* means touch that is subtle and can be easily located in the skin. Conversely, *crude touch* is more easily identified but is more difficult to locate on the skin than discriminative touch.

Meissner Corpuscle. Also called *tactile corpuscle,* this receptor mediates sensations of discriminative touch such as light versus deep pressure, as well as low-frequency vibration. Meissner corpuscles are most numerous in hairless areas such as nipples, fingertips, and lips.

Ruffini Corpuscle. Located in the dermis, Ruffini corpuscles alert us when the skin comes into contact with deep or continuous pressure. They adapt slowly and permit us to stay in contact with grasped objects. The ability to clutch a pencil or pen in your hand for long periods and still be able to feel it depends on these receptors. Some references indicate that these corpuscles are secondary thermoreceptors, detecting temperatures ranging from 85° to 120° F, so they are often called *heat receptors.*

Pacinian Corpuscle. Located in the deeper dermal layers, primarily in the hands and feet and in many joint capsules, these receptors respond quickly to crude and deep pressure, vibration, and stretch, and receive proprioceptive information about joint position. Pacinian corpuscles adapt quickly to stimuli; for this reason, they respond only when the stimulus is first applied.

Krause End Bulb. These receptors are found widely distributed in mucous membranes, more so than in the skin. Because of this arrangement, they are also called *mucocutaneous corpuscles.* They are involved in discriminatory touch and low-frequency vibration. Some references indicate that these receptors are secondary thermoreceptors, detecting temperatures below 65° F, so they are often called *cold receptors.*

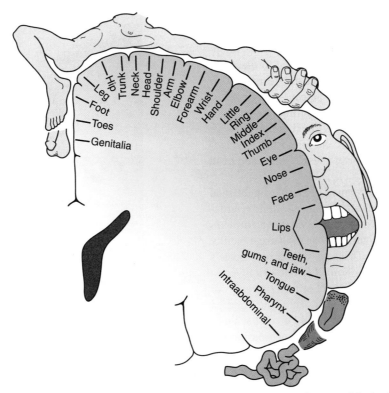

FIGURE 22-5 The *homunculus*, or little man, in the postcentral gyrus of the brain.

Merkel Disk. Located in the epidermis, these receptors respond to light touch and discriminative touch.

Hair Root Plexus. Also called *hair follicle receptors,* these structures are light-touch receptors that detect hair movement and resemble a web of receptors wrapping around hair follicles. They may alert us to slight breezes or intrusive insects crawling on our skin.

▌MINI-LAB

Take the bottom of a clear glass and press it into the heel of your hand. Describe the color changes and possible explanation for these changes. What would happen to the skin cells if the pressure were prolonged? How does this experiment reflect what happens to the skin when clients are bedridden? How can massage, with its circulatory effects, aid in preventing decubitus ulcers (bedsores)?

ⓔvolve *Using the Evolve website, access the chapter-related activity "Tournament of Terminology" to review structures of the skin. Use it for review or as a study guide for upcoming tests.* ▪

PIONEERS IN TOUCH RESEARCH

Many doctors, nurses, biochemists, and psychologists have developed studies on the effects of touch. These studies address physical, intellectual, psychological, and emotional themes. Several studies discussed here are considered groundbreaking and fundamental. These include brief summaries from research that focus on touch. As you read them and draw your own conclusions, apply the concepts you develop to your attitude about massage and to your role as therapist. Be sure to read current research on the effects of touch and massage.

Rene Spitz and Wayne Dennis

Both Spitz and Dennis studied children in orphanages in different parts of the world (e.g., Lebanon, the United States).

Dr. Rene A. Spitz (1887-1974), a Hungarian psychiatrist and pioneer in touch deprivation research, explored the development (or lack of development) of institutionalized children. In a 1945 study, Spitz followed the social development of babies who, for various reasons, were removed from their mothers early in life. Some children were placed with foster families while others were raised in institutions such as orphanages and nursing homes. The orphanages and nursing home lacked a family-like environment. More than a third of these children died. A large percentage were still living in institutions after 40 years. All survivors experienced some form of developmental delay. Spitz claimed that these individuals were depressed. This condition is now considered an attachment disorder.

In another study, Spitz observed young children in an orphanage who were fed and kept clean but who received no consistent affection from a sole caregiver. The long-standing absence of emotional warmth took an enormous toll on the children, primarily on their emotional development but also on their physical growth and development. Of 91 such babies he observed, 27 died in their first year of life, followed by 7 more the second year. In other such homes for children, up to 90 percent died in early infancy. Babies who did survive in institutions were classified as "hopeless." Spitz concluded that providing only for a baby's physical needs is not sufficient for normal development. Touch was essential to normal development and even to survival.

In the 1950s, Dr. Wayne Dennis (1905-1976) published his findings on what was then called infant and child retardation. His research was based on his experience at an orphanage in Beirut, Lebanon. He found that the orphanage facility was more than adequate, but because of the orphanage's meager funding, personnel was limited to one employee to 10 infants. The children were taken out of the cribs only for feedings, diaper changing, and a daily bath. The children remained in the crib until they began to pull up on the sides. From that point, they were placed in a playpen during the daylight hours with two other children. Opportunities for touch were very limited. A large number of these children died, even though they were receiving adequate nutrition and hygiene. The children who did survive were often dwarfed or deformed.

The explanation Dennis gave for his findings of *marasmus* (wasting away) combined with the tragic death rates in the Lebanese orphanages was touch deprivation and lack of physical stimulation and learning opportunities. The employees were providing their physical needs, but did not have time to hold and caress the infants. When aides were hired to rock and sing to the infants, mortality rates dropped 70%.

> ⊜volve   *Log on to the Evolve website to see a photo of Rene Spitz, and a child affected with marasmus. This is the condition that infants in Lebanese orphanages had in Wayne Dennis' study. Locate similar studies that feature touch as an important element in human (and mammalian) growth and development.* ∎

Harry Harlow

In 1958, Dr. Harry Harlow (1906-1981), another pioneer in touch research, conducted experiments at the University of Wisconsin that involved the isolation of infant monkeys from their mothers. Initially, the infants protested by crying. When nothing changed, they became depressed, engaging in self-stimulating behaviors, such as rocking. These infant monkeys valued tactile stimulation more than they did nourishment. Harlow created two artificial surrogate "mothers." One was a bare wire sculpture of a monkey that housed a bottle of formula. The other was a fur-covered wire monkey that felt and smelled like other monkeys, but offered no

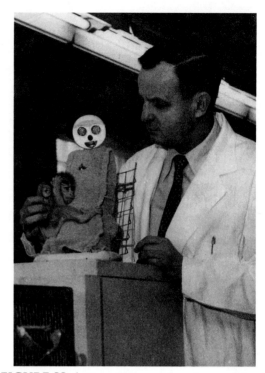

FIGURE 22-6 Harry Harlow and monkey participant.

food. The infant monkeys preferred to cling to the "mother" who provided a semblance of physical contact without nourishment rather than to the wire models that provided food (Figure 22-6).

As these monkeys grew older, they developed violent and self-mutilating behaviors. Most of the juvenile and adult monkeys did not groom themselves. Their sexual organs developed normally, but they did not exhibit normal sexual behaviors. It seemed that lack of touch during their early developmental years impaired them emotionally, socially, and sexually.

Dysfunctional behaviors continued even after the female monkeys become mothers themselves. They often refused mating, becoming hostile and aggressive when approached. The monkeys that did mate rejected or harmed their young.

Abraham Maslow

In the 1960s, Dr. Abraham Maslow (1908-1970), a renowned psychologist, placed the needs of human beings in a sequential order, from the most basic and concrete to the most ideal and abstract (Figure 22-7). He believed that these needs directed all human behavior and, as these needs are met, other needs of the hierarchy begin to emerge until the individual reaches what he terms self-actualization. Maslow called this progression the *Theory of Human Motivation.*

Maslow stated that humans have basic needs, beginning from the concrete, biologic needs of food and water to abstract needs of self-actualization. Maslow characterized the self-actualized person as self-accepting, striving to help

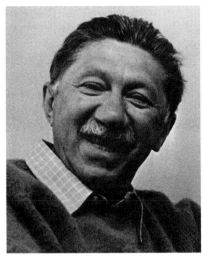

FIGURE 22-7 Abraham Maslow.

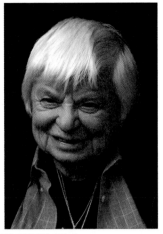

FIGURE 22-8 Delores Krieger.

BOX 22-2

Hierarchy of Human Needs

1. Survival (food and water)
2. Safety (shelter and clothing)
3. Touching, skin contact
4. Attention
5. Mirroring and echoing
6. Guidance
7. Listening
8. Being genuine
9. Participating
10. Acceptance
11. Opportunity to grieve losses and to grow
12. Support
13. Loyalty and trust
14. Accomplishment
15. Altering one's state of consciousness, transcending the ordinary
16. Sexuality
17. Enjoyment or fun
18. Freedom
19. Nurturing
20. Unconditional love (including connection with a Higher Power)

Compiled by Dr. Charles Whitfield from works by Glasser, 1985; Maslow, 1962; Miller, 1981; Weil, 1973.

Delores Krieger

In the 1970s Dr. Delores Krieger (1935-present), a professor at New York University, became interested in touch healing (Figure 22-8). She was fascinated with the idea that intent was highly important in healing touch.

Through Krieger's research a tangible relationship emerged between touching and healing. In Krieger's study, when a healthy person placed his hands on or near an ill person for 10 to 15 minutes with the intent to heal, hemoglobin levels were increased. Hemoglobin is the oxygen-carrying molecule in red blood cells. The technique that emerged from her work is referred to as *healing touch* or *therapeutic touch*.

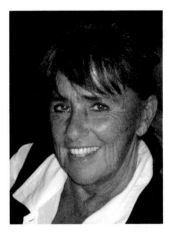

FIGURE 22-9 Tiffany Field.

Tiffany Field

Dr. Tiffany Field, professor of pediatrics, psychology, and psychiatry at the University of Miami School of Medicine, began a research project in 1986 to study the effects of massage on 40 premature babies (Figure 22-9). Half of the group was massaged three times a day for 15 minutes for 10 days. The massaged infants gained 47% more weight. They spent less time in the hospital than the babies who were not

others, and engaging in activities that will help him or her achieve the highest potential. His model was later redesigned, with the help of other psychologists, to a more comprehensive list of human needs (Box 22-2). It is interesting to note that touching and skin contact are ranked very high on the list, just below the individual's needs for shelter. Many massage therapists attest to the fact that clients often receive massage to get their touch needs met.

massaged, even though both groups of babies had the same number of feedings and averaged the same intake per feeding. The massaged babies were also more active and alert and left the hospital six days earlier than non-massaged babies. The massaged babies were also more socially active and more responsive, and had better coordination and motor skills, compared with the nonmassaged babies.

In 1992 Dr. Field formally established the Touch Research Institute (TRI) at the University of Miami School of Medicine through a start-up grant from Johnson & Johnson. The TRI is devoted solely to the study of touch and its application in both science and medicine. Research efforts continue today. The TRI has researched the effects of massage therapy in all stages of life, from newborns to senior citizens. In these studies, the TRI has shown that touch therapy has many positive effects on health and well-being.

> *"Writing a novel is like driving a car at night.*
> *You can see only as far as your headlights,*
> *but you can make the whole trip that way."*
> —E. L. Doctorow

DERMATOLOGIC PATHOLOGIES

Bacterial Skin Infections

Acne. Acne is an inflammatory bacterial infection of hair follicles and their associated sebaceous glands. It is marked by the presence of pimples with localized redness. Acne laden skin often appears greasy. Scars may develop if the condition becomes chronic.

Massage over the infected area is contraindicated.

Impetigo. Impetigo is a bacterial infection that occurs mainly around the mouth, nose, and hands (Figure 22-10). The infection is highly contagious and is easily spread by direct contact or by handling contaminated objects such as eating utensils, toothbrushes, towels, and bed (or massage) linens.

Massage is postponed until the affected area has completely healed as impetigo is highly contagious.

Folliculitis. Folliculitis is an infection that occurs when bacteria (usually staphylococci) enter hair follicles damaged by friction, such as from shaving or clothing. It can occur anywhere in hair-bearing skin, but is seen mainly in the groin, axillae, or the bearded areas of males. It often resembles acne.

Local massage is contraindicated because massage will further irritate follicles, which would increase inflammation.

Boils. Boils, or furuncles, are infected skin glands or hair follicles. Pain increases as the boil enlarges (which can be as large as a golf ball). Eventually, the abscess bursts. Once drainage occurs, the boil heals. This sequence of events takes about 2 weeks.

Local massage is contraindicated because massage will make the inflammation worse and may spread the infection.

Fungal Skin Infections

Ringworm. Ringworm is a fungal infection of the skin. This condition usually affects nonhairy parts of the face, trunk, and limbs (Figure 22-11). Ringworm is characterized by red, raised, round or oval scaling areas, creating a ringed appearance.

Since ringworm is contagious, massage is contraindicated until lesions have completely disappeared.

Athlete's Foot. Athlete's foot is a fungal infection of the foot. It is characterized by skin discoloration with a ridge of red tissue. The skin may flake, crack, and bleed, or ooze clear fluid. The infected foot often appears dry and has an unpleasant or musty odor.

Massage over the infected area is contraindicated. Although athlete's foot is not easily spread by contact with infected linens, treat massage linens as contaminated.

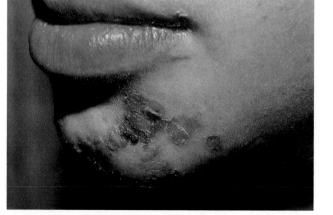

FIGURE 22-10 Impetigo.

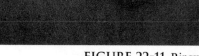

FIGURE 22-11 Ringworm.

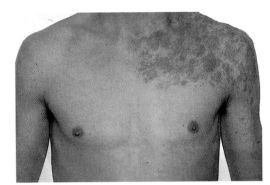

FIGURE 22-12 Shingles.

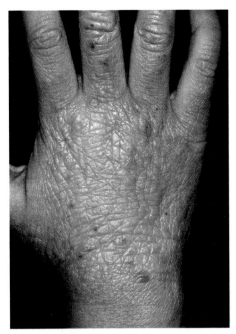

FIGURE 22-13 Eczema.

Viral Skin Infections

Cold Sores. Cold sores (fever blisters, herpes simplex) are recurrent viral infections that affect skin and mucous membranes. They most often affect the area around the mouth. Cold sores are highly contagious and may be spread by direct contact or indirectly through contact with contaminated items such as razors, linens, and eating utensils. Lesions tend to recur because the virus lies dormant in sensory nerve cells that correspond to the site of infection. Reactivation of the virus can be triggered by exposure to sunlight or wind or the presence of another infection, such as the common cold (hence the name "cold sores"), or by fever (hence the name "fever blisters"), hormonal changes that occur during menstruation and pregnancy, as well as stress and anxiety.

Massage is postponed until lesions have completely disappeared as cold sores are highly contagious.

Shingles. Shingles, or herpes zoster, is an acute, localized reactivation of a past viral infection (varicella or chickenpox). Initial symptoms are tingling, pricking, or numbness followed by eruptions of painful vesicles in a bandlike pattern (Figure 22-12). Lesions erupt, crust over, and fall off after 7 to 10 days of their debut. Shingles is contagious to persons who have not had chickenpox, and contact with the fluid in the vesicles should be avoided as it contains the virus. The infected person should avoid contact with anyone who has not had chickenpox, as the virus is contagious to them.

Massage should be postponed until the client has completely healed.

Warts. Warts are small benign masses resulting from rapid cell growth. Warts may occur anywhere on the body, but most are located on the hands (common or palmar warts), feet (plantar warts), face and legs (flat warts), or genitals (genital warts). Warts are caused by human papillomavirus (HVP). Warts tend to recur.

Local massage is contraindicated because warts are contagious. Be sure to treat massage linens as contaminated.

Inflammatory Skin Conditions

Eczema. Eczema is a chronic type of dermatitis. Eczema is most often found on the hands, scalp, face, nape of the neck, or creases of the elbow and knees, and ankles and feet. Eczema is characterized by dry skin that is scaly, leathery, or crusty (Figure 22-13). This condition is not contagious and has no known cause; some cases are related to allergic reactions.

Massage over affected areas is contraindicated if skin is broken. Adjust pressure in areas that are sensitive. Some clients do best with a hypoallergenic product. Do not add essential oils to the lubricant because it could provoke an adverse skin reaction. Obtain permission before touching affected areas as some clients may not want these areas touched.

Psoriasis. Psoriasis is a chronic skin disorder where the proliferation rate of epidermal cells is greatly accelerated. Instead of skin renewing every month, it occurs every few days. Because old skin cells do not slough off quickly, they build up in thick patches (Figure 22-14). Episodes of exacerbation and remission are noted; exacerbations are related to trauma and emotional stress. Psoriasis is not contagious. Although the cause of psoriasis is unknown, the immune system and genetics play a part in the activation of psoriasis.

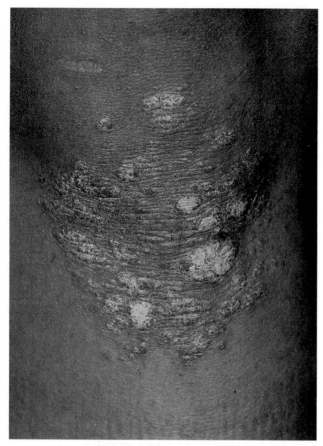

FIGURE 22-14 Psoriasis.

Hypersensitive areas or areas of inflammation or broken skin should be avoided. Pressure should be adjusted in areas that are sensitive. Some clients do best with a hypoallergenic product. Obtain permission before touching affected areas as some clients may not want these areas touched.

Contact Dermatitis. Contact dermatitis is inflammation of the skin. The two main types of contact dermatitis are irritant and allergic, so named for their causative agents (irritating substances or allergens).

Ask where the contact dermatitis is located and how widespread the area is. If the affected area is small (e.g., confined to one hand or elbow), avoid massage to that area or to the entire limb. If the affected area is large and the condition widespread (e.g., across the back), postpone massage until the skin has completely healed. Ask your client to preview the ingredient list of any massage lubricants you might use to be sure it does not contain substances to which your client is allergic, or use a hypoallergenic product. Ask your client about allergies to latex before using latex gloves.

Seborrhea. Seborrhea, or seborrheic dermatitis, is a chronic inflammatory condition of sebaceous glands marked by an increase in the amount of and changes in these secretions.

Naturally, it occurs in areas with the greatest number of sebaceous glands, such as the scalp, eyebrows, eyelids, and sides of nose, area behind the ears, axillae, and middle of the chest. Seborrhea is not contagious and has no known cause. Many affected persons experience periods of exacerbation and remission.

Hypersensitive areas should be avoided. Pressure should be adjusted in areas that are sensitive. Use a thin lotion rather than oil or cream.

Rosacea. Rosacea is a progressive, inflammatory skin disease characterized by persistent skin redness, dryness, warmth, and swelling. Red bumps and pustules appear, resembling teenage acne. Typically only the middle third of the face is affected (i.e., nose, cheeks, chin). Rosacea is not contagious and has no known cause.

Hypersensitive areas or areas of inflammation should be avoided. Pressure should be adjusted in areas that are sensitive.

Lice and Mites

Lice. A louse is a wingless parasite that lives its entire life cycle on a single human host and depends on its blood for survival. Lice are spread by physical contact with an infected person and through contaminated items such as towels, combs and brushes, pillowcases, and hats. The most common sign of lice is the presence of *nits* (egg sacs) on the hair shaft, on the body, or in clothing. Nits appear as oval, white to yellow pinpoint specks.

Massage is contraindicated because lice are contagious and can be transmitted by contact with an infected person or infected personal items.

Scabies. Scabies infestation is caused by a burrowing parasitic mite called *Sarcoptes scabiei*. Scabies is spread by close physical contact and by contaminated towels, combs and brushes, and clothing. The most common sign is a rash of thin, tiny, light brown lines called a *scabies trail*, often with tiny blisters. reddened skin, and intense itching.

Massage is contraindicated because scabies is contagious and can be transmitted by contact with an infected person or infected personal items.

Skin Injuries

Bruises. A bruise, or contusion, is an injury that does not break the skin. It is usually caused by trauma. Bruises usually appear within 24 hours of the incident and are characterized by swelling, discoloration, local tenderness, and pain. Bruises are also a side effect of certain medications (Warfarin, long-term corticosteroid use) or a sign of vitamin C deficiency or of disease (leukemia, hepatitis). Bruise-like purple-blue marks on the elderly are called senile purpura.

Local massage is contraindicated until the bruise begins to turn greenish-yellow. At this time, gentle stroking of the area may relieve pain and encourage blood flow. If bruising is seen in an elderly client (senile purpura), lighter and more perpendicular pressure is indicated to avoid further damage to fragile tissues.

Burns. A burn is an injury that causes damage to the epidermis, dermis, and/or the subcutaneous layer (hypodermis). There are three degrees of burn severity, depending on the depth of injury.

A *first-degree burn* damages only the epidermis. The area is painful, red, and swollen and typically heals in 3 to 4 days. A *second-degree burn* involves both the epidermis and upper layers of the dermis. Some signs and symptoms are swelling, redness, blistering, and pain (these burns are the most painful). A *third-degree burn* destroys the epidermis, dermis, hair follicles, and associated glands, and may extend to the subcutaneous tissue and underlying soft tissue. The skin becomes leathery, white or blackened and charred, but is numb as a consequence of nerve damage. Because of injury to local lymphatics, there is little swelling.

Avoid massage over the affected area until it has completely healed. Once healed, skin rolling and frictional movements can be used over the burn scar to loosen any adhesions and to increase local circulation (this includes area of healed skin grafts). Pressure should be reduced in areas that are sensitive or numb.

Stretch Marks. Stretch marks are from tearing, thinning, or overstretching of skin. They are most commonly located on the breasts, hips, thighs, buttocks, and abdomen. Stretch marks are usually from extreme stretching of the skin such as occurs from pregnancy and sudden weight gain.

Lighter-than-normal pressure is indicated over stretch marks. Massage will not reduce stretch marks because they are not due to a buildup of scar tissue.

Scars. A scar is a mark left on damaged skin after it is healed. It is essentially fibrotic tissue that replaces normal skin tissue after injury.

There are two types of abnormal scars, hypertrophic and keloid scars. Both types of scars are the result of excess collagen production, which causes the scar to be raised above the surrounding skin. *Hypertrophic scars,* which are more common than keloid scars, do not grow beyond the boundaries of the original wound. *Keloid scars* extend beyond the wound site.

Avoid massage over the affected area until it has completely healed. Afterward, scar mobilization is permissible and may help to break up excess fibrosis. Staying within the client's pain tolerance, cross-fiber, circular, and chucking friction can be applied directly to the scar. Be sure to mobilize tissue toward the scar rather than away from it to avoid overstretching the healed tissue.

Decubitus Ulcers. Decubitus ulcers are localized areas of dead skin that can extend to the epidermis, dermis, subcutaneous tissue, or all the way to underlying bones and joints. They are caused by local ischemia of an area that has been subjected to sustained pressure.

Decubitus ulcers are classified in four stages from stage I (least extensive) to stage IV (most extensive).

Postpone massage if the ulcer is emitting a discharge or has a foul odor because these are signs of infection. Otherwise, local massage is contraindicated within a 4-inch radius around the ulcer's edge. Gentle massage using gliding strokes in a wide area encircling the ulcer may increase local blood flow, so long as the 4-inch rule is respected.

CHAT ROOM

Transdermal patches are used for a variety of reasons such as hormone replacement therapy and to manage high blood pressure or pain. Because the massage lubricant will weaken the adhesive, avoid its use up to 2 inches around the patch area.

SPOTLIGHT ON RESEARCH

Research suggests that massage therapy may:
- Improve scar tissue healing
- Increase skin temperature
- Contribute to the skin health
- Decrease symptoms of eczema and other skin conditions
- Be helpful in treating or preventing bed sores
- Reduce stress that may exacerbate certain dermatologic conditions
- Improve hand function, strength, skin pliability, and a reduction in contracture in persons with scleroderma
- Reduce pain during débridement (skin brushing) of burns and increase range of motion in burned scarred tissue

E-RESOURCES

⊝volve

http://evolve.elsevier.com/Salvo/MassageTherapy
- Chapter challenge
- Flash cards
- Photo gallery
- Weblinks

BIBLIOGRAPHY

Abrahams P, Marks S, Hutchings R: *McMinn's color atlas of human anatomy,* St Louis, 2003, Mosby.

Applegate EJ: *The anatomy and physiology learning system,* ed 3, Philadelphia, 2006, Saunders.

Beers MH, Berkow R: *The Merck manual of diagnosis and therapy*, Whitehouse Station, NJ, 2006, Merck Research Laboratories.

Clarke AM, Clarke AD: *Early experience: myth and evidence*, London, 1979, Open Books.

Como D, editor: *Mosby's medical, nursing, and allied health dictionary*, ed 6, St Louis, 2002, Mosby.

Crawley J, Van De Graaff KM: *A photographic atlas for anatomy and physiology*, Englewood, Colo, 2002, Morton.

Damjanov I: *Pathophysiology for the health-related professions*, ed 3, Philadelphia, 2006, Saunders.

Ferri FF: *2003 Ferri's clinical advisor, instant diagnosis and treatment*, St Louis, 2003, Mosby.

Frazier MS, Drzymkowski JW: *Essentials of human diseases and conditions*, ed 3, Philadelphia, 2004, Saunders.

Fritz S: *Massage online for essential sciences for therapeutic massage*, ed 3, St Louis, 2010, Mosby.

Gerson J: *STD textbook for professional estheticians*, ed 9, Albany, NY, 2003, Delmar Learning.

Goldberg S: *Clinical anatomy made ridiculously simple*, Miami, 2004, Medmaster.

Gould BE: *Pathophysiology for the health professions*, ed 3, Philadelphia, 2006, Saunders.

Grafelman T: *Graf's anatomy and physiology guide for the massage therapist*, Aurora, Colo, 1998, DG Publishing.

Guyton A: *Human physiology and mechanisms of disease*, ed 6, Philadelphia, 1996, Saunders.

Haubrich WS: *Medical meanings: a glossary of word origins*, New York, 1984, Harcourt Brace Jovanovich.

Huether SE, McCance KL: *Understanding pathophysiology*, ed 3, St Louis, 2004, Mosby.

Jacob S, Francone C: *Elements of anatomy and physiology*, Philadelphia, 1989, Saunders.

Juhan D: *Job's body: a handbook for bodyworkers*, ed 3, Barrington, NY, 2003, Station Hill Press.

Kalat JW: *Biological psychology*, ed 8, Belmont, Calif, 2003, Wadsworth.

Kapit W, Elson LM: *The anatomy coloring book*, ed 3, New York, 2002, Benjamin Cummings.

Kapit W, Macey R, Meisami E: *The physiology coloring book*, ed 2, New York, 1999, HarperCollins.

Kendall F, McCreary E: *Muscles: testing and function*, Baltimore, 1983, Williams & Wilkins.

Kordish M, Dickson S: *Introduction to basic human anatomy*, Lake Charles, La, 1985, McNeese State University.

Krieger D: Therapeutic touch: the imprimatur of nursing, *Am J Nurs* 75(5):784-787, 1975.

Kumar V, Abbas A, Fausto N: *Robbins and Cotran physiologic basis of disease*, ed 7, St Louis, 2005, Mosby.

Marieb EN: *Essentials of human anatomy and physiology*, ed 8, New York, 2005, Benjamin Cummings.

Martini FH, Bartholomew EF: *Essentials of anatomy and physiology*, ed 3, New York, 2003, Benjamin/Cummings.

McAleer N: *The body almanac*, Garden City, NY, 1985, Doubleday.

McCance K, Huether S: *Pathophysiology: the biological basis for disease in adults and children*, St Louis, 2006, Mosby.

Merck manual, ed 17, Whitehouse Station, NJ, 1998, Merck Co.

Montagu A: *Touching: the human significance of the skin*, ed 2, New York, 1978, Harper & Row.

Moore KL: *Clinically oriented anatomy*, ed 5, Baltimore, 2005, Lippincott Williams & Wilkins.

Netter FH: *Atlas of human anatomy*, ed 3, Teterboro, NJ, 2003, Icon Learning Systems.

Newton D: *Pathology for massage therapists*, ed 2, Portland, Ore, 1995, Simran.

Olsen A, McHose C: *Bodystories: a guide to experiential anatomy*, Barrytown, NY, 1991, Station Hill Press.

Premkumar K: *Pathology A to Z: a handbook for massage therapists*, Baltimore, 1999, Lippincott Williams & Wilkins.

Salvo SG: *Mosby's pathology for massage therapists*, ed 2, St Louis, 2009, Mosby.

Skin Cancer Foundation: *The ABCDs of moles and melanomas*, New York, 2005, The Foundation.

Solomon EP, Phillips GA: *Understanding human anatomy and physiology*, Philadelphia, 1987, Saunders.

Thibodeau G, Patton K: *Anatomy and physiology*, ed 6, St Louis, 2006, Mosby.

Thibodeau G, Patton K: *Structure and function of the body*, ed 12, St Louis, 2004, Mosby.

Tortora GJ: *Introduction to the human body: the essentials of anatomy and physiology*, ed 3, New York, 1994, HarperCollins.

Tortora GJ, Derreckson B: *Principles of human anatomy and physiology*, ed 11, New York, 2006, John Wiley & Sons.

Venes D, Thomas CL, Taber CW: *Taber's cyclopedic medical dictionary*, ed 20, Philadelphia, 2005, FA Davis.

MATCHING I

Place the letter of the answer next to the term or phrase that best describes it.

A. Arrector pili
B. Dermis
C. Epidermis
D. Hair follicles

E. Integumentary
F. Keratin
G. Meissner corpuscle
H. Melanocytes

I. Pacinian corpuscle
J. Sebaceous glands
K. Subcutaneous layer
L. Sudoriferous glands

_____ 1. Receptor that mediates sensations of discriminative touch such as light versus deep pressure

_____ 2. A tough, fibrous protein located in the epidermis that provides protection by waterproofing the skin

_____ 3. System that includes skin and its appendages such as hair, nails, and glands

_____ 4. Glands that help regulate body temperatures and eliminate wastes

_____ 5. Specialized cells in the epidermis that produce melanin or pigment

_____ 6. Tiny muscles that pull hair upright

_____ 7. True skin; made of connective tissue and blood vessels, nerve receptors, hair follicles, muscles and glands

_____ 8. Loose connective tissue layer that connects the dermis to underlying structures

_____ 9. Receptor that responds quickly to crude and deep pressure, and perceives proprioceptive information about joint position

_____ 10. Glands that secrete a fatty substance, lubricating both hair and the epidermis

_____ 11. Outer region of the skin; composed of epithelial tissue

_____ 12. Structure that can become irritated during a massage because of allergies, hair pulling, and inadequate amounts of lubricant

MATCHING II

Place the letter of the answer next to the term or phrase that best describes it.

A. Carotene
B. Cyanosis
C. Elastin fibers
D. Hyperemia

E. Melanin
F. Pallor
G. Postcentral gyrus
H. Scar

I. Stratum germinativum
J. Stratum lucidum
K. Vitamin D
L. Langerhan cells

_____ 1. Redness of the skin due to excessive blood flow

_____ 2. Epidermal layer found only in the thick skin of the palms and soles

_____ 3. Epidermal cells that play a role in immunity

_____ 4. Area of the brain that houses the sensation of touch

_____ 5. Term that denotes paleness of skin

_____ 6. Substance that can give skin a yellow-golden color

_____ 7. Connective tissue component in the dermis that gives skin its elasticity and resilience

_____ 8. Skin pigment that helps serve as a protective shield from the damaging effects of sunlight

_____ 9. Connective tissue that forms when the skin is injured

_____ 10. Vitamin synthesized in the skin with exposure to UV rays in sunlight

_____ 11. Term used to describe a blue or purple cast to skin

_____ 12. Deepest epidermal layer; undergoes continuous cell division and generates all other layers

CASE STUDY

If It Itches, Scratch It

Contessa had been working at a very chic midtown salon doing massages on their upscale clientele for approximately 4 years. One of her regulars was Julia, wife of a prominent local attorney and stay-at-home mom to three kids. Julia, who also receives other salon services, came in faithfully every week for a 90-minute massage.

Contessa usually spent the first hour massaging Julia's back while Julia was prone and then turned her supine for the last 30 minutes. Julia

usually napped when she was face down, but she liked to spend the last 30 minutes chatting. As they were talking about kids and parenting, Julia suddenly exclaimed, "Oh! I almost forgot, please save the last 5 minutes or so for a scalp massage. My oldest daughter, Jill, came home with head lice, and ever since then, I can't stop thinking about it, and the very thought makes my head itch. I think Jill got them when she went to spend the night with one of the girls in her dance class."

CASE STUDY—cont'd

As Contessa began to comply with Julia's request for a scalp massage, she realized that nits were attached to some of Julia's own hair shafts. Contessa finished the massage without saying anything. She knew that she should tell Julia, but she was afraid of ruining the relaxation effect of the massage, afraid of Julia's reaction, and afraid of losing her as a client. If you were Contessa, how might you have approached Julia with the news?

Should Contessa share the information with the other employees at the salon, especially Julia's hairdresser?

What steps does Contessa need to take as far as sanitizing her table, linens, and face rest?

If you were Julia, how might you have received the news that you were infested with head lice?

CRITICAL THINKING

How do skin conditions (pathologies) affect the way you conduct a massage therapy session? How do the client and the massage therapist interact for a successful massage therapy session?

CHAPTER 23

Nervous System

"My green thumb came only as a result of the mistakes I made while learning to see things from the plant's point of view."
—H. Fred Ale

LEARNING OBJECTIVES

After completing this chapter, the student should be able to:

- List anatomic structures and describe the physiologic processes of the nervous system.
- Discuss basic organization of the nervous system, outlining structures in both the central and the peripheral nervous systems.
- Contrast and compare the somatic and autonomic divisions of the peripheral nervous system.
- Outline types of cells found in the nervous system.
- Describe properties found in neurons.
- Label parts of a neuron.
- Identify connective tissue structures within nerves.
- Classify neurons according to their function.
- Discuss nerve impulses, including resting and action potentials.
- Contrast and compare continuous and saltatory conductions.
- Identify synaptic structures and outline the steps in synaptic transmission.
- Define neurotransmitters, giving examples of each.
- List structures, functions, and characteristics of the central nervous system.
- Identify structures, functions, and characteristics of the peripheral nervous system.
- Contrast and compare parasympathetic and sympathetic divisions of the autonomic nervous system, listing the physiologic effects of each.
- Discuss the senses.
- Name and discuss receptors.
- Name types of pathologic conditions of the nervous system, giving characteristics and massage considerations for each.

http://evolve.elsevier.com/Salvo/MassageTherapy

INTRODUCTION

The human body uses two systems to monitor and stimulate changes needed to maintain homeostasis. The endocrine system, which is discussed in the next chapter, responds more slowly and uses hormones as chemical messengers to cause physiologic changes. The nervous system responds to changes more rapidly and uses nerve impulses to cause physiologic changes.

But it is the nervous system that is the body's master control and communications system; it also monitors and regulates many aspects of the endocrine system. Every thought, action, and sensation reflects nerve activity. We are what our brain has experienced. If all past sensory input could be completely erased, we would be unable to walk, talk, or communicate; we would remember no pain or pleasure.

This chapter examines both the structure and function of the nervous tissue. It begins with an overview of nerves, progresses to nerve impulses and synaptic transmissions, and then examines divisions of the nervous system itself. Finally, the chapter reviews specialized nerve receptors that provide the senses and pathologic conditions of the nervous system, some of which may affect the application of massage.

ANATOMY

Basic structures and components of the nervous system are:
- Brain
- Spinal cord
- Cranial nerves
- Spinal nerves
- Cerebrospinal fluid
- Meninges
- Sense organs
- Neurotransmitters

PHYSIOLOGY

Functions of the nervous system are:

Sensory input. Sensory receptors detect changes, or stimuli, inside the body, such as lowered blood sugar levels, or outside the body, such as an increase in temperature. Receptors carry nerve impulses into the spinal cord and brain.

Interpretive functions. The spinal cord and brain integrate sensory information. They analyze it, store some of it, and decide on appropriate responses.

Motor output. Motor neurons carry nerve impulses from the brain and spinal cord to smooth muscle, cardiac muscle, skeletal muscle, and glands.

Higher mental functioning and emotional responsiveness. The nervous system is also responsible for mental processes (i.e., cognition and memory) and emotional responses (i.e., joy, excitement, anger, anxiety).

IT'S ALL GREEK TO ME

arachnoid	*Gr.* spider; shaped
autonomic	*Gr.* self; law
axon	*Gr.* axis
baroreceptor	*Gr.* weight; *L.* to receive
Broca area	Broca, French surgeon (1824-1880)
cauda equina	*L.* tail-like; horse
cerebellum	*L.* little brain
cerebrum	*L.* brain
chemoreceptor	*Gr.* chemical; *L.* to receive
cochlea	*L.* snail shell
conduction	*L.* to lead together
corpus callosum	*L.* body; hard or callused
cortex	*L.* bark or rind
cyton	*Gr.* cell
dendrites	*Gr.* treelike
diencephalon	*Gr.* two or second; brain
dura mater	*L.* hard or tough; mother
encephalic	*Gr.* brain
filum terminale	*L.* threadlike; at the end
ganglion	*Gr.* knot
gyri	*Gr.* circle
incus	*L.* anvil
internuncial	*L.* between; together, amid; messenger
intrafusal	*L.* within; spindle
macula	*L.* spot
mechanoreceptor	*Gr.* machine; *L.* to receive
medulla oblongata	*L.* marrow or middle; long
meninges	*Gr.* membrane
myelin	*Gr.* marrow
neurilemma	*Gr.* sinew; husk
neuro	*Gr.* sinew
neuroglia	*Gr.* sinew; glue
neurotransmitter	*Gr.* sinew; *L.* a sending across
nociceptor	*L.* hurt; to receive
node of Ranvier	Ranvier, French pathologist (1835-1922)
oligodendrocyte	*Gr.* little; tree; cell
parasympathetic	*Gr.* by the side of, sympathetic
photoreceptor	*Gr.* light; *L.* to receive
pia mater	*L.* tender, soft; mother
plexus	*L.* braid
presbyopia	*Gr.* old man; eye
proprioceptor	*L.* one's own; a receiver

pons	*L.* bridge
reciprocal inhibition	*L.* to move backward; to restrain
reflex	*L.* bent back
retina	*L.* a net
saltatory	*L.* to dance or leap
Schwann cell	Schwann, German anatomist (1810-1882)
soma	*Gr.* body
stapes	*L.* stirrup
stimuli	*L.* to incite
sulci	*L.* groove or furrow
summation	*L.* total
sympathetic	*Gr.* to feel with
synapse	*Gr.* to join
thalamus	*Gr.* chamber
thermoreceptor	*Gr.* heat; *L.* to receive
tympanic	*Gr.* drum
vagus	*L.* wandering
Wernicke area	Wernicke, German neurologist (1848-1905)

Gr., Greek; *L.*, Latin.

BASIC ORGANIZATION

The nervous system has two basic divisions, the central and peripheral nervous systems (Figure 23-1).

Central Nervous System

The central nervous system (CNS) occupies a central or medial position. It is primarily concerned with interpreting incoming sensory information and issuing instructions in the form of motor responses. It is also the center for thoughts and emotional experiences. The major components of the CNS are the brain (cerebrum, cerebellum, diencephalon, and brainstem), meninges, cerebrospinal fluid, and spinal cord. These structures are surrounded by bones of the skull and spinal column.

Peripheral Nervous System

The peripheral nervous system (PNS) is composed of cranial and spinal nerves emerging from the CNS. Cranial nerves exit the brain, and spinal nerves exit the spinal cord. The PNS has 43 pairs of nerves: 12 pairs of cranial nerves and 31 pairs of spinal nerves. The PNS can be further subdivided into the somatic nervous system and the autonomic nervous system.

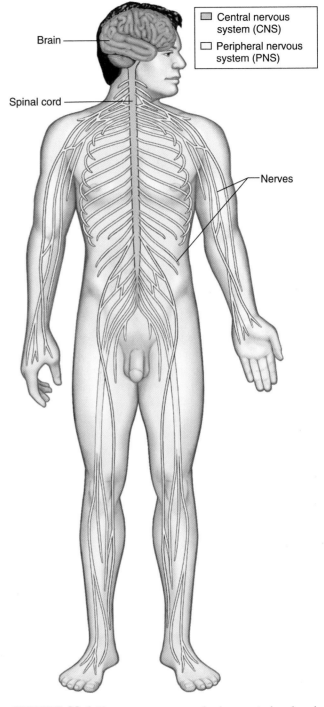

FIGURE 23-1 Nervous system organization; central and peripheral divisions.

Somatic Nervous System. The somatic nervous system (SNS) contains receptors that transmit information from bones, muscles, joints, and skin, as well as from receptors of the special senses, such as vision, hearing, taste, and smell. Motor neurons in the SNS carry impulses from the CNS to skeletal muscles. Because these responses can be consciously controlled, they are considered voluntary.

Autonomic Nervous System. The autonomic nervous system (ANS) is an involuntary system that supplies impulses to smooth muscle, cardiac (heart) muscle, and glands. The ANS consists of *sympathetic* and *parasympathetic* divisions, each possessing complementary responses. For example, if the sympathetic nervous system increases heart rate during times of need, the parasympathetic nervous system returns it to a resting heart rate when the demand has passed. The two divisions of the PNS are discussed later.

The nervous system is made up of billions of cells called neurons and supporting cells called neuroglial cells.

⊖volve *Log onto Evolve and study for exams with online activities and flash cards* ∎

CELLS OF THE NERVOUS SYSTEM

Neuroglia

Neuroglia, or glia, is connective tissue that supports, nourishes, protects, insulates, and organizes neurons. Because it is not neural tissue, neuroglia is unable to transmit impulses. However, these cells are able to replicate themselves through cell division. For this reason, most brain tumors arise from neuroglia. Neuroglia are smaller and more numerous than neurons. In fact, more than 50% of the CNS is made up of these cells.

There are six types of glial cells; four types are located in the CNS (astrocytes, ependymocytes, microglial cells and oligodendrocytes), and two are located in the PNS (satellite cells and Schwann cells).

Supporting cells of the CNS are:

Astrocyte. Needed for structural support of delicate CNS neurons and is part of the blood-brain barrier.

Ependymocyte. Also called ependymal cells, these cells line cranial ventricles and the central canal of the spinal cord. These cells produce, secrete, and assist in the circulation of cerebrospinal fluid (CSF).

Microglia. Specialized macrophages that protects neurons by destroying pathogens and removing dead tissue.

Oligodendrocyte. Forms a myelin sheath that surrounds some axons in the CNS.

The following supporting cells of the PNS are very similar and differ mainly because of their location.

Schwann Cell. Also called a neurolemmocyte, this cell forms a myelin sheath that surrounds only axons in the PNS (Figure 23-2). The outer layer of this sheath is called the neurilemma.

Satellite Cell. Needed for structural support of the PNS and are found surrounding neuron cell bodies within ganglia. Ganglia are knotlike masses of neural cell bodies in the PNS.

Neurons

The human body contains an estimated 100 billion neurons. **Neurons** are basic impulse-conducting cells possessing specialized properties:

Excitability – The ability to respond to a stimulus and convert it to a nerve impulse.

Conductibility – The ability to conduct or transmit the impulses to other neurons, muscles, and glands.

Secretion – For a neuron to conduct an impulse, it must secrete chemicals called neurotransmitters.

Parts of a Neuron. Neurons vary widely in shape and size, but they all have three basic parts: cell body, dendrite, and an axon (see Figure 23-2).

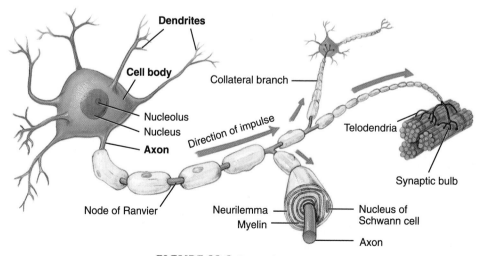

FIGURE 23-2 Parts of a neuron.

Cell Body – The **cell body,** or cyton, contains the nucleus, ribosomes, and other organelles. Neural cell bodies are gray matter of the nervous system. In the brain, gray matter is found on the outer region, or cortex, and in the central region of the brain. In the spinal cord, gray matter is centrally located and forms regions called horns.

Dendrite – **Dendrites** are typically short, narrow, and highly branched extensions of the neuron. These extensions receive and transmit stimuli toward the cell body.

Axon – **Axons** carry nerve impulses away from the cell body toward another neuron, muscle cell, or gland. Long axons are often referred to as the nerve fibers. Axons may possess infrequent branches, called collaterals.

Several structures are associated with axons.

Telodendria. These clusters of short, fine filaments are located on the ends of axons.

Synaptic bulb. At the end of each telodendron are small budlike structures called synaptic bulbs, which contain synaptic vesicles.

Synaptic vesicles. Within each synaptic bulb are saclike structures called vesicles. These contain chemicals called neurotransmitters (see Figure 23-5).

Myelin sheath. Myelin sheaths are fatty layers of tissue surrounding most axons in the PNS. This insulating structure prevents nerve impulses from leakage to adjacent neurons and also increases the speed of the impulse.

MOSHE FELDENKRAIS, DSc

Born: May 6, 1904; died: July 1, 1984

"We settle for so little! As long as we can get by, we let it go at that."

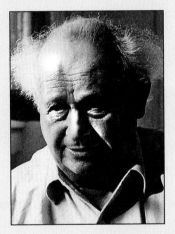

Moshe Feldenkrais obtained his doctorate in science and degrees in both mechanical and electrical engineering and proceeded to work on the French atomic research program and the British antisubmarine program. As a boy of 16 in Palestine, Feldenkrais was part of a group called the Haganah, which means self-defense force. They learned some basic jujitsu. At this time in his life, Feldenkrais realized that the only way to learn was to start at the beginning—with the first move.

"And I built this system of defense for any sort of attack where the first movement is not what you think to do, what you decide to do, but what you actually do when you are frightened. And I said, 'All right, let's see now, we will train the people so that the end of their first spontaneous movement is where we must start.'"

—Moshe on Moshe on the Martial Arts, *Feldenkrais Journal 12*, Issue 2

Feldenkrais published an instructional book on the subject, which gained him admission to his first judo exhibition. The Japanese minister of education, and founder of judo, Jigaro Kano, rather taken by Feldenkrais and what he had accomplished without any formal training, asked him to introduce judo to Europe. Feldenkrais refused, explaining he was unable to devote himself to such an enterprise and continue his university studies at the same time, but the minister was determined. Soon everyone involved agreed that an expert would come to France and work with Feldenkrais when time would allow.

Thus Feldenkrais became one of the first Europeans to hold a black belt in judo. He was also a fierce soccer player.

A soccer injury flared up during the German invasion of France and prompted him to use both his martial arts experience and his engineering and mechanical background to explore the relationship between the nervous system and body function. (A 50/50 chance that surgery would correct the problem was not worth it to Feldenkrais.)

The result of his work is pure genius, but his philosophy became his legacy. He believed in and made a difference to the potential of humankind. He helped men and women become more themselves. He saw the infinite possibilities because he, as did Descartes, viewed the human being as a tabula rasa, or blank slate.

*Reprinted in Embodied Wisdom: The Collected Articles and Interviews of Moshe Feldenkrais, by Moshe Feldenkrais (edited by Elizabeth Berlnger, North Atlantic Books, 2010).

Continued

MOSHE FELDENKRAIS, DSc (*continued*)

*"The problem is that much of what we have learned is harmful to our system because it was learned in childhood, when immediate dependence on others distorted our real needs. Long-standing habitual action feels right. Training a body to be perfect in all the possible forms and configurations of its members changes not only the strength and flexibility of the skeleton and muscles, but makes a profound and beneficial change in the self-image and quality of the direction of the self."**

—Moshe Feldenkrais, *Mind and Body*

Feldenkrais believed that habitual patterns are imprinted in the nervous system, good or bad, but that verbally directed exercises and manipulation could help the brain and body learn movements that would free bodily limitations and instill our natural birthright, a sense of grace.

Feldenkrais' methods led to what might be considered incredible results. People with multiple sclerosis and cerebral palsy gained a new lease on life, and athletes without any obvious physical limitations sought his therapy.

A typical session consists of an instructor leading a group in various exercises or manipulating an individual through small, repeated movements. This system creates a new awareness or spatial reality, which the brain recognizes as being immediately right or better than the original impeded movement.

The sensations experienced in these sessions bring into focus the tension and stress that make our movement inefficient and prepare us to learn new patterns that permit the body to function at a level much closer to its full human potential. Feldenkrais was big on the concept of learning. He thought it was the gift of life, inextricably tied to personal growth and the key to a healthy body and mind.

*"My way of learning, my way of dealing with people is to find out, for that person who wants it, what sort of accomplishment is possible for that person. People can learn to move and walk and stand differently, but they have given up because they think it's too late now, that the growth process has been completed, that they can't learn something new, that they don't have the time or ability. You don't have to go back to being a baby in order to function properly. You can, at any time of your life, rewire yourself, provided I can convince you that there is nothing permanent or compulsive in your system, except what you believe to be so."**

—Moshe Feldenkrais and Will Shutz,
Movement and the Mind

*Reprinted in *Embodied Wisdom: The Collected Articles and Interviews of Moshe Feldenkrais,* by Moshe Feldenkrais (edited by Elizabeth Berlnger, North Atlantic Books, 2010).

Myelin sheaths are formed by Schwann cells, creating a tight covering around the axon. The outer layer of the sheath is called the neurolemma. Myelin sheaths are white in color; therefore myelinated axons are known as white matter.

Nodes of Ranvier. These structures are gaps located at intervals along myelinated axons. Nerve impulses can jump from one node to another, increasing the speed of the impulse (i.e., saltatory conduction featured later).

CHAT ROOM

A mnemonic device for remembering that axons carry impulses away from the cell body is that both *A*xon and *A*way begin with the letter *A*.

Connective Tissues: Neurons to Nerves

Nerves, like muscles, are protected by a series of connective tissue layers. And similar to muscles, neural connective tissues have the same prefixes: endo-, peri-, and epi-.

Each individual neuron is wrapped by a connective tissue layer called *endoneurium*. Bundles of neurons, known as fascicles, are wrapped by *perineurium*. This important connective tissue layer allows for nerve vascularization. Within the fascicle, lymph fills the spaces between the connective tissue–wrapped neurons. A nerve is formed by several fasciculi bound by a connective tissue layer called *epineurium* (Figure 23-3). Fat fills the spaces between connective tissue–wrapped fasciculi.

To review:

Neuron (nerve cell) → nerve fascicle (bundles of neurons) → nerve (bundles of fasciculi)

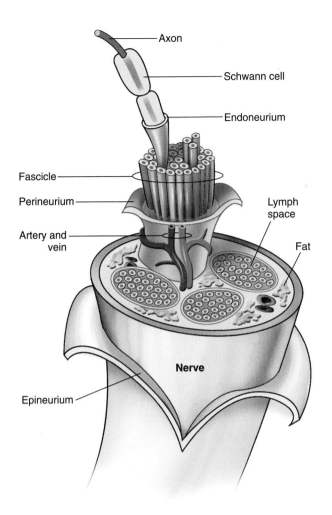

FIGURE 23-3 A nerve.

Endoneurium (wraps neurons) → perineurium (wraps nerve fascicles) → epineurium (wraps nerves)

CLASSIFICATION OF NERVES

Nerves can be classified as sensory, interneurons, or motor. These classifications are based on the direction the impulse is traveling.

Sensory (Afferent) Nerves. Sensory nerves are said to be afferent because they carry impulses to the CNS. Some sensory nerves are close to the skin's surface such as Meissner corpuscles (see Chapter 22). Some lie within the body such as proprioceptors (discussed later).

Interneurons. Interneurons, or association nerves, are found between sensory and motor neurons and they participate in integrative functions. Most neurons are interneurons and are located in the brain and spinal cord.

Motor (Efferent) Nerves. Motor nerves are classified as efferent, which means that they carry impulses from the CNS to activate or inhibit muscles or glands. The muscles or glands that efferent neurons act on are called *effectors.*

NERVE IMPULSES

Neural cell membranes possess the potential, or opportunity, to conduct a nerve impulse. When they are not conducting nerve impulses, they are said to be in a resting state. A **nerve impulse** is an electrical signal that conveys information along a neuron. It consists of a series of events that create an electrical charge inside the cell, moving it from a negative (polarized) resting state to a positive (depolarized) state and back to a negative (repolarized) resting state.

Action Potential

An **action potential** is a brief series of events in which the electrical membrane of a nerve cell changes to conduct an impulse. These changes are caused by movement of charged particles, or ions, across the cell membrane (Figure 23-4). Let us look at membrane potentials in more detail.

Polarization. Polarization describes a neuron's resting membrane potential. During this state, the inside of the neuron bears a negative charge and the outside bears a positive charge. As long as the neuron is polarized, the cell is resting and not transmitting an impulse.

The mechanism that produces and maintains polarization of the neural membrane is called the **sodium-potassium pump.** The membrane transports sodium ions (Na^+) and potassium ions (K^+) in opposite directions at an unequal rate. It moves three Na^+ out of the cell for every two K^+ it moves into the cell (3 : 2). As this pump operates, very little sodium enters the cell.

The concentration of Na^+ outside creates a positive (+) charge, and the concentration of K^+ inside creates a negative (−) charge. The charge differential is said to be polarized.

Depolarization. When a neuron is stimulated, the interior of the cell changes from negative to positive, or depolarizes. During this state, sodium ion channels open, allowing them to flow into the cell.

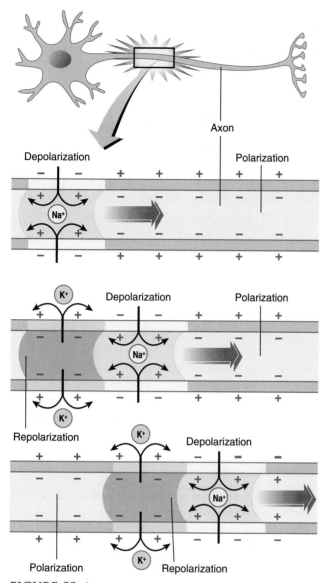

FIGURE 23-4 Nerve impulse: Polarization (*blue area*), depolarization (*yellow area*), and repolarization (*purple area*).

Positively charged sodium ions flow in this direction because they are electrically attracted to the negative charge inside the cell. The migration of sodium ions into the cell continues as long as the channels remain open. This causes the polarity of the cell to reverse, or become positive, owing to the increased presence of positive sodium ions. This occurs in segments down the axon (see Figure 23-4), much like a line of dominoes; the ripple of current travels the length of the neuron until it reaches its destination.

Impulses are conducted along the membrane at maximum capacity without fluctuations in membrane potential and without any decrease in magnitude. The impulse will continue until it reaches the end of the neuron. Nerve transmission never moves back up the neuron, which would restimulate the region from which it just came. These principles are referred to as the **all-or-none response**.

Repolarization. Very quickly, the neuron resumes its resting, or polarized, state. This occurs using several mechanisms. First, the membrane once again becomes impermeable to sodium ions, which closes the sodium ion channels. Potassium ions are electrically repelled by the (now) high concentration of positively charged sodium ions inside of the cell. Potassium ion channels open and allow potassium to flow out of the cell. As potassium ions leave the cell, the membrane repolarizes. The exterior of the cell once again becomes positively charged and the interior resumes its negative charge by means of the sodium potassium pump mentioned previously.

Neurons must be repolarized to be stimulated again. The inability to accept another stimulus until it repolarizes is referred to as **refractory**. The refractory period is its unresponsive period.

Therefore, the nerve impulse is simply a matter of ions changing places, which creates the electrical charge along the neural membrane.

Conduction and Impulse Speed

There are two types of nerve impulse conduction: along unmyelinated axons and along myelinated axons. Nerve impulses conducted along myelinated axons are the faster of the two.

Continuous Conduction. Nerve impulse conduction along unmyelinated axons is called **continuous conduction.**

Saltatory Conduction. Nerve impulse conduction along myelinated axons is called **saltatory conduction.** When nerve impulses reach a myelinated axon, the impulses are able to jump along the length of an axon from one node of Ranvier to the next. The ability of an impulse to jump across the length of the axon greatly increases the speed of conduction. The term saltatory comes from the Latin word *saltare,* meaning "to leap." Another term for myelinated axons is fast-conducting nerve fibers.

The fastest nerve fibers, such as those that innervate the skeletal muscles, can conduct impulses up to approximately 130 meters per second (close to 300 miles per hour). The slowest fibers, such as sensory receptors in the skin, may conduct impulses at only 0.5 meter per second (little more than 1 mile per hour).

⊖volve *To see an image of saltatory conduction or how nerve impulses are transmitted on myelinated axon, look up the course materials for Chapter 23 on the Evolve website.* ■

SYNAPSE

The junction between two neurons or between a neuron and a muscle or gland is called a **synapse** (Figure 23-5). Nerve

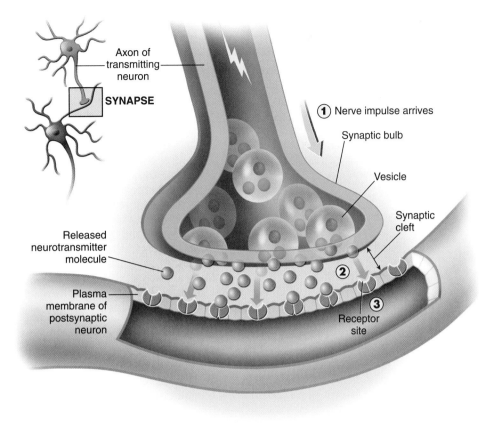

Axon of
transmitting
neuron

SYNAPSE

(1) Nerve impulse arrives

Synaptic bulb

Vesicle

Synaptic
cleft

Released
neurotransmitter
molecule

(2)

(3)

Plasma
membrane of
postsynaptic
neuron

Receptor
site

FIGURE 23-5 Synapse: structures and transmission.

impulses are transmitted across the synapse through the action of neurotransmitters.

Synaptic Structures

A synapse is made up of three primary structures.

Synaptic Bulb (Presynaptic Neuron). Located on the ends of axons are small budlike structures called synaptic bulbs, which contain synaptic vesicles. Each vesicle is filled with chemicals called neurotransmitters (see later discussion).

Synaptic Cleft. The space between the synaptic bulb and the plasma membrane of the postsynaptic neuron is called the synaptic cleft or synaptic gap.

Plasma Membrane (Postsynaptic Neuron). The plasma membranes found on dendrites of postsynaptic neurons contain receptor sites. These serve as binding sites for neurotransmitters released from presynaptic vesicles.

Synaptic Transmission

Synaptic transmission is a one-way process. Let us examine the process in three steps (see Figure 23-5).

1. A nerve impulse travels down an axon to a synaptic bulb. Nerve impulses cannot cross synaptic clefts; instead, neurotransmitters are released from vesicles within the synaptic bulb.
2. Neurotransmitters travel across the synaptic cleft toward postsynaptic neuron's plasma membrane.
3. The neurotransmitters bind with receptor sites on the postsynaptic neuron, which brings about a response by the postsynaptic neuron. The response may be either excitatory or inhibitory, depending on the neurotransmitter eliciting the response. This means that either the impulse will be continued or it will be stopped.

The action of neurotransmitters does not persist for a long time because the neurotransmitter is continuously removed from the synaptic cleft by either enzymes or **reuptake** (the drawing up of a substance by the presynaptic neuron).

Neurotransmitters

Neurotransmitters are a collective term for chemical messengers involved in impulse transmission; it is how neurons talk to each other and to muscles and glands. Recall that these chemicals are stored in vesicles and released during synaptic transmission.

Neurotransmitters can be either excitatory or inhibitory. Excitatory neurotransmitters decrease the membrane

TABLE 23-1 Examples of Neurotransmitters

NEUROTRANSMITTER	LOCATION	FUNCTION
Acetylcholine (ACh)	Found in neuromuscular junctions and in many parts of the brain	Can be excitatory or inhibitory; vital for stimulating muscle contraction; also involved with memory
Epinephrine	Found in several areas of the CNS and in the sympathetic division of the ANS	Can be excitatory or inhibitory; mediates the "fight or flight" response; hormonelike action when secreted by the adrenal medulla
Norepinephrine	Found in several areas of the CNS and in the sympathetic division on the ANS	Similar to epinephrine, can be excitatory or inhibitory; also a hormone secreted by the adrenal medulla. This hormone mediates several physiologic and metabolic responses related to sympathetic arousal (fight or flight); also involved in dreaming, mood regulation, and emotional responses
Dopamine	Found in the brain and ANS	Mostly inhibitory and involved in emotions, moods, and motor control regulation; also implicated in attention and learning
Serotonin	Found in several regions of the CNS	Mostly inhibitory and important for sensory perception, mood regulation, and normal sleep
Histamine	Found in the brain	Mostly excitatory and involved in emotions, body temperature regulation, and water balance; histamine stimulates inflammatory responses when not acting as a neurotransmitter
Enkephalins	Found in several regions of the CNS, the retina, and the intestinal tract	Mostly inhibitory and action is similar to that of opiates as a pain-reducing agent
Endorphins	Found in several regions of the CNS, the retina, and the intestinal tract	Mostly inhibitory and action is similar to that of opiates as a pain-reducing agent
Gamma-aminobutyric acid (GABA)	Found in the brain	Mostly inhibitory
Substance P	Found in the brain, spinal cord, pain pathways, and the intestinal tract	Mostly excitatory and transmits pain information

potential (the charge difference across the membrane), thereby allowing the impulse to be continued. Inhibitory neurotransmitters increase the membrane potential to the point that the impulse cannot be continued.

The most common neurotransmitter is acetylcholine (ACh). Other neurotransmitters include epinephrine, norepinephrine, serotonin, dopamine, gamma-aminobutyric acid (GABA), and endorphins. See Table 23-1 for a list of neurotransmitters.

CHAT ROOM

Catecholamines are a chemical family containing norepinephrine, epinephrine, and dopamine. The major functions of catecholamines include excitation and inhibition of certain muscles, cardiac excitation, metabolic action, and endocrine action. Catecholamines act directly on the sympathetic nervous system.

CENTRAL NERVOUS SYSTEM

The brain and spinal cord together make up the CNS. The brain is housed inside the skull and the spinal cord is housed inside the vertebral column. In addition to bony protection, the brain and spinal cord are protected by connective tissue membranes called meninges and cerebrospinal fluid.

BRAIN

One of the largest organs in the body, the brain contains an estimated 100 billion neurons. The brain is where information is fused into character and behavior.

Brain cells use only glucose as an energy source, and this glucose cannot be stored as glycogen, unlike glucose stored by liver or muscle cells. Glucose breaks down only by aerobic respiration; thus the brain needs a continuous supply of both glucose and oxygen. The brain uses approximately 20% of the body's oxygen intake.

The brain consists of four main parts: (1) cerebrum, (2) diencephalon, (3) cerebellum, and (4) brain stem (Figure 23-6).

CEREBRUM

Shaped like a boxing glove, the cerebrum is the largest part of the brain. This structure is where sensations (e.g., vision, smell, taste, body movements) are consciously perceived, where skeletal muscle motor movements are initiated, and where emotional and intellectual processes occur. This area is also where decisions are made. Sensory areas interpret sensory input, and motor areas control muscular movement. Language centers that interpret written and spoken words, as well as initiating speech, are located in the cerebrum. The *limbic system* within the cerebrum governs emotional aspects

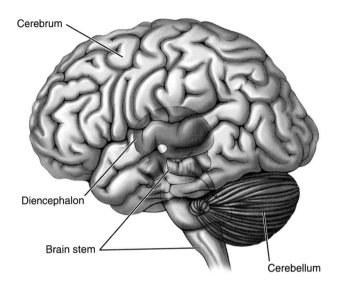

Cerebrum

Diencephalon

Brain stem

Cerebellum

FIGURE 23-6 Main parts of the brain.

of behavior needed for survival, such as sexual feelings, rage, and docility.

The *cerebral cortex* is a thin gray layer covering the outer region of the cerebrum. White matter, which constitutes most of the cerebrum, lies beneath the cerebral cortex.

The brain's topography is characterized by grooves and elevated ridges. *Sulci* are grooves in the outer layer of the cerebral cortex. These structures separate the cerebrum into lobes (see later discussion). A *fissure* is a deep sulcus. *Gyri* are elevated ridges of tissue.

CHAT ROOM

Throughout the cerebrum's white matter are patches of gray matter called *basal ganglia*. These areas assist in motor control (including facial expression). Dopamine is largely responsible for basal ganglia activity. Dopamine depletion produces symptoms of rigidity, tremors, and uncoordinated and slower-than-normal movement, such as seen in Parkinson disease.

Hemispheres

The *longitudinal fissure* separates the cerebrum into *left* and *right cerebral hemispheres*. Connecting the hemispheres are large fibrous bundles of transverse fibers, the *corpus callosum*, which provides a communication pathway for impulses to move from one hemisphere to the other.

Hemispheric Specialization. Left and right cerebral hemispheres are similar in appearance. However, research indicates that they possess specialized functions. These differences were discovered mainly through examination of patients who underwent surgery in an attempt to control

seizures by severing the corpus callosum. The following hemispheric differences were noted.

Left Hemisphere – The left hemisphere specializes in language, both receptive and expressive. It also governs many mathematical abilities, as well as reasoning and analytical skills.

Right Hemisphere – The right hemisphere specializes in perception of sounds, such as melodies; art; and emotional expression. The right hemisphere appears to be superior in regard to perceiving and visualizing spatial relationships.

Despite the specializations of each cerebral hemisphere, both sides of a normal person's brain communicate with each other via the corpus callosum to accomplish many complex functions.

Lobes

Each hemisphere contains four lobes (Figure 23-7). They are named for the overlying skull bone.

Frontal Lobe. The frontal lobe regulates motor output, cognition, and speech production (Broca's area; typically the left hemisphere only). The frontal lobe contains the *prefrontal cortex*, which is connected directly to the limbic system making up what is known as the *corticolimbic system*. The prefrontal cortex acts as the executive controller of this system, where emotions are processed.

The *central sulcus* is located between the frontal and parietal lobes. Located anterior to the central sulcus is an area called the *precentral gyrus*. This area controls voluntary movements and is also called the "primary motor area." Of interest is that the larger the area of brain tissue, the more complex the movement (Figure 23-8).

Parietal Lobe. Parietal lobes receive information about proprioception (a sense of where your body is), reading, and taste. This area also governs sensory input (namely the skin and muscles).

Located posterior to the central sulcus is the *postcentral gyrus*. Because it receives sensory information, this area is also called the "primary somatosensory area." Like the precentral gyrus, the larger the area, the more receptors found in the corresponding part of the body (see Figure 22-5). The hands, face, lips, jaw, and tongue take up approximately 80% of this neural space.

Temporal Lobe. Temporal lobes house auditory and olfactory areas and the Wernicke area. The latter area is critical to language comprehension, which is typically in the left hemisphere only.

The *lateral fissure* separates the temporal lobe and the frontal and parietal lobes.

Occipital Lobe. The occipital lobe contain centers for visual input.

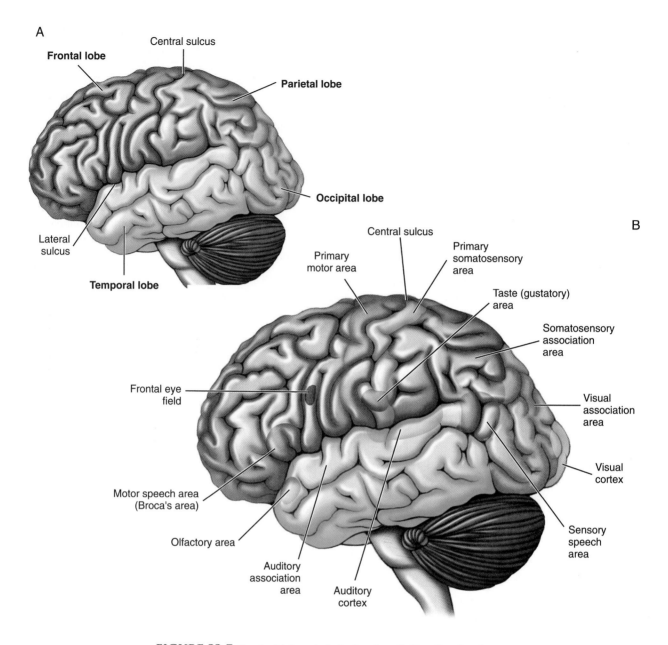

FIGURE 23-7 Cerebral lobes. **A,** Lobe location. **B,** Functional regions.

Brain Waves and States of Consciousness

In this discussion, *consciousness* is the degree of mental alertness and responsiveness. The cerebral cortex regulates levels of consciousness and these levels can be recorded by an electroencephalogram (EEG) as brain wave patterns. Scientists have noted that these patterns are linked to states of consciousness. These brain wave patterns are classified based on their frequency and amplitude. *Frequency* is the number of waves per second, measured in hertz (Hz). *Amplitude* refers to voltage. Brain waves and their associated states of consciousness and are identified by Greek letters. Listed in order of frequency from fastest to slowest, these brain wave patterns are beta, alpha, theta, and delta.

Beta. The beta state (13 to 30 Hz) is associated with wakeful consciousness and mental activity. Attention is focused on external surroundings, and rational thinking, with occasional thought patterns. High-intensity beta waves are associated with extreme stress. Beta waves are busy waves. Dreaming while sleeping (rapid eye movement [REM]) appears as beta waves.

Alpha. Alpha state (8 to 12 Hz), in contrast with beta, is a relaxed state. The subject is awake but calm and inattentive. Alpha activity is also associated with creative processes, and meditation.

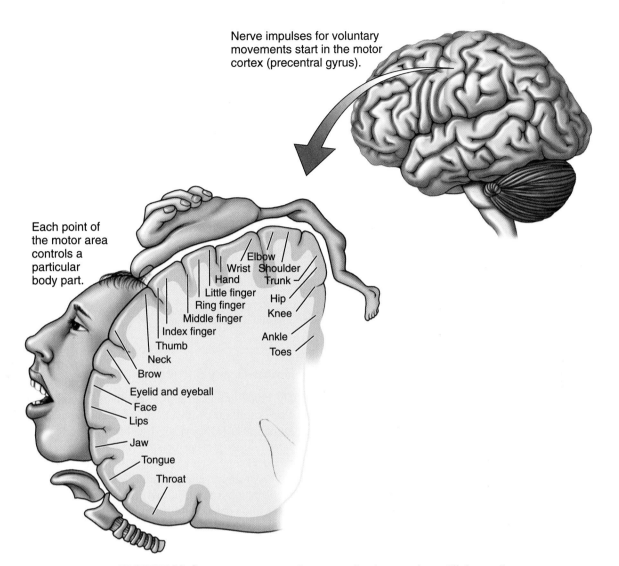

Nerve impulses for voluntary movements start in the motor cortex (precentral gyrus).

Each point of the motor area controls a particular body part.

Elbow
Wrist Shoulder
Hand Trunk
Little finger
Ring finger Hip
Middle finger Knee
Index finger
Thumb Ankle
Neck Toes
Brow
Eyelid and eyeball
Face
Lips
Jaw
Tongue
Throat

FIGURE 23-8 Precentral gyrus and corresponding homunculus or "little man."

Theta. Theta state (4 to 8 Hz) is associated with drowsiness, dreamlike awareness, collective subconscious, and out-of-body experiences. This state of consciousness is used in hypnosis to access deep-rooted memories.

Delta. Delta state (0.5 to 4 Hz) patterns are deep sleep waves from which the subject is not easily aroused.

DIENCEPHALON

Located in the center of the brain, the diencephalon houses two primary structures: the thalamus and the hypothalamus (Figure 23-9). Included in the diencephalon are structures such as pituitary and pineal glands.

Thalamus. The thalamus, which is nearly 80% of the diencephalon, relays sensory information (except olfaction) to appropriate parts of the cerebrum.

Hypothalamus. The hypothalamus regulates the ANS and endocrine system by governing the pituitary. The hypothalamus also controls behavioral patterns and the 24-hour cycle called the *circadian rhythm*. The hypothalamus controls hunger, thirst, anger, aggression, hormones, sexual behavior, temperature, and sleep patterns, and along with the reticular activating system, it maintains consciousness.

The **pituitary** is connected to the hypothalamus by a slender stalk (infundibulum) and sits in the sella turcica of the sphenoid bone. The **pineal** is located below the corpus callosum. Although its function is not clear, the pineal gland produces and secretes the hormone melatonin. Both of these glands are discussed in Chapter 24.

CEREBELLUM

The cerebellum is a cauliflower-shaped structure located posterior and inferior to the cerebrum. The cerebellum is the

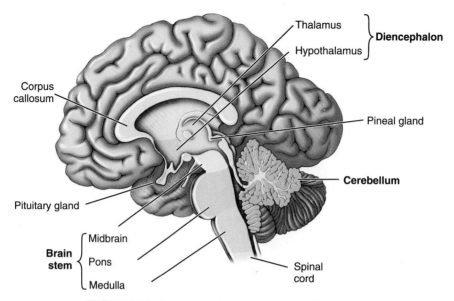

FIGURE 23-9 Diencephalon, cerebellum, and brainstem.

second largest part of the brain and is concerned with muscle tone, coordinates complex movements, and regulates posture and balance (see Figure 23-9).

BRAINSTEM

The brainstem is continuous with the spinal cord and has three main divisions: mid-brain, pons, and medulla oblongata (see Figure 23-9). Structures associated with the *reticular activating system* are found throughout the entire brain stem. This system functions in waking the person up from sleep and maintaining consciousness.

Mid-brain. The midbrain conducts nerve impulses from the cerebrum to the pons and sensory impulses from the spinal cord to the thalamus. It also helps control movements of the eyes, head, and neck in response to visual and auditory stimuli.

Pons. The pons bridges the cerebellum and cerebrum with the spinal cord.

Medulla Oblongata. The most inferior portion of the brainstem, the medulla oblongata conducts sensory and motor impulses between other parts of the brain and the spinal cord. The medulla, often considered the most vital part of the brain, contains the respiratory, cardiovascular, and vasomotor centers. The medulla also controls gastric secretions and reflexes, such as sweating, sneezing, swallowing, and vomiting.

The medulla oblongata contains much of the crossing over fibers that cause the left cerebral hemisphere's association with the body's right side and vise versa. This crossing over is called *decussation*.

Blood-Brain Barrier

The blood-brain barrier is a selective semipermeable wall of blood capillaries with a thick basement membrane and neuroglial cells (astrocytes). The function of the blood-brain barrier is to prevent or slow down the passage of some chemical compounds and disease-causing organisms such as viruses from traveling from the blood into the CNS. Blood itself contains chemicals that can damage neurons; if neurons come into contact with blood, they die.

SPINAL CORD

The spinal cord exits the skull through the foramen magnum and extends to approximately the second lumbar (L2) region. In addition to being an integrating center, the spinal cord acts as an information highway. It conveys sensory information from peripheral nerves to the brain and motor information from the brain to peripheral nerves.

Two enlargements are located in the length of the spinal cord: one in the cervical region and one in the lumbar region (Figure 23-10). The lower ends of the cord fan out, resembling a horse's tail, and form a structure appropriately called the *cauda equina*. The lower portion of the spinal cord is marked by threadlike fibrous extension called the *filum terminale*, which is anchored to the coccyx.

A cross section of the spinal cord reveals white matter on the periphery surrounding gray matter (H-shaped) in the deeper region. In the center of the spinal cord is a structure properly named the *central canal*, which runs the entire length and contains circulating CSF.

Horns. The sides of the H in the gray matter are called *horns*, which are divided into the anterior, lateral, and posterior horns.

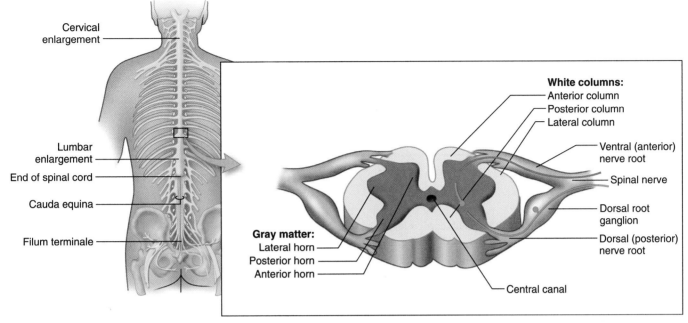

FIGURE 23-10 Spinal cord.

Columns. White matter is organized into regions called *columns*. There are anterior, lateral, and posterior columns.

Tracts. Within the spinal cord is a collection of nerves running up and down in columns called *tracts*. Tracts are divided into two categories: ascending and descending. Sensory or afferent impulses travel up the cord to the brain on ascending tracts, and motor or efferent impulses travel down and out of the cord on descending tracts.

Meninges

Connective tissue coverings deep in the skull and spine surrounding the brain and spinal cord are called meninges. In between each layer is a fluid-filled space (Figure 23-11).

Pia Mater. The innermost layer, the pia mater, is delicate, transparent, and vascular and is attached to the surface of the CNS.

Arachnoid. The middle layer, the arachnoid or arachnoid mater, forms a loose covering around the CNS.

Between the pia mater and arachnoid is the *subarachnoid space*. It is filled with CSF and an arrangement of collagen and elastic fibers that resemble a spider's web. These extensions extend into the arachnoid.

Dura Mater. The outermost layer, the thick and dense dura mater, lies against bone and contains a double layer of connective tissue, with the outer layer resembling

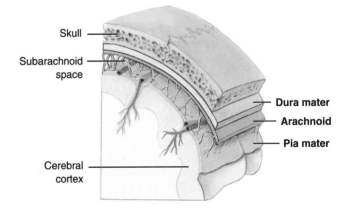

FIGURE 23-11 Meninges in the skull region.

periosteum. Dura mater surrounding the brain dips down between the cerebral hemispheres, creating the *falx cerebri*; dips across between the cerebrum and cerebellum, creating the *tentorium cerebelli*; and dips down between the paired cerebellar hemispheres to create the *falx cerebelli*.

The *subdural space*, filled with circulating serous fluid, lies between dura mater and arachnoid.

The *epidural space* lies between the dura and the vertebral canal. This space, which is the safest place for injections such as saddle blocks, contains adipose tissue, connective tissue, and blood vessels.

Cerebrospinal Fluid

Circulating around the brain and spinal cord within the subarachnoid space is a clear fluid called **cerebrospinal fluid** (CSF). This fluid is derived from blood and supplies tissues of the brain and spinal cord with oxygen and nutrients, and carries away wastes. It also acts as a shock absorber.

After CSF circulates through cavities within the brain and spinal cord, it is reabsorbed into the bloodstream. CSF is sensitive to glucose and electrolyte balance and to changes in the carbon dioxide content.

> *"I happen to feel that the degree of a person's intelligence is directly reflected by the number of conflicting attitudes she can bring to bear on the same topic."*
> —Lisa Alter

PERIPHERAL NERVOUS SYSTEM

All nervous tissue outside the central nervous system is considered part of the peripheral nervous system or PNS. Nerves arising from the brain are called *cranial nerves*; there are 12 pairs of them. Nerves arising from the spinal cord are called *spinal nerves*; there are 31 pairs of them. Most of the peripheral nerves have sensory and motor neurons within them.

Cranial Nerves

The 12 pairs of cranial nerves emerge from the inferior surface of the brain and are named by Roman numerals (I though XII) or by the area(s) they supply (Figure 23-12):

CN I: Olfactory. Senses smell.
CN II: Optic. Employs vision.
CN III: Oculomotor. Moves eyeballs and eyelids. Constricts pupils.
CN IV: Trochlear. Moves eyeballs.
CN V: Trigeminal. Contains three branches; pain, temperature, and motor innervation for muscles of mastication.
CN VI: Abducens. Moves eyeballs.

CN VII: Facial. Facial expression and produces both saliva and tears.
CN VIII: Vestibulocochlear. Auditory or acoustic and conveys messages of equilibrium and hearing.
CN IX: Glossopharyngeal. Produces saliva and employs taste and swallowing.
CN X: Vagus. Receives sensations from external ear and external auditory canal and thoracic and abdominal organs. Aids digestion. Regulates heart activity.
CN XI: Accessory or spinal accessory. Controls the tongue for speech and swallowing. Innervates trapezius and sternocleidomastoid muscles.
CN XII: Hypoglossal. Moves the tongue for speech and swallowing.

Spinal Nerves

The spinal cord consists of 31 segments, each of which gives rise to a pair of spinal nerves. Beginning at the top of the cord are 8 cervical nerves, 12 thoracic nerves, 5 lumbar nerves, 5 sacral nerves, and 1 coccygeal nerve (Figure 23-13). Spinal nerves exit the spine through tiny holes in the vertebrae called *foramina.*

Nerve Roots. Each pair of spinal nerves joins the spinal column at two points called roots; one on the left and another on the right. Each spinal nerve has a *ventral (anterior) nerve root* and a *dorsal (posterior) nerve root* (see Figure 23-10). The ventral nerve root contains motor neurons, and the dorsal nerve root, contains sensory neurons. Hence, all spinal nerves have sensory and motor components.

Ganglion. A cluster of nerve cell bodies located in the PNS is called a **ganglion.** Most ganglia are located next to the spinal cord. The dorsal nerve root of the spinal nerve contains a cluster of sensory nerve cell bodies called the *dorsal root ganglion* (see Figure 23-10).

When a spinal nerve exits the spinal cord, it divides into two branches: (1) *anterior ramus* and (2) *posterior ramus.* Anterior rami innervate the extremities, lateral and anterior trunk, and superficial back muscles. Posterior rami innervate the skin and deep back muscles.

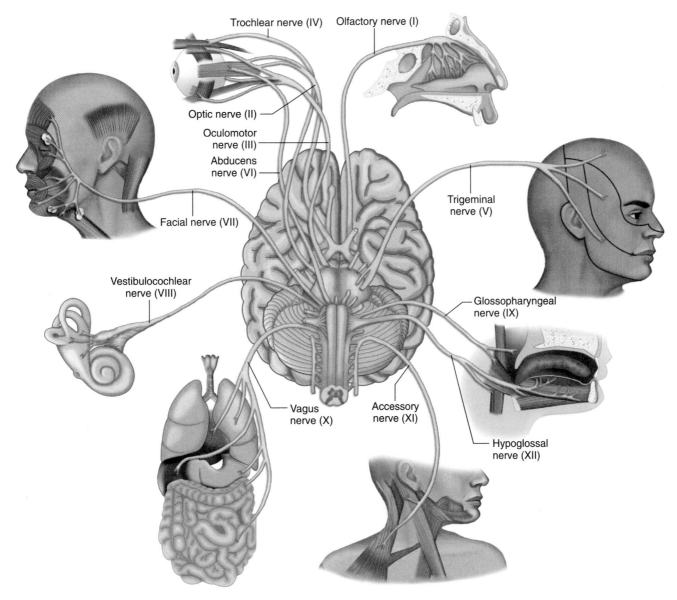

FIGURE 23-12 Cranial nerves.

Nerve Plexuses

A network of intersecting nerves in the PNS is called **plexus.** The body contains many plexuses; the major ones are the (see Figure 23-13):

Cervical Plexus (C1-C5). Supplies skin and muscles of the head, neck, and shoulders. Supplies the diaphragm.

Brachial Plexus (C5-T1). Supplies skin and muscles of the upper extremity.

Lumbosacral Plexus (L1-S4). Supplies skin and muscles of the abdomen, lower back, genitalis, and lower extremities.

Dermatomes

A **dermatome** is an area of skin that a specific sensory nerve root supplies. Dermatomes are named for the particular nerve it serves. For example, the C6 dermatome is innervated by the spinal nerve C6.

Dermatomes are roughly the same from person to person, although sometimes an overlap in innervation is found between adjacent dermatomes. The distribution of these nerves is called a dermatome map (Figure 23-14).

Myotomes

Similar to a dermatome, a **myotome** is a group of skeletal muscles innervated by a single spinal segment. Some overlap

Plexuses

Spinal nerves

Cervical plexus

Brachial plexus

Axillary nerve

Phrenic nerve

Musculo-
cutaneous nerve

Radial nerve

Median nerve

Ulnar nerve

Cauda equina

*Lumbosacral
plexus*

Sciatic nerve

Femoral nerve

Tibial nerve

Common peroneal
nerve

C1
C2
C3
C4
C5
C6
C7
C8
T1
T2
T3
T4
T5
T6
T7
T8
T9
T10
T11
T12
L1
L2
L3
L4
L5
S1
S2
S3
S4
S5
CO1

Cervical (8)

Thoracic (12)

Lumbar (5)

Sacral (5)

Coccygeal (1)

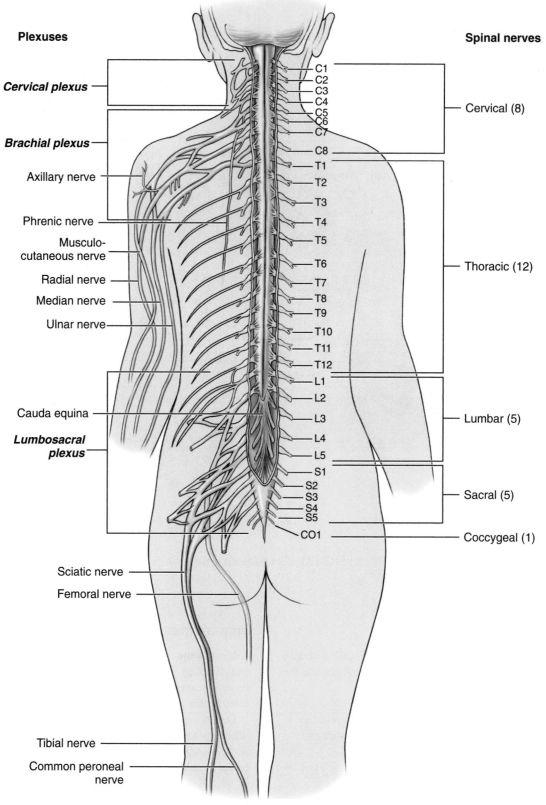

FIGURE 23-13 Spinal nerves.

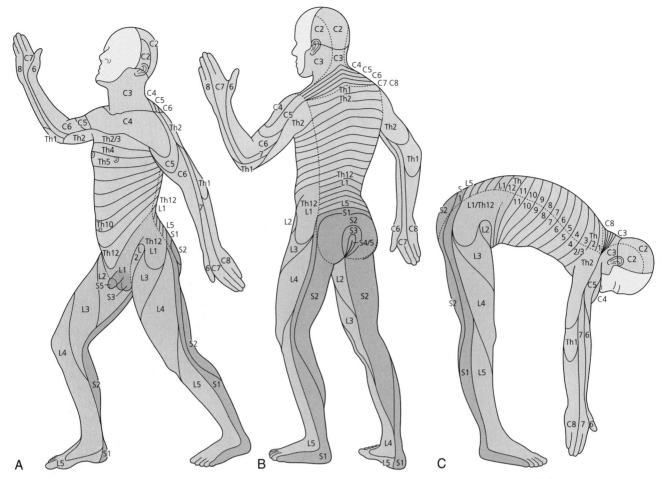

FIGURE 23-14 Dermatome map. **A,** Anterolateral view. **B,** Posterolateral view. **C,** Lateral view.

exists among myotomes. Figure 23-15 illustrates movements produced by skeletal muscles innervated by specific spinal nerves, indicated by arrows. The distribution of these nerves is called a myotome map.

Reflexes

A **reflex** is an involuntary, predictable response to a stimulus. Reflexes are essentially a protective reaction. Some spinal reflexes are responsible for contraction of skeletal muscles, such as the patellar reflex that occurs when the patellar tendon is tapped with a rubber hammer (i.e., knee-jerk) (Figure 23-16).

There are many kinds of reflexes such as spinal reflexes as just described. Other reflexes help to maintain homeostasis through coughing, sneezing, blinking, and correcting heart rate, respiratory rate, and blood pressure.

Reflexes involve a neurologic unit called a reflex arc. While the neuron represents the nervous system's simplest structural unit, the reflex arc is the simplest functional unit. The **reflex arc** carries a stimulus impulse to the spinal cord where it connects with a motor neuron that carries the reflex

impulse back to an appropriate muscle or gland (called an effector).

When certain stimuli (e.g., contact with direct heat) enter a sensory nerve, it travels into the posterior horn of the spinal cord and generates a response from a motor nerve. This causes retraction from the injurious stimuli. Information about the event does not reach the brain until after the reflex response occurs.

Other spinal reflexes, such as stretch reflexes governed by muscle spindles and Golgi tendon organs, are discussed later in this chapter.

An abnormal arc, or *physiopathologic reflex arc*, is caused by increased stimuli or an increase in the amount of sensory information entering the cord. These increases may be the result of pain from an accident, emotional stress, or biomechanical dysfunction such as poor posture. For instance, poor posture may cause increased muscle tonus, which in turn causes vasoconstriction, which causes ischemia. This, in turn, causes pain. Trigger points often form in these tissues. Pain from trigger points may referred to adjacent tissues, causing them to tighten up in response, and a cycle of pain continues. This circumstance is an example of a physiopathologic reflex arc.

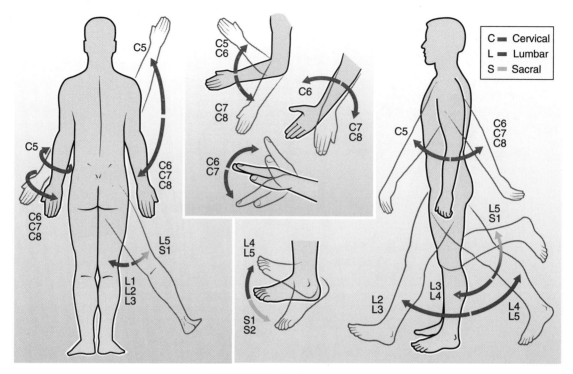

FIGURE 23-15 Myotome map.

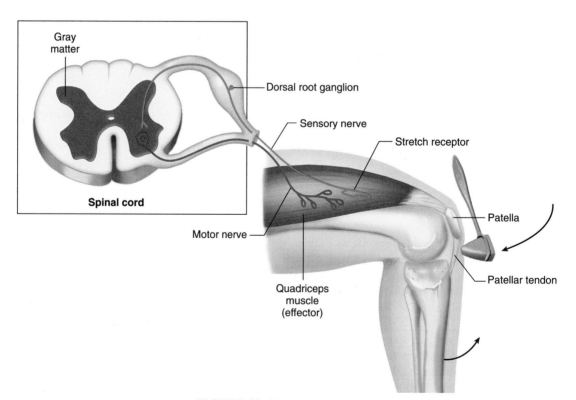

FIGURE 23-16 Patellar reflex.

CHAT ROOM

Massage therapy aids in breaking the physiopathologic reflex arc and helps reestablish equilibrium and a normal reflex arc. As the tissues are warmed, fascia, which encases muscle, is softened, allowing them to lengthen more easily. As muscles lengthen, intra-joint pressure is decreased. Massage may increase local circulation of blood. Massage may also stimulate the release of natural painkillers, such as endorphins. Massage may also inhibit the sensation of pain via gate control theory (see Chapter 6), in which the experience of one type of sensation (e.g., pressure, cold, heat) can act to exclude the experience of another (e.g., pain) that are all vying for the same "gate" or entrance to the CNS.

AUTONOMIC NERVOUS SYSTEM

The ANS innervates cardiac and smooth muscles, as well as glands. By this, the ANS regulates heart and respiration rate, blood circulation, body temperature, gastrointestinal activity, and many other body functions (Figure 23-17). The hypothalamus regulates the activity of the ANS.

Divisions. Within the ANS are two divisions: sympathetic nervous system and parasympathetic nervous system. The effects of these two systems are most often opposed; one system excites, and the other system inhibits. This relationship controls organs in a way to maintain homeostasis (Table 23-2). In some cases, the effects of both systems are complementary. For example, penile erection occurs during parasympathetic arousal and ejaculation occurs during sympathetic arousal.

Dual Innervation. Most organs and body structures are innervated by both sympathetic and parasympathetic divisions. This is called dual innervation. Some structures have only sympathetic innervation (adrenal glands and blood vessels); some structures have only parasympathetic innervation (lacrimal apparatus). In extreme fear, both systems may act simultaneously, producing involuntary emptying of the bladder and rectum and a generalized sympathetic response.

"I have been twenty-five for four years, and I shall stay there for another four. Then I'll be twenty-seven for a while. I intend to grow old gracefully."
—Zsa Zsa Gabor as Jane Avril in "Moulin Rouge"

Parasympathetic Nervous System

The nickname of the parasympathetic division is the "rest-and-digest division"; it dominates at rest and supports body functions that conserve and restore body energy, such as digestion. Because the parasympathetic nervous system is most active under calm conditions and stimulates visceral organs for normal functions as it maintains homeostasis, it is also referred to as the "housekeeping system." Body processes in parasympathetic mode include salivation, urination, digestive processes, defecation, and storing nutrients to be used later.

Fibers of the parasympathetic nervous system occupy spaces at the spinal cord level S2 to S4 and cranial nerves III, VII, IX, and X (see Figure 23-17). For this reason, the parasympathetic nervous system is often called *craniosacral outflow.*

TABLE 23-2 Various Autonomic Responses

SYMPATHETIC ACTIVITY	PARASYMPATHETIC ACTIVITY
Increases heart rate and strength of contraction	Decreases heart rate and strength of contraction
Increases respiratory rate	Maintains resting respiratory rate
Facilitates bronchiolar dilation	Facilitates bronchial constriction
Releases glucose from liver; raises blood sugar	Non-applicable
Facilitates blood vessel constriction (skin and viscera); raises blood pressure and loss of skin color	Non-applicable
Facilitates blood vessel dilation (skeletal muscles and heart)	Facilitates coronary blood vessel dilation; no effect on skeletal muscle blood vessels
Facilitates blood vessel dilation of external genitalia, causing erection	Facilitates blood vessel contraction of external genitalia
Facilitates pupillary dilation; accommodates far vision	Facilitates pupillary constriction; accommodates near vision
Increases perspiration	Non-applicable
No effect on tearing of eyes	Stimulates tearing of eyes
Inhibits salivation	Stimulates salivation
Inhibits pancreatic secretions	Stimulates pancreatic secretions and that of insulin
Decreases gastrointestinal motility (inhibits digestion)	Increases gastrointestinal motility
Facilitates constriction of gastrointestinal tract sphincters	Facilitates relaxation of gastrointestinal tract sphincters
Inhibits urination	Stimulates urination
Facilitates stimulation of adrenal glands to release epinephrine and norepinephrine	Non-applicable

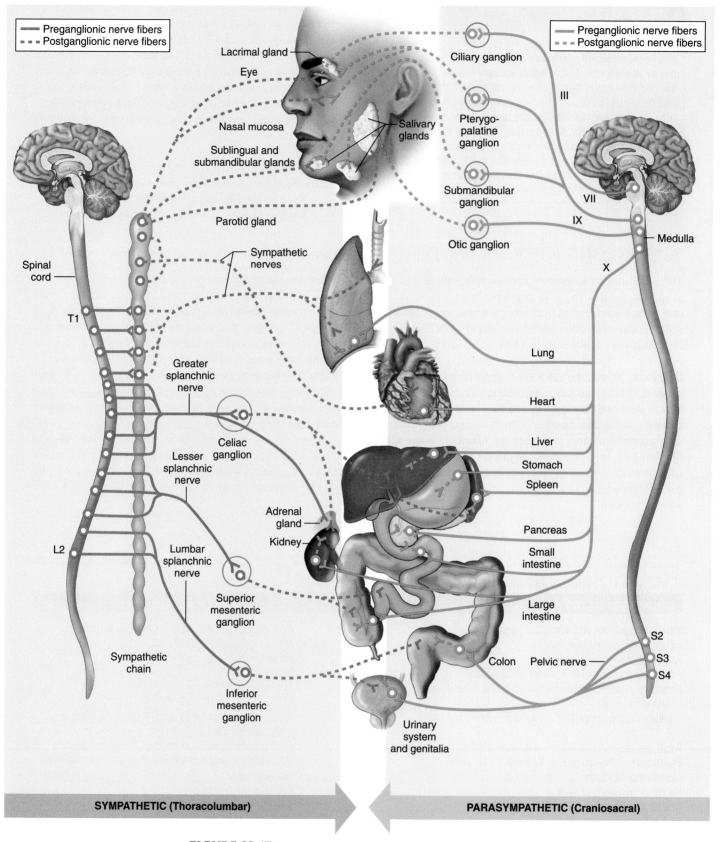

FIGURE 23-17 Autonomic nervous system: divisions and pathways.

During stressful situations, the sympathetic nervous system narrows the perceptual field to facilitate the fight-or-flight response. In contrast, during times of rest and relaxation, the parasympathetic nervous system broadens the perceptual field. One gift of parasympathetic response that occurs during a massage is that, in the client's relaxed state, he or she can often contemplate additional options or solutions to life's challenges.

Sympathetic Nervous System

The sympathetic division overrides the parasympathetic division during physical exertion or emotional stress; thus the set of responses for this division has the nickname of the "fight-or-flight" or "stress" response. Sympathetic responses require body energy. Effects include pupil dilation; increased in heart rate, force of heart contraction, and in blood pressure; dilation of airways; and constriction of blood vessels in the digestive tract so more blood can be moved to dilated blood vessels in skeletal muscles and the heart. All reactions of the sympathetic division occur quickly. Processes that are not needed for meeting the stressful situation, such as secretions and movements of the digestive tract, are suppressed (see Box 23-1: Self-Awareness and Massage Therapy).

Nerves of this division cause the adrenal gland to secrete epinephrine, which sustains the actions of the sympathetic nervous system through the use of hormones.

Most of the cell bodies of the sympathetic system lie in a paravertebral chain of ganglia at the level of T1 to L2 (see Figure 23-17). For this reason, the sympathetic nervous system is often called *thoracolumbar outflow*.

SENSES

The five senses are touch, taste, smell, vision, and hearing. The senses help us experience our environment. Receptors located in their respective organs, arise from ectoderm, the cellular layer from which the brain and spinal cord arise (see Chapter 18). The Greek philosopher Aristotle was the first to discuss the five senses. Four of the five senses reside in the head and are called *special senses*. Touch, which involves the skin, is known as a *general sense*.

Touch

The sense of touch is an amalgamation of many receptors found in the skin. The skin can perceive many sensations, including temperature pressure, pain, and movement. Indeed, touch is not one sense but many. Touch and touch receptors are discussed in Chapter 22. Receptors that detect temperature are called *thermoreceptors* and receptors that detect pressure and movement are called *mechanoreceptors*. These receptors are discussed later.

BOX 23-1

Self-Awareness and Massage Therapy

When we are around someone who is anxious, we often become anxious as well. When we are around someone who is calm, we often become calm. We can mirror the emotions, or internal environment, of others and they can be our mirrors. This phenomenon of shared experience is called *intersubjectivity*.

Conscious awareness of our emotions and internal environment, no matter how it is generated, is the first step toward modifying them when needed. Sensations most easily noticed are cardiac and respiration rates and muscle tension. This sensory awareness, called *interoceptive awareness*, can be developed while participating in activities such as martial arts, yoga, meditation, and mindfulness.

So what can you do when you notice your heart is racing or feel a lump in your throat during a massage? All the aforementioned experiences are signs of sympathetic arousal. While the first step is awareness, the next step is to invite relaxation by activating the relaxation response or parasympathetic response. Slow deep breaths will help you relax. Thinking pleasant thoughts or visualizing relaxing scenery may also facilitate relaxation.

Because of the intersubjective response, you can help your client relax more fully when you are relaxed. Conversely, your client can perceive when you are preoccupied such as thinking about tonight's dinner plans or the phone call you forgot to make.

Periodically throughout the massage, note how your body is feeling. If you notice tension, try to release it. Use a method that works for you. Because when you are more fully relaxed, you can be more present with your client. This is a great gift to give to our clients and to ourselves.

Touch is the most primitive of all sensations. Among the many studies that have been conducted, touch is the earliest sense to become functional in the human embryo. When the embryo is less than 6 weeks of age, measuring less than an inch long from crown to rump, light stroking of the upper lip or wings of the nose will cause bending of the neck and trunk away from the source of stimulation. At this stage of gestation, neither the eyes nor ears have developed.

Taste

Mediated by taste buds or gustatory organs, taste is a collection of chemoreceptors concentrated in projections on the tongue called *papillae*. Within each papilla are taste hairs extending from taste pores (Figure 23-18).

These hairs are attached to a taste cell that supports the chemoreceptors, which become aroused when a molecule of a particular size and shape enters the receptor site, similar to a lock-and-key mechanism. The taste cell is located in the taste bud surrounded by supporting cells.

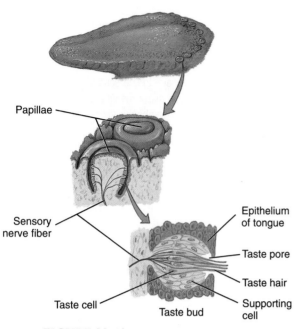

FIGURE 23-18 Taste buds on the tongue.

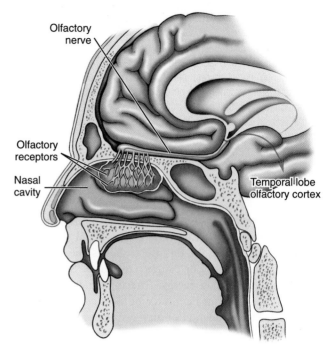

FIGURE 23-19 Structures involved in smell.

There are five primary tastes; salty, sweet, bitter, sour, and savory. Most of these are localized in specific regions on the tongue. However, taste discernment is a combination of impulses from many taste receptors. The input from one receptor means little without the combined information from other receptors, just as the letter K is relatively meaningless without surrounding letters to form a word.

Taste is strongly influenced by smell. Tasting food without scent molecules is difficult (e.g., cold food does not have as much taste as hot food). A condition such as a head cold often interferes with the sense of smell, so that taste is inhibited.

Smell

Smell, or olfaction, uses chemoreceptors to detect odors. Olfactory chemoreceptors are found in the superior nasal cavity, and their dendritic extensions are located in nasal mucosa. Inhalation forces airborne molecules to the mucosa, where they dissolve and come into contact with receptors. Once certain chemical molecules fit into the corresponding receptor site, nerve impulses are created and sent to the olfactory bulb, to the olfactory nerve, and then to the temporal lobe of the cerebrum (Figure 23-19).

Research suggests that humans can detect between 7 and 32 primary odors; for example, ether, camphor, musk, floral, mint, pungent, and putrid. Smell plays an important role in sexual behavior for most mammals and is the sense linked most strongly to memories.

Vision

Vision uses photoreceptors (rods and cones) that are located in the eye. Light enters the eye through the pupil (opening in the center of the iris) and strikes the retina, which is essentially a membranous screen composed of delicate nervous tissue at the rear of the eye (Figure 23-20).

Photoreceptors within the retina convert light energy into nerve impulses, which are transmitted to the brain through the optic nerve. A point near the thalamus and hypothalamus where portions of each optic nerve cross over is called the optic chiasm. A blind spot exists where the optic nerve exits the retina, but this does not affect vision because of the existence of two eyes, and the blind spots do not coincide with each other.

CHAT ROOM

Terms of Sight

Astigmatism: Condition in which the eyeball is not spherical; thus images and light rays striking the retina are not clearly focused. This defect may cause eye discomfort related to blurred vision.

Emmetropia: Normal vision

Hyperopia: Farsightedness, or difficulty seeing objects that are nearby

Myopia: Nearsightedness, or difficulty seeing objects that are farther away

Presbyopia: Farsightedness that often develops with advancing age

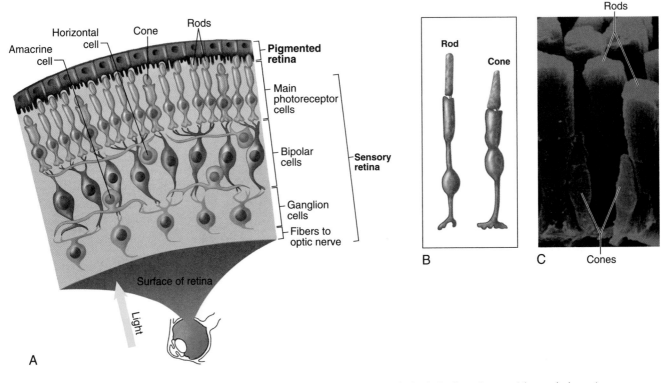

FIGURE 23-20 Vision. **A,** The retina. **B,** Rods and cones (illustration). **C,** Rods and cones (electronic image).

Hearing

Hearing is achieved by detection of sound waves or vibrations via mechanoreceptors. Sound waves hit the tympanic membrane (eardrum) at the back of the auditory canal. The membrane, which separates the outer ear from the middle ear, vibrates as a drum at the same frequency as sound waves striking the membrane. These waves are transmitted through three small bones (ossicles) in the middle ear: (1) malleus (hammer), (2) incus (anvil), and (3) stapes (stirrup). Bones within the ear are the smallest in the body. The vibration of these bones is relayed to the oval window.

The oval window is a membrane that covers the opening to a coiled, fluid-filled cavity (cochlea) of the inner ear. From here, sound waves travel through fluid in the cochlear duct (endolymph). Within the cochlea are three fluid-filled semicircular canals. Waves of fluid are interpreted as sound (Figure 23-21).

Two characteristics of sound are pitch and volume. *Pitch* is the quality of a tone or sound, which depends on vibration speed; slow vibrations produce deep sounds, and fast vibrations produce high sounds. The ability to hear high-pitched sounds may decline with age. *Volume* is the loudness of sound and can change without altering pitch.

Ears also play a large part in balance and equilibrium. Within the semicircular canals are gel-filled sacs containing special mechanoreceptors that resemble hair cells. When these sacs are turned to a new position, hair cells bend. This action results in an impulse to the vestibulocochlear nerve, notifying the brain of a change in position.

TYPES OF RECEPTORS

Special receptors detect certain types of sensory information. These receptors can be classified two ways. One is by where the stimuli is located (e.g., inside versus outside the body). The second is by the type of stimuli they detect (e.g., light, temperature).

Receptors Classified by Location of Stimuli

Exteroceptors. Receptors located in skin, mucous membranes, and sense organs, responding to stimuli, such as touch, pressure, or sound, that originates outside the body.

Proprioceptors. Receptors located in skin, ears, muscles, tendons, joints, and fascia that respond to movement and body position.

Interoceptors. Also known as *visceroceptors,* receptors located in the viscera that respond to stimuli, such as digestion, excretion, and blood pressure, originating within the body.

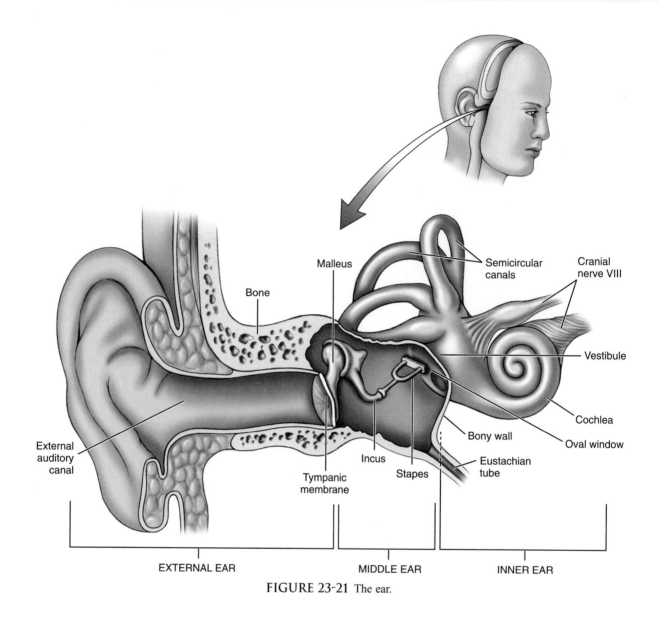

FIGURE 23-21 The ear.

Receptors Classified by Type of Stimuli they Detect

Receptors can also be classified by the stimuli they detect such as pressure, light, heat, pain, or various chemicals. These types of receptors include chemoreceptors, mechanoreceptors, thermoreceptors, photoreceptors, and nociceptors.

Receptors often exhibit a functional mechanism called adaptation. When a stimulus is constant, over time, **adaptation**, a decrease in sensitivity to a prolonged stimulus, may occur. Adaptation tends to be rapid for pressure, touch, and smell. We become accustomed to the weight of our clothes during the day, and an odor that offended us when we first entered the room typically is no longer detected later.

Adaptation occurs slowly with pain and body position. This characteristic is a protective mechanism preventing us from becoming accustomed to severe pain or from keeping our bodies in awkward, potentially harmful body positions.

Chemoreceptors. Located in the nose, tongue, within some arterial walls, and in the medulla oblongata, chemoreceptors are activated by chemical stimuli to detect smells, tastes, and changes in blood chemistry.

Chemoreceptors within arterial walls and in the medulla are sensitive to changes in pH and carbon dioxide concentration. If oxygen levels are lowered or carbon dioxide is high, the chemoreceptors stimulate the medulla oblongata to increase respiration rate.

Mechanoreceptors. Mechanoreceptors respond to mechanical stimuli and are found in skin, blood vessels, ears, muscles, tendons, joints, and fascia. They detect sensations such as pressure (including blood pressure), vibration (the onset and removal of pressure), stretching, muscular contraction, proprioception, sound, and equilibrium.

Pressure Receptors. Examples are Meissner, Ruffini, and Pacinian corpuscles and Krause end bulbs. Also included are Merkel disks and the hair root plexus. These receptors are discussed in Chapter 22.

Stretch Receptors. These include muscle spindles, Golgi tendon organs, and baroreceptors.

Muscle Spindles – Stretch-sensitive receptors wrapped around intrafusal muscle fibers that monitor changes in muscle length, as well as the rate of this change (Figure 23-22). When muscles are stretched rapidly or are overstretched (ballistic stretch), muscle spindles are activated and cause reflexive contraction. Referred to as a *myotatic stretch reflex*, this action guards against tissue damage by counteracting sudden muscle lengthening.

> ### CHAT ROOM
>
> A therapist may use the myotatic stretch reflex when strengthening a weak antagonist. For example, if a client has rounded shoulders, then the pectoralis major may be tight, whereas the rhomboids are weak. During treatment, use hacking tapotement across the fibers of the rhomboids to create minute muscle contractions. Using weight training, strengthening of the rhomboids may pull the shoulders back for a more balanced posture.

Golgi Tendon Organs – Located at musculotendinous junctions are Golgi tendon organs that are activated by both tension and slow stretch (Figure 23-23). If tension is too great, motor neurons are inhibited. Referred to as an *inverse stretch reflex* or *tendon reflex*, this protective mechanism helps ensure that muscles do not contract too strongly and damage their tendons. Stimulation of Golgi tendon organs inhibits contraction throughout the entire muscle.

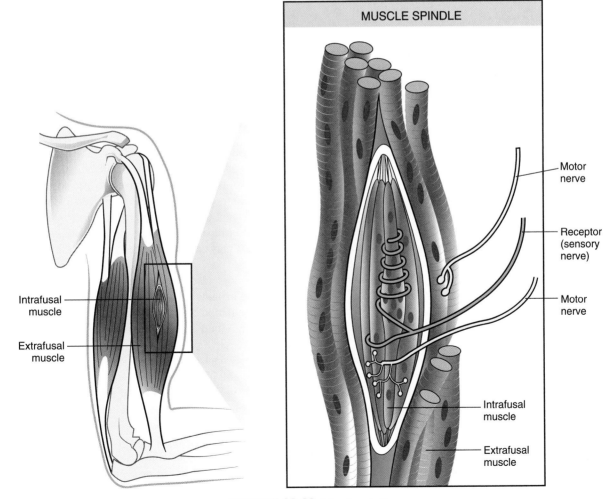

MUSCLE SPINDLE

Intrafusal muscle

Extrafusal muscle

Motor nerve

Receptor (sensory nerve)

Motor nerve

Intrafusal muscle

Extrafusal muscle

FIGURE 23-22 Muscle spindle.

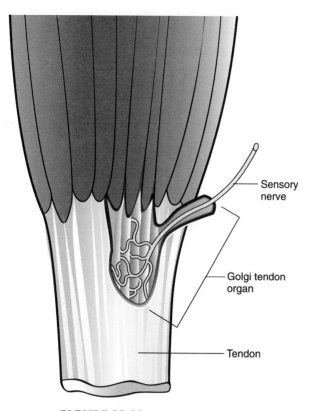

FIGURE 23-23 Golgi tendon organ.

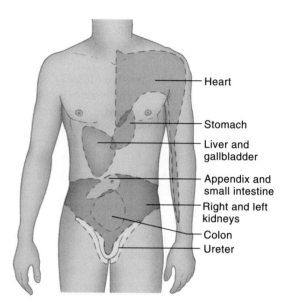

FIGURE 23-24 Referred pain patterns.

CHAT ROOM

The tendon reflex may also be used during massage treatment. Plucking the tendons perpendicularly tricks the Golgi tendon organs into thinking a load is present and reduces muscular tension. This technique, also called the transverse tendon technique (triple T), enhances muscular relaxation by inhibiting contraction.

Baroreceptors – These receptors detect blood pressure by monitoring the amount of stretch exerted on certain arterial walls, namely carotid arteries and the aortic arch. When needed, impulses are relayed to the vasomotor center in the medulla oblongata, which seeks to restore normal blood pressure.

Photoreceptors. Photoreceptors are sensitive to light and are located in the retina of the eye. The two types are rods and cones. The retina, which is essentially a membranous extension of the optic nerve, contains more than 100 million rods and 3 million cones.

Rods – These slender rodlike projections are sensitive to dim light and shades of black, white, and gray. Note how difficult it is to determine color and detail in dim light.

Cones – These structures are needed for color vision; they are short and thick with blunt projections. Most cones are found in the center of the retina, where few rod cells are located. This area of the retina is designated for acute,

detailed vision partly because blood vessels do not exist there so color vision is not hindered.

Cones and rods function in a similar way. Three variations of cones exist, and each is sensitive to a different light wavelength (blue, red, and green). Combinations of these three colors give us an entire color spectrum. If all color pigments are activated, then white is perceived; if no color pigments are activated, then black is seen.

Nociceptors. Also referred to as *free nerve endings*, nociceptors detect pain and are located in almost every tissue of the body, but are concentrated in skin. The brain lacks nociceptors; however, other tissues of the cranium, such as the meninges and blood vessels, have a large supply of them.

Nociceptors serve a protective function and rarely adapt. If they adapted to pain stimuli, then pain would stop being sensed, and irreparable damage might result. In some cases, nociceptors may continue to fire even after the painful stimulus is removed.

Nociceptors also respond to stimuli that cause tissue damage, to irritants (e.g., ones released by injured cells), and to overstimulation or excessive stimuli (e.g., excessive heat, bright light, loud sound, intense mechanical stimulation such as excessive pressure).

Pain may cause reflexive withdrawal of the involved body segments. Pain may cause sympathetic arousal, such as changes in heartbeat and blood pressure.

In most instances, pain is felt at the point of stimulation. However, a client may have *referred pain*, which can be experienced as sensations such as tingling, numbness, itching, aching, heat, or cold. Visceral pain may be sensed in the area over the organ or projected to another area of the body (Figure 23-24). In many instances, the same spinal segment (Hilton's law—Box 23-2) innervates these

BOX 23-2

Neurologic Laws

Arndt's Law
Rudolf Arndt, German Psychiatrist, 1835-1900
Weak stimuli excite physiologic activity, moderately strong ones favor it, strong ones retard it, and very strong ones arrest it.

Arndt's law applies to physiologic effects of stress and relaxation (massage). Strong stimuli, such as pain and trigger point formation, may disrupt normal functioning. Muscle tonus may become increased, digestive functions may be inhibited, and blood pressure may rise. Massage, being a weak but pleasurable stimulus, helps return the body to homeostasis.

Davis' Law
If muscle ends are brought closer together, the pull of tonus is increased, thereby shortening the muscle, which may even cause hypertrophy. If muscle ends are separated beyond normal, then tonus is lessened or lost, thereby weakening the muscle.

Davis' law is an example of the body, preferring balance to extremes and can be observed in various situations. The increase in muscle tonus gained by weight lifting is the result of repetitive contractions. However, chronic shortening contractions can produce spasms, such as a muscle that remains in a shortened position for extended periods (e.g., sleeping on the stomach with ankles in full extension, wearing shoes with high heels).

The opposite extreme can occur when muscles have been overstretched in an accident, exceeding their normal limit (e.g., whiplash). The microtrauma of tearing many muscle fibers often causes a loss of strength and increase in muscle flaccidity. These scenarios can be addressed effectively with massage and joint mobilizations.

Hilton's Law
John Hilton, English Surgeon, 1804-1878
A nerve trunk that supplies a joint also supplies the muscles of the joint and the skin over the insertions of such muscles.

Hilton's law is significant for massage therapists, especially when combined with Arndt's law. Each nerve trunk supplies both sensory information and motor control for joints, muscles, vessels, skin, and organs in a given area. Pain in this area results in a physiopathologic reflex arc, which generates a spontaneous increase in motor impulses, sending impulses of pain to the cord. The increased motor stimuli cause vasoconstriction, a decrease in visceral function, an increase in muscular tonus, and an increase in intrajoint pressure. Arndt's law states that strong stimuli retard or arrest physiologic activity.

The advantage of Hilton's law for massage therapists is that massage not only produces the direct effects of increasing local circulation, relaxing muscle, and calming stimulated nerves, but also has an indirect effect of interrupting the physiopathologic reflex arc. As the pain subsides because of disruption of strong stimuli, normal function returns.

Pfluger's Laws
Eduard Friederich Wilhelm Pfluger, German Physiologist, 1829-1910
Although not specifically stated, Pflugers' laws are progressive in nature and dependent on the degree of nerve irritation. Progressive refers to the fact that these laws are experienced in order—that is, a client begins by experiencing the law of unilaterality and, if the cause of the irritating stimulus is left untreated, can proceed through each succeeding law until the law of generalization is reached. This concept does not mean that every client experiences the effects of all five laws; recognize that progression is dependent on the degree of nerve irritation. Clients with minor injuries may experience only the law of unilaterality, whereas others may progress to the law of symmetry, the law of intensity, and so on.

Law of Unilaterality
If a mild irritation is applied to one or more sensory nerves, then the movement takes place usually on one side only—the side that is irritated.

The word movement in Pflugers' laws refers primarily to motor reflexes responding to stimuli. Increased tonus occurs on the side of the body reporting pain or injury first. Motor reflexes tighten muscles on the affected side and limit range of motion as protective mechanisms; this may prevent further injury. Constriction of vessels prevents internal bleeding in muscular tears.

Law of Symmetry
If the stimulation is sufficiently increased, then motor reaction is exhibited not only by the irritated side but also in similar muscles on the opposite side of the body.

When an injury is left untreated on one side of the body, symptoms begin to migrate to the opposite side. Spasms in the right levator scapula, if not addressed, increase in intensity. Eventually, the body seeks to reduce some sensory input (pain) by directing it to motor nerves on the opposite side of the body. The result is a general increase in tonus of the left levator scapula and other muscles innervated by the same nerve.

Law of Intensity
Reflex movements are usually more intense on the side of irritation. At times, the movements of the opposite side equal them in intensity, but they are usually less pronounced.

Pfluger law of intensity states that irritation (pain) increases in intensity on both sides of the body, but the pain is greater on the initial side of irritation.

Law of Radiation
If the excitation continues to increase, then it is propagated upward, and reactions take place through centrifugal nerves coming from the cord segments higher up.

Continued

BOX 23-2, cont'd

Again, if left untreated, discomfort grows, and the client proceeds from one law to the next. The body seeks to dissipate more sensory input (pain), directing it to motor nerves higher up the cord, such as a tight shoulder muscles radiating to neck muscles.

Law of Generalization
When the irritation becomes very intense, it is propagated in the medulla oblongata, which becomes a focus from which stimuli radiate to all parts of the cord, causing a general increase of tonus in all muscles of the body.

This law is represented by chronic pain in a client who has a long-standing history of pain and limited range of motion. The law of generalization seldom applies to something similar to a tight levator and is usually reserved for clients with problems such as chronic lower back pain. Once the medulla is involved, the internuncial pool of the entire spinal cord is excited, causing pain and increased tonus to all muscles. Clients with chronic pain may experience severe headaches, neck and shoulder stiffness, arm pain, and lower back pain. The goal of massage is to reduce sensory stimulation and muscle tonus to a point at which the client's discomfort level begins to back down the scale of Pfluger's laws and symptoms abate. Hydrotherapy, in conjunction with massage, is an excellent modality for clients who have advanced to this stage of pain.

Sherrington's Law
Sir Charles Scott Sherrington, English Physician, 1857-1952
When a muscle receives a nerve impulse to contract, its antagonist simultaneously receives an impulse to relax.

Sherrington's law is also known as *reciprocal inhibition.* Moving would be difficult if all muscles contracted at the same time. In fact, if opposing muscles were both able to contract simultaneously, weaker muscles might be torn. Reciprocal inhibition ensures that when an agonist is creating movement, the antagonist cooperates by relaxing

and elongating. In a client with normal neurologic function, these two impulses occur simultaneously.

Massage therapists can apply this principle to turn off messages of contraction in acute muscle cramps. For example, when hamstrings are experiencing a muscle cramp, the cramp might be relieved by forcibly contracting their antagonists, the quadriceps femoris. This task is best accomplished through active resistance (isometric contraction). Maintain contraction for 10 to 20 seconds; then release. Repeat three times.

This law is applied in techniques of proprioceptive neuromuscular facilitation.

Law of Facilitation
When an impulse has passed once through a certain set of neurons to the exclusion of others, it tends to take the same course on future occasions, and each time it traverses this path, the resistance is less.

The repetition of a particular action ingrains a habit between brain and muscle. Pain from postural distortions and improper movement patterns is often habitual. The best way to break a bad habit is to replace it with a good one. Massage helps reprogram nerves by giving them new information via experience. The client can move differently because he or she has felt something different during the session. The form of massage used really does not matter, so long as it is not perceived as painful to the client because pain triggers a protective response.

A client with a first-degree tear of the right supraspinatus may not be able to raise the right arm above shoulder level. Even after the tear has healed, previous experience of pain and limited movement prevents full range of motion. However, if the therapist treats the injury with massage and passively ranges the arm without going through the pain barrier, then the brain is reprogrammed to accept the movement pattern once again. By repeating passive movements several times, neural messages cross certain synapses repeatedly. The message can then easily begin taking that particular route in the future.

---

areas. For example, the pain of angina may cause pain down the left arm resulting from a common spinal nerve connection.

Thermoreceptors. Located immediately under the skin, these receptors include two types of free nerve endings: those that detect cold and those that detect heat. Cold receptors are 10 times more numerous than heat receptors and are stimulated by lowering temperatures. Rising temperatures stimulate heat receptors. Once the temperature falls below 10° C (50° F) or rises above 45° C (113° F), nociceptors rather than thermoreceptors are activated.

NEUROLOGIC PATHOLOGIES

Central Nervous System Disorders

Seizure Disorder. Seizure disorders are characterized by explosive episodes of uncontrolled and excessive electrical

activity in the brain, called a seizure. A seizure may be subtle and consist of abnormal sensations, or it may produce overt involuntary repetitive movements and loss of consciousness. Once a seizure begins, it cannot be stopped. It can be triggered by physical stimuli, loud noises, bright lights, or stress. See Chapter 9 for procedural suggestions if your client has a seizure.

If the condition is not being medically supervised, postpone massage until medical clearance is given because this situation increases the likelihood of serious complications. If your client is under medical supervision, massage can proceed. Ask about known triggers, and avoid them during the session. For example, if certain odors can trigger a seizure, avoid using essential oils.

Spinal Cord Injury. Spinal cord injuries result from damage to the vertebrae and neural tissues, causing paralysis distal to the area of insult. The area of spinal insult determines the type of paralysis. *Quadriplegia* is due to injury to the cervical area and results in paralysis of the trunk and all four extremities. *Paraplegia* is due to injury to the lower thoracic or upper lumbar area and results in paralysis of the lower trunk and legs.

If your client is recovering from the injury, obtain medical clearance for massage. Otherwise, modify massage according to the disability, which may include being wheelchair-bound.

Attention Deficit–Hyperactivity Disorder. Attention deficit–hyperactivity disorder (ADHD) is a neurologic disorder in which the affected person displays an array of behaviors associated with inattentiveness, hyperactivity, and impulsivity. Adults with this condition claim that their biggest aggravations are the inability to focus and to prioritize, leading to missed deadlines and forgotten appointments and social events.

Shorter-than-normal sessions are best. You are likely to face challenges ranging from excessive fidgeting and talking during the massage to missed appointments and forgotten wallets. On one hand, tolerance is advisable; on the other, too much tolerance may lead to unenforced office policies. When working with children with ADHD, teaching parents how to massage is best. This approach makes massage more accessible and gives parents a tool to help the child relax and focus.

Autism. Autism is a syndrome of social withdrawal and obsessive behavior. He or she may avoid eye contact and have an aversion to touching and cuddling. The person may engage in repetitive motions (spinning, rocking), exhibit a compulsion for sameness, have a narrow interest range, and possess a superior memory of certain facts (U.S. presidents, for example).

Use firm gliding and compressive strokes applied with full hand contact. Sessions are brief (10 to 15 minutes). If the child is showing any signs of intolerance, discontinue massage and try again another day. In most circumstances, teaching the parents how to massage the child is best, which makes massage more accessible and gives parents a tool to communicate affection.

Neurodegenerative Diseases

Alzheimer Disease. Alzheimer disease is a progressive degenerative disease of the brain that produces a typical profile of mental deterioration. The clinical picture includes loss of memory, inability to concentrate, lack of reasoning, apathy, and personality changes.

Tailor the massage to the stage of disease, with few adjustments needed in earlier stages to significant modifications required for later stages. Later-stage adjustments may include a light, slow massage of short duration or even a gentle foot massage. Be willing to adjust your technique according to the client's wishes, which might change abruptly. Tolerance of

behavior is needed, given that these individuals experience personality changes that become worse over time.

Parkinson Disease. Parkinson disease is a progressive disorder that produces a syndrome of abnormal movements. The classic triad of signs is tremors, rigidity, and slowness of voluntary movements. The person is unable to maintain an upright position, resulting in a standing posture that is stooped. Activities such as getting out of a chair or rolling over from a supine position to a lateral or prone position can be quite challenging. Eventually the face takes on a masklike appearance, lacking expression.

Massage is best performed in a position that your client can easily assume, which may be lying down or sitting. Gentle, slow massage of shorter-than-normal duration is indicated. The goal is to reduce rigidity. Symptoms may be reduced, although only temporarily.

Multiple Sclerosis. Multiple sclerosis (MS) is progressive demyelination of neurons in the brain and spinal cord, as well as cranial nerves (especially the optic nerve). Loss of myelin ultimately leads to scarring and plaque formation; this interferes with nerve impulse transmission (both motor and sensory nerves). MS worsens throughout the person's life, with periods of remission and exacerbation (also called relapses or flare-ups). With each exacerbation, additional areas of the CNS are affected.

Massage is contraindicated during periods of exacerbation. While the client is in remission, massage may be performed. Assess your client at every visit because symptoms may change daily. If your client is fatigued, reduce treatment time to 30 minutes, and use lighter-than-normal pressure. Because nerve transmission is reduced, you cannot completely rely on client feedback regarding pressure, and injury can occur with aggressively applied techniques; caution is merited.

Vascular Disorders

Transient Ischemic Attack. Transient ischemic attacks (TIAs) are brief episodes of impaired brain functioning caused by temporary ischemia. Symptoms include visual disturbances, speech difficulties, and difficulty understanding others. The episode lasts from a few seconds to hours, with symptoms gradually subsiding. Complete recovery occurs within 24 hours with no residual neurologic dysfunction.

Massage is appropriate for clients who have had a TIA.

Stroke. A stroke, cerebrovascular accident, or brain attack is a sudden disruption of cerebral blood flow. This disruption causes death of brain tissue, most often leading to brain damage or, in some cases, coma and death. If the person survives the event, complications depend on the location of the stroke and range from mild to severe with resultant hemiplegia (paralysis on one side of the body).

Massage can be performed during the rehabilitation process after obtaining medical clearance. Massage strokes should be slow, superficial, soothing, and rhythmic. The first few massages should be brief (not more than 30 minutes) and scheduled for only a couple of times per week so as to prevent overtiring your client. Treatments can gradually be increased to 1 hour.

Migraine Headache. Migraine headaches are severe and recurrent headaches, often completely incapacitating, and are accompanied by symptoms such as visual disturbances and nausea. Migraines are often provoked by a trigger factor such as hunger, alcohol (namely red wine), or hormonal changes (menstruation, ovulation, contraceptive use). Migraine headaches, called attacks, can last from 6 to 48 hours, and a prolonged recovery period often ensues.

Because of severe pain and nausea, massage is postponed until your client has completely recovered. Additionally, a client experiencing a migraine would not likely want a massage.

Peripheral Nerve Disorders

Trigeminal Neuralgia. Trigeminal neuralgia (TN), also called tic douloureux, is characterized by excruciating episodic pain in areas supplied by the trigeminal nerve (cranial nerve V). Attacks may be spontaneous or triggered by mechanical stimulation such as touching the face (as while shaving), chewing, drinking, speaking, and brushing teeth. Pain usually lasts from a few seconds to several hours.

Postpone massage during the attack. If your client has had TN, avoid the face and scalp so as to prevent triggering another one. Also, avoid the prone position because pressure from the table or face cushion may trigger an attack.

Bell Palsy. Bell palsy is a condition of the facial nerve (cranial nerve VII) causing weakness or paralysis of facial muscles on one side of the face. Paralysis may be so severe that the person may not be able to open or close an eye; one side of the mouth may droop. When this occurs, the person is unable to smile, whistle, or grimace or control salivation on the affected side.

Light gliding strokes on the face, directed upward, can be helpful. Light kneading, percussion, and vibration may help stimulate flaccid muscles.

Peripheral Neuropathy. Peripheral neuropathy is inflammation or degeneration of the PNS leading to loss of sensations and movement difficulties. The affected area may be numb or tingly or feel unusually hot or cold. Pain may or may not be present. Symptoms often begin in distal body regions (hands and feet) and progress proximally. Neuropathies may be complications of diseases such as Raynaud

disease, MS, and diabetes or it may develop after a surgical procedure.

Avoid hypersensitive areas. Because of reduced sensation, your client may be unable to give accurate feedback about pressure so reduce pressure over affected areas. When applying stretching or joint mobilizations, use caution.

Bulging and Herniated Disks. A *herniated disk* involves protrusion of the nucleus pulposus (gelatinous inner component) through a tear in the annulus fibrosus (tough, outer ring). A *bulging disk* is similar to a herniated disk but is less severe because the nucleus pulposus remains contained within the annular wall. A common location for both conditions is the lumbosacral area. Symptoms include severe, sharp pain that may worsen with movement. Pain may radiate and produce paresthesia.

Observe your client. If he or she is in severe pain while performing tasks related to getting a massage (removing a jacket, sitting in a chair, climbing on a massage table), postpone massage until a day when pain is less severe. Otherwise, reduce pressure over affected areas and avoid techniques involving mobilization of the affected spinal region. Because you cannot rely on client feedback regarding pressure in areas of paresthesia, injury may occur from aggressive techniques; caution is merited.

Sciatica. Inflammation of the sciatic nerve, or sciatica, refers to pain that originates in the lower back or hip and may radiate down the thigh and leg. Most often, sciatica is a symptom of another condition such as bulging or herniated disk, rather than its own diagnosis. Paresthesia is common.

Modify massage according to the cause. For example, if sciatica is caused by a herniated disk and your client arrives in severe pain, massage may need to be postponed. Because you cannot rely on client feedback regarding pressure in areas of paresthesia, injury can occur from aggressively applied techniques; caution is merited.

Thoracic Outlet Syndrome. Thoracic outlet syndrome is caused by compression of the brachial plexus and subclavian artery (also known as the neurovascular bundle). Hypertonus of scalenes or the pectoralis minor may either pull the first rib upward (reducing the area between the first rib and the clavicle) or compress the neurovascular bundle into the rib cage. Symptoms include pain and paresthesia down the arm on the affected side; some people have pain in the chest and neck.

If the area is swollen, elevate it above the level of the heart and use gentle superficial gliding strokes. Be sure to massage the proximal area first (arm before forearm). If edema is not present, massage can be performed. Be sure to address the scalenes, pectoralis minor, and muscles of the shoulder and arm within the client's tolerance.

Carpal Tunnel Syndrome. Carpal tunnel syndrome results from medial nerve compression within the carpal tunnel (see Figure 21-10). Symptoms include pain and paresthesia in the lateral side of affected hand and fingers. Common causes are repetitive wrist movements combined with compression and direct trauma.

If the area is inflamed (swollen, red, warm to the touch), local massage is contraindicated. Otherwise, massage the muscles of the forearm and palm, within the client's tolerance.

SPOTLIGHT ON RESEARCH

Research suggests that massage therapy may:

- Increase serotonin and dopamine, important chemicals relating to depression, pain, fatigue, and other conditions
- Decrease motor neuron pool excitability
- Improve sleep
- Decrease stress, depression, and anxiety
- Activate parasympathetic response and increase relaxation
- Enhance brain wave activity
- Improve cognitive and memory functioning
- Reduce spasticity, increase muscle flexibility and motor function
- Improve social interaction in persons with cerebral palsy
- Improve functional abilities, range of motion, and muscle strength in persons with spinal cord injury
- Reduce pain and increase nerve conduction velocity in persons with carpal tunnel syndrome
- Decrease fidgeting and improve mood in persons with attention deficit–hyperactivity disorder
- Reduce touch aversion and other stereotypic behaviors in persons with autism
- Reduce agitation, resisting, and other stereotypic behaviors in persons with dementia and Alzheimer disease
- Improve daily functioning and improve sleep in persons with Parkinson disease
- Decrease anxiety and depression and improve self-esteem and body image in persons with multiple sclerosis

E-RESOURCES

evolve

http://evolve.elsevier.com/Salvo/MassageTherapy
- Chapter challenge
- Flash cards
- Photo gallery
- Educational animations
- Additional information
- Weblinks

BIBLIOGRAPHY

Abrahams P, Marks S, Hutchings R: *McMinn's color atlas of human anatomy*, St Louis, 2003, Mosby.

Applegate EJ: *The anatomy and physiology learning system*, ed 3, Philadelphia, 2006, Saunders.

Beers MH, Berkow R: *The Merck manual of diagnosis and therapy*, Whitehouse Station, NJ, 2006, Merck Research Laboratories.

Como D, editor: *Mosby's medical, nursing, and allied health dictionary*, ed 6, St Louis, 2002, Mosby.

Crawley J, Van De Graaff KM: *A photographic atlas for anatomy and physiology*, Englewood, Colo, 2002, Morton.

Crooks R, Stein J: *Psychology: science, behavior, and life*, ed 3, Philadelphia, 1993, Harcourt College Publishers.

Damjanov I: *Pathophysiology for the health-related professions*, ed 3, Philadelphia, 2006, Saunders.

Ferri FF: *2003 Ferri's clinical advisor, instant diagnosis and treatment*, St Louis, 2003, Mosby.

Frazier MS, Drzymkowski JW: *Essentials of human diseases and conditions*, ed 3, Philadelphia, 2004, Saunders.

Goldberg S: *Clinical anatomy made ridiculously simple*, Miami, 2004, Medmaster.

Gould BE: *Pathophysiology for the health professions*, ed 3, Philadelphia, 2006, Saunders.

Grafelman T: *Graf's anatomy and physiology guide for the massage therapist*, Aurora, Colo, 1998, DG Publishing.

Gray H: *Gray's anatomy*, ed 29, Philadelphia, 1974, Running Press.

Guyton A: *Human physiology and mechanisms of disease*, ed 6, Philadelphia, 1996, Saunders.

Haubrich WS: *Medical meanings: a glossary of word origins*, New York, 1984, Harcourt Brace Jovanovich.

Huether SE, McCance KL: *Understanding pathophysiology*, ed 3, St Louis, 2004, Mosby.

Jacob S, Francone C: *Elements of anatomy and physiology*, Philadelphia, 1989, Saunders.

Juhan D: *Job's body: a handbook for bodyworkers*, ed 3, Barrington, NY, 2003, Station Hill Press.

Kalat JW: *Biological psychology*, ed 8, Belmont, Calif, 2003, Wadsworth.

Kapit W, Elson LM: *The anatomy coloring book*, ed 3, New York, 2002, Benjamin Cummings.

Kordish M, Dickson S: *Introduction to basic human anatomy*, Lake Charles, La, 1995, McNeese State University.

Kumar V, Abbas A, Fausto N: *Robbins and Cotran physiologic basis of disease*, ed 7, St Louis, 2005, Mosby.

Marieb EN: *Essentials of human anatomy and physiology*, ed 8, New York, 2005, Benjamin Cummings.

Martini FH, Bartholomew EF: *Essentials of anatomy and physiology*, ed 3, New York, 2003, Benjamin Cummings.

McAleer N: *The body almanac*, Garden City, NY, 1985, Doubleday.

McAtee R: *Facilitated stretching*, ed 2, Colorado Springs, Colo, 1999, Human Kinetics.

McCance K, Huether S: *Pathophysiology: the biological basis for disease in adults and children*, St Louis, 2006, Mosby.

Melzack R, Wall PD: *The challenge of pain*, New York, 1996, Basic Books.

Merck manual, ed 17, Whitehouse Station, NJ, 1998, Merck Co.

Moore KL: *Clinically oriented anatomy*, ed 5, Baltimore, 2005, Lippincott Williams & Wilkins.

Netter FH: *Atlas of human anatomy*, ed 3, Teterboro, NJ, 2003, Icon Learning Systems.

Newton D: *Pathology for massage therapists*, ed 2, Portland, Ore, 1995, Simran.

Premkumar K: *Pathology A to Z, a handbook for massage therapists*, Baltimore, 1999, Lippincott Williams & Wilkins.

Salvo SG: *Mosby's pathology for massage therapists*, ed 2, St Louis, 2009, Mosby.

Solomon EP, Phillips GA: *Understanding human anatomy and physiology*, Philadelphia, 1987, Saunders.

St John P: *St John neuromuscular therapy seminars, manual I*, Largo, Fla, 1995, self-published.

Thibodeau G, Patton K: *Anatomy and physiology*, ed 6, St Louis, 2006, Mosby.

Thibodeau G, Patton K: *Structure and function of the body*, ed 12, St Louis, 2004, Mosby.

Tortora GJ: *Introduction to the human body: the essentials of anatomy and physiology*, ed 5, Hoboken, NJ, 2000, John Wiley & Sons.

Tortora GJ, Grabowksi SR: *Principles of anatomy and physiology*, ed 11, New York, 2005, John Wiley & Sons.

Travell JG, Simons D: *Myofascial pain and dysfunction, the trigger point manual*, Baltimore, 1992, Lippincott Williams & Wilkins.

Venes D, Thomas CL, Taber CW: *Taber's cyclopedic medical dictionary*, ed 20, Philadelphia, 2005, FA Davis.

Voss DE, Ionta MK, Myers BJ: *Proprioceptive neuromuscular facilitation*, Philadelphia, 1985, Harper & Row.

MATCHING I

Place the letter of the answer next to the term or phrase that best describes it.

A. Autonomic nervous system
B. Axon
C. Central nervous system
D. Dendrite
E. Myelin sheath
F. Nerve
G. Neurons
H. Parasympathetic
I. Peripheral nervous system
J. Somatic nervous system
K. Sympathetic
L. Synapse

_____ 1. Bundles of neurons held together by several layers of connective tissue

_____ 2. Division of the autonomic nervous system responsible for the body's alarm reaction; also known as thoracolumbar outflow

_____ 3. Impulse-conducting cells that possess properties of excitability and conductibility

_____ 4. Division of the peripheral nervous system that carries sensory impulses from the bones, muscles, joints, skin, and carries motor impulses from the central nervous system out to skeletal muscles

_____ 5. Cell extension that transmits impulses away from the cell body

_____ 6. Division of the nervous system that includes the brain, spinal cord, cerebrospinal fluid, and meninges

_____ 7. Division of the peripheral nervous system that is involuntary and supplies smooth muscles, heart muscle, skin, special senses, some proprioceptors, organs, and glands

_____ 8. Junction between two neurons or between a neuron and a muscle or gland

_____ 9. Extensions of a nerve cell that receive and transmit stimuli toward the cell body

_____ 10. Division of the autonomic nervous system involved with the relaxation response; also known as craniosacral outflow

_____ 11. Fatty layers of tissue that provides insulation around some axons and increase the speed of impulse conduction

_____ 12. Division of the nervous system that includes cranial and spinal nerves

MATCHING II

Place the letter of the answer next to the term or phrase that best describes it.

A. Cerebellum
B. Cerebrum
C. Dermatome
D. Golgi tendon organ

E. Hypothalamus
F. Medulla oblongata
G. Muscle spindle
H. Myotome

I. Nerve impulse
J. Nociceptor
K. Proprioceptor
L. Reflex arc

_____ 1. Electrical signal that conveys information along a neuron

_____ 2. Stretch receptor activated by both tension and excessive stretch, responding by inhibiting motor neurons

_____ 3. Area of the brain that regulates the autonomic nervous and endocrine systems, controls behavioral patterns, circadian rhythm, hunger, thirst, body temperature, and sleep patterns

_____ 4. Carries a stimulus to the spinal cord where it connects with a motor neuron that carries the reflex impulse back to an appropriate effector such as a muscle or gland

_____ 5. Area of skin that a specific sensory nerve root serves

_____ 6. Receptor that detects pain

_____ 7. Stretch receptor that monitor changes in muscle length, as well as the rate of this change, responding by causing reflexive contraction

_____ 8. Part of the brainstem containing respiratory, cardiovascular, and vasomotor centers

_____ 9. Part of the brain where sensations are consciously perceived, where skeletal muscle motor movements are initiated, and where emotional and intellectual processes occur

_____ 10. Receptor located in skin, ears, muscles, tendons, joints, and fascia that responds to movement and body position

_____ 11. Group of skeletal muscles innervated by a single spinal segment

_____ 12. Part of the brain that governs muscle tone, coordinates complex movements, and regulates posture and balance

MATCHING III

Place the letter of the answer next to the term or phrase that best describes it.

A. Adaptation
G. Meninges
B. Alpha
H. Motor

C. Cerebrospinal fluid
I. Neurotransmitters
D. Delta
J. Plexus

E. Depolarization
K. Polarization
F. Ganglion
L. Sensory

_____ 1. Fluid circulating around the brain and spinal cord

_____ 2. A neuron's resting membrane potential; the inside of the neuron is negatively charged and the outside is positively charged

_____ 3. Connective tissue membranes surrounding the brain and spinal cord

_____ 4. Deep sleep brain waves from which a person is not easily aroused

_____ 5. Decrease in sensitivity to a prolonged stimulus

_____ 6. Occurs when a neuron is stimulated; the interior of the cell changes from negative to positive

_____ 7. Network of intersecting nerves in the peripheral nervous system

_____ 8. Type of nerve that carries impulses to the central nervous system

_____ 9. Chemicals involved in nerve impulse transmission across a synapse

_____ 10. Cluster of nerve cell bodies in the peripheral nervous system

_____ 11. Brain wave pattern present when the subject is awake but relaxed and nonattentive

_____ 12. Type of nerve that carries impulses from the central nervous system to activate or inhibit muscles or glands

CASE STUDY

Roll Up Your Sleeves

Ronald is a regular client who enjoys his weekly massage. A few months ago, he was diagnosed with carpal tunnel syndrome of his right wrist.

When he comes for his appointment this week, you noticed that he used his left hand rather than his right to open the office door. During the assessment, he states that the area is painful and tender to the touch. You ask him to remove his jacket and pull up his right sleeve. You notice the area is slightly swollen. When you palpate the area, it feels overly warm.

How should you proceed? Include your rationale.

CRITICAL THINKING

A new client arrives with her caregiver. Before you have had a chance to talk or review her medical history, you notice that she appears to be paralyzed on her left side. What is a likely explanation for this condition?

CHAPTER 24

Endocrine System

> *"Controlled hysteria is what's required. To exist constantly in a state of controlled hysteria. It's agony. But everyone has agony. The difference is that I try to take my agony home and teach it to sing."*
> —Arthur Miller

LEARNING OBJECTIVES

After completing this chapter, the student should be able to:

- Contrast and compare exocrine and endocrine glands.
- List the anatomic structures and describe the physiologic properties of the endocrine system.
- Define hormones and describe types of hormonal control systems.
- Identify specific endocrine glands and their hormonal secretions.
- Name organs that possess endocrine cells and their hormonal secretions.
- Name types of pathologic conditions of the endocrine system, giving characteristics of and massage considerations for each.

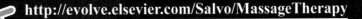

http://evolve.elsevier.com/Salvo/MassageTherapy

INTRODUCTION

The endocrine system works along with the nervous system to coordinate most body system functions. Whereas the nervous system uses neural impulses to communicate, the endocrine system uses chemical messengers called *hormones*. The endocrine system regulates processes that continue for relatively long periods, and its effects are more widespread than those of the nervous system (Figure 24-1).

The two types of glands of the body are exocrine and endocrine. **Exocrine glands** secrete their products into ducts that open to body cavities, the hollow center of an organ, or onto the surface of the body. Examples of exocrine glands are sudoriferous (secretes perspiration), sebaceous (secretes oil), and ceruminous (secretes ear wax). Other exocrine glands are salivary and other digestive glands, which secrete enzymes into various locations of the gastrointestinal tract.

Endocrine glands, or *ductless glands,* have specialized cells that produce hormones. Most hormones are released in one part of the body and travel through the bloodstream, affecting cells in other parts of the body. Some hormones do not enter the bloodstream but work on neighboring cells instead.

Compared with other body systems, which are made up of fairly large organs, the glands of the endocrine system are small. Although the total weight of all of the endocrine glands is less than 0.5 lb, normal functioning of these glands is vital to the body process. This becomes apparent when hormone levels are too low or too high; drastic changes in metabolism occur when hormonal levels are out of balance (Figure 24-2).

ANATOMY

Basic components to the endocrine system are:
- Hormones
- Hypothalamus
- Pituitary
- Pineal
- Thyroid
- Parathyroids
- Thymus
- Adrenals
- Pancreatic islets
- Ovaries
- Testes

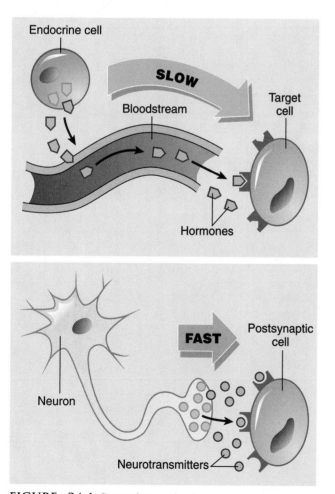

FIGURE 24-1 Comparing endocrine and nervous system functions.

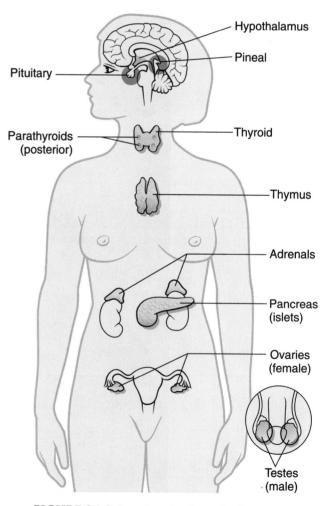

FIGURE 24-2 Location of major endocrine glands.

Also included in this chapter are organs that possess endocrine cells or act as temporary endocrine glands:

- Placenta
- Gastric and intestinal mucosa
- Heart
- Fat cells

PHYSIOLOGY

The functions of the endocrine system are:

- Produces and secretes hormones
- Regulates metabolic activities such as growth and development
- Regulates the activity of other organs and glands, as well as smooth and cardiac muscle
- Assists the body to adapt during times of stress, such as infection, trauma, dehydration, emotional stress, and starvation
- Regulates the chemical composition and volume of body fluids (intracellular and extracellular)
- Contributes to the reproductive process

HORMONES

Hormones are the chemical messengers of the endocrine system. These secretions act as catalysts in biochemical reactions and in the regulation of physiologic activity of body cells. The word hormone means to "set in motion" or "to arouse." Because hormones circulate in blood, they have the potential to come into contact with every cell type. However, hormones *do not affect* every cell they encounter. Each type of hormone is specifically programmed to seek out a certain cell, called a *target cell* (see Figure 24-1). These target cells contain *receptor sites,* which are chemically compatible with their corresponding hormone. When the hormone comes into contact with a receptor site on the target cell, they lock together like puzzle pieces. This produces the desired effect, which may be either an increase or a decrease in the target cell's primary metabolic function (Table 24-1).

Prostaglandins

Prostaglandins, or *local hormones*, are produced by many tissues and generally act near their site of secretion. Prostaglandins help to regulate smooth muscle contractions and inflammatory responses. Prostaglandins are also thought to increase the sensitivity of nerve receptors that detect pain. Medications such as aspirin and ibuprofen block prostaglandins and are therefore used to relieve pain and inflammation.

Hormonal Control Mechanisms

Generally, negative-feedback systems, other hormones, and the nervous system regulate hormonal secretions.

Negative Feedback. Most hormone levels in the body are regulated by a negative-feedback system. Information about hormone levels is relayed back to the endocrine gland, and the gland responds by secreting more or less hormone. This process is known as the negative-feedback system because the stimulus triggers the negative, or opposite, response. For example, when the level of calcium in the bloodstream is low, it triggers an increase of parathyroid hormone from the parathyroids. This releases stored calcium from bones into the bloodstream. This increase continues until the level of calcium exceeds the target value or becomes higher; the parathyroids then respond by decreasing production.

Another example of a negative-feedback system involves thyroid hormone from the thyroid gland. Thyroid hormones regulate metabolism. When metabolic needs are low, less thyroid hormone is secreted; when metabolic needs are higher, more thyroid hormones are secreted.

Hormonal Control. Hormones themselves can stimulate or inhibit the release of other hormones. The hypothalamus regulates the function of the anterior pituitary gland by the production of releasing or inhibiting hormones.

Neural Control. Some hormones are secreted as a result of neural stimulation, the most classic example being the release of epinephrine and norepinephrine from the adrenal medulla.

The adrenal medulla receives signals from the sympathetic nervous system during the stress response (see Chapter 23). The adrenal medulla responds by releasing epinephrine and norepinephrine into the bloodstream. This action helps maintain the fight-or-flight response.

Neural control systems have a faster response time than negative-feedback or hormonal control systems. Hormone release from the posterior pituitary is controlled by neural impulses from the hypothalamus.

IT'S ALL GREEK TO ME

adenohypophysis	*Gr.* gland; below; to grow
adrenal	*L.* kidney
antidiuretic	*Gr.* against; urine; production
endocrine	*Gr.* within; to separate
exocrine	*Gr.* away from; to separate
hormone	*Gr.* to excite, arouse, urge on
oxytocin	*Gr.* swift; childbirth
pancreas	*Gr.* all flesh
pineal	*L.* pine cone
suprarenal	*L.* above; kidney
thyroid	*Gr.* shield; shaped

Gr., Greek; *L.,* Latin.

TABLE 24-1 Major Hormones

HORMONE	GLAND	PRIMARY ACTION(S)
Adrenocorticotropic hormone (ACTH)	Anterior pituitary	Stimulates the adrenal cortex to secrete hormones, especially cortisol
Aldosterone	Adrenal cortex	Regulates blood volume and blood pressure and helps maintain proper mineral balance
Androgens	Adrenal cortex	Assists in the development of secondary sex characteristics
Antidiuretic hormone (ADH)	Posterior pituitary	Decreases urine production and raises blood pressure
Calcitonin (CT)	Thyroid	Decreases blood calcium levels
Cortisol (hydrocortisone)	Adrenal cortex	Assists in protein synthesis during times of stress and has an antiinflammatory effect
Epinephrine (adrenaline)	Adrenal medulla	Enhances and prolongs sympathetic arousal
Estrogen	Ovaries; placenta during pregnancy	Development of female secondary sex characteristics; assists in the development and release of the ovum at ovulation; and stimulates proliferation and thickening of the uterine lining in anticipation of implantation of a fertilized ovum
Follicle-stimulating hormone (FSH)	Anterior pituitary	Women: stimulates estrogen production and ovarian follicle development; men: stimulates sperm production
Glucagon	Pancreas	Increases blood glucose levels
Growth hormone (GH)	Anterior pituitary	Stimulates protein synthesis for muscle and bone growth, maintenance and repair; plays a role in metabolism
Insulin	Pancreas	Decreases blood glucose levels
Luteinizing hormone (LH)	Anterior pituitary	Women: stimulates the release of estrogens and progesterone, ovulation, and development of the corpus luteum; men: stimulates testosterone production
Melanocyte-stimulating hormone (MSH)	Intermediate pituitary	Increases skin pigmentation
Melatonin	Pineal	Controls the growth and development of sexual organs
Norepinephrine (noradrenaline)	Adrenal medulla	Enhances and prolongs sympathetic arousal
Oxytocin (OT)	Posterior pituitary	Stimulates uterine contractions and milk expression from mammary glands
Parathyroid hormone (PTH)	Parathyroids	Increases blood calcium levels
Progesterone	Ovaries; placenta during pregnancy	Maintains the uterine lining for implantation and pregnancy
Prolactin (PRL)	Anterior pituitary	Stimulates milk production from mammary glands
Relaxin	Ovaries; placenta during pregnancy	Relaxes the uterus to facilitate implantation; during pregnancy, it increases flexibility of the pubic symphysis and helps the cervix dilate, assisting in fetal delivery
T3 (triiodothyronine)	Thyroid	Controls metabolism and regulates growth and development
T4 (tetraiodothyronine or thyroxine)	Thyroid	Controls metabolism and regulates growth and development
Testosterone	Testes	Promotes secondary male sex characteristics, libido, and sperm production
Thymopoietin	Thymus	Stimulates T cell maturation
Thymosin	Thymus	Stimulates T cell maturation
Thyroid-stimulating hormone (TSH)	Anterior pituitary	Stimulates the thyroid to synthesize and secrete its hormones
Thyrotropin-releasing hormone	Hypothalamus	Stimulates the release of thyroid-stimulating hormone

HYPOTHALAMUS

As mentioned previously, the hypothalamus can stimulate or inhibit the release of pituitary hormones. For example, thyrotropin-releasing hormone of the hypothalamus *stimulates* the release of thyroid-stimulating hormone by the anterior pituitary. The thyroid-stimulating hormone then stimulates the release of thyroid hormones by the thyroid. A different hypothalamic hormone, somatostatin, *inhibits* the release of thyroid-stimulating hormone.

Hypophyseal Portal System

Hormones secreted by the hypothalamus travel through a complex network of small blood vessels called the hypophyseal portal system (hypophysis is another term for pituitary). This system carries hormones from the hypothalamus directly to the anterior pituitary.

A portal system is an arrangement of two capillary beds connected by veins. This way, hormones secreted by the hypothalamus do not have to travel to the heart and back before affecting the anterior pituitary. It is a special passageway.

"If you think you are too small to be effective, you have never been in bed with a mosquito."
—Anonymous

PITUITARY

The pituitary sits in the sella turcica of the sphenoid bone and extends from the hypothalamus by a stalklike structure known as the *infundibulum*. Approximately the size of a small grape, the pituitary is protected on all sides by bone and is considered to be the most protected gland in the body. The pituitary consists of an anterior and a posterior lobe and a small intermediate lobe.

The pituitary was once known as the master gland because its hormones control and stimulate other glands to produce and secrete their hormones (Figure 24-3). However, the pituitary itself has a master—the hypothalamus, which sends hormones and nerve impulses to control secretions of the pituitary; therefore the hypothalamus is the true master gland.

Anterior Lobe

Also known as the *adenohypophysis,* the anterior lobe of the pituitary constitutes approximately 75% of the total weight of the entire gland. Of the nine hormones secreted by the pituitary, six are produced by the anterior lobe. The anterior lobe and the hypothalamus are interconnected by the hypophyseal portal system (mentioned previously).

Adrenocorticotropic Hormone (ACTH). Stimulates the adrenal cortex to secrete hormones, especially cortisol.

Growth Hormone (GH). Stimulates protein synthesis for muscle and bone growth, maintenance and repair, and plays a role in metabolism.

Thyroid-Stimulating Hormone (TSH). Stimulates the thyroid to synthesize and secrete its hormones.

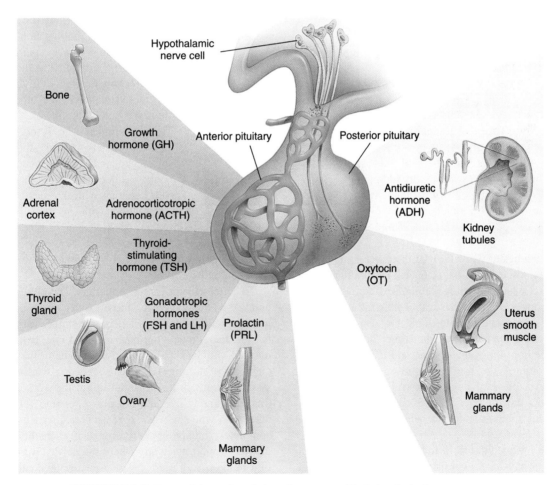

FIGURE 24-3 Some of the major pituitary hormones with their principal target organs.

Follicle-Stimulating Hormone (FSH). Women: stimulates estrogen production and development of ovarian follicle; men: stimulates sperm production in the testes. This hormone and luteinizing hormone (LH) featured next, together are collectively called *gonadotropic hormones.*

Luteinizing Hormone (LH). Women: stimulates the release of estrogens and progesterone, ovulation, and development of the corpus luteum; men: stimulates production of testosterone.

Prolactin (PRL). Together with other hormones, promotes milk production by the mammary glands.

Intermediate Lobe

Melanocyte-stimulating Hormone (MSH). Increases skin pigmentation by stimulating the synthesis and release of melanin from skin/hair.

Posterior Lobe

Also known as the *neurohypophysis,* the posterior lobe of the pituitary is not technically an endocrine gland because it does not produce the hormones it releases. Rather, it stores and releases hormones produced by the hypothalamus.

JANET TRAVELL, MD

Born: December 17, 1901; died: August 1, 1997

"It is obvious that our potential for optimal health depends not alone on the pathology of disease, but on the fiber of our personalities."

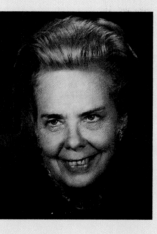

At the 1949 American Medical Association (AMA) convention, a renowned British rheumatologist and author was introduced to Dr. Janet Travell. His response was, "Oooh! Dr. Travell! Soooo, you're the Trigger Queen."

Most massage therapists today are familiar with Travell's groundbreaking work, but mapping previously uncharted patterns of pain is only part of this extraordinary woman's legacy. In addition to her unceasing study of the human body, she was a poet, a mother, and the first female physician in the White House.

As a youngster, Travell loved the process of learning but especially enjoyed the sciences. Her mother taught her basket making, tooling leather, sewing, tatting lace, and knitting. Her father was responsible for teaching her how to shoot—and how to think. He also showed her how to make the best use of her time. "Over and over, he pointed out the value of time and the importance of concentration," she has been quoted as saying. "If I could do a piece of homework well in 15 minutes, I should not dawdle over it for 30. I learned to shut out extraneous matters and to accelerate the pace of my thinking."

Travell wanted to follow in her father's footsteps and become a physician "because he was a magician, and everything he did was wonderful." It did not surprise Travell when she learned through her mother that her father regularly set off giant firecrackers in the fireplace at 3 AM. "I think that he must have been born with a firecracker in one hand and a lighted match in the other," she wrote in her autobiography.

Travell completed tasks too quickly to suit one of her medical school professors. Again and again, he accused her of hurrying through her dissection. Travell came up with the idea of doing the dissection with her left hand to slow her down enough to match the speed of the rest of the students. Not only did this appease her professor, she also delighted at her newfound ambidexterity.

To better balance career and family, Travell scaled her practice of medicine back to part time. However, it did not really slow her down much; she simply earned less money. Jack Powell, her husband, said that, before they married, he had thought carefully about the consequences of starting a life with someone whose career made her quite different from most of the women of her time. He knew he could not make her into something other than who she was, so he accepted her wholly and completely, including her rigorous daily schedule, offering her support when and where she needed it the most. In a reunion address 45 years after her medical school

Antidiuretic Hormone (ADH). Decreases urine production by promoting the reabsorption of water in kidney tubules. Also constricts blood vessels, which raises blood pressure. Alcohol consumption inhibits secretion of ADH, thereby increasing urine production.

Oxytocin (OT). Stimulates uterine contractions and milk expression from mammary glands during lactation. A synthetic version of OT, pitocin, is used to stimulate labor in pregnant women.

PINEAL

The pineal gland, or *pineal body,* is a pinecone-shaped structure located on the posterior aspect of the brain's diencephalon region (see Figure 24-2). The pineal produces and secretes the hormone melatonin.

Melatonin. Involved in the control of biorhythms (the body's 24-hour cycle) and in the growth and development of sexual organs. When injected into the body, melatonin produces drowsiness and inhibits the secretion of LH.

JANET TRAVELL, MD (*continued*)

graduation, Travell commended him and the importance of the man behind every successful woman.

Travell's part-time schedule did give her the freedom to practice at home. Her initial investigation into muscular pain rose out of this additional time to do research, her father's physical medicine experience, and her own shoulder injury at age 38.

When working in a cardiac clinic, Travell had also treated patients with life-threatening pulmonary disease. Common among both the heart and the lung patients were complaints of persistent, acute pain in the shoulder area. Travell came up with enough published findings, mostly from outside the United States, to begin her own study.

Travell researched, ignored skeptics, looked at muscle tissue under a microscope, injected, poked, prodded, and sprayed but did not even stop there. She recognized the role of body mechanics and quizzed patients about how they stood, worked, or turned. She discovered that muscles have memory and can stay contracted for long periods. She found evidence of existing myofascial pain from old injuries that responded to trigger point therapy. Although the prevailing protocol in her time was heat for sore muscles, she successfully experimented with the use of cold. She developed a method for painless needle injections and even meandered into chair design for a time. She was a *whole-body practitioner* who listened carefully to her patients, preached preventive medicine, and made pain go away, even for those whose pain had been diagnosed for years as psychosomatic by stumped physicians.

Travell bemoaned the fact that so many of us are willing to accept average health. With this intense dedication and track record for success, not surprisingly, word of her reputation reached the young Senator John F. Kennedy, for whom Travell has been credited with getting into good enough shape to launch a presidential race. In return, he appointed her White House physician. After his assassination, Travell remained on staff at President Lyndon Johnson's request. During her tenure in the position, she missed only 1 day because of illness. "Although my health was not a problem, I took the precautions of having thorough medical checkups and of taking a sensible dose of regular exercise," she stated in her autobiography. On her departure, the Johnsons presented her with a token of their appreciation—a framed "Prescription for Happiness" that stated at the top, "OFFICE HOURS DAY & NIGHT." "That indeed had been my life," she said in the book she later named after the plaque, "and my happiness was founded on hard work."

Travell left the White House in 1965, and although she was 64, she was in no way considering retirement. She published her autobiography in 1968, and in 1992, she and David G. Simons published *The Trigger Point Manuals.*

Wilson describes her mother as "a true humanitarian who wanted to solve the pain problems of as many people as she could and didn't stop answering letters and reading her journals until a few weeks before her death at [age] 95, on August 1, 1997." Richard and Kathryn Weiner of the American Academy of Pain Management wrote a tribute to Travell that included the following line: "She loved those whom she encountered and in return received that special gift of knowing that her life mattered."

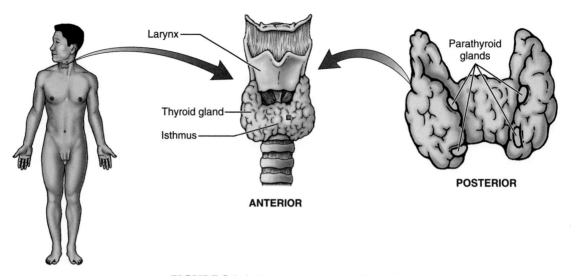

FIGURE 24-4 Thyroid and parathyroid glands.

THYROID

Located at the base of the throat is the butterfly-shaped thyroid (Figure 24-4). The thyroid consists of two lobes and is connected in the center by a mass of tissue known as the *isthmus*.

T3 (Triiodothyronine) and T4 (Tetraiodothyronine [Thyroxine]). Control the metabolic rate and regulate growth and development. These hormones, which are often collectively called *thyroid hormones* (TH), consist of an amino acid bound to iodine; therefore they cannot be made without iodine. Some good sources of iodine are iodized salt and seafood.

Calcitonin (CT). Decreases blood calcium levels (hypocalcemic) by stimulating osteoblasts to increase calcium storage in bones. CT production decreases in older adults, which may explain why many elderly people experience an increase in the decalcification of bones.

PARATHYROID

Usually four in number, the tiny parathyroids are located on the posterolateral surface of the thyroid lobes. *Para-* means "next to" or "alongside of."

Parathyroid Hormone (PTH). Increases blood calcium (hypercalcemic) by breaking down bone and releasing calcium into the blood. This is accomplished by stimulating osteoclast activity. PTH also increases calcium reabsorption from urine and the intestines back into the blood, to raise blood calcium levels.

THYMUS

The thymus is a located posterior to the sternum (see Figure 24-2). Although it is a lymphatic organ, it secretes hormones and thus possesses an endocrine role. Large in infancy, the thymus reaches its maximum size at puberty; it then atrophies and is replaced by adipose tissue in adulthood.

Thymosin and Thymopoietin. Stimulates the maturation of the T cells (specialized lymphocytes involved in immune response).

ADRENALS

The adrenals (suprarenals) are located superior to each kidney and are among the most vascular glands in the body. These important glands are divided into two regions, each possessing two types of tissue. Each tissue type produces different hormones (Figure 24-5).

Adrenal Cortex

The adrenal cortex is the outer region. It arises from the embryonic tissue endoderm, which is similar to that of the kidneys. The adrenal cortex secretes three steroids: glucocorticoids (primarily cortisol), mineralocorticoids (primarily aldosterone), and sex hormones (primarily adrenal estrogens [female hormones] and androgens [male hormones]). *Glucocorticoids* affect carbohydrate, protein, and fat metabolism, converting them to fuel for energy when needed. *Mineralocorticoids* cause the kidneys to reabsorb water and sodium and to excrete potassium; this action helps to regulate fluid and electrolyte balances.

Cortisol (Hydrocortisone). Cortisol is a stress hormone. During times of stress, this hormone helps ensure that glucose, lipids, and amino acids are available for cells to use for energy and protein synthesis. It also has an antiinflammatory effect. For this reason, cortisol is used as an antiinflammatory medication.

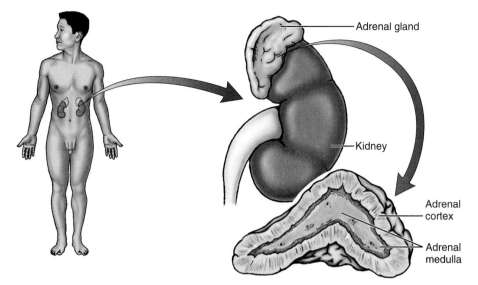

FIGURE 24-5 Adrenal glands.

Aldosterone. Aldosterone stimulates the kidneys to conserve sodium and excrete potassium in urine. Because of this, aldosterone is referred to as the *salt-retaining hormone.* Aldosterone also helps regulate blood volume and blood pressure while helping to maintain proper mineral balance.

Sex Hormones. Androgens (primarily testosterone) assist in the development of secondary sex characteristics. Estrogens secreted by the ovaries usually mask the effects of estrogens secreted by the adrenal cortex. Because of this, adrenal estrogens are physiologically insignificant.

> ### CHAT ROOM
> One way to remember the three hormones of the adrenal cortex are the three Ss—*S*ugar (glucocorticoids), *S*alt (mineralocorticoids), and *S*ex (sex hormones).

Adrenal Medulla

The adrenal medulla is the inner region, which arises from ectoderm. Hormones of the adrenal medulla, also called *neurohormones,* mimic the effects of the sympathetic nervous system and account for the sudden emergency energy required for the stress response.

Epinephrine (Adrenaline). Enhances and prolongs sympathetic arousal, or fight or flight response, of the nervous system.

Norepinephrine (Noradrenaline). Enhances and prolongs sympathetic arousal of the nervous system.

> ### CHAT ROOM
> To memorize the hormones of the adrenal medulla, use the following mnemonic: *a*drenal *m*edulla produces *e*pinephrine and *n*orepinephrine (AMEN).

PANCREATIC ISLETS

The pancreas is located inferior to the stomach and is both endocrine and exocrine. Within the pancreas are more than 1 million islands of specialized cells called the **islets of Langerhans**, or **pancreatic islets.** These contain alpha cells, which secrete glucagon, and beta cells, which secrete insulin (see Figure 29-9). These pancreatic hormones help regulate carbohydrate metabolism (Figure 24-6). Other pancreatic hormones are somatostatin and pancreatic polypeptides. *Somatostatin* inhibits the release of other gastrointestinal hormones. The exact function of *pancreatic polypeptides* is uncertain, but they seem to influence absorption in the digestive tract.

Insulin. Decreases blood glucose levels (hypoglycemic) by causing cells in the liver, muscle, and adipose tissue to take up glucose. The liver and muscle cells store glucose as glycogen. Insulin, secreted by **beta cells,** is the only hormone that decreases blood glucose levels. Because digestive enzymes deactivate this hormone, it cannot be administered orally. If a person requires insulin, then it must be given by injection.

Glucagon. Increases blood glucose levels causing hyperglycemia. Glucagon, secreted by the **alpha cells,** is

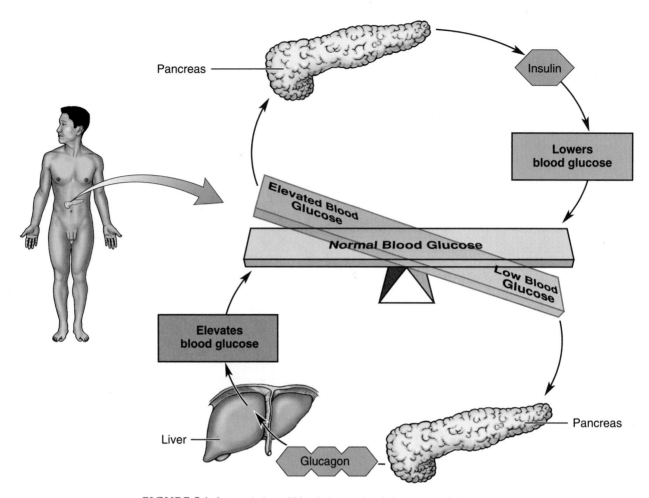

FIGURE 24-6 Regulation of blood glucose levels by pancreatic hormones.

stimulated by low glucose blood levels, causing the liver and the skeletal muscles to break down stored glycogen into glucose.

OVARIES

The ovaries are located in the abdominopelvic area of the female body (see Figure 24-2). The ovaries produce progesterone and estrogens, which are responsible for regulating the menstrual cycle and secondary sexual characteristics that occur at puberty. These characteristics include distribution of adipose tissue in the breasts, hips, and abdomen; a wide pelvis; and pubic and axillary hair. These hormones are also involved in maintaining pregnancy (discussed in Chapter 25). Other ovarian hormones are relaxin and inhibin. *Relaxin* relaxes the uterus to facilitate implantation. (During pregnancy, relaxin is also produced by the placenta, as discussed later on). *Inhibin* inhibits the secretion of FSH and LH.

Estrogens. These hormones are responsible for development of female secondary sex characteristics. Estrogens, along with luteinizing hormone (LH) secreted by the anterior pituitary, promote the development and release of the ovum from the ovary at the time of ovulation. Estrogens also stimulate the uterine lining to proliferate and thicken in anticipation of a fertilized ovum. Estrogens are also produced in the placenta during pregnancy.

Progesterone. Progesterone maintains the uterine lining for implantation and pregnancy. Progesterone also slightly elevates body temperature, creating an incubating effect. One cause of spontaneous abortion (miscarriage) is a drop in progesterone levels. Progesterone is also produced in the placenta.

CHAT ROOM

In 1960 the U.S. Food and Drug Administration approved the first oral contraceptive, Enovid. It was manufactured and distributed that same year. More than 9 million women in the United States and Europe use contraceptives every year.

Most oral contraceptives contain estrogens and progesterone. These hormones inhibit ovulation by suppressing FSH and LH.

TESTES

The testes are located in the male scrotum (see Figure 24-2). Scattered between testicular tubules are the **interstitial cells (of Leydig)**. These cells produce androgens (male sex hormones); the principal androgen is testosterone. Androgens are also secreted in small amounts by the adrenal cortex.

Testosterone. Testosterone stimulates sperm production and secondary sex characteristics in the male. It is involved in arousing libido (sex drive).

> *"Every artist was an amateur."*
> —Ralph Waldo Emerson

ORGANS THAT POSSESS ENDOCRINE CELLS

The glands discussed previously make up the endocrine system, but numerous hormone-secreting cells are scattered in organs throughout the body.

Placenta

The placenta, which is a reproductive organ, also serves as a temporary endocrine gland (see Figure 25-11). In additional to the hormones listed below, estrogens and progesterone are also secreted by the placenta.

Human Chorionic Gonadotropin (hCG). This is called the pregnancy hormone because it is present in maternal blood and urine. hCG stimulates the ovaries to secrete estrogen and progesterone and to decrease lymphocyte activation. Both factors are important in preparing the uterus for fetal implantation.

Relaxin. Facilitates implantation by relaxing the uterus; softens connective tissue in pregnant women, especially the pelvic ligaments, for fetal delivery; helps dilate the cervix during labor and delivery. Relaxin is also produced in the ovaries.

CHAT ROOM

Because relaxin loosens connective tissue during pregnancy, all joint mobilization and stretching activities must be kept to a minimum and performed with caution.

Gastric and Intestinal Mucosa

Gastrin. This hormone initiates the production and secretion of gastric juices and stimulates bile and pancreatic enzyme emissions into the small intestines.

Cholecystokinin. Cholecystokinin stimulates the gallbladder to release bile and the pancreas to secrete enzymes.

Secretin. Secretin stimulates the pancreas to secrete an alkaline liquid that neutralizes acidic chyme, thereby facilitating the action of the intestinal enzymes. Secretin has a limited effect on the production of bile.

Heart

Atrial Natriuretic Hormone (ANH). This hormone is released when pressure-sensitive receptors in the right atrium become overstretched. This hormone triggers urine production (diuresis), thereby decreasing blood volume in an attempt to reduce blood pressure. In regard to increasing urine production, ANH is an antagonist to antidiuretic hormone and aldosterone.

Fat Cells

Leptin. Plays a key role in regulating energy (appetite and metabolism), perhaps signaled by how much fat is stored by the body.

Resistin. Increases blood glucose levels (potentially inducing hyperglycemia) by reducing insulin sensitivity.

ENDOCRINE PATHOLOGIES

Diseases of the Thyroid

Goiter. Enlargement of the thyroid is called a goiter. Goiters are caused by various hyperthyroid and hypothyroid conditions, which may occur in puberty, during pregnancy, or in response to iodine deficiency. In countries where dietary iodine intake is inadequate, goiters are more prevalent.

Avoid the throat because the pressure of massage may damage tissues. If your client is not comfortable lying prone, perform the massage with the person in the supine or side-lying position.

Hypothyroidism/Myxedema. An underactive thyroid, termed hypothyroidism, may lead to thyroid hormone deficiency. When hypothyroidism is diagnosed in adulthood, it is called *myxedema.* It develops slowly over many months or years. Hypothyroidism is marked by fatigue and lethargy, muscle weakness, slowed metabolic rate, cold intolerance, weight gain, and slowed mental processes.

Ask your client about his or her vitality. If your client is vital, then vigorous massage can be performed, within the client's tolerance. If not, reduce treatment time to 30 minutes, and use lighter-than-normal pressure. If your client chills easily, use a warm blanket over your sheet or a towel drape.

Diabetes Mellitus

Type 1. Type 1 diabetes occurs when the pancreatic beta cells that produce insulin become damaged or destroyed, creating a lack of insulin. The affected person becomes dependent on insulin. Treatment consists of a lifelong commitment to monitoring blood sugar, taking insulin injections, regular exercise, and maintaining weight through controlled caloric intake.

Avoid vigorous massage over recent injection sites for 24 hours. Sites of frequent injections may be bruised or have layers of hardened fascia. These areas may respond to deep stroking or frictional movements, as long as the 24-hour rule is respected.

Type 2. Type 2 diabetes is caused by a decrease in insulin production or insulin resistance by body cells or both. Most cases are related to central obesity and sedentary lifestyle. A strong genetic link also exists. Type 2 diabetes accounts for more than 90% of all cases. In contrast with persons with type 1 diabetes, persons with type 2 diabetes can often be treated with oral medications. In rare cases, the person with type 2 diabetes simply does not produce enough insulin. Insulin injections are needed along with oral medications.

Common complications of long-term diabetes include neuropathy and skin ulcers. These two conditions can be a dangerous combination because your client may have an ulcer on the foot but cannot feel it, which may lead to life-threatening infections and possible amputation. Other complications are atherosclerosis, peripheral arterial disease, hypertension, diabetic retinopathy and cataracts, periodontal disease, and kidney and heart diseases.

Query your client about any disease complications (e.g., reduced sensations, skin ulcers) and modify the massage accordingly.

Suggest that your client eat a meal within 2 to 3 hours or has a good snack no more than 1 hour before the massage to help prevent a drop in blood sugar. Ask if your client carries glucose tablets or gel and, if so, where they are in case they are needed quickly during a hypoglycemic episode. Be sure to keep a form of simple sugar in the office (orange juice, regular [not diet] soda, or tube of cake frosting), which may be needed in this event. See Chapter 9 for more information regarding hypoglycemia as a medical emergency.

Diseases of the Adrenal Cortex

Cushing Disease/Syndrome. Cushing disease is characterized by excessive amounts of cortisol in the blood (hypercortisolism). Most often, it is caused by a pituitary tumor that stimulates excessive production of adrenocorticotropic hormone (ACTH), resulting in hypercortisolism.

The affected person develops a round face (called moon facies), acne, puffy eyes, ruddy complexion, thinning scalp hair, and growth of facial hair in women. The skin becomes thin and fragile and is easily bruised. Wound healing is poor, and the person is prone to infection.

Cushing syndrome is characterized by excessive amounts of cortisol in the blood, most often from prolonged and excessive use of high-dose cortisone drugs. These drugs include prednisone, dexamethasone (Decadron), and methylprednisolone (Medrol). Cushing syndrome is more common than Cushing disease because of the use of corticosteroids as treatment for many autoimmune diseases. Signs and symptoms of Cushing syndrome are the same as for Cushing disease.

Ask your client about his or her vitality. If your client is vital, then vigorous massage can be performed, within the client's tolerance. If not, reduce treatment time to 30 minutes, and use lighter-than-normal pressure. Find out about bone fragility. This information will help determine what regions merit reduced pressure because of fracture susceptibility regardless of reported vitality. Because of skin thinning, use adequate amounts of lubricant to reduce skin drag.

Addison Disease. Addison disease is caused by chronic adrenal insufficiency leading to underproduction of cortisol (hypocortisolism). Addison disease is often the result of autoimmune processes, local or general infection, or adrenal cancer. Addison disease is characterized by general weakness, fatigue, and dizziness with fainting. Other signs and symptoms are hyperpigmentation of the skin and mucous membranes (called bronzing) and cold intolerance.

Ask your client about his or her vitality. If your client is vital, then vigorous massage can be performed, within the client's tolerance. If not, reduce treatment time to 30 minutes, and use lighter-than-normal pressure. If your client chills easily, use a warm blanket over your sheet or towel drape. If your client experiences dizziness when getting up from the massage table, be ready to assist.

---

evolve   There are numerous activities and animations on the Evolve website that accompanies this text. Be sure to check out the animation on insulin. ∎

SPOTLIGHT ON RESEARCH

Research suggests that massage therapy may:
- Influence levels of multiple hormones
- Influence production/absorption of insulin
- Influence other massage outcomes and effects
- Decrease glucose levels to normal range and improve dietary compliance in persons with diabetes
- Produce changes in hormones related to pregnancy, labor, and postpartum depression

E-RESOURCES

evolve

http://evolve.elsevier.com/Salvo/MassageTherapy

- Chapter challenge
- Flash cards
- Photo gallery
- Educational animations
- Weblinks

BIBLIOGRAPHY

Abrahams P, Marks S, Hutchings R: *McMinn's color atlas of human anatomy*, St Louis, 2003, Mosby.

Applegate EJ: *The anatomy and physiology learning system*, ed 3, Philadelphia, 2006, Saunders.

Beers MH, Berkow R: *The Merck manual of diagnosis and therapy*, Whitehouse Station, NJ, 2006, Merck Research Laboratories.

Crawley J, Van De Graaff KM: *A photographic atlas for anatomy and physiology*, Englewood, Colo, 2002, Morton.

Como D, editor: *Mosby's medical, nursing, and allied health dictionary*, ed 6, St Louis, 2002, Mosby.

Ferri FF: *2003 Ferri's clinical advisor, instant diagnosis and treatment*, St Louis, 2003, Mosby.

Guyton A: *Human physiology and mechanisms of disease*, ed 6, Philadelphia, 1996, WB Saunders.

Haubrich WS: *Medical meanings: a glossary of word origins*, Philadelphia, 1997, American College of Physicians.

Herlihy B: *The human body in health and illness*, ed 3, St Louis, 2007, Saunders.

Huether SE, McCance KL: *Understanding pathophysiology*, ed 3, St Louis, 2004, Mosby.

Jacob S, Francone C: *Elements of anatomy and physiology*, Philadelphia, 1989, WB Saunders.

Kalat JW: *Biological psychology*, ed 8, Belmont, Calif, 2003, Wadsworth.

Kapit W, Elson LM: *The anatomy coloring book*, ed 3, New York, 2002, Benjamin Cummings.

Kordish M, Dickson S: *Introduction to basic human anatomy*, Lake Charles, La, 1985, McNeese State University.

Kumar V, Abbas A, Fausto N: *Robbins and Cotran physiologic basis of disease*, ed 7, St Louis, 2005, Mosby.

Marieb EN: *Essentials of human anatomy and physiology*, ed 8, New York, 2005, Benjamin Cummings.

Martini FH, Bartholomew EF: *Essentials of anatomy and physiology*, ed 3, New York, 2003, Benjamin Cummings.

McAleer N: *The body almanac*, Garden City, NY, 1985, Doubleday.

McCance K, Huether S: *Pathophysiology: the biological basis for disease in adults and children*, St Louis, 2006, Mosby.

Merck manual, ed 17, Whitehouse Station, NJ, 1998, Merck Co.

Netter FH: *Atlas of human anatomy*, ed 3, Teterboro, NJ, 2003, Icon Learning Systems.

Newton D: *Pathology for massage therapists*, ed 2, Portland, Ore, 1995, Simran.

Premkumar K: *Pathology A to Z, a handbook for massage therapists*, Baltimore, 1999, Lippincott Williams & Wilkins.

Salvo SG: *Mosby's pathology for massage therapists*, ed 2, St Louis, 2009, Mosby.

Solomon EP, Phillips GA: *Understanding human anatomy and physiology*, Philadelphia, 1987, WB Saunders.

Thibodeau G, Patton K: *Anatomy and physiology*, ed 7, St Louis, 2009, Mosby.

Thibodeau G, Patton K: *Structure and function of the body*, ed 12, St Louis, 2004, Mosby.

Tortora GJ: *Introduction to the human body: the essentials of anatomy and physiology*, ed 5, Hoboken, NJ, 2000, John Wiley & Sons.

Tortora GJ, Grabowksi SR: *Principles of anatomy and physiology*, ed 11, New York, 2005, John Wiley & Sons.

Venes D, Thomas CL, Taber CW: *Taber's cyclopedic medical dictionary*, ed 20, Philadelphia, 2005, FA Davis.

MATCHING I

Place the letter of the gland next to the term or phrase that best describes it.

A. Adrenal cortex
B. Adrenal medulla
C. Anterior pituitary
D. Hypothalamus

E. Ovaries
F. Pancreas
G. Parathyroids
H. Pineal

I. Placenta
J. Posterior pituitary
K. Testes
L. Thymus

_____ 1. Secretes hormones insulin and glucagon

_____ 2. Secretes hormones that stimulate T cell maturation

_____ 3. Secretes parathyroid hormone

_____ 4. Controls secretions of the anterior pituitary through hormones, controls secretions of the posterior pituitary through nerve impulses

_____ 5. Secretes hormones estrogen and progesterone

_____ 6. Secretes antidiuretic hormone

_____ 7. Secretes prolactin

_____ 8. Secretes relaxin during pregnancy

_____ 9. Secretes testosterone

_____ 10. Secretes cortisol

_____ 11. Secretes melatonin

_____ 12. Secretes epinephrine and norepinephrine

MATCHING II

Place the letter of the hormone next to the term or phrase that best describes it.

A. Adrenocorticotropic hormone
B. Antidiuretic hormone
C. Calcitonin
D. Epinephrine and norepinephrine

E. Glucagon
F. Growth hormone
G. Insulin
H. Luteinizing hormone

I. Oxytocin
J. Prolactin
K. Testosterone
L. Thyroid hormones

_____ 1. Stimulates protein synthesis for muscle and bone growth, maintenance, and repair

_____ 2. Promotes secondary male sex characteristics, libido, and sperm production

_____ 3. Controls metabolism and regulates growth and development

_____ 4. Stimulates uterine contractions and milk expression from mammary glands

_____ 5. Enhances and prolongs sympathetic arousal

_____ 6. Decreases urine production and raises blood pressure

_____ 7. Stimulates the release of estrogens and progesterone, and ovulation in women; stimulates testosterone production in men

_____ 8. Decreases blood glucose levels

_____ 9. Increases blood glucose levels

_____ 10. Stimulates the adrenal cortex to secrete hormones, especially cortisol

_____ 11. Decreases blood calcium levels

_____ 12. Stimulates mammary glands to produce milk

CASE STUDY

Blood Sugar See-Saw

Steve is a 48-year-old man who works as a business executive for a financial institution. About 4 years ago, he was diagnosed with diabetes. He takes several medications to control his blood sugar, cholesterol levels, and hypertension. Because of the economic climate, he has been negligent about exercise. Fast food is what is on his menu most meals.

Steve arrives at 4 PM for his weekly appointment. During his intake, he mentions an area on his right foot that is painful. He also mentions that he was extremely busy and that he missed lunch, as well as his medication this morning. He is looking forward to his massage today. He stands up and walks toward the massage room, pulling off his necktie in the process.

How do you proceed?

CRITICAL THINKING

One of your clients is a type 2 diabetic who has recently been placed on insulin injection therapy. During her massage, she interrupts you and says she needs to take a break to eat something. After having a chance to eat the snack she brought along and rest for awhile, she apologizes for the interruption and says she is feeling much better. What probably happened here?

Reproductive System

LEARNING OBJECTIVES

After completing this chapter, the student should be able to:

- List basic anatomic structures and describe physiologic processes of the reproductive system.
- Identify structures of the male reproductive system.
- Name structures of the female reproductive system.
- Discuss the menstrual cycle.
- Outline aspects of sexual intercourse between men and women.
- Identify stages fertilization, trimesters of pregnancy, and stages of childbirth.
- Discuss inheritance and dominant and recessive gene expression.
- Identify pathologic conditions related to the reproductive system, pregnancy, and sexually transmitted infections, and ascertain their massage modifications.

INTRODUCTION

The reproductive system contains the organs and processes needed for sexual reproduction. **Sexual reproduction** is the process by which sex cells known as spermatozoa (*singular,* spermatozoon) from males and oocytes from females unite to produce offspring for the survival of the species and pass on hereditary traits from one generation to the next. The male and female gonads, or testes and ovaries, produce these sex cells and the hormones necessary for proper human growth, development, and maintenance, and for the normal functioning of reproductive organs.

Both male and female reproductive systems contribute to these events. However, the female reproductive organs assume responsibility for the developing young, as well as for birth, and providing nourishment for the young through lactation and breast-feeding.

ANATOMY

Basic anatomic structures of the reproductive system are:
- Gonads (testes in men, ovaries in women)
- Gametes or sex cells (spermatozoon in men, oocyte in women)
- Ducts (spermatic duct in men [epididymis, vas deferens, ejaculatory duct, urethra], fallopian tubes in women)
- Male accessory sex glands (prostate, bulbourethral, seminal vesicles)
- Male organs (penis and scrotal sac)
- Female organs and accessory glands (uterus, vagina, and breasts)

PHYSIOLOGY

The functions of the reproductive system are:
- **Produce offspring.** As with most higher forms of life, human beings reproduce sexually. This process allows new individuals of a species to be produced and genetic material to be passed from one generation to the next.
- **Release hormones.** Many reproductive structures release hormones that regulate reproduction and other body processes.

IT'S ALL GREEK TO ME

Term	Meaning
bulbourethral glands	*L.* swollen root
cervix	*L.* neck
chromosome	*Gr.* color; body
corpus albicans	*L.* body; white
corpus luteum	*L.* body; yellow
Cowper gland	William Cowper, English surgeon, 1666-1709
cremaster	*Gr.* hanging
ejaculation	*L.* to hurl or throw out
embryo	*Gr.* in, to grow
epididymis	*Gr.* upon; pair
Fallopian tubes	Gabriele Fallopio, Italian anatomist (1523-1562)
fertilization	*L.* fruitful
fetus	*L.* fruitful
gametes	*Gr.* to marry
gene	*Gr.* to produce
glans	*Gr.* acorn
gonads	*Gr.* seed
hymen	*Gr.* membrane
inheritance	*L.* within; to inherit
interstitial cells of Leydig	Franz von Leydig, German anatomist (1821-1908)
labia	*L.* lips
lactation	*L.* milk; process
mammary	*L.* breast
mons pubis	*L.* mountain; grown-up or hair
morula	*L.* mulberry or blackberry
mutation	*L.* to change
oocyte	*Gr.* egg; cell
ovum	*L.* egg
placenta	*L.* cake
prostate	*Gr.* standing before
rugae	*L.* ridge
scrotum	*L.* a bag
semen	*L.* seed
seminiferous	*L.* seed; to bear
seminal vesicles	*L.* seed; bladder
spermatozoon	*Gr.* seed; life
testis	*L.* to bear witness
uterus	*L.* womb
vagina	*L.* sheath
vas deferens	*L.* to lead; to carry away
vulva	*L.* a covering
zygote	*Gr.* yoke

Gr., Greek; *L.,* Latin.

MALE REPRODUCTIVE SYSTEM

The male reproductive system consists of primary reproductive organs called the testes and a duct system to help transport male sex cells called sperm out of the body. Male accessory glands secrete fluids that help to nourish sperm. Organs that facilitate these events are the scrotum and the penis (Figure 25-1).

Testes

Testes, or testicles, are paired oval glands enclosed in an external sac, the scrotum. The testes are the site of sperm production. *Seminiferous tubules* within the testes produce sperm.

Interstitial cells of Leydig within the testes produce testosterone. Testosterone is converted into the hormone dihydrotestosterone (DHT). DHT is 10 times stronger than testosterone. Luteinizing hormone (LH) from the anterior pituitary stimulates testosterone production. Follicle-stimulating hormone (FSH) from the anterior pituitary and testosterone controls spermatogenesis.

Testosterone and DHT are also responsible for the development of the male sex organs and secondary male characteristic changes that appear at puberty. These changes include widening of the shoulders and narrowing of the hips, appearance of facial, axillary, pubic, and chest hair, and the enlargement of the larynx, which contributes to deepening of the male voice.

Spermatic Duct

The duct system in the male reproductive system is called the *spermatic duct*. It includes the epididymis, vas deferens, ejaculatory duct, and the urethra. Each duct listed is a pair, except the urethra, of which only one is present.

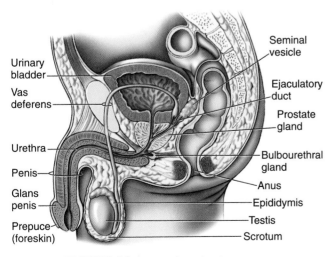

Urinary bladder
Vas deferens
Urethra
Penis
Glans penis
Prepuce (foreskin)
Seminal vesicle
Ejaculatory duct
Prostate gland
Bulbourethral gland
Anus
Epididymis
Testis
Scrotum

FIGURE 25-1 Male reproductive organs.

Epididymis. The epididymis is located in the posterior testes and connects each testicle to its vas deferens. The epididymis is the site for final sperm maturation.

Vas Deferens. The vas deferens (also called the ductus deferens and seminal duct) runs from the epididymis into the pelvic cavity, where it loops over the side and down the posterior surface of the urinary bladder. The vas deferens carries sperm from the epididymis to the ejaculatory duct in anticipation of ejaculation. A portion of this tube is surgically removed and closed off during a sterilization procedure called a *vasectomy*.

Ejaculatory Duct. The ejaculatory duct passes through the prostate to join the urethra.

Urethra. The urethra, located below the bladder, transports both semen and urine. The urethra passes through the prostate and the penis. On ejaculation, semen flows through the urethra to the outside of the body.

Male Accessory Glands

The male accessory glands secrete the liquid portion of the semen. These glands possess ducts that conduct the fluids they secrete into the urethra.

Prostate. The prostate surrounds the urethra as it exits the bladder. Its alkaline secretions make up approximately 25% of semen volume. Semen needs to be alkaline to neutralize the acidic environment of the vagina. The prostate also prevents the flow of urine during ejaculation.

Bulbourethral Glands. The bulbourethral glands, or Cowper glands, are a pea-sized pair of glands located on either side of the prostate. Their secretions make up approximately 5% of semen volume.

Seminal Vesicles. Seminal vesicles are located at the base of the bladder. Their secretions, containing proteins, enzymes, fructose, mucus, and vitamin C, make up approximately 60% of semen volume.

Penis

The penis is composed of erectile tissues. The end of the penis, or *glans penis*, is covered with a loose flap of skin called the *prepuce*, or *foreskin*. This foreskin often is removed in a surgical procedure called *circumcision*.

Under sexual stimulation, penile arteries dilate, and large quantities of blood enter penile sinuses, resulting in erection. A sphincter at the base of the urinary bladder closes during ejaculation to prevent mixing acidic urine with semen in the urethra; this also prevents semen from entering the bladder. During ejaculation, the penis deposits semen out of the body.

Scrotum

The scrotum is the divided pouch that supports the testes. The sac is made of thin, loose, usually wrinkled skin that hangs down behind the penis. The scrotal skin contains hairs and numerous sebaceous glands, which give the scrotum a characteristic odor.

The primary function of the scrotum is temperature regulation to facilitate sperm production and survival (approximately 4° F cooler than normal body temperature). The cremaster muscle draws the testes closer to or away from the body, depending on ambient temperature.

Sperm and Semen

Male sex cells, called **sperm** or *spermatozoa*, carry genetic information from the male that produced them (Figure 25-2). Sperm cell production, or *spermatogenesis*, begins during puberty and continues throughout life. Each day, a man makes millions of sperm.

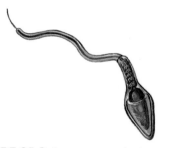

FIGURE 25-2 Spermatozoon (male sex cell).

Semen is a thick, milky mixture of sperm (10%) and seminal fluid (90%). Seminal fluid consists of secretions from male sex glands (i.e., prostate and bulbourethral glands, seminal vesicles). Seminal fluid is a transport medium and source of nutrients for sperm. Between 50 and 100 billion sperm cells are found in each cubic centimeter of semen; any level lower than 50 million is regarded as clinically sterile.

Male External Genitalia

Male external genitalia include the scrotum and penis.

FEMALE REPRODUCTIVE SYSTEM

The primary reproductive organs in women are the ovaries. Secondary organs include the fallopian tubes, uterus, cervix, vagina, and the vulva (mons pubis, labia majora and minora, and clitoris) (Figure 25-3). Female breasts are also considered accessory reproductive glands because they produce and secrete the milk that will feed the young.

Ovaries

The ovaries are a pair of almond-shaped glands located lateral to the uterus in the pelvic cavity. Each ovary contains numerous fluid filled sacs called *ovarian (Graafian) follicles*. Each follicle contains immature *oocytes* or unfertilized eggs. When a female is born, her ovaries contain all the oocytes she will ever have; their maturation is arrested until puberty. Beginning at puberty, hormones stimulate usually one oocyte, but sometimes more, to mature. A mature oocyte

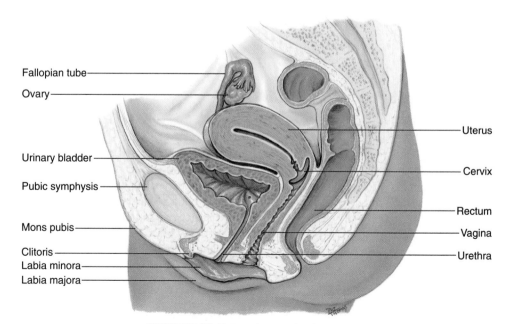

FIGURE 25-3 Female reproductive organs.

TIFFANY FIELD, PhD

"The best pioneers are the ones actually out there doing massage. They get devotees just from having put their hands on them. That's what keeps the field alive and moving."

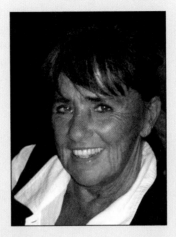

Tiffany Field has always been a woman on the move. As the daughter of an insurance executive and a teacher, she lived in 12 different places when she was growing up, but now she's found her home and her life's calling—on the beach in Hollywood, Florida.

She is not a massage therapist, and she has not developed any particular massage method or technique; however, her work has dramatically affected the credibility of the profession. Tiffany Field is a professor of pediatrics, psychology, and psychiatry, and she is the director of the University of Miami School of Medicine's Touch Research Institute (TRI). TRI was established in 1992 and is the only center in the world devoted solely to the study of touch and its applications in science and medicine.

According to an article in *Massage Therapy Journal* by Mirka Knaster, Field holds a doctorate in developmental psychology and has 25 years of research experience, with numerous publishing credits, awards, and research grants. She has written for 50 professional journals and retains membership in more than a dozen professional organizations.

TRI evolved after her team's research findings supported touch as a factor that increased birth weight in premature infants. Premature infants who receive massage put on weight faster and leave the hospital earlier. With 470,000 premature births in the United States each year, that could add up to $7.05 billion in annual savings. The potential for Field's research and the cost-cutting measures earned the grant money to explore touch therapy further.

Some of the work being examined at TRI is particularly groundbreaking. Still considered by many a contraindication for massage, an ongoing breast cancer study shows an increase in natural killer cells (cells that kill cancer cells) and a decrease in other pathologies after massage. In a society that values scientific proof, such findings could eventually make massage therapy a component of mainstream medicine.

Field has a hectic schedule that involves lots of travel for fund-raising, overseeing projects, and writing grant proposals. To unwind, she swims daily; practices yoga, ballet, and tai chi when she has spare time; and of course she gets a massage whenever she can.

For over a decade, Field has probably been one of the most instrumental people in helping gain respect for massage therapy and advises new massage therapists to "join a group practice to learn the ropes of operating a business."

---

is called an *ovum*. During ovulation, the follicle ruptures and releases an ovum. This cycle of maturing oocytes continues from menarche (first menstruation) until menopause (when ovarian functions cease).

The ovaries produce the hormones progesterone, estrogens, relaxin, and inhibin. Progesterone and estrogens are responsible for regulating the menstrual cycle and development of the secondary sexual characteristics that appear at puberty. These characteristics include distribution of adipose tissue in the breasts, hips, and abdomen; a wide pelvis; and pubic and axillary hair.

Fallopian Tubes

The fallopian tubes, or *oviducts*, extend laterally from the uterus. Each tube serves as a passage through which ova (*singular*, ovum) move toward the uterus. The fallopian tubes are the site of fertilization for most ova.

Uterus

The uterus, or womb, is a hollow, muscular, pear-shaped organ that receives the fertilized ovum and allows the

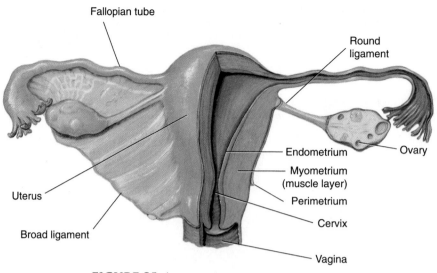

FIGURE 25-4 Uterus, fallopian tubes, and vagina.

embryo to grow and develop into a fetus during pregnancy and from which menses flow if no pregnancy takes place (Figure 25-4).

The uterus contains three layers. The inner lining, the *endometrium*, is shed each month during menstruation. The *myometrium* is the middle muscular layer. During childbirth, uterine contractions push the fetus into the vagina. The *perimetrium* is the outer layer.

The uterus has three parts. The *body* contains a hollow cavity; the walls of the cavity touch unless the woman is pregnant. The *fundus* is the uppermost portion. The lower, narrow portion is the *cervix*, which opens into the vagina.

CHAT ROOM

Cells of the uterine cervix are scraped for a Papanicolaou (Pap) smear. A Pap smear aims to screen for precancerous or cancer cells, which are usually caused by sexually transmitted human papillomaviruses. Women should undergo a Pap smear exam 3 years after starting vaginal intercourse or at age 21. Pap smears are reliable in detecting cervical cancer more than 90% of the time.

Vagina

The vagina is a canal that receives sperm from the male and serves as the birth canal. It extends from the cervix to outside the body. The vagina is actually a potential space; its walls possess transverse folds called *rugae*, which permit expansion for intercourse and childbirth. A thin membrane may be found, called the *hymen*, which may partially cover the opening.

On either side of the vaginal opening are located *Bartholin glands*. They produce mucus for lubrication during intercourse and are equivalent to the bulbourethral glands in men. During orgasm, the muscular layer of the vagina contracts, moving semen toward the cervix.

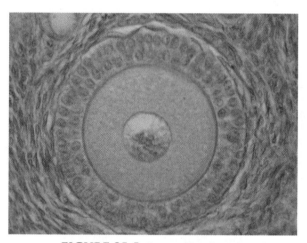

FIGURE 25-5 Oocyte (female egg).

CHAT ROOM

The *perineum* is the diamond-shaped area between thighs and buttocks in both men and women that contains the external genitalia and anus. If the vagina is too small to accommodate the head of the emerging fetus, then the perineum between the vagina and anus may tear. In this case, an episiotomy may be performed. An episiotomy is a small incision made in perineal skin and underlying tissues just before delivery. It usually is required for forceps delivery, performed electively to prevent tearing of the perineum, to hasten or facilitate delivery of the baby, or to prevent overstretching of perineal muscles and related tissue.

Oocyte to Ovum

Female sex cells, called **oocytes** or eggs, carry genetic information from the woman who produced them (Figure 25-5). Oocytes mature within ovarian follicles and one (or sometimes more) is released during ovulation. Hormones that assist in maturation are the FSH and LH. Both FSH and LH are secreted by the anterior pituitary.

An **ovum** is a mature oocyte that has ovulated. The ovum travels down the fallopian tube toward the uterus. If fertilization occurs, the ovum (now called the *zygote*) implants in the uterine lining. If fertilization does not occur, the ovum is flushed out during menses.

Female External Genitalia

The **vulva** is the external genitalia in women. It consists of the labia majora and minora, and the clitoris, and the mons pubis.

Labia Majora. The labia majora are two folds of skin extending from the mons pubis; they are equivalent to the scrotum in men. The labia majora contain adipose tissue and oil and sweat glands and are covered with pubic hair.

Labia Minora. The labia minora are two folds of skin inside the labia majora and contain numerous oil glands.

Clitoris. The clitoris is a small cylindrical mass of erectile tissue and nerves located at the anterior junction of the labia minora. A small layer of foreskin is formed at the point where the labia minora unite and cover the body of the clitoris. The clitoris and the glans penis in men are equivalent structures. The clitoris enlarges upon tactile stimulation and assumes a role in sexual excitement.

Mons Pubis. The mons pubis, which cushions the symphysis pubis, is a mound of fatty tissue that becomes covered with hair during puberty.

Female Breasts

Female breasts, or mammary glands, produce and secrete milk after pregnancy. They lie over the pectoris major and serratus anterior muscles. Each gland consists of 15 to 20 lobules arranged radially. Each lobule has a system of ducts for the passage of milk to the nipple. The pigmented area around the nipple is the *areola*. The outer portion of the breast is mostly adipose tissue (Figure 25-6). Milk production, which is under hormonal control, is called *lactation*. Pituitary hormones prolactin and oxytocin regulate milk production and expression respectively.

> *"A loving person lives in a loving world.*
> *A hostile person lives in a hostile world:*
> *everyone you meet is your mirror."*
> —Ken Keyes, Jr.

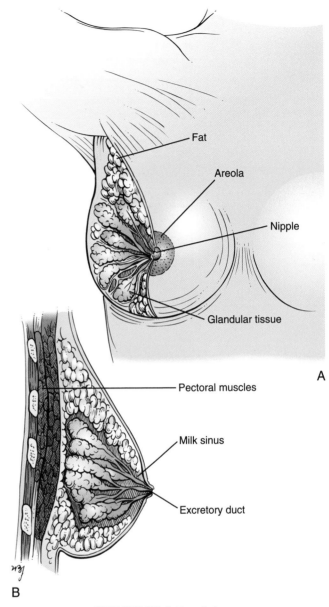

Fat

Areola

Nipple

Glandular tissue

A

Pectoral muscles

Milk sinus

Excretory duct

B

FIGURE 25-6 Female breast.

MENSTRUAL CYCLE

A series of hormonal events, called the **menstrual cycle,** begins at puberty and occurs approximately every 28 days. Also called the *reproductive* or *fertility cycle,* this cycle is divided into three phases: the follicular phase (days 1 to 13); ovulation (day 14); and the luteal phase (days 15 to 28) (Figure 25-7). In brief, the uterine lining sheds: then re-grows, proliferates, and is maintained for several days; then sheds again at menstruation. This monthly cycle usually continues until menopause, unless interrupted by pregnancy, disease, or stress.

Menstruation is the periodic discharge of built-up endometrial lining from the non-pregnant uterus. The discharge, called *menses,* contains between 50 and 150 ml of blood, tissue fluid, mucus, and epithelial cells of the uterine lining.

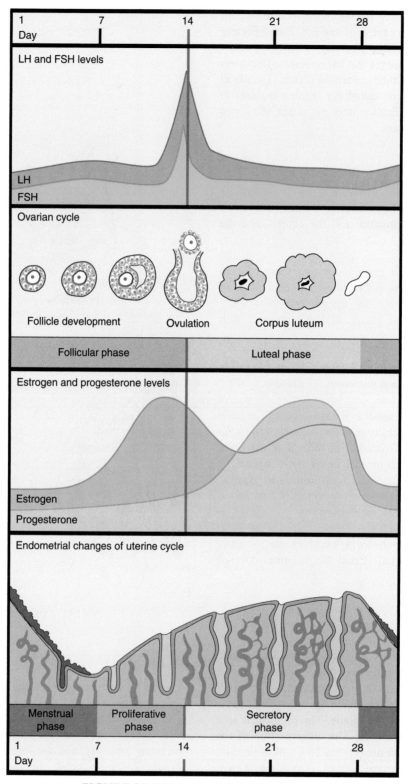

FIGURE 25-7 The menstrual cycle.

Menstruation is caused by a sudden reduction in estrogens and progesterone, which, in turn, causes constriction of uterine arteries and death of the internal lining. As a result, patchy areas of bleeding develop, and small portions of the lining detach. Menstruation lasts approximately 5 days.

Follicular Phase

The follicular phase begins with menstruation (the first day of menstruation is day one of the menstrual cycle). During menstruation, ovarian follicles begin to develop.

As follicles develop, FSH secreted by the anterior pituitary assist the secretion of estrogens by the ovaries. These estrogens, along with LH secreted by the anterior pituitary, promote the development and release of the ovum at the time of ovulation. Estrogens also stimulate the uterine lining to proliferate and thicken in anticipation of a fertilized ovum.

Ovulation

Ovulation occurs about day 14 in a 28-day cycle. A surge of LH causes rupture of an ovarian follicle and release of the ovum. This ovum then travels down the fallopian tube toward the uterus. The collapsed follicle develops into the *corpus luteum*. If the ovum is fertilized by sperm, hormone secretion by the corpus luteum will cease only after the placenta develops and takes over hormone secretion. If the ovum is not fertilized, the corpus luteum remains functional for about 10 days, and then regresses into a *corpus albicans*, which is primarily scar tissue (Figure 25-8).

Luteal Phase

The luteal phase occurs from day 15 to day 28. The corpus luteum secretes estrogens and progesterone, which maintain the uterine lining for implantation and pregnancy. Progesterone also slightly elevates body temperature, creating an incubating effect. Other ovarian hormones involved in this phase are relaxin and inhibin. Relaxin relaxes the uterus to

facilitate implantation. Inhibin inhibits the secretion of FSH and LH.

If the ovum is not fertilized, hormone levels decrease. This causes the endometrium to shrink and die, leading to menstruation. The unfertilized egg is then flushed out of the body with menses.

SEXUAL INTERCOURSE

Presented next is a brief discussion of sexual intercourse.

Men

Erection. Erection is enlargement and stiffening of the penis initiated by stimuli such as anticipation, memory, visual stimuli, or touch. Arteries dilate and fill penile sinuses with blood.

Lubrication. Bulbourethral glands secrete mucus through the urethra. However, the female vagina produces the major portion of lubricating mucus needed for comfortable intercourse.

Orgasm. Tactile stimulation of the penis brings about propulsion of sperm into the urethra and release of seminal fluids from male accessory glands. Impulses from the spinal cord stimulate muscles at the base of the penis to expel semen from the urethra outside the male body; this is called *ejaculation.* Ejaculation is accompanied by increases in respiration, pulse, and blood pressure, and a pleasurable sensation associated with orgasm (or climax).

Women

Erection. Stimulation of the female external genitalia results in clitoral erection and widespread sexual arousal (dependent on both psychologic and tactile responses).

Lubrication. Cervical lining and Bartholin glands produce mucus.

Orgasm. Orgasm occurs as genital stimulation reaches maximal intensity. It increases respiration, pulse, and blood pressure, and muscular contractions of reproductive organs, which aid in fertilization of the ovum. Female orgasm differs from male orgasm by the possibility of multiple orgasms of variable intensity, with accompanying pleasurable sensations.

Semen liquifies approximately 15 minutes after it is deposited within the vagina. If sexual intercourse occurs during ovulation, this liquifaction allows sperm to swim up a thread of female mucus, leading to the awaiting ovum. This voyage is aided by uterine contractions to move sperm toward the fallopian tubes, where fertilization occurs.

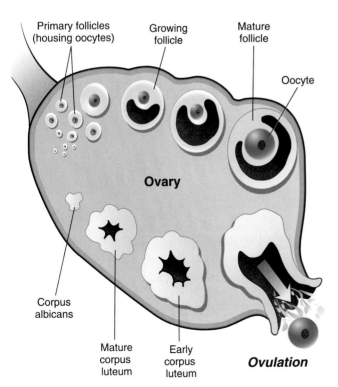

FIGURE 25-8 Stages of ovarian follicle development.

FERTILIZATION

Fertilization is the penetration of the ovum by a spermatozoon. This process occurs approximately 24 hours after ovulation. The fertilized ovum, or *zygote*, contains genetic information from each parent. The number of chromosomes in each ovum and each spermatozoon is one half that of all other body cells. When the sperm fertilizes the egg, the resulting offspring must contain the same number of chromosomes as the parent cells. The ovum contains one X (female) chromosome. Sperm contains either an X (female) or a Y (male) chromosome, so the male determines the sex of the offspring.

Approximately 36 hours after fertilization, the zygote undergoes division to form two cells; cells divide again to form four cells, then eight, then 16, and so forth. Although the number of cells increase, the size of the zygote does not. Finally, a solid mass of tiny cells, the *morula*, is formed 3 to 4 days after fertilization. The solid mass eventually becomes a hollow fluid-filled ball of cells called the *blastocyst*. During this process, the conceptus continues to be swept through the fallopian tube and enters the uterus about day 7 after fertilization, where it implants (Figure 25-9). The result is pregnancy. The uterus nourishes the fertilized egg through stages of growth and development. If the pregnancy is successful, it ends in the birth of a viable infant.

⊖volve *To view a zygote, an embryo in the earliest stages of human development, log on to your student account from the Evolve website and access the materials for Chapter 23. Keep in mind that, in actuality, a zygote is smaller than the period at the end of this sentence.* ∎

*"Love slays what we have been that
we may be what we were not."*
—Saint Augustine

PREGNANCY

Pregnancy is the sequence of events that includes implantation and embryonic and fetal growth and ends in birth. The process of gestation takes approximately 10 lunar months (40 weeks, 9 calendar months, or approximately 266 days). Pregnancy and is divided into trimesters (Figure 25-10).

First Trimester

The first trimester is considered the *time of the embryo* because this is when most embryonic development occurs and the pregnant woman experiences few structural changes.

By day 14, a connecting stalk forms; this structure will later develop into the umbilical cord. By day 16, the inner

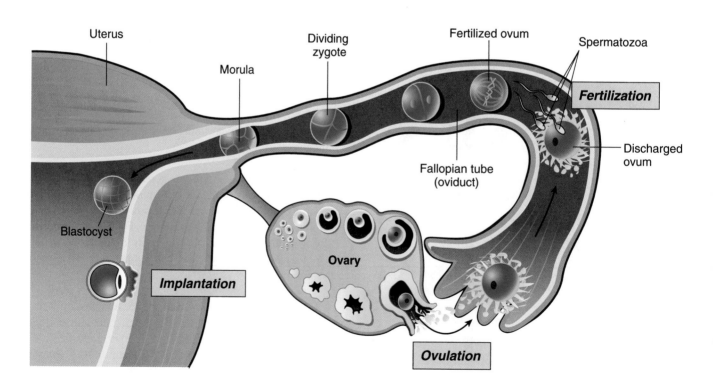

FIGURE 25-9 Ovulation, fertilization, and implantation.

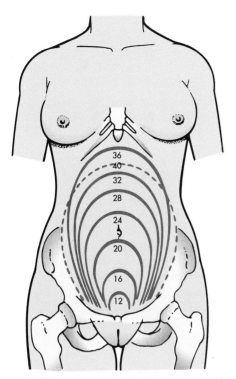

FIGURE 25-10 Uterine growth during pregnancy. Numbers are weeks of pregnancy.

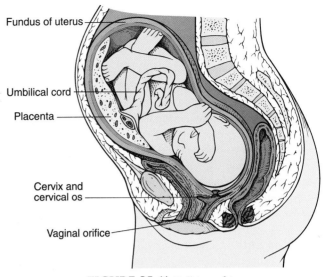

FIGURE 25-11 Full-term fetus.

cell mass of the blastocyte begins to differentiate into three primary germ layers. From superficial to deep, these layers are *ectoderm*, *mesoderm*, and *endoderm* (see Figure 18-8). These layers will develop into all tissues and organs of the body. Fluid-filled spaces form and produce the amnion and yolk sacs. The yolk sac is temporary and provides nutrients to the developing embryonic disk.

By day 24, the embryonic disk has developed into a curved embryo with a definitive head and "tail" surrounded by amniotic fluid. The gastrointestinal tract, brain, and heart begin to develop. Fingerlike projections, called the *chorionic villi*, will grow into the uterine lining and absorb nourishment from the mother for the embryo.

After 8 weeks, the baby is termed a *fetus*. For the remaining 32 weeks of pregnancy, organs grow rapidly, and the fetus takes on a human appearance. The fetus is contained within the fluid-filled amniotic cavity and is joined to the placenta by the umbilical cord.

Placenta. By 8 weeks, a section of the chorionic villi will develop into the placenta, which allows the developing fetus and the mother to exchange nutrients and wastes; it also secretes hormones required to maintain the pregnancy. The placenta serves as a spongelike filter system that allows only small molecules (e.g., glucose, oxygen, nitrogen) to enter. Blood cells are too large to pass through the filter. Unfortunately, many drugs, alcohol, viruses (e.g., rubella, human immunodeficiency virus), and other toxic substances can pass through.

Human Chorionic Gonadotropin. The developing embryo secretes human chorionic gonadotropin (hCG), stimulating the continual production of estrogens and progesterone, which enables the uterus to maintain pregnancy. The corpus luteum secretes increasing amounts of progesterone. Pregnancy tests detect the presence of hCG in the mother's urine.

Relaxin. During pregnancy, the ovaries and placenta produce large amounts of relaxin. This hormone increases flexibility of the pubic symphysis and helps the cervix dilate, assisting in fetal delivery.

Second Trimester

The mother begins to "show" and she should feel the baby move by the end of the second trimester. The former embryo is now a fetus and grows to approximately 11 inches in length and weighs about 1.5 lb.

Third Trimester

The last trimester finds the mother-to-be heavy with the baby, and postural changes are evident. The fetus grows to about 20 inches in length and between 5 and 9 lbs in weight (Figure 25-11). The mother may experience occasional, preparatory contractions in which the uterus hardens and then returns to normal. Colostrum, the early form of breast milk, may leak from the breasts.

Childbirth

For normal childbirth to occur, the uterus contracts forcefully during a complex process called *labor*. Labor begins after the fetus reaches a gestational age of approximately 40 weeks (10 lunar months). There are three stages of labor.

First Stage: Dilation of the Cervix. This stage is the time from the onset of labor to complete cervical dilation (10 cm or 4 inches). Rupture of the amniotic sac often occurs during this stage.

Second Stage: Expulsion of the Fetus. This stage is the time from complete cervical dilation, the fetal journey down the vagina, and welcome of the newborn by the parents.

Third Stage: Expulsion of the Placenta. The placenta, or *afterbirth*, is then expelled by uterine contractions. These contractions also constrict any blood vessels that were torn during delivery to prevent hemorrhage. The mother and the newborn can now rest.

Cesarean Birth. A cesarean section, or C-section, is a surgical procedure that removes the fetus through the abdominal wall. In some instances, the pregnant woman knows in advance that she will deliver her child by cesarean section. In others, it is used as an emergency procedure to save the life of the baby and/or the mother.

Lactation

The secretion and ejection of milk by the mammary glands is called *lactation*. This process is facilitated by the pituitary hormones prolactin (milk production) and oxytocin (milk expression). During late pregnancy and the first few days after birth, the mammary glands secrete fluid called *colostrum* (first milk). True breast milk appears at approximately the fourth day post partum. Breast milk contains antibodies that protect the infant from disease during the first few months of life.

INHERITANCE

Both traits and conditions are passed from one generation to another through sexual reproduction. The expression of this genetic material is called **inheritance**. The study of inheritance is *genetics*.

Every cell in the body except eggs and sperm contains 23 pairs, or 46 chromosomes. An egg and a sperm each have only 23 unpaired chromosomes because they will potentially unite, combining their chromosomes for a total of 46 chromosomes (23 pairs) in the fertilized egg.

Each chromosome contains a chemical called *deoxyribonucleic acid* (DNA), which appears as a small-coiled string. Different sections of the DNA strand code for the production of substances called *enzymes* (and other functional proteins or polypeptides). A section of DNA on a chromosome that codes for a specific enzyme is called a **gene**.

When reproduction occurs, the offspring receives 23 chromosomes from the father and a corresponding 23 from the mother. As mentioned previously, they join together in the fertilized egg to reestablish 23 pairs of chromosomes. Combinations of these chromosomes control our traits (e.g.,

hair and eye color, blood type). Sometimes mistakes, or *mutations*, occur in our gene-coding system so that an incorrect message is sent to the cells. This can result in something mild such as an eye color different from either parent all the way to serious defects in the body's structure or function. Mutations can occur spontaneously, or they can be passed through generations. Mutations happen all the time, many without our knowing.

Two different kinds of genetic diseases are chromosomal and gene diseases. *Chromosomal diseases* are caused by having too many or not enough chromosomes or by having a broken or missing piece of a chromosome. Examples include trisomy 21 or Down syndrome (three No. 21 chromosomes) and Turner syndrome (only one X chromosome). *Genetic diseases* are caused by a mistake in the DNA code of a particular gene on a particular chromosome. Examples include Huntington disease, cystic fibrosis, sickle cell disease, muscular dystrophy, and spina bifida. Expressions of these diseases vary, depending on whether the mutation occurred on a dominant gene, a recessive gene, or a sex chromosome (the X or Y chromosome).

Dominant and Recessive Genes

When genes pair, sometimes one gene dominates over its corresponding gene. This leads to a greater likelihood of its traits being expressed and the other gene's traits not being expressed. For example, the gene for brown eyes is usually dominant over the gene for blue eyes. The gene for brown eyes is dominant; the gene for blue eyes is recessive. Usually the only way a person can have blue eyes is if he or she has both genes for blue eyes. If the individual receives a gene for brown eyes from one parent and a gene for blue eyes from the other parent, he or she is likely to have brown eyes, unless a mutation has occurred.

REPRODUCTIVE PATHOLOGIES, CONDITIONS, AND SEXUALLY TRANSMITTED INFECTIONS

Prostatic Pathologies

Benign Prostatic Hyperplasia. Benign prostatic hyperplasia (or hypertrophy) is an enlargement of the prostate gland. It is nonmalignant and noninflammatory. Signs and symptoms include increased urinary urgency, hesitancy in starting flow, weak urine stream, postvoiding dribbling, and incomplete bladder emptying, which leads to urinary frequency.

Suggest use of the toilet before massage as a comfort measure and be prepared for a toilet break during the session.

Prostatitis. Prostatitis is inflammation of the prostate. Types are acute bacterial, chronic bacterial, and asymptomatic inflammatory prostatitis. In all types, the affected person experiences frequent and urgent urination as well as symptoms of urinary tract infection (i.e., low-grade fever and fatigue, painful urination).

If your client has fever, postpone massage until he has been fever-free for 48 hours. Then, avoid the lower abdomen if pressure causes uneasiness or discomfort. Suggest use of the toilet before massage as a comfort measure and be prepared for a toilet break during the session.

Female Conditions

Menstruation. Menstruation is characterized by the sloughing off of endometrial tissue from a nonpregnant uterus. The only sign related to menstruation is bloody vaginal discharge. Products used to absorb menses include sanitary pads, tampons, and menstrual cups. Abdominopelvic pain is a common symptom, which may refer to the lower back. Some women experience headaches and water retention.

Avoid the abdomen or use only gently gliding strokes over this area if the client is experiencing abdominopelvic discomfort. Because she will be wearing some kind of feminine protection (pads or tampons), she may choose to leave her undergarments on during the massage. Deep gliding, kneading, and deep friction on the quadratus lumborum, the paraspinals, latissimus dorsi, thighs, and possibly the gluteals may be helpful.

Menopause. Menopause is the cessation of menstruation. This signifies the end of a woman's reproductive period. American women typically reach menopause between the ages of 48 and 55. Along with lighter flow and less frequent periods, women may experience mood swings such as irritability, anxiety, and depression. Hot flashes are a frequent complaint (80%), with their duration lasting from 1 to 5 minutes. Other signs and symptoms include vaginal and general skin dryness, night sweats, and sleep disturbance. Menopause may be induced with surgical removal of the ovaries and/or uterus or with chemotherapy.

Use an emollient lubricant to alleviate dry skin. Because of the prevalence of hot flashes, avoid overheating by limiting the use of blankets and flannel sheets as drape material and use a thinner, cooler fabric instead. Consider uncovering the client's arms and feet or use a cool washcloth over her forehead or across the base of her neck to help her feel comfortable.

Pathologies of the Female Reproductive System

Premenstrual Syndrome. Premenstrual syndrome is a cluster of symptoms that occur before menstruation and are relieved by its onset. More common complaints are weight gain, edema, bloating, breast tenderness, headaches, muscle and joint pain, and acne flare-ups. Emotional symptoms range from irritability and restlessness to fatigue and depression.

Devise a treatment plan according to the client's symptoms. For example, headaches may be relieved by head, neck, and shoulder massage. Position her for comfort to address any breast tenderness, which may include using supportive cushions.

Dysmenorrhea. Painful menstruation, or dysmenorrhea, is the most frequent gynecologic problem, occurring occasionally in almost all menstruating women. The discomfort usually begins just before, or at the start of, menstruation and usually lasts from 1 to 2 days. The most common symptom is abdominopelvic cramps.

Ascertain the location and severity of the pain. In most cases, it is best to avoid the abdomen as pressure may exacerbate symptoms. Keep in mind that if your client has severe cramps before or during the massage treatment, then she may not feel up to receiving massage.

Endometriosis. Endometriosis is the presence of functioning endometrial tissue outside the uterus. The most common sites are the fallopian tubes and ovaries, but such tissue has been found throughout the body. This displaced tissue responds to the hormonal fluctuations of the menstrual cycle (it proliferates, breaks down, and is expelled with bleeding in normal menses). This tissue causes localized inflammation and pain.

Abdominal massage is contraindicated if pressure causes pain. If your client is dealing with infertility issues, consider making a referral to a mental health counselor or fertility specialist.

Uterine Fibroids. Uterine fibroids are benign tumors composed largely of smooth muscle and fibrous tissue. Most are discovered during pelvic ultrasound examinations. In most cases, fibroids are asymptomatic. When signs do occur, it is often heavy bleeding during menstruation.

Avoid the abdomen if pressure causes pain.

Ovarian Cysts. Ovarian cysts, which are fluid-filled sacs within the ovary, are common in women during their reproductive years. Most cysts are associated with the menstrual cycle. Large ovarian cysts may cause menstrual irregularities, abdominopelvic pain, swelling, and symptoms related to pressure on the bladder or colon such as urinary frequency, urgency, and constipation

Avoid the abdomen if pressure causes pain. Inquire about presenting symptoms and make appropriate modifications (e.g., suggest a toilet break).

Polycystic Ovary Syndrome. With polycystic ovary syndrome (PCOS), the ovaries enlarge bilaterally while becoming studded with multiple cysts. This condition is the leading cause of infertility in the United States. Symptoms are menstrual irregularities, abdominopelvic pain, and painful intercourse. Some women experience referred pain in the midabdomen or low back (true with ovarian cysts, too). Young women will often have acne, facial hair, excessive body hair, and infertility.

Inquire about presenting symptoms. Avoid the abdomen if pressure causes pain. If lower back pain is actually referred pain from PCOS, it will not be relieved by massage. This should be reflected in the treatment plan and conveyed to your client.

Vaginal Yeast Infection. Yeast infection is caused by a yeastlike fungus called *Candida albicans.* Common manifestations are a thick creamy or curdlike vaginal discharge, foul odor, local itching, redness, and swelling. It can also cause painful urination. Yeast infections can occur after immunosuppression (following antibiotic therapy, diabetes mellitus, AIDS, and chemotherapy).

There are no special massage considerations for women who have yeast infections.

Conditions of Female Breasts

Fibrocystic Breast Change. Fibrocystic breast change is the presence of nodules in breast tissue. It is so common in premenopausal and perimenopausal women, and not related to a pathologic process, that many health care providers prefer the term fibrocystic breast change over fibrocystic breast disease. The affected person often indicates that the breasts feel heavy or full. This condition tends to be cyclic and is often worse before menstruation.

Position the client for comfort to address breast tenderness, which may include using supportive cushions. Refer to the Evolve site for more information on addressing fibrocystic breast changes with massage.

Mastitis. Mastitis is inflammation of the breast; usually only one breast is affected. Most cases of mastitis are associated with lactation (breast-feeding) and are most often found during the first 2 to 3 weeks (but the condition can occur anytime). Infection usually enters through a skin laceration acquired during infant sucking. The breast is swollen and the skin is red and warm to the touch.

There is a painful, localized mass accompanied by enlarged axillary lymph nodes, and the person may have a fever.

If your client has a fever, postpone massage until she has been fever-free for 48 hours. Otherwise, massage can be performed, while avoiding her upper body until signs of localized infection have resolved (heat, redness, pain, swelling).

Pregnancy Pathologies

Pregnancy is discussed as a special population in Chapter 11.

Abortion. Abortion is the premature termination of pregnancy. Miscellaneous signs and symptoms are severe abdominopelvic and lower back pain, cramping, and vaginal bleeding. There are three types of abortion:

- Spontaneous abortion: Also called a miscarriage, the involuntary termination of pregnancy up to 20 weeks gestation or below a fetal weight of 500 g. About 20% of all pregnancies terminate in spontaneous abortion.
- Therapeutic abortion: Pregnancy is terminated because its progression is harmful to the women's health (e.g., ectopic pregnancy).
- Elective abortion: The woman does not wish to be pregnant.

Massage is contraindicated with the presence of any symptoms of miscarriage. Afterward, avoid the abdomen if pressure causes pain. Be prepared to emotionally support your client as she may be grieving.

Preeclampsia and Eclampsia. Preeclampsia is a state of persistent elevated blood pressure (typically 140/90 mm Hg on two or more occasions) with protein in the urine. It most often develops in the last half of pregnancy and resolves after delivery. Generalized edema is common. Pitting edema may occur in the legs. If left uncontrolled, preeclampsia can lead to damaged retinal or renal blood vessels, as well as compromised fetal blood flow, liver abnormalities, bleeding disorders, and seizures (eclampsia). Preeclampsia is also called pregnancy-induced hypertension or toxemia.

Eclampsia is a severe form of preeclampsia that involves seizures. It is extremely rare (less than 1% of all pregnancies). If eclampsia is allowed to progress, possible consequences may include placental abruption, pulmonary edema, and maternal and fetal death.

Massage is postponed until the condition has been resolved or the child is born, and the mother has fully recovered.

Gestational Diabetes Mellitus. Gestational diabetes mellitus (GDM) is a form of glucose intolerance that develops in some women during pregnancy. It is most often diagnosed during the second trimester. Hormones produced by the placenta may block insulin's action, causing GDM. Some women are asymptomatic, whereas others demonstrate the cardinal signs of diabetes mellitus: excessive urination, excessive thirst, and excessive hunger. Insulin injections are often required.

Avoid vigorous massage over sites of recent injection for 24 hours. Suggest that the client eat a meal within 2 to 3 hours or have a good snack no more than 1 hour before the massage to help prevent a drop in blood sugar. Ask her if she carries glucose tablets or gel and, if so, where they are in case they are needed quickly during a hypoglycemic episode (see Chapter 9 for more information).

Sexually Transmitted Infections

Chlamydia. Chlamydia is a bacterial infection of the urogenital tract. It is the most common sexually transmitted bacterial infection in the United States and is called the silent sexually transmitted infection (STI) because symptoms may be slow to develop or absent and transmission can occur without the person's knowledge (25% of men and 30% of women never develop symptoms). When signs and symptoms do occur, they include vaginal discharge, localized burning, and itching in women and penile discharge and painful urination, as well as localized burning and itching, in men.

Postpone massage until after your client has completed antibiotic therapy.

Gonorrhea. Gonorrhea is a bacterial infection of the urogenital tract, but it also can involve the pharynx, eyes, and rectum. Transmission occurs through sexual activity (genital, oral, anal) or from an infected pregnant woman to her baby during vaginal delivery. Men exhibit signs and symptoms more frequently than women; these include penile discharge with frequent and painful urination. In women, manifestations include thick vaginal discharge with localized burning and itching. Both men and women may be asymptomatic.

Postpone massage until after your client has completed antibiotic therapy.

Syphilis. Syphilis is a systemic bacterial infection. It is most often transmitted by contact with infected body fluids (semen, vaginal secretions, blood) or by contact with an active lesion through broken skin. It can also spread through the transplacental route while the infected mother is pregnant. The main sign in primary stages is the formation of a painless, highly contagious skin lesion called a *chancre*. It forms at the site of bacterial invasion (usually the male or female genitalia) about 3 weeks after exposure, and then disappears in a few weeks.

Postpone massage until after your client has completed antibiotic therapy.

Genital Herpes. Genital herpes is a viral infection that features painful itchy skin lesions in the genital area. These lesions may also occur on the buttocks or inner thighs and even the mouth area. Genital herpes is a chronic and incurable disease with cycles of flare-ups (called *outbreaks*) and remissions. Outbreaks occur on the average of 5 to 8 times per year, but may be as frequent as every month or as rare as every few years.

Postpone massage if your client has a fever. Massage can be performed after he or she has been fever-free for at least 48 hours. As we do not massage genitals, massage can be performed on clients with genital herpes while avoiding skin lesions and the buttocks or medial thighs (lesions may be present in these areas). Because the virus may be shed during active and inactive periods, treat the massage linens as infectious.

Genital Warts. Genital warts are soft, skin-colored single or clustered growths and are most often located on the genitalia, perineal, and perianal areas. They can develop in the mouth or throat of a person who has had orogenital contact with an infected person. Most genital warts are painless, but they may cause discomfort depending on their size, number, and location.

As we do not massage genitals, there are no special massage considerations for a client with genital warts. Treat massage linens as infectious.

SPOTLIGHT ON RESEARCH

Research suggests that massage therapy may:
- Improve mood, and decrease anxiety, pain, and water retention in persons with premenstrual syndrome
- Decrease anxiety and reduce obstetric and postnatal complications in women
- Reduce labor pains in pregnant women
- Reduce postpartum depression and promote better parent-child interaction

E-RESOURCES

evolve

http://evolve.elsevier.com/Salvo/MassageTherapy

- Chapter challenge
- Flash cards
- Photo gallery
- Educational animations
- Additional information
- Weblinks

BIBLIOGRAPHY

Abrahams P, Marks S, Hutchings R: *McMinn's color atlas of human anatomy*, St Louis, 2003, Mosby.

Applegate EJ: *The anatomy and physiology learning system*, ed 3, Philadelphia, 2006, Saunders.

Beers MH, Berkow R: *The Merck manual of diagnosis and therapy*, Whitehouse Station, NJ, 2006, Merck Research Laboratories.

Como D, editor: *Mosby's medical, nursing, and allied health dictionary*, ed 6, St Louis, 2002, Mosby.

Crawley J, Van De Graaff KM: *A photographic atlas for anatomy and physiology*, Englewood, Colo, 2002, Morton.

Damjanov I: *Pathophysiology for the health-related professions*, ed 3, Philadelphia, 2006, Saunders.

Ferri FF: *2003 Ferri's clinical advisor, instant diagnosis and treatment*, St Louis, 2003, Mosby.

Frazier MS, Drzymkowski JW: *Essentials of human diseases and conditions*, ed 3, Philadelphia, 2004, Saunders.

Fritz S: *Massage online for essential sciences for therapeutic massage*, ed 3, St Louis, 2010, Mosby.

Gould BE: *Pathophysiology for the health professions*, ed 3, Philadelphia, 2006, Saunders.

Gray H, Pick TP, Howden R: *Gray's anatomy*, ed 29, Philadelphia, 1974, Running Press.

Haubrich WS: *Medical meanings: a glossary of word origins*, New York, 1984, Harcourt Brace Jovanovich.

Huether SE, McCance KL: *Understanding pathophysiology*, ed 3, St Louis, 2004, Mosby.

Jacob S, Francone C: *Elements of anatomy and physiology*, Philadelphia, 1989, WB Saunders.

Kapit W, Elson LM: *The anatomy coloring book*, ed 3, New York, 2002, Benjamin Cummings.

Kordish M, Dickson S: *Introduction to basic human anatomy*, Lake Charles, La, 1995, McNeese State University Press.

Kumar V, Abbas A, Fausto N: *Robbins and Cotran physiologic basis of disease*, ed 7, St Louis, 2005, Mosby.

Marieb EN: *Essentials of human anatomy and physiology*, ed 8, New York, 2005, Benjamin Cummings.

Marieb EN: *Human anatomy and physiology*, ed 7, New York, 2000, Benjamin Cummings.

Martini FH, Bartholomew EF: *Essentials of anatomy and physiology*, ed 3, New York, 2003, Benjamin Cummings.

McAleer N: *The body almanac*, Garden City, NY, 1985, Doubleday.

McCance K, Huether S: *Pathophysiology: the biological basis for disease in adults and children*, St Louis, 2006, Mosby.

Merck manual, ed 17, Whitehouse Station, NJ, 1998, Merck and Co.

Moore KL: *Clinically oriented anatomy*, ed 5, Baltimore, 2005, Lippincott Williams & Wilkins.

Netter FH: *Atlas of human anatomy*, ed 3, Teterboro, NJ, 2003, Icon Learning Systems.

Newton D: *Pathology for massage therapists*, ed 2, Portland, Ore, 1995, Simran.

Premkumar K: *Pathology A to Z, a handbook for massage therapists*, Baltimore, 1999, Lippincott Williams & Wilkins.

Salvo SG: *Mosby's pathology for massage therapists*, ed 2, St Louis, 2009, Mosby.

Solomon EP, Phillips GA: *Understanding human anatomy and physiology*, Philadelphia, 1987, Saunders.

Thibodeau G, Patton K: *Anatomy and physiology*, ed 6, St Louis, 2006, Mosby.

Thibodeau G, Patton K: *Structure and function of the body*, ed 12, St Louis, 2004, Mosby.

Tortora GJ: *Introduction to the human body: the essentials of anatomy and physiology*, ed 5, Hoboken, NJ, 2000, John Wiley & Sons.

Tortora GJ, Grabowksi SR: *Principles of anatomy and physiology*, ed 11, New York, 2005, John Wiley & Sons.

MATCHING I

Place the letter of the answer next to the term or phrase that best describes it.

A. Epididymis
B. Gametes
C. Gonads
D. Interstitial cells of Leydig

E. Penis
F. Prostate
G. Scrotum
H. Semen

I. Sexual reproduction
J. Spermatozoon
K. Testes
L. Urethra

_____ 1. Male and female sex cells

_____ 2. Process of uniting male and female sex cells to produce offspring

_____ 3. Cells within the testes that produce testosterone

_____ 4. Structure that deposits semen out of the body during ejaculation

_____ 5. Paired oval glands within the scrotum

_____ 6. Convoluted and tightly coiled portion of the spermatic duct that houses sperm during final maturation

_____ 7. Male sex cells that carry genetic information from the man who produces them

_____ 8. Pouch that supports the testes

_____ 9. Passageway for semen and urine in males

_____ 10. General term to denote the testes in men and ovaries in women

_____ 11. Gland that secretes approximately 25% of semen volume and prevents the flow of urine during ejaculation

_____ 12. Thick, milky fluid that is a mixture of sperm and seminal fluid

MATCHING II

Place the letter of the answer next to the term or phrase that best describes it.

A. Cervix
B. Fallopian tubes
C. Follicular phase
D. Luteal phase

E. Menopause
F. Menstrual cycle
G. Menstruation
H. Oocytes

I. Ovaries
J. Ovulation
K. Uterus
L. Vagina

_____ 1. Cessation of ovarian hormone function and menstruation in the females

_____ 2. Canal that extends from the female cervix to the outside of the body

_____ 3. Paired almond-shaped glands located lateral the uterus

_____ 4. Periodic discharge of endometrial tissue from the non-pregnant uterus

_____ 5. Series of events in which the uterine lining sheds, then re-grows, proliferates, is maintained for several days, then sheds again at menstruation

_____ 6. Female sex cells that carry genetic information from the woman who produced them

_____ 7. Hollow organ in which a fertilized ovum implants and a fetus develops and from which menses flow

_____ 8. Lower, narrow portion of the uterus that opens into the vagina

_____ 9. Menstrual cycle phase in which the uterine lining is maintained and the uterus relaxes to facilitate possible implantation and pregnancy

_____ 10. Tubes that serve as passages for ova traveling toward the uterus

_____ 11. Menstrual cycle phase characterized by the releases of a mature oocyte

_____ 12. Menstrual cycle phase in which the uterine lining becomes thick and vascular in anticipation of a fertilized ovum

CASE STUDY

A Personal Matter

Melinda is a healthy, 24-year-old athlete. She initially came seeking treatment for lower back pain that likely developed as a result of compensating patterns following a knee injury. Paul, her massage therapist, was able to relieve Melinda's symptoms, allowing her to get back to her normal activities, and she has continued to see him for maintenance related to the injury and general relaxation ever since. In fact, Melinda was so impressed and grateful for Paul's skill that she single-handedly increased his client list by 10%. Melinda knows a lot of people!

Today Melinda explained that she felt like she needed a full-body massage. She hasn't felt any back or knee pain since their last session 3 weeks ago. She stated that she has been feeling tired for the past few days, and has had general body aches. She joked that it was probably because she recently began dating a new fellow, who she really likes, and they'd been going out a lot. He could be the one!

Paul noticed that she squirmed in her chair, seemingly unable to find a comfortable position. When she finished her paperwork, Paul asked if she wanted to use the bathroom before they began. "NO!" she yelped, as if the question frightened her. She apologized for the outburst and explained that she'd been drinking less water because urinating is uncomfortable. She said that she thought she might have a yeast infection, and would see her doctor tomorrow if the symptoms didn't go away.

Paul entered the room when Melinda was ready and began warming her tissues through the sheets. When he laid his hands on her bare skin, he noticed that she felt warm. He asked if she'd had a fever, and she said she didn't think so, but that she often feels warm when she is overly tired. She squirmed a bit on the table, and adjusted her underwear. At that point, Paul began to wonder if the symptoms Melinda suspected were a yeast infection might actually be an initial outbreak of herpes.

As a professional, how should Paul proceed with this session?

Would suggesting the possibility of herpes violate Melinda's privacy?

Would discussing herpes with Melinda constitute an action outside of Paul's scope of practice?

If he decides to discuss his concern with Melinda, how can he approach this sensitive issue?

If Melinda denies the possibility of having herpes, but Paul is still concerned, what should he do?

CRITICAL THINKING

Is it appropriate to ask a client who has genital herpes or genital warts to leave undergarments on (if they are worn)? What do you think and why?

CHAPTER 26

Cardiovascular System

"Be a lamp, a lifeboat, or a ladder."

—Rumi

LEARNING OBJECTIVES

After completing this chapter, the student should be able to:

- List basic anatomy and describe the physiology of the cardiovascular system.
- Describe the blood's characteristics, components (plasma and blood cells), and blood types.
- Discuss the layers within the heart's wall, its chambers, valves, and coronary vessels.
- Trace the flow of blood through the heart.
- Discuss the heart's conduction system, defining important terms.
- Explain how the sounds of the heart are produced.
- List types of blood vessels, identifying characteristics of each.
- Name major arteries and veins.
- Discuss blood pressure.
- Describe the primary paths of blood circulation.
- Name cardiovascular pathologies and state appropriate massage modifications.

INTRODUCTION

The body is 60% to 80% fluid (by volume). This fluid requires circulation to maintain the body's health. The cardiovascular system and the lymphatic system are responsible for fluid movement and health maintenance. Both systems are regarded as *pick-up and delivery* systems because their primary function is transportation. The cardiovascular system consists of the blood, heart, and blood vessels. The heart pumps oxygen and nutrient-rich blood through arteries and arterioles. Oxygen and nutrients in the blood leave small capillaries and enter body tissues. Carbon dioxide and metabolic wastes leave tissues and enter the capillaries. Oxygen depleted blood travels through venules and veins on their way to the lungs, liver, and kidneys. The lungs eliminate carbon dioxide during exhalation; the liver and kidneys either alter or eliminate other wastes.

ANATOMY

Basic anatomy of the cardiovascular system is:
- Blood
- Blood vessels such as arteries, veins, and capillaries
- Heart

PHYSIOLOGY

The functions of the cardiovascular system are:
- **Transportation.** Substances that are transported include respiratory gases, nutrients from the digestive tract, antibodies, waste materials, and hormones from endocrine glands, as well as transportation of heat from active muscles to the skin, where the heat can be dissipated.
- **Protection.** The body is protected through disease-fighting white blood cells and the removal of impurities and pathogens.
- **Combat hemorrhage.** This is accomplished by clotting mechanisms, which prevent the loss of body fluids from damaged vessels.

BLOOD

Blood transports nutrients to, and waste products from, individual cells. **Blood** is a fluid medium containing formed elements and liquid plasma. Formed elements are erythrocytes (red blood cells), leukocytes (white blood cells), and thrombocytes (platelets) (Figure 26-1). Blood is classified as a liquid connective tissue and is essential for human life because tissues can get oxygen and nutrients only from its blood supply. Under normal circumstances, a blood cell makes a round trip through the circulatory system every 60 seconds.

Blood makes up approximately 8% of total body weight (Figure 26-2). Blood volume in the average-size person is approximately 5 L, which equals 6 quarts or 12 pints. In an

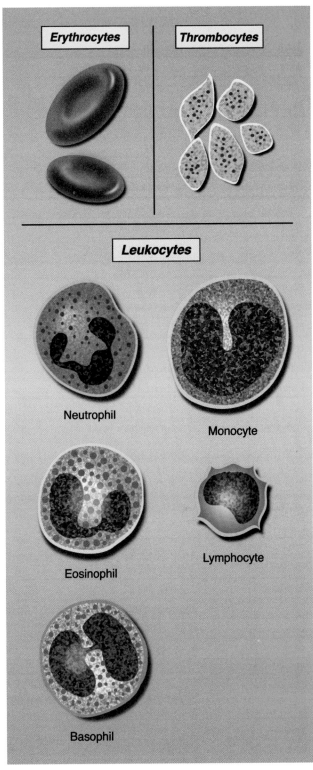

FIGURE 26-1 Types of blood cells.

adult, blood cells form mainly in red bone marrow. The process of blood cell development is called *hematopoiesis*.

Blood is a viscous fluid that is thicker and more adhesive than water and its pH is slightly alkaline. The color of blood varies from bright scarlet red to dull maroon, depending on oxygen content. Blood is slightly warmer than normal body

IT'S ALL GREEK TO ME

Term	Meaning
aorta	*Gr.* a strap; to suspend
atrium	*L.* corridor
bicuspid	*L.* two; pointed
brady	*Gr.* slow
capillary	*L.* hairlike
cardio, cardia	*Gr.* heart
chordae tendineae	*Gr.* cordlike; *L.* tendon
coagulation	*L.* to curdle
coronary	*L.* shaped like a crown or circle
cyanosis	*Gr.* dark blue; condition
diastole	*Gr.* to expand
edema	*Gr.* swelling
erythrocyte	*Gr.* red; cell
fibrinogen	*L.* fiber; *Gr.* to produce
hemoglobin	*Gr.* blood; *L.* globe
hemorrhage	*Gr.* blood; to burst forth
hemostasis	*Gr.* blood; stopping
intima	*L.* innermost
ischemia	*Gr.* to hold back blood
leukocytes	*Gr.* white; cell
lumen	*L.* light
mitral	*L.* headdress
plasma	*Gr.* a thing formed
platelet	*Fr.* flat
Purkinje fibers	Purkyně, Czech anatomist (1787-1869)
saphenous	*Gr.* the hidden
semilunar	*L.* half; moon
sphygmomanometer	*Gr.* pulse; thin; measure
systole	*Gr.* contraction
tachy	*Gr.* rapid, fast, or swift
thrombocyte	*Gr.* clot; cell
tricuspid	*Gr.* three; *L.* pointed
tunica	*L.* a tunic
vascular	*L.* a vessel or duct
vasoconstriction	*L.* vessel; a binder
vasodilation	*L.* vessel; to widen
vena cava	*L.* vein; cavity
ventricle	*L.* little belly

Fr., French; *Gr.*, Greek; *L.*, Latin.

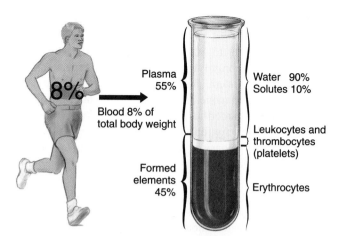

FIGURE 26-2 Composition of blood.

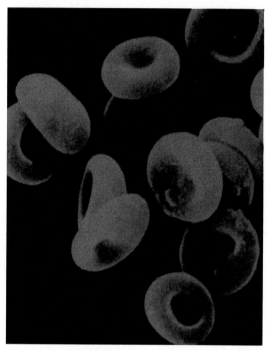

FIGURE 26-3 Erythrocytes.

temperature (approximately 100° F). Whole blood is blood from which no constituents have been removed. This includes red blood cells, white blood cells, platelets, or plasma.

Components of Blood

Erythrocytes. Erythrocytes, also known as red blood cells (RBCs) or red corpuscles, make up more than 90% of blood cells. The primary function of **erythrocytes** is to transport oxygen to cells. RBCs do not have a nucleus, which keeps these cells from reproducing or carrying out extensive metabolic activities (Figure 26-3). The life span of an erythrocyte is approximately 120 days, after which it begins to fragment, and the remains are eliminated by the spleen and liver.

Erythrocytes are biconcave (with raised edges and a flattened middle) to allow greater surface area for more efficient diffusion of oxygen and for movement ease through tiny capillaries (minute blood vessels).

Erythrocytes are occupied by a pigment called **hemoglobin**, giving blood its characteristic red color. Hemoglobin, an iron-based protein, combines temporarily with oxygen and carbon dioxide so that these gases can be transported and then released. Hemoglobin carries oxygen or carbon dioxide, but not both, at any given time. Special proteins on the surfaces of RBCs determine the different blood types (A, B, AB, or O). See next section for more information.

Leukocytes. **Leukocytes,** also known as white blood cells (WBCs) or white corpuscles, serve as part of the body's immune system by protecting the body from invading pathogens and by removing dead cells and substances. Whenever WBCs mobilize for action, the body doubles their production within a short time. Think of these cells as the blood's defensive mobile army. WBCs begin to mobilize and destroy invaders using *phagocytosis* and *pinocytosis* (see Chapter 18). The life span of WBCs ranges from a few hours to a few days to several years.

Types of leukocytes include neutrophils, eosinophils, basophils, monocytes, and lymphocytes (see Figure 26-1). Some WBCs combat irritants by producing *histamine*, a compound released in allergic, inflammatory reactions that, in extreme cases, causes dilation of capillaries, decreased blood pressure, and constriction of smooth muscles of the bronchi. Other WBCs produce antibodies. Antibodies are produced in response to specific foreign substances such as bacteria, viruses, or cells of an incompatible blood type.

Thrombocytes. Also known as *platelets*, **thrombocytes** are fragmented cells that are important in blood clotting or coagulation. Their jagged shape helps them adhere to torn surfaces easily, such as occurs in a damaged blood vessel. The life span of a thrombocyte is approximately 10 days.

The clotting process starts when a vessel is damaged and it takes only a few minutes to form a blood clot. *Coagulation*, or clot formation, is the process of transforming fibrinogen in plasma into fibrin threads that trap red blood cells and then tighten into a clot (Figure 26-4). Calcium and vitamin K are also needed during this process. Once a clot is formed, it goes through a process of retraction (tightening) that draws the injured area of the vessel wall closer together for repair, and then reduces and stops blood loss. At the time a clot is formed, an enzyme is formed, which has the ability to slowly dissolve the clot over time when healing is complete.

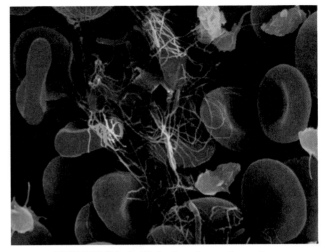

FIGURE 26-4 Fibrin threads creating a clot.

To review blood cells:
- Erythrocytes (RBCs) transport oxygen and carbon dioxide.
- Leukocytes (WBCs) fight disease (the body's mobile army).
- Thrombocytes (platelets) clot blood.

---

evolve *Log on to the Evolve website to access a visual representation of blood clotting mechanisms. Be sure to reread the explanation above to review the main processes involved in both the blood and the blood vessel.* ∎

Plasma. **Plasma** is a straw-colored liquid that helps transport blood cells. Approximately 55% of blood is plasma, but plasma itself is 90% water and 10% solutes (chemicals such as sodium, potassium, and chloride dissolved in a solution). One substance, *fibrinogen*, functions in blood clotting. When necessary, fibrinogen is converted to *fibrin* to begin the process of blood clotting. Fibrin forms a network of fibers; this fibrous mesh traps red blood cells, platelets, and fluid (see Figure 26-4). The mesh then contracts to form a clot, which seals the damaged blood vessel. Other solutes include plasma proteins, hormones, enzymes, and wastes.

TABLE 26-1 ABO Blood Groups

| | | | PEOPLE WITH THIS BLOOD TYPE | |
BLOOD TYPE	ANTIGEN (RBC MEMBRANE)	ANTIBODY (PLASMA)	CAN RECEIVE BLOOD FROM	CAN DONATE BLOOD TO
A (40%)	A antigen	Anti-B antibodies	A, O	A, AB
B (10%)	B antigen	Anti-A antibodies	B, O	B, AB
AB* (4%)	A antigen / B antigen	No antibodies	A, B, AB, O	AB
O† (46%)	No antigen	Both anti-A and anti-B antibodies	O	O, A, B, AB

*Type AB blood characterizes the universal recipient.
†Type O blood characterizes the universal donor.

Blood Types

The most common blood typing system is the ABO system, which uses the absence or presence of proteins to classify blood groups. The surfaces of RBCs contain genetically determined proteins called *antigens*. Two blood antigens are A and B. Additionally, blood plasma contains the antibody against the antigen not present on the RBC.

- **Type A.** Presence of antigen A; antibodies against antigen B
- **Type B.** Presence of antigen B; antibodies against antigen A
- **Type AB.** Presence of antigens A and B; no antibodies
- **Type O.** Absence of both antigens; presence of antibodies against both antigens A and B (Table 26-1)

When a foreign red blood cell is introduced to the body, its corresponding antibody recognizes it as being nonself and attacks it. This invasion may occur in blood transfusion if the body is given the wrong blood type. If a person with type A blood is given type B or type AB blood, then the recipient's body recognizes the type B antigens as a foreign protein, attacks it, clumps them together, and slices them open. Widespread inflammatory response occurs, and the iron released from the sliced open hemoglobin can cause organ failure. Blood transfusions must be made using compatible blood types because mismatching can cause severe medical problems or death.

Because type AB has no antibodies, a person with this blood type can receive all other blood types and is referred to as a **universal recipient**.

Because Type O has no antigens and does not react to any other blood types, a person with this blood type is referred to as a **universal donor**.

Rh Factor. The Rh factor is an antigenic substance present in erythrocytes of 85% of the population. A person who has the Rh factor is Rh positive (Rh^+) and a person lacking Rh factor is Rh negative (Rh^-). If a person who is Rh^- receives blood that is Rh^+, antibodies attack the foreign antigen. Rh^+ infants may be exposed to antibodies to the factor produced in the Rh^- mother's blood, resulting in the destruction of RBCs in the infant's blood. Because of medical advances, this situation is now rarely life-threatening for the infant. Rh factor was first identified in the blood of a rhesus (Rh) monkey.

HEART

The **heart** is a hollow, muscular organ about the size of a clenched fist. It is located in the mediastinum (space between

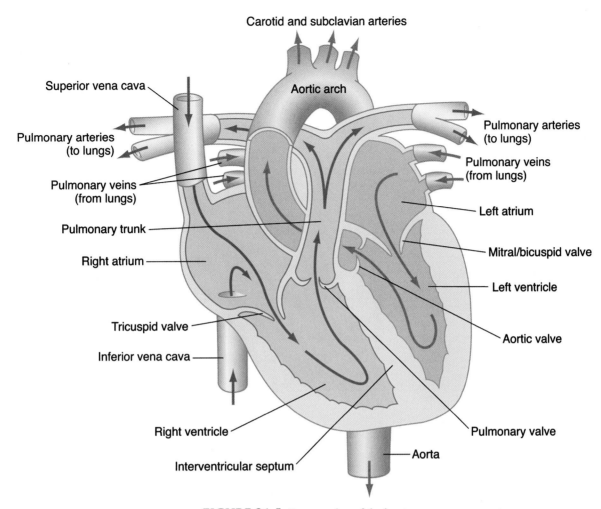

FIGURE 26-5 Cross section of the heart.

the lungs and behind the sternum). The pericardium surrounds the heart and secretes a lubricating fluid that prevents friction. The heart wall has three layers: the myocardium, epicardium, and endocardium. Four hollow chambers are present within the heart: two atria (superior chambers) and two ventricles (inferior chambers). A partition called a septum separates the ventricles and extends up between the atria (Figure 26-5).

The two sides of the heart (left and right) function as a double pump: The right side pumps oxygen-depleted blood to the lungs, whereas the left side pumps oxygen-rich blood out to the rest of the body. Pumping blood is the heart's primary function. Heart valves open and shut to keep blood on its course. A healthy heart continually pumps blood for an average of 72 beats per minute in a resting person.

Heart Wall

As stated previously, surrounding the heart is a double-layered sac called the *pericardium*. Serous fluid is found between the outer parietal layer and the inner visceral layer. This fluid functions to decrease friction as the heart beats.

The heart wall possesses the following three layers: (1) epicardium, (2) myocardium, and (3) endocardium (Figure 26-6). The *epicardium* is a thin outer connective tissue layer. This protective layer possesses adipose tissue and the blood vessels that nourish the heart (coronary vessels). The *myocardium* is the thick muscular layer that makes up the bulk of the heart wall. Contraction of the myocardium forces blood out of the ventricles (see Chapter 11 for a discussion of cardiac muscle). The *endocardium* is the thin, inner lining and is continuous with the endothelial lining of the heart chambers and blood vessels, as well as the valves of the heart.

"Hippocrates had no means of recognizing the heart as a pump, because there was no such item in his world, and no such word in his vocabulary."
—Guido Majno, MD

Heart Chambers

The heart is subdivided into four chambers that receive and pump blood. The superior chambers are called the right and

JOHN F. BARNES, PT, LMT, NCTMB

Born: February 3, 1939

"The master therapist is real, calm, nonjudgmental, intelligent, sensitive, strong yet flexible, supportive, compassionate, empathic, and joyful."

One of the major differences between *myofascial release* and many other forms of bodywork is that, at its best, it allows the therapist to bring more to the table. It is systematic, physiologically grounded, and intuitive without apology. John F. Barnes, PT, LMT, developer of the John F. Barnes Myofascial Release Approach, is a physical therapist and teacher of the highest caliber who values a wide range of modalities such as the work of Ida Rolf, Milton Trager, John Upledger, and Paul St. John.

Barnes's father died when he was 3 years of age, and he was raised by his mother. He remembers enjoying being alone in the forest and learning to be so quiet that the wildlife would venture out. He studied karate and learned about the role of *Qi*. As a junior in high school, Barnes knew he wanted to be a physical therapist. He graduated from the University of Pennsylvania as a Physical Therapist in 1960 and is licensed in Pennsylvania, Arizona, New Jersey, Delaware, Colorado and Hawaii.

With warm eyes, a burly build, and a full beard, Barnes resembles those who live in a log cabin and love nature—and he does. He as been called an old soul and does not scoff at the label. He does not believe in assembly-line quick fixes. How could he? He knows how insidious pain can be.

As a teen, Barnes was lifting weights and could not recover from a deep squat, so he attempted a back roll and landed on his tailbone with an extra 300 pounds to boot. Not long after, his back locked up just as he was about to kiss a girl. He did not pay much attention to his condition; he was young and charged on, until a skiing accident left him in worse condition. Surgery helped, but the pain left an indelible scar.

Robert Calvert, founder of *Massage Magazine*, quotes Barnes as saying, "I don't really mean this should happen, but in a way, every physician or therapist should be severely injured, and not just hurt for a week or two or a month, but a couple years. It's a whole different story when you are a prisoner in your own body. I felt broken, and I was broken. It was a horrible, horrible experience."

---

left **atria** (*singular*, atrium) and take in blood through large veins and then pump it to the inferior chambers. Atria are separated by the *interatrial septum*.

The lower chambers, or right and left **ventricles**, pump blood to the body's organs and tissues. Thick ventricular walls are separated by the *interventricular septum*.

Heart Valves

Heart valves are flaps of endothelium located between the chambers of the heart and between the ventricles and some of the great vessels (see Blood Vessels, next section). These valves regulate blood flow through the heart and keep blood moving in one direction. These valves include the atrioventricular and the semilunar valves.

The *atrioventricular valves*, or AV valves, allow blood to flow into the ventricles (Figure 26-7). The **bicuspid** or **mitral valve** (left atrioventricular valve) is located between the left atrium and the left ventricle. The **tricuspid valve** (right atrioventricular valve) is located between the right atrium and the right ventricle. As their names imply, the bicuspid (mitral) valve has two flaps or cusps, and the tricuspid valve has three. These valves are held in place by tendonlike cords called *chordae tendineae*, which attach to the heart wall by *papillary muscles*.

The *semilunar valves* allow blood to flow out of the ventricles into the aorta and pulmonary trunk. The **aortic valve** (left semilunar valve) is located between the left ventricle and the aorta. The **pulmonary valve** (right semilunar valve) is located between the pulmonary trunk and the right ventricle. As the name suggests, each semilunar valve consists of half moon-shaped cusps, named for the vessels to which they lead.

Heart Sounds. Closure of the valves produces the two characteristic sounds of the heart beat: "lubb-dubb." The

JOHN F. BARNES, PT, LMT, NCTMB (*continued*)

Yet another injury led Barnes to explore alternative therapies. He began to blend experience with principles from different disciplines and discovered how fascia and energy flow are connected. Myofascial release is based on understanding the role of fascia, a web of interconnected tissue that travels the body without interruption. It surrounds individual cells, organs, and systems and then wraps it up in one huge package, head to toe. This network is the communication medium from cell to cell and organ to organ. Trauma, surgery, or inflammation can change the consistency of the web, solidifying and shortening fibers and blocking the flow of messages that are necessary for homeostasis. This web, if pulled too tightly in one place, can leave other areas restricted, creating crushing pressure on nerves, muscles, organs, and bones.

As a physical therapist and massage therapist, Barnes's style had always been focused, slow, and rhythmic. He did not know he was treating the fascial system, per se, until he attended a physicians' course on connective tissue. He then began to see and treat the interrelationship of the whole body—including the mind or spirit—rather than isolated areas or conditions. This shift in thinking enhanced the results of his work and stirred up emotions.. As his work evolved, so did Barnes.

Barnes started teaching other people his form of bodywork in the mid-1970s. His teaching begins by reawakening the therapist's ability to *feel* what is happening with the body. Then he teaches the techniques to evaluate and release restricted areas in a systematic way.

Even with such a systematic and comprehensive approach, Barnes is realistic about results. Therapists do not *fix* clients; they offer tools for change in the form of bodywork and also in *mindwork*. When you get down to it, therapists cannot help clients unless they are ready to help themselves. Barnes's advice for new massage therapists is to continue learning advanced methods after graduation. Simply reading about a bodywork concept or a basic introduction to a modality is insufficient to practice it successfully and, in some cases, may lead to bad habits or faulty techniques. Barnes suggests learning as many forms of bodywork as possible to adapt to the wide range of client needs.

John F. Barnes lectures internationally, presenting the "John F. Barnes Myofascial Release Approach" seminar series and "Advances in Spinal Diagnosis and Treatment for the 21st Century," for the American Back Society's symposiums. He has written two books: *Myofascial Release: The Search for Excellence* and *Healing Ancient Wounds: The Renegade's Wisdom* as well as numerous articles. Massage Magazine also named him one of the most influential persons in the therapeutic profession in the last century. John F. Barnes is president of the Myofascial Release Treatment Center in Paoli, PA and Therapy on the Rocks in Sedona, AZ.

---

first low-pitched "lubb" sound is generated by the turbulence of blood when the AV valves (mitral and tricuspid) close. The second higher-pitched "dubb" sound is caused by the turbulence of blood when the semilunar valves (aortic and pulmonary semilunar) close. Extra sounds such as those resulting from faulty valves are referred to as *murmurs*. Heart sounds can be heard through a stethoscope.

Coronary Vessels

The heart has its own blood supply provided by the coronary vessels. These vessels lie in grooves between the atria and ventricles and between the two ventricles. Coronary arteries originate at the base of the aorta and supply oxygenated blood to the myocardium. Coronary veins return blood to the right atrium through the coronary sinus. If any coronary artery is unable to supply sufficient blood to the myocardium, a myocardial infarction (heart attack) can result. See the Cardiovascular Pathologies section for more information.

Blood Flow Through the Heart

Blood moves into and out of the heart in three well-coordinated and timed stages.

During *stage I*, oxygen-depleted blood enters the superior and inferior vena cava and flows into the right atrium. When the right atrium is full, it empties through the tricuspid valve into the right ventricle.

During *stage II*, the right ventricle contracts and pushes blood through the pulmonary valve into the pulmonary trunk. The pulmonary trunk then divides into the left and right pulmonary arteries, which take blood to each lung (these are the only arteries in the body that carry deoxygenated blood). Four pulmonary veins leave the lungs and carry oxygen-rich blood back to the left atrium (these are the only veins in the body that carry oxygenated blood).

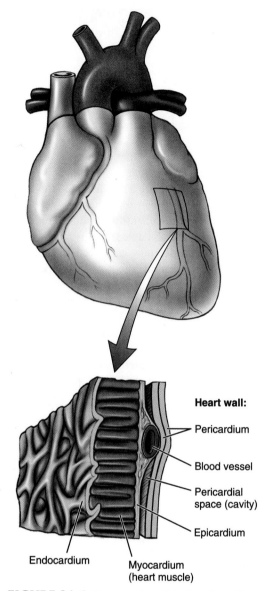

Heart wall:

Pericardium

Blood vessel

Pericardial space (cavity)

Epicardium

Endocardium

Myocardium (heart muscle)

FIGURE 26-6 Cross section of the heart's wall.

Blood leaves the left atrium and passes through to the left ventricle through the mitral valve during *stage III*. The left ventricle contracts and pushes blood through the aortic valve into the aorta and descending aorta and to all parts of the body except the lungs.

Stage I and stage III occur at the same time.

Heart's Conduction System

The coordinated rhythm of the heart's beat is controlled by an intrinsic electrical system. This conduction system initiates and moves impulses through the myocardium. The heart also has the ability to generate its own independent muscle contraction without outside innervation. This is called autorhythmicity. The conduction system includes the *sinoatrial node* (SA node) and the *atrioventricular node* (AV

node), the *atrioventricular bundle* (AV bundle or bundle of His), and the *Purkinje fibers* (Figure 26-8).

The SA node lies on the posterior wall of the right atrium and initiates the cardiac impulse, stimulating both the right and left atria to contract simultaneously. This pushes blood into the ventricles. The SA node fires an impulse 60 to 100 times a minute. Because the firing of the SA node sets the rate at which the heart beats, it is called the *pacemaker*.

The impulse from the SA node then travels to the AV node, then down through the AV bundle (located in the interventricular septum), and then around to the Purkinje fibers (located along the side of the ventricles). This pathway allows both ventricles to contract simultaneously, ejecting blood into the pulmonary trunk and the aorta.

To review:
- The SA node fires, causing the atria to contract and fill the ventricles with blood.
- The signal then travels to the AV node—
  - Then to the AV bundle
  - Then to the Purkinje fibers
- The ventricles contract to eject blood into the arteries.

Heart rhythm can be checked by an *electrocardiogram* (ECG), which monitors the electrical changes in the heart. If difficulties within the SA or AV node develop, physicians can implant a device known as a pacemaker to assist or initiate the signal.

The autonomic nervous system can affect rate of the rhythm and force of contraction through sympathetic and parasympathetic activation.

Cardiac Cycle. The cardiac cycle is the sequence of events related to the flow of blood that occurs from the beginning of one heartbeat to the beginning of the next. The cardiac cycle consists of two ventricular phases. The first phase is called systole and the second phase is called diastole.
- During **systole**, the ventricles contract and eject blood.
- During **diastole**, the ventricles relax and fill with blood.

Although the heart does have atrial diastole and systole, the stronger ventricular actions are used for identification of the cardiac cycle.

Heart Rate. Heart rate is the number of cardiac cycles that occur in 1 minute. The average healthy person has a heart rate of 60 to 80 cycles, or beats, per minute.

Stroke Volume. Stroke volume is the amount of blood pumped from the left ventricle with each beat. Stroke volume helps determine cardiac output. Because stroke volume decreases in certain heart conditions and diseases, stroke volume correlates with cardiac function.

Cardiac Output. Cardiac output is the product of stroke volume times the heart rate. Under normal condition, average cardiac output is 5 L of blood. During exercise or times of stress, output may increase to 20 L or more to accommodate the increased need for oxygen.

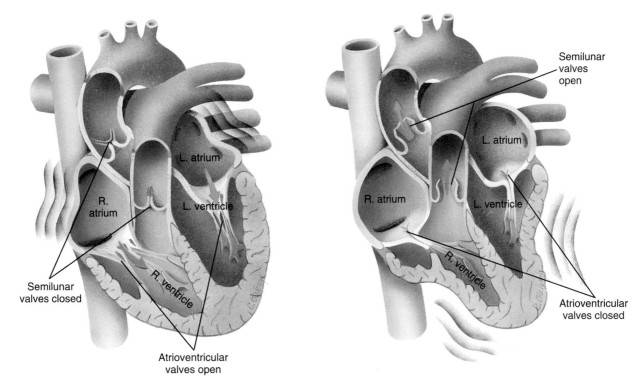

FIGURE 26-7 Heart's chambers and valves during the cardiac cycle. The green arrow represents the flow of oxygenated blood; the yellow arrow represents the flow of deoxygenated blood.

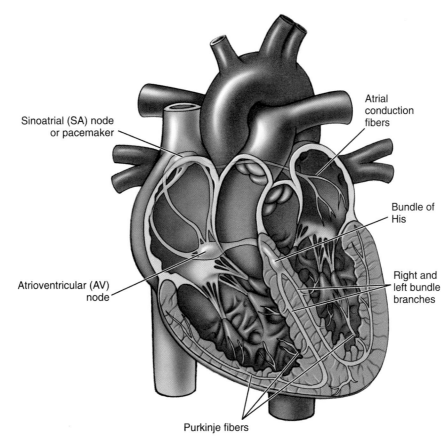

FIGURE 26-8 Heart's conduction system.

"A man is only as old as his arteries."
—Pierre Cabanis, French physician

BLOOD VESSELS

Blood vessels are a closed network of tubes connected to the heart that transport blood to cells of the body. These blood vessels are divided into three main groups based on their structure and function: (1) arteries, (2) veins, and (3) capillaries. These vessels are the body's highway system; they are comparable to hollow streets.

The walls of both arteries and veins possess three layers (tunics). The innermost layer is called the *tunica interna,* which is endothelium fused with a small quantity of elastic connective tissue. The middle layer is the *tunica media,* which contains quantities of both connective tissue and smooth muscle. The outer layer, possessing mostly dense connective tissue, is the *tunica externa* (Figure 26-9). Large blood vessels have their own blood supply called the *vasa vasorum,* which means "vessels of the vessels," and are located in the tunica externa.

The space within arteries and veins can change the diameter. The open space within a tube is called the *lumen.* **Vasodilation** occurs when the lumen enlarges. **Vasoconstriction** occurs when the lumen becomes narrower. Either change can be initiated by (1) *direct nerve stimulation* from the vasomotor center located in the medulla oblongata and (2) *local reflex response* resulting from a stimulus such as pressure (e.g., massage) or temperature (e.g., heat or cold application).

Increased local blood flow is called **hyperemia,** which causes the skin to become reddened and warm. This condition often occurs during massage or heat application. Local abnormal decrease in blood flow is called **ischemia** and is often marked by pain and tissue dysfunction. Ischemia occurs when blood flow is disturbed, such as by blockage or severe, abnormal vasoconstriction.

Arteries

Arteries are vessels that move blood away from the heart. Blood within the arteries is oxygenated. The pulmonary arteries are the only arteries that carries deoxygenated blood from the heart to the lungs. Because arteries are closer to the pumping action of the heart, their walls are considerably thicker and stronger (compared with veins) to withstand higher blood pressure. Arteries continue to branch off into smaller and thinner vessels, becoming **arterioles,** as they lose their two outer layers. When these vessels possess only a single layer, they are called *capillaries.*

CHAT ROOM

A mnemonic device to help you remember that arteries carry blood away from the heart is that both *arteries* and *away* begin with the letter *A.*

Pulse. **Pulse** is the expansion effect that occurs when the left ventricle contracts, producing a wave of blood that surges through and expands arterial walls. This wave can be felt in the arteries located near the surface of the body or where they lie over bone or other firm tissue. Each pulse point is named for the body region in which it is located.

The common pulse points are detailed in the following list (Figure 26-10).
- **Temporal artery:** anterior to the ear; temple region
- **Facial artery:** inferior to the corner of the mouth
- **Common carotid artery:** sides of the throat
- **Axillary artery:** armpit region
- **Brachial artery:** antecubital region
- **Radial artery:** lateral aspect of the wrist
- **Femoral artery:** crease between lower abdomen and upper thigh
- **Popliteal artery:** posterior knee
- **Posterior tibial artery:** behind medial malleolus
- **Dorsalis pedis artery:** anterior medial foot

MINI-LAB

Using the diagram of pulse points, locate these areas on a partner or on yourself. Note that firm pressure must be used to feel the pulse. When feeling the pulse, avoid using your thumb or index finger because each contains its own pulse.

CHAT ROOM

Avoid deep prolonged pressure on the specific pulse location.

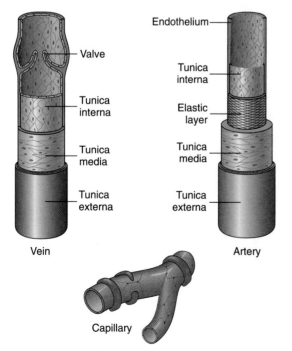

Vein

Endothelium

Valve

Tunica interna

Tunica media

Tunica externa

Tunica interna

Elastic layer

Tunica media

Tunica externa

Artery

Capillary

FIGURE 26-9 Blood vessel wall layers.

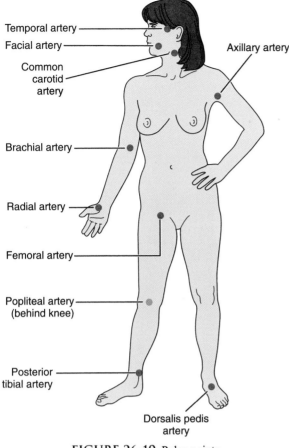

FIGURE 26-10 Pulse points.

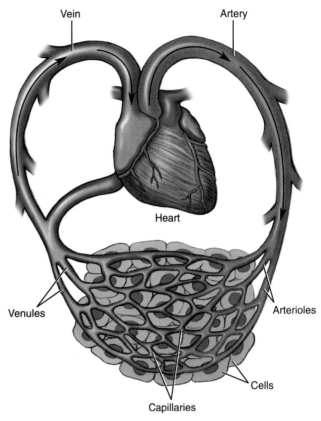

FIGURE 26-11 Blood circulation through arteries, veins, and capillaries.

Capillaries

Capillaries are located between arterioles and venules and have thin, permeable membranes. Capillaries are the functional unit of the cardiovascular system as exchange of gases, nutrients, and wastes occur across its cell walls (see Figure 26-9). Movement of blood in capillaries is the slowest of all the vessels, and its flow is intermittent, which ensures maximum contact time between blood and tissue. Flow of blood through the capillary bed is referred to as the *microcirculation*. The actual exchange of gases at the capillary level is called internal or tissue respiration (see Chapter 28).

Some tissues have a more abundant network of capillaries than others. For example, dense connective tissue such as in ligaments has a poor capillary network compared with heart, kidney, and liver tissue. Areas that are avascular (without blood vessels) are cartilage, epidermis, hair, nails, and lens and cornea of the eye.

Veins

Veins return deoxygenated blood to the heart. Venous walls are thinner (they contain less smooth muscle) and collapse more easily than arteries. Unlike arteries, no pulse is felt in veins. Veins have a large diameter and thus offer less resistance to blood flow (see Figure 26-9). The venous system begins at the capillary level, with vessels that start out small. Smaller veins are called **venules**. These vessels gradually become larger until they reach the heart (Figure 26-11). The pulmonary veins are the only veins that carry oxygenated blood, to the heart from the lungs.

Some veins, especially in the arms and legs, have internal folds in the endothelial lining that function as valves, allowing blood to flow only toward the heart.

CHAT ROOM

The veins are generally located superficially and near the skeletal muscles so that muscular contraction can assist venous blood flow. This is why massage movements are performed centripetally (toward the center; to assist the veins in their function).

Venous Return. Maintaining adequate venous return is vital because cardiac output is influenced by cardiac input (or venous return). Veins return blood to the heart passively and, especially in the lower extremities, the blood is fighting against gravity to return to the heart. This is why elevating the feet increases venous return. Several mechanisms exist to help venous return.

Venomotor Tone – Another mechanism involves venomotor tone. Venomotor tone is the degree of smooth muscle contraction in the venous wall. This mechanism is under

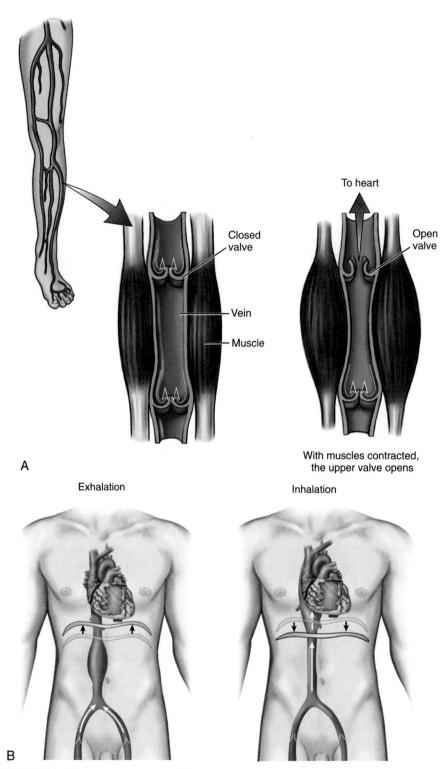

FIGURE 26-12 Venous pump mechanisms. **A,** Skeletal muscle pump. **B,** Respiratory pump.

control of the sympathetic nervous system. Changes in venomotor tone can increase or decrease venous circulation capacity and thus partially compensate for variations in blood volume. A lack of venomotor tone might make you dizzy when sitting or standing up suddenly because blood volume shifts briefly from the head and neck region.

Skeletal Muscle Pump – The skeletal muscle pump occurs when skeletal muscles contract and squeeze venous walls; this moves blood toward the heart (Figure 26-12, *A*). The more frequent and powerful these rhythmic contractions are, the more efficient their action. However, sustained contractions impede blood flow.

Respiratory Pump – The blood in veins flows down a pressure gradient, or from an area of higher pressure to lower pressure. Pressure changes in the thorax and abdomen during breathing also press against venous walls, assisting venous return. This is called the respiratory pump (Figure 26-12, *B*). During inhalation, the thoracic cavity enlarges mainly owing to the lowering of the diaphragm, and the pressure within the veins in the thoracic cavity decreases. The abdominal cavity correspondingly becomes smaller, increasing the pressure within its veins. A pressure gradient has been set up—it is lower in the thoracic cavity and higher in the abdominal cavity. During exhalation, the thoracic cavity becomes smaller and the pressure in its veins decreases; the abdominal cavity becomes larger and the pressure in its veins increases. Venous blood naturally flows from the area of higher pressure to the area of lower pressure, or from the abdominal veins into the thoracic veins.

Naming of Arteries and Veins

Names of most arteries and veins are derived from the structures they lie over or the organs they serve. The *femoral artery* and *vein*, for example, lie over the femur. The *renal artery* and *vein* serve the kidneys. The names of many arteries and veins change as they enter into and pass through certain areas of the body (e.g., the axillary artery becomes the brachial artery as it moves down the arm).

Arteries and veins are found on both sides of the body and are identified as right and left (e.g., right and left common carotid arteries).

Major Arteries

Major arteries are (Figure 26-13):

Brachiocephalic. The brachiocephalic artery becomes the common carotid artery and the subclavian artery.

Subclavian. The subclavian artery, located beneath the clavicle, supplies the upper extremities.

Common carotid. The common carotid arteries, located in the throat, branch to become the external and internal carotid arteries. The common carotid arteries are sites for important pulse points as well as structures avoided during massage. See Chat Room box below.

Axillary. The subclavian artery becomes the axillary artery at the clavicle. The axillary artery has a pulse point.

Brachial. The axillary artery becomes the brachial artery near the head of the humerus. The brachial artery divides at the elbow region into the ulnar and radial arteries. The brachial artery is an important artery for measuring blood pressure and has a pulse point.

CHAT ROOM

Common Carotid Artery

The carotid arteries are located in the throat area just posterolateral to the sternocleidomastoid muscle. Massage to the carotid arteries is avoided for several reasons. (1) If there is any blockage in the artery, massage might dislodge a clot and cause a stroke or other complications. Since the blockage may be undiagnosed, it best to err on the side of caution. (2) Pressure receptors called baroreceptors are located within the carotid sinus (small dilation at the beginning of the internal carotid artery). Massage stimulates the carotid sinus reflex, slows heart rate, and reduces blood pressure. This may be used in certain medical situations (e.g., atrial flutter, atrial tachycardia) by physicians, with ECG monitoring. But this procedure is outside of a massage therapist's scope of practice.

However, massage therapists often massage the sternocleidomastoid muscle. Before massaging this muscle, be sure to grasp it and elevate it slightly. This will move it away from the carotid artery; the artery will have a pulse.

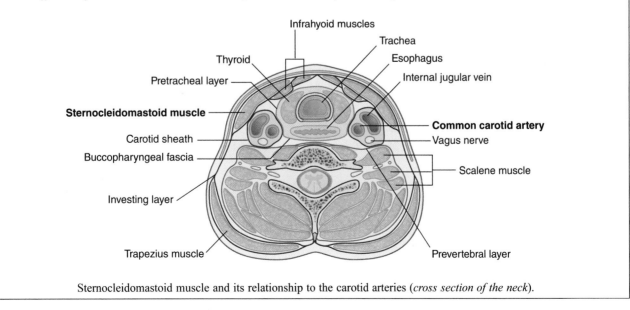

Sternocleidomastoid muscle and its relationship to the carotid arteries (*cross section of the neck*).

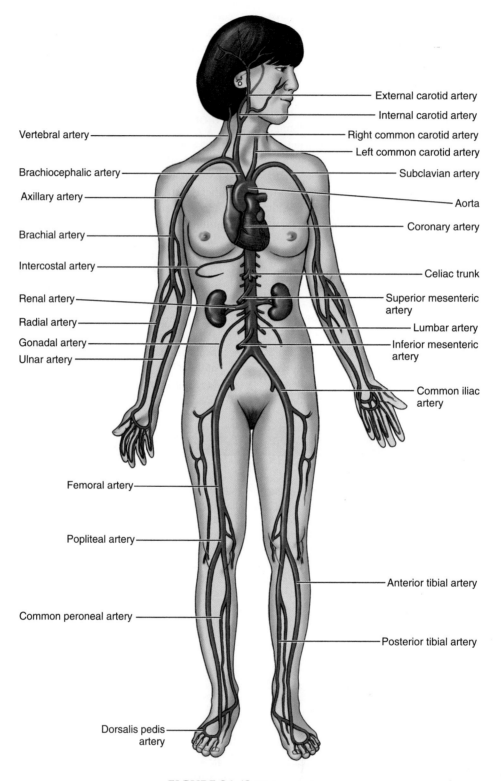

External carotid artery

Internal carotid artery

Right common carotid artery

Left common carotid artery

Vertebral artery

Brachiocephalic artery

Axillary artery

Subclavian artery

Aorta

Coronary artery

Brachial artery

Intercostal artery

Celiac trunk

Renal artery

Superior mesenteric artery

Radial artery

Lumbar artery

Gonadal artery

Inferior mesenteric artery

Ulnar artery

Common iliac artery

Femoral artery

Popliteal artery

Anterior tibial artery

Common peroneal artery

Posterior tibial artery

Dorsalis pedis artery

FIGURE 26-13 Major arteries.

Ulnar. The ulnar artery lies deep and medial in the forearm.

Radial. The radial artery lies more superficial and lateral in the forearm. The radial artery also has a pulse point.

Aorta. The aorta is the largest artery and contains several branches, which include the aortic arch, the thoracic aorta, and the abdominal aorta (Figure 26-14). The thoracic aorta and the abdominal aorta are collectively called the descending aorta.

CHAT ROOM

Abdominal Aorta

When using deep pressure on the psoas major muscle through the abdominal wall, approach the lumbar spine laterally to avoid the abdominal aorta. A strong pulse arises from this artery; so any area where a strong pulse is felt should be avoided. Deep pressure may compromise an abdominal aortic aneurysm and since this condition may be undiagnosed, it is best to err on the side of caution.

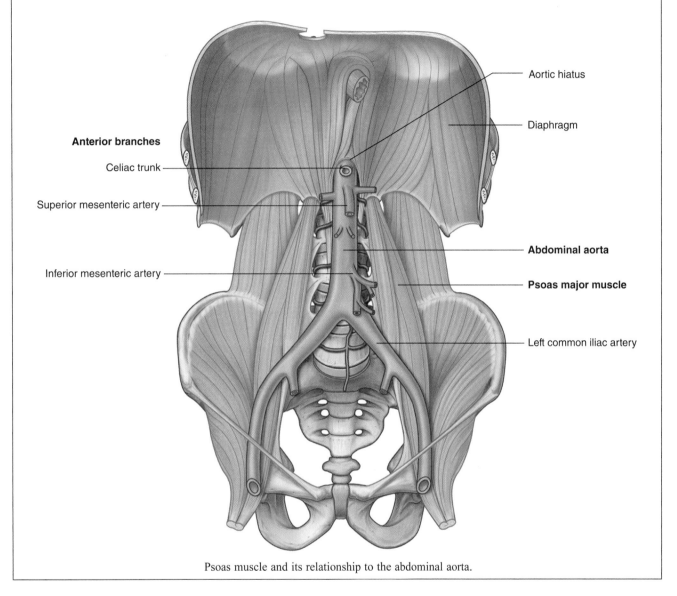

Psoas muscle and its relationship to the abdominal aorta.

Aortic arch. The aortic arch emerges from the left ventricle and gives rise to three arteries; the brachiocephalic artery, the left common carotid, and the left subclavian artery. Then it descends to become the thoracic aorta.

Thoracic aorta. The thoracic aorta extends from the aortic arch to the diaphragm.

Abdominal aorta. The abdominal aorta extends from the diaphragm till its bifurcation. The newly formed branches are the common iliac arteries. The abdominal aorta is a structure that should be avoided during massage. See Chat Room box on p. 686.

Femoral. The femoral artery lies superficially just below the groin and then descends posteriorly through the adductor muscles. The femoral artery has a pulse point.

Popliteal. When the femoral artery emerges behind the knee, it becomes the popliteal artery. The popliteal artery has a pulse point.

Anterior and posterior tibial. The popliteal artery then divides to become the anterior and posterior tibial arteries. The posterior tibial artery has a pulse point.

Dorsalis pedis. The anterior tibial artery becomes the dorsalis pedis artery on the dorsal aspect of the foot. The dorsalis pedis artery has a pulse point.

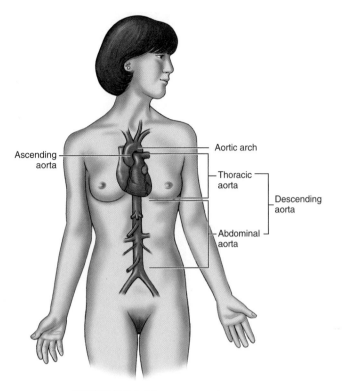

Ascending aorta

Aortic arch

Thoracic aorta

Descending aorta

Abdominal aorta

FIGURE 26-14 Branches of the aorta.

Major Veins

The body's major veins include (Figure 26-15):

Jugular. The right and left external jugular veins drain blood from the face, head, and neck and empty into the subclavian veins. Venous drainage from the brain is accomplished by the internal jugular veins, which then join the subclavian veins.

Subclavian. The subclavian veins join the internal jugular veins to become the brachiocephalic vein. These are important for use in intravenous infusion (hemodialysis and chemotherapy).

Superior vena cava. The superior vena cava empties into the right atrium.

Inferior vena cava. The inferior vena cava drains blood from the abdominal viscera into the right atrium.

Great saphenous. The great saphenous vein ascends medially from the foot up the leg to the thigh and drains into the femoral vein. These can become chronically dilated in some persons and develop into varicose veins. They may also become inflamed, leading to formation of blood clots—a condition known as thrombophlebitis.

CHAT ROOM

When applying deep gliding pressure over a superficial leg vein, always move from a distal point to a proximal point, or you may promote development of varicosities. Varicose veins, or damaged veins, lack a sufficient valve system.

BLOOD PRESSURE

The amount of pressure exerted by the blood on the blood vessel walls is called **blood pressure**. The maximal pressure, called *systolic pressure*, occurs when the left ventricle contracts. *Diastolic pressure*, which is the lowest pressure, occurs when the left ventricle relaxes. Systole and diastole were introduced during the previous discussion of the cardiac cycle. Blood forced into the aorta during systole sets up a pressure wave that travels along the arteries and expands arterial walls.

Blood pressure is measured with a blood pressure cuff (sphygmomanometer). Blood pressure depends on numerous factors, such as a person's size. The average newborn has a blood pressure of 90/60 mm Hg. At 15 years of age, the average blood pressure is about 120/60 mm Hg. An average, healthy young adult has a blood pressure of 120/80 mm Hg. A pressure above 140/90 mm Hg is considered high blood pressure (hypertension). Hypertension is regarded as a disease. See the section on cardiovascular pathologies later in the chapter for more information.

"Wise men learn much from fools. Wise guys don't."
—Michel de Montaigne

PATHS OF BLOOD CIRCULATION

The cardiovascular system contains two paths or circuits based on the areas of the body that are served: (1) pulmonary and (2) systemic (Figure 26-16). In a resting body, 75% of blood volume is located within the systemic system and 25% in the pulmonary system. Looking more closely at blood volume within the systemic system; 20% is arterial, 75% is venous, and the rest is found in the capillaries.

Pulmonary Circuit

The purpose of the pulmonary circuit is to replenish the oxygen supply of the blood and to eliminate gaseous wastes. To accomplish this, the **pulmonary circuit** brings deoxygenated blood from the right ventricle to the alveoli of the lungs to release carbon dioxide and regain oxygen. Oxygenated blood returns to the left atrium of the heart and moves into the systemic circuit with the contraction of the left ventricle.

The pulmonary arteries carry blood away from the heart and the pulmonary veins carry blood back to the heart, but the oxygen content of the blood is reversed—that is, the pulmonary arteries carry deoxygenated blood and the pulmonary veins carry oxygenated blood.

Systemic Circuit

The function of the systemic circuit is to bring nutrients and oxygen to all systems of the body and to carry waste

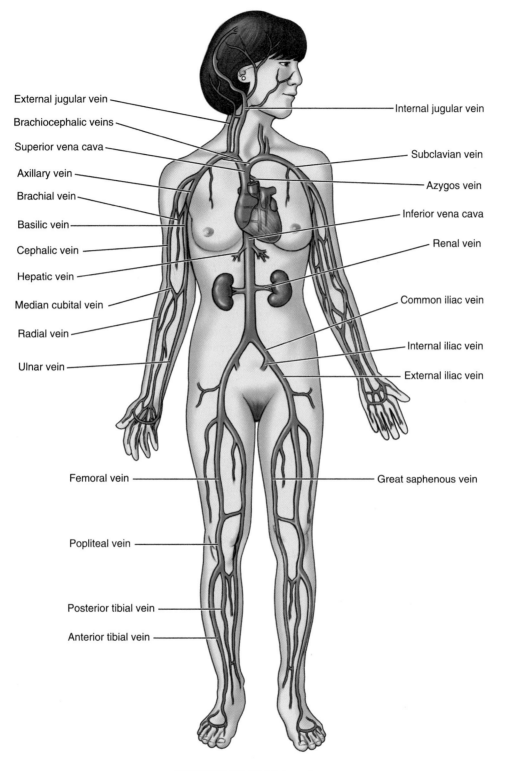

External jugular vein

Brachiocephalic veins

Superior vena cava

Axillary vein

Brachial vein

Basilic vein

Cephalic vein

Hepatic vein

Median cubital vein

Radial vein

Ulnar vein

Femoral vein

Popliteal vein

Posterior tibial vein

Anterior tibial vein

Internal jugular vein

Subclavian vein

Azygos vein

Inferior vena cava

Renal vein

Common iliac vein

Internal iliac vein

External iliac vein

Great saphenous vein

FIGURE 26-15 Major veins.

materials from the tissues for elimination. So the **systemic circuit** brings oxygenated blood from the left ventricle through numerous arteries into the capillaries. From here, blood moves back through the veins and returns the now deoxygenated blood to the right atrium to enter the pulmonary circuit.

Hepatic Portal System. Within the systemic circuit are venous portal systems that begin and end in veins (i.e., without arteries or capillaries).

These systems are present in the brain pituitary and abdomen. The portal system located in the abdomen is called the *hepatic portal system*; it moves products of digestion to

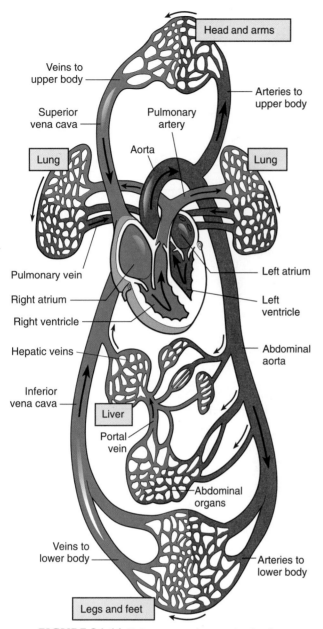

FIGURE 26-16 Pulmonary and systemic circuits.

the liver (hence the name hepatic). Portal blood contains substances absorbed by the stomach and intestine.

Because the liver is a key organ involved in maintaining the proper glucose, fat, and protein concentrations in the blood, the hepatic portal system allows the blood from the digestive organs to detour through the liver to process these substances before they enter the general circulation (Figure 26-17).

The other venous portal system is located between the hypothalamus and the anterior pituitary of the brain.

CARDIOVASCULAR PATHOLOGIES

Disorders of Blood

Anemia. Anemia is a decrease in the number of functional RBCs or their hemoglobin. This impairs the blood's ability to carry oxygen to body cells. Types of select anemias are *iron deficiency* (most common), *pernicious* (malabsorption of vitamin B_{12}), *folic acid deficiency*, *sickle cell* (genetic defect that causes sickle-shaped RBCs), and *aplastic* (from bone marrow failure).

Find out which type of anemia your client has. Medical clearance is needed for severe types (sickle cell and aplastic). If your client chills easily, place a warm blanket over the sheet drape.

If your client is fatigued, reduce treatment time to 30 minutes, and use lighter-than-normal pressure.

Thrombosis. Thrombosis, or blood clot formation, is the transformation of fluid blood into a gelatinous mass. Thrombi form to prevent excess blood loss from broken blood vessels. After the vessel heals, thrombi dissolve.

When thrombosis occurs in a damaged, but intact vessel, the formed thrombus attaches to the vessel wall (or heart wall). Thrombi do not cause symptoms until affected vessels become occluded. A piece of a thrombus can break off and be transported by the bloodstream. The floating mass is called an *embolus*. If an embolus occludes a blood vessel, the condition is called an *embolism*.

If your client is at risk for thrombosis (such as recent surgery), deep pressure and vigorous massage should be avoided on lower extremities. Apply these restrictions for 10 days after your client is ambulatory.

Disorders of the Heart

Angina Pectoris. Angina pectoris is sudden chest pain from a temporary reduced blood supply to the heart. The episode is often called an *angina attack*. It is usually caused by coronary artery disease and may be triggered by emotional stress, cold temperatures, or physical exertion such as exercise, climbing stairs, or running. Nausea, disorientation, fatigue, shortness of breath, anxiety, and profuse sweating may accompany the attack. Once the attack is over, normal blood flow resumes and the heart muscle remains undamaged.

Because sudden exposure to cold can bring on an attack, keep your client warm with a blanket over the sheet drape and avoid cryotherapy. Ask your client to have necessary medications easily accessible (e.g., nitroglycerin) in case of an attack during the massage.

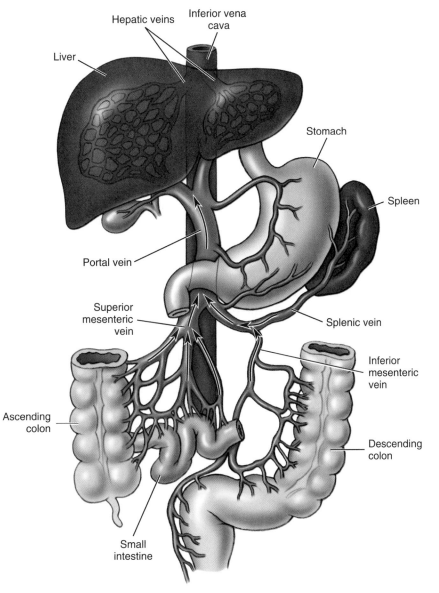

FIGURE 26-17 Hepatic portal system.

Arrhythmias. Any deviation from normal heartbeat or rhythm is called arrhythmia. This term encompasses abnormally fast or slow rhythms, as well as irregular rhythms.

Also called irregular heartbeats, arrhythmias are common and usually harmless and do not always indicate disease. Arrhythmias are classified by rate of contraction or where they originate. Types include:

- *Bradycardia.* Abnormally slow heartbeat (<50 or 60 beats/min). This condition is common in well-trained endurance athletes or persons on certain medications such as beta blockers, or during sleep.
- *Tachycardia.* Excessively rapid heartbeat (>100 beats/min). This condition is normal during fever, during and immediately after exercise, or during periods of anxiety and excitement.

- *Atrial fibrillation.* Atria quiver instead of producing a single, forceful contraction. This condition mainly affects people with hypertension or other heart problems; it is seldom life-threatening but can lead to more serious conditions, such as stroke.
- *Ventricular fibrillation.* Also called V-fib. Ventricles quiver instead of producing a single, forceful contraction. Often triggered by a heart attack, it causes the person to quickly lose consciousness. If left untreated, V-fib results in rapid death.

If your client has shortness of breath, avoid the prone position and elevate the upper body while supine. If your client is fatigued, reduce treatment time to 30 minutes, and use lighter-than-normal pressure. V-fib is obviously an emergency requiring immediate medical attention.

Congestive Heart Failure. Congestive heart failure (CHF) refers to the heart's inability to pump blood to meet the body's demands. CHF is usually caused by an underlying condition such as heart problems (previous myocardial infarction, valve defects) or results from increased demands on the heart (long-standing hypertension). Other causes are lung disease (chronic bronchitis, emphysema) and diseases that contribute to heart failure (diabetes, severe anemia). CHF may occur as an acute episode, but it is usually a chronic condition with possible acute exacerbations. Signs and symptoms include shortness of breath (even when the person is lying down), fatigue, dizziness, and tachycardia. Significant edema of the lower extremities may occur.

Acute CHF represents a medical emergency. Massage is postponed until the condition resolves and medical clearance is given. If pitting edema is present in chronic CHF, avoid the area. If your client is fatigued, reduce treatment time to 30 minutes, and use lighter-than-normal pressure. If shortness of breath occurs, avoid the prone position and elevate the upper body while the client is supine.

Myocardial Infarction. A myocardial infarction (MI), or heart attack, is death of heart muscle from interrupted blood supply and prolonged ischemia. Cardiac tissues die in about 20 minutes.

MIs are usually caused by occluded coronary arteries from (1) thrombus build-up of atherosclerosis, or (2) thromboemboli. The area supplied by the occluded artery is often destroyed by infarction.

MI is a medical emergency requiring immediate medical attention. If your client has had a MI, find out when it occurred and how well recovery is proceeding. If the MI is recent and your client is weak and debilitated, clearance from the client's physician is essential. If cleared for massage, a lighter-than-normal massage of shorter duration is indicated. If your client is further along in the recovery and has regained most of his or her strength, medical clearance is recommended and massage with moderate pressure is indicated. If your client has completely recovered and regained all of his or her strength, a more vigorous massage can be performed.

Diseases of Arteries

Peripheral Arterial Disease. Peripheral arterial disease (PAD) is caused by atherosclerosis of the extremities, which leads to reduced blood flow. In most individuals, PAD affects vessels in the legs and feet. An early symptom is intermittent calf pain that initially subsides with rest but becomes more severe with time and is not relieved by rest. Other symptoms are weakness, numbness, and fatigue in the legs. The skin over the affected area may be pale, cyanotic, or shiny, feel cold to the touch; and lack hair. The nails are often thick and malformed.

Because of the possibility of clot formation, avoid affected area (usually lower extremities). If stents were used to treat the affected vessels, adapt the massage according to restrictions placed on the client by his or her physician. For example, if your client has been instructed to avoid sharply bending a joint, avoid joint mobilizations to that joint.

Hypertension. Hypertension is a disorder of intermittent or sustained elevated blood pressure.

Hypertension is known as the *silent killer*, meaning that there are no symptoms in early stages and diagnosis may not occur until complications arise. For example, over time, untreated high blood pressure can damage arterial walls (leading to or accelerating atherosclerosis), cause vessels walls to dilate or tear (forming aneurysms), and damage organs (from sustained ischemia). Targeted organs are the kidneys, retinas, and brain. The heart may enlarge from a sustained workload; CHF is a frequent consequence of hypertension.

Ascertain if and how the condition is controlled. Clients whose hypertension is not under control by diet, regular exercise, or medications should not receive massage owing to the likelihood of unmonitored severe complications. Medical clearance is needed. If the condition is under control, your client may experience dizzy spells as a common side effect of antihypertensive medications; instruct him or her to move slowly and carefully and be ready to assist.

Aneurysm. An aneurysm is a localized weakness in a blood vessel wall that may bulge outward.

These areas may leak blood or rupture, resulting in hemorrhage and possible death. Most aneurysms are asymptomatic until they rupture, with the affected person exhibiting signs of hypovolemic shock for abdominal and thoracic aneurysms. Headaches or stroke may accompany cerebral aneurysms.

Obtain medical clearance before massaging a client with a diagnosed aneurysm. Once this is obtained, avoid the affected area (such as the abdomen).

Orthostatic Hypotension. Also called a *dizzy spell*, orthostatic hypotension is a sudden drop in blood pressure when moving from a lying or sitting position to an upright or standing position, causing a loss of balance. Orthostatic hypotension is caused by gravity-induced blood pooling in the lower extremities. Causes include medication use (antihypertensives, diuretics, antidepressants), dehydration (nursing mothers, being outside on a hot day), prolonged immobility, venous pooling from pregnancy, and extensive varicosities. The affected person may be weak and confused, have blurred vision, and experience dizziness or fainting.

Because massage often lowers blood pressure temporarily, remind your clients (especially elderly clients) to sit up for a moment before standing so that blood pressure can adjust to postural changes. Also remind your client to move slowly rather than quickly; the client may require assistance.

Raynaud Disease.   Raynaud disease is a cycle of periodic temporary, but severe, vasospasms in superficial tissues of the fingers and toes. During the beginning of an attack, small and medium-size arteries contract in a disordered manner, causing temporary ischemia. Skin in the affected area turns white and then blue, followed by paresthesias (sensations of tingling, pricking, pins-and-needles, or numbness.). As circulation is restored, the affected area turns purplish red followed by pain that may sting or throb. The condition can also affect the tip of the nose, parts of the ears, parts of the cheek, and tongue. Attacks are often precipitated by cold weather, emotional stress, or smoking (nicotine is a powerful vasoconstrictor).

During attacks, avoid the affected area. Between attacks, massage is indicated and may improve local circulation and reduce stress. Be sure to use a blanket over the sheet drape to prevent chilling. All forms of cryotherapy, including ice packs, are contraindicated.

Diseases of Veins

Phlebitis/Thrombophlebitis.   Phlebitis is inflammation of the veins. If this condition is accompanied by a thrombus formation, it is called *thrombophlebitis.* Thrombophlebitis of deep veins is called *deep vein thrombosis* (DVT). Venous stasis (slowed blood flow in the veins, usually in the legs) is the most common cause and results from prolonged inactivity, such as being bedridden or sitting or standing for long periods. The affected area is painful and tender; it is often swollen and can be either hot or cold to the touch.

Avoid the affected area until the risk of thrombus has been eliminated (as determined by a physician) and the condition has resolved.

Varicose Veins.   Varicose veins are veins that have become dilated from excess blood as a result of incompetent valves. Once they are dilated, they tend to remain so. Pregnancy, particularly multiple pregnancies, can result in varicose veins because of the pressure exerted by the uterus on the femoral veins. This pressure results in increased venous pressure, ultimately damaging the venous valves. Also, prolonged inactivity such as sitting or standing causes pressure within leg veins to be slightly elevated. This, along with the effects of gravity, causes vessel walls to dilate. When this effect occurs, venous valves no longer seal properly, allowing blood to pool. The ankles may swell. As the condition progresses, veins may appear bluish purple in color and feel hard to the touch.

Avoid the affected area if pressure causes pain or there is a history of clot formation. Clients with severe varicosities may benefit from massage. During massage, place the legs on soft bolsters to raise them above the level of the heart. Massage should be geared toward increasing blood flow. Perform massage proximal to the affected area first; for example, massage the thigh before the leg. This encourages venous return.

SPOTLIGHT ON RESEARCH

Research suggests that massage therapy may:
- Increase capillary flow rate, blood viscosity, and filtration rate
- Increase blood flow to the skin and muscular tissue
- Increase blood oxygen saturation levels
- Increase surface tissue temperatures of the treated and adjacent areas
- Increase red and white blood cell and platelet counts
- Decrease heart rate, blood pressure, and heart rate variability
- Decrease diastolic and systolic blood pressure in persons with hypertension

---

E-RESOURCES

⊖volve

http://evolve.elsevier.com/Salvo/MassageTherapy

- Chapter challenge
- Flash cards
- Photo gallery
- Educational animations
- Weblinks

BIBLIOGRAPHY

Abrahams P, Marks S, Hutchings R: *McMinn's color atlas of human anatomy,* St Louis, 2003, Mosby.

Applegate EJ: *The anatomy and physiology learning system,* ed 3, Philadelphia, 2006, Saunders.

Beers MH, Berkow R: *The Merck manual of diagnosis and therapy,* Whitehouse Station, NJ, 2006, Merck Research Laboratories.

Calenda E: Personal communication, 2010.

Crawley J, Van De Graaff KM: *A photographic atlas for anatomy and physiology,* Englewood, Colo, 2002, Morton.

Como D, editor: *Mosby's medical, nursing, and allied health dictionary,* ed 6, St Louis, 2002, Mosby.

Damjanov I: *Pathophysiology for the health-related professions,* ed 3, Philadelphia, 2006, Saunders.

Ferri FF: *2003 Ferri's clinical advisor, instant diagnosis and treatment,* St Louis, 2003, Mosby.

Frazier MS, Drzymkowski JW: *Essentials of human diseases and conditions*, ed 3, Philadelphia, 2004, Saunders.

Fritz S: *Essential sciences for therapeutic massage*, ed 3, St Louis, 2009, Mosby.

Fritz S: *Fundamentals of therapeutic massage*, ed 4, St Louis, 2009, Mosby.

Gould BE: *Pathophysiology for the health professions*, ed 3, Philadelphia, 2006, Saunders.

Gray H, Pickering P, Howden R: *Gray's anatomy*, ed 29, Philadelphia, 1974, Running Press.

Guyton A: *Human physiology and mechanisms of disease*, ed 6, Philadelphia, 1996, WB Saunders.

Haubrich WS: *Medical meanings: a glossary of word origins*, New York, 1984, Harcourt Brace Jovanovich.

Huether SE, McCance KL: *Understanding pathophysiology*, ed 3, St Louis, 2004, Mosby.

Jacob S, Francone C: *Elements of anatomy and physiology*, Philadelphia, 1989, Saunders.

Kalat JW: *Biological psychology*, ed 8, Belmont, Calif, 2003, Wadsworth.

Kapit W, Elson LM: *The anatomy coloring book*, ed 3, New York, 2002, Benjamin Cummings.

Kumar V, Abbas A, Fausto N: *Robbins and Cotran physiologic basis of disease*, ed 7, St Louis, 2005, Mosby.

Lowe W: Personal communication, 2010.

Marieb EN: *Essentials of human anatomy and physiology*, ed 8, New York, 2005, Benjamin Cummings.

Martini FH, Bartholomew EF: *Essentials of anatomy and physiology*, ed 3, New York, 2003, Benjamin Cummings.

McAleer N: *The body almanac*, Garden City, NY, 1985, Doubleday.

McCance K, Huether S: *Pathophysiology: the biological basis for disease in adults and children*, St Louis, 2006, Mosby.

Merck manual, ed 17, Whitehouse Station, NJ, 1998, Merck and Co.

Moore KL: *Clinically oriented anatomy*, ed 5, Baltimore, 2005, Lippincott Williams & Wilkins.

Netter FH: *Atlas of human anatomy*, ed 3, Teterboro, NJ, 2003, Icon Learning Systems.

Newton D: *Pathology for massage therapists*, ed 2, Portland, Ore, 1995, Simran.

Premkumar K: *Pathology A to Z, a handbook for massage therapists*, Baltimore, 1999, Lippincott Williams & Wilkins.

Salvo SG: *Mosby's pathology for massage therapists*, ed 2, St Louis, 2009, Mosby.

Solomon EP, Phillips GA: *Understanding human anatomy and physiology*, Philadelphia, 1987, Saunders.

Thibodeau G, Patton K: *Anatomy and physiology*, ed 6, St Louis, 2006, Mosby.

Thibodeau G, Patton K: *Structure and function of the body*, ed 12, St Louis, 2004, Mosby.

Tortora GJ: *Introduction to the human body: the essentials of anatomy and physiology*, ed 5, Hoboken, NJ, 2000, John Wiley & Sons.

Tortora GJ, Grabowksi SR: *Principles of anatomy and physiology*, ed 11, New York, 2005, John Wiley & Sons.

Travell JG, Simons D: *Myofascial pain and dysfunction, the trigger point manual*, Baltimore, 1992, Lippincott Williams & Wilkins.

Venes D, Thomas CL, Taber CW: *Taber's cyclopedic medical dictionary*, ed 20, Philadelphia, 2005, FA Davis.

MATCHING I

Place the letter of the answer next to the term or phrase that best describes it.

A. Atria
B. Blood
C. Blood pressure
D. Erythrocytes

E. Hematopoiesis
F. Hemoglobin
G. Leukocytes
H. Plasma

I. Thrombocytes
J. Type AB
K. Type O
L. Ventricles

_____ 1. Universal blood donor

_____ 2. Process of blood cell development

_____ 3. Term synonymous with platelets; involved in blood clotting

_____ 4. Red blood cells; transports oxygen to cells

_____ 5. Fluid medium containing formed elements and liquid plasma

_____ 6. Universal blood recipient

_____ 7. Superior chambers of the heart

_____ 8. Pressure exerted by blood on blood vessel walls

_____ 9. Iron-based protein that primarily transports oxygen and some carbon dioxide

_____ 10. Straw-colored liquid in blood

_____ 11. Inferior chambers of the heart

_____ 12. White blood cells; serve as part of the body's immune system

MATCHING II

Place the letter of the answer next to the term or phrase that best describes it.

A. Aorta
B. Arteries
C. Bicuspid valve
D. Cardiac output

E. Carotid
F. Conduction system
G. Myocardium
H. Pericardium

I. Systemic circuit
J. Tricuspid valve
K. Vasodilation
L. Veins

_____ 1. Thick muscular heart layer

_____ 2. Vessels that return deoxygenated blood back to the heart

_____ 3. Heart's intrinsic electrical system that helps initiate and coordinate heart rhythm

_____ 4. Vessels that move oxygenated blood away from the heart

_____ 5. Largest artery of the body

_____ 6. Valve located between the left atrium and the left ventricle

_____ 7. Superficial artery in the throat region

_____ 8. Valve located between the right atrium and the right ventricle

_____ 9. Path of blood from the left ventricle out to the tissues and then back through the veins to the right atrium

_____ 10. Term used to describe enlargement of the vascular lumen

_____ 11. Sac that surrounds the heart

_____ 12. Amount of blood ejected from the left ventricle each minute

CASE STUDY

Congestive Heart Failure

Andre is a 55-year-old man who survived a heart attack a little over a year ago. About 4 months back, he was released by his cardiologist and began receiving weekly massages.

Over his left pectoralis major muscle, he has a pacemaker that was placed there 3 months ago.

Andre swims three times a week and is current on his meds.

When Andre arrives for his appointment today, he looks a little tired and pale.

During the intake, he states that he is fatigued, and you both decide that a 30-minute massage is best. After the massage, if Andre wishes to nap on the table, that would be fine because your next appointment is not for another 3 hours.

After he has readied himself for the massage, you enter the room and begin with him supine just in case he experiences shortness of breath.

As you pull back the sheet to place a bolster beneath his knees, you notice swelling around his ankles. You press your thumb into the skin and as you pull your hand back to examine the area, and your thumbprint remains for about 10 seconds.

What modifications, if any, are needed?

CRITICAL THINKING

When performing massage, why is it important to consider the underlying vasculature and the factors that can affect blood and lymph flow?

CHAPTER 27

Lymphatic System and Immunity

"When an ordinary man attains knowledge, he becomes a sage. When a sage attains knowledge, he becomes an ordinary man."

—Zen saying

LEARNING OBJECTIVES

After completing this chapter, the student should be able to:

* List anatomic structures and describe the physiologic processes of the lymphatic system.
* Trace lymph flow from the lymphatic capillaries to the major lymphatic ducts.
* Discuss nonspecific and specific immunity.
* Describe immune system dysfunctions, such as immune deficiency, hypersensitivity, and autoimmune disease.
* Name lymphatic and immune pathologies, giving characteristics of and massage considerations for each.

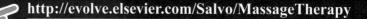

INTRODUCTION

The lymphatic system is a one-way system composed of lymph, lymph vessels, and specialized tissues, glands, nodes, and organs. Lymph moves from the tissues through a series of vessels and ends in the cardiovascular system. The lymphatic system helps maintain fluid balance, supports the transport of nutrients within the body, and has disease-fighting functions. This chapter explores the lymphatic system and the body's immunologic responses.

ANATOMY

The lymphatic system consists of:
- Lymph
- Lymph vessels
- Lymph glands (e.g., thymus)
- Lymphatic organs (e.g., spleen)
- Lymph nodes
- Lymphocytes

PHYSIOLOGY

The functions of the lymphatic system are as follows:
- **Transportation.** The lymphatic system transports dietary proteins, lipids and lipid-soluble vitamins (i.e., A, D, E, and K) from the digestive tract to the blood. Lipids and lipid-soluble vitamins are large molecules that cannot be taken up by blood capillaries. Instead, they are taken up by specialized lymphatic capillaries within the digestive tract called *lacteals*.
- **Immune response.** The lymphatic system also plays an active role in immune defenses.
- **Maintains homeostasis.** The lymphatic system helps to maintain homeostasis through collecting accumulated tissue fluid and returning it to blood circulation. This process also maintains blood volume and pressure and prevents swelling (edema).

LYMPH

Lymph is the nearly colorless fluid found in lymphatic vessels. It is chemically similar to blood plasma and contains numerous white blood cells, proteins, and fats.

LYMPH VESSELS

Lymphatic vessels, or lymphatics, include lymph capillaries, lymph vessels, lymphatic trunks, and two main lymphatic ducts (Figure 27-1).

Lymph Capillaries

Also called *initial lymphatic vessels*, lymph capillaries, are tiny open-ended vessels located in tissue spaces

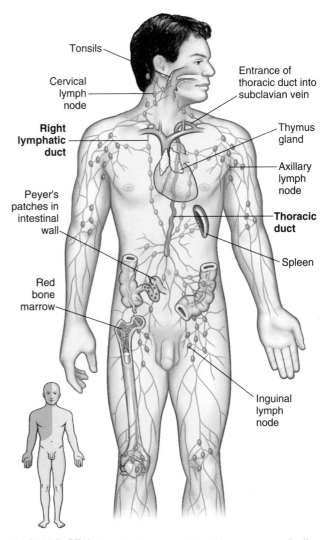

FIGURE 27-1 Lymphatic system. Inset figure: green shading indicates area drained by right lymphatic duct. Blue shading indicates area drained by thoracic duct.

throughout most of the body (except for the brain, spinal cord, and cornea). These vessels have a structure similar to that of blood capillaries, but they are larger and more permeable.

Lymph Vessels

Lymph capillaries become larger and are called lymph vessels. Compared with veins, lymphatic vessels have thinner walls and more valves. These valves open in only one direction, permitting fluid to flow only toward the center of the body.

Lymphatic Trunks

Lymphatic vessels join to form larger lymphatic vessels called lymphatic trunks.

Lymphatic Ducts

Lymphatic trunks join to form one of two regionally draining lymphatic ducts. These are the right lymphatic and the thoracic duct.

Right Lymphatic Duct. Drains lymph from the right arm and the right side of the head and the right half of the thorax into the right subclavian vein.

Thoracic Duct. Drains lymph from all remaining parts of the body into the left subclavian vein. The thoracic duct begins at the *cisterna chyli* (i.e., lymphatic sac located between the abdominal aorta and L2) and lies anterior to the thoracic vertebrae.

LYMPHATIC STRUCTURES

Primary lymphatic structures are the bone marrow and thymus. These structures are also known as *generative lymphatic organs* because they produce and mature lymphocytes.

Secondary lymphatic structures include the spleen, lymph nodes, and mucosa-associated lymphoid tissue (tonsils, Peyer patches, appendix). These secondary lymphatic structures are populated by lymphocytes from the bone marrow and the thymus.

Bone Marrow

Bone marrow, located in the hollow cavity of bones, produces blood cells, such as red blood cells and white blood

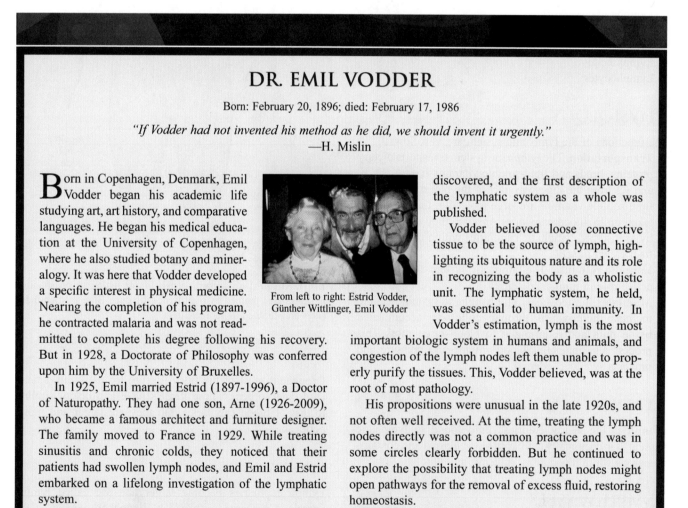

DR. EMIL VODDER

Born: February 20, 1896; died: February 17, 1986

"If Vodder had not invented his method as he did, we should invent it urgently."
—H. Mislin

Born in Copenhagen, Denmark, Emil Vodder began his academic life studying art, art history, and comparative languages. He began his medical education at the University of Copenhagen, where he also studied botany and mineralogy. It was here that Vodder developed a specific interest in physical medicine. Nearing the completion of his program, he contracted malaria and was not readmitted to complete his degree following his recovery. But in 1928, a Doctorate of Philosophy was conferred upon him by the University of Bruxelles.

In 1925, Emil married Estrid (1897-1996), a Doctor of Naturopathy. They had one son, Arne (1926-2009), who became a famous architect and furniture designer. The family moved to France in 1929. While treating sinusitis and chronic colds, they noticed that their patients had swollen lymph nodes, and Emil and Estrid embarked on a lifelong investigation of the lymphatic system.

Emil's research began with papers written hundreds of years earlier, when many discoveries about the lymphatic system were made by scientists including Gaspare Aselli, Jean Pecquet, Olof Rudbeck, and Thomas Bartholin. During that era, the system of lymphatic vessels and lymph circulation—the cisterna chyli, the path between the thoracic duct and venous arch—were

From left to right: Estrid Vodder, Günther Wittlinger, Emil Vodder

discovered, and the first description of the lymphatic system as a whole was published.

Vodder believed loose connective tissue to be the source of lymph, highlighting its ubiquitous nature and its role in recognizing the body as a wholistic unit. The lymphatic system, he held, was essential to human immunity. In Vodder's estimation, lymph is the most important biologic system in humans and animals, and congestion of the lymph nodes left them unable to properly purify the tissues. This, Vodder believed, was at the root of most pathology.

His propositions were unusual in the late 1920s, and not often well received. At the time, treating the lymph nodes directly was not a common practice and was in some circles clearly forbidden. But he continued to explore the possibility that treating lymph nodes might open pathways for the removal of excess fluid, restoring homeostasis.

While some had previously discovered that manual pressure, bandaging and pumping were helpful to reduce edema, it was the investigations of Emil and Estrid Vodder that lead to the development of the gentle, rhythmic lymphatic drainage techniques commonly used today. From Emil Vodder's combination of careful scrutiny of the anatomic etchings of the anatomy and cells (WBCs). **Lymphocytes** are a type of WBC that comprises approximately 25% of the total WBC count. Some lymphocytes produced in bone marrow also mature there and are called B cells (B = Bone marrow). Other lymphocytes travel to the thymus and mature there, becoming T cells (T = thymus).

Thymus

Also an endocrine gland, the **thymus** is located behind the sternum. As stated previously, the thymus receives immature T cells. Once mature, T cells as well as B cells both travel to secondary lymphatic structures, such as lymph nodes, appendix, and tonsils. The thymus is most prominent in the newborn and begins to atrophy after puberty, becoming only a small lymphoid remnant in the adult. The hormones thymosin and thymopoietin are produced by the thymus. These hormones play a role in immunity because they stimulate the production and activation of T cells.

Spleen

The largest lymphatic organ, the dark purple **spleen** lies within the left lateral rib cage (between the ninth and eleventh ribs) just posterior to the stomach. The spleen stores lymphocytes, releasing them in immune responses. WBCs called *macrophages* destroy worn-out red blood cells, as well as destroy harmful microorganisms. The spleen serves as a blood reservoir and can release small amounts of blood into the circulation during times of emergency or blood loss.

DR. EMIL VODDER (*continued*)

physiology of the lymphatic system, and countless practical applications, he developed a protocol of superficial circular strokes, gentle pumping and light pressure to decongest lymph nodes. As more and more of his patients' conditions resolved, Vodder began to realize that he may have found a successful treatment for conditions ranging from acne to migraines.

During a 1936 congress in Paris, Vodder presented his theories. These were published in Santé Pour Tous under the title *Le drainage lymphatique, une nouvelle méthode thérapeutique (Lymphatic drainage, a new therapeutic method)*. They were not immediately embraced, possibly because Vodder was not a physician or licensed physical or massage therapist. In addition, there was concern in the medical community that addressing the lymph nodes directly would cause toxins to spread throughout the body. Despite the cool reception of their work, Emil and Estrid continued to study and practice this new technique, presenting their theories as opportunities arose.

When World War II began, the Vodders returned to their home in Copenhagen. While the war may have slowed their progress in presenting their inspiring discoveries, it also gave them time to perfect the practice. Shortly following the end of the war, Vodder began receiving invitations to teach his method of lymphatic drainage throughout Europe. But a perceived lack of evidence thwarted the adoption of this practice by the larger medical community.

In the 1960s the German Dr. Johannes Asdonk took great interest in Vodder's work. As a result, a list of indications, contraindications, and cautions for the use of Vodder's method of lymphatic therapy was established on the basis of statistical results from more than 2,000 case studies. In 1967 the Vodders, along with Dr. Asdonk and Günther Wittlinger, founded The Association of Dr. Vodder's Manual Lymphatic Drainage and held the first congress addressing the subject.

In 1976 Swiss professor H. Mislin published his research titled *Active Contractility of the Lymphangion and Coordination of Lymphangion Chains*. His research into the mechanical characteristics of lymphangions, the functional units of lymph vessels, supported Vodder's theories that stimulation of these vessels increases the rate and amplitude of pulsation, increasing efficiency. Mislin's work underscored that Vodder's method of reducing edemas is an effective method for resolving health problems related to insufficient filtering of interstitial fluids.

Vodder was awarded the Röhrbach-Medal by the German Massage and Physical Therapy Association in 1985. He died in February 1986, just shy of his eightieth birthday. His wife, Estrid, died in 1996, just shy of her one-hundredth birthday. Few have had such a profound impact on the full spectrum of manual therapy as Drs. Emil and Estrid Vodder. Today, there are numerous schools devoted to the instruction of Vodder's manual lymphatic drainage. His treatments continue to be widely used by physical therapists, and massage therapists, and are increasingly prescribed by physicians to treat a wide variety of acute and chronic conditions.

Lymph Nodes

Lymph nodes are bean-shaped structures located along lymph vessels. As lymph flows, it passes through one or more lymph nodes before entering the bloodstream.

Lymph nodes are the only place where lymph is filtered. These structures serve as powerful defense stations that help protect the body from invaders. Lymph nodes house phagocytes and lymphocytes (both B and T cells) that destroy pathogens in lymph. The structure of the lymph node slows lymph flow through them, providing time to filter and remove pathogens (Figure 27-2). During periods of infection, lymph nodes may enlarge in response to their disease-fighting activity. Superficial lymph nodes are:

Inguinal Nodes. Located in the groin.

Axillary Nodes. Located in the axillae.

Cervical Nodes. Located in the neck.

Mucosa-Associated Lymphoid Tissue

Mucosa-associated lymph tissue (MALT) is small masses of lymph tissue in which lymphocytes are produced or reproduced (i.e., cloned). MALT is positioned strategically to protect the respiratory and gastrointestinal tracts from pathogens and other foreign material. Most MALTs are small and solitary, but some are found in large clusters and include:

Tonsils. Located in the oral cavity and pharynx and include the adenoids, palatine, and lingual tonsils.

Peyer Patches. Seen in the lower portion of the small intestine (ileum) and are also called *intestinal tonsils.*

Vermiform Appendix. Attached to the first part of the large intestine (cecum).

> *"For peace of mind, resign as general manager of the universe."*
> —Larry Eisenberg

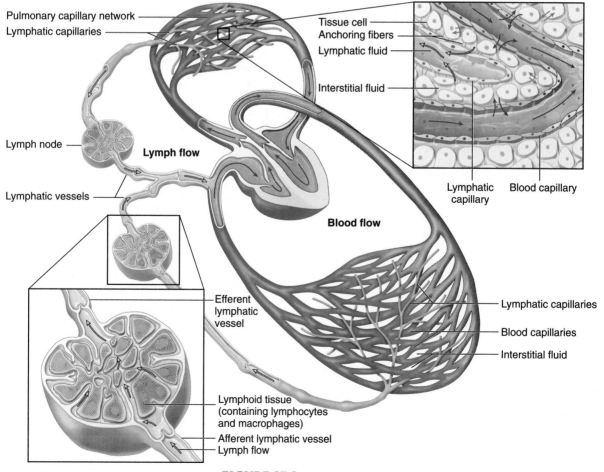

FIGURE 27-2 Flow of lymph.

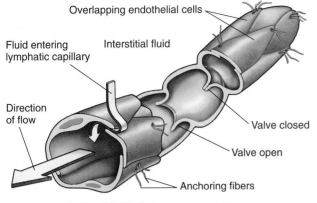

FIGURE 27-3 Lymphatic capillary.

LYMPH FLOW

Lymph starts out as interstitial fluid. As fluid enters a lymph capillary, a flap valve prevents it from returning to interstitial spaces (Figure 27-3). Lymph from lymph capillaries moves into lymph vessels, which become progressively larger. Lymph moves slowly when compared with blood flow and flows in only one direction. Periodically along its path, lymph flows through lymph nodes where it is filtered.

Lymph converges into either the right lymphatic duct or the thoracic duct. The right lymphatic duct drains only the right side of the head and neck, the right upper extremity, and the right half of the upper trunk and delivers the lymph to the right subclavian vein. The thoracic duct drains lymph from the rest of the body and delivers the lymph to the left subclavian vein (see Figure 27-1).

The movement of lymph is also known as *lymphatic drainage*.

Lymphatic Pump

Without a muscular pump such as the heart to assist flow, lymph moves only through pressure gradients from external sources exerted on its vessel walls (Figure 27-4). This pressure can come from:
- The milking action of skeletal muscle contractions against vessel walls.
- Pressure changes in the thorax and abdomen during breathing.
- Pulling of the skin and fascia during movement.

Additionally, smooth muscle in the wall of lymphatic vessels contracts to move lymph from one section of the vessel to the next.

Lymphatics are also found on the soles and the palms. The rhythmic pumping of walking and grasping facilitate lymphatic flow.

IMMUNITY

Immunity is a complex reaction that involves all body systems as they join together to destroy and eliminate

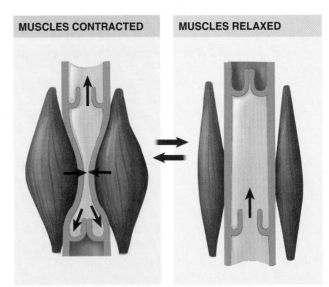

FIGURE 27-4 Lymphatic pump.

CHAT ROOM

Lymphatic Massage

Muscle tension and binding by connective tissues put pressure on the lymph vessels and may restrict them, interfering with efficient drainage. Massage can normalize muscle tension and improve connective tissue pliability. As the muscles relax and connective tissue has more space, lymph vessels open. Specialized application of massage can be effective in increasing lymph removal from stagnant or edematous tissue.

Pressure and Direction. Massage that uses light pressure to drag skin significantly increases superficial lymph movement. Crosswise and lengthwise stretching of lymph vessels' anchoring filaments opens the lymph capillaries, thus allowing interstitial fluid to enter the lymphatic system (see Figure 27-3). Be sure to apply massage strokes in the direction of normal lymphatic flow, thus enhancing lymph drainage. In the extremities, lymph generally moves toward the groin or to the axillae. Because lymph capillary plexuses are present on the bottoms of the feet, rhythmic compression on the soles also enhances lymph flow.

Lymphatic massage mechanically stimulates lymph flow by following lymphatic routes. Light pressure is used to pull on skin and superficial connective tissues. This ultimately opens up lymphatic capillaries. The focus of pressure is on the dermis (just below the surface layer of skin but above the muscles). Too much pressure squeezes lymphatic capillaries closed. Rhythmic, gentle, passive and active joint movement, and rhythmic muscle contraction can also assist lymphatic drainage. These actions reproduce the way the body normally pumps lymph. Ask the client to assist the process by breathing slowly and deeply; this stimulates lymph flow.

When possible, position the area to be treated above the heart so gravity can assist drainage.

Precautions. When applying these techniques, avoid excessive increases in lymph flow in persons who have heart or kidney conditions. The venous system must accommodate the load of lymphatic fluid delivered to the subclavian veins. When your client has a heart or kidney condition, these systems are already overloaded. Significantly increasing the amount of fluid moving into the cardiovascular system could place excessive strain on the heart and kidneys.

pathogens, foreign substances, or toxic materials. Thus, the "immune system" is not actually an organ system but a functional system that draws on structures and processes of other organs, tissues, and cells, as well as chemicals produced by them to protect the body. The two major mechanisms of immunity are nonspecific and specific.

Nonspecific Immunity

Also called *innate immunity*, nonspecific immunity is a set of responses that provide a more general defense by simply acting against a wide variety of organisms recognized as "nonself" or foreign to the body. Primary cells involved in nonspecific immunity are epithelium (skin and mucosa), phagocytic WBCs (neutrophils, macrophages), and natural killer cells. Cellular and inflammatory responses are also aspects of nonspecific immunity. In addition to these, fever destroys many disease-producing organisms.

Specific Immunity

Also called *adaptive immunity*, specific immunity recognizes specific threats and respond by launching an attack against them, and if/when they reappear. Primary cells involved in specific immunity are lymphocytes called T cells and B cells. As you may recall, lymphocytes are types of WBCs. Specific immunity can be acquired either *naturally* (from simple exposure) or *artificially* (from introducing substances into the body to stimulate immune responses [e.g., vaccinations]). Specific immune responses develop quickly, but not as quickly as nonspecific responses, because the latter types are already in place and can attack the threat when presented.

Additional information on nonspecific and specific immunity is featured next.

NONSPECIFIC IMMUNITY

Physical Barriers, Chemical Barriers, and Reflexes

Nonspecific immunity can involve barriers, such as intact skin and mucosae, or reflexes, such as coughing and vomiting. These responses can be affected by diet, mental health, environment, and metabolism.

Skin. Intact skin is a physical protective barrier. Sebum produced by oil glands has antibacterial properties. Skin also has limited protection from ultraviolet radiation due to melanin production, or skin pigmentation.

Mouth. Sticky mucus and saliva trap microorganisms, allowing them to be swallowed and disposed of in the digestive tract. Saliva contains lysozyme, an enzyme with antibacterial properties. Located in the back of

the mouth and throat, tonsils are also part of the body's defenses.

Stomach. Gastric juices, which contain hydrochloric acid, kill most organisms entering the digestive tract. Vomiting is also a defense mechanism because it rids the body of irritants and toxins.

Intestines. Small and large intestines possess an intestinal flora, which contributes to normal function. The intestines are supplied liberally with MALT throughout their length. Like vomiting, diarrhea can also be considered a defense mechanism, although in most instances it occurs far too late in the course of infection to be of much benefit.

Genitourinary Tract. Downward flow of urine washes out the urethra and protects against many ascending infections. Vaginal secretions help to maintain an acidic environment, creating an inhospitable environment for many pathogens.

Respiratory Tract. Nose hairs prevent insects and large particles from entering the upper respiratory tract. These particles can also be removed by sneezing. Mucus traps smaller particles and moves them to the digestive tract to be destroyed. The trachea and bronchi are lined with cilia that trap debris. Cilia can propel a stream of mucus away from the lungs and toward the pharynx to be swallowed or expectorated. Organisms that reach the lungs are destroyed or inactivated by resident macrophages. Lungs are supplied with lymph nodes that act as another filter. Coughing is a defensive reflex that removes particles or excess mucus in the lower respiratory tract.

Eyes and Ears. Tears contain high levels of lysozyme, which has antibacterial properties. Blinking is a reflex that eliminates irritants. Cerumen, or ear wax, provides a sticky barrier to foreign agents entering the ear canal.

Cellular Responses

Cellular responses involve the actions of nonspecific immunity cells. These include how certain WBCs phagocytize, or surround and destroy, pathogens. Some WBCs, such as eosinophils, release chemicals that slow or halt inflammatory responses. Mast cells (located in connective tissue) release chemicals that initiate inflammation. Complementary proteins found in blood combine to create substances that destroy bacteria. Interferons are produced by T cells and are antiviral proteins that help protect uninfected cells.

Natural killer cells, a subset of lymphocytes, attack and kill abnormal cells such as tumor cells and virus-infected cells during their initial developmental stage, before the immune system is activated.

Other chemical responders include inflammatory mediators.

Inflammation

Inflammation is a sequence of events that seeks to destroy pathogens and aid in tissue repair (see Figures 18-15 and 18-16).

Cardinal signs and symptoms of inflammation can be remembered by the acronym SHARP, which stands for:

- **S**welling
- **H**eat
- **A** loss of function
- **R**edness
- **P**ain

The inflammatory response begins with vasodilation and migration of WBCs to the site. Vasodilation increases local circulation; thus an increase in heat and redness occurs. Cells release histamines and kinins; these chemicals sustain vasodilation and increase permeability in the walls of local blood capillaries. These changes allow blood plasma to cross into the interstitial spaces. This excess fluid causes swelling, which results in increased tissue pressure, thereby causing pain. The sensation of pain, combined with swelling and muscle splinting, limits motion, producing a loss of function.

Shortly after the inflammatory response is activated, migrated white blood cells engulf cellular debris, foreign matter, and pathogens. Interstitial fluids cleanse the area and dilute toxic materials. Clotting proteins located in blood assemble a clot to seal any breaks in vessel walls, to form partitions, and to help isolate the area. Most inflammatory responses conclude between day 4 and 6 of the initial inflammatory response.

It is important to note that inflammation is not synonymous with infection. *Infection* occurs when pathogens reside in/on the body. *Inflammation* is the body's response to a pathogen or insult to tissues such as by trauma.

> *"We should be careful to get out of an experience all the wisdom that is in it. Not like the cat that sits down on a hot stove lid. She will never sit down on a hot stove lid again. And that is well; but also, she will never sit down on a cold one anymore."*
> —Mark Twain

SPECIFIC IMMUNITY

Specific immunity involves diverse but specific responses to invaders deploying specialized lymphocytes; B cells and T cells. Once these lymphocytes are fully developed, they travel to areas of lymphatic tissues.

When T cells and B cells come into contact with a pathogen, they are activated for that specific pathogen. This interaction can occur in three main ways. One way is for the pathogen to travel through the lymph to a lymph node. Another way is for the pathogen to travel through the blood to the lymphatic tissue in the spleen. The third way is for

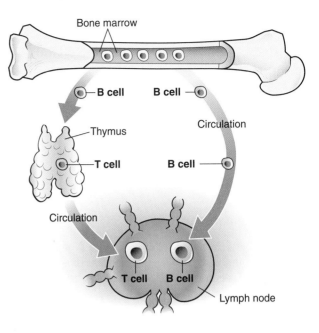

FIGURE 27-5 Development of B and T cells.

the pathogen to penetrate mucous membranes and come in contact with the embedded lymphatic nodules. Once activated, T cells and B cells clone themselves by the thousands, which accounts for the swelling of lymph nodes during infection.

T Cells

T cells begin as B cells migrating from bone marrow and travel to the thymus, where they complete their maturation (Figure 27-5). They recognize pathogens and respond by releasing inflammatory and toxic substances. Specialized T cells, called CD4$^+$ cells, initiate immune responses. Other cells, called CD8$^+$ cells, suppress the response. Some T cells develop into memory cells and handle pathogenic reexposure.

B Cells

B cells grow and mature in the bone marrow. These cells produce antibodies, which circulate in body fluids such as blood and lymph. Their antibodies inactivate pathogens as they come across them. Some B cells, like T cells, become memory cells and handle reexposure.

IMMUNE SYSTEM DYSFUNCTIONS

Dysfunctions of the immune system can occur in several ways and include immune deficiencies, hypersensitivities, or autoimmune diseases.

Immune Deficiency

Immune deficiency, or immunosuppression, occurs when the body is unable to launch a proper immune response. The body becomes more susceptible to diseases. Some immune deficiencies are present at birth, but most arise later in life, such as happens with acquired immunodeficiency syndrome (AIDS). Diabetes causes mild immune suppression. The immune system in elderly people is often weaker than in younger individuals. Chronic stress also suppresses the immune system.

Hypersensitivity

Hypersensitivity reactions are altered immunologic responses to otherwise harmless substances. These reactions may be immediate or delayed. There are four basic types of hypersensitivity.

Type I. This encompasses allergic reactions such as hay fever, allergic sinusitis, allergic contact dermatitis, food allergies, and anaphylaxis. Most hypersensitivity reactions are type I. Because of this, most health care professions use the term *allergy* to indicate type I hypersensitivity.

Type II. This includes tissue-specific reactions such as ABO blood incompatibility and some drug and graft or transplant reactions.

Type III. These are immune complex–mediated reactions such as seen in systemic lupus erythematosus and some dietary reactions such as to gluten (wheat).

Type IV. Type IV reactions are cell-mediated reactions, such as those seen in cases of irritant contact dermatitis (poison ivy, metals) and some graft or transplant reactions.

Autoimmune Disease

In autoimmune diseases, T and B cells are unable to distinguish the body's own tissues from something that is foreign to the body. These cells then attack normal tissues. For instance, in rheumatoid arthritis, the immune system attacks the synovial lining of joints. In multiple sclerosis, the immune system attacks the myelin sheath around neurons in the central nervous system. In type 1 diabetes mellitus, the immune system attacks the insulin-producing cells of the pancreas.

LYMPHATIC AND IMMUNE PATHOLOGIES

Because the lymphatic system is involved in inflammatory, circulatory, and cancer disorders, diseases limited to the lymphatic system are few. The ones included in this section are edema/lymphedema and enlarged lymph nodes. Massage considerations are tailored for therapists without advanced training in lymphatic massage. Therapists with advanced training will be able to identify both workable and nonworkable conditions and make appropriate decisions including the administration of specialized protocols.

Disorders of the Lymphatic System

Edema/Lymphedema. *Edema* is the abnormal accumulation of fluids due to a sluggish or overloaded lymph transport system. Skin over the swollen area may be pale or reddish pink in color; it may appear shiny and tight.

Edema can also be pitting or nonpitting. *Pitting edema* is used to describe edema that leaves a pit or dent in a swollen area once the skin is compressed for a few seconds and released; the edematous tissue rebounds slowly. *Nonpitting edema* does not leave a dent after it is compressed and released. Most edema is nonpitting.

Edema may be caused by prolonged inactivity or a high salt intake. Some medications can cause mild edema (corticosteroids, nonsteroidal antiinflammatories, and hormone replacement). Heart, liver, and kidney diseases often have edema as one of their presenting signs. Edema is often associated with injuries, as well as local or systemic inflammatory processes. In this case, signs of inflammation such as redness, heat, and pain may also be present.

You may hear the terms lymphedema and edema used interchangeably. Both are conditions that involve swelling, but they have very different causes. *Lymphedema* is abnormal accumulation of fluids specifically caused by an obstruction in lymph flow or a decreased number of lymph vessels, which results in swelling. Lymphedema is essentially mechanical failure of the lymphatic system. On the other hand, edema is abnormal accumulation of fluids from a sluggish or overloaded lymph transport system. Edema represents a problem with fluid accumulation rather than fluid obstruction. Lymphedema is usually caused by a condition such as an infection, chronic inflammation, or tumors. It can also be from medical procedures that damage or remove lymph nodes. The latter may occur in cases of cancer treatments, such as surgery and radiation therapy.

Avoid the area if it is red and warm as these are signs of inflammation. Also avoid the area if the client indicates that it tends to swell, especially in cases of past surgery or radiation therapy. Otherwise, avoid vigorous massage and aggressive techniques such as friction as they may cause a localized inflammatory response and increase swelling. Place the noninflamed swollen area on cushions to raise it above the level of the heart. Use only gentle superficial gliding strokes applied centripetally. Massage proximal to the swollen area first if it is located on the extremities. All forms of thermotherapy are contraindicated because it can increase swelling.

Enlarged Lymph Nodes. Enlarged lymph nodes may indicate an underlying local or systemic infection. If the cause is systemic infection, other signs and symptoms may be present, such as chills, fever, fatigue, loss of appetite, and headaches. When palpated, enlarged lymph nodes feel hard, similar to a tablet or capsule under the skin. The skin over the lymph nodes may be red or hot, and the limb distal to the affected area or areas may be edematous.

If the condition is accompanied by a systemic disease, massage is postponed until the disease has resolved. Otherwise, treat as a local contraindication.

Disorders of Immunity

In general, immune disorders represent an immune malfunction and may generate a hypersensitive reaction (allergy), an autoimmune disease, or an immunodeficiency disorder.

Allergy. Allergies, or hypersensitivity reactions, are altered immunologic responses to otherwise harmless substances. These reactions may be immediate or delayed. Common allergic reactions include hay fever, allergic sinusitis, and contact dermatitis.

Massage can be performed so long as the client is not experiencing any acute allergic reaction or difficulty breathing. Before massage, ascertain allergens to which the client is sensitive and eliminate them from the massage area. Avoid aromatherapy and any scent that may trigger an allergic reaction in susceptible clients.

Chronic Fatigue Syndrome. Chronic fatigue syndrome (CFS) is characterized by prolonged and severe tiredness and disabling fatigue. Fatigue is not relieved by rest and may worsen with physical or mental activity. Along with persistent fatigue, the person may also experience confusion and memory deficits, sleep disturbance, influenza-like signs and symptoms, such as low-grade fever, sore throat, headache, and unexplained muscle soreness.

Because symptoms vary daily, ask about current symptoms and adjust the massage accordingly. If your client is feeling overly fatigued, reduce treatment time to 30 minutes, and use lighter-than-normal pressure.

Systemic Lupus Erythematosus. Systemic lupus erythematosus (SLE), also called lupus, is a chronic autoimmune, inflammatory disease in which connective tissue is under attack. It commonly affects skin, bones and joints, nerves, kidneys, lungs, and other organs. Lupus is the most common autoimmune disease, with periods of remission and exacerbation (typical with all autoimmune diseases). A rash may develop on the face, spreading from one cheek across the nose on to the other cheek, and is called a butterfly rash or malar rash. Fever, enlarged lymph nodes, and extreme fatigue may be noted. Fever is often the first sign of exacerbation.

Massage is contraindicated during periods of exacerbation or when fever is present. During periods of remission, a gentle full-body massage is indicated, avoiding skin rashes. Because symptoms vary daily, ask about current symptoms and adjust the massage accordingly.

Acquired Immunodeficiency Syndrome. Acquired immunodeficiency syndrome, or AIDS, is an infectious viral disease that causes progressive impairment of the immune system. This impairment creates increased susceptibility to infections and malignant tumors. A person is considered HIV-positive when blood tests positive for the virus, even if the infected person has few, if any, symptoms. The person has AIDS when the immune system has weakened to the point at which he or she has had at least three opportunistic diseases, or T cell blood count below 200 cells per milliliter (normal range is between 600 and 1200 cells per millilter). AIDS is the final stage (stage 4) of HIV infection. The average time from exposure to development of AIDS is just over 10 years.

AIDS is caused by a human immunodeficiency virus (HIV). HIV attacks specific T cells, called $CD4^+$ cells, using them as host cells in HIV replication. This leads to their decreased number and function. T cells, in general, are the body's safeguard against pathogens and tumors. HIV is found in body fluids of infected persons. Blood contains the highest concentration, with semen next and then breast milk and vaginal secretions. Tears, sweat, saliva, and urine do not contain enough of the virus to cause infection. The virus can survive up to 15 days at room temperature in the medium of a body fluid but is inactivated at temperatures over 140°F (60°C). It is also inactivated by disinfectants, such as alcohol and household bleach.

The virus is most readily spread by direct contact with blood or semen of an infected person. Sexual contact with an infected person is the primary means of transmission. It is also transmitted by sharing needles or syringes with an infected person or, less commonly, through transfusions of infected blood or blood clotting factors. HIV can be spread by transplacental route, during birth, or post partum from breast milk. HIV cannot be transmitted by simple or casual contact with an infected person. Intact skin is adequate protection from the virus.

Antibodies against HIV appear rapidly after infection through blood products (within 2 to 10 weeks). When the virus is transmitted by sexual activity, the antibodies may not appear for 6 to 14 months. The time period between infection and the appearance of antibodies is known as the *window*. This creates an opportunity of an infected person to transmit the virus unknowingly because the presence of these antibodies helps determine diagnosis.

Approximately 2 to 4 weeks after the initial HIV infection, between 80% and 90% of persons develop *acute retroviral syndrome* (ARS). Common signs and symptoms of ARS are fever, sore throat, enlarged lymph nodes, muscle and joint pains, and night sweats. These disease manifestations last between 3 to 14 days. During this time, most affected people who visit a medical facility will be misdiagnosed as having a common infectious disease (such as influenza) with the same symptoms.

Clinical stage 1 is marked by a period of asymptomatic infection. During clinical stages 2 and 3, more general signs and symptoms of HIV infection appear, such as unexplained weight loss, diarrhea, fatigue, night sweats, enlarged lymph nodes, fungal infections, and recurrent respiratory infections. Immunodeficiency is now more evident and marked by frequent or opportunistic infections. T cell count plummets, and the person enters the final stage of infection. In the final stage, called stage 4 or AIDS, infections become more prominent and more serious, which eventually lead to death.

Inquire about areas that need to be avoided, including skin lesions, enlarged lymph nodes, and the most recent site of blood work. Inquire about your client's vitality. (Can he or she climb a flight of stairs without feeling out of breath? If not, reduce treatment time to 30 minutes, and use lighter-than-normal pressure.) In general, individuals who are HIV positive can typically tolerate a more vigorous massage, and individuals with AIDS cannot.

Ask about any secondary diseases (e.g., shingles, tuberculosis, lymphoma) and address them in the treatment plan. Because the immune system of a HIV-infected client is not fully functional, your client is more susceptible to contacting infections through simple exposure. You are a greater health hazard to an HIV-infected client than an infected client is to you. If you know or suspect that you have contracted an infection (e.g., a cold, the flu), reschedule the massage for the client's benefit.

SPOTLIGHT ON RESEARCH

Research suggests that massage therapy may:

- Assist in lymphatic drainage
- Decrease edema
- Reduce edema and lymphedema
- Increase killer T cells and other markers of healthy immune system function
- Promote increases in lymphocyte levels
- Promote immune system health and function and overall well-being through combined mechanical, physiologic, and psychologic therapeutic effects
- Decrease fatigue and other symptoms in persons with chronic fatigue syndrome
- Reduce anxiety and stress and increased natural killer cell activity in persons who were HIV-positive

E-RESOURCES

Evolve

http://evolve.elsevier.com/Salvo/MassageTherapy

- Chapter challenge
- Flash cards
- Photo gallery
- Educational animations
- Weblinks

BIBLIOGRAPHY

Abrahams P, Marks S, Hutchings R: *McMinn's color atlas of human anatomy*, St Louis, 2003, Mosby.

Applegate EJ: *The anatomy and physiology learning system*, ed 3, Philadelphia, 2006, Saunders.

Beers MH, Berkow R: *The Merck manual of diagnosis and therapy*, Whitehouse Station, NJ, 2006, Merck Research Laboratories.

Chikly B: *Silent waves: theory and practice of lymph drainage therapy, an osteopathic lymphatic technique*, ed 2, Portland, Ore, 2002, IHH Publishing.

Crawley J, Van De Graaff KM: *A photographic atlas for anatomy and physiology*, Englewood, Colo, 2002, Morton.

Como D, editor: *Mosby's medical, nursing, and allied health dictionary*, ed 6, St Louis, 2002, Mosby.

Damjanov I: *Pathophysiology for the health-related professions*, ed 3, Philadelphia, 2006, Saunders.

Dr Vodder School: *Manual lymph drainage history* (website): http://www.vodderschool.com/manual_lymph_drainage_history. Accessed January 11, 2010.

Dr Vodder School: *Emil Vodder – his life and his life work* (website): http://www.vodderschool.com/emil_vodder_life_work_article. Accessed January 11, 2010.

Eliska O, Eliskova M: Are peripheral lymphatics damaged by high pressure manual massage? *Lymphology* 28:21-30, 1995.

Ferri FF: *2003 Ferri's clinical advisor, instant diagnosis and treatment*, St Louis, 2003, Mosby.

Foeldi M: *Foldi's textbook of lymphology for physicians, and lymphedema therapist*, ed 2, St Louis, 2007, Mosby/Elsevier.

Frazier MS, Drzymkowski JW: *Essentials of human diseases and conditions*, ed 3, Philadelphia, 2004, Saunders.

Fritz S: *Essential sciences for therapeutic massage*, ed 3, St Louis, 2009, Mosby.

Fritz S: *Fundamentals of therapeutic massage*, ed 4, St Louis, 2009, Mosby.

Gould BE: *Pathophysiology for the health professions*, ed 3, Philadelphia, 2006, Saunders.

Gray H, Pickering P, Howden R: *Gray's anatomy*, ed 29, Philadelphia, 1974, Running Press.

Guyton A: *Human physiology and mechanisms of disease*, ed 6, Philadelphia, 1996, Saunders.

Haubrich WS: *Medical meanings: a glossary of word origins*, New York, 1984, Harcourt Brace Jovanovich.

Huether SE, McCance KL: *Understanding pathophysiology*, ed 3, St Louis, 2004, Mosby.

Jacob S, Francone C: *Elements of anatomy and physiology*, Philadelphia, 1989, Saunders.

Kalat JW: *Biological psychology*, ed 8, Belmont, Calif, 2003, Wadsworth.

Kapit W, Elson LM: *The anatomy coloring book*, ed 3, New York, 2002, Benjamin Cummings.

Kumar V, Abbas A, Fausto N: *Robbins and Cotran physiologic basis of disease*, ed 7, St Louis, 2005, Mosby.

Marieb EN: *Essentials of human anatomy and physiology*, ed 8, New York, 2005, Benjamin Cummings.

Martini FH, Bartholomew EF: *Essentials of anatomy and physiology*, ed 3, New York, 2003, Benjamin Cummings.

McAleer N: *The body almanac*, Garden City, NY, 1985, Doubleday.

McCance K, Huether S: *Pathophysiology: the biological basis for disease in adults and children*, St Louis, 2006, Mosby.

Merck manual, ed 17, Whitehouse Station, NJ, 1998, Merck and Co.

Moore KL: *Clinically oriented anatomy*, ed 5, Baltimore, 2005, Lippincott Williams & Wilkins.

Netter FH: *Atlas of human anatomy*, ed 3, Teterboro, NJ, 2003, Icon Learning Systems.

Newton D: *Pathology for massage therapists*, ed 2, Portland, Ore, 1995, Simran.

Premkumar K: *Pathology A to Z, a handbook for massage therapists*, Baltimore, 1999, Lippincott Williams & Wilkins.

Salvo SG: *Mosby's pathology for massage therapists*, ed 2, St Louis, 2009, Mosby.

Solomon EP, Phillips GA: *Understanding human anatomy and physiology*, Philadelphia, 1987, WB Saunders.

Thibodeau G, Patton K: *Anatomy and physiology*, ed 6, St Louis, 2006, Mosby.

Thibodeau G, Patton K: *Structure and function of the body*, ed 12, St Louis, 2004, Mosby.

Tortora GJ: *Introduction to the human body: the essentials of anatomy and physiology*, ed 5, Hoboken, NJ, 2000, John Wiley & Sons.

Tortora GJ, Grabowksi SR: *Principles of anatomy and physiology*, ed 11, New York, 2005, John Wiley & Sons.

Travell JG, Simons D: *Myofascial pain and dysfunction, the trigger point manual*, Baltimore, 1992, Lippincott Williams & Wilkins.

Venes D, Thomas CL, Taber CW: *Taber's cyclopedic medical dictionary*, ed 20, Philadelphia, 2005, FA Davis.

Vodder's Manual Lymphatic Drainage (website): http://www.drainagelymphatique.info/VodderMLD.html. Accessed January 11, 2010.

Wiley Online Library: *The Vodder school: the Vodder method* (website): http://www3.interscience.wiley.com/journal/75501211/abstract. Accessed January 11, 2010.

MATCHING I

Place the letter of the answer next to the term or phrase that best describes it.

A. Cervical
B. Cisterna chyli
C. Inguinal
D. Lymph

E. Lymph nodes
F. Peyer patches
G. Right lymphatic duct
H. Spleen

I. Thoracic duct
J. Thymus
K. Tonsils
L. Vermiform appendix

_____ 1. Term for lymph nodes located in the groin area

_____ 2. Duct that drains lymph from the right arm, right side of head, and right half of thorax into the right subclavian vein

_____ 3. Lymphatic tissue located in the lower portion of the small intestine

_____ 4. Groups of specialized lymph tissues located in the oral cavity and pharynx

_____ 5. Structures located along lymph vessels that filter lymph

_____ 6. Term for lymph nodes located in the neck region

_____ 7. Lymphatic structure attached to the cecum of the large intestines

_____ 8. Fluid found in lymphatic vessels

_____ 9. Duct that drains lymph from the majority of the body into the left subclavian vein

_____ 10. Largest lymphatic organ

_____ 11. Lymphatic sac located between the abdominal aorta and second lumbar region; inferior portion of the thoracic duct

_____ 12. Lymph gland located behind the sternum that is also an endocrine gland

MATCHING II

Place the letter of the answer next to the term or phrase that best describes it.

A. Autoimmune diseases
B. B cells
C. Bone marrow and thymus
D. Hypersensitivity

E. Immunity
F. Lymph capillaries
G. Lymph vessels
H. Lymphatic drainage

I. Lymphocytes
J. Nonspecific immunity
K. Specific immunity
L. T cells

_____ 1. These cell types include CD4+ cells and CD8+ cells

_____ 2. Type of immunity that includes skin and mucosa, phagocytic white blood cells, natural killer cells, inflammation, and fever

_____ 3. Type of disease that involves the body's attacking its own normal tissue because it thinks it is foreign

_____ 4. Cell type that includes T cells and B cells

_____ 5. Term used to describe allergic reactions, blood incompatibility, and contact dermatitis

_____ 6. Term used to describe the movement of lymph

_____ 7. Type of immunity that involves activation of T cells and B cells for a particular pathogen and then attacking it

_____ 8. Vessels that have thin walls and more valves compared with veins

_____ 9. Generative lymphatic structures; produce precursors of all lymphocytes

_____ 10. General term used to describe complex reactions that involves all body systems as they join together to eliminate pathogens, foreign substances, or toxic materials

_____ 11. Tiny open-ended vessels located in tissue spaces throughout the body except for the brain, spinal cord, and cornea

_____ 12. Cells that produce antibodies, which circulate in body fluids such as blood and lymph

CASE STUDY

Lupus

Judy is a client referred to you by a local lupus support group. She was diagnosed with systemic lupus erythematosus when she was in her late 20s. That was about 5 years ago.

Since Judy is quite familiar with the disease, she calls you to make an appointment when her condition is in remission. She requests an appointment right away, since it is impossible to predict how long the remission state will last.

You can see her today at 4 PM.

Judy arrives with a big smile. She walked a mile this morning and swam a few laps after lunch. Good vitality? Check.

You inquire about any skin rashes; she shows you a reddish, slightly raised rash over her cheeks and across her nose.

Judy also brushes her fingertips between her left and right clavicles and says that there is also a rash there. Check.

What are some treatment guidelines that are appropriate for Judy today?

CRITICAL THINKING

During a massage session, you notice that the lymph nodes in your client's neck, armpits, and groin are swollen. Should you continue the massage as usual, alter the routine, or stop entirely? What guides your decision?

CHAPTER 28

Respiratory System

"Life is known only by those who have found a way to be comfortable with change and the unknown. Given the nature of life, there may be no security, but only adventure."

—Rachel Naomi Remen

LEARNING OBJECTIVES

After completing this chapter, the student should be able to:

- List basic anatomy and describe physiology of the respiratory system.
- Explain the mechanisms of breathing, both for inhalation and exhalation.
- Define factors that control normal breathing and abnormal breathing patterns.
- Contrast and compare internal and external respiration.
- Describe reflexes that affect breathing.
- Name types of pathologic conditions of the respiratory system, giving characteristics of and massage considerations for each.

INTRODUCTION

Breathing has long been the inspiration of poets and philosophers. Books are filled with references such as *his dying breath, her breath rose and fell, his breath quickened,* and *he breathed life into them.* Breath and the breathing process are synonymous with life itself. Breathing is the most easily observable of the body's vital signs. Through respiration, we take in new air, extract oxygen from it, and expel carbon dioxide and other waste gases back into the atmosphere. Every cell of the body needs oxygen, and delivery is accomplished by way of the bloodstream. The respiratory and cardiovascular systems work together to provide oxygen to the tissues and remove metabolic wastes away. Failure of either system has the same effects on the body, including disruption of homeostasis and rapid cell death from oxygen deprivation.

The respiratory system also functions in smell (olfaction) and speech production, and helps maintain homeostasis. Respiration and breathing are used in the expression of emotion, such as laughing, crying, bursts of anger and frustration, fear and anxiety, and sighs of relief.

Respiration is the movement of air in and out of the lungs. It is also the exchange of oxygen and carbon dioxide between the lungs and the blood (external respiration) and the blood and the body tissues (internal respiration). **Breathing** is a mechanical action of inhalation (inspiration) and exhalation (expiration) that draws oxygen into the lungs and then releases carbon dioxide into the atmosphere. On average, adults breathe 12 to 16 times per minute.

ANATOMY

The organs of respiration are divided into the upper and lower respiratory tracts. The upper respiratory tract consists of the:
- Nose and nasal cavity
- Pharynx
- Larynx

The lower respiratory tract consists of the:
- Trachea
- Bronchi and bronchioles
- Alveoli
- Lungs

The diaphragm, the main muscle of respiration, and the sinuses are also studied in this system.

PHYSIOLOGY

The functions of the respiratory system include the following:
- **Exchange of gases:** Oxygen and carbon dioxide exchange is the primary function of the respiratory system (Figure 28-1). This gas exchange occurs in the lungs and through the capillary walls.
- **Olfaction:** *Olfaction* refers to the sense of smell. It is through the act of inhalation that we detect scents.
- **Sound production:** Sound production occurs by air moving over the vocal cords. This action, combined with movements of the lips, facial muscles, and tongue, forms words and produces speech.
- **Maintenance of homeostasis:** The respiratory system helps maintain oxygen levels in the blood. It also helps maintain homeostasis through the elimination of wastes (e.g., carbon dioxide, heat). Excess carbon dioxide in the blood can lead to dangerously acidic conditions. The act of breathing helps regulate blood pH.

UPPER RESPIRATORY TRACT

Nose

The **nose** is the port of entry for air and the beginning of the air conduction pathway. The nose is divided into external and internal portions. What we see and feel as the external structure of the nose is mostly cartilage. The upper third, or bridge, of the nose is formed by two small nasal bones.

The nostrils are called *anterior* or *external nares* (*singular,* naris). Air enters the external nares via inhalation and then passes across nasal hairs, which trap particles and foreign materials. Air then flows into the nasal cavity.

Nasal Cavity

Immediately within the nose is the nasal cavity. The **nasal cavity** is separated into left and right halves by a septum. The upper portion of the nasal cavity contains three ridges called *conchae* that extend out of each lateral wall of the nasal cavity (Figure 28-2). The grooved passageway between each conchae is called a *meatus.* The inferior meatus terminates just above two funnel-shaped orifices called the *posterior* or *internal nares.* Air flows from the nasal cavity down the throat.

As air passes through the nasal cavity, it is warmed by superficial blood vessels and moistened by mucosal secretions.

Tiny particles that make it past the nasal hairs are trapped by sticky mucus. Tiny hairlike projections of the mucosae called *cilia* also trap foreign particles, which are transported to the throat where they are either swallowed or coughed out through the mouth. Because of these collective functions, the nasal cavity is often referred to as the "air-conditioning chambers."

Because the nasal mucosa has such a rich blood supply, nosebleeds, or *epistaxis,* often occur as a result of blows to the nose, weak blood vessels, or high blood pressure. Although they are dramatic, nosebleeds are seldom serious.

Olfaction. Olfaction refers to the sense of smell. Through the act of inhalation, scent molecules enter the nose and

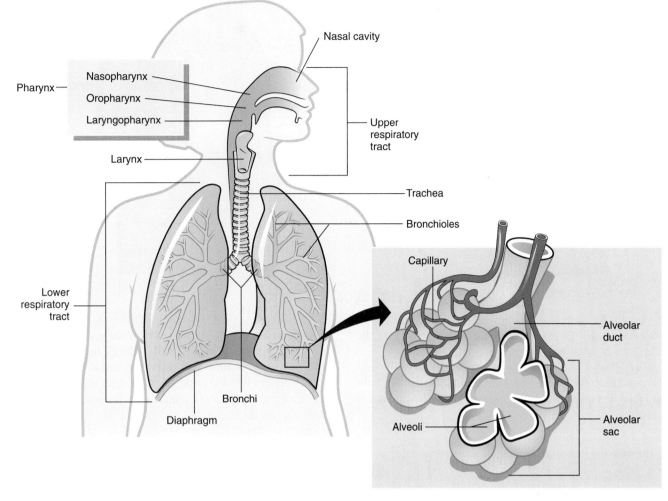

FIGURE 28-1 The respiratory system.

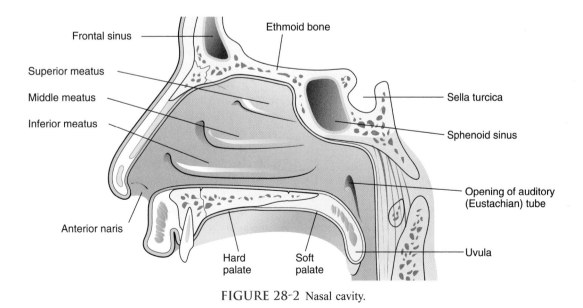

FIGURE 28-2 Nasal cavity.

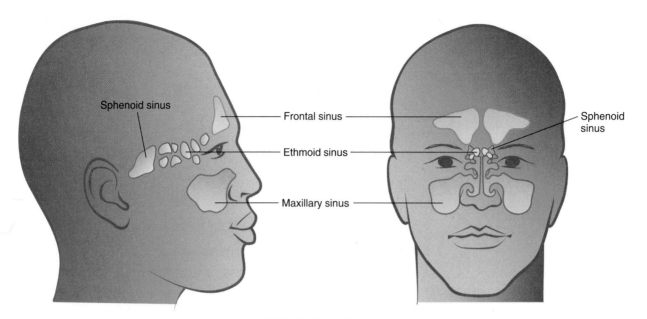

FIGURE 28-3 Sinuses.

are forced against ends of the olfactory nerves (one of the 12 pairs of cranial nerves).

The olfactory nerves lie in the upper third of both nasal cavities. The olfactory nerves connect to the olfactory bulb and then to the cerebral cortex, which interprets scent nerve impulses.

IT'S ALL GREEK TO ME

Term	Meaning
alveoli	*L.* little hollow
apnea	*Gr.* not; breathing
auditory	*L.* to hear
bronchus	*Gr.* windpipe
cilia	*L.* hairlike
conchae	*Gr.* shell
Eustachian	Bartolomeo Eustachio, Italian anatomist (1524-1574)
glottis	*Gr.* back of the tongue
meatus	*L.* passage
olfaction	*L.* to smell
phrenic	*Gr.* diaphragm
pleura	*Gr.* rib; side
pneumo, pneum	*Gr.* air; lungs
pulmo	*L.* lung
trachea	*Gr.* rough
ventilation	*L.* to air
volitional	*L.* will

Gr., Greek; *L.*, Latin.

Sinuses. The sinuses, or paranasal sinuses, are four groups of air-filled cavities in the skull. Sinuses lighten the head and act as resonance chambers for sound. Because the sinuses opens into the nasal cavity, sinuses are prone to the same infections. Sinuses are named for the bones near which they are located (Figure 28-3):
- Frontal sinus
- Sphenoidal sinus
- Ethmoidal sinus
- Maxillary sinus

Pharynx

The **pharynx,** or throat, is a muscular tube approximately 5 inches long that is shared by the respiratory and the digestive systems. Located anterior to the cervical vertebrae, the pharynx extends from behind the nasal cavity (nasopharynx) to the back of the oral cavity (oropharynx) and down to the larynx (laryngopharynx).

The *nasopharynx* contains openings to the Eustachian tubes, which help to equalize pressure in the head, nose, and pharynx. Because of this close proximity, respiratory infections can easily lead to middle ear infections and vice versa.

The *oropharynx* is the portion of the throat that you can see. It contains the tonsils, which help our immune system by protecting against inhaled or ingested pathogens (Figure 28-4).

The *laryngopharynx* begins at the hyoid bone and separates into the esophagus and larynx. Thus, it functions as a pathway for the respiratory and digestive tracts.

Larynx

The **larynx,** or voice box, connects the pharynx to the trachea. The larynx produces sound, while the lips and the tongue create speech.

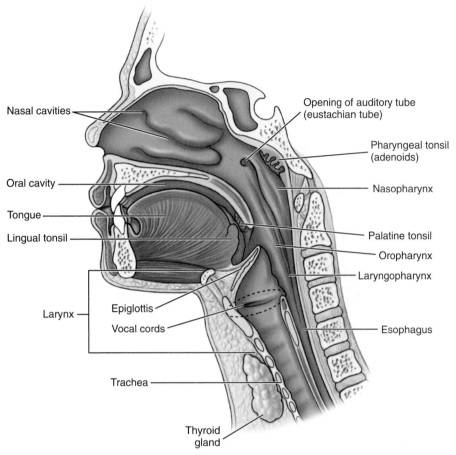

Nasal cavities

Oral cavity

Tongue

Lingual tonsil

Larynx
Epiglottis
Vocal cords

Trachea

Thyroid
gland

Opening of auditory tube
(eustachian tube)

Pharyngeal tonsil
(adenoids)

Nasopharynx

Palatine tonsil

Oropharynx

Laryngopharynx

Esophagus

FIGURE 28-4 Upper respiratory tract.

The larynx consists of single and paired cartilages, ligaments, connective tissue, muscles, and the vocal cords. The single cartilages are the epiglottis, cricoid, and thyroid (Adam's apple), which is the largest. One of the single laryngeal cartilages, the *epiglottis*, closes the trachea during swallowing (deglutition), preventing food from entering the lower respiratory passageways. Because of this function, the epiglottis is referred to as the *guardian of the airways*. The three paired cartilages (arytenoid, corniculate, and cuneiform) attach to and support the vocal cords.

Air passes over the vocal cords, causing vibration and producing sound. In high-pitched sounds, the glottis is narrower and the vocal cords are more tense, whereas in low-pitched sounds, the glottis is wider and the vocal cords are more relaxed.

⊖volve   *One of the interesting things about going to massage school is learning about the human body. To view a photograph of a set of vocal cords, log on to the Evolve website for* Massage Therapy: Principles and Practice, *ed 4, and go to Chapter 28. While there, explore other items of interest for this chapter.* ■

"All things share the same breath."
—Chief Sealth, Duwamish tribe, 1885

LOWER RESPIRATORY TRACT

Trachea

The **trachea,** or windpipe connects the larynx with the bronchi. Located anterior to the esophagus, the trachea measures approximately 9 to 10 inches long and consists of 16 to 21 half-ring hyaline cartilages. These half-ring cartilages serve a dual purpose. The incomplete sections of the ring allow the esophagus to expand into the trachea when a food bolus is swallowed (Figure 28-5). The rings also keep the tracheal wall from collapsing during pressure changes that occur during breathing. The trachea bifurcates at its base into two primary (left and right) bronchi.

Bronchi and Bronchioles

The right and left primary **bronchi** are the large air-conduction passageways leading from the trachea to each lung. The bronchi have the same structural framework as the trachea except that bronchi have more smooth muscle. The right primary bronchus is wider and has a slightly steeper downward angle than the left; because of this feature, foreign bodies more often lodge on the right side.

Each primary bronchus enters the lungs on its respective side, branching out, and becoming smaller (similar to a tree

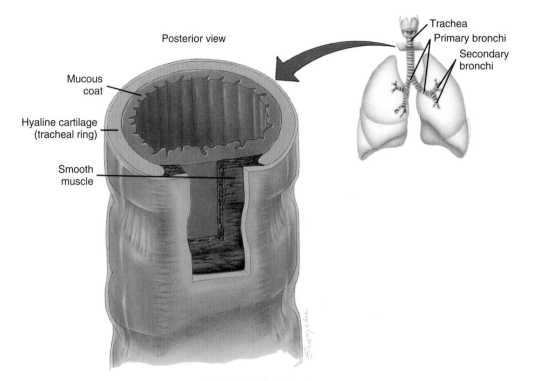

Posterior view

Mucous coat

Hyaline cartilage (tracheal ring)

Smooth muscle

Trachea
Primary bronchi
Secondary bronchi

FIGURE 28-5 Trachea.

trunk and branches). The amount of cartilage within the tube lining gradually decreases until only smooth muscle remains. At that point the tubes are about 1 mm in diameter; they are now called the **bronchioles,** which terminate in the air sacs, or alveoli.

Alveoli

Alveoli, located in the lungs, are tiny sacs surrounded by capillaries and are attached to alveolar ducts. Groups of alveoli are *alveolar sacs*, which resemble a cluster of grapes. Each alveolus is made of single-layer epithelial tissue; this feature makes gas exchange possible. The walls are so thin that imagining their thinness is difficult, but a sheet of notepaper is much thicker. Adult lungs contain approximately 300 to 600 million alveoli, providing an immense surface area of approximately 1000 square feet (ft^2), roughly the area of a handball court. Superficial to the alveoli are numerous capillaries, so many that 900 ml of blood are able to participate in gas exchange at any given time (see Figure 28-1).

Each alveolus is coated with a fluid containing surfactants. *Surfactants* assist in the exchange of gas by stabilizing the alveolus and reducing surface tension. The alveoli are like little balloons. When they deflate, their walls collapse inward and, without surfactants, would stick together, making reinflation difficult. Lungs are the last organs to develop in utero. Infants born prematurely (before 28 gestational weeks) may not have produced enough surfactants for their alveoli to expand properly. Medical advances have done much to rectify this problem.

Lungs

The two **lungs** are the primary organs of respiration (Figure 28-6). They are spongy, elastic, highly vascular structures separated into different lobes. The lungs extend from the diaphragm to just above the clavicles and lie against the interior portion of the ribcage. Although the lungs fill most of the thoracic cavity, they weigh less than 1 lb each. The inferior surface of the lungs is broad and concave to match the shape of the superior surface of the diaphragm. The right lung has three lobes; the left lung has two lobes. A depression called the *cardiac notch* is located in the left lung to accommodate the heart.

The lungs are lined by two pleural membranes. One membrane (visceral pleura) is attached to the lung; the other (parietal pleura) is connected to the mediastinum and internal chest wall. Between these double membranes is a serous fluid. The lubricating fluid helps to reduce friction between the two layers as we breathe.

External respiration takes place in the lungs across the respiratory (alveolar) membrane.

Diaphragm

The **diaphragm** is a dome-shaped muscle that separates the thoracic cavity from the abdominal cavity and is the main muscle of respiration. The diaphragm attaches to the internal chest wall, back of the xyphoid process, and the internal surfaces of the lower six costal cartilages and their adjoining ribs before inserting into its central tendon. The diaphragm

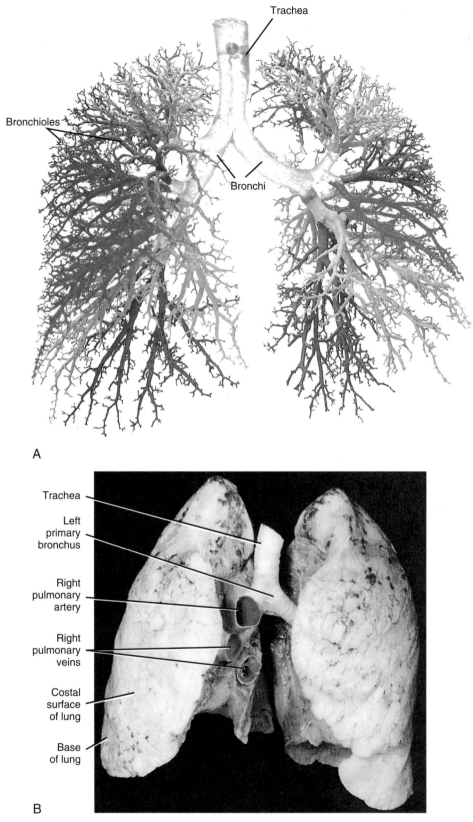

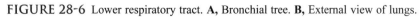

FIGURE 28-6 Lower respiratory tract. **A,** Bronchial tree. **B,** External view of lungs.

ROBERT TISSERAND

Born: November 11, 1948

*"Love what you do. Enjoy listening to people. It can be hard work,
but the potential for helping people is tremendous."*

Robert Tisserand, author and aroma-therapist, was born in London to a father who made baskets and a mother who "did a little of this and that, but mostly raised three kids." Luckily for his "mum," the two girls were not quite as inquisitive as Tisserand, who shares his first "taste" of the aromatherapy experience. "Curiously, I did actually drink a bottle of perfume when I was about 2 years old. My father bought it for my mother in a flea market in Paris in 1945, so the perfume would have been about 5 years old at the time. It was called *Creme de Zofali*. I survived, but the bottle has not."

Considering that it is often the smell and not the taste of foods that makes them appealing, it is easy to understand why a little boy would not think twice before turning up a bottle of perfume. However, aromas affect more than our appetites. Odors of certain plants have been used to dedicate newborns, banish evil spirits, guide dearly departed souls to the other side, and heal all manner of ills in between. Long before frankincense and myrrh were offered to the Christ child, Egyptian physicians were using it in their practices. Greek mythology includes stories regarding the healing properties of aromatic plants, and Romans enjoyed massage with wonderfully scented and unbelievably expensive oils.

What has become a popular trend in the last few years was an academic area of study as far back as the Middle Ages. During this time, essential oils were classified according to the four elements or humors, the degree of *hotness* or *coldness*, and by the shape or color of the plant from which it was derived. For example, lungwort resembles lungs; therefore it was used for the respiratory system. Blue is a calming color; thus plants with blue flowers were considered to have sedative properties. This way of cataloging plant essences was called the *doctrine of signatures*. Astronomy also helped play a role in organizing certain scents. Late in the sixteenth century, Nicholas Culpepper, an astrological physician, associated oils with planetary characteristics. For instance, ylang-ylang is identified as having Venus properties because it has a strong, sweet odor and a slightly yellow tint and is considered an aphrodisiac.

---

contains opening for the passage of the descending aorta, inferior vena cava, and the esophagus (see Figure 16-172).

As the diaphragm contracts and moves downward during inhalation, the thoracic cavity enlarges, creating a vacuum that sucks air into the lungs. As the diaphragm relaxes during exhalation, it arches upward, allowing the lungs to deflate, and the elastic recoil of the alveoli pushes out air.

CHAT ROOM

Because the diaphragm never stops contracting, the potential for trigger point development is tremendous. Tightening of the diaphragm's fibers can cause torquing of the ribcage around the spine and central tendon, thus limiting the efficiency of inhalation. Some ribcage mobilizations and diaphragmatic releases can potentially increase the lung's vital capacity.

In review, air is conducted by the following pathway of structures:

Nose
↓
Nasal cavity
↓
Pharynx
↓
Larynx
↓
Trachea
↓
Bronchi
↓
Bronchioles
↓
Alveoli

ROBERT TISSERAND (*continued*)

The first people to dispense aromatics were the priests. They were the first perfumers or what we would call an *aromatherapists* today. Physicians picked up the practice soon thereafter.

Although aromatherapy (the use of plant-derived essential oils) has been widely used in England for some time, only recently did its climb in popularity start in the United States. Lately, massage therapists are learning more about how aromatherapy can benefit their practices. At the very least, aromatherapy adds another sensory-pleasing dimension to the experience of receiving a massage. However, because of the strong connection between our sense of smell and mood, it can also add other benefits. For instance, lavender is thought to be calming. On the other end of the spectrum, mints and citrus oils have an energizing effect. Mixed with oil or lotion, essential essences are considered by many people to work magic on a myriad of maladies, from clogged sinuses to diarrhea. Aromatherapy can also be ingested (only by trained aromatherapists) for treatment of some ailments.

When asked which five essential oils are most important for massage therapists to always have on hand, Tisserand hesitates, pointing out that, ideally, no limit should be made. However, if choosing only five is necessary, then he recommends eucalyptus, lavender, rosemary, geranium, and ylang-ylang. He also advises therapists to practice the craft in as professional a manner as possible, experiment, and attend some type of training

in aromatherapy. Massage therapists should also be aware that some oils do have contraindications. For example, a popular essential oil for muscular aches and pains, bergamot, can cause photosensitivity.

Tisserand's "taste" for aromatherapy piqued around 1967 at age 19, when he attended a lecture on the subject along with his mother. She bought a book and had it signed by the speaker, Dr. Jean Valnet. A couple of years later, Tisserand became interested in bodywork and did some training in that area. He soon made a conscious decision to pursue a career in aromatherapy. "Not for the money," he laughs, "or I would have given up a long time ago. Basically, I starved for 20 years."

Today, Tisserand teaches others the art of aromatherapy. He has also developed Tisserand essential oil products and distributes them all over the world. His works include the quintessential *The Art of Aromatherapy* (Beekman, 1977), *Aromatherapy to Heal and Tend the Body* (Lotus Light, 1996), and *Essential Oil Safety* (Churchill Livingstone, 1995). Tisserand travels and lectures as an industry consultant.

Tisserand still has his mother's signed copy of Valnet's French aromatherapy book, and after 30 years of hard work, audiences flock to his seminars worldwide, buy his books, seek his advice, and ask for his signature. The little boy who could not resist his mother's bottle of flea market perfume is finally able to sit back and enjoy the sweet smell of success.

BREATHING

Breathing is a mechanical action consisting of two phases, inhalation (inspiration) and exhalation (expiration). These phases are the result of nerve stimulation, muscle contraction, and differences between the pressure in the lungs and the atmospheric pressure outside the lungs.

Inhalation

When we inhale, the diaphragm contracts and moves down. The external intercostal muscles located between the ribs contract to lift the lower portion of the ribcage up and out (Figure 28-7, *A*). This causes pressure in the lungs to be slightly lower compared to atmospheric pressure. As a result, air moves from an area of higher pressure (the atmosphere) to an area of lower pressure (the lungs).

Inhalation, an autonomic nervous system process, can be intensified such as during exercise or it can be forced. Forced inhalation requires additional muscular contraction by the sternocleidomastoid, scalenes, and pectoralis minor. These muscles are regarded as accessory muscles of respiration.

The ease with which the thorax and lungs are able to stretch during inhalation is called *compliance*. The tendency of the thorax and lungs to return to their pre-inhalation size is called *elastic recoil*. See Box 28-1 for terms related to pulmonary volume.

Exhalation

During exhalation, muscles and the diaphragm relax, which deceases the size of the ribcage and lungs (Figure 28-7, *B*). This causes pressure in the lungs to become slightly higher compared to atmospheric pressure. As a result, air moves

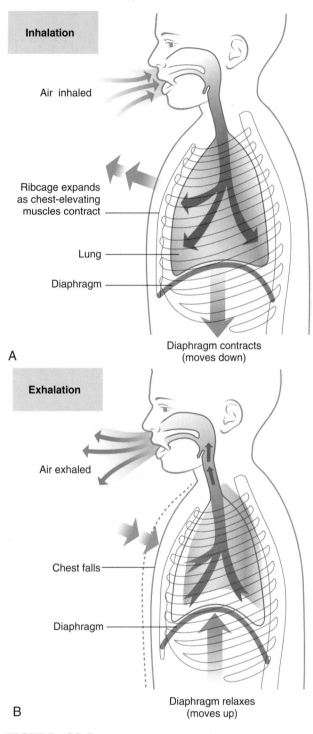

Inhalation

Air inhaled

Ribcage expands as chest-elevating muscles contract

Lung

Diaphragm

Diaphragm contracts (moves down)

A

Exhalation

Air exhaled

Chest falls

Diaphragm

Diaphragm relaxes (moves up)

B

FIGURE 28-7 Mechanisms of breathing. **A,** Inhalation; **B,** Exhalation.

from an area of higher pressure (the lungs) to an area of lower pressure (the atmosphere).

Exhalation, similar to inhalation, can also be forced. Forced exhalation is an active process, using voluntary muscular contractions of the internal intercostal and abdominal muscles.

BOX 28-1

Pulmonary Volumes

Breathing in and out results in different pulmonary volumes of air inside the lungs. These volumes are often used as guidelines in health assessments.

Tidal volume. Amount of air inhaled and exhaled in a single breath during normal breathing, usually while the person is resting.

Inspiratory reserve. Amount of air the person can inhale forcefully after normal tidal volume inspiration.

Expiratory reserve. Amount of air the person can exhale forcefully after a normal exhalation.

Residual volume. Amount of air that remains in the lungs and passageways after a maximal expiration.

Vital capacity. Total of the tidal volume, inspiratory reserve volume, and expiratory reserve volume. In the normal, healthy adult lung, vital capacity usually ranges from 3.5 to 5.5 L of air.

Age, gender, physical fitness, and disease affect vital capacity and expiratory reserve volumes.

Control of Breathing

At rest, adults breathe approximately 12 to 16 times a minute; children breathe twice as fast as adults.

The neurologic respiratory center in the brain's medulla oblongata controls breathing. Impulses travel down the phrenic nerve to the diaphragm. These impulses are also sent to other muscles of respiration.

Several factors help regulate breathing. For example, the brain can modify breathing patterns during laughing or crying and can initiate volitional breathing. *Volitional*, or voluntary, breathing allows you to hold your breath while swimming under water and to take deep breaths to project your voice during public speaking. However, if you control your breath by rapid breathing (hyperventilation), or if you hold your breath too long, you will become unconscious. How long the breath is held is limited by carbon dioxide buildup in the blood.

An increase in body temperature (e.g., fever, exercise) increases respiration, whereas a decrease in body temperature (e.g., hypothermia, jumping into cool water) decreases respiration. Emotions alter the rate of respiration. Fear, grief, and shock slow the rate, whereas excitement, anger, and sexual arousal cause an increase. Chemoreceptors and baroceptors also send nerve impulses to the brain and alter respiration.

Terms indicating abnormal breathing patterns are listed in Box 28-2.

CHAT ROOM

If an individual lives to be age 72, then he or she will have taken more than 530 million breaths of air.

BOX 28-2

Terms Used to Describe Abnormal Breathing Patterns

Hyperpnea: Fast breathing
Tachypnea: Rapid, but shallow breathing
Bradypnea: Slow breathing
Dyspnea: Labored or difficult breathing
Apnea: Absence of normal, spontaneous breathing

MINI-LAB

Using a tape measure, note the change in circumference as you measure the ribcage during inspiration and expiration. Measure other parts of the body, such as the upper and lower ribs and abdomen.

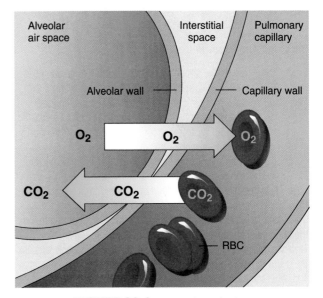

FIGURE 28-8 External respiration.

*"How people treat you is their karma;
how you react is yours."*
—Wayne Dyer

EXTERNAL AND INTERNAL RESPIRATION

The main functions of the respiratory process are to supply the body with oxygen and dispose of carbon dioxide. Cells need oxygen to sustain life. Respiration occurs through two distinct processes: (1) external respiration and (2) internal respiration. Each cell participates in absorption of oxygen and removal of carbon dioxide in connection with these processes.

This process takes place by *diffusion*, or the tendency of molecules to move from an area of high concentration to an area of low concentration.

External Respiration

External respiration, or *pulmonary respiration*, is gas exchange in the lungs. It occurs between blood in capillaries and air in the alveoli that came from the external environment.

Pulmonary arteries transport the body's oxygen-depleted blood to the lungs. Carbon dioxide diffuses from the bloodstream and travels across the respiratory (alveolar) membrane to be released during exhalation. Oxygen then diffuses in the opposite direction, going from the air inside the lungs, across the alveolar (respiratory) membrane, and then binding to the hemoglobin molecule in red blood cells. Oxygen is then transported by the bloodstream to cells throughout the body (Figure 28-8).

Internal Respiration

Internal respiration, or *tissue respiration*, is the gas exchange between blood and the body's tissues.

The pulmonary veins return oxygenated blood to the heart. It then travels throughout the body via systemic blood vessels. While blood is in the capillaries, oxygen moves across the vessel wall to enter cells. Carbon dioxide then diffuses in the opposite direction, going from the cells through the capillary wall and into red blood cells in the bloodstream. Oxygen-depleted blood is then transported to the lungs, where removal of carbon dioxide occurs.

---

e*volve* *The difference between internal and external respiration is often a difficult concept for students to grasp. Because most people learn best visually, a diagram is located on the Evolve website materials for this chapter. I've drawn this image on the board for years and was delighted to find it in a textbook.* ■

REFLEXES THAT AFFECT BREATHING

Some reflexes that can affect breathing are featured next.

Sneeze

Sneezing is a forceful involuntary expulsion of air through the nose and mouth to clear the *upper respiratory passageways*. Most sneezes occur as a result of irritation of the respiratory lining by foreign particles such as dust or pollen.

CHAT ROOM

Massage and Breathing

Notice the wave of the client's breathing movements during the massage. When possible, apply pressure during your client's exhalation and release pressure on the inhalation. This technique not only gives a sense of rhythm to your massage strokes but also uses the client's natural ability to relax during an exhalation to enhance the effectiveness of your work.

Encourage your client to breathe properly during the massage. *While your client is supine*, place your hand just below his or her navel. Ask the client to take a deep breath and to allow his or her belly to elevate your hand. Occasionally, a simple goal such as using the breath to move the therapist's hand helps the client understand the abdominal changes that occur while breathing. *While your client is prone*, place your hand on the small of his or her back and ask the client to take a deep breath, elevating your hand during inhalation. After instructing your client how to breathe for relaxation, teach him or her to use this simple technique when feeling stressed or fatigued.

These types of lessons help teach clients how to relax and how to become aware of their bodies.

⊖volve   *To see an illustration of a breathing wave, log on to the Evolve website and click on Breathing Wave in Chapter 28. Note both the functional and dysfunctional patterns.* ∎

Cough

Coughing is a sudden expulsion of air to clear the *lower respiratory passageways* of irritants or foreign materials. Coughing is a protective reflex but can be voluntarily induced or inhibited. The act of coughing occurs after a brief inhalation. Abdominal muscles contract, which forces air out of the lungs during exhalation. Productive coughing helps clear the respiratory tract.

Hiccup

Hiccups, or hiccoughs, are intermittent involuntary contractions of the diaphragm followed by a spasmodic closure of the vocal cords. The sound occurs when inhaled air hits the closed vocal cords. Hiccups have a variety of causes that appear to be linked to irritation of gastrointestinal sensory nerve endings.

Yawn

A yawn is a very deep inhalation initiated by opening the mouth wide. Some researchers believe that yawning is triggered by the need to increase the oxygen content and decrease carbon dioxide in the blood or as a result of drowsiness, boredom, or depression, but the precise cause is unknown.

CHAT ROOM

Breathing and Relaxation

Breathing not only reflects our physiologic and psychologic states but also creates them. Actors have known this for many years. When their character was anxious, actors use shallow, rapid breaths to help them become anxious. Conversely, when a scene requires their character to appear calm and relaxed, they use slow, deep breaths to bring them to a state of relaxation. Massage therapists use breathing techniques themselves while they are giving a massage and often teach these techniques to their clients.

The most effective type of breathing to produce relaxation is deep, slow abdominal or diaphragmatic breathing. During deep breathing, the muscles of the abdominal wall expand when the diaphragm moves down during inhalation; the abdominal contents get a massage as they are compressed and released.

When we breathe deeply, it is a total body experience. Deep breathing can ease pain, relax tension, or introduce much-needed energy into the body. Shallow breathing does not encourage relaxation and can create tension in the neck and shoulders.

Breathing creates and reflects our emotional sphere; therefore deep, full breaths positively affect the free expression of our feelings. Restrictive breathing tends to constrict our expressions and wall off our feelings; we feel disconnected from the world around us.

The rhythm of breathing can give us an indication of how we feel about our surroundings. If we observe a slight pause before inhalation, then this may announce a fear of new experiences. People inevitably stop breathing in an attempt to prevent something from happening. Clients hold their breath during a massage when the pressure is uncomfortable. A slight pause before exhalation may indicate a fear of the client's own personal expression.

Imagine that the air around you has a fluid quality. As you inhale, the bottom portion of your lungs fills up first, similar to a glass of water. This filling causes a depression of the diaphragm and an expansion of the abdomen and thorax. As air fills the upper lungs, the ribcage expands on all sides. The spine also moves to accommodate the expansion. To complete your inhalation, puff out your cheeks and tightly close your lips. Allow your breath to burst out of your lips and exhale through your mouth, nose, or both. Although exhalation is typically a passive event, you may force air out of your lungs by contracting your abdominal muscles and "kissing your belly button to your spine." As you breathe, you should feel your body, especially your spine, ribs, and abdomen, move. Subtle movements may be felt in the extremities.

Children and most animals breathe with their bellies. Observe a sleeping cat or a child. The belly moves in a wave during breathing. On mornings when you can wake up naturally (without an alarm), notice how you are breathing; you will probably be doing abdominal breathing. Encourage your body to breathe this way throughout the day.

RESPIRATORY PATHOLOGIES

Upper Respiratory Tract Infections

Common Cold. Common colds are acute viral infections of the upper respiratory tract, usually confined to the nose and throat. It is contagious and can spread through airborne droplets or by touching infected objects, then touching the nose or mouth. Signs and symptoms include coughing, sneezing, watery eyes, nasal congestion and thick yellow discharge, headache, sore throat, and hoarseness. Slight fever (102°F) and chills may accompany a cold. Other names for a common cold are head cold and infectious rhinitis.

Postpone massage until the client has completely recovered, usually 5 days from disease onset.

Sinusitis. Sinusitis is inflammation of the sinuses. As inflamed mucosa swells and respiratory secretions buildup, the person often experiences headaches and facial pain, which intensifies when bending over. The person has difficulty breathing through the nose. Fever often accompanies acute cases, but not chronic cases.

Postpone massage if the client is experiencing fever. Once the client has been fever-free for 48 hours, he or she may receive massage. For chronic sinusitis, avoid the prone position if pressure of the face cushion is uncomfortable or if the client has breathing difficulty. While the client is supine, use a semireclining position. Deep localized friction applied over the sinuses may help to reduce pain.

Pharyngitis. Also called sore throat, pharyngitis is inflammation of the pharynx. Most often, pharyngitis is a sign of a disease (e.g., common cold, sinusitis, influenza) and not a disease itself. Strep throat, a type of pharyngitis, is due to the bacterium *Streptococcus*. Other causes of pharyngitis are irritation from nasal secretions and inhaled irritants (e.g., cigarette smoke). Pharyngitis is also caused from throat strain from yelling, as might happen during sports events.

Ascertain from your client the cause of the pharyngitis. If pharyngitis is due to infection, postpone massage until the infection has completely resolved and your client is symptom-free for at least 48 hours. For noninfective causes of pharyngitis, massage can be performed.

Laryngitis. Laryngitis is inflammation of the larynx. Most often, respiratory infections are the cause of laryngitis. Other causes are irritation from voice strain such as yelling during sports events or from reflux of stomach acids seen in gastroesophageal reflux disease (GERD). The main symptoms of laryngitis are hoarseness and loss of voice.

Ascertain from your client the cause of the laryngitis. If it is due to an infectious disease, postpone massage until the condition has resolved and your client has been symptom-free for 48 hours. If the laryngitis is not caused by infection, massage can be performed. Do not require your client to talk extensively. Perhaps ask questions and suggest that the client shake or nod his or her head in response, or use an alternative communication method.

Hay Fever. Hay fever, or allergic rhinitis, is hypersensitivity of the nasal mucosa to allergens. An acute allergic attack is characterized by sudden bouts of sneezing, swelling, and profuse watery discharge of the nasal mucosa, with itching and watering of the eyes. During an allergy attack, a bronchodilator may be used to help open the airways.

Postpone massage if your client is experiencing an acute allergic attack. Before massage, ascertain what allergens your client is sensitive to, and eliminate them from the massage area. Side-lying and semireclining positions are preferred if your client is concerned about ease of breathing or has difficulty breathing in the prone position. Avoid aromatherapy and any scent that may trigger hay fever; this includes scented soaps and deodorants (chamomile is a form of ragweed). If your client uses a bronchodilator, ask the person have it handy in the event of an allergy attack.

Influenza. Influenza, or flu, is an acute, highly contagious viral disease of the upper respiratory tract. The virus is transmitted by infected droplets or touching infected objects (e.g., doorknobs, phones, computer keyboards, shopping cart handles) and then touching the nose or mouth.

Influenza is characterized by sudden onset of signs and symptoms such as chills, fever (temperatures can be as high as 104°F), and sore throat. Fever lasting more than 5 days may indicate a secondary infection, such as pneumonia.

Massage is contraindicated as influenza is contagious. Postpone massage until the condition has resolved and the client has been symptom-free for 48 hours.

Infectious Mononucleosis. Infectious mononucleosis, or mono, is a contagious respiratory infection. It is most commonly transmitted by contaminated saliva (i.e., kissing) or respiratory droplets, and by touching infected objects (doorknobs, phones, computer keyboards, shopping cart handles), then touching the nose or mouth.

Massage is contraindicated until the client has completely recovered and is cleared for massage by his or her physician.

Lower Respiratory Tract Infections

Pneumonia. Pneumonia is a lung infection. In 75% of cases, the cause of pneumonia is bacteria. Viruses, fungi, protozoa, or parasites may also cause the disease. In the United States, pneumonia is the most common cause of death from infectious disease and the sixth leading cause of death. The most commonly affected persons are older adults, infants, and immunocompromised individuals.

Massage is postponed until your client has completely recovered.

Chronic Obstructive Pulmonary Diseases

Asthma. Asthma is a chronic, inflammatory disorder of the airways characterized by bronchial obstruction in susceptible persons. Asthma is also classified as an allergic disorder. Immediate treatment during an asthma attack involves the use of inhaled medications that relax smooth muscle in the bronchi and reopen the airways.

Before massage, ascertain what allergens your client is sensitive to and eliminate them from the massage area. If your client uses a bronchodilator, ask the person to have it handy in the event of an asthma attack. Side-lying and semi-reclining positions are preferred if your client is concerned about ease of breathing.

Bronchitis. Inflammation of the bronchial mucosa with resultant swelling and mucus hypersecretion is called bronchitis. There are two types: acute and chronic. Acute bronchitis usually follows a viral upper respiratory tract infection; acute cases resolve along with the respiratory infection. The most common type, chronic bronchitis, is usually caused from chronic exposure to cigarette smoke.

Massage is contraindicated if your client has acute bronchitis. Once your client with acute bronchitis has been symptom-free for 48 hours, he or she may receive massage. If your client has chronic bronchitis, side-lying and semi-reclining positions are preferred if he or she is concerned about ease of breathing.

Emphysema. Emphysema involves permanent enlargement of lower airways accompanied by destruction of alveolar walls. Pulmonary obstruction results from destroyed lung tissue rather than mucus production and inflammation (as seen in asthma and chronic bronchitis). Because there is no excess mucus production, there is little coughing and modest, if any, sputum production.

Avoid the prone position if your client is concerned about or is experiencing breathing difficulties. In these cases, use a side-lying and semi-reclining position while your client is supine.

Obstructive Sleep Apnea. A condition rather than a disease, apnea is temporary cessation of breathing (usually lasting 15 seconds) or absence of spontaneous breathing. The most common type of sleep apnea is obstructive sleep apnea (OSA). Relaxed muscles and tongue block the airway while the person is lying down and asleep. Obstruction can also be the result of mucus buildup from chronic obstructive pulmonary disease. While the affected person is sleeping, carbon dioxide levels slowly build up in the blood. The brain senses changes in blood chemistry and rouses the person to breathe normally. The person may wake up as many as 20 to 30 times an hour and may or may not be aware of waking frequency.

Ask your client what positions he or she usually sleeps in. Use the preferred position for the major portion of the massage.

CHAT ROOM

Cigarette smoking eventually destroys alveoli and reduces gas exchange in the lungs. Smoking also destroys respiratory cilia that remove particles in the nasal cavity and respiratory tract. As cilia die and the respiratory lining becomes irritated, the body produces excess mucus to trap the foreign particles in the cigarette smoke and to protect these delicate membranes. This circumstance is why smokers often cough (trying to expel the extra mucus).

Smoking can also inhibit macrophage cells, which increases the likelihood of respiratory infections. The excess mucus is also a breeding ground for bacteria. Hence smokers tend to be sick more often than nonsmokers. Many respiratory diseases are related to cigarette smoking, including passive smoking or "second-hand smoking." These diseases include chronic obstructive pulmonary disease.

SPOTLIGHT ON RESEARCH

Research suggests that massage therapy may:
- Increase peak flow and vital capacity in persons with chronic obstructive pulmonary disease, asthma, and cystic fibrosis

E-RESOURCES

⊝volve

http://evolve.elsevier.com/Salvo/MassageTherapy

- Chapter challenge
- Flash cards
- Photo gallery
- Educational animations
- Weblinks

BIBLIOGRAPHY

Abrahams P, Marks S, Hutchings R: *McMinn's color atlas of human anatomy*, St Louis, 2003, Mosby.

Applegate EJ: *The anatomy and physiology learning system*, ed 3, Philadelphia, 2006, Saunders.

Beers MH, Berkow R: *The Merck manual of diagnosis and therapy*, Whitehouse Station, NJ, 2006, Merck Research Laboratories.

Como D, editor: *Mosby's medical, nursing, and allied health dictionary*, ed 6, St Louis, 2002, Mosby.

Crawley J, Van De Graaff KM: *A photographic atlas for anatomy and physiology*, Englewood, Colo, 2002, Morton.

Damjanov I: *Pathophysiology for the health-related professions*, ed 3, Philadelphia, 2006, Saunders.

Ferri FF: *2003 Ferri's clinical advisor, instant diagnosis and treatment*, St Louis, 2003, Mosby.

Ford CW: *Where healing waters meet: touching mind and emotions through the body*, Barrytown, NY, 1992, Station Hill Press.

Fritz S: *Essential sciences for therapeutic massage*, ed 3, St Louis, 2009, Mosby.

Fritz S: *Fundamentals of therapeutic massage*, ed 4, St Louis, 2009, Mosby.

Fritz S: *Massage online for essential sciences for therapeutic massage*, ed 3, St Louis, 2010, Mosby.

Gray H, Pick TP, Howden R: *Gray's anatomy*, ed 29, Philadelphia, 1974, Running Press.

Haubrich WS: *Medical meanings: a glossary of word origins*, New York, 1984, Harcourt Brace Jovanovich.

Huether SE, McCance KL: *Understanding pathophysiology*, ed 3, St Louis, 2004, Mosby.

Jacob S, Francone C: *Elements of anatomy and physiology*, Philadelphia, 1989, WB Saunders.

Kalat JW: *Biological psychology*, ed 8, Belmont, Calif, 2003, Wadsworth.

Kapit W, Elson LM: *The anatomy coloring book*, ed 3, New York, 2002, Benjamin Cummings.

Kordish M, Dickson S: *Introduction to basic human anatomy*, Lake Charles, La, 1995, McNeese State University.

Kumar V, Abbas A, Fausto N: *Robbins and Cotran physiologic basis of disease*, ed 7, St Louis, 2005, Mosby.

Marieb EN: *Essentials of human anatomy and physiology*, ed 8, New York, 2005, Benjamin Cummings.

Martini FH, Bartholomew EF: *Essentials of anatomy and physiology*, ed 3, New York, 2003, Benjamin Cummings.

McAleer N: *The body almanac*, Garden City, NY, 1985, Doubleday.

McCance K, Huether S: *Pathophysiology: the biological basis for disease in adults and children*, St Louis, 2006, Mosby.

Merck manual, ed 17, Whitehouse Station, NJ, 1998, Merck and Co.

Moore KL: *Clinically oriented anatomy*, ed 5, Baltimore, 2005, Lippincott Williams & Wilkins.

Netter FH: *Atlas of human anatomy*, ed 3, Teterboro, NJ, 2003, Icon Learning Systems.

Newton D: *Pathology for massage therapists*, ed 2, Portland, Ore, 1995, Simran.

Premkumar K: *Pathology A to Z, a handbook for massage therapists*, Baltimore, 1999, Lippincott Williams & Wilkins.

Salvo SG: *Mosby's pathology for massage therapists*, ed 2, St Louis, 2009, Mosby.

Solomon EP, Phillips GA: *Understanding human anatomy and physiology*, Philadelphia, 1987, WB Saunders.

Thibodeau G, Patton K: *Anatomy and physiology*, ed 6, St Louis, 2006, Mosby.

Thibodeau G, Patton K: *Structure and function of the body*, ed 12, St Louis, 2004, Mosby.

Tortora GJ: *Introduction to the human body: the essentials of anatomy and physiology*, ed 5, Hoboken, NJ, 2000, John Wiley & Sons.

Tortora GJ, Grabowksi SR: *Principles of anatomy and physiology*, ed 11, New York, 2005, John Wiley & Sons.

Venes D, Thomas CL, Taber CW: *Taber's cyclopedic medical dictionary*, ed 20, Philadelphia, 2005, FA Davis.

MATCHING I

Place the letter of the answer next to the term or phrase that best describes it.

A. Alveoli
B. Breathing
C. Bronchi
D. Diaphragm
E. Epiglottis
F. Larynx
G. Lungs
H. Nasal cavity
I. Pharynx
J. Respiration
K. Sinuses
L. Trachea

_____ 1. Area that is referred to as the air-conditioning chamber

_____ 2. Main muscle of respiration

_____ 3. Paired organs of respiration

_____ 4. Term synonymous with windpipe

_____ 5. Term synonymous with throat; tube shared by respiratory and digestive systems

_____ 6. Mechanical action that draws oxygen into the lungs and releases carbon dioxide into the atmosphere; includes inhalation and exhalation

_____ 7. Closes the trachea during swallowing; referred to as the guardian of the airways

_____ 8. The exchange of oxygen and carbon dioxide between lungs and blood and the blood and body tissues

_____ 9. Air-conduction passageways leading to each lung

_____ 10. Tiny sacs surrounded by capillaries

_____ 11. Term synonymous with voice box; houses the vocal cords

_____ 12. Air-containing cavities in the skull

MATCHING II

Place the letter of the answer next to the term or phrase that best describes it.

A. Apnea
B. Compliance
C. Elastic recoil
D. Epistaxis

E. Exhalation
F. External respiration
G. Inhalation
H. Internal respiration

I. Olfaction
J. Surfactants
K. Tidal volume
L. Vital capacity

_____ 1. Amount of air inhaled and exhaled in a single breath during normal breathing

_____ 2. Process of expelling air from the lungs

_____ 3. Sense of smell

_____ 4. Substance that assist in the exchange of gas by stabilizing the alveolus and reducing surface tension

_____ 5. Absence of normal, spontaneous breathing

_____ 6. Process of drawing air into the lungs

_____ 7. Total amount of air that can be forcibly inspired and expired from the lungs in one breath

_____ 8. Tendency of the thorax and lungs to return to their pre-inhalation size

_____ 9. Gas exchange between blood and body tissues

_____ 10. Gas exchange between blood in capillaries and air in the alveoli that came from the external environment

_____ 11. Medical term for nosebleed

_____ 12. Ease with which the thorax and lungs are able to stretch during inhalation

CASE STUDY

Gesundheit

It was Monday morning. Wanda had not felt like her usual self as she headed to her massage therapy office. She decided that her sluggishness and stuffy nose were caused by the dusting she had done over the weekend as she spring cleaned her condo. She also felt excited as she was in the process of fixing up her condo. In fact, she had booked a full day of clients for some extra spending money for the redecorating.

At about 11 AM, Wanda began her third client of the day, a middle-aged man named Randy. As she exerted herself against his stubborn back muscles, Wanda suddenly felt worse. Her stuffy nose turned to sniffles, and she began to feel flushed. All at once, her nose began to run, not just a slight drip that could be sniffed away, but steady streams of mucus.

"Your hands sure are warm!" observed Randy. Wanda was glad Randy was lying prone where he could not witness her wiping her nose against her sleeve. But this was not a suitable remedy for her sudden illness.

What should Wanda do now? Do you think she is contagious? If so, what are her obligations to herself and to her clients?

Should Wanda excuse herself from the room and try to clear her nasal passages, take some medication, and finish Randy's massage? How do you think Randy will respond to an ill therapist who wants to finish the massage?

Should Wanda end the massage before the appointment is over? If so, should she charge Randy for the incomplete session? What might she tell Randy if this is what she has decided to do?

How should Wanda handle her other clients for this day? Cancel them or see if she can make it through some of her other appointments?

CRITICAL THINKING

Why is it important for massage therapists to include assessment questions during intake about possible respiratory conditions clients might have?

CHAPTER 29

Digestive System

"Be careful about reading health books. You may die of a misprint."
—Mark Twain

LEARNING OBJECTIVES

After completing this chapter, the student should be able to:

- List anatomic structures and describe the physiologic processes related to the digestive system.
- Discuss the peritoneum.
- Identify specific divisions of the gastrointestinal tract, including the oral cavity, pharynx, esophagus, stomach, and small and large intestines.
- Name the accessory organs of digestion and discuss their functions.
- Name types of pathologic conditions of the gastrointestinal tract and give the massage considerations for each.

INTRODUCTION

People consume more than 40 tons of food in an average lifetime. The digestive system provides processes by which molecules are broken down into a state more easily used by body cells. Essentially, the digestive process is a *disassembly line*. The digestive process consumes metabolic resources, but fortunately it produces more energy than it uses.

The Nervous System chapter explained the two divisions of the autonomic nervous system: sympathetic and parasympathetic. Digestive functions are initiated by the parasympathetic division of the nervous system. Because digestion requires an expenditure of energy, it occurs primarily during periods of low activity. The body can then reallocate energy that would normally be spent on muscular activity and route it to the digestive system. Because of this, activation of the parasympathetic nervous system is also known by the nickname *rest and digest*. Stress and emotional responses serve to slow digestion because they stimulate the sympathetic nervous system. People in high-stress or high-responsibility positions are more likely than others to have problems with ulcers, heartburn, colitis, irritable bowel syndrome, and constipation because of frequent disruption of the digestive process.

The digestive system is primarily a long tube with accessory organs and glands. It starts at the mouth, extends through the body, and ends at the anus (Figure 29-1). The tube is known as the **gastrointestinal (GI) tract** or the **alimentary canal**.

ANATOMY

Basic anatomy of the digestive system includes the GI tract, accessory organs, and glands.

The GI tract consists of the:
- Oral cavity
- Pharynx
- Esophagus
- Stomach
- Small intestine
- Large intestine

Accessory organs and glands include the:
- Salivary glands
- Pancreas
- Liver
- Gallbladder

PHYSIOLOGY

The functions of the digestive system are:
- **Ingestion.** The process of orally taking materials into the body is called ingestion (eating and drinking).
- **Digestion.** Digestion is the series of mechanical and chemical processes that occur as food is broken down into simple molecules. *Mechanical digestion* includes

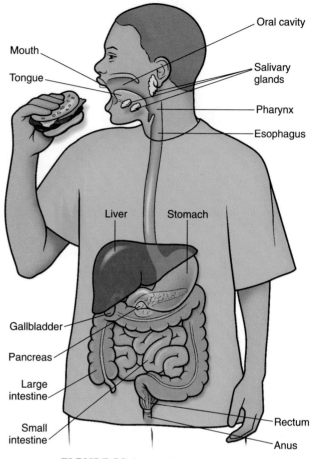

FIGURE 29-1 The digestive system.

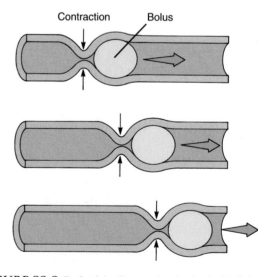

FIGURE 29-2 Peristalsis. Contraction begins behind the bolus.

chewing, churning in the stomach, and the mixing movements of the intestinal tract. These movements, which include **peristalsis** (rhythmic contractions of the GI tract), serve to mix and propel products of digestion along the tube (Figure 29-2). *Chemical digestion* includes the effects of acids, bases, and enzymes that are released into the digestive tract in response to food. Chemical digestion is the more significant of the two.

- **Absorption.** Absorption is the process by which simple molecules from the digestive tract are moved into the bloodstream or lymph vessels and then into the body's cells.
- **Defecation.** The process of eliminating indigestible or unabsorbed material from the body is called defecation.

These functions can also be seen as the four steps of the digestive process (ingestion [first step], digestion [second step], absorption [third step], and defecation [final step]).

IT'S ALL GREEK TO ME

Term	Meaning
amylase	*Gr.* starch; enzyme
bolus	*Gr.* a lump
Brunner glands	Brunner, Swiss anatomist (1653-1727)
cecum	*L.* blindness
chyme	*Gr.* juice
deglutition	*L.* to swallow
duodenum	*L.* 12 fingers (refers to its length)
enzyme	*Gr.* leaven
gingiva	*L.* gums
gustatory	*L.* to taste
haustra	*L.* to draw, drink
hepato	*Gr.* liver
ileum	*L.* twisted
jejunum	*L.* empty
lacteal	*L.* of milk
mastication	*L.* to chew
mesentery	*Gr.* middle; intestine
omentum	*L.* a covering or apron
peristaltic	*Gr.* around; contraction
plicae circulares	*L.* a fold; a little ring
pylorus	*Gr.* gatekeeper
rectum	*L.* straight
rugae	*L.* a crease or fold
sacchar	*Gr.* sugar
sigmoid	The Greek letter *sigma*, meaning S-shaped
sphincter	*Gr.* a binder
sphincter of Oddi	Oddi, Italian physician (1864-1913)
taenia coli	*L.* tape; colon
tonsils	*L.* almond
vermiform appendix	*L.* wormlike; hanger-on
villi	*L.* tuft of hair

Gr., Greek; *L.*, Latin.

PERITONEUM

The abdomen, or abdominal cavity, contains the major organs of digestion. This cavity is enveloped by a large serous membrane called the **peritoneum**. Within the peritoneum are blood vessels, lymph vessels, and nerves. The peritoneum contains two main layers. The layer lying against the body wall is the *parietal peritoneum*; the layer surrounding each abdominal organ is called the *visceral peritoneum*. Some organs, such as the pancreas and kidneys, lie behind the peritoneum and so are considered *retroperitoneal*.

A fluid-filled space (the peritoneal cavity) lies between these two layers and contains serous fluid, which lubricates the viscera and allows layers of the peritoneum to slide across each other.

Sections of the peritoneum include the mesenteries, and greater and lesser omentum (Figure 29-3). These structures are discussed later in the section on the small intestine.

ORAL CAVITY

Also known as the *mouth*, the **oral cavity** is the first portion of the gastrointestinal tract. The oral cavity contains the tongue, teeth, gums, and openings from the salivary glands.

Here, food is mechanically chewed *(masticated)*, chemically broken down, and mixed with saliva. Chewing is aided

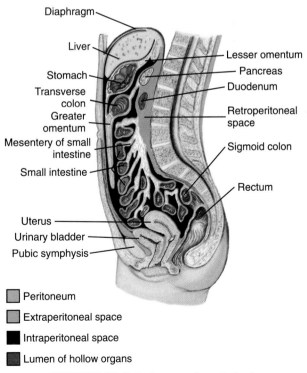

Diaphragm
Liver
Stomach
Transverse colon
Greater omentum
Mesentery of small intestine
Small intestine
Uterus
Urinary bladder
Pubic symphysis

Lesser omentum
Pancreas
Duodenum
Retroperitoneal space
Sigmoid colon
Rectum

☐ Peritoneum
☐ Extraperitoneal space
■ Intraperitoneal space
■ Lumen of hollow organs

FIGURE 29-3 Peritoneum (lateral view).

by the tongue. This process turns food into a **bolus** (soft ball of chewed food), which is ready for swallowing *(deglutition)*. With the exception of several medications (e.g., nitroglycerin), no absorption takes place in the oral cavity.

Tongue. The **tongue** is a large, strong muscle that mixes food particles with saliva and directs the bolus toward the back of the throat. Nestled in spherical pockets on the superior and lateral surfaces of the tongue are the *taste buds* (gustatory organs), which are chemoreceptors that detect the primary tastes of sweet, sour, bitter, salty, and savoriness.

Taste is most often the response of many receptors, not just those located on the tongue. For example, receptors for smell found in the superior portion of the nasal cavity play a significant role in taste.

Teeth. **Teeth** are accessory structures used to bite off and mechanically break up larger pieces of food into smaller ones that can be swallowed. Within the adult mouth are 32 secondary (permanent) teeth. Children possess only 20 primary (deciduous) teeth that are usually shed between the ages of 6 and 12 years. Enamel, the hardest substance in the body, covers each tooth. Teeth are classified according to shape and function: incisors, cuspids (canines), bicuspids (premolars), and multicuspids (molars). The third molars are also called *wisdom teeth* because they erupt when a person is old enough to be "wise" (usually between the ages of 17 and 25).

Salivary Glands. The three paired **salivary glands** are the (1) the *submandibular glands*, (2) the *sublingual glands*, and (3) the large *parotid glands*.

Secretions

These glands secrete saliva, a clear, viscous fluid that helps keep the oral mucosa moist and lubricates food so that it is easier to swallow. Saliva contains water, mucus, organic salts, and digestive enzymes. An **enzyme** is a catalyst that accelerates chemical reactions. *Salivary amylase*, a digestive enzyme found in saliva, breaks down carbohydrates. *Lingual lipase*, secreted by glands located near the tongue, breaks lipids down into glycerol and fatty acids. Smell, sight, taste, and the thought of food stimulate the production of saliva.

PHARYNX

The **pharynx**, or throat, receives the food bolus from the mouth and transports it and liquids to the esophagus during swallowing. The pharynx also conducts air during breathing. The pharynx is divided into three sections.

The *nasopharynx* contains openings to the Eustachian tubes, which help to equalize pressure in the head, nose,

and pharynx. Because of this close proximity, respiratory infections can easily lead to middle ear infections and vice versa.

The *oropharynx* is the portion of the throat that you can see. It contains the tonsils, which help our immune system by protecting against inhaled or ingested pathogens.

The *laryngopharynx* begins at the hyoid bone and separates into the esophagus and larynx. Thus it functions as a pathway for the respiratory and digestive tracts.

ESOPHAGUS

The **esophagus,** located behind the trachea, is a muscular tube extending from the pharynx to the stomach by passing through the diaphragm. The esophageal lining secretes mucus to aid in the transport of food.

At the point of attachment between the esophagus and the stomach is a thickened region called the *lower esophageal sphincter*. A **sphincter** is a ring of muscle that remains contracted or closed until triggered to relax and open. The trigger for relaxation of the lower esophageal sphincter is most often food traveling down the esophagus and approaching the stomach. Several other sphincters are located along the GI tract.

STOMACH

The **stomach** is a J-shaped, saclike organ that is essentially an enlargement of the gastrointestinal tract bound at both ends by sphincters. The superior sphincter, located between the esophagus and stomach, is the *lower esophageal sphincter* (mentioned previously). The *pyloric sphincter* is located between the stomach and small intestine (Figure 29-4).

The stomach receives the bolus and with the addition of gastric juice, breaks it down into a semiliquid substance called **chyme**.

When empty, the stomach is approximately the size of a large sausage. Depending on body size, the stomach, when full, can hold up to 1 gallon of food. The stomach's lining contains folds called *rugae* that enable it to expand as food is ingested. The only substances that are absorbed by the lining of the stomach are water, some minerals, alcohol, and some medications such as aspirin.

The pyloric sphincter opens periodically to allow chyme to enter the small intestine. The process of moving chyme into the small intestine may take up to 4 hours; thus the stomach also serves as both a storage tank and digestive chamber. Because of this slow release of chyme into the small intestines, the body is able to maintain energy needs with only two or three meals a day, instead of requiring a steady supply of food, as grazing animals and birds do.

JOEY ERWIN MAZZERA

Born: February 7, 1976

"If you can't get outside of your own garbage, you will never be able to handle anyone else's."

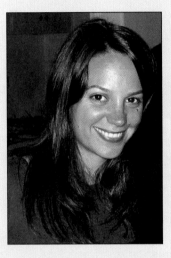

Joey Erwin Mazzera was born in California in 1976. Mazzera went to massage school with the idea of pursuing oncology massage firmly planted in her mind. The American Cancer Society estimates that more than 10 million patients with cancer are in the United States, but for Mazzera, this number is more personal. Instead of a statistic, she sees the face of her stepfather and uncle, both of whom died of cancer. Cancer still remains a part of her everyday life, owing to several more friends and family members being diagnosed recently.

Erwin studied at the California College of Physical Arts in Huntington Beach, California, before receiving her Holistic Health Practitioner's Certificate in 2003. As a student, she spent a great deal of time outside the classroom, learning as much as she could about the practice of oncology massage. A decade ago, Mazzera noted, "There seemed to be a conservative approach to oncology massage," and she had difficulty locating instruction in a field that was at the time predominantly closed to patients with cancer.

Today, this taboo is changing. Mazzera had the chance to put her oncology lessons in practice at a weekend retreat for patients with breast cancer. She served as one of a small group of massage therapists on hand to give therapy sessions. Mazzera remembers one client in particular who would ultimately shape and define her passion for oncology massage.

"One woman had so many tumors taken out and so many complications, her body looked like a road map of scars. She was so uncomfortable and in so much pain and just wanted massage," Mazzera said. As her hands went to work, Mazzera said she was able to feel the woman changing under her touch. They both cried. The woman told her that nobody had touched her like that for years.

That moment was a turning point in Mazzera's career. She no longer felt fear of sickness or dying but rather had a renewed interest in bringing the healing powers of massage to patients with cancer. Today, Mazzera is excited about the future of her profession and hopes that others will follow in her footsteps.

"Lose your fear," she says. "People are scared of scars, sickness, tubes, and bags. It's messy and it's dirty and it's stinky, but when you get the really challenging cases … those are my favorites."

Mazzera recently received her MS in Traditional Chinese Medicine at the American College of Traditional Chinese Medicine in San Francisco. She is now a licensed acupuncturist still focusing on oncology support. She currently volunteers doing hospice massage for the Emeryville Hospice and Visiting Nurse Association in California.

When the waters rose in New Orleans after hurricane Katrina, Mazzera was there. When the floods subsided, she was back, ready to rebuild. As a pioneer in the practice of oncology massage, Mazzera hopes to always be on the cutting edge in her field.

Secretions

Glands within the walls of the stomach secrete the hormone gastrin and gastric juices, which contain hydrochloric acid, enzymes, mucus, and water.

Gastrin, produced by *G cells*, initiates the secretion of gastric juice and stimulates bile and pancreatic enzyme emissions into the small intestines (Table 29-1).

The *parietal cells* located in the stomach produce *intrinsic factor*, a substance required for the absorption of vitamin B_{12}. The parietal cells also produce *hydrochloric acid*, a compound of hydrogen and chlorine, which breaks down protein and activates many gastric enzymes. Hydrochloric acid, which kills bacteria and other pathogens, is so powerful that it can eat through wood.

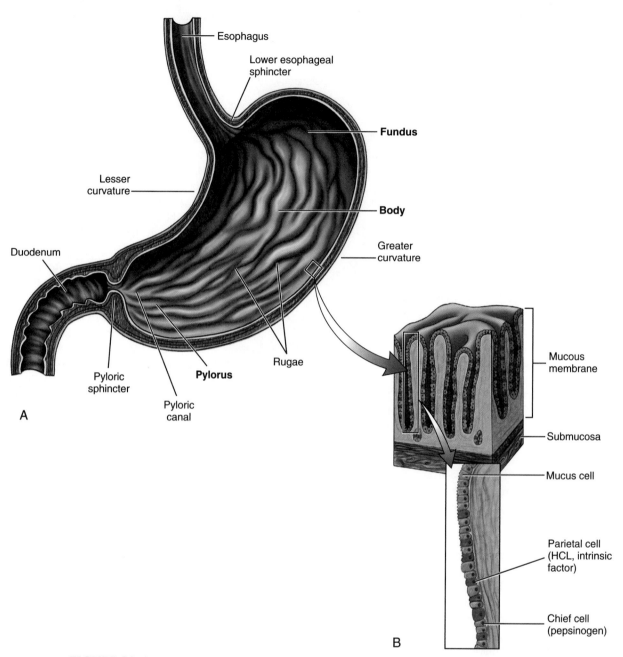

FIGURE 29-4 Stomach. **A,** Structures of the stomach. **B,** Cross section of the stomach's lining.

CHAT ROOM

Chief cells produce the enzyme *pepsinogen*, which is a precursor to pepsin. *Pepsin* is secreted in an inactive form to prevent the stomach's lining from eroding from pepsin's protein digestion. Pepsinogen converts to pepsin when it comes into contact with hydrochloric acid and begins the chemical digestion of proteins.

The gastric lining is also protected from enzymes and acids by a thick layer of mucus.

Chymosin (renin), an enzyme found in the gastric juices of infants, is used to aid in milk curdling and is made commercially to produce cheese.

What is hunger? Is it the need for food and energy? Heredity? Several theories exist, but most likely it is a primordial reflex from days past, when there were no stable sources of food. Another idea is that hunger is experienced when the body detects a low level of blood sugar or a combined reduction of all available digestible foods. Additionally, the hypothalamus appears to regulate the sensation of hunger and the feeling of *satiety* (fullness). People, when asked why they eat, cite a variety of reasons besides hunger, such as loneliness, depression, or boredom. It is most likely a combination of several physiologic and psychologic events, some of which can cause pathologic eating disorders later in life.

TABLE 29-1 Substances Affecting Digestion

NAME AND SUBSTANCE	LOCATION PRODUCED	ACTION(S)
Bile (emulsifier)	Liver	Physically breaks apart large fat globules into smaller ones
Carboxypeptidase (enzyme)	Pancreas	Breaks down proteins
Cholecystokinin (hormone)	Small intestine	Stimulates the release of bile from the gallbladder and the secretion of pancreatic enzymes
Chymosin/rennin (enzyme)	Stomach (infants only)	Aids in milk curdling
Chymotrypsin (enzyme)	Pancreas	Breaks down proteins
Enterocrinin (hormone)	Small intestine	Stimulates the flow of intestinal juice
Enterokinase (enzyme)	Small intestine	Activates protein enzyme secretion from pancreas
Gastrin (hormone)	Stomach (G cells)	Initiates production and secretion of gastric juice; stimulates release of bile and pancreatic enzymes into the small intestines
Hydrochloric acid (compound)	Stomach (parietal cells)	Breaks down protein and activates gastric enzymes
Intrinsic factor (substance)	Stomach (parietal cells)	Promotes absorption of vitamin B_{12} from the small intestine into the bloodstream
Lactase (enzyme)	Small intestine	Promotes carbohydrate digestion
Lingual lipase (enzyme)	Oral cavity	Breaks lipids down into glycerol and fatty acids
Maltase (enzyme)	Small intestine	Promotes carbohydrate digestion
Pancreatic amylase (enzyme)	Pancreas	Converts polysaccharides into disaccharides
Pancreatic lipase (enzyme)	Pancreas	Converts triglycerides into monoglycerides and fatty acids
Pepsinogen/pepsin (precursor/enzyme)	Stomach (chief cells)	Begins chemical digestion of proteins by converting them into peptides
Peptidase (enzyme)	Small intestine	Promotes the digestion of proteins
Salivary amylase/ptyalin (enzyme)	Salivary glands	Begins carbohydrate digestion
Secretin (hormone)	Small intestine	Stimulates the production and secretion of pancreatic enzymes
Sucrase (enzyme)	Small intestine	Promotes carbohydrate digestion
Trypsinogen/trypsin (precursor/enzyme)	Pancreas	Breaks protein into smaller chains of amino acids

SMALL INTESTINE

The **small intestine** (small bowel) is the longest portion of the GI tract. This coiled tube is bound at both ends by sphincters; the proximal sphincter is the *pyloric sphincter* (located between the stomach and the small intestine) and the distal sphincter is the *ileocecal sphincter* (located between the small and large intestine).

The lumen of the small intestine possesses circular folds—*plicae circulares*. The lumen also contains numerous *villi*, which are fingerlike projections that house blood and lymph capillaries (Figure 29-5). *Microvilli* are present along the surface of the villi, giving the intestines a velvety appearance (brush border). All three structures (i.e., plicae circulares, villi, and microvilli) assist absorption by increasing surface area.

Mucus-producing *goblet cells* are found in the spaces between some of the villi. Lymph capillaries within the villi are called *lacteals*, which assist in the absorption of fat.

Ninety percent of nutrient absorption occurs in the length of the small intestine; the other 10% occurs in the stomach and large intestine (Figure 29-6).

The divisions of the small intestine, from beginning to end, are (1) the duodenum, (2) the jejunum, and (3) the ileum.

Duodenum. The shortest portion, making up the first 10 to 12 inches of the small intestine, is called the duodenum. It contains ducts from the liver, gallbladder, and pancreas. The *sphincter of Oddi* regulates the flow of secretions from these organs. The *major duodenal papilla* is a dilation formed by the juncture of the pancreatic and common bile ducts (see Figure 29-8).

Jejunum. The jejunum continues from the duodenum for the next 7 to 8 feet. The walls of the jejunum are slightly thicker than those of the ileum, and the jejunum possesses a smaller lumen. The villi are larger in this section, presumably to increase absorption.

Ileum. The last 12 feet of the small intestine is called the ileum. The ileum terminates at the ileocecal sphincter (or valve). This section contains numerous clusters of lacteals to enhance fat absorption.

Secretions

Brunner's glands (duodenal glands) secrete alkaline mucus. Other intestinal glands secrete intestinal juices containing digestive enzymes, such as enterokinase, peptidase, maltase, sucrase, and lactase. These enzymes promote protein and carbohydrate digestion. Hormones secreted by the intestinal mucosa are enterocrinin, cholecystokinin, and secretin. *Enterocrinin* stimulates the flow of intestinal juice, and *cholecystokinin* stimulates contraction of the gallbladder and pancreatic enzyme secretion. *Secretin* stimulates the

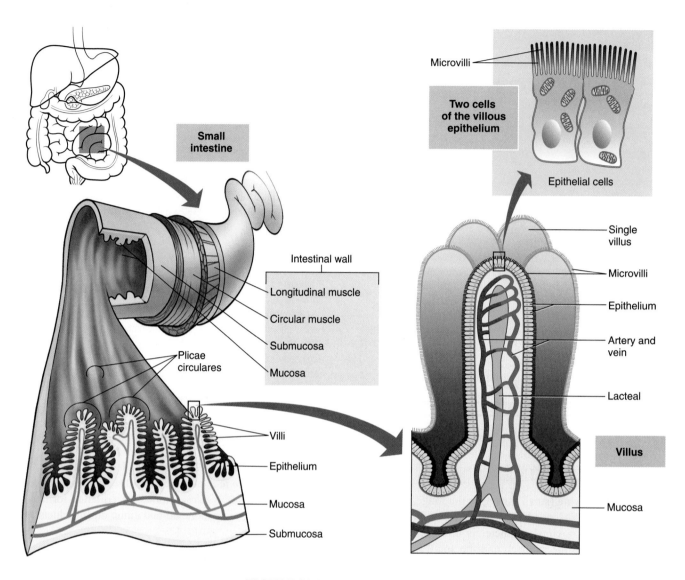

FIGURE 29-5 Small intestinal wall.

pancreas to secrete an alkaline liquid that neutralizes the acid chyme, facilitating the action of the intestinal enzymes (see Table 29-1).

Mesenteries

All divisions of the small intestines are connected to each other and to the posterior abdominal wall by sections of the peritoneum called the *mesenteries* (see Figure 29-3). The mesenteries make up a large, fan-shaped structure consisting of two omentums. The *greater omentum* extends from the stomach and duodenum to the transverse colon. Fat stored in the greater omentum accounts for much of the girth in obesity. The *lesser omentum* extends from the stomach and the duodenum to the liver.

CHAT ROOM

Many gastrointestinal diseases have a strong connection with stress. The digestive system is highly responsive to fluctuations in the autonomic nervous system. Chronic sympathetic arousal can lead to hypersecretion or hyposecretion of digestive enzymes and changes in peristalsis. The latter can lead to chronic constipation or hyperactive gut. Research indicates that stress management and soothing massage induces relaxation by stimulation of the parasympathetic nervous system, which increases gastric motility.

⊖volve *View a close-up cutaway of the intestines featuring its numerous villi in Chapter 29. It is easy to imagine that "it takes a villus" to deal with the absorption issues in the small intestines.* ■

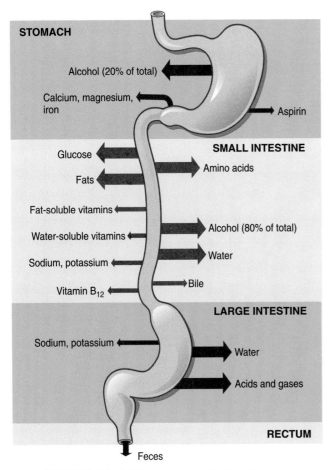

STOMACH

Alcohol (20% of total) ←

Calcium, magnesium, iron ←

→ Aspirin

SMALL INTESTINE

Glucose ←
→ Amino acids

Fats ←

Fat-soluble vitamins ←

Water-soluble vitamins ←
→ Alcohol (80% of total)

Sodium, potassium ←
→ Water

Vitamin B$_{12}$ ←
→ Bile

LARGE INTESTINE

Sodium, potassium ←
→ Water

→ Acids and gases

RECTUM

Feces

FIGURE 29-6 Absorption sites in digestive tract.

LARGE INTESTINE

The **large intestine** (colon) is the final route that undigested and unabsorbed food takes before it is eliminated by the body. It also forms and stores feces until defecation. The large intestine begins at the ileocecal *sphincter* (located between the small and large intestine) and ends with the *anal sphincter*.

The large intestine is characterized by taeniae coli and haustra. Thick, longitudinal bands called *taeniae coli* resemble a thread-gathering fabric. The gathers, or tucks, along the length of the colon make a series of pouches, called *haustra*. Once filled, these pouches contract to push the contents to the next haustrum. The large intestine consists of the cecum; the ascending, transverse, descending, and sigmoid colon; rectum; and anus (Figure 29-7).

The large intestine absorbs water and electrolytes and helps in the manufacture of certain vitamins.

Cecum. The first section of the colon, the *cecum*, is a small saclike structure located in the right lower quadrant of the abdomen. The cecum receives the digested matter from the ileum. Suspended from and opening into the inferior

portion of the cecum is the *vermiform appendix*. It is about 3 inches in length and contains lymphatic tissue (see Chapter 27).

Ascending Colon. The next segment is the *ascending colon*, which continues from the cecum upward and curves toward the left just beneath the liver. This curve is called the *hepatic (right colic) flexure*.

Transverse Colon. After the hepatic flexure, the colon moves horizontally from right to left, draping to form the *transverse colon*. Just beneath the spleen, it turns downward. The downward curve is called the *splenic (left colic) flexure*.

Descending Colon. The *descending colon* extends from the splenic flexure to about the top of the iliac crest. Here, the descending colon turns back toward the right at the *sigmoid flexure*.

Sigmoid Colon. The S-shaped *sigmoid colon* begins at the sigmoid flexure and continues to the middle of the abdomen, where it joins the *rectum*.

Rectum. The *rectum* is essentially a straight continuation of the sigmoid colon, beginning at about the level of S3 and terminates at the *anus*. This section contains approximately three circular folds that overlap when empty and expand as the rectum fills with feces. The main function of the rectum is temporary storage of feces.

Defecation – As feces fill the rectum, the anal sphincter distends, stimulating pressure-sensitive receptors and initiating the defecation reflex. During defecation, the levator ani muscle raises the anus to eliminate feces. Feces, or stool, is excrement from the GI tract formed in the intestine and released through the anus. Feces consist of indigestible foodstuffs, water, bacteria, and cells sloughed off the walls of the large intestine.

If the defecation reflex is suppressed, then it may dissipate, and it may be hours before the desire to defecate returns. If the urge to defecate is chronically suppressed, then copious amounts of water are absorbed from the colon, and constipation may result.

Secretions

The lining of the large intestine does not produce digestive enzymes; instead, it produces mucus that allows the developing feces to move more easily.

ⓔvolve   *Here's your opportunity to see food's "trail's end." An image of the rectum and anus is located on the Evolve website. Note how the valves go from convoluted to straight before a defecation reflex is experienced.* ∎

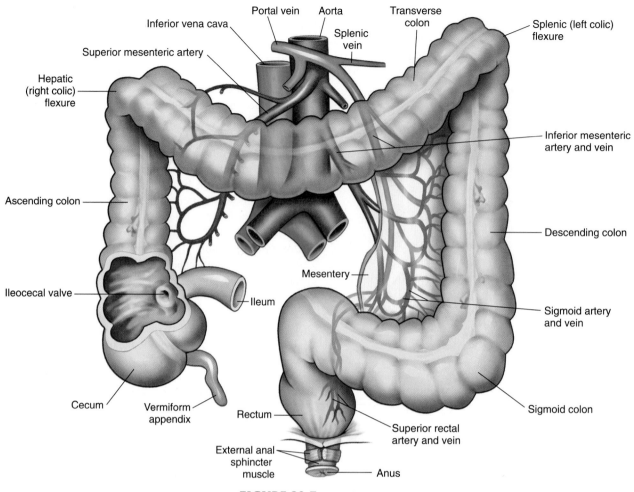

FIGURE 29-7 Large intestine.

"The body tells the story. It is, in fact, a living autobiography."
—Elaine Mayland

ACCESSORY ORGANS

The accessory digestive organs produce substances that aid digestion in the small intestines. They are the liver, gallbladder, and pancreas (Figure 29-8). The digestive substances produced and secreted by these organs continue the chemical digestion of food.

LIVER

The **liver** is the largest and most complex internal organ in the body (weighing approximately 3 lb) and lies beneath the diaphragm. The liver has many important functions, including:

- Metabolizes amino acids (building blocks of protein)
- Removes glucose from the blood and stores it as glycogen when levels are high, converting it back to glucose when levels are low
- Breaks down fatty acids and stores the fat as fuel for later use
- Produces plasma proteins and fibrinogens (blood clotting substances)
- Produces antibodies
- Stores nutrients: iron, copper, and vitamins A, B_{12}, D, E, and K

- Detoxifies the blood by removing toxins, drugs, and hormones
- Destroys old red blood cells and platelets

Secretions

In its digestive functions, the liver secretes *bile*. Produced from the hemoglobin in old red blood cells, bile is not an enzyme but an emulsifier. It physically breaks apart large fat globules into smaller ones, which provides a larger surface area for the fat-digesting enzymes to work. Bile gives urine and the stool their characteristic colors. Bile enters the left and right *hepatic ducts*, which join to form the *common bile duct* that leads to the duodenum of the small intestine.

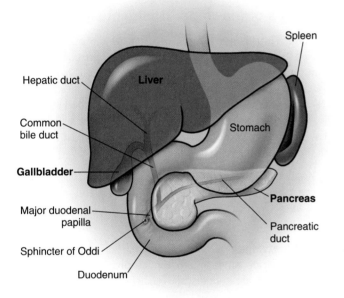

FIGURE 29-8 Accessory digestive organs.

GALLBLADDER

The **gallbladder** is a pear-shaped sac that lies on the inferior surface of the liver. The gallbladder stores and concentrates bile produced by the liver. The *sphincter of Oddi* controls the release of bile acids into the duodenum.

PANCREAS

The **pancreas**, a carrot-shaped organ located behind the stomach, is connected to the duodenum by ducts. The most important digestive gland, the pancreas produces enzymes that break down all categories of digestible foods, including proteins, carbohydrates, and fats.

The pancreas also functions as an endocrine gland. Pancreatic islets, which are scattered throughout the pancreas, produce and secrete hormones, including insulin, which regulates the uptake of glucose from the blood.

Secretions

In its digestive functions, the pancreas secretes enzymes called pancreatic juices. *Acini cells* that produce these enzymes. The pancreatic duct runs the length of the organ and empties pancreatic enzymes into the duodenum (Figure 29-9). Pancreatic enzymes are secreted in an alkaline fluid to neutralize the acid chyme from the stomach.

The pancreas produces approximately 1.0 to 1.5 quarts of digestive enzymes per day, including trypsinogen, chymotrypsin, carboxypeptidase, pancreatic amylase, and pancreatic lipase. *Trypsinogen*, a protein-splitting enzyme, is converted to *trypsin* when it enters the duodenum. Trypsin, activated by the intestinal enzyme enterokinase, breaks protein into peptides before their conversion to amino acids. *Chymotrypsin* and *carboxypeptidase* assist in the breakdown of proteins. *Pancreatic amylase* converts polysaccharides into disaccharides (maltose, sucrose, and lactose). *Pancreatic lipase* helps convert fats into fatty acids.

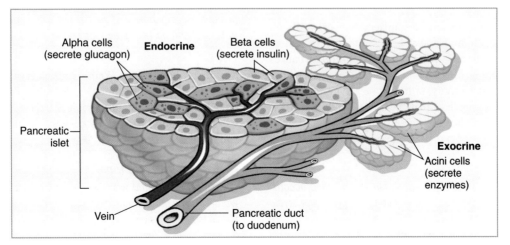

FIGURE 29-9 Exocrine cells of the pancreas and their relationship to endocrine cells.

GASTROINTESTINAL PATHOLOGIES

General Dysfunctions of the Gastrointestinal Tract

Nausea. Nausea is an unpleasant subjective experience often leading to the urge to, or act of, vomiting. Nausea has many causes, including motion sicknesses, early pregnancy, heart attack, emotional stress, migraines, cancer treatments, and gastrointestinal (GI) infections. Some terms used to describe nausea are "sick to my stomach," "upset stomach," "queasiness," and "butterflies in my stomach."

Query your client regarding the reasons for the nausea, and then decide how to proceed. For example, if nausea is caused by a migraine headache or GI infections, it is best to postpone massage until the condition has resolved. However, for nausea caused by emotional stress or cancer treatment, massage is appropriate and often beneficial. In these cases, use a semireclining position, and avoid pressure and speed that rock the client.

Constipation. Constipation is infrequent or difficult passing of stool. Normal bowel habits range from two to three evacuations per day to three per week. Common causes of constipation are insufficient intake of fluid or dietary fiber and lack of physical activity, or it may be a symptom manifestation in diseases such as irritable bowel syndrome (IBS) and diverticulitis. Medication side effects may reduce bowel motility and can lead to constipation (particularly with narcotics).

Ascertain the cause of the constipation and proceed accordingly. For example, if the cause is irritable bowel syndrome, avoid the abdomen if pressure causes pain. Otherwise, abdominal massage can help relieve constipation by stimulating forward movement of intestinal contents.

Diarrhea. The frequent passing of unformed, loose, watery stools is called diarrhea. Diarrhea can be acute (lasting a few days) or chronic (lasting a few weeks or longer), depending on the cause. Most acute cases of diarrhea are caused by viruses, parasites, or bacteria (especially *Escherichia coli*). Possible reasons for chronic diarrhea include Crohn disease, ulcerative colitis, celiac disease, and IBS. Other causes of diarrhea include stress, diet, medication side effects (particularly antibiotics and hypoglycemics), and use of artificial sweeteners (sorbitol and mannitol).

Ascertain the cause of the diarrhea. In cases of acute diarrhea, postpone massage until your client is symptom-free for 48 hours. In cases of chronic diarrhea, avoid the lower abdomen if pressure causes uneasiness or discomfort. Suggest use of the toilet before massage as a comfort measure and be prepared for a toilet break during the session.

Diseases of the Upper Gastrointestinal Tract

Thrush. Thrush is a fungal infection of the oral mucosa caused by *Candida albicans*. It is characterized by soft, white to yellow, curdlike patches in the mouth, inside the cheek and on the tongue and gums. These patches, which resemble cottage cheese, create a sensation of food sticking to the mouth and they are slightly painful when wiped off, leaving a raw bleeding surface. The smell of yeast may be on the breath.

Avoid massage to lower portion of the face (e.g., cheeks, jaw). If your client complains of facial pain while prone, avoid this position.

Gastroesophageal Reflux Disease. Periodic regurgitation of gastric contents into the esophagus is known as gastroesophageal reflux disease (GERD). The most common symptom of GERD is heartburn that worsens when lying down. Heartburn occurs within 30 to 60 minutes after eating or at night.

If your client indicates that the upper abdomen is sensitive, avoid the area. While he or she is supine, use a semireclining position. Recommend that your client avoid eating a heavy meal at least 2 and up to 3 hours before the scheduled appointment.

Peptic Ulcer Disease. Peptic ulcer disease involves ulcerations of the mucosal lining in sections of the GI tract that are exposed to acidic gastric juice. Peptic ulcers are named by their location, such as esophageal ulcers, gastric ulcers, and duodenal ulcers.

Avoid the abdomen if the area is sensitive to pressure. Ask about pain associated with food intake. If pain is reduced afterward, suggest that a small meal or snack be eaten before massage. If pain is more pronounced after mealtime, recommend not eating a heavy meal at least 2 and up to 3 hours before the scheduled appointment.

Diseases of the Lower Gastrointestinal Tract

Diverticulosis. Diverticulosis is a condition characterized by the presence of diverticula in the colon wall. These are outpouchings in the colon wall, and once formed, they do not go away. Their development is associated with decreased dietary fiber, leading to irregular bowel habits. Symptoms include mild abdominal discomfort, nausea, flatulence, and difficulty in defecation with alternating constipation and diarrhea.

If your client indicates that the abdomen is sensitive, avoid the area. Position the client for comfort.

Diverticulitis. When diverticula become infected or inflamed, the condition is called diverticulitis. Feces can enter diverticula and become infected. The most common symptom of diverticulitis is abdominal pain with distention. The person often has difficulty defecating, with alternating constipation and diarrhea. In cases in which infection is present, the person may have fever, chills, nausea, and vomiting.

Diverticulitis is a disorder requiring immediate medical attention. Massage is postponed until the condition has resolved.

Irritable Bowel Syndrome. IBS is characterized by abnormal muscular contraction in the colon wall. Main symptoms include abdominal pain, bloating, and nausea, with either constipation or diarrhea, or both. Affected individuals often suffer with depression and anxiety, which worsen IBS symptoms.

If your client indicates that the abdomen is sensitive, avoid the area. If the person in nauseated, use a semireclining position, and avoid pressure and speed that rock the client. Because many cases of IBS are related to stress, massage is indicated, especially treatments that promote relaxation.

Ulcerative Colitis. Ulcerative colitis is inflammation of the colon with the formation of ulcers. Cases of ulcerative colitis usually begin with bouts of diarrhea, rectal bleeding, and abdominal pain. Chronic diarrhea may lead to problems with dehydration, fatigue, weight loss, and hemorrhoids. Most affected persons experience periods of exacerbation and remission.

Avoid the abdomen. Because periods of exacerbation are linked to stress, massage is indicated when the condition is in remission. Use techniques that promote relaxation. If your client is fatigued, reduce treatment time to 30 minutes, and use lighter-than-normal pressure.

Crohn Disease. Crohn disease is inflammation affecting any part of the GI tract and can extend through all of its layers. Diarrhea is the most common sign. Chronic diarrhea may lead to problems with dehydration, fatigue, weight loss, and hemorrhoids. Thirty percent of persons also have low-grade fever. Most affected persons experience periods of exacerbation and remission.

Avoid the abdomen. Because periods of exacerbation are linked to stress, massage is indicated when the condition is in remission. Use techniques that promote relaxation. If your client is fatigued, reduce treatment time to 30 minutes, and use lighter-than-normal pressure.

Appendicitis. The combination of inflammation and infection of the vermiform appendix is called appendicitis. Epigastric or umbilical pain is the typical presenting symptom; the pain is vague at first and then shifts to the lower right quadrant of the abdomen (McBurney point). The affected person may experience loss of appetite, become nauseated, vomit, and have fever. The pain usually increases over a period of 6 to 12 hours and eventually becomes severe. Abdominal muscle guarding and rebound tenderness are common findings.

Appendicitis is a medical emergency requiring immediate medical attention. Massage is postponed until the condition resolves.

Diseases of the Liver and Gallbladder

Viral Hepatitis. Hepatitis is inflammation of the liver. There are several forms (e.g., viral, alcoholic, drug-induced, obstructive). The most common form is viral hepatitis. Viral hepatitis types are named for letters, such as hepatitis A, B, and C. Hepatitis B, which is most often transmitted by sexual contact, is the most prevalent. Disease manifestations of viral hepatitis range from mild with no symptoms to pain in the upper right quadrant, low-grade fever, and occasional headache. Persons with viral hepatitis may bruise easily from decreased production of blood-clotting factors by the liver. Some people develop jaundice, especially in advanced cases.

The appropriateness of massage is determined by your client's symptoms. For example, if fever or jaundice is present, massage is contraindicated. If you decide massage is appropriate, avoid the abdomen. Use lighter-than-normal pressure if your client bruises easily. If your client is fatigued, reduce treatment time to 30 minutes, and use lighter-than-normal pressure.

Cirrhosis. Cirrhosis is a progressive liver disease that destroys liver cells. The damage is irreversible. Initial signs and symptoms include loss of appetite, weight loss, nausea, anemia, fatigue, and diarrhea. Legs become edematous as the disease progresses. Persons with cirrhosis may bruise easily from decreased production of blood-clotting factors by the liver.

Massage is contraindicated in later stages, indicated by the presence of jaundice. Massage in earlier stages is indicated, avoiding massage over the abdomen or over areas of pitting edema. Use lighter-than-normal pressure if your client bruises easily. If your client is feeling fatigued, reduce treatment time to 30 minutes, and use lighter-than-normal pressure.

Gallstones. Forty percent of the time, the presence of gallstones is unknown and a person is asymptomatic until the stone causes an obstruction. At first, symptoms mimic indigestion and include heartburn, flatulence, bloating, and belching. Symptoms then progress to nausea, vomiting, and abdominal pain. Pain may radiate to the midupper back and right shoulder. The pain decreases as the stone is passed.

If the symptoms are severe, massage is contraindicated. If the pain is less severe or absent, massage is indicated while avoiding the abdomen.

Disorders of Nutrient Intake

Anorexia Nervosa. Classified as both an eating disorder and a psychiatric disorder, anorexia nervosa is the refusal to maintain normal body weight for age and height. The affected person weighs at least 15% less than expected. Not only does the person show signs of extreme weight loss and emaciation (skeleton-like appearance), but he or she also may experience abdominal pain, fatigue, dizziness, anemia, and heart arrhythmias. Other signs and symptoms are constipation, dry skin, thin hair, brittle nails, and cold intolerance.

Massage can be a helpful adjunct to counseling, and a gentle, nurturing massage can help improve your client's self-image. Be sure to keep your client covered with both a sheet drape and warm blanket as he or she is prone to feeling chilly. Use an emollient lubricant to alleviate dry skin. If your client is fatigued, reduce treatment time to 30 minutes and use lighter-than-normal pressure. Some individuals are uncomfortable with their bodies and may elect not to disrobe; be prepared to work through clothes. Also, be aware that clients with anorexia nervosa may be very sensitive to any comments about their body so they are best avoided.

Bulimia. Bulimia is characterized by an insatiable craving for food resulting in episodes of continuous eating (binge eating or bingeing) followed by recurrent inappropriate compensatory behaviors to prevent weight gain. These activities include self-induced vomiting called purging (primary method); misuse of laxatives, diuretics, and enemas; excessive exercise, and fasting. During episodes of binge eating, food that are high in calories are usually preferred and are ingested within a very short amount of time. The person also often feels guilt and shame associated with bulimic behaviors.

Massage can be a helpful adjunct to counseling, and a gentle, nurturing massage can improve your client's self-image. Use an emollient lubricant to alleviate dry skin. If your client is overly fatigued, reduce treatment time to 30 minutes and use lighter-than-normal pressure. Some individuals with bulimia are uncomfortable with their bodies and may elect not to disrobe; be prepared to work through clothes.

Obesity. Obesity is characterized by an abnormal increase in the proportion of fat cells, primarily in subcutaneous and visceral tissues of the body. An individual is regarded as obese when his or her body mass index (BMI) is greater than 30 kg/m^2. BMI is calculated as weight (in kilograms), divided by height (in meters squared). Obesity is most often the result of excessive caloric intake in relation to calories burned through physical activity. BMI calculators are found easily by searching the Internet.

Some clients feel uncomfortable within their bodies and may elect not to disrobe; be willing to work through clothing. Consider lowering the massage table height. Use a semireclining position while your client is supine and limit the time spent in the prone position if your client is concerned about ease of breathing. Other suggestions are found in Chapter 11.

SPOTLIGHT ON RESEARCH

Research suggests that massage therapy may:
- Increase gastric motility in persons with constipation

"In dwelling, live close to the ground. In thinking, keep it simple. In conflict, be fair and generous. In governing, don't control. In work, do what you enjoy. In family life, be completely present."
—Tao Te Ching

E-RESOURCES

⊜volve

http://evolve.elsevier.com/Salvo/MassageTherapy
- Chapter challenge
- Flash cards
- Photo gallery
- Educational animations
- Weblinks

BIBLIOGRAPHY

Abrahams P, Marks S, Hutchings R: *McMinn's color atlas of human anatomy*, St Louis, 2003, Mosby.

Applegate EJ: *The anatomy and physiology learning system*, ed 3, Philadelphia, 2006, Saunders.

Beers MH, Berkow R: *The Merck manual of diagnosis and therapy*, Whitehouse Station, NJ, 2006, Merck Research Laboratories.

Como D, editor: *Mosby's medical, nursing, and allied health dictionary*, ed 6, St Louis, 2002, Mosby.

Crawley J, Van De Graaff KM: *A photographic atlas for anatomy and physiology*, Englewood, Colo, 2002, Morton.

Crooks R, Stein J: *Psychology: science, behavior, and life*, New York, 1990, Harcourt College Publishers.

Damjanov I: *Pathophysiology for the health-related professions*, ed 3, Philadelphia, 2006, Saunders.

Ferri FF: *2003 Ferri's clinical advisor, instant diagnosis and treatment*, St Louis, 2003, Mosby.

Frazier MS, Drzymkowski JW: *Essentials of human diseases and conditions*, ed 3, Philadelphia, 2004, Saunders.

Fritz S: *Massage online for essential sciences for therapeutic massage*, ed 3, St Louis, 2010, Mosby.

Goldberg S: *Clinical anatomy made ridiculously simple*, Miami, 1984, Medmaster.

Gould BE: *Pathophysiology for the health professions*, ed 3, Philadelphia, 2006, Saunders.

Haubrich WS: *Medical meanings: a glossary of word origins*, New York, 1984, Harcourt Brace Jovanovich.

Huether SE, McCance KL: *Understanding pathophysiology*, ed 3, St Louis, 2004, Mosby.

Jacob S, Francone C: *Elements of anatomy and physiology*, Philadelphia, 1989, WB Saunders.

Kalat JW: *Biological psychology*, ed 8, Belmont, Calif, 2003, Wadsworth.

Kapit W, Elson LM: *The anatomy coloring book*, ed 3, New York, 2002, Benjamin Cummings.

Kordish M, Dickson S: *Introduction to basic human anatomy*, Lake Charles, La, 1995, McNeese State University.

Kumar V, Abbas A, Fausto N: *Robbins and Cotran physiologic basis of disease*, ed 7, St Louis, 2005, Mosby.

Marieb EN: *Essentials of human anatomy and physiology*, ed 8, New York, 2005, Benjamin Cummings.

Martini FH, Bartholomew EF: *Essentials of anatomy and physiology*, ed 3, New York, 2003, Benjamin Cummings.

McAleer N: *The body almanac*, Garden City, NY, 1985, Doubleday.

McCance K, Huether S: *Pathophysiology: the biological basis for disease in adults and children*, St Louis, 2006, Mosby.

Merck manual, ed 17, Whitehouse Station, NJ, 1998, Merck and Co.

Moore KL: *Clinically oriented anatomy*, ed 5, Baltimore, 2005, Lippincott Williams & Wilkins.

Newton D: *Pathology for massage therapists*, ed 2, Portland, Ore, 1995, Simran.

Premkumar K: *Pathology A to Z, a handbook for massage therapists*, Baltimore, 1999, Lippincott Williams & Wilkins.

Salvo SG: *Mosby's pathology for massage therapists*, ed 2, St Louis, 2009, Mosby.

Solomon EP, Phillips GA: *Understanding human anatomy and physiology*, Philadelphia, 1987, WB Saunders.

Thibodeau G, Patton K: *Anatomy and physiology*, ed 6, St Louis, 2006, Mosby.

Thibodeau G, Patton K: *Structure and function of the body*, ed 12, St Louis, 2004, Mosby.

Tortora GJ: *Introduction to the human body: the essentials of anatomy and physiology*, ed 5, Hoboken, NJ, 2000, John Wiley & Sons.

Tortora GJ, Grabowksi SR: *Principles of anatomy and physiology*, ed 11, New York, 2005, John Wiley & Sons.

Venes D, Thomas CL, Taber CW: *Taber's cyclopedic medical dictionary*, ed 20, Philadelphia, 2005, FA Davis.

MATCHING I

Place the letter of the answer next to the term or phrase that best describes it.

A. Absorption
B. Defecation
C. Deglutition
D. Digestion

E. Esophagus
F. Gastrointestinal tract
G. Ingestion
H. Mastication

I. Peristalsis
J. Peritoneum
K. Salivary glands
L. Stomach

_____ 1. Glands that secrete a clear, viscous fluid that helps keep oral mucosa moist, as well as lubricating food so that it is easier to swallow

_____ 2. Muscular tube that extends from the pharynx to the stomach

_____ 3. Term synonymous with chewing

_____ 4. Large serous membrane that envelopes the abdominal cavity and major digestive organs

_____ 5. Term synonymous with swallowing

_____ 6. Process of orally taking materials into the body

_____ 7. Hollow organ located between the lower esophageal sphincter and the pyloric sphincter

_____ 8. Process of eliminating indigestible or unabsorbed material from the body

_____ 9. Rhythmic muscular contraction that mixes and propels products of digestion along the gastrointestinal tract

_____ 10. Process by which molecules from the digestive tract move into the bloodstream or lymph vessels, and then into cells

_____ 11. Long tube that starts at the mouth, extends through the body, and ends at the anus

_____ 12. Mechanical and chemical processes that break food down into simple molecules

MATCHING II

Place the letter of the answer next to the term or phrase that best describes it.

A. Amylase
B. Gallbladder
C. Ileocecal
D. Large intestine

E. Lipase
F. Liver
G. Pancreas
H. Pepsinogen/pepsin

I. Pyloric
J. Rugae
K. Small intestine
L. Villi

_____ 1. Gland that produces enzymes that break down all categories of digestible foods, including proteins, carbohydrates, and fats

_____ 2. Hollow organ that stores bile

_____ 3. Digestive enzyme produced by the stomach's chief cells that break down proteins

_____ 4. Fingerlike projections located in the small intestine that house blood and lymph capillaries

_____ 5. Sphincter located between the small and large intestine

_____ 6. Sphincter located between the stomach and small intestine

_____ 7. Area of the gastrointestinal tract that contains the cecum and rectum

_____ 8. Area of the gastrointestinal tract that contains the duodenum, jejunum, and ileum

_____ 9. Digestive enzyme that breaks down carbohydrates

_____ 10. Folds in the stomach's lining enabling it to expand as food is ingested

_____ 11. Digestive organ that secretes bile

_____ 12. Digestive enzyme that breaks down lipids into glycerol and fatty acids

CASE STUDY

Oh No, Not Now

Sandy arrives at your office at 4:45 for her 5 PM massage appointment.

She is a 29-year-old white woman who just found out she is pregnant.

After she fills out the intake form, Sandy heads for the restroom and does not return for about 10 minutes.

During the interview, Sandy says that she has diarrhea and some cramping today, "but that's normal with IBS, you know," she adds.

Because of her pregnancy, her doctor took her off her medications. What is an appropriate treatment plan for Sandy?

CRITICAL THINKING

You've probably heard someone tell a picky eater not to worry about food combinations because "it all ends up in the same place." What are the shortcomings of this assertion?

CHAPTER 30

Urinary System

"One doesn't discover
new lands without
consenting to lose sight
of the shore for a very
long time."

—Andre Gide

LEARNING OBJECTIVES

After completing this chapter, the student should be able to:

- List anatomic structures and physiologic processes of the urinary system.
- Describe the kidneys, including their two regions.
- Name and describe parts of a nephron and the collecting ducts.
- Define parts of the juxtaglomerular apparatus and discuss its importance.
- Identify blood vessels and describe blood flow through the kidneys.
- Explain the filtration process.
- List and describe the urinary system's accessory structures, such as the ureters, urinary bladder, and urethra.
- Explain what urine is and what influences its production and secretion.
- Identify and discuss fluid imbalances.
- Name types of urinary pathologies, giving characteristics and massage considerations for each.

INTRODUCTION

The human body is a complex machine and, as such, does not perform properly if wastes from fuel consumption and other processes are not removed. Cells of the body metabolize nutrients, which produce wastes such as nitrogen, ammonia, and urea. These are toxic to the body. Sodium chloride, sodium sulfate, phosphate, hydrogen molecules, ions, and other substances also accumulate as a result of metabolic activities. All of these waste materials must be excreted from the body for homeostasis to be maintained and for metabolism to function optimally.

Excretion of waste products is such a large task that no single body system can handle it alone.

Several systems contribute to waste elimination—the respiratory, integumentary, and digestive systems, as well as the urinary system.

The kidneys within the urinary system filter waste products from the blood and produce urine. It travels through the ureters and down into the urinary bladder, which contains it until expelling it out of the body through the urethra. **Voiding,** or **micturition,** is the act of urination.

ANATOMY

Basic anatomy of the urinary system is:
- Kidneys
- Ureters
- Urethra
- Urinary bladder

PHYSIOLOGY

The functions of the urinary system are:
- **Eliminates wastes and foreign substances.** Waste products produced by metabolism and foreign substances (drug metabolites, environmental toxins) are eliminated.
- **Regulates chemical composition of blood.** The kidneys possess cells that monitor the acid-base balance of the blood. Wastes are filtered from the blood, substances such as glucose, sodium, vitamins, and minerals are reabsorbed to adjust the blood's chemical composition.
- **Regulates blood pH.** Mechanisms in the kidney assist with the regulation of blood pH by eliminating acids and ions.
- **Regulates blood volume and fluid balance.** The kidneys adjust blood volume by conserving or eliminating water. In this way, both the blood volume and the body's fluid balance are altered.
- **Regulates blood pressure.** The kidneys continuously monitor blood pressure and help maintain it within normal range by secreting an enzyme that stimulates

vasoconstriction. Blood pressure is also kept in balance by the regulation of blood volume. Blood pressure is complex and also involves interaction of the circulatory, endocrine, and nervous systems. Problems within one or several of these systems can cause blood pressure abnormalities.
- **Maintains homeostasis.** Because they remove wastes, regulate the blood's chemical composition and blood volume, and by maintain fluid balance and blood pressure, the kidneys have the title of *major homeostatic organs of the body.* Cells and tissues are making wastes constantly as byproducts of metabolism. If these wastes are not removed quickly, they build up, potentially resulting in cell, tissue, and even organ failure. In fact, malfunction of the kidneys causes dangerous changes in blood composition, which may lead to death.

KIDNEYS

The **kidneys** are the two reddish-brown organs located bilaterally at or about the spinal level of T11 to L3 (Figure 30-1). They are lima bean–shaped organs (convex laterally and concave medially) and are approximately the size of a bar of bath soap.

The indentation on the medial side of the kidneys is where the renal arteries, veins, and the ureters enter and exit. Both kidneys lie behind the peritoneum (or retroperitoneally). On top of each kidney is an adrenal gland.

The kidneys are surrounded by a fibrous capsule and are imbedded in adipose tissue, which both serve as a barrier against trauma and the spread of infection. Because of the presence of the liver, the kidney on the right side of the body is slightly lower than the one on the left.

The principal organs of the urinary system, the kidneys process blood and form urine to be excreted. In the average person, the kidneys filter about 180 L of blood and produce about 1 L of urine per day. Each kidney is a separate, functioning organ. If one kidney is removed, the other will then increase its filtering capacity so that it will filter at 80% of the capacity of two normal kidneys.

Kidney Regions

Each kidney is divided into regions (Figure 30-2). The cortex and medulla contain approximately 1 million nephrons, specialized tube-shaped structures that filter, reabsorb, and excrete substances to form urine.

Cortex. The outer region of the kidney. The nephron's glomerulus and Bowman's capsule is located in the renal cortex.

Medulla. The inner region of the kidney. The nephron's loop of Henle is located in the renal medulla.

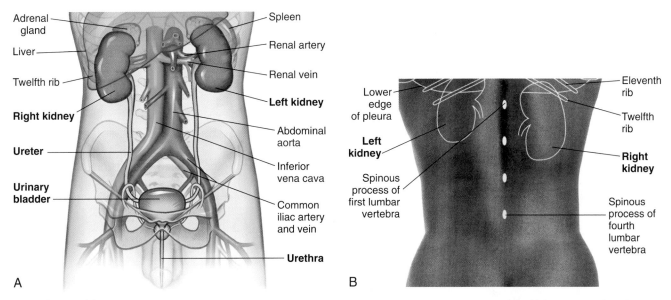

FIGURE 30-1 The urinary system. **A,** General urinary structure (anterior view) and **(B)** location of the kidneys (posterior view).

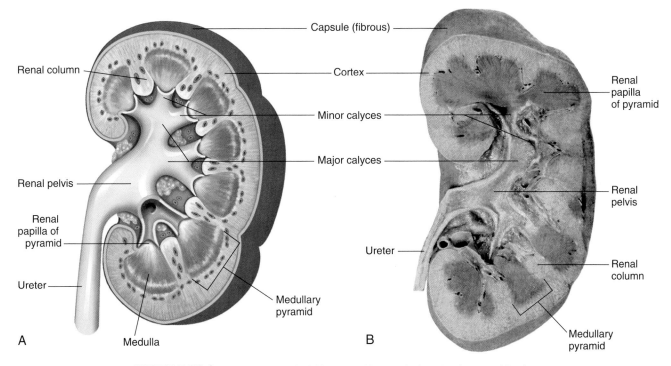

FIGURE 30-2 Cross section of a kidney. **A,** Illustrated view. **B,** Photographic view.

NEPHRON

The kidneys are composed of filtering units called **nephrons**. Approximately 1.25 million nephrons are found in each kidney, and 85% of all them are located almost entirely in the renal cortex. The remainder lie in the renal medulla. The nephron has three main parts: (1) the glomerulus; (2) Bowman's capsule; and (3) the renal tubule (Figure 30-3).

Glomerulus

The glomerulus is a small cluster of blood vessels within Bowman's capsules. Between the glomerulus and Bowman's capsule is a filtration membrane (also called the glomerular basement membrane). This membrane contains pores through which substances are filtered out of the blood. Blood cells and proteins are too large to fit through the filtration membrane in a normally functioning kidney. Blood pressure is the force responsible for filtration.

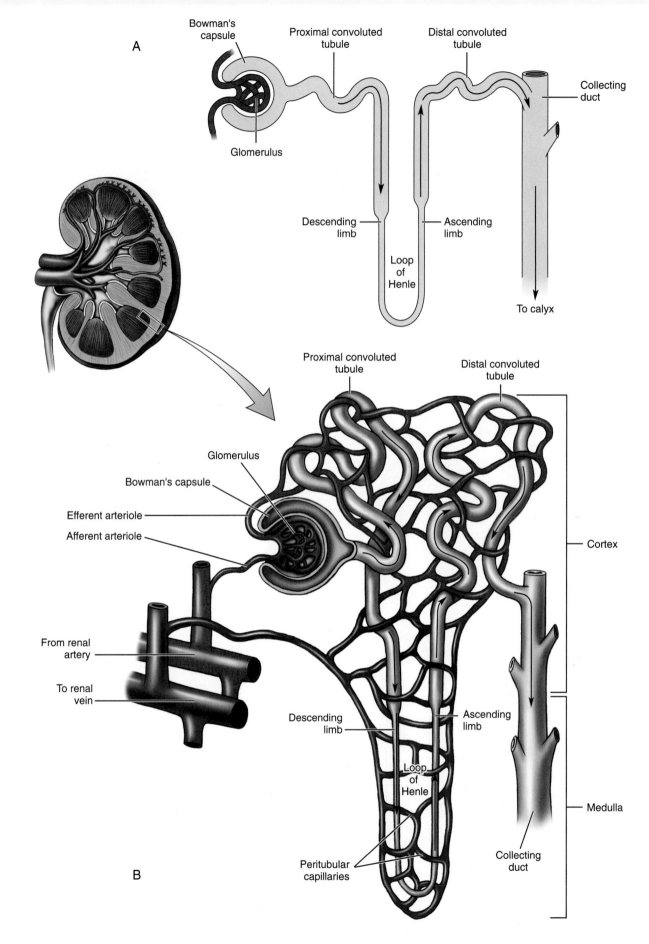

FIGURE 30-3 A nephron's tubular and vascular network. **A,** A nephron's fluid flow. **B,** Nephron and surrounding peritubular capillaries.

Bowman's Capsule

The hollow cup-shaped mouth of a nephron is called Bowman's capsule. **Filtrate** (fluid filtered by the kidneys) is collected in Bowman's capsule then transported to the renal tubule.

Bowman's capsule and the glomerulus are often collectively referred to as the *renal corpuscle.*

Renal Tubules

The renal tubule is part of the nephron leading from Bowman's capsule. This is where collected wastes and fluids become urine. As filtrate travels through the renal tubule, some substances such as certain ions and water are moved back into the blood, while other substances such as additional wastes remain as filtrate.

Parts of the renal tubule are the *proximal convoluted tubule,* the *loop of Henle,* and the *distal convoluted tubule.* An important structure, the juxtaglomerular apparatus, is found at the point where the afferent arteriole touches part of the distal convoluted tubule (see next section).

Numerous collecting tubules organize themselves into a dozen or so distant triangular wedges called *medullary pyramids.* Cortical tissue located between the medullary pyramids are called the *renal columns.*

Distal tubules of several nephrons connect to one collecting duct. Collecting ducts join larger ducts and become the *renal papillae,* located at the narrow base of each pyramid.

Each renal papilla protrudes into a small, cuplike structure called a *calyx.* Several minor calyces join to form a major calyx. These structures combine together to form a large collection reservoir called the *renal pelvis,* which is the upper region of the ureter. The following diagram represents how fluids flow in the nephron.

Bowman's capsule
↓
Renal tubule
↓
Collecting duct
↓
Renal papilla
↓
Minor calyx
↓
Major calyx
↓
Renal pelvis
↓
Ureter

JUXTAGLOMERULAR APPARATUS

Given that blood pressure is the force behind filtration, the kidneys are equipped with cells that measure blood pressure; the juxtaglomerular apparatus (Figure 30-4). Within the juxtaglomerular apparatus are two important structures: (1) the juxtaglomerular cells and (2) the macula densa.

Juxtaglomerular Cells

Juxtaglomerular cells are located in the afferent arteriole. These cells contain renin granules that act as mechanoreceptors (receptors detecting pressure). Juxtaglomerular cells assist in maintaining blood pressure by secreting an enzyme called *renin* when blood pressure drops. Renin converts angiotensinogen from the liver into angiotensin I. Angiotensin I, when transported through the lungs, becomes angiotensin II. Angiotensin II causes the secretion of aldosterone from the adrenal cortex, a hormone that increases sodium and water reabsorption. This action increases blood volume and blood pressure. This pathway is called the *renin-angiotensin-aldosterone system.*

⊖volve *The renin-angiotensin-aldosterone system is essential to understand because many medications used to treat high blood pressure act on this system as inhibitors. Log on to the Evolve website to see a schematic drawing of this mechanism.* ∎

Macula Densa

The macula densa is located in the ascending limb of the Henle loop and contains dense, tightly packed cells that

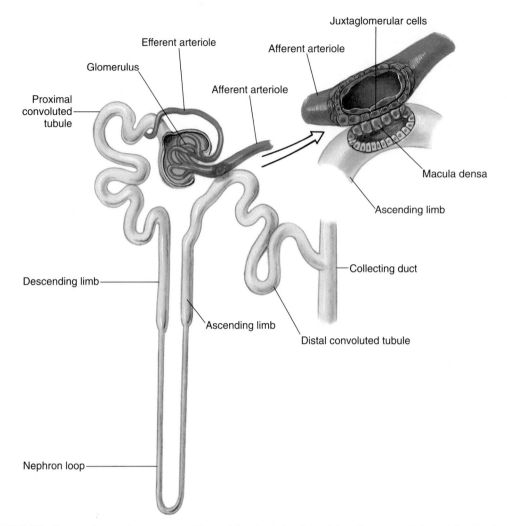

FIGURE 30-4 Juxtaglomerular apparatus. The positional relationship of the afferent arteriole and the distal tubule.

are chemoreceptors (receptors detecting chemicals), sensing the concentration of the filtrate as it passes through the renal tubule. The cells of the macula densa respond to a decrease in sodium by releasing prostaglandins (hormonelike substances), which also stimulates renin secretion. You already know how renin affects blood pressure.

In review, the juxtaglomerular cells monitor changes in blood pressure in the afferent arteriole, and the macula densa monitors the concentration of the filtrate in the renal tubule. Both respond by secreting renin.

BLOOD VESSELS AND BLOOD FLOW IN THE KIDNEYS

Oxygen-rich blood enters the kidneys via the renal artery. As the renal artery enters the kidney, the artery narrows, becoming the *afferent arteriole*. The afferent arteriole branches into a small cluster of fine capillaries within Bowman's capsule called the *glomerulus*.

At this juncture, blood leaves the glomerulus and flows into *efferent arterioles* (not into venules). Blood from the

efferent arterioles moves into the *peritubular capillaries*. The placement of an arteriole between two capillary beds (glomerulus and peritubular capillaries) is unique and found only in the kidney. The peritubular capillaries surround the renal tubule. This is where most reabsorption of substances in the filtrate back into the blood occurs, and where additional substances in the blood are added to the filtrate. Blood from the peritubular capillaries then joins the venous system first through the *renal venules*, then the *renal vein*, and finally the *inferior vena cava* (see Figure 30-3, *B*). To review, the sequence of blood in the kidneys is as follows:

Renal artery

↓

Afferent arteriole

↓

Glomerulus

↓

Efferent arteriole

↓

Peritubular capillaries

↓

JAN SCHWARTZ

Born: May 12, 1947

"Be the change you want to see in the world."

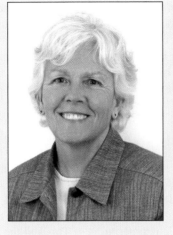

Jan Schwartz fell into a career in massage therapy, but that has not kept her from making her mark in the industry. Today, Schwartz is widely recognized for her efforts to advance educational standards for massage therapists.

Schwartz was born in Pennsylvania in 1947. She attended Rutgers University and graduated with a bachelor's degree in economics. After a long career with Dale Carnegie, Schwartz was ready for what she called "the proverbial get out of corporate life."

Schwartz moved to Tucson, Arizona, in 1992 with her partner. "As we drove up Sixth Avenue, I saw the Desert Institute of the Healing Arts and we stopped. I went in and found out they were a school of massage therapy and I thought, oh, I could do that for a year," recalls Schwartz.

What started out as 1 year turned to 14 with the Desert Institute. After completing her training, Schwartz stayed on as the admissions director for 3 years and spent 7 years as the school's education director.

While with the Desert Institute, Schwartz also spent time in the classroom, teaching injury management and rehabilitation classes. An avid runner and cyclist, Schwartz dealt with the common aches and pains that come with dedicated athleticism for her entire life. Schwartz has completed the 100-mile Tour de Tucson quite a few times and competed in the Kona half-marathon. A bad hamstring injury from cycling that plagued her for 6 years gave Schwartz intimate knowledge from which to teach.

"I love teaching, I like being able to transfer knowledge and demonstrate application to other people. I like to witness the excitement when people start to get it," Schwartz said.

After the Desert Institute, Schwartz worked with Cortiva Institute, an education company that boasted nine massage therapy schools in 11 different locations around the country. Schwartz took the job with Cortiva to help shape the future of massage therapy. She codeveloped, from the ground up, a 750-hour curriculum with a 250 hour add-on program for those schools who wanted to continue to teach 1000 hours. She is constantly looking for ways to improve the educational standards and teaching practices for massage therapists.

Schwartz says, "One of the shortcomings of vocational education in this country is that there's the mistaken idea that if you can do something well you can then teach something well and the profession of teaching requires a certain skill set that isn't conveyed when you learn massage therapy."

Schwartz served on the Commission of Massage Therapy Accreditation for five years and was Chair for three. She was recognized by the American Massage Therapy Association for outstanding leadership and distinguished service in 2002 and 2005. Currently, she is on the Board of the Academic Consortium for Complementary and Alternative Health Care and on the Board of Trustees of the Massage Therapy Foundation.

After completing her master's degree at Prescott College in 2009, Schwartz began a business with Whitney Lowe, Education and Training Solutions. They create and host online education programs for continuing education providers and for schools. She says, "I love my new job, it allows me to continue my work to improve educational standards and teaching practices for massage therapy in new and exciting ways."

Renal venule
↓
Renal vein
↓
Inferior vena cava

CHAT ROOM

The entire blood supply of the body passes through the kidneys every 3 minutes. At rest, a fourth to a fifth of the body's blood can be found in the kidneys. In fact, the body's entire blood volume is filtered 65 times in a 24-hour period.

FILTRATION PROCESS

Initially, the kidneys filter out materials that are both needed and unneeded. Many necessary nutrients and molecules are reabsorbed back into the blood before they are excreted in urine. This takes place in a three-step process.

Filtration

The first step in this process is called filtration. Here, blood enters the glomerulus. Water and small solids in the blood pass through the filtration membrane and enter Bowman's capsule and renal tubule. Proteins and blood cells that are too large to cross the membrane remain in the bloodstream. This process is so efficient that approximately 45 gallons (180 L) of filtrate is produced in a 24-hour day. Not all of this water is excreted as urine. Most of it is reabsorbed back into the blood.

Reabsorption

Approximately 99% of the removed fluids along with much-needed substances such as glucose and amino acids are reabsorbed and moved back into the bloodstream. This process occurs in the length of the renal tubule into peritubular capillaries.

Tubular Secretion

Before filtrate leaves the body as urine, the kidneys have one more opportunity to adjust its composition. During this stage, some substances are moved in the opposite direction; from the peritubular capillaries into the renal tubules for excretion. Tubular secretions rid the body of toxic compounds to regulate blood pH.

⊖volve   *As simplistic as this system may seem, the filtration process is one of the hardest concepts to teach because it is just short of a miracle. Posted on the Evolve website under Chapter 30 are illustrated steps of the filtration process. Log on to your student account to view it and other important materials.* ∎

"All feelings, both positive and unpleasant, come out of the same faucet. To turn down the faucet on pain is to slow the flow of pleasant feelings as well."
—Gay and Kathlyn Hendricks

URETERS

The **ureters** are two slender, hollow tubes extending from the renal pelvis of the kidneys to the urinary bladder. As the bladder fills, the distal portion of the ureter compresses, preventing a reverse flow of urine.

URINARY BLADDER

The **urinary bladder** is a hollow, muscular organ and a reservoir for urine. The bladder is located in the pelvis behind the pubic symphysis (Figure 30-5). In women, the bladder sits anterior to the vagina and posterior to the uterus (see Figure 25-3), whereas in men, it just superior to the prostate (see Figure 25-1). The bladder contains openings for two ureters and the urethra (discussed next).

The urinary bladder becomes filled with and then is emptied of urine. To allow for expansion, it contains folds in its interior lining called *rugae*. When the bladder is distended, the signal to void occurs.

URETHRA

The **urethra** is a narrow tube that transports urine from the urinary bladder out of the body during voiding (micturition, urination). The male urethra extends through the prostate; both urine and semen travel down this tube.

In females, the path of the urethra is between the vaginal opening and the clitoris and functions only to pass urine. The female urethra is relatively short (about 1.5 inches). This and the fact that the female urinary orifice is close to the anal opening may account for the much higher incidence of urinary tract infections in women.

CHAT ROOM

If water loss exceeds 5% to 10% of total body weight, serious dehydration results. A 20% loss of water is often fatal. Common causes of water loss are infection, fever, severe burns, and diarrhea.

URINE

Urine is concentrated filtrate from the kidneys that is 96% water and 4% dissolved wastes (e.g., urea, creatinine, uric acid, sodium chloride, potassium, sulfates, phosphates, drug residue). Urine tends to be slightly acidic and has a normal amber color. The more concentrated the urine is, the darker its color will be. Abnormal constituents in urine may include albumin, glucose, red blood cells (uremia), white blood cells, bilirubin, kidney stones, and bacteria.

Micturition, or *voiding,* begins with a voluntary relaxation of the external sphincter muscle of the bladder.

The average adult produces 1 L of urine per day. Chemical, nervous, and even physical factors can affect the amount of urine produced and excreted by the body. An example of a chemical factor is the consumption of caffeine in coffee, tea, and many carbonated beverages. Stimulating the production of urine, these drinks have a diuretic effect on the urinary system. A *diuretic* is a substance that promotes the formation and excretion of urine. Alcohol also has a diuretic effect because it inhibits the secretion of antidiuretic hormone (discussed in the next section).

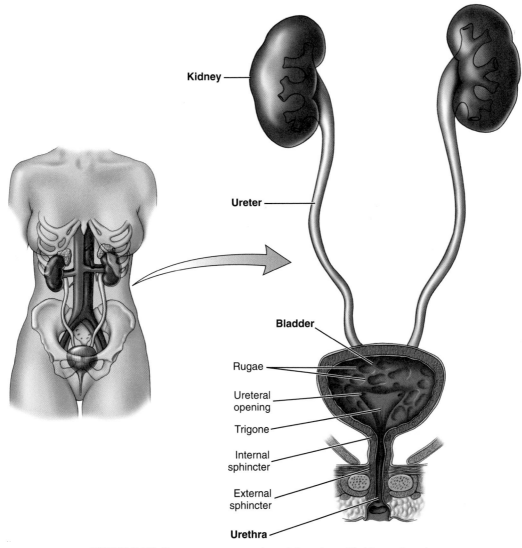

Kidney

Ureter

Bladder

Rugae

Ureteral opening

Trigone

Internal sphincter

External sphincter

Urethra

FIGURE 30-5 Ureters, cross section of the urinary bladder, and urethra.

FLUID BALANCE

For the body to maintain homeostasis, input of water and electrolytes must be balanced by output. The fluid, or water, content of the body ranges from 40% to 60% of its total weight. The total water of the body can be subdivided into two major compartments: extracellular fluids and intracellular fluids. *Extracellular fluids* consist of plasma, interstitial fluid, lymph, and transcellular fluid. These fluids provide a constant environment for cells and help in the transportation of substances to and from them. *Intracellular fluids* lie within cells and facilitate chemical reactions that maintain life. Most body fluid is intracellular (Figure 30-6).

The key to fluid balance lies with the secretion of hormones. *Antidiuretic hormone* (ADH) secreted by the pituitary regulates the balance of water in the body. If the bloodstream becomes concentrated as a result of the loss of water through sweat or urination, ADH is released, which stimulates the kidneys to reabsorb more water. If blood is

too dilute, ADH secretion is inhibited and the kidneys produce more urine. The hormone *aldosterone,* (produced in the adrenal cortex) works in concert with ADH to maintain homeostasis of body fluids. Production of these hormones will also vary depending on how much fluid the person is taking in.

Additionally, specialized cells located in the atrial walls of the heart produce *atrial natriuretic hormone* (ANH). This hormone decreases sodium by triggering urine production, or *diuresis,* which additionally decreases blood volume and blood pressure. In this regard, ANH is an antagonist to ADH and aldosterone.

Fluid regulation is essential to homeostasis. If water or electrolyte levels rise or fall beyond normal limits, many body functions fail to proceed at their normal rates. Dehydration is an example of a fluid imbalance. Maintaining normal pH levels is also important for normal body functioning because small changes in pH can produce major changes in metabolism.

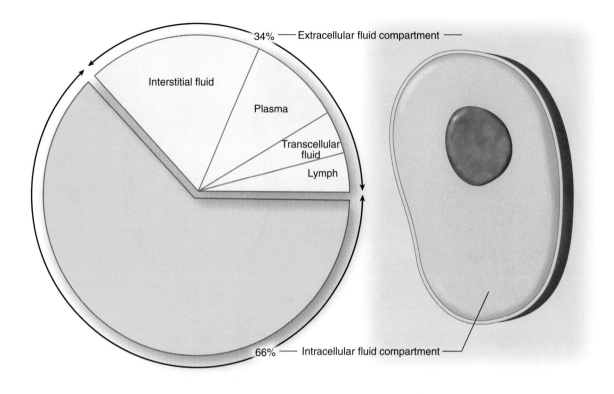

FIGURE 30-6 Distribution of fluids within the body.

FLUID IMBALANCE

Fluid imbalance can occur in many ways. These include problems with urine production, inadequate fluid intake, inadequate ADH production, diabetes mellitus, and lymph blockage.

Dehydration can occur when water is unavailable or with conditions such as severe diarrhea or vomiting and excessive sweating. Edema, or swelling, can occur with the accumulation of excess fluids in interstitial compartments. In some cases, fluid imbalance causes severe health problems and even death.

Turgor

If you suspect that your client is dehydrated, check his or her skin turgor. *Turgor* is skin resiliency, which decreases during dehydration. To test turgor, grasp the skin for a few seconds, and then release. If the skin rebounds quickly, your client has good skin turgor. If this produces a tent, your client has poor skin turgor and may be dehydrated. Common places to assess skin turgor are over the back of the hand, lower arm, and abdomen. Keep in mind that many elderly people have decreased skin elasticity, so wrinkled, loose skin on the back of the hand should not be mistaken for poor turgor.

Edema

Edema is abnormal accumulation of fluids. Kidney, heart, and liver diseases often have edema as one of their presenting signs. Edema is often associated with injuries or surgeries, as well as local or systemic inflammatory processes. Edema can also be pitting or nonpitting. *Pitting edema* is used to describe edema that leaves a pit or dent in a swollen area once the skin is compressed for a few seconds and released; the edematous tissue rebounds slowly. Most edema is nonpitting. See Chapter 27 for more information on edema.

URINARY PATHOLOGIES

Kidney Disorders

Kidney Stones. Stones found in the kidney, renal pelvis, or ureters are called kidney stones. Some are asymptomatic and pass unnoticed. When a stone lodges, the affected person experiences sudden severe flank pain. Pain may be accompanied by nausea, vomiting, fever and chills, bloating, blood or pus in the urine, or a foul odor in the urine.

Massage is contraindicated during the acute phase, indicated by signs and symptoms listed above. Once the stone has passed or has been addressed via medical procedures, massage is indicated. Also, if your client has a history of kidney stones but none currently, massage may be performed while avoiding vigorous percussion over the kidneys (because recurrence is so common).

Polycystic Kidney Disease. Polycystic kidney disease (PKD) is a slowly progressive disease wherein the kidneys become riddled with thousands of multiple grapelike cysts. PKD is one of the most common genetic disorders in the United States.

Clearance from your client's health care provider is essential before providing massage to the person with PKD. Once this has been obtained, avoid deep pressure over the lumbar and abdominopelvic areas. Recommend that the client void before the massage begins.

Kidney Failure. Kidney failure is inability of the kidneys to adequately perform their functions. There are two main types: acute and chronic. With *acute renal failure*, there is an abrupt and severe reduction in kidney function, usually within hours. However, most people who acquire acute renal failure are already hospitalized, particularly those in intensive care, so treatment is usually expedient. *Chronic renal failure*, often caused by diabetes and untreated high blood pressure, is usually not suspected until kidney function has decreased to less than 25% of normal.

Acute renal failure is a medical emergency requiring immediate medical attention. Massage is postponed until the condition resolves. For cases of chronic renal failure, medical clearance must be obtained. Then, massage with lighter-than-normal pressure and for no longer than 20 minutes is indicated. Be sure to address other medical conditions, such as diabetes, in the

treatment plan. Clients should be advised to drink plenty of water before and after their massage.

Disorders of the Bladder and Urinary Tract

Bladder Infection. Bladder infection, or cystitis, is often characterized by pain in the suprapubic region or lower back, burning and pain during urination, blood in urine, or cloudy urine with a foul odor. Bladder infection is also marked by urinary urgency and frequency. Elderly people may not have the typical symptoms, but instead complain of only lower back pain, or mild nausea. Bacteria such as *E. coli* present in feces can be transported to the female urethra as a result of improper toilet habits (i.e., wiping from back to front rather than front to back).

Position your client for comfort and avoid massage over the lumbar and abdominopelvic areas if pressure causes pain or discomfort. Suggest use of the toilet before massage as a comfort measure and be prepared for a toilet break during the session.

Urinary Incontinence. Loss of voluntary bladder control is called urinary incontinence. The most common type is *stress incontinence*: The affected person laughs or sneezes, and urine leaks through the bladder sphincter without the feeling of prior urgency. This can also occur during late-stage pregnancy or during physical exertion such as lifting or running. Many elderly who are affected by stress incontinence use absorbent pads.

Avoid the abdominopelvic region if pressure causes distress or discomfort. Suggest use of the toilet before massage as a comfort measure and be prepared for a toilet break during the session.

E-RESOURCES

(e)volve

http://evolve.elsevier.com/Salvo/MassageTherapy

- Chapter challenge
- Flash cards
- Photo gallery
- Educational animations
- Weblinks

BIBLIOGRAPHY

Abrahams P, Marks S, Hutchings R: *McMinn's color atlas of human anatomy*, St Louis, 2003, Mosby.

Applegate EJ: *The anatomy and physiology learning system*, ed 3, Philadelphia, 2006, Saunders.

Beers MH, Berkow R: *The Merck manual of diagnosis and therapy*, Whitehouse Station, NJ, 2006, Merck Research Laboratories.

Como D, editor: *Mosby's medical, nursing, and allied health dictionary*, ed 6, St Louis, 2002, Mosby.

Crawley J, Van De Graaff KM: *A photographic atlas for anatomy and physiology*, Englewood, Colo, 2002, Morton.

Damjanov I: *Pathophysiology for the health-related professions*, ed 3, Philadelphia, 2006, Saunders.

Ferri FF: *2003 Ferri's clinical advisor, instant diagnosis and treatment*, St Louis, 2003, Mosby.

Goldberg S: *Clinical anatomy made ridiculously simple*, Miami, 2004, Medmaster.

Gould BE: *Pathophysiology for the health professions*, ed 3, Philadelphia, 2006, Saunders.

Gray H, Pick TP, Howden R: *Gray's anatomy*, ed 29, Philadelphia, 1974, Running Press.

Guyton A: *Human physiology and mechanisms of disease*, ed 6, Philadelphia, 1996, WB Saunders.

Haubrich WS: *Medical meanings: a glossary of word origins*, New York, 1984, Harcourt Brace Jovanovich.

Huether SE, McCance KL: *Understanding pathophysiology*, ed 3, St Louis, 2004, Mosby.

Jacob S, Francone C: *Elements of anatomy and physiology*, Philadelphia, 1989, Saunders.

Kapit W, Elson LM: *The anatomy coloring book*, ed 3, New York, 2002, Benjamin Cummings.

Kordish M, Dickson S: *Introduction to basic human anatomy*, Lake Charles, La, 1995, McNeese State University.

Kumar V, Abbas A, Fausto N: *Robbins and Cotran physiologic basis of disease*, ed 7, St Louis, 2005, Mosby.

Marieb EN: *Essentials of human anatomy and physiology*, ed 8, New York, 2005, Benjamin Cummings.

Martini FH, Bartholomew EF: *Essentials of anatomy and physiology*, ed 3, New York, 2003, Benjamin Cummings.

McAleer N: *The body almanac*, Garden City, NY, 1985, Doubleday.

McCance K, Huether S: *Pathophysiology: the biological basis for disease in adults and children*, St Louis, 2006, Mosby.

Merck manual, ed 17, Whitehouse Station, NJ, 1998, Merck and Co.

Moore KL: *Clinically oriented anatomy*, ed 5, Baltimore, 2005, Lippincott Williams & Wilkins.

Netter FH: *Atlas of human anatomy*, ed 3, Teterboro, NJ, 2003, Icon Learning Systems.

Newton D: *Pathology for massage therapists*, ed 2, Portland, Ore, 1995, Simran.

Premkumar K: *Pathology A to Z, a handbook for massage therapists*, Baltimore, 1999, Lippincott Williams & Wilkins.

Salvo SG: *Mosby's pathology for massage therapists*, ed 2, St Louis, 2009, Mosby.

Solomon EP, Phillips GA: *Understanding human anatomy and physiology*, Philadelphia, 1987, WB Saunders.

Thibodeau G, Patton K: *Anatomy and physiology*, ed 6, St Louis, 2006, Mosby.

Thibodeau G, Patton K: *Structure and function of the body*, ed 12, St Louis, 2004, Mosby.

Tortora GJ: *Introduction to the human body: the essentials of anatomy and physiology*, ed 5, Hoboken, NJ, 2000, John Wiley & Sons.

Tortora GJ, Grabowksi SR: *Principles of anatomy and physiology*, ed 11, New York, 2005, John Wiley & Sons.

Venes D, Thomas CL, Taber CW: *Taber's cyclopedic medical dictionary*, ed 20, Philadelphia, 2005, FA Davis.

MATCHING I

Place the letter of the answer next to the term or phrase that best describes it.

A. Cortex
B. Densa
C. Juxtaglomerular apparatus
D. Kidneys

E. Medulla
F. Nephron
G. Pelvis
H. Retroperitoneal

I. Ureters
J. Urethra
K. Urinary bladder
L. Urine

_____ 1. Term that means behind the abdominal peritoneum

_____ 2. Basic filtering unit of the kidney

_____ 3. Outer region of the kidney

_____ 4. Tube that transports urine from the urinary bladder out of the body during urination

_____ 5. Upper region of the ureter and large collection reservoir

_____ 6. Bean-shaped pair of urinary system organs

_____ 7. Muscular, hollow organ providing a temporary storage for urine

_____ 8. Two slender tubes that transport urine from the kidneys to the urinary bladder

_____ 9. Inner region of the kidney

_____ 10. Area within the kidney that monitors blood pressure

_____ 11. Structure that monitors the concentration of the filtrate in the renal tubule; macula _____.

_____ 12. Concentrated filtrate from the kidneys

MATCHING II

Place the letter of the answer next to the term or phrase that best describes it.

A. Aldosterone
B. Antidiuretic hormone
C. Blood pressure
D. Bowman's capsule
E. Edema

F. Filtrate
G. Glomerulus
H. Micturition
I. Peritubular capillaries
J. Renal tubule

K. Renin-angiotensin-aldosterone system
L. Turgor

_____ 1. Abnormal accumulation of fluids

_____ 2. Blood vessels that surround the renal tubule

_____ 3. Term used to describe skin resiliency; decreases during dehydration

_____ 4. Pituitary hormone that stimulates the kidneys to reabsorb more water

_____ 5. Nephronic structure that collects filtered fluids in the glomerulus, then transports these fluids to the renal tubule

_____ 6. Term used to describe the fluid filtered from blood within the kidneys

_____ 7. Mechanism that increases blood volume and blood pressure when kidneys detect a drop in blood pressure

_____ 8. Area in the nephron where ions and water move from the filtrate back to the blood and substances are added to the filtrate from the blood

_____ 9. Force or pressure responsible for filtration in the glomerulus

_____ 10. Term synonymous with urination

_____ 11. Hormone of the adrenal cortex that promotes the retention of sodium, which stimulates the reabsorption of water back into the blood

_____ 12. Nephron structure formed by a small cluster of blood vessels

CASE STUDY

Time Out for Tom

Tom is a 26-year-old man with a history of recurrent kidney stones. He is currently in college and is working two jobs to help support his wife and newborn daughter. His parents bought him a massage to give him an opportunity to relax.

When Tom arrives at your office for his scheduled appointment, he asks to use the toilet. Afterward, he walks back into the office and apologizes for the awful smell. During Tom's intake, he complains of lower back pain, which he would like you to focus on. He also states that he

has gained a few pounds this week. You complete the intake and begin to escort him to the massage room. He asks if he could use the toilet once more. He returns from the toilet, but this time you notice that his face looks a little flushed.

Do you proceed with the massage? What are appropriate modifications you might implement for him?

If not, why?

CRITICAL THINKING

Many massage therapists state that tapotement/percussion should be avoided over the kidney area of the lower back. Explain that precaution and state whether you feel it is valid or not.

APPENDIX: SOAP NOTES

Sandy Grover Mason, BA, LMBT 4403, CMT, AMTA, NCTMB

Why Use SOAP Notes?

SOAP charting is your best option any time extensive documentation is necessary and is therefore the preferred chart for outcome-based massage, and for schools or therapists whose focus is a medical massage setting. The SOAP notes record client symptoms, functional limitations, and specific soft-tissue pain sources such as trigger points, inflammation, hypertonicities, etc.—basically any details pertaining to a client who has health problems that benefit from massage therapy. It is also the preferred documentation for a therapist when a doctor has referred a patient for treatment, or when insurance is involved in reimbursement for services. Considering that these situations are becoming more common, one can see why SOAP is widely used and is perhaps the most universal form among health care practitioners. If your massage business is geared toward work within the medical community, then you may consider SOAP to be your ideal choice for session documentation.

In the case where your client has been referred to you by a doctor, physical therapist, chiropractor, or other health care professional, the massage therapist should keep in mind that referring providers usually have a specific outcome in mind for their patient and will be expecting a report documenting progress toward this outcome. This should cue the therapist to perform a thorough assessment before and after treatment, and to clarify priorities with the client to reach a mutual agreement regarding goals for the client's health. It is helpful for everyone involved if the documentation process addresses the reason for the initial referral, and is in accordance with accepted practices and standards for the basic SOAP format. In the event that insurance is involved, the therapist should be aware that reimbursement is typically based solely on medical necessity and may be allowed only for treatment of the specific area of injury, *not* for full body massage. A SOAP chart is the proper document for evidence of need, as well as proof of measurable results from the session. Your records should include information regarding reduction of pain, change in posture, increase in range of motion or mobility and effects on activities of daily living (ADLs).

The primary advantages to charting with SOAP notes:

- Documentation: A SOAP chart is a legal document, defensible in court. Clear, precise, detailed notes on each session are the best form of protection, both for the therapist and the client.
- Communication: SOAP is the most common documentation form among health care practitioners; misunderstandings or breakdowns in communication within a health care team can be minimized by using this format.

- Clarity and brevity: Using the SOAP format and abbreviations helps minimize strain on your hands from writing or typing out full sentences. It also organizes every session the same way, and makes retrieving information from previous sessions quick and easy.
- Taking the burden off the therapist: The massage therapist using SOAP will not have to remember what applications or techniques were used, or what worked well in a session and what did not; they simply refer to the chart before beginning work with a client.
- Professionalism: By keeping all records well-documented, maintaining clear communication with other health providers, and keeping the therapist quickly and easily updated with all pertinent past information (from their own sessions or the work of other professionals), SOAP can help a massage therapist maintain a professional demeanor throughout their career.

What is a SOAP Note?

SOAP is an acronym for **S**ubjective, **O**bjective, **A**pplication, and **P**lan. Descriptions of what type of information a therapist should record in each section of the chart follow. At the end of this Appendix there are example forms—both blank and completed—and a list of common abbreviations used on the form. Be as specific as possible when documenting these items to demonstrate a measurable or quantifiable result.

Flexibility

There may exist slight alterations in exact categorization from one professional clinic to another regarding how a therapist can best customize their SOAP documentation. This is common in the medical field, and thus usually part of the orientation of a new therapist. Specific instructions regarding placement of information on the SOAP form will be given. Understanding the basics and intentions of SOAP notes gives a massage therapist a solid base from which they can alter certain details according to the demands of the professional setting in which they are operating.

An example of where one office may differ from another: Once the session is complete, the therapist should record which treatments seem to be effective and which do not; and whereas one office/hospital may prefer this information to be included as Objective information (as it is considered the therapist's observation), another may wish it to be recorded in Assessment, as part of what was noted during a session, or even Plan, as information to be remembered and included

Continued on p. 753

SOAP NOTES

Client: _____   **Client DOB:** _____

Therapist: _____   **Date:** _____

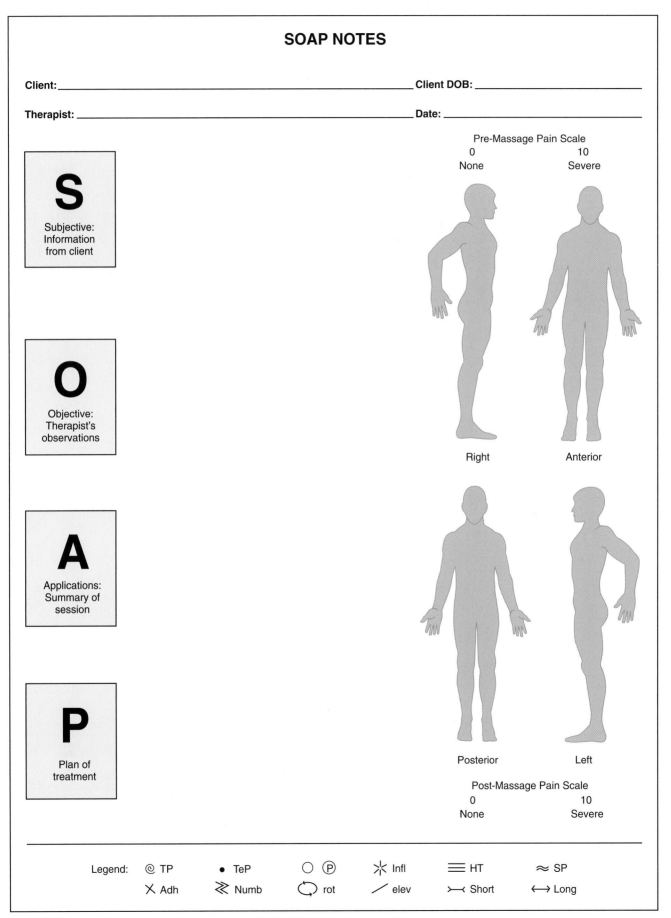

S

Subjective:
Information
from client

O

Objective:
Therapist's
observations

A

Applications:
Summary of
session

P

Plan of
treatment

Pre-Massage Pain Scale
0   10
None   Severe

Right   Anterior

Posterior   Left

Post-Massage Pain Scale
0   10
None   Severe

Legend: @ TP   • TeP   ○ ℗   ✳ Infl   ≡ HT   ≈ SP
          ✕ Adh   ≷ Numb   ↻ rot   ╱ elev   ⊁ Short   ↔ Long

Blank SOAP note documentation.

SOAP NOTES FOR THERAPEUTIC MASSAGE

Client: __John Doe__   Therapist: __Mary Therapist, LMT__

Date: __5/10/12__   Session Type: __SW/DT/MFR__   Duration: __60 min__

Pre-Massage Pain Scale

0 -------- (7) ---- 10
None   Severe

S Information from client

Ct. c/o (R) sh. (P) 2° yard work
Rec't surgery @ (L) ACL
~ 1 week; seeks ↓(P) + ≡

O Assessment by therapist

↓ AROM @ (R) AC joint; ≡ @ (R) trap
TP's @ (R) mid- + post.delts; ct.
prefers MFR @ (R) ↑ trap, Fx @
(R) delts

Right   Front

A Summary of session

FB SW w/o (L) knee 2° contra;
DT @ (R) sh. girdle, conc. MFR
@ (R) ↑ trap, Fx @ (R) mid +
post delts. ↑ PROM post sess,
Δ (P) from 7 to 3

P Treatment plan

↑ H₂O intake post sess; return for
60 min sess @ 2 weeks.
HW: AROM (R) sh, stretches +
moist heat after work

Back   Left

Post-Massage Pain Scale

0 --(3)------------ 10
None   Severe

Legend: ⊚ TP   • TeP   ○ (P)   ✳ Infl   ≡ HT   ≈ SP
✕ Adh   ≋ Numb   ⟲ rot   ╱ elev   ⊁ Short   ⟷ Long

Mary Therapist

Completed SOAP note documentation.

in future session plans. The beauty of SOAP is that, although broadly universal, it is also flexible in the realm of specifics, and can be adapted to the demands of a given situation. If you are a new hire, any agency will communicate clearly to you their customized, preferred style, and as long as you understand the basics of SOAP, you will be able to adapt to whatever the expressed needs may be.

- **Subjective** = Symptoms. In this first section, the therapist records information from the client—what the client says, their feelings, and his or her past and present symptoms. It includes information from the initial interview, health history and intake form, how the condition started, what the client feels makes the condition worsen or improve. It also includes the client's initial statements regarding treatment goals for the session. If a pain scale is used, the client's beginning self-assessment numbers are entered here. In the Subjective category, it is appropriate and often useful to quote the client directly (e.g., "Client stated, 'I feel a burning sensation when I move my wrist.'"). The therapist may choose to begin making notes in this section during the client interview, before the session work begins, to most accurately record the client's phrasing. It is wise to consider the techniques outlined in Chapter 10 for all documentation processes, and use skills such as active listening, thorough review of the health intake form with the client, asking inquisitive questions, and encouraging the client to become more self-aware to best pinpoint their own needs. Consider all aspects of a client's experience, and do your best to communicate clearly. When completed, the subjective section should represent clearly the client's opinion of his or her condition.

- **Objective** = Signs. Items entered here include what the therapist observes from the intake interview and forms, conclusions from functional tests and assessments, what the therapist measures and palpates, and whether the condition might be acute or chronic. The therapist may note any lack of symmetry; the client's posture, movement, skin texture, and breathing; areas of guarding or splinting; and evidence of scar tissue. If the chart contains a human outline, the symbols delineated on the form would be considered Objective information. Basically, the Objective section should reflect the therapist's thoughts and conclusions from the Subjective material, the therapist's understanding of agreed-upon treatment goals, and the initial design of the massage session.

- **Application**
  - *Nonmassage settings*: Medical terminology and abbreviations can vary slightly, not only from one profession to another (e.g., physical therapy vs. occupational therapy), but also within professions (as from one medical doctor's practice to another). In general, however, medical professionals use this section of SOAP to read "Assessment," and this would be the place they would usually insert a physician's diagnosis of the patient's condition.
  - *Massage therapists*: In the massage therapy arena, it is outside the therapist's scope of practice to diagnose, and often a therapist will perform work on a client who has not previously been diagnosed by a physician. Therefore, the more common use of this section, which we term "Application," is to list what actions were performed during the session. This includes which specific massage techniques were used, and the postsession results. If a pain scale is being used, the client's postsession self-assessment numbers may be entered here. Client responses may be noted here; session goals reviewed and evaluated; and changes, progress, or regress noted.

- **Plan** = Homework and future session goals. Here the therapist will record any suggestions, recommendations, nutrition information, stretches, or exercises given to the client once the massage session is completed (the beginning therapist should remember to keep recommendations and client homework within your scope of practice and consistent with state law). The therapist should note what techniques should be repeated or added next session, and if follow-up sessions are agreed upon, the number and dates will also be entered here. Record the timing and frequency of future massages planned, in accordance with the perceived progress, measurable outcomes, and the client's budget. It is also helpful to state goals, short term or long term, in relation to the desired outcome.

If you are working independently in your own practice, SOAP notes provide the flexibility to use them as you prefer; however, be consistent. Using the example filled-out form, if you record the effectiveness of certain treatments in the Objective-section of the form, be sure to record it in the same place for other clients as well. This will provide clarity to you, as well as to anyone who may need to review your SOAP notes in the future.

Updating Records

SOAP notes are ideal for detailed reporting, but they can also be abbreviated for updating visits, or if a series of sessions ends up focusing solely on relaxation or stress reduction. Whether the sessions require more extensive notes, as in the initial visit or the continuation of outcome-based treatment massage sessions, or more truncated charts, such as follow-up sessions (when the session format is anticipated to be very similar to the one that preceded it), the therapist should continue to carefully document everything that happens during the massage. It is not uncommon to have two types of SOAP notes: a longer version for initial intakes and periodic reviews and a shorter version for regular sessions.

SUMMARY

Although SOAP charting is not the only option for the massage therapist, it is most appropriate for proper documentation when the therapist's practice is oriented toward outcome-based massage, or is frequently oriented toward a medical setting. It can also be used by any therapist during times, whether normal or infrequent, when a client has been referred by a medical provider or other health care professional, or when insurance reimbursement may be involved in the session. Careful attention to detail; clear, concise communication; proper use of abbreviations; and objective, professional comments are key to productive use of the SOAP format, and, when used accordingly, SOAP notes can be a true asset to any massage therapist.

BIBLIOGRAPHY

Beck MF: *Theory and practice of therapeutic massage*, ed 4, Florence, Ky, 2006, Delmar Cengage Learning, pp. 373-376.

Fritz S: *Business and professional skills for massage therapists*, St Louis, 2010, Mosby, 2010, p. 115.

Fritz S: *Mosby's fundamentals of therapeutic massage*, ed 4, St Louis, 2009, Mosby, pp 110-113.

Fritz S: *Mosby's massage therapy review*, St Louis, 2002, Mosby, pp 118-119.

Fritz S: *Sports & exercise massage—comprehensive care in athletics, fitness & rehabilitation*, St Louis, 2005, Mosby, p. 162.

Fritz S, Grosenbach MJ: *Mosby's essential sciences for therapeutic massage*, ed 3, St Louis, 2009, Mobsy, pp 56-57.

Simons DC, Travell JC, Simons LS: *Travell & Simons' myofascial pain and dysfunction—the trigger point manual, vol 1. Upper half of body*, ed 2, Philadelphia, Lippincott Williams & Wilkins, 1998, pp 9-12, 97-99.

Stone PS: *Therapeutic reflexology—a step-by-step guide to professional competence*, Upper Saddle River, NJ, 2011, Prentice Hall, p. 63.

Thompson DL: *Hands heal; communication, documentation and insurance billing for panual therapists*, ed 3, Philadelphia, 2006, Lippincott Williams & Wilkins, pp. 121-153, 270, 273.

GLOSSARY

Abdominal   Relating to the abdomen or the superior region of the abdominopelvic cavity

Abdominopelvic cavity   Body cavity that contains the abdominal and pelvic organs

Abduction   Movement away from the median plane

Absolute contraindication   Factor or condition for which receiving massage would put the therapist or the client at health risk or the client's condition could be made worse

Absorption   Process by which products of digestion move into the bloodstream or lymph vessels and then into cells

Abstract   Summary of a research article and findings

Accounting   Art of interpreting, measuring, and describing economic activity

Accounts payable   Money a business owes to suppliers

Accounts receivable   Money owed to a business

Acetabulum   Hip socket with the ilium, ischium, and pubic bones contributing equally to its makeup

Acetylcholine   Neurotransmitter involved in muscle contraction

Actin   Protein molecules within a muscle cell that contain binding sites used during skeletal muscle contraction; help make up thin myofilaments

Acromial   Relating to the top of the shoulder

Action potential   Brief series of events in which the electrical membrane of a nerve cell changes to conduct an impulse

Active-assisted movements   Client actively performs the movement while the therapist assists; see *Active movements*

Active movements   Client actively performs the movement after the therapist describes or demonstrates it; types are *active-assisted* and *active-resisted* movements

Active-resisted movements   Client actively performs the movement while the therapist resists it; see *Active movements*

Active transport   Movement of atoms and molecules against the concentration gradient from low levels to high levels

Active trigger point   Trigger point that causes symptoms such as pain, even at rest

Acupoint   See *Tsubo*

Acupressure   See *Sustained pressure*

Acute disease   Disease with abrupt onset of severe symptoms that run a brief course (less than 6 months) and then resolve or, in some cases, bring death

Acute pain   Normal, predicted physiologic response to an adverse stimulus, often trauma; the affected area may be inflamed

Adaptation   Decrease in sensitivity to a prolonged stimulus

Addiction   Persistent, compulsive dependence on a behavior or substance

Adduction   Movement toward the median plane

Adenosine triphosphate (ATP)   The body's energy molecule

Adhesion   Abnormal tissue that can restrict the normal movement between tissues, limiting the strength and motion of the body

Adipose tissue   Connective tissue specialized for fat storage

Adrenal cortex   Outer region of the adrenals; secretes glucocorticoids, mineralocorticoids, and sex hormones

Adrenal glands   Glands located superior to each kidney; also called the *suprarenals*

Adrenal medulla   Inner region of the adrenals; secretes epinephrine and norepinephrine

Adrenaline   See *Epinephrine*

Adrenocorticotropic hormone (ACTH)   Pituitary hormone that stimulates the adrenal cortex to secrete hormones, especially cortisol

Advertising   Making a business noticeable to the public by developing a message and using forms of media to deliver that message, usually at a cost

Afferent   See *Sensory*

Agnis   In Ayurveda, enzymes that assist in the digestion and assimilation of food

Agonist   See *Prime Mover*

Aldosterone   Adrenal hormone that stimulates kidneys to conserve sodium, which results in water retention in the blood; also helps maintain proper mineral balance

All-or-none response   Physiologic response whereby each individual muscle fiber, when sufficiently stimulated, contracts to its fullest extent or not at all; also refers to the fact that impulses are conducted along a neuron's membrane at maximum capacity without fluctuations in membrane potential and without any decrease in magnitude

Alpha cell   Pancreatic cell that produces the hormone glucagon

Alveoli   Tiny sacs attached to alveolar ducts within the lungs; site of oxygen and carbon dioxide exchange between the blood and the air in the lungs

Amino acids   Components that make up protein; commonly referred to as the "building blocks" of protein

Amma   Ancient Chinese style of massage regarded as the original massage technique and the precursor to all other therapies—manual and energetic

Amphiarthrosis joint   Joint that is slightly movable; also called a *cartilaginous joint*

Amylase   Digestive enzyme that breaks down carbohydrates

Anabolism   Constructive phase of metabolism in which smaller, simpler molecules are built up into larger molecules

Analgesics   Agents that reduce pain

Analytical research   In-depth investigations into complex issues and mechanisms

Anatomic position   Standard body position used in Western medicine, with the body upright and facing forward, arms at the sides, palms facing forward, thumbs to the side, feet about hip distance apart, and toes pointing forward

Anatomy   Study of the structures of the human body and their positional relationship to one another

Androgens   Sex hormones produced by the adrenal cortex that assist in the development of secondary sex characteristics

Antagonist   Muscle that must relax and lengthen or eccentrically contract and lengthen to allow actions of the agonist to occur

Antebrachial   Relating to the forearm area between the wrist and elbow

Antecubital   Relating to the front of the elbow or the bend of the elbow

Anterior   Pertaining to the front side of a structure; also called *ventral*

Anterior pelvic tilt   Movement of the pelvis in which the ilium is tilted forward

Antidiuretic hormone (ADH, vasopressin)   Pituitary hormone that promotes water retention

Anus   Terminal end of the gastrointestinal tract through which the feces are released from the body

Aortic valve   Valve between the left ventricle and the aorta; also called the left *semilunar valve*

Aponeurosis   Broad, flat tendon; attaches skeletal muscle to bone, another muscle, or skin

Arachnoid   Middle meningeal layer; forms a loose, weblike covering around the central nervous system

Archer stance   See *Bow stance*

Aromatherapy   Use of plant-derived essential oils for therapeutic purposes; also called *essential oil therapy*

Arrector pili   Tiny muscles attached to hair follicles that contract to pull the hair upright

Arrhythmia   Any deviation from a normal heart beat or rhythm

Arteriole   Small-sized arteries

Artery   Vessel that carries blood away from the heart to the tissues of the body

Articular cartilage   Hyaline cartilage covering an epiphysis

Articulation (arthrosis)   Joint; where bones join together

Ascending colon   The portion of the large intestine that extends from the cecum to the hepatic flexure

Asclepiades   Founder of the group of ancient Greek physicians residing in Rome known as the Methodists, who restricted their treatments to bathing, diet, massage, and a few drugs

Asclepius   Ancient Greek physician who was believed to have evolved into a god who was responsible for the emerging medical profession; his holy snake and staff are the symbol of the medical profession

Asian bodywork therapy   The use of traditional Asian techniques and strategies to treat the human body, mind, and spirit (this includes the electromagnetic or energetic fields that surround, infuse, and bring that body to life)

Assessment   Process involved in appraising a client's condition based on subjective reporting and objective findings

Assets   Economic resources that offer value to a business

Association neuron   See *Interneuron*

Astrocyte   Neuroglial cell used for structural support of central nervous system's neurons; part of the blood-brain barrier

Atrial natriuretic hormone   Hormone secreted by the heart that decreases blood volume and blood pressure

Atrium   Superior heart chamber

Autoimmune disease   Disease marked by the body's inability to distinguish its own tissues from something foreign to the body

Autonomic nervous system   Division of peripheral nervous system supplying impulses to smooth muscle, cardiac muscle, and glands; has sympathetic and parasympathetic divisions

Avascular   Lacking blood vessels

Avicenna (980-1037)   Name by which Persian physician Abu-Ali al-Husayn ibn-Sina was known in the West; authored numerous books, notably his *Canon of Medicine* that compiled all the theoretical and practical medical knowledge of his time; the text makes numerous references to the use of massage

Axillary   Relating to the armpit

Axon   Neural extension that carries nerve impulses away from the neuron toward another neuron, a muscle cell, or gland

Ayurveda   India's traditional healing modality; a science of health and medicine designed to maintain or improve health through the use of dietary modification, massage, yoga, and herbal preparations

Balance sheet   A summary of a business's assets and liabilities and the owner's equity at an exact point in time, usually at the end of a quarter or a fiscal year

Ball-and-socket (multiaxial/triaxial) joint   Joint permitting all movements except gliding; offers the greatest range of motion

Ballistic stretching   Uses a bouncing motion; is not preferred because it stimulates muscle spindles

Balneology   Art and science of bathing for therapeutic and relaxation purposes

Baroreceptor   Detects blood pressure by monitoring the amount of stretch exerted on certain arterial walls, namely carotid arteries and the aortic arch

Bartering   The practice of providing goods or services for other goods or services without the exchange of money

Basal ganglia   Patches of gray matter throughout the cerebrum's white matter that assist in motor control, including facial expression

Basic research   Seeks to find fundamental information at the molecular, cellular, or tissue level and is typically conducted in a laboratory

Benign tumor   Noncancerous tumor

Beta cell   Pancreatic cell that produces the hormone insulin

Biarticular   Term used to describe muscles that cross two joints, acting on both joints

Bicuspid valve   See *Mitral valve*

Bile   Emulsifies fat; produced in the liver and stored in the gallbladder

Birth canal   See *Vagina*

Blood   Liquid connective tissue composed of plasma, erythrocytes, leukocytes, and platelets

Blood pressure   Pressure exerted by blood on the blood vessel walls

Blood-brain barrier   Selective semipermeable wall of blood capillaries that prevents or slows down the passage of some chemical compounds and disease-causing organisms into the central nervous system

Body mechanics   The use of postural techniques, foot stances, leverage techniques, and other elements to deliver massage therapy and related bodywork methods with efficiency and the least amount of trauma to the therapist

Body polish   Method of exfoliation using a fine, grainy substance

Body scrub   Method of exfoliation using a coarse, grainy substance

Body shampoo   Method of gently scrubbing the skin using a cloth or brush dipped in warm, soapy water

Bodywork   Generic term used to describe any therapeutic or personal self-development practice that may include massage, healing touch, movement, or energetic work

Bolster   Propping device, such as a pillow or cushion, that assists client comfort by supporting and enabling proper alignment of individual joints that, in turn, helps muscles relax; can be commercially manufactured or can be a rolled-up towel or blanket

Bond   Loan in which an investor is the lender, and the borrowers range from the government, municipalities, and corporations;

in exchange for the lender's money, the borrower agrees to pay interest at a predetermined rate

Bonding   Solid connection between the parent and child that nourishes the infant on a core level

Bone   Connective tissue that consists of compact bone, spongy bone, collagenous fibers, and mineral salts

Bony marking   Place on bones where muscles, tendons, and ligaments attach or where nerve and blood vessels pass

Borelli, Giovanni Alfonso (1608-1679)   Italian anatomist who carried out extensive anatomic dissections and analyzed the phenomenon of muscle contraction

Boundary   Parameter indicating a border or limit; delineates differences between clients and massage therapists; clarifies each person's role in the therapeutic relationship such as individual responsibilities, expectations, and limitations

Bow stance   Stance used when the therapist proceeds from one point to the next along the client's body, with the therapist's feet placed on the floor in a 30- to 50-degree angle, one pointing straight forward *(lead foot—pointing in the direction of movement)* and the other pointing toward the side *(trailing foot)*

Bowman's capsule   Hollow cup-shaped mouth of a nephron

Brachial   Relating to the part of the arm between the shoulder and the elbow

Bradycardia   Slow heart rate (<50 or 60 beats per minute)

Brain   Central nervous system organ that contains an estimated 100 billion neurons; divided into four major regions: cerebrum, diencephalon, cerebellum, and brain stem

Brainstem   Part of the brain that is continuous with the spinal cord; has three main divisions: mid-brain, pons, and medulla oblongata

Breast   A mammary gland that produces and secretes milk after pregnancy

Breathing   A mechanical action consisting of two phases: inhalation (inspiration) and exhalation (expiration)

Bright, Timothy (c. 1551-1615)   British Renaissance–era physician who taught and published material on the use of baths, exercise, and massage to restore health

Bronchi   Passageways from the trachea to each lung; branch into smaller passageways called *bronchioles*

Bronchiole   Smaller branches of the bronchi

Brunner's gland   Duodenal gland that secretes alkaline mucus

Buccal   Relating to the lower cheek

Bulbourethral (Cowper's) gland   Gland located on either side of the prostate that secretes an alkaline substance, making up approximately 5% of semen volume

Burnout   The condition of being tired of, or unhappy with, one's work

Bursa   Collapsed saclike structure with an interior lining of synovial membrane; contains synovial fluid

Business personal property insurance   Insurance that covers the cost of business property such as a desk, massage table, chairs, and stereo equipment in a business location

Business plan   Tool to gather data to answer questions related to aspects of a current or prospective business; includes personal information, general description of the business, services, fees and pricing, competition, location and operations, and management and personnel

Calcaneal   Relating to the heel of the foot

Calcitonin   Thyroid hormone that decreases blood calcium by stimulating osteoblasts to increase calcium storage in bones

Calf (sural)   Relating to the posterior leg

Calorie (kilocalorie)   Unit of energy-producing potential in food; it is equal to the heat energy needed to raise the temperature of 1 kg of water by $1°$ C

Calyx   Cuplike structure protruding from the renal papilla in the kidney; minor calyces join to form a major calyx that leads to the renal pelvis

Cancer   Disease characterized by abnormal cells that possess uncontrollable cell division, lack programmed cells death, and can accumulate into masses called tumors

Capillary   Vessel between an arteriole and a venule; possesses a thin, permeable membrane for efficient gas exchange with tissues

Carbohydrate   Also known as starches and sugars; classified according to molecular structure as mono-, di-, and polysaccharides

Cardiac cycle   Sequence of events related to the flow of blood that occurs from the beginning of one heart beat to the beginning of the next

Cardiac output   Product of stroke volume times the heart rate

Carpal   Relating to the wrist

Carrier oil   Oil used to dilute and suspend one or more essential oils

Cartilage   Avascular, tough, protective connective tissue found chiefly in the thorax, joints, and some rigid tubes of the body (trachea, larynx)

Cartilaginous joint   See *Amphiarthrosis*

Cash flow   Movement of money into and out of a business

Catabolism   Destructive phase of metabolism in which larger, more complex molecules are converted to smaller, simpler molecules

Catecholamines   Chemical family containing norepinephrine, epinephrine, and dopamine; major functions include excitation and inhibition of certain muscles, cardiac excitation, metabolic action, and endocrine action

Caudal   See *Inferior*

Cautionary site   Certain area of the body containing structures that, when massaged, may negatively impact the client's health; also called *endangerment site*

Cavity   A hollow space within a larger structure

Cecum   A small, saclike structure that is the first section of the large intestine

Cell   Fundamental unit of all living organisms and the simplest form of life that can exist as a self-sustaining unit

Cell body   Main region of the neuron containing the nucleus, ribosomes, and other organelles

Cell membrane   Semipermeable membrane that separates cytoplasm from the surrounding external environment

Celsus, Aulus   Ancient Roman writer who cited the Asclepiades treatise on friction (massage) in his own writings on friction

Centeredness   Mental, emotional, and physical states of consciousness in which the therapist's mind is cleared and he or she is experiencing the present moment; may also include feeling the presence of God, nature, or a higher power, and feeling like being part of a larger whole

Central   See *Deep*

Central nervous system   Body system that includes the brain, meninges, cerebrospinal fluid, and spinal cord

Centripetally   Toward the center

Cephalad   See *Superior*

Cephalic   Pertaining to the head area

Cerebellum   Second largest part of the brain; located posterior and inferior to the cerebrum; involved with muscle tone, coordination of skeletal muscles and balance, and control of fine and gross motor movements

Cerebral cortex   Thin, gray layer covering the outer portion of the cerebrum

Cerebrospinal fluid   Fluid circulating around the brain and spinal cord within the subarachnoid space; supplies oxygen and nutrients, carries away wastes, and acts as a shock absorber

Cerebrum   Largest part of the brain, where vision, smell, taste, and body movements are consciously perceived, where skeletal muscle movements are initiated, and where emotional and intellectual processes occur

Certification   The voluntary process by which a nongovernmental organization grants certification to an individual who possesses certain skills or abilities relevant to a field of practice

Cervical   Relating to the neck area

Chain of infection   Series of events that occur during the invasion of pathogens; includes infectious agent, reservoir, portal of exit, transmission, portal of entry, and host susceptibility

Chakras   In Ayurveda, seven energy centers in the body that receive, process, and distribute energy, and keep the spiritual, mental, emotional, and physical health of the body in balance

Channels   In traditional Chinese medicine, pathways and vessels through which chi (ki) flows; the connection of the material body to the nonmaterial part of the body; channels distribute, balance, and connect the chi (ki) of the interior organs with the surface or exterior of the body (also called meridians)

Chemoreceptor   Activated by chemical stimuli; detects smells, tastes, and changes in blood chemistry

Chi   See *Ki*

Chief cell   Stomach's exocrine cell that produces pepsinogen, a precursor to pepsin

Cholecystokinin   Hormone produced by the intestinal mucosa that stimulates the gallbladder to release bile and the pancreas to secrete enzymes

Chromosomal diseases   Caused by having too many or not enough chromosomes, or by having a broken or missing piece of a chromosome

Chromosomes   Structures in the nucleus of cells that contain DNA, the cell's genetic material

Chronic disease   Disease that develops slowly and lasts 6 months or longer, in some cases, a lifetime; no cure is known

Chronic pain   Pain that persists for a longer period of time than expected for the condition

Circumduction   Cone-shaped range of motion that occurs when the distal end moves in a circle and the proximal end is fixed

Class-1 lever   Lever in which the fulcrum is positioned between the pull and the load—similar to a seesaw or a pair of scissors

Class-2 lever   Lever in which the fulcrum is at one end, the load is in the middle, and the pull is at the opposite end—similar to a wheelbarrow

Class-3 lever   Lever in which the fulcrum is at one end, the pull is located in the center, and the load is at the opposite end—similar to using a shovel

Clavicular   Relating to the collar bone

Client abuse   Physical or emotional harm sustained from deliberate acts of the massage therapist

Client neglect   Unintentional physical or emotional harm that the client sustains resulting from insensitivity or lack of knowledge

Clinical massage   Involves the use of specific focused techniques that, when applied properly, reduce reported signs and symptoms and improve function

Clinical (applied) research   Uses investigations, or research studies, to examine questions on a functional level

Clitoris   Small cylindrical mass of erectile tissue with nerves; located at the anterior junction of the labia minora

Coccygeal   Relating to the bottom of the spinal column or the upper region of the gluteal cleft

Code of ethics   Set of guiding moral principles that members of particular professions are expected to follow

Cold mitten friction   See *Cold towel friction*

Cold towel friction   Ice application through towels dipped in icy water and applied to the body with friction movements

Collagen   Long strands of protein that are the main component of connective tissue

Collecting duct   Structure made up of the distal tubules of several nephrons; joins several larger ducts to become the renal papilla

Communicable disease   Contagious disease; caused by pathogens

Communication   Act of exchanging information through words, actions, behaviors, body language, and feelings

Compact bone   Forms the hard outer shell of all bones and a portion of the shaft bulk of long bones; provides protection, support, and resistance to stress of weight and movement

Compress   Wet cloth that has had water wrung from it and is applied to the skin's surface

Compression   Nongliding technique of sustained pressure or a sequence of rhythmic, alternating pressures

Concentric contraction   Type of isotonic contraction when contraction results in shortening of a muscle

Conduction   Exchange of thermal energy while the body's surface is in direct contact with the thermal agent or conductor

Confidentiality   Nondisclosure of privileged information

Congenital disorder   Disorder that is present at birth

Connective tissue   Tissue that is the most abundant and diverse; connects, supports, transports, and defends

Contamination   Results from effective exposure and successful transfer of pathogens

Continuity   In massage, refers to the uninterrupted flow of strokes and to the unbroken transition from one stroke to the next

Continuous conduction   Nerve impulse conduction along unmyelinated axons

Control group   A group that is not treated in a research study

Contract   Written voluntary agreement between two or more parties, enforceable by law, that communicates expectations, duties, and responsibilities

Contraindication   Presence of a disease or physical condition that makes it unsafe to treat a particular client in the usual manner

Contralateral   Related to opposite sides of the body

Contrast method   Combining heat and cold in the same treatment

Convection   Transfer of heat energy through movement of air or liquid

Conversion   One energy source changing or converting into a heat energy source as it passes into the body

Coronal plane   See *Frontal plane*

Coronal suture   Suture that separates the frontal bone from the parietal bones

Corporation   A business entity that is granted a charter recognizing it as a separate legal entity having its own privileges and liabilities distinct from its members

Corpus callosum   Transverse fibers that connect and provide a communicative pathway between the two cerebral hemispheres

Cortical (cortex)   Outer region of an organ or structure

Cortisol (hydrocortisone)   Stress hormone; glucocorticoid that ensures that glucose, lipids, and amino acids are available for cells to use for energy and protein synthesis; also has an anti-inflammatory effect

Costal   Relating to the ribs

Coulter, John S.   American physician who in 1926 became the first full-time academic physician in the field of physical medicine

Countertransference   Term for when a massage therapist brings unresolved emotional issues or personal needs into the therapeutic relationship

Coxal   Relating to the hip

Cranial   Relating to the upper skull

Cranial nerve   Nerve originating in the brain

Cranial   See *Superior*

Crepitus   Noisy discharge produced by the body that may resemble a cracking sound

Cross-contamination   Passing of microorganisms from one source to another

Crude touch   Touch that is more easily identified but is more difficult to locate on the skin than discriminative touch

Crural   Relating to the leg between the knee and ankle

Cryokinetics   Cold therapy combined with joint movement

Cryotherapy   External therapeutic application of cold

Cubital   Relating to the elbow

Cun   In traditional Chinese medicine, the body inch unit; the width of the client's own thumb knuckle

Cupping   In Asian bodywork therapy, a method in which a warmed cup is placed upside down directly on the skin, creating a vacuum that suctions the skin to relieve energy stagnation

Curriculum vitae   See *Resume*

Cutaneous membrane   Membrane that covers the entire surface of the body; the skin

Cuticle   Tough ridge of skin that grows out over the nail from its base

Cyanosis   Blue or purple cast to the skin

Cytoplasm   Gel-like fluid within the cell membrane in which organelles float

Dan tien   A point in the hara located three finger-widths' distance below the navel described as the center of focused power and action; it is where all movement of the body originates

Day spa   Spa providing beauty, health, and therapeutic treatments on a day-use basis with no overnight accommodations

Debt-to-income ratio   The relationship, stated as a percentage, between monthly gross income and monthly payments on loans, including payments made on a home, car, and credit cards

Decoction   Tea made from boiling parts of a plant, usually bark, roots, or seeds

Deep   Pertaining to or situated at a center of the body; also called central

Deep vein thrombosis (DVT)   Blood clots in deep leg veins

Defecation   Process of eliminating indigestible or unabsorbed material from the body

Deficiency disease   Disease caused by a lack of dietary vitamins, minerals, or nutrients; can also result from inability to properly digest or absorb a particular nutrient

Degenerative disease   Disease in which an organ or its function deteriorates over time

Deglutition   Swallowing

Delayed-onset muscle soreness   Soreness felt 8 to 14 hours after activity, often reaching a peak after 48 hours

Deltoid   Relating to the curve of the shoulder and upper arm formed by the deltoid muscle; a shoulder muscle

Dendrite   Short, narrow, neural extensions that receive and transmit stimuli toward the neuron's cell body

Depolarization   Occurs when a neuron is stimulated; the interior of the cell changes from negative to positive

Deoxyribonucleic acid (DNA)   Chemical within chromosomes that code for the production of specific enzymes and other functional proteins or polypeptides; a section on a chromosome that codes for a specific enzyme is called a *gene*

Depreciation   The process of spreading the deduction for the cost of an asset over time

Depression   Lowering or dropping a body part, moving inferiorly

Dermatome   Area of skin served by a specific sensory nerve root

Dermis   Inner region of the skin; contains blood vessels, sensory nerve receptors, hair follicles, muscles, sweat and oil glands, and connective tissue

Descending colon   The portion of the colon that extends from the splenic flexure to the sigmoid flexure

Descriptive research   Includes survey and interview studies

Destination spa   Spa offering onsite overnight accommodations, spa services, physical fitness and wellness elements, educational programming, and spa cuisine

Dhatus   In Ayurveda, the tissues of the human body; there are seven dhatus. Dhatus, doshas (psychophysic elements and forces) and three malas (waste products) make up the human body

Diagnosing   Science and skill of distinguishing diseases or disorders from each other; performed by qualified health care professionals

Diaphragm   Main muscle of respiration and structure separating the thoracic cavity from the abdominal cavity

Diaphysis   Cylindrical shaft of a long bone

Diarthrosis joint   Freely movable joint; also called a *synovial joint*

Diastole   Phase of the cardiac cycle when the ventricles relax and fill with blood

Diastolic pressure   Lowest pressure in blood pressure measurement; occurs when the left ventricle relaxes

Diencephalon   Part of the brain that houses the thalamus and the hypothalamus; also includes the pituitary and pineal glands

Diet   Food and drink consumed to supply the processes of nutrition

Diffusion   Movement of molecules from an area of high concentration to an area of low concentration, a process that continues until the distribution of particulates is equal in all areas

Digestion Mechanical and chemical processes that occur as food is broken down into simple molecules

Digital (phalangeal) Relating to fingers or toes

Disability Physical or mental impairment that substantially limits or restricts the condition, manner, or duration under which an average person in the population can perform a major life activity, such as walking, seeing, hearing, speaking, breathing, learning, working, or self-care

Disability insurance Insurance that provides income in the event a person cannot work as a result of a disability such as an illness or injury

Disclosure Honest and open sharing of personal knowledge, as well as ideas and insights

Discriminative touch Touch that is subtle and can be easily located in the skin

Disease Illness characterized by signs and symptoms

Disorder A condition of functional abnormality

Distal Farther from the point of reference; term used when referencing the extremities

Diureses Urine production

Diuretic Substance that promotes the formation and excretion of urine

Dividend Portion of a company's profits distributed at regular intervals to its shareholders

Documentation Process of providing written or digitized information of client care

Dopamine Neurotransmitter involved in emotions, moods, regulating motor control, attention, and learning

Dorsal See *Posterior*

Dorsal cavity Cavity located on the posterior aspect of the body; further divided into the cranial and spinal cavities

Dorsiflexion Flexing the ankle dorsally so that the toes are moving toward the shin

Dorsum Top of the foot

Doshas In Ayurveda, psychophysic elements and forces that, along with the seven dhatus (tissues) and three malas (waste products), make up the human body; doshas are made up of five basic elements: earth, air, fire, water, and space or ether; the three active doshas, or tri-doshas, are vata (wind), pitta (bile), and kapha (phlegm)

Draping Covering the body with cloth to provide a professional atmosphere, support the client's need for emotional privacy (modesty) and sense of security, and provide warmth, while allowing access to individual parts of the client's body

Dual innervation Innervation by both the sympathetic and parasympathetic divisions

Dual relationships Massage therapist having more than one relationship with a client; more than just a therapeutic relationship

Ductus deferens See *Vas deferens*

Duodenum First portion of the small intestine

Dura mater Outermost meningeal layer; thick, dense, lies against bone, and contains a double layer of connective tissue, with the other layer resembling periosteum

Duration In massage, the length of the massage session, or the length of time massage is performed on a given area

Eccentric contraction Type of isotonic contraction occurring when contraction results in lengthening of a muscle

Ectoderm Outermost embryonic cell layer; gives rise to structures of the nervous system, including the special senses, the mucosa of the mouth and anus, the epidermis and epidermal tissues

Edema Abnormal accumulation of fluids in body tissue

Effectors The muscles or glands that motor neurons act on

Efferent See *Motor*

Effleurage Application of gliding movements that are repeated and follow the contours of the body

Ejaculatory duct Tube that transports sperm from the vas deferens to the urethra during ejaculation

Elastin Protein in connective tissue that returns to its original length after being stretched

Electrocardiogram (ECG or EKG) Recording of the electrical activity of the heart

Electroencephalogram (EEG) Recording of brain wave patterns

Elevation Raising or lifting a body part; moving superiorly

Ellipsoidal/condyloid (biaxial) joint Joint with movement limited to flexion, extension, abduction, and adduction

Empirical Measurable and verifiable via the senses

Emulsifier Substance that physically breaks apart fat globules into smaller ones, which provides a larger surface area for fat-digesting enzymes to work

Endangerment site See *Cautionary site*

End-feel A restriction of motion at the end of passive joint mobilization or stretching; types of restrictions include joint structures (i.e., hard end-feel) and myofascial elements (i.e., soft end-feel)

Endochondral (cartilaginous) ossification Bone formation from cartilage; found in most bones of the body

Endocrine gland Ductless gland that produces hormones

Endocytosis Process that moves large particles across the cell membrane into the cell; includes phagocytosis and pinocytosis

Endoderm Innermost embryonic cell layer; gives rise to the lining of the gastrointestinal and respiratory tracts and most of the internal organs and their coverings

Endoneurium Connective tissue layer that wraps each individual neuron

Endomysium Connective tissue layer that surrounds individual muscle fibers

Endoplasmic reticulum Complex network of membranous channels within the cytoplasm that aid in protein and lipid synthesis and assist in the transportation of these materials from one part of the cell to another

Endorphin Neurotransmitter that functions as an opiate to block pain

Enkephalin Similar to endorphin (see *Endorphin*)

Enzyme Catalyst that accelerates chemical reactions

Ependymocyte Neuroglial cell that lines cranial ventricles and the central canal of the spinal cord; produces, secretes, and assists in the circulation of cerebrospinal fluid

Epidermis Outer region of the skin; composed of epithelial tissue

Epididymis Tightly coiled duct located on the posterior border of the testes; site for final sperm maturation

Epidural space Space between the dura mater and the vertebral canal; filled with adipose tissue, connective tissue, and blood vessels

Epiglottis One of the laryngeal cartilages that close the trachea during swallowing to prevent food from entering the inferior respiratory passageways

Epimysium   Connective tissue layer surrounding an entire muscle

Epinephrine (adrenaline)   Neurotransmitter located in several areas of the central nervous system and in the sympathetic division of the autonomic nervous system; can be excitatory or inhibitory; also a hormone secreted by the adrenal medulla

Epineurium   Connective tissue layer that bounds several fasciculi together, forming a nerve

Epiphyseal line   Replaces the epiphyseal plate when bone growth is complete in mature bone

Epiphyseal disk   Thin layer of cartilage between epiphysis and diaphysis where new bone is formed in immature bone; also known as growth plate or epiphyseal plate

Epiphysis   End of a long bone

Epithelial tissue   Tissue that lines or covers the body's external surface (skin); internal organs; blood vessels; body cavities; and the digestive, respiratory, urinary, and reproductive tracts

Equity   The difference between total assets and liabilities; also called *net worth*

Errors and omission insurance   See *Professional liability insurance*

Erythrocyte   Red blood cell; transports oxygen and carbon dioxide

Esophagus   Muscular tube that connects the pharynx to the stomach

Essential nutrient   A nutrient that is either produced by the body in insufficient amounts or not at all; must be obtained by the foods consumed

Essential oil   Concentrated essence of one or more aromatic plants

Essential oil therapy   See *Aromatherapy*

Estrogens   Hormones responsible for female secondary sex characteristics; promote the development and release of the ovum from the ovary at ovulation; stimulate the uterine lining to proliferate and thicken in anticipation of a fertilized ovum

Evaporation   Transfer of heat through the process of changing a liquid into a vapor

Eversion   Elevation of the lateral edge of the foot so that the sole is turned outward (or laterally)

Exacerbation   Increase in the severity of a disease's signs and symptoms

Excursion   In massage, the distance traveled during the length of a massage stroke

Exfoliation   Any treatment in which the client's skin is stimulated by abrasion

Exocrine gland   Gland that secretes products into ducts that open into body cavities, the hollow center of an organ, or onto the body's surface

Exocytosis   Process by which material is released from a cell's interior

Expiration (exhalation)   Process of expelling air from the lungs

Extension   Straightening or increasing the angle of a joint

External   Nearest the outside of a body cavity

External respiration   Gas exchange in the lungs; occurs between blood in capillaries and air in the alveoli

Exteroceptor   Receptor located in the skin, mucous membranes, and sense organs; responds to stimuli originating from outside of the body

Extracellular fluids   Fluids found outside cells; consist of plasma, interstitial fluid, and lymph and transcellular fluid

Facial   Relating to the face

Facilitated diffusion   Special type of diffusion that uses a carrier protein or channels to facilitate the diffusion process

Fallopian tube   Tube extending laterally from the ovary to the uterus; serves as a passageway for an ovum; site of fertilization

Fascia   A type of connective tissue; superficial fascia is immediately deep to the skin, and deep fascia surrounds muscles, holds them together, and separates them into functioning groups

Fasciculi   Groups of muscle fibers or neurons; singular form is *fasciculus*

Fats   Subgroup of lipids called triglycerides; at room temperature, unsaturated fats are liquid and saturated fats are solid

Femoral   Relating to the thigh between the hip and the knee

Fertilization   Penetration of the ovum by the spermatozoon

Fibroblasts   Stem cells that are precursors for cells specializing in tissue healing and metabolism

Fibrous joint   See *Synarthrosis*

Filtrate   Resulting fluid filtered from the blood in the nephron of the kidney; after processing, it becomes urine

Filtration   Movement of particles across the cellular membrane as a result of pressure

Financial portfolio   All the various investments held by an individual investor

Five phases   In traditional Chinese medicine, the dynamic state of chi (ki) expressed as earth, wood, fire, metal, and water; also known as the *five elements*

Fixator   Specialized synergistic muscles that act as stabilizers

Flank   Relating to the lateral trunk

Flaccid   Skeletal muscles with less tone than normal

Flexion   Bending or decreasing the angle of a joint

Follicle-stimulating hormone (FSH)   Pituitary hormone that stimulates estrogen production and ovarian follicle development in women, and sperm production in men

Fomentation pack   Hot pack

Free nerve endings   See *Nociceptor*

Frequency   In massage, the rate at which massage strokes are repeated in a given time frame

Friction   Performed by rubbing one surface over another in several directions; can be applied superficially with hands gliding over the skin or deeply while moving skin across underlying tissue layers (this is called *deep friction*)

Frontal   Relating to the forehead

Frontal lobe   Cerebral lobe regulating motor output, cognition, and speech production (Broca's area; typically the left hemisphere only)

Frontal plane   Plane that passes through the body side to side, creating anterior and posterior sections; also called a *coronal plane*

Fu   In traditional Chinese medicine, refers to the yang, more hollow organs such as the small intestine, gallbladder, large intestine, bladder, triple heater, and stomach

G cells   Stomach's endocrine cells that secrete the hormone gastrin

Gait   The manner in which a person moves on foot, such as in walking or running

Galen of Pergamon (c. 130-200 AD)   Roman physician who combined and unified Greek medical knowledge; his system dominated Western medicine until relatively recent times

Gallbladder   Hollow organ located on the inferior surface of the liver; stores bile

Gametes Male and female sex cells; spermatozoon and oocytes

Ganglion Cluster of nerve cell bodies located in the peripheral nervous system

Gastrin Hormone secreted by the stomach that initiates the production and secretion of gastric juices and stimulates bile and pancreatic enzyme emissions into the small intestines

Gastrointestinal (GI) tract Muscular passageway of the digestive system; leads from the mouth to the anus; also known as the alimentary canal

Gate control theory Theory that multiple nerve impulses compete for the same gate into the spinal cord; the impulse that hits the gate first wins, and the gate then closes and prevents or inhibits other nerve impulses from entering

Gel state Thick, gelatinous state of the ground substance in fascia

Gene Section of deoxyribonucleic acid on a chromosome that codes for a specific enzyme

General liability insurance Insurance that covers liability costs that are a result of bodily injury, property damage, and personal injury incurred while the client is on the massage therapist's premises; also called *premise liability insurance*

Genetic disease Disease caused by an abnormal genetic code

Genetics Study of inheritance

General partnership A business in which members share equally in decision making, profit sharing, and personal liability

Geriatric Refers to someone who is 70 years of age or older

Gliding/planar (triaxial) joint Joint with movement limited to gliding or planar movements but movement may be permitted in all planes

Glomerulus In the nephron, a small ball of fine capillaries within Bowman's capsule

Glucagon Pancreatic hormone that increases blood glucose levels

Gluteal (buttock) Relating to the curve of the buttocks formed by the gluteal muscles

Golgi body Series of four to six horizontal membranous sacs that pack and store proteins and lipids until needed

Golgi tendon organ Receptor located at musculotendinous junction; detects tension and excessive stretch, causing the nervous system to respond by inhibiting contraction

Gonads Primary reproductive organs; testes in men and ovaries in women

Graham, Douglas O. American physician and Swedish massage practitioner who authored several works on the history of massage between 1874 and 1925

Greater omentum Part of the mesentery that extends from the stomach and duodenum to the transverse colon

Gross income Money a person or business makes before subtracting expenses and/or taxes

Growth hormone (GH) Pituitary hormone that stimulates protein synthesis for muscle and bone growth and maintenance and repair, and that plays a role in metabolism

Gua-Sha In Asian bodywork therapy, a skin-scraping technique that helps to expel excess heat or remove energy stagnation

Gustatory organ Taste bud

Hair root plexus (hair follicle receptor) Receptor that responds to light touch and hair movement

Hallux Great toe

Handicap Refers to a limitation or a barrier

Hara In Japanese, the lower abdomen

Harvey, William (1578-1657) British anatomist who demonstrated that blood circulation in animals is impelled by the beat of the heart through arteries and veins

Haustra Series of pouches in the large intestine; formed by contractions of taenia coli; haustrum is singular

Haversian canal Minute vascular canal that runs longitudinally through a bone

Health Condition of physical, mental, and social well-being with the absence of disease

Health questionnaire See *Intake form*

Heart Hollow, muscular organ that pumps and circulates blood throughout the body

Heart rate The number of cardiac cycles (heart beats) that occur in 1 minute

Hematopoiesis See *Hemopoiesis*

Hemoglobin Red respiratory pigment in an erythrocyte; carries oxygen or carbon dioxide, but not both, at any given time

Hemopoiesis Blood cell production; also called *hematopoiesis*

Hepatic (right colic) flexure A bend of the colon just beneath the liver

Hepatic portal system Circuit that collects blood from the digestive organs and delivers it to the liver for processing and storage

High-risk pregnancies Pregnancies that put the mother, the developing fetus, or both at higher-than-normal risk for complications during or after the pregnancy and birth

Hinge (monoaxial) joint Joint limited to flexion and extension

Hippocrates of Cos (c. 460-375 BC) Greek physician; considered the father of modern Western medicine; he was a fine clinician, founder of a medical school, author of numerous books, and a proponent of massage

Histamine Neurotransmitter involved in emotions and regulation of body temperature, water balance, and stimulation of inflammatory responses

Homeostasis Constancy of the body's internal environment; it represents a relatively stable condition within a very limited range

Homolateral See *Ipsilateral*

Horizontal plane See *Transverse plane*

Hormone Glandular secretion that acts as a catalyst in biochemical reactions and regulates the physiological activity of other cells

Horse stance Stance used when the therapist applies strokes that traverse relatively short distances; both of the therapist's feet are placed on the floor a little more than hip-width distance apart, with toes pointing forward

Host Organisms in which pathogens reside

Hotel spa See *Resort spa*

Human chorionic gonadotropin (hCG) Placental hormone that stimulates estrogen and progesterone; can be detected in the urine to determine pregnancy

Hunting response Cycles of vasodilation and vasoconstriction associated with cold application

Hyaline cartilage Type of cartilage that is elastic, rubbery, and smooth; covers articulating ends of bones; connects ribs to the sternum; and supports the nose, trachea, and part of the larynx

Hydrotherapy Internal and external therapeutic use of water and complementary agents

Hygiene Collective principles of health preservation

Hyperemia Excessive blood flow

Hypodermis See *Subcutaneous layer*

Hypoglycemia   Low blood sugar; may occur in clients who have diabetes mellitus

Hypothalamus   Part of the diencephalon that governs and regulates the autonomic nervous system and pituitary gland; also controls hunger, thirst, temperature, anger and aggression, release of hormones, sexual behavior, sleep patterns, and consciousness

Hypothesis   Expected result of a research study based on background research and knowledge

Hypoxemia   Excessive amounts of deoxygenated blood

Ice immersion   Type of bath that involves soaking the affected area in icy water

Ice massage   Ice applied using circular friction

Ileocecal sphincter   Sphincter located between the small and large intestine

Ileum   Final portion of the small intestine

Immediate muscle soreness   Experienced during or shortly after exercise or activity, disappearing as soon as the person has rested and blood flow returns to normal

Immersion bath   Type of bath that involves soaking the body or affected area; types of immersion baths include whirlpools, spas, hot tubs, foot baths, and underwater massage

Immunity   Reaction that involves all body systems as they join together to destroy and eliminate pathogens, foreign substances, or toxic materials

Income tax   Tax paid on the net income (or profits) earned by a person or a business

Independent variables   Things that the researcher controls or manipulates in a research study

Infection   The period after disease transmission; pathogens use host resources to multiply

Inferior   Situated below or toward the tail end; also called *caudal*

Inflammation   Protective mechanism in response to tissue damage that serves to stabilize the injured area, contain infection, and initiate the healing process for damaged tissue

Informed consent   Permission from a client to accept treatment after he or she has been informed of the risks, benefits, and consequences of the techniques and procedure(s)

Infusion   Tea made from steeping the parts of a plant, usually the stems and leaves

Ingestion   The process of taking materials into the body orally

Ingham, Eunice (1889-1974)   Mother of reflexology; a physiotherapist who popularized reflexology in North America

Inguinal (groin)   Relating to the area between the thigh and abdomen

Inheritance   Expression of genetic material

Insertion   Tendinous muscle attachment on the more movable bone or other structure

Inspiration (inhalation)   Process of drawing air into the lungs

Insulin   Pancreatic hormone that decreases blood glucose levels

Internal respiration   Gas exchange between blood and the body tissues; also called tissue respiration

Intimacy   Close personal association in which choice, mutuality, reciprocity, trust, and delight exist

Intake form   Form filled out by the client before the first massage session; includes the client's personal information and contact information, as well as health and medical histories; also called a *health questionnaire*

Intention   In massage, a consciously sought goal that defines the purpose of the session

Internal   Nearest the inside (within) of a body cavity

Internal (tissue) respiration   Gas exchange between blood and the body's tissues

Interneuron   Neuron between a sensory and motor neuron; participates in integrative functions; also known as an *association neuron*

Interoceptive awareness   Being aware of one's own visceral sensations such as heart movement and respiratory rate

Interoceptor   Receptor located in the viscera; responds to stimuli, such as digestion, excretion, and blood pressure, originating within the body

Interosseous membrane   Membrane that interconnects select bones by attaching to their periosteum; also provides muscle attachment; also known as the *interosseous ligament*

Interstitial cells of Leydig   Endocrine cells located in the testes that produce testosterone

Intersubjectivity   Nonverbal communication between two people

Intracellular fluids   Fluids within cells

Intramembranous ossification   Bone formation from membranes; found in flat bone development

Inventory   Unsold retail items that a business has in stock

Inversion   Elevation of the medial edge of the foot so that the sole is turned inward (or medially)

Ipsilateral   Related to the same side of the body; also called *homolateral*

Ischemia   Lack of blood flow

Ischemic compression   See *Sustained pressure*

Islets of Langerhans (pancreatic islets)   Islands of endocrine cells located on the pancreas; secrete insulin and glucagon

Isometric contraction   Contraction in which muscle length remains the same while muscle tension increases

Isotonic contraction   Contraction in which muscle tone or tension remains the same as the length of the muscle changes

Jejunum   Intermediate portion of the small intestine

Jitsu   Japanese term that means full, yang, excess, or too much ki; also means the quality of the ki such as responsive, sluggish, soft, hard, expansive, or contractive

Joint   Where bones come together or join; also called articulation or arthrosis

Joint capsule   Double-layered structure around a synovial joint; the outer layer is fibrous and forms ligaments, and the inner layer is the synovial membrane

Joint cavity   Space with a joint capsule; lined with a synovial membrane and filled with synovial fluid

Joint mobilizations   Moving a joint through its full normal range of motion

Jump sign   Spontaneous reaction of pain or discomfort that causes a client to wince, jump, or verbalize at the application of pressure

Juxtaglomerular apparatus   Structure within the kidney that measures blood pressure; located where the afferent arteriole touches part of the distal convoluted tubule, and consists of the juxtaglomerular cells and the macula densa

Juxtaglomerular cell   Structure located in the afferent arteriole that assists in maintaining blood pressure by secreting renin when blood pressure drops

Kapha   In Ayurveda, dosha made up of the elements of earth and water

Kellogg, John Harvey (1852-1943)   American who wrote numerous articles and books on massage and helped popularize massage in the United States

Keratinocyte   Epidermal cell that produces keratin, a protein that waterproofs the skin

Ki   In Japanese, the energy or life force that creates and binds together all things and phenomena existing in the universe; this includes everything that manifests physically in nature and in the human body, as well as the emotions, thoughts, and spirit

Kidneys   Principal organs of the urinary system located in the upper lumbar region; they process blood and form urine to be excreted

Kinesiology   Study of human motion

Kneipp, Father Sebastian (1821-1897)   Father of hydrotherapy; possessed exceptional knowledge and skill in using water to heal the ailments that afflicted his community; these treatments are known collectively as Kneipp therapy and are still used today

Krause end bulb   Receptor involved in discriminatory touch and low-frequency vibration; may also detect cold

Kyo   Japanese term that means empty, yin, depleted, or not enough ki

Labia majora   Two folds of skin extending inferiorly and posteriorly from the mons pubis; covered with pubic hair in adult women

Labia minora   Two folds of skin inside the labia majora containing numerous oil glands

Labor   Process the body undergoes to expel a fetus; includes dilation of the cervix, expulsion of the fetus, and expulsion of the placenta

Lactation   Milk production

Lacteal   Lymph capillary located within a villus of the small intestines; assist in the absorption of fat

Lambdoidal suture   Suture that separates the parietal bones from the occipital bone

Langerhans cell   Epidermal cell that trigger immunologic reactions

Large intestine (colon)   Final section of the gastrointestinal tract that undigested and unabsorbed food takes before the body eliminates it; also forms and stores feces until defecation

Larynx   Connects the pharynx to the trachea; houses the vocal cords; also known as the *voice box*

Latent trigger point   Trigger point that does not cause referred pain or other sensations until direct pressure is applied

Lateral   Oriented farther away from the midline of the body

Lateral deviation   Side-to-side movement in the transverse plane

Lesion   Any noticeable or measurable deviation from normal healthy tissue

Lesser omentum   Part of the mesentery that extends from the stomach and duodenum to the liver

Leukocyte   White blood cell; serves as part of the body's immune system

Liabilities   Debts owed by a person or business

Licensure   A mandatory process in which a license is granted and permission given to perform an activity

Limited liability partnership   A business in which a member or members can limit their liability to their equity in the company and are not held liable for another partner's misconduct or negligence

Limited partnership   A business in which a member or members may be silent (also called a *silent partner*) and do not actively participate in business management, but still receive profit and is liable only up to the amount of personal investment

Ling, Pehr Henrik (1776-1839)   Swedish physiologist and gymnastics instructor; considered the father of Swedish massage; developed his own system of medical gymnastics and exercise, known as the Ling System, Swedish Movements, and the Swedish Movement Cure; a component of Ling's system was massage

Liniment   Not really a lubricant; used as an analgesic and to create the sensation of heat and sometimes cold

Lipase   Digestive enzyme that breaks lipids down into glycerol and fatty acids

Liver   Organ located in the upper right quadrant of the abdominal cavity; largest and most complex internal organ; filters toxins, produces bile, metabolizes nutrients, and produces plasma proteins

Local contraindication   A situation in which massage can be administered safely while avoiding an area of the body

Local disease   Disease affecting only one area of the body, such as a foot fungus

Local twitch response   Reflexive impulse that causes the affected muscle or an adjacent muscle to fire or twitch spontaneously; characteristic of trigger points

Loop of Henle   Section of the renal tubule just past the proximal convoluted tubule that consists of a descending limb, a hairpin turn, and an ascending limb

Lower esophageal sphincter   Sphincter located between the esophagus and stomach

Lucas-Championnière, Just (1843-1913)   French physician who advocated the use of massage and passive-motion exercises after certain injuries

Lumbar   Relating to loin or lower back between the ribs and the hips

Lumen   Inside space of a tubular structure, such as that inside of an artery or the intestines

Lung   Organ of respiration; extends from the diaphragm to just above the clavicles

Lunge position   See *Bow stance*

Luteinizing hormone (LH)   Pituitary hormone that stimulates the release of estrogens and progesterone and ovulation in women, and testosterone production in men

Lymph   Liquid connective tissue that is part of the lymphatic system

Lymph capillary   Tiny, open-ended channel located in tissue space throughout most of the body

Lymph vessel   Larger vessels than lymph capillaries; have thinner walls and more valves than veins; have lymph nodes situated along them

Lymph node   Bean-shaped structures located along lymph vessels; filters lymph; houses phagocytes and lymphocytes that destroy pathogens and other foreign substances in the lymph before it returns to the blood

Lymphatic trunk   Made up of large vessels into which lymph is drained from the lymph vessels

Lymphocyte   Type of white blood cell; can be either a B cell or T cell

Lysosome   Organelle containing digestive enzymes to engulf and digest pathogens and cellular debris

Macula densa   Structure located in the distal convoluted tubule of Henle with cells that sense the concentration of filtrate as it passes through the tubule; respond to a decrease in sodium by releasing prostaglandins, which stimulate renin secretion

Major duodenal papilla   Site of entry for secretions from the pancreas, liver, and gallbladder into the duodenum

Malas   In Ayurveda, the waste products of the human body

Malignant tumor   Cancerous tumor

Malpractice insurance   See *Professional liability insurance*

Mammary (pectoral)   Relating to the breast/super anterior thorax

Mammary gland   See *Breast*

Mandibular   Relating to the lower jaw

Marketing   Ideas, strategies, and activities to aid in attracting and retaining clients

Massage therapy   Manual and scientific manipulation of the soft tissues of the body for the purpose of establishing or maintaining good health and promoting wellness

Mastication   Chewing

Mechanoreceptor   Receptor that detects pressure and movement; found in the skin, blood vessels, ears, muscles, tendons, joints, and fascia; detects pressure, blood pressure, vibration, stretching, muscular contraction, proprioception, sound, and equilibrium

Media   Methods of mass communication

Medial   Oriented toward or near the midline of the body

Median plane   See *Midsagittal plane*

Mediastinal   Pertaining to the area between the lungs

Medical release form   A form the client completes (in writing) to authorize the release of any of his or her medical or personal information to a third party

Medical spa   Spa providing medical and wellness care in an environment that integrates spa services

Medulla oblongata   Part of the brainstem that conducts sensory and motor impulses between other parts of the brain and the spinal cord; also contains the respiratory, cardiovascular, and vasomotor centers

Medullary (medulla)   Inner region of an organ or structure

Medullary cavity   Hollow space within the center of a long bone's diaphysis

Medullary pyramid   Structure made by numerous collecting tubules; appears as a distant triangular wedge in the kidney

Meissner (tactile) corpuscle   Receptor that mediates sensations of discriminative touch such as light versus deep pressure, as well as low-frequency vibration

Melanocyte   Epidermal cell that produces melanin, a pigment that contributes to skin color and decreases the amount of ultraviolet light that can penetrate into the deeper layers of the skin

Melanocyte-stimulating hormone (MSH)   Pituitary hormone that increases skin pigmentation by stimulating the synthesis and release of melanin from melanocytes

Melatonin   Pineal gland hormone responsible for the control of biorhythms (the body's 24-hour cycle), and in the growth and development of sexual organs

Membrane   Thin, soft, pliable sheets of tissue that cover the body, line tubes or body cavities, cover organs, and separate one part of a cavity from another

Meninges   Connective tissue coverings surrounding the brain and spinal cord

Meniscus   Fibrocartilage pads found in select joints such as the knee and job; helps the joint move smoothly and serves as a shock absorber; plural form is *menisci*

Menstrual cycle   A cycle of hormonal events that lasts approximately 28 days; it begins at puberty and lasts through a woman's childbearing years, ending at menopause; the cycle, which lasts for about 28 days, begins with ovulation, which causes the uterine lining to grow, proliferate, and maintain itself for several days in anticipation of implantation of a fertilized egg; if no implantation occurs, the uterine lining sheds, which signals the onset of menstruation; the cycle then repeats itself; also called the *reproductive cycle* or *fertility cycle*

Menstruation   Periodic discharge of built-up endometrial lining from the non-pregnant uterus

Mental   In anatomy, relating to the chin

Mercuriale, Girolamo (1530-1606)   Italian Renaissance–era physician who wrote *De Arte Gymnastica,* considered to be the first book written in the field of sports medicine; the book compiled the history of gymnastics up to that time

Meridians   See *Channels*

Merkel disk   Receptor that responds to light touch and discriminative touch

Mesentery   Section of the peritoneum consisting of the two omenta (greater and lesser)

Mesoderm   Middle embryonic cell layer; gives rise to muscles, bones, and connective tissues of the body

Metabolic disease   Disease caused by abnormal metabolic processes and disruption of homeostasis

Metabolic rate   Overall rate at which metabolic reactions use energy

Metabolism   Total of all physical and chemical processes that occur in an organism

Metaphysis   Growth portion of a bone; located where the diaphysis and epiphysis connect

Metastasis   Spreading of cancerous cells

Mezger, Johann (1817-1983)   Dutch physician who was responsible for making massage a fundamental component of physical rehabilitation; also credited for the introduction of French terminology into the massage profession

Microglia   Neuroglial cell protecting the central nervous system by destroying pathogens and removing dead neural tissue

Micromassage   See *Ultrasound*

Micturition   See *Urination*

Mid-brain   Part of the brain stem that conducts nerve impulses from the cerebrum to the pons and conducts sensory impulses from the spinal cord to the thalamus

Midsagittal plane   Plane that runs longitudinally or vertically down the body, anterior to posterior, dividing the body into equal right and left sections

Minerals   Chemical agents found in nature; vital in regulating many body functions; divided into macro (bulk) minerals such as calcium and micro (trace) minerals such as iron

Mission statement   Statement of purpose that briefly and succinctly defines a type of business and its objective

Mitochondria   Sites of cellular respiration, providing most of a cell's adenosine triphosphate (ATP)

Mitral valve   Valve located between the left atrium and left ventricle; also called the *bicuspid valve* and the *left atrioventricular valve*

Mons pubis   Mound of adipose tissue covered by skin and pubic hair, cushioning the pubic symphysis

Motor   Term for a nerve that carries impulses from the central nervous system to activate or inhibit a muscle or gland

Motor neuron   Neuron that sends a nerve impulse to a muscle cell

Motor unit   Single motor neuron plus all the muscle fibers it innervates

Moxibustion In Asian bodywork therapy, stimulation of acupoints with heat from burning the herb mugwort (moxa) applied above or on the acupoints

Mucosal-associated lymphoid tissue Small masses of lymph tissue in respiratory and digestive tracts; made up of the tonsils, Peyer patches, and vermiform appendix

Mucous membranes Membranes that line openings to the outside of the body (e.g., nasal membranes)

Multiarticular Term used to describe muscles that cross more than two joints, acting on all joints crossed

Muscle fatigue Loss of muscle strength or endurance felt after strenuous physical activity

Muscle fiber Threadlike muscle cell

Muscle spindle Stretch receptor located within the muscle belly; detects sudden stretching, causing the nervous system to respond by reflexively contracting the muscle

Muscle tissue Tissue that produces movement of the body; has the ability to contract, elongate, and return to its original shape after movement; types are smooth, cardiac, and skeletal muscle

Muscle tone Continued partial contraction of skeletal muscle; also called *tonus*

Mutual fund Contains many types of securities, but mostly stocks

Mutation Mistakes in the gene coding system

Myelin sheath Fatty tissue layer surrounding most axons in the peripheral nervous system; insulates the neuron and increases nerve impulse speed

Myocardium Thick muscular layer that makes up the bulk of the heart wall; its contraction forces blood out of the ventricles

Myofascial Referring to skeletal muscles and their related fascia

Myofascial release Group of manual techniques used to reduce fascial restrictions

Myofibrils Thin strands within each muscle fiber; contain myofilaments

Myofilaments Thick and thin protein strands within each sarcomere; consist of actin and myosin

Myoglobin Red respiratory pigment in muscle cells; similar to hemoglobin in red blood cells

Myosin Protein molecules within a muscle cell that attach to actin during skeletal muscle contraction; make up the bulk of thick myofilaments

Myotome Group of skeletal muscles innervated by a single spinal segment

Nadis In Ayurveda, channels in which prana energy flows

Nail Compact keratinized cells that form the thin hard plates found on the distal surfaces of the fingers and toes

Nail bed Skin beneath the nail

Nail body Main and most visible part of the nail

Nail root Place where nail production takes place

Nasal Relating to the nose

Nasal cavity Cavity just behind the nose

Negative feedback system Mechanism that triggers the negative, or opposite, response

Nephron Kidney's filtering unit; contains three main parts: glomerulus, Bowman's capsule, and renal tubule

Nerve Fascicles of neurons held together by epineurium

Nerve impulse An electrical signal that conveys information along a neuron

Nerve root Attachment of a spinal nerve to the spinal column; the ventral nerve root contains motor neurons, and the dorsal nerve root contains sensory neurons

Nervous tissue Tissue that has the ability to detect and transmit electrical signals by converting stimuli into nerve impulses

Net income The amount of money a person or business has left after subtracting expenses and taxes

Net worth See *Equity*

Neuroglia Connective tissue that supports, nourishes, protects, insulates, and organizes neurons

Neuromuscular junction Junction between a motor neuron and a motor end plate

Neuron Impulse-conducting cell possessing excitability and conductibility

Neurotransmitters Collective term for chemical messengers involved in nerve impulse transmission; can be either excitatory or inhibitory

Nissen, Hartvig (1857-1924) Prominent early practitioner of Swedish massage in the United States; helped popularize Ling's methods with his numerous publications

Nociceptor Receptor that detects pain; also called *free nerve ending*

Nodes of Ranvier Gaps along myelinated axons; increase speed of a nerve impulse by allowing the impulse to jump from one node to another

Nonspecific immunity Nonspecific response to invading pathogens; includes intact skin and mucous membranes, saliva, gastric juices, vomiting, urine flow, certain white blood cells, and inflammation

Norepinephrine (noradrenaline) See *Epinephrine*

Nose Port of entry for air and the beginning of the air conduction pathway

Nuchal Relating to the posterior neck

Nucleus Cell organelle that houses DNA; control center of the cell, directing nearly all metabolic activities

Nutrient A substance that provides nourishment and affects metabolic processes such as cell growth and repair

Nutrition The manner in which the body takes in and uses, or assimilates, food

Objective data Measurable and quantitative information obtained by the therapist through empirical means

Occipital Relating to the back lower part of the skull

Occipital lobe Cerebral lobe that contains centers for visual input

Occupational license A business license required to operate any kind of business

Olecranal Relation to the back of the elbow

Olfactory Sense of smell

Oligodendrocyte Neuroglial cell that forms a myelin sheath around some axons in the central nervous system

Oocyte Female sex cell; also called *unfertilized egg*

Opposition Movement in which the tip of the thumb comes into contact with the tip of any other digit on the same hand

Oral Relating to the mouth

Oral cavity First portion of the gastrointestinal tract; also known as the *mouth*

Orbital (ophthalmic) Relating to the eye

Organ Complex structures of two or more tissue types performing a specific function

Organelle Cellular structures that possess distinct structures and functions; made up of the nucleus, ribosomes, endoplasmic reticulum, Golgi body, mitochondria, and lysosomes

Organism Living entities composed of several organ systems

Organ system Related organs with complementary functions that perform certain tasks

Origin Tendinous muscle attachment on the less movable bone or other structure

Osmosis Movement of a pure solvent such as water from an area of low concentration (most dilute) to an area of high concentration (least dilute); movement will continue until the two concentrations equalize

Ossification Process of bone development that begins between the sixth and seventh week of embryonic life and continues throughout adulthood

Osteoblast Bone-forming cell found just beneath the periosteum

Osteoclast Bone-destroying cell found in the lining of the medullary cavity; breaks down bone tissue to maintain blood calcium levels

Osteocyte Mature bone cell

Otic (auricular) Relating to the ear

Outcome (dependent variables) Specific measurements, such as heart rate or blood flow, after a massage treatment that can be measured in a research study

Ovary Gland located in the superior part of the pelvic cavity, lateral to the uterus; houses developing oocytes within the follicles and produces the hormones progesterone and estrogen

Oviduct See *Fallopian tube*

Ovum Female oocyte that has been released by the ovary; a mature oocyte

Oxytocin (OT) Pituitary hormone that stimulates uterine contractions during labor and milk expression from mammary glands during lactation

Pacinian corpuscle Receptor that responds to crude and deep pressure, vibration, and stretch, and perceives proprioceptive information about joint position

Pain cycle Painful stimuli resulting in muscle contraction and localized muscle splinting or guarding, which restricts movement and decreases local circulation; subsequent swelling creates more pain as local nerves are compressed; muscle splinting is then intensified and the cycle repeats itself

Palliative care Care that seeks to improve the quality of life by relieving symptoms and reducing suffering; also called *comfort care*

Pallor Paleness of the skin

Palmar (volar) Relating to the anterior surface of the hand

Palpation Touching with purpose and intent

Pancreas Organ located inferior to the stomach; both an endocrine gland that secretes insulin and glucagon, and an exocrine gland that secretes enzymes that break down proteins, carbohydrates, and fats

Pancreatic islets See *Islets of Langerhans*

Paracelsus (1493-1541) Name by which Swiss physician Philippus von Hohenheim was generally known; he laid the foundation of chemical pharmacology

Paraffin bath Body dip in a heated waxy mixture

Parasite Organism living in or on a host organism and relying on that host for nourishment, sometimes to the detriment of the host organism's health

Parasympathetic division Part of the autonomic nervous system that conserves the body's energy resources; also known as the *rest-and-digest division* and the *craniosacral outflow*

Parathyroids Glands located on the posterolateral surface of the thyroid; usually four in number; secrete parathyroid hormone (PTH)

Parathyroid hormone (PTH) Hormone that increases blood calcium by stimulating osteoclast activity to break down bone and release calcium into the blood, and increases calcium reabsorption from urine and the intestines back into the blood

Paré, Ambroise (c. 1510-1590) French military surgeon who, in addition to inventing several surgical instruments, was among the earliest modern physicians to discuss the therapeutic effects of massage, especially in orthopedic surgery cases

Parietal cell Stomach's exocrine cell that produces intrinsic factor and hydrochloric acid

Parietal lobe Cerebral lobe that receives information about proprioception, reading, and taste, and governs somatosensory input (namely the skin and muscles)

Partnership A business owned by two or more people working together with a common goal

Passive movements Client relaxes or is passive while the therapist performs the movement on the client

Patellar Relating to the kneecap

Pathogen Infectious agent capable of causing disease

Pathology Study of disease

Pectoral Relating to the upper anterior thorax

Pedal Relating to the foot or feet

Pediatric Refers to young people between 3 and 18 years of age

Peer review Process where subject matter experts assess the quality of a study, grant, or manuscript

Pelvic Relating to the pelvis or inferior region of the abdominopelvic cavity

Pelvic girdle Pairing of the ilium, ischium, and pubis

Pelvic tilt Anterior or posterior tilting of the entire pelvis in the frontal plane around a mediolateral axis

Penis Male structure that excretes semen outside of the body

Pepsin Digestive enzyme secreted by the stomach that breaks down proteins

Pericardium Tissue that surrounds the heart and secretes a lubricating fluid that prevents friction

Perineal Relates to the region between the anus and the genitals

Perineurium Connective tissue layer that binds neurons into a fascicle

Periosteum Fibrous sheath surrounding the bone's shaft containing blood and lymphatic vessels, nerves, and bone-forming cells for growth and fracture healing

Peripheral See *Superficial*

Peripheral nervous system Composed of the cranial and spinal nerves emerging from the central nervous system

Peristalsis Wavelike contractions that mix and propel materials in the gastrointestinal tract

Peritoneum Serous membrane of the abdominal cavity that surrounds the organs within it

Perimysium Connective tissue layer that surrounds fasciculi in muscles

Periosteum Fibrous, dense, vascular tissue sheath that surrounds the diaphysis of a long bone

Petty cash Cash used to pay for incidental expenses; usually set up and treated like a separate account from a business's main account

Pétrissage Lifting soft tissues vertically and then compressing and releasing them; the compression is accomplished by either squeezing or rolling the tissues before releasing, using rhythmic alternating pressures

Peyer patches Groups of lymphatic tissue in the lower portion of the ileum

Phagocytosis Process by which specialized cells ingest harmful microorganisms and cellular debris, break them down, and expel the harmless remains back into the body

Pharynx Muscular tube shared by respiratory and digestive systems; also known as the *throat*

Phasic muscle A muscle that provides movement

Photoreceptor Receptor that is sensitive to light; photoreceptors in the eye are rods and cones

Physical rehabilitation Process used after illness, injury, or surgery to help the affected individual regain as much function and self-sufficiency as possible

Physiology Study of how the body and its individual parts function in normal body processes

Pia mater Innermost meningeal layer; delicate, transparent, and attached to the surface of the central nervous system

Pineal gland Gland located on the posterior aspect of the brain's diencephalon; produces and secretes the hormone melatonin; also known as the pineal body

Pinocytosis Process by which specialized cells engulf liquids and draw them into the cell

Pitta In Ayurveda, dosha made up of the elements fire and water

Pitting edema Edema that leaves a pit or dent in a swollen area once the skin is compressed for a few seconds and released; the edematous tissue rebounds slowly

Pituitary Bilobed gland that extends from the hypothalamus; its hormones control and stimulate other glands to produce and secrete their hormones

Pivot (monoaxial) joint Joint with movement limited to rotation

Placebo Sham treatment

Placebo effect Change in a research study participant's condition from thinking that he or she is receiving a beneficial treatment

Placenta Organ formed against the uterine lining that allows the developing embryo and the mother to exchange nutrients and wastes; also secretes hormones required to maintain the pregnancy

Plan of care See *Treatment plan*

Plane A flat surface determined by three points in space such as height, depth, and width

Plantar (volar) Relating to the bottom, or sole, of the foot

Plantar flexion Extension of the ankle such that the toes are pointing downward, increasing the ankle angle anteriorly

Plasma Liquid portion of blood

Plasma membrane See *Cell membrane*

Platelet See *Thrombocyte*

Plexus Network of intersecting nerves in the peripheral nervous system

Plicae circulares Circular folds located in the lumen of the small intestine

Polarization Describes a neuron's resting membrane potential; the inside of the neuron bears a negative charge and the outside bears a positive charge

Pollex Thumb

Pons Part of the brainstem that relays nerve impulses from one side of the cerebellum to another

Pool plunge Type of bath that consists of a brief dip in a cold, deep water pool

Popliteal Relating to the posterior knee

Posterior Pertaining to the back of a structure; also called *dorsal*

Posterior pelvic tilt Movement of the pelvis in which the ilia are tilted backward

Postural muscle A muscle that helps to maintain the body's posture or vertical position

Posture How the body distributes itself in relation to gravity over a base or bases of support

Poultice Packs in which products, such as mustard, are spread between layers of cloth and applied hot to provide heat or counterirritation

Prakriti In Ayurveda, a person's unique constitution, or one's innate, natural state

Prana In Ayurveda, the energy of the body, mind, and spirit

Preceptor Someone who guides a massage therapist during his or her clinical practice

Pregnancy Also known as the *gestational process*, the sequence of events, including implantation and embryonic and fetal growth, that ends in birth; normal pregnancy is divided into three trimesters of three months each

Premise liability insurance See *General liability insurance*

Prescription A physician's order for medication, medical treatments, or medical devices

Press release A short, written piece used to inform the public on local events

Prime mover Muscle responsible for causing a specific or desired action; also called the *agonist*

Professionalism The adherence to a set of values and obligations, formally agreed codes of conduct, and reasonable expectations of clients, colleagues, and coworkers

Professional liability insurance Insurance that covers professional activities; also called *malpractice insurance* and *errors and omission insurance*

Profit and loss statement Summary of income and expenses over a fixed period, indicating whether the business made a profit or sustained a loss

Progesterone Hormone that maintains the uterine lining for implantation and pregnancy

Prolactin (PRL) Pituitary hormone that, with other hormones, promotes milk production of the mammary glands

Pronation Medial (inward) rotation of the forearm so that the palm is turned down

Prone position Lying face down

Proposal Written idea put forward for consideration, discussion, or adoption

Proprioceptor Receptor located in the skin, ears, muscles, tendons, joints, and fascia; responds to movement and body position

Prostaglandins Local hormones; produce many tissues and generally act near their site of secretion

Prostate Gland located inferior to the urinary bladder that produces an alkaline secretion, making up approximately 25% of semen volume

Protein Structure composed of chains of amino acids

Protraction Movement forward or anteriorly

Proximal Nearer to the point of reference; term used when referring to the extremities

Pubic Related to the region of the pubic symphysis or genital area

Publicity   Free media exposure

Pubococcygeus exercises   Regimen of isometric exercises involving voluntary contractions of the muscles of the pelvic diaphragm and perineum; formerly called *Kegel exercises*

Pulmonary circuit   Circuit that brings deoxygenated blood from the right ventricle of the heart to the lungs to release carbon dioxide and regain oxygen, then transports the oxygenated blood to the left atrium

Pulmonary valve   Valve between the right ventricle and the pulmonary trunk; also called the *right semilunar valve*

Pulse   Expansion effect of arteries that occurs when the left ventricle contracts and produces a wave of blood that surges through and expands arterial walls

Pyloric sphincter   Sphincter located between the stomach and small intestine

Qi   See *Ki*

Qualitative research   Research that seeks to understand processes that underlie various behavioral patterns; revolves around words and themes

Quantitative research   Research that measures variables numerically; revolves around numbers rather than words

Radiation   Transfer of heat energy in rays

Range of motion   Movement around a joint or set of joints

Recruitment   Process of motor unit activation based on muscular contraction needs

Rectum   Section of the large intestine between the sigmoid colon and the anal canal

Referral form   A form produced by the massage therapist and filled out by a health care provider authorizing massage therapy treatment

Referred pain phenomenon   Tendency of a trigger point to refer pain to a target area associated with the particular point; sensations include not only pain but tingling, numbness, and burning

Reflex   Involuntary, predictable response to a stimulus

Reflex arc   Carries a stimulus impulse to the spinal cord where it connects with a motor neuron that carries the reflex impulse back to an appropriate muscle or gland (effector)

Reflex points   In reflexology, points that correspond to the body's organs and structures

Reflexology   Method of stimulating life force through applied pressure on reflex points located on the hands, ears, face, and feet

Refractory   The inability of a neuron to accept another stimulus until it repolarizes

Registration   The state granting the privilege to participate in a particular profession maintains an official registry or record, listing the names of persons in an occupation who have satisfied specific requirements

Relaxin   Placental hormone facilitating implantation of fertilized ovum and softening of connective tissue in pregnant women

Reliability   Ability of a test to yield the same results on repeated trials

Remission   Period of partial or complete disappearance of symptoms occurring with the disease process

Renal pelvis   Large urine collection reservoir within the kidney; forms the upper region of a ureter

Renal tubule   Small tube within the nephron through which filtrate flows as it is being processed; subdivided into the proximal and distal tubule and the loop of Henle

Renin   Substance secreted by the juxtaglomerular cells that initiates the renin-angiotensin-aldosterone system, which eventually increases blood volume and blood pressure

Renin-angiotensin-aldosterone system   Enzyme and hormone pathway initiated by the secretion of renin by juxtaglomerular cells in the kidney when blood pressure drops; ultimately results in the secretion of aldosterone, a hormone that increases sodium and water reabsorption from the filtrate back into the blood, causing blood volume and, therefore, blood pressure to increase

Repetitive strain injuries (RSIs)   Self-inflicted injuries related to poor biomechanics, including general posture, sporting movements, and work habits; also known as *repetitive motion injuries*

Repolarization   Term for a neuron resuming its resting, or polarized, state

Reservoir   Source of infection that may lead to disease

Research literacy   Ability to locate, read, and understand research literature

Resort spa   Spa located within a resort or hotel that provides spa services, fitness and wellness components, and spa cuisine

Respiration   Movement of air into and out of the lungs

Résumé   An autobiographical sketch that documents a person's achievements, including occupational, avocational, academic, and personal information; also called *curriculum vitae* (CV)

Retina   Nervous tissue membrane of the eye continuous with the optic nerve; where rods and cones are located

Retinacula   Bandagelike retaining bands of connective tissue found primarily around the elbows, knees, ankles, and wrists; may also act as a pulley for tendons; singular is retinaculum

Retraction   Movement backward or posteriorly

Retroperitoneal   Term used to describe organs behind the abdominal peritoneum

Reuptake   Drawing up of neurotransmitters in the synapse by the pre-synaptic neuron

Rhazes (c. 850-932)   Name by which Persian physician Abu Bakr Muhammad ibn-Zakariya al-Razi was known in the West; wrote an encyclopedic work that discussed Greek, Roman, and Arabic medical practices, including massage

Rhythm   In massage, the regularity of technique application

Ribosome   Small granules of ribonucleic acid and protein in the cytoplasm that synthesize protein for use within the cell and produce other proteins that are exported outside of the cell

Right lymphatic duct   Lymphatic trunk that drains the right arm and the right side of the head and the right half of the thorax into the right subclavian vein

Rotation   Circular movement when a bone moves around its own central axis

Rubefacient   Agents that redden the skin as the ingredients cause irritation

Ruffini corpuscle   Receptor that mediates deep or continuous pressure; they adapt slowly and permit the body to stay in contact with grasped objects; may also detect heat

Rugae   Folds in the interior lining of the stomach, urinary bladder, and vagina

Sacral   Relating to the sacrum of the spinal column

Sacroiliac   Relating to the region between the sacrum and the pelvic bone

Saddle (biaxial) joint   Joint allowing the movements of flexion, extension, abduction, adduction, opposition, reposition, and circumduction

Sagittal plane Plane passing through the body parallel to the midsagittal plane

Sagittal suture Suture that joins the two parietal bones

Sales tax permit Required to sell products; allows the collection of sales tax on products sold

Saliva Fluid secreted by salivary and mucous glands in the mouth; contains digestive enzymes that break down lipids and carbohydrates

Saltatory conduction Nerve impulse conduction along myelinated axons; the impulses are able to jump along the length of an axon from one node of Ranvier, greatly increasing the speed of conduction

Sample population Group of individuals whose characteristics fit the experimental inclusion criteria for a research study

Sanitation Application of measures to promote a healthy, disease-free environment

Sarcolemma Muscle cell membrane

Sarcomere A muscle's contractile unit; found within myofibrils

Sarcoplasm Muscle cell cytoplasm

Sarcoplasmic reticulum A fluid-filled system of sacs similar to endoplasmic reticulum; stores and releases calcium ions

Satellite cell Cell that provides structural support of neurons in the peripheral nervous system; found only in surrounding neuron cell bodies within ganglia

Sauna Dry heat treatment in a wood-lined room with temperatures ranging from 160° to 210° F with 10% to 20% humidity

Scapular Relating to the shoulder blade

Schwann cell Cell that forms a myelin sheath surrounding axons in the peripheral nervous system

Scientific method Accepted process or standards that define the protocols used to create new knowledge through research

Scope of practice Outlines the activities and procedures that can be performed by licensed members of a profession

Scotch hose Handheld hose that sprays strong jets of water over the client's body

Scrotum Pouch that holds the testes

Seated massage Type of massage developed by David Palmer, whose vision was to make massage therapy safe, convenient, and affordable for anyone, anywhere, anytime

Sebaceous (oil) gland Skin gland that secretes sebum (oil) to lubricate both the hair and the epidermis

Secretin Hormone produced by the intestinal mucosa that stimulates the pancreas to secrete an alkaline liquid that neutralizes the acid chyme and facilitates the action of intestinal enzymes

Securities Instruments that represent financial value

Sedation In shiatsu, a technique that disperses excess ki in a tsubo

Seizure Change in behavior caused by an explosive episode of uncontrolled and excessive electrical activity in the brain; may be subtle and consist of abnormal sensations, or it may produce overt involuntary repetitive movements and loss of consciousness

Seizure disorders Characterized by explosive episodes of uncontrolled and excessive electrical activity in the brain; this activity results in a sudden change in a behavior called a seizure

Self-disclosure Massage therapist revealing his or her thoughts, feelings, and personal history to the client

Self-employment tax The full amount of Social Security and Medicare taxes owed from a self-employed person

Semen Thick, milky, alkaline fluid that is a mixture of sperm (10%) and seminal fluid (90%)

Seminal duct See *Vas deferens*

Seminal vesicles Located at the base of the urinary bladder; their secretions are a thick alkaline fluid that makes up a large porttion of semen volume

Seminiferous tubules Tightly coiled tubes within the testes that produce sperm

Semipermeable Term meaning that some materials can pass freely, whereas others cannot

Semireclining position Position in which the upper body is elevated while supine

Sensory Term for receptors that detect sensations or a nerve that carries impulses into the central nervous system; also called *afferent*

Sequence In the massage, the arrangement or order of massage strokes

Serotonin Neurotransmitter important for sensory perception, mood regulation, and normal sleep

Serous membrane Membrane that lines closed body cavities that do not open to the outside of the body

Sexual misconduct Sexual contact between a massage therapist and a client or any sexualizing of the therapeutic relationship

Sexual reproduction Process by which male and female sex cells unite to produce offspring

Shiatsu Japanese Asian bodywork therapy that uses pressure on the surface of the skin along energy channels to restore, maintain, or balance the harmonic flow of energy throughout the body-mind-spirit

Shirodhara Ayurvedic treatment that delivers a steady stream of oil over the client's forehead to achieve deep relaxation

Shoulder girdle Pairing of the clavicle and scapula

Side-lying position Lying on the right or left side

Sigmoid colon The S-shaped part of the colon in between the sigmoid flexure and the rectum

Sigmoid flexure The backward right turn the descending colon takes to connect with the sigmoid colon

Signs Objective changes in the body that can be observed and measured such as edema, fever, and high blood pressure

Sliding filament mechanism Model of muscle contraction in which thin filaments sliding toward the sarcomeres center shorten the muscle fiber

Small intestine Longest section of the gastrointestinal tract; situated in the central abdomen; consists of the duodenum, jejunum, and ileum

Social networking sites A broad expanse of generally free websites that connect a community of people together

Sol state Thin, fluid state of the ground substance in fascia

Sole proprietorship A business with a single owner

Sodium-potassium pump Mechanism used to maintain the resting potential of a neural cell membrane; moves Na^+ out of the cell and K^+ into the cell

Somatic nervous system Division of peripheral nervous system that transmits information from bones, muscles, joints, skin, and special senses of vision, hearing, taste, and smell into the central nervous system, and carries impulses from the central nervous system to skeletal muscles

Somatic reflex Reflex that is responsible for contraction of skeletal muscles

Spa Term for a place where water therapies are administered

Spa therapies   Variety of body treatments administered in spas that may incorporate massage, but use water as the heart of the spa experience

Spasm   Abnormal sustained muscle contraction

Spastic   Skeletal muscle with more than normal tone

Specific immunity   Body's response to invaders; T cells and B cells become activated for a specific pathogen after they come in contact with it and then destroy it

Speed   In massage, the rate at which massage movements are applied; how rapidly or slowly the therapist's hands are moving

Sperm   Male sex cell; also called spermatozoon (single sperm cell) and spermatozoa (multiple sperm cells)

Spermatic duct   Duct system in the male reproductive system that includes the epididymis, vas deferens, ejaculatory duct, and urethra

Spermatogenesis   Sperm cell production

Spermatozoon   Male sex cell; also called sperm and spermatozoa (multiple sperm cells)

Sphincter   Ring of muscle that remains contracted or closed until it is triggered to relax and open

Sphincter of Oddi   Sphincter regulating the flow of secretions from the pancreas, liver, and gallbladder into the duodenum

Spinal cord   Structure that exits the skull through the foramen magnum and extends to approximately the second lumbar region; functions as an integrating center and an information highway between the brain and the periphery

Spinal nerve   Nerve originating from the spinal cord

Spleen   Largest lymphatic organ; located within the left lateral rib cage just posterior to the stomach; stores lymphocytes, releasing them during immune responses

Splenic (left colic) flexure   The downward curve the colon takes just beneath the spleen

Spongy (cancellous) bone   Lattice of thin beams of bone within bones; lightens the bone and is filled with red marrow

Squamosal suture   Suture located where the parietal bones and temporal bones meet

Srotas   In Ayurveda, the vessels or channels of the body through which all substances circulate

Standards of practice   Guiding principles by which members of a particular organization conduct their day-to-day professional responsibilities

Standard precautions   Centers for Disease Control and Prevention (CDC) guidelines that represent a wide range of infection control measures such as glove use when touching mucous membranes and hand sanitation; developed in 1996 from the original CDC universal precautions

Static stretching   Stretching performed slowly and rhythmically, and that does not cause muscle contraction

Steam bath   Heat treatment in a ceramic-tiled room filled with water vapor at 105° to 120° F

Stem cell   Unspecialized cell that can become any of a number of different types of cells

Steroid hormone   Hormones that derive from cholesterol

Stock   Type of security issued in the form of shares

Stomach   Organ that is an enlargement of the gastrointestinal tract, bound at both ends by sphincters; breaks bolus of food down into chyme; secretes the digestive enzyme that breaks down proteins

Stress   Response of the body to any demand placed on it. It can be emotional, mental, physical, or chemical, all of which require a response from the body

Stretching   Method that lengthens and elongates soft tissues

Stroke volume   Amount of blood ejected from the left ventricle with each beat

Subacute pain   Condition in which the client appears to be well but is experiencing symptoms such as pain and discomfort

Subarachnoid space   Space between the pia mater and the arachnoid; filled with cerebrospinal fluid

Subcutaneous layer   Layer beneath the dermis but not a true layer of skin; consists of loose connective tissue, fat, and nerve receptors; also called the *hypodermis* and *superficial fascia*

Subdural space   Space between the arachnoid and the dura mater; filled with serous fluid

Subjective data   Information learned from the client or the client's family and friends; includes most written information obtained on the intake form and information gathered during conversation

Sudoriferous (sweat) gland   Skin gland that secretes sweat in response to excess heat

Superficial   Pertaining to the outside surface, periphery, or surrounding the external area of a structure; also called *peripheral*

Superficial fascia   See *Subcutaneous layer*

Superior   Situated above or toward the head end; also called *cranial* and *cephalad*

Supination   Lateral (outward) rotation of the forearm so that the palm is turned up

Supine hypotensive syndrome   Dizziness experienced from a sudden drop in blood pressure as major abdominal blood vessels are being compressed while the affected person is lying supine; most often, the compression is caused by a large, pregnant uterus

Supine position   Lying on the back

Sustained pressure   Held pressure usually applied with a finger or thumb, elbow, or a hand-held tool; displaces fluids in the tissues being compressed, spreads muscle fibers, and relieves muscle spasms; also sometimes called *acupressure* or *ischemic compression*

Swedish gymnastics   Part of the Ling system; a therapeutic system that, by influencing movements, would overcome discomfort that had arisen through abnormal conditions; consisted of passive, active, and duplicated movements; massage was a component

Swedish massage   Term for the therapy that developed out of Swedish gymnastics; Ling blended massage with physiology and, shortly thereafter, this new emphasis resulted in Swedish massage

Swiss shower   Has one large showerhead on the ceiling and multiple showerheads positioned vertically on each of the three walls

Sympathetic division   Part of the autonomic nervous system that spends the body's energy resources during physical exertion or emotional stress; also known as the *"fight-or-flight" response* and the *thoracolumbar outflow*

Symptoms   Subjective changes in the body that cannot be measured and are only aware to the person experiencing them (e.g., headaches, pain, anxiety)

Synapse   Junction between two neurons or between a neuron and a muscle or gland

Synaptic cleft   Space between the synaptic bulb and the plasma membrane of the postsynaptic neuron, muscle cell, or gland; also called the *synaptic gap*

Synaptic end bulb Small budlike structure on the ends of telodendra; contains synaptic vesicles

Synaptic vesicle Saclike structure located within the synaptic bulbs that contain neurotransmitters

Synarthrosis joint Joint with movement that is extremely limited; also called a *fibrous joint*

Syndrome Group of signs and symptoms that present a pattern defining a particular disease or abnormality

Synergist Muscle that aids movement by contracting at the same time as prime movers

Synovial fluid Viscous fluid secreted by synovial membranes; provides nutrition and lubrication

Synovial joint See *Diarthrosis*

Synovial membrane Membrane that line cavities of freely moving joints

Synovial (tendon) sheath Tubelike structure lined with synovial membrane that surround long tendons

Systemic circuit Circuit that brings oxygenated blood from the left ventricle of the heart through numerous arteries into the capillaries, then moves it through the veins and returns the now deoxygenated blood to the right atrium of the heart

Systemic disease Disease affecting large parts of the body or the entire body

Systolic pressure Maximal pressure in blood pressure measurement; occurs when the left ventricle contracts

T3 and T4 See *Thyroid hormones*

T-tubule Runs transversely across the sarcoplasmic reticulum, forming inward channels; transports stored calcium ions from the sarcoplasmic reticulum into the interior of the muscle cell

Tachycardia Rapid heart rate (>100 beats per minute)

Taenia coli Thick, longitudinal bands along the large intestine that make haustra

Tai Ji In traditional Chinese medicine, the familiar black and white icon that symbolizes the interaction of Yin and Yang

Tapotement Repetitive staccato striking movements of the hands, moving either simultaneously or alternately

Target cell Cell containing receptor sites that are chemically compatible with their corresponding hormone

Tarsal Relating to the ankle

Taylor, Charles Fayette and George Henry American physicians who were brothers; they introduced the Swedish movement system into the United States and helped popularize Ling's methods

Telodendria Clusters of short, fine filaments located at the end of each axon

Temporal Relating to the side of the skull

Temporal lobe Cerebral lobe that houses auditory and olfactory areas and the Wernicke area (critical to language comprehension; typically in the left hemisphere only)

Tender point Specific spots on the body that elicit pain and discomfort where compressed; these points do not refer pain

Tendon Cordlike structure anchoring the end of a muscle to a bone

Tetraiodothyronine (T4, thyroxine) See *Thyroid hormones*

Testes (Testicles) Glands that are the site of sperm and testosterone production

Testosterone Hormone that promotes secondary male sex characteristics, libido, and sperm production

Thalamus Part of the diencephalon that relays sensory information (except olfaction) to appropriate parts of the cerebrum

Thalassotherapy Use of sea and marine products, primarily seaweed

Therapeutic relationship The relationship between a therapist and client that seeks to support the client's therapeutic goals; regardless of its length, the therapeutic relationship serves the needs and interests of the client

Thermogenesis Heat production through skeletal muscle contraction

Thermoreceptor Receptor that detects temperature changes

Thermotherapy External therapeutic application of heat

Thixotropy Fascia's ability to change the physical state of its ground substance in the matrix from a gel to a sol state and vice versa

Thoracic Relating to chest between the neck and the diaphragm

Thoracic cavity Contains the heart and lungs

Thoracic duct Lymphatic trunk that drains most of the body's lymph into the left subclavian vein

Thrombocyte Platelet; prevents blood loss through clotting mechanisms

Thymopoietin See *Thymosin*

Thymosin Along with thymopoietin, thymus hormone that stimulates the maturation of T cells

Thymus Bilobed gland posterior to the sternum; secretes thymosin and thymopoietin, which stimulate the production and activation of T cells

Thyroid Bilobed gland located at base of the throat, posterior and inferior to the larynx; secretes the hormones T3 (triiodothyronine), T4 (tetraiodothyronine [thyroxine]), and calcitonin

Thyroid hormones T3 (triiodothyronine) and T4 (tetraiodothyronine [thyroxine]); control the metabolic rate, and regulate growth and development

Thyroid-stimulating hormone (TH) Pituitary hormone that stimulates the thyroid to synthesize and secrete its hormones

Thyroxine (T4, tetraiodothyronine) See *Thyroid hormones*

Tissot, Simon André (1728-1797) French writer who published several works on gymnastic exercises that recommended massage for various diseases and gave indications for its use

Tissue Group of similar cells that act together to perform a specific function; the four major tissue types are epithelial, connective, muscle, and nerve

Tonification In shiatsu, a technique that draws ki toward a particular tsubo

Tonsils Group of lymph tissue embedded in the oral cavity and pharynx

Tonus See Muscle tone

Trachea Tube that connects the larynx with the bronchi; anterior to the esophagus; also known as the *windpipe*

Transcytosis Process in which substances are moved into, through, and out of a cell by transport vesicles

Transference Term for when a client transfers feelings, thoughts, and behaviors related to a significant person in his or her early life (e.g., parents) onto the therapist

Transverse colon The horizontal portion of the large intestine between the hepatic and splenic flexures

Transverse plane Plane that passes through the body to create superior and inferior sections; also called a horizontal plane

Treatment plan The therapist's strategy used to help the client achieve his or her goals; also called *plan of care*

Treatment planning The documented process of planning a client's treatment or course of treatment; it takes into account the client's therapeutic goals or reasons for seeking massage therapy, his or her current health status, information gathered on a completed intake form, answers to questions asked by the therapist, palpation of tissues, and assessment procedures such as for range of motion, gait, and posture

Tricuspid valve Valve located between the right atrium and the right ventricle; also called the *right atrioventricular valve*

Tri-doshas See *Doshas*

Trigger point Localized areas of hyperirritability; when pressed, may refer sensations (usually pain) to other areas of the body

Triiodothyronine (T3) See *Thyroid hormones*

Tsubo Japanese term for specific points along the channels at which the energy concentrates and surfaces as vortices of ki

Turgor Skin resiliency; decreases during dehydration

Ultrasound Acoustic mechanical vibration of high frequency that produces thermal and nonthermal effects; therapeutic ultrasound is referred to as *micromassage*

Umbilical Relating to the navel

Unconditional positive regard Respect for another that does not depend on his or her behavior; valuing the other because his or her humanity warrants care

Uniarticular Term used to describe muscles that cross one joint

Universal donor Person who has blood type O; this blood type can be donated to all of the blood types

Universal precautions Guidelines developed by the Centers for Disease Control and Prevention (CDC) in response to 1991 federal legislation that requires all health care providers adhere to a plan that helps prevent transmission of blood-borne pathogens; under universal precautions, blood and certain body fluids of all patients are considered potentially infectious

Universal recipient Person who has blood type AB; this blood type can receive all other blood types

Ureter Slender hollow tube transporting urine formed by the kidney to the urinary bladder

Urethra Narrow tube that transports urine from the urinary bladder out of the body during urination

Urinary bladder Hollow, muscular organ that is a storage reservoir for urine; located in the pelvis behind the symphysis pubis

Urination Release of urine from the urinary bladder to outside of the body; also called *micturition* and *voiding*

Urine Concentrated filtrate from the kidneys that is 96% water and 4% dissolved wastes

Uterus Hollow, pear-shaped organ in which the fertilized ovum implants, the fetus develops, and from which menses flow; also called the *womb*

Vagina Canal extending from the uterine cervix to outside the body; passageway for menstrual flow and childbirth; receptacle for the penis during sexual intercourse

Vas deferens Tube that runs from the epididymis into the pelvic cavity where it loops over the side and down the posterior surface of the urinary bladder; carries sperm from the epididymis to the ejaculatory duct; also called the *ductus deferens* and the *seminal duct*

Vasoconstriction Narrowing of the vascular lumen's diameter

Vasodilation Enlargement of the vascular lumen's diameter

Vata In Ayurveda, the dosha composed of the elements air and space

Vector transmission Involves stings or bites from insects and/or animals that act as intermediaries of disease exchange between two or more hosts

Vehicle transmission Occurs when infectious organisms are transmitted in or on a common vehicle or source such as food and water or objects such as computer keyboards or doorknobs

Vein Vessel that carries blood toward the heart

Ventral See *Anterior*

Ventral cavity Body cavity located on the anterior aspect of the body; further divided into the thoracic and abdominopelvic cavities

Ventricle Inferior heart chamber

Venule Small-sized veins that connect with capillaries

Vertebral Relating to vertebrae of the spinal column

Vesalius, Andreas (1514-1564) Flemish physician who wrote *De Humani Corporis Fabrica* (1543), considered one of the most important studies in the history of medicine

Vibration Shaking, quivering, trembling, or rocking movements applied with the fingers, full hand, or an appliance

Vichy shower Taken while the client reclines on a special table as jets of water spray from a horizontal bar with multiple downfacing showerheads along its length

Villi Fingerlike projections on the plicae circulares in the small intestine

Vision statement A statement that embraces the desires a person has for his or her business

Vital substances In traditional Chinese medicine, they are qi (ki), essence, blood, body fluids, and Spirit

Vitamins Essential for metabolic reactions in the body; water-soluble vitamins (B vitamins and vitamin C) are absorbed easily and excreted within hours; fat-soluble vitamins (vitamins A, D, E, and K) are absorbed slowly and often reside in the liver and fat cells

Vocal cords Cords located in the larynx used for voice production

Voiding See *Urination*

Volkmann canal Canals that run horizontally through a bone, connecting Haversian canals

Vulva Female external genitalia that include the mons pubis, labia majora and labia minora, and the clitoris

Warrior stance See *Horse stance*

Watsu Combination of water and shiatsu

Wellness Expression of health in which an individual is aware of, chooses, and practices healthy choices, creating a more successful and balanced life

Womb See *Uterus*

Zang/Fu In traditional Chinese medicine, the organ systems, divided into Yin and Yang; includes the physical organs and associated channels as well as the emotional, mental, and spiritual aspects of human existence

Zang In traditional Chinese medicine, refers to organs that are the Yin, more solid organs such as the heart, liver, lungs, kidney, pericardium, and spleen

Zone According to reflexology, what the body's energy travels through; used to map reflex points

Zygomatic Relating to the upper cheek

Zygote Fertilized ovum

ILLUSTRATION CREDITS

Chapter 1

Pehr Henrik Ling photo: Courtesy of Armand Dedrick Maanum, the last Master-Master Masseur-Teacher of the Sjuk Gymnastiken Passiva Rorelser Massage of Pehr Henrik Ling

Figure 1-2 Courtesy U.S. National Library of Medicine, Bethesda, Maryland

Figure 1-3 1921 "Autobiography" by Hartvig Nissen.

Figure 1-4 © Judi Calvert

Chapter 2

Nina McIntosh photo: From Associated Bodywork and Massage Professionals, *A Tribute to Nina McIntosh*, http://www.abmp.com/news/a-tribute-to-nina-mcintosh/

Chapter 4

Figure 4-1 Copyright 2006 John Keith. Image from Bigstock.com

Figure 4-2 University of Nebraska–Lincoln. Illustration of the Wellness Model, 2009. http://wellness.unl.edu/wellness_model.shtml

Figure 4-5 Adapted from http://www.fda.gov

Figure 4-6 Image courtesy of http://www.mypyramid.gov

Chapter 9

David Lauterstein photo: © David Lauterstein. Portrait by Larissa Nicole Rogers, Spirit Essence Photography.

Figure 9-1 From Perry AG: *Clinical nursing skills and techniques*, ed 7. St. Louis, 2009, Elsevier.

Figure 9-4 From Ignatavicius DD, Workman ML: *Medical-surgical nursing: patient-centered collaborative care*, Single Volume, ed 6, St. Louis, 2010, Saunders.

Chapter 10

Milton Trager photo: Courtesy Trager Institute, Mill Valley, California

Figure 10-1 From Adler/Towne/Holt, Rinehart and Winston, Inc. *Looking Out, Looking In*, 7E. ©1993 Wadsworth, a part of Cengage Learning, Inc. Reproduced by Permission. www.cengage.com/permissions

Figure 10-5 From Hockenberry MJ, Wilson D: *Wong's essentials of pediatric nursing*, ed 8, St. Louis, 2009, Mosby. Used with permission. Copyright Mosby.

Chapter 11

Figure 11-1 From Seidel, HM et al: *Mosby's guide to physical examination*, ed 7, St. Louis, 2011, Elsevier.

Figure 11-3 From Lowdermilk D, Cashion MC, Perry S: *Maternity and women's health care*, ed 10, St. Louis, 2012, Mosby.

Figure 11-11 Comstock Images/Getty Images

Chapter 12

Figure 12-1 Bath and North East Somerset Council

Figures 12-2A, 12-8, 12-9 Courtesy TouchAmerica, Hillsborough, North Carolina

Figure 12-7 Courtesy Golden Ratio, Emigrant, Montana

Figure 12-15 © Petra Tsekos

Figure 12-16 © Chelsea Anne Breaux, 2011

Chapter 13

Figure 13-1 Courtesy International Institute of Reflexology

Figure 13-3 Norman L: *Feet first: a guide to foot reflexology*, New York, 1998, Simon & Schuster.

Chapter 14

Figure 14-1 Reprinted from *Best Practice & Research Clinical Rheumatology*, Vol 21/Issue 2, Cummings M, Baldry P, Regional myofascial pain: diagnosis and management, pages 367-387, April 2007, with permission from Elsevier.

Figure 14-7 Modified from Neumann DA: *Kinesiology of the musculoskeletal system: foundations for rehabilitation*. St. Louis, 2010, Mosby.

Chapter 16

Figures 16-3, 16-18 From Anderson SK: *The practice of shiatsu*. St. Louis, 2008, Mosby.

Figures 16-5 through 16-17 Modified from Anderson SK: *The practice of shiatsu*. St. Louis, 2008, Mosby.

Chapter 18

Deane Juhan photo: © Karen Zurlinden Photography

Figure 18-1 From Patton KT, Thibodeau GA: *Anatomy & physiology*, ed 7, St. Louis, 2010, Mosby. (Barbara Cousins)

Figures 18-5, 18-6A-C, 18-9, 18-10, 18-14, 18-21AB From Herlihy B: *The human body in health and illness*, ed 4, St. Louis, 2011, Mosby.

Figure 18-8 From Thibodeau GA, Patton KT: *Anatomy & physiology*, ed 6, St. Louis, 2007, Mosby.

Figures 18-16, 18-23AB From Patton KT, Thibodeau GA: *Anatomy & physiology*, ed 7, St. Louis, 2010, Mosby.
Figures 18-11, 18-12, 18-13 © Dennis Strete
Figure 18-15 Reprinted by permission of Professor Peter Cull, London University.

Chapter 19

Ida Rolf photo: Courtesy Rolf Institute, Boulder, Colorado (Photo by David Kirk Campbell).
Figure 19-1 From Patton KT, Thibodeau GA: *Anatomy & physiology*, ed 7, St. Louis, 2010, Mosby.
Figure 19-2AB, 19-3 From Herlihy B: *The human body in health and illness*, ed 4, St. Louis, 2011, Mosby.

Chapter 20

Figures 20-1, 20-4, 20-7, 20-8AB, 20-9A-C Modified from Patton KT, Thibodeau GA: *Anatomy & physiology*, ed 7, St. Louis, 2010, Mosby.
Figure 20-3A-C Modified from Patton KT, Thibodeau GA: *Anatomy & physiology*, ed 7, St. Louis, 2010, Mosby.
Figure 20-10AB Adapted from Muscolino JE: *Kinesiology*, St. Louis, 2006, Mosby.

Chapter 21

Figures 21-1, 21-40, 21-41AB From Herlihy B: *The human body in health and illness*, ed 4, St. Louis, 2011, Saunders.
Figures 21-2, 21-3, 21-4A-C, 21-6, 21-7, 21-8, 21-9, 21-10AB, 21-11, 21-12AB, 21-13, 21-16, 21-17, 21-18A-D, 21-22, 21-23, 21-24, 21-25AB, 21-26AB Modified from Drake RL, Vogl AW, Mitchell AWM: *Gray's anatomy for students*, ed 2, Philadelphia, 2010, Churchill Livingstone.
Figures 21-5A,B, 21-14A,B, 21-15, 21-19, 21-20 From Patton KT, Thibodeau GA: *Anatomy & physiology*, ed 7, St. Louis, 2010, Mosby.
Figure 21-21 Modified from Leonard PC: *Building a medical vocabulary*, ed 7, St. Louis, 2009, Saunders.
Figure 21-38AB From Muscolino JE: *Kinesiology*, ed 2, St. Louis, 2011, Mosby.
Figures 21-42AB, 21-48A,B, 21-51AB, 21-59AB, 21-68AB, 21-87AB, 21-88, 21-91, 21-98, 21-103, 21-109, 21-116, 21-120, 21-121AB, 21-134AB, 21-135, 21-139AB, 21-145, 21-153, 21-158AB, 21-164, 21-171 Modified from Muscolino J: *Muscular system manual: the skeletal muscles of the human body*, ed 3, St. Louis, 2010, Mosby.
Figures 21-43A,B, 21-44, 21-45, 21-46, 21-47, 21-49, 21-50, 21-52, 21-53, 21-54, 21-55, 21-56, 21-57, 21-58, 21-60, 21-61, 21-62, 21-63, 21-64, 21-65, 21-66, 21-67, 21-69, 21-70, 21-71, 21-72, 21-73, 21-74, 21-75, 21-76, 21-77, 21-78, 21-79, 21-80, 21-81, 21-82, 21-83, 21-84, 21-85, 21-86, 21-89, 21-90, 21-92, 21-93, 21-94, 21-95, 21-96, 21-97, 21-99, 21-100, 21-101, 21-102, 21-104,

21-105, 21-106, 21-107, 21-108, 21-110, 21-111, 21-112, 21-113, 21-114, 21-115, 21-117, 21-118, 21-119, 21-122, 21-123AB, 21-124, 21-125, 21-126, 21-127, 21-128, 21-129, 21-130, 21-131, 21-132, 21-133, 21-136, 21-137, 21-138, 21-140, 21-141, 21-142, 21-143, 21-144, 21-146, 21-147, 21-148, 21-149, 21-150, 21-151, 21-152, 21-154, 21-155, 21-156, 21-157, 21-159, 21-160, 21-161, 21-162, 21-163, 21-165, 21-166, 21-167, 21-168, 21-169, 21-170, 21-172, 21-173, 21-174, 21-175, 21-176 From Muscolino J: *Muscular system manual: the skeletal muscles of the human body*, ed 2, St. Louis, 2005, Mosby.

Chapter 22

Figure 22-6 Courtesy Harlow Primate Laboratory, University of Wisconsin, Madison, Wisconsin
Figure 22-7 Courtesy Corbis, Inc. © Bettmann
Figure 22-8 Courtesy Katharine J. Wilmering
Figure 22-9 Courtesy Tiffany Field
Figure 22-10 From Lookingbill D, Marks J: *Principles of dermatology*, ed 3, Philadelphia, 2000, Saunders.
Figure 22-11 From Callen J, Greer K, Hood A, et al: *Color atlas of dermatology*, ed 2, Philadelphia, 2000, Saunders.
Figure 22-12 Forbes CD, Jackson WF: *Color atlas and Text of Clinical Medicine*, ed 3, Edinburgh, 2003, Mosby Ltd.
Figures 22-13, 22-14 From Habif: *Clinical dermatology: a color guide to diagnosis and therapy*, ed 4, St. Louis, 2004, Mosby.

Chapter 23

Moshe Feldenkrais photo: © International Feldenkrais Federation Archive
Figures 23-1, 23-10, 23-12, 23-16, 23-17, 23-20AB, 23-24 From Patton KT, Thibodeau GA: *Anatomy & physiology*, ed 7, St. Louis, 2010, Mosby.
Figures 23-2, 23-11, 23-18 From Applegate E: *The anatomy and physiology learning system*, ed 4, St. Louis, 2011, Saunders.
Figures 23-6, 23-7AB, 23-8, 23-9, 23-13, 23-19, 23-21 From Herlihy B: *The human body in health and illness*, ed 4, St. Louis, 2011, Saunders.
Figures 23-14A-C From Habif: *Clinical dermatology: a color guide to diagnosis and therapy*, ed 5, St. Louis, 2010, Mosby.
Figures 23-20C Courtesy Dr. Scott Mittman, Johns Hopkins Hospital, Baltimore, MD.

Chapter 24

Figure 24-3 From Thibodeau GA, Patton KT: *Anatomy & physiology*, ed 6, St. Louis, 2007, Mosby.
Figures 24-4, 24-5, 24-6 Modified from Herlihy B: *The human body in health and illness*, ed 4, St. Louis, 2011, Saunders.

Chapter 25

Tiffany Field photo: © Tiffany Field
Unn. Figure, 25-10 From Seidel, HM: *Mosby's guide to physical examination*, ed 7, St. Louis, 2011, Mosby.
Figure 25-1 From Herlihy B: *The human body in health and illness*, ed 4, St. Louis, 2011, Saunders.
Figure 25-2, 25-3, 25-4, 25-7 From Applegate E: *The anatomy and physiology learning system*, ed 4, St. Louis, 2011, Saunders.
Figure 25-5 From Patton KT, Thibodeau GA: *Anatomy & physiology*, ed 7, St. Louis, 2010, Mosby.
Figure 25-6 From Swartz MH: *Textbook of physical diagnosis: history and examination*, ed 6, Philadelphia, 2010, Saunders.
Figure 25-11 From Frazier MS, Drzymkowski JW: *Essentials of human disease and conditions,* ed 4, St. Louis, 2009, Saunders.

Chapter 26

Table 26-1, Figures 26-6, 26-10, 26-11, 26-12A, 26-13, 26-14, 26-15, 26-17 From Herlihy B: *The human body in health and illness*, ed 4, St. Louis, 2011, Saunders.
Figures 26-8 From Herlihy B: *The human body in health and illness*, ed 3, St. Louis, 2007, Saunders.
Figure 26-2 From Applegate E: *The anatomy and physiology learning system*, ed 4, St. Louis, 2011, Saunders.
Figure 26-3 From Bevelander G, Ramaley JA: *Essentials of histology*, ed 8, St. Louis, 1979, Mosby.
Figure 26-4 Copyright Dennis Kunkel Microscopy, Inc.
Figures 26-7, 26-12B Modified from Patton KT, Thibodeau GA: *Anatomy & physiology*, ed 7, St. Louis, 2010, Mosby.
Unn. Figures From Drake RL et al: *Gray's Anatomy for Students*, ed 2, Philadelphia, 2010, Churchill Livingstone.

Chapter 27

Emil Vodder photo: © Georg Thieme Verlag, Stuttgart
Figures 27-1, 27-2, 27-3 From Patton KT, Thibodeau GA: *Anatomy & physiology*, ed 7, St. Louis, 2010, Mosby.

Figure 27-4 Adapted from McCance K, Huether S: *Pathophysiology*, ed 4, St. Louis, 2002, Mosby in Patton KT, Thibodeau GA: *Anatomy & physiology*, ed 7, St. Louis, 2010, Mosby.

Chapter 28

Figure 28-4 From Herlihy B: *The human body in health and illness*, ed 4, St. Louis, 2011, Saunders.
Figure 28-5 From Thibodeau GA, Patton KT: *Anatomy & physiology*, ed 6, St. Louis, 2007, Mosby.
Figure 28-6A From Abrahams P, Boon J, Spratt J, Hutchings R: *McMinn's clinical atlas of human anatomy*, ed 6, Philadelphia, 2008, Mosby.
Figure 28-6B From Vidic B, Suarez FR: *Photographic atlas of the human body*, St. Louis, 1984, Mosby.

Chapter 29

Figures 29-2, 29-3, 29-7 From Thibodeau GA, Patton KT: *Anatomy & physiology*, ed 6, St. Louis, 2007, Mosby.
Figure 29-4 From Herlihy B: *The human body in health and illness*, ed 4, St. Louis, 2011, Saunders.
Figure 29-9 Barbara Cousins, modified from Thibodeau GA, Patton KT: *Structure & function of the body*, ed 13, St. Louis, 2008, Mosby.

Chapter 30

Figures 30-1A, 30-4 From Applegate E: *The anatomy and physiology learning system*, ed 4, St. Louis, 2011, Saunders.
Figures 30-1B, 30-2B From Abrahams P, Hutchings RT, Marks SC: *McMinn's color atlas of human anatomy*, ed 4, St. Louis, 1999, Mosby.
Figure 30-2A From Brundage DJ: *Renal disorders*, St. Louis, 1992, Mosby.
Figures 30-3A,B, 30-5 From Herlihy B: *The human body in health and illness*, ed 4, St. Louis, 2011, Saunders.
Figure 30-6 From Patton KT, Thibodeau GA: *Anatomy & physiology*, ed 7, St. Louis, 2010, Mosby.

SHORT BIOGRAPHY INDEX

INDEX